Blood tests requiring immediate transport of the specimen

ABO blood typing
Acetylcholine receptor antibodies
Acid phosphatase
ACTH, plasma
Activated partial thromboplastin time
Aldosterone
Alkaline phosphatase
Ammonia, plasma
Androstenedione
Angiotensin-converting enzyme
Antibodies to extractable nuclear antigen
Antibody screening test
Antidiuretic hormone
Antiglobulin, direct (direct Coombs')
Arginine test
Arterial blood gas analysis
Aspartate aminotransferase
Bilirubin, serum
Calcitonin, plasma
Carbon dioxide, total
Carcinoembryonic antigen
Catecholamines, plasma
Ceruloplasmin, serum
Cholesterol, total
Cholinesterase
Coagulation, extrinsic system
Coagulation, intrinsic system
Cold agglutinins
Complement assays
Cortisol
Creatine, serum
Creatine kinase
Creatinine, serum
Crossmatching
Cryoglobulins
Erythrocyte sedimentation rate
Erythrocyte total porphyrins
Estrogen, serum
Euglobulin lysis time
Febrile agglutination tests
Fibrin split products
Fibrinogen, plasma
Folic acid, serum
Fungal serology
Galactose-1-phosphate uridyltransferase

Gastrin, serum
Glucose, fasting plasma
Glucose, plasma, 2-hour postprandial
Glucose tolerance, oral
Growth hormone, serum
Growth hormone suppression
Heinz bodies
Hematocrit
Human chorionic gonadotropin, serum
Human placental lactogen, serum
Hydroxybutyric dehydrogenase
Immune complex assays, serum
Immunoglobulins G, A, and M
Insulin, serum
Insulin tolerance
Iron, serum
Iron-binding capacity, total
Isocitrate dehydrogenase
Lactate dehydrogenase
Lactic acid and pyruvic acid (lactate and pyruvate)
Lipoprotein-cholesterol fractionation
Lymphocyte transformation
Manganese, serum
Microbiology culture
Neonatal thyroid-stimulating hormone
Parathyroid hormone, serum
Phenylalanine, serum (Guthrie test)
Phospholipids
Plasma thrombin time
Plasminogen
Progesterone, plasma
Prothrombin consumption time
Prothrombin time
Renin, plasma
Rh typing
Serum glucagon
T- and B-lymphocyte counts
Transferrin, serum
Triglycerides
Vitamin A and carotene, serum
Vitamin B_{12}, serum
Vitamin C, plasma
Zinc, serum

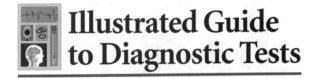

Illustrated Guide to Diagnostic Tests

Second Edition

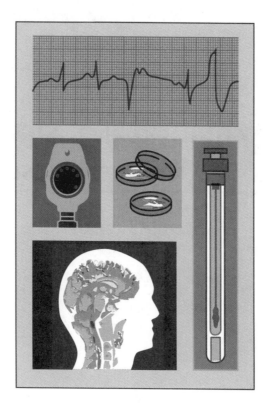

Illustrated Guide to Diagnostic Tests

Second Edition

Springhouse Corporation
Springhouse, Pennsylvania

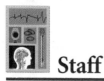

Staff

Executive Director
Matthew Cahill

Editorial Director
Patricia Dwyer Schull, RN, MSN

Art Director
John Hubbard

Clinical Project Manager
Judith Schilling McCann, RN, MSN

Senior Editor
H. Nancy Holmes

Clinical Editor
Beverly Tscheschlog

Editors
Doris Weinstock, Jane V. Cray, Peter Johnson, Jeanette Moss

Copy Editors
Cynthia C. Breuninger (manager), Diane Armento, Karen C. Comerford, Stacey Ann Follin, Brenna H. Mayer

Designers
Arlene Putterman (associate art director), Lesley Weissman-Cook (book designer), Amy Litz

Illustrators
Jackie Facciolo, Jean Gardner, Robert Neumann

Typography
Diane Paluba (manager), Joyce Rossi Biletz, Phyllis Marron, Valerie Rosenberger

Manufacturing
Deborah C. Meiris (manager), T.A. Landis

Production Coordinator
Margaret Rastiello

Editorial Assistants
Carol Caputo, Beverly Lane, Mary Madden

Printed in the United States of America.

IGDT2 - 020198

A member of the Reed Elsevier plc group

Library of Congress Cataloging-in-Publication Data
Illustrated guide to diagnostic tests. -- 2nd ed.
    p. cm.
    Includes bibliographical references and index.
    1. Diagnosis. 2. Nursing.
I. Springhouse Corporation.
[DNLM: 1. Diagnosis--nurses' instruction.
WB 141 I29 1997]
RC71.I44 1997
616.07'5--dc21
DNLM/DLC   96-45274
ISBN 0-87434-882-X (alk. paper)   CIP

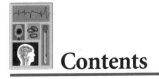

Contents

SECTION I: BLOOD TESTS

Chapter 1

Hematology

Chapter 2

Hemostasis

Chapter 3

Blood gases and electrolytes

Chapter 4

Enzymes

Chapter 5

Hormones

SECTION V: BODY SYSTEM TESTS

SECTION VI: MISCELLANEOUS TESTS

SECTION VII: APPENDICES AND INDEX

Contributors and consultants

Charol Abrams, MS, MT(ASCP)SH, CLS(NCA), CLSp(H)
CLS Consultant
Philadelphia

Kathryn A. Altergott, RN, BSN
Radiology Nurse Supervisor
Good Samaritan Regional Medical Center
Phoenix, Ariz.
Desert Samaritan Medical Center
Mesa, Ariz.

Patrice Blanchard, RDCS
Echocardiography Lab Technician
Doylestown (Pa.) Hospital

Michelle Clugston, RCVT
Cardiovascular Technician
Doylestown (Pa.) Hospital

Joan T. Converse, MA, MT(ASCP), CLS(NCA)
Education Coordinator, Biochemistry and MLT
Mayo Medical Center
Rochester, Minn.

Jane Curnow, CRN, MSN, CNA
Physician Affiliations Director
Misericordia Hospital
Philadelphia

Eileen DeCristofano, RN
Case Manager
Aetna/U.S. Healthcare
Blue Bell, Pa.

Ellen Digan, MA, MT(ASCP)
Professor of Biology and Coordinator of MLT Program
Manchester (Conn.) Community-Technical College

Nancy M. Flynn, RN,C, MSN
Clinical Nursing Educator
Bryn Mawr (Pa.) Hospital

Marna J. Fontana, RN, BSN
Samaritan Health Services
Phoenix, Ariz.

Ellie Z. Franges, RN, MSN, CCRN, CNRN
Director of Neuroscience Services
Sacred Heart Hospital
Allentown, Pa.

Pamela Weston Gitschier, MT, MS
Independent Consultant
Breinigsville, Pa.

Debra R. Hanna, RN, MSN, CNRN
Assistant Director of Nursing
Bergen Pines County Hospital
Paramus, N.J.

Connie S. Heflin, RN, MSN
Professor
Paducah (Ky.) Community College

Pamela Hockett, RN, BSN, OCN, CRNI
Parenteral Service Coordinator
El Camino Hospital
Mountain View, Calif.

Karen Jeffers, RN,C, MA
Director of Nursing Staff Development
Chestnut Hill Hospital
Philadelphia

Michel E. Lloyd, MT(ASCP), SBB
Technical Coordinator, Blood Bank
St. Luke's Hospital
Bethlehem, Pa.

Andrea Marino, RN, BSN, CCRN
Staff Nurse CCU
Allegheny University Medical Center
Elkins Park (Pa.) Campus

Carol McLimans, MA, MT(ASCP), SM
Program Director, Medical Laboratory Technician Program
Mayo Foundation
Rochester, Minn.

Barbara Ann Moyer, RN, EdD
Education Nurse Specialist
Lehigh Valley Hospital
Allentown, Pa.
Assistant Professor
Allentown College of St. Francis de Sales
Center Valley, Pa.

Kathleen M. Murtaugh, BS, MT(ASCP)
Independent Consultant and Med Tech
Generalist
Doylestown (Pa.) Hospital

Nancy Novitski-Runta, RN, BSN, CCRN
Medical-Surgical Staff Development
Educator
North Penn Hospital
Lansdale, Pa.

Catherine Paradiso, RN, MS, CCRN
Clinical Nurse Specialist
St. Vincent's Medical Center of Richmond
Staten Island, N.Y.

Judith E. Peterson, RN, CNII
Nursing Staff
Good Samaritan Regional Medical
Center
Phoenix, Ariz.

Ruth Pfeiffer, RTN
Nuclear Medicine Technician
Doylestown (Pa.) Hospital

Linda T. Raichle, PhD, MT(ASCP)
Laboratory Training Advisor
Exton, Pa.

Dorothy L. Rhoads, RN,C, MSN, CRNP
Ob/Gyn Nurse Practitioner
Willow Grove, Pa.

Teresa A. Richardson, BS, MT, MLT(AMT)
Medical Technologist
St. Luke's Quakertown (Pa.) Hospital

Sharon Rimmer, RDMS
Ultrasound Technician
Doylestown (Pa.) Hospital

Bethany Schroeder, RN, MFA, MS
Manager of Staff Development and
Specialty Nursing
MidPeninsula Home Care and Hospice
Services, Inc.
Mountain View, Calif.

Daniele Shollenberger, RN, MSN
Clinical Process Development Coordinator, Care Management Systems
Lehigh Valley Hospital
Allentown, Pa.

Joan Simpson, MS, MT(ASCP)
Consultant
Mansfield Center, Conn.

Marian J. Spirk, RN, MSN, CNSN
Clinical Nurse Specialist–Nutrition
Lehigh Valley Hospital
Allentown, Pa.

Johanna K. Stiesmeyer, RN, MS, CCRN
Clinical Consultant
Nursing Educational Services
Placitas, N. Mex.

LeAnn Tatman, RN, BSN
Assistant Nurse Manager
University of Iowa Hospital and Clinics
Iowa City

Deborah Porter Thornton, MEd
Independent Consultant
Newton Grove, N.C.

Debbie Thorrick, RDMS
Ultrasound Technician
Doylestown (Pa.) Hospital

Rachelle Trauger, RCVT
Cardiovascular Technician
Doylestown (Pa.) Hospital

Jay W. Wilborn, CLS, MEd
MLT-AD Program Director
Garland County Community College
Hot Springs, Ariz.

Cynthia Williams, BS, MT(ASCP), SI(ASCP)
Medical Technologist
St. Luke's Hospital
Bethlehem, Pa.

Patricia Zander-Hubing, BS, RTR
Clinical Chief Technologist
University of Iowa Hospital and Clinics
Iowa City

Foreword

Every year, technological advances and scientific discoveries lead to the creation of new and often complex diagnostic tests and, sometimes, to the modification of existing tests. A major nursing challenge is keeping abreast of these changes and the impact they have on patient care.

The newly revised edition of *Illustrated Guide to Diagnostic Tests* will help you meet this challenge. Among the important new tests that will influence your practice, it features two groundbreaking tests for Alzheimer's disease, bone densitometry, stereotactic breast biopsy, hysteroscopy, and radiopharmaceutical myocardial perfusion imaging. With more than 550 laboratory and diagnostic tests and hundreds of illustrations, photos, charts, and tables, this comprehensive volume gives you the information you need to ensure the safe completion of diagnostic procedures and to understand the implications of test results.

This thoroughly updated reference is organized into five major sections that include virtually all available diagnostic tests, from routine procedures, such as complete blood count and urinalysis, to the very latest new tests. A special introductory section, *Collection techniques*, summarizes recommended procedures for obtaining and handling blood and urine samples--the two most widely used laboratory specimens.

Section I (Chapters 1 to 11) presents tests that are performed on a blood sample. Section II (Chapters 12 to 17) contains tests that require a urine specimen. The tests in Section III (Chapters 18 and 19) involve histology, microbiology, and parasitology. Those in Section IV (Chapters 20 to 22) are divided by body organ (thyroid, eye, and ear), and those in Section V (Chapters 23 to 29) are classified by body system. The final section (Chapter 30) covers miscellaneous procedures, including skin tests. Each chapter begins with an introduction that discusses all the tests that follow, including explanations of their uses, summaries of test methods, and additional information where applicable, such as anatomy and physiology.

Each test entry follows the same easy-to-use format, beginning with a brief introductory explanation of the test. This is followed by *Purpose*, which lists the indications for the test, and *Patient preparation*, which provides guidelines for preparing the patient both physically and psychologically. (Where applicable, some entries also list the equipment that's necessary to perform the test.) *Procedure* describes the test in detail, including, when appropriate, the nurse's role. *Precautions* lists contraindications, factors that are necessary to ensure the test's accuracy--such as prompt transport of specimens--and adverse reactions to watch for after the test. Next, *Normal findings* or *Reference values* (for tests whose results are expressed in numerical values) provides normal results for each test. (Be aware that numerical values may vary by laboratory and method and are provided as a general guide.) *Implications of abnormal findings* highlights possible abnormal results and their clinical significance, and *Post-test care* discusses nursing actions needed to help the patient resume pretest activities or diet or deal with the adverse effects of the test. Finally, *Interfering factors* lists points that can invalidate the test or make interpretation difficult.

Throughout the volume, the *Nursing alert* logo points out potentially hazardous steps in procedures and offers practical advice on how to deal with--or prevent--a problem.

At the end of the book are five invaluable appendices, beginning with a guide to commonly used medical abbreviations and a guide to color-top collection tubes. *Quick-reference guide to laboratory test results* summarizes normal adult, pediatric, and geriatric values in a 10-page section that's color-tabbed for fast access. *Patient guide to test preparation* provides 14 pages of teaching aids to prepare your patients for specific procedures, such as cardiac catheterization. *Illustrated guide to home testing* is an 11-page collection of teaching aids that explain how to perform specific tests, such as pregnancy and HIV detection tests, accurately at home.

Even the end pages of this updated reference are packed with useful information--crisis values of laboratory tests, blood tests requiring immediate specimen transport, and normal values for some of the most commonly performed laboratory tests.

From routine blood collection to the newest and most complex imaging procedures, the second edition of *Illustrated Guide to Diagnostic Tests* has it all. No practicing nurse can afford to be without it.

John J. Shane, M.D.
Chairman, Department of Pathology
Lehigh Valley Hospital
Allentown, Pa.

Clinical Professor of Pathology
Allegheny University Hospitals
Philadelphia

Clinical Professor of Pathology
Pennsylvania State University
Hershey Medical Center
Hershey, Pa.

Collection techniques:
Blood and urine samples

Blood

The type of blood sample that's required for a test — whole blood, plasma, or serum — depends on the nature of the test. *Whole blood* — containing all blood elements — is the sample of choice for blood gas analysis, determination of hemoglobin derivatives, and measurement of red blood cell constituents. In addition, most routine hematologic studies, such as complete blood count, erythrocyte sedimentation rate, reticulocyte and platelet counts, and the osmotic fragility test, require whole blood samples.

Plasma is the liquid part of whole blood, which contains all the blood proteins; *serum* is the liquid that remains after whole blood clots. Plasma and serum samples, which contain most of the physiologically and clinically significant substances found in blood, are used for most biochemical, immunologic, and coagulation studies. They also provide electrolyte evaluation, enzyme analysis, glucose concentration, protein determination, and bilirubin level.

Venous, arterial, and capillary blood

Venous blood returns to the heart through the veins. It carries a high concentration of carbon dioxide from the cells back to the lungs for exhalation. Because venous blood represents physiologic conditions throughout the body and is relatively easy to obtain, it's used for most laboratory procedures.

Arterial blood, replenished with oxygen from the lungs, leaves the heart through the arteries to distribute nutrients throughout the capillary network. Although an arterial puncture increases the risks of hematoma and arterial spasm, arterial blood samples are necessary for determining pH, partial pressure of arterial oxygen, partial pressure of carbon dioxide, and oxygen saturation.

Capillary, or peripheral, blood does the real work of the circulatory system — exchanging fluids, nutrients, and wastes between blood and tissues. Capillary blood samples are most useful for such studies as hemoglobin and hematocrit determinations; blood smears; microtechniques for clinical chemistry; and platelet, red blood cell, and white blood cell counts requiring only small amounts of blood. (See *Common arterial and venous puncture sites*, page xvi.)

Quantities and containers

The most recent guidelines from the Centers for Disease Control and Prevention (CDC) mandate that gloves always be worn when obtaining and handling blood and urine specimens as well as any other body fluid. (See *Standard precautions*, pages xvii to xix.)

Sample quantities needed for diagnostic studies depend on the laboratory, available equipment, and the type of test. Some laboratories, for example, use automated analyzer systems that require a serum sample of 100 µl or less; others use manual systems that require a larger amount. The desired sample quantity determines the collection procedure and the type and size of the container. A single venipuncture with a conventional glass or disposable plastic syringe can provide 10 ml of blood — sufficient for many hematologic, immunologic,

(Text continues on page xix.)

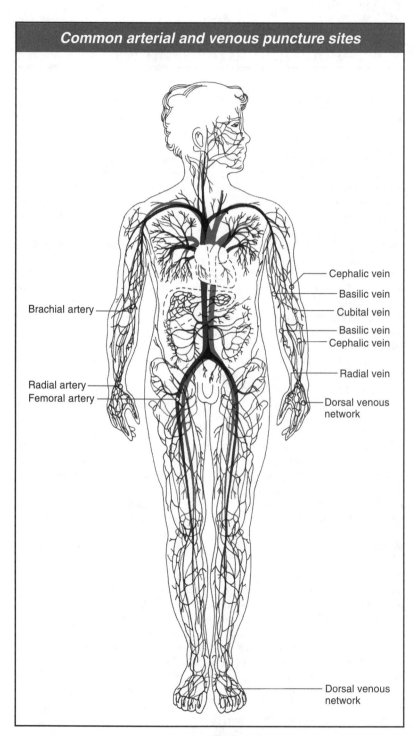

Common arterial and venous puncture sites

Brachial artery

Radial artery
Femoral artery

Cephalic vein
Basilic vein
Cubital vein
Basilic vein
Cephalic vein

Radial vein

Dorsal venous
network

Dorsal venous
network

Standard precautions

The Centers for Disease Control and Prevention (CDC) and the Hospital Infection Control Practices Advisory Committee have developed two categories of guidelines for preventing the transmission of nosocomial infections. These latest guidelines — *standard precautions* and *transmission-based precautions* — have replaced the previous *universal precautions* and *category-specific guidelines.* The transmission-based precautions are further divided into three types, based on the mode of transmission: *airborne precautions, droplet precautions, and contact precautions.*

Standard precautions are designed to decrease the risk of transmitting organisms from both recognized and unrecognized sources of infection in hospitals. They should be followed at all times, with every patient.

Standard precautions combine the major features of the former universal precautions, which were developed in response to the increasing incidence of human immunodeficiency virus (HIV), hepatitis B virus (HBV), and other blood-borne diseases, and the former *body-substance isolation precautions,* which were developed to reduce the risk of pathogen transmission from moist body surfaces. Because standard precautions reduce the risk of transmitting blood-borne and other pathogens, many patients with diseases that previously required category-specific or disease-specific isolation precautions now require only standard precautions.

The specific substances covered by standard precautions include blood and all other body excretions, except sweat, even if blood is not visible. Standard precautions should also be followed in the presence of nonintact skin or exposed mucous membranes.

Transmission-based precautions should be followed — in addition to standard precautions — whenever a patient is known or suspected to be infected with a highly contagious and epidemiologically important pathogen that is transmitted by air, by droplets, or by contact with dry skin or other contaminated surfaces. Examples include the pathogens that cause measles (transmitted by air), influenza (transmitted by droplets), and GI, respiratory, skin, and wound infections (transmitted by contact).

Transmission-based precautions replace all previous categories of isolation precautions, including strict isolation, contact isolation, respiratory isolation, enteric precautions, and drainage and secretion precautions, as well as other disease-specific precautions. One or more transmission-based precautions may be combined when a patient has a disease with multiple modes of transmission.

Equipment
Gloves, masks, goggles, or face shields ✦ gowns or aprons ✦ resuscitation masks ✦ bags for specimens ✦ 1:10 dilution of bleach to water (mixed daily) or hospital-strength disinfectant certified effective against HIV and HBV.

Implementation
■ Wash your hands immediately if they become contaminated with blood or body fluids; also wash them before and after patient care and after removing gloves (as shown at top of next page). Hand washing retards the growth of organisms on your skin.

(continued)

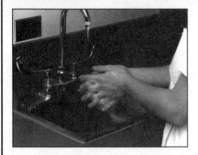

■ Wear a gown and face shield (or goggles and a mask) during procedures that are likely to generate droplets of blood or body fluid, such as surgery, endoscopic procedures, and dialysis (as shown below).

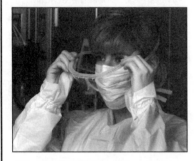

■ Wear gloves if you will, or could, come in contact with blood, specimens, tissue, body fluids, or excretions as well as contaminated surfaces or objects (as shown below). Change your gloves between patient contacts to prevent cross-contamination.

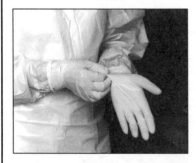

■ Handle used needles and other sharp implements carefully. Do not bend or break them, reinsert them into their original sheaths, or handle them unnecessarily. Discard them intact immediately after use in a sharps biohazard container. These measures reduce the risk of accidental injury or infection.

■ Notify your employee health provider immediately about all needle-stick injuries, mucosal splashes, and contamination of open wounds with blood or body fluids to allow investigation of the accident and appropriate care and documentation.

■ Properly label all specimens collected from patients, and place them in plastic biohazard bags at the collection site.

■ Promptly clean all blood and body fluids with a 1:10 dilution of bleach to water (mixed daily) or with an approved hospital-strength disinfectant that's effective against HIV and HBV.

■ Disposable food trays and dishes are not necessary.

■ If you have an exudative lesion, avoid all direct patient contact until the condition has resolved and you've been cleared by your employee health provider. Intact skin is your best defense against infection.

Special considerations

Standard precautions are intended to supplement — not replace — recommendations for routine infection control, such as hand washing and wearing gloves.

Keep mouthpieces, resuscitation bags, and other ventilation devices nearby to minimize the need for emergency mouth-to-mouth resuscitation, thus reducing the risk of exposure to body fluids.

Because precautions can't be specified for every clinical situation, you must use your judgment in individual cases. If your job requires you to be exposed to blood, make sure you receive an HBV vaccine.

Complications
Failure to follow standard precautions may lead to exposure to blood-borne diseases and all the complications they may incur.

---

chemical, and coagulation tests, but hardly enough for a series of tests.

To avoid multiple venipunctures when tests require a large blood sample, use an evacuated tube system (Vacutainer, Corvac) with interchangeable glass tubes, optional draw capacities, and a selection of additives. Evacuated tubes are commercially prepared with or without additives (indicated by their color-coded stoppers) and with enough vacuum to draw a predetermined blood volume (2 to 20 ml per tube). (See *Guide to color-top collection tubes* in the appendices.)

Microanalysis of minute amounts of capillary blood collected with micropipettes or glass capillary tubes allows numerous hematologic and routine laboratory studies to be performed on infants, children, and patients with severe burns or poor veins. Micropipettes are color-coded by sample capacity and hold 30 to 50 µl of whole blood; glass capillary tubes hold 80 to 130 µl of serum or plasma.

Equipment
For venipuncture: gloves ✦ tourniquet ✦ 70% alcohol or povidone-iodine solution ✦ sterile syringes or evacuated tubes ✦ sterile needle (20G or 21G for forearm; 25G for wrist, hand, or ankle and for children) ✦ color-coded tubes with appropriate additives ✦ identification labels ✦ small adhesive bandage ✦ sterile 2" x 2" gauze pads.

For arterial blood: gloves ✦ 10-ml luer-lock glass syringe ✦ 1-ml ampule heparin ✦ 20G 1½" short-bevel needle ✦ 23G 1" short-bevel needle ✦ rubber stopper or cork ✦ antiseptic swabs ✦ 70% alcohol or povidone-iodine solution ✦ sterile 2" x 2" gauze pads ✦ tape or adhesive bandage ✦ iced specimen container ✦ labels (for syringe and specimen bag) for patient's name, doctor's name, hospital number, date, collection time, and details of oxygen therapy.

For capillary blood: gloves ✦ sterile, disposable blood lancet ✦ sterile 2" x 2" gauze pads ✦ 70% alcohol or povidone-iodine solution ✦ glass slides, heparinized capillary tubes, or pipettes ✦ appropriate solutions.

Venous sample
The nature of the test and the patient's age and condition determine the appropriate blood sample, collection site, and technique. Most tests require a venous sample. Although a relatively simple procedure, venipuncture must be performed carefully to avoid hemolysis or hemoconcentration of the sample, to prevent hematoma formation, and to prevent damage to the patient's veins. (See *How to collect a venous sample,* page xx.) Label all test tubes clearly with the patient's name, date, and collection time.

Select a venipuncture site. The most common site is the antecubital fossa area; other sites are the wrist and the dorsum of the hand or foot. When drawing the sample at bedside, instruct the patient to lie on his back, with his head slightly elevated and his arms rest-

How to collect a venous sample

Gather the necessary equipment. Wash your hands thoroughly and apply gloves. Screw the Vacutainer needle into the sleeve (as shown).

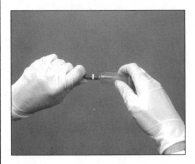

Select a venipuncture site, usually the antecubital fossa. Apply a soft rubber tourniquet above the venipuncture site. Then, using a circular motion, clean the area first with povidone-iodine solution (as shown) and then with alcohol.

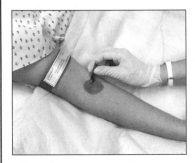

Remove the needle cover from the Vacutainer needle. With the bevel facing up, insert the needle into the patient's vein at a 15-degree angle (as shown).

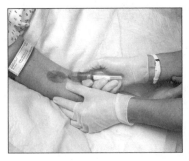

When a drop of blood appears just inside the needle holder, gently push the Vacutainer tube into the needle sleeve, so the blood enters the tube. Try to keep the needle still to prevent it from penetrating the patient's vein. When the tube is filled, remove the tourniquet.

If another specimen is needed, gently remove the filled Vacutainer tube and place another tube into the needle. When collection is complete, remove the tourniquet and place a 1" x 1" gauze pad over the venipuncture site (as shown), apply direct pressure, and remove the needle.

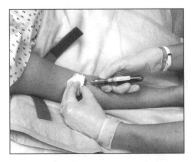

After 2 to 3 minutes, cover the site with an adhesive bandage.

Safeguards for venipuncture

- Make sure the patient is adequately supported in case of syncope.
- To avoid injecting air into a vein when using a syringe to withdraw a sample, first make sure that the plunger is fully depressed.
- Avoid drawing blood from an arm or leg used for I.V. infusion of blood, dextrose, or electrolyte solutions because this dilutes the blood sample. If you must collect blood near an I.V site, choose a location below it.
- For easier identification of veins in patients with tortuous or sclerosed veins or veins damaged by repeated venipuncture, antimicrobial therapy, or chemotherapy, apply warm, wet compresses 15 minutes before attempting venipuncture.

- If you are not successful after two attempts, ask another nurse to do the venipuncture.
- When you can't find a vein quickly, release the tourniquet temporarily to avoid tissue necrosis and circulation problems.
- Be sure to insert the needle at the correct angle to reduce the risk of puncturing the opposite wall of the vein and causing a hematoma.
- Always release the tourniquet before withdrawing the needle to prevent a hematoma. When drawing multiple samples, release the tourniquet within 1 minute after beginning to draw blood to prevent a hemoconcentration sample.

ing at his sides. When drawing blood from an ambulatory patient, have him sit in a chair, with his arm supported on an armrest or a table. Restrain small children if necessary.

Always wash your hands and put on gloves before drawing a blood sample. When using an evacuated tube, attach the needle to the holder before applying the tourniquet. Unless cautioned otherwise, apply a soft rubber tourniquet above the puncture site to increase venous pressure, which makes the veins more prominent. Make sure the tourniquet is snug but not constrictive. If the patient's veins appear distinct, you may not need to apply a tourniquet. Using a tourniquet for a patient with large, distended, and highly visible veins increases the risk of hematoma. Do the venipuncture below all I.V. sites or in the opposite arm. Instruct the patient to make a fist several times to enlarge the veins. Select a vein by palpation and inspection. If you can't feel a vein distinct-

ly, *don't* attempt the venipuncture. (See *Safeguards for venipuncture*.)

Working in a circular motion from the center outward, clean the puncture site with alcohol or povidone-iodine solution, and dry it with a gauze pad. If you must touch the cleaned puncture site again to relocate the vein, palpate with an antiseptically clean finger, and wipe the area again with an alcohol pad. Draw the skin tautly over the vein by pressing just below the puncture site with your thumb to keep the vein from moving.

Hold the syringe or tube with the needle bevel up and the shaft parallel to the path of the vein at a 15-degree angle to the arm. Enter the vein with a single direct puncture of the skin and vein wall. If you use a syringe, venous blood will appear in the hub. Withdraw the blood slowly, gently pulling on the syringe to create steady suction until you obtain the desired amount. If you're using an evacuated tube, when a drop of blood appears just inside the needle holder, grasp the needle holder securely and push down on the collection tube until the needle punctures the rubber stopper; blood will then flow into the tube automatically. When the tube is filled, remove it; if you're drawing multiple samples, repeat the procedure with additional tubes.

To prevent stasis, release the tourniquet as soon as you establish adequate blood flow. If the flow is sluggish, you may want to leave the tourniquet in place longer. However, always remove the tourniquet before withdrawing the needle.

After drawing the sample, ask the patient to open his fist as soon as you collect the desired amount. Release the tourniquet. Place a gauze pad over the puncture site; then withdraw the needle slowly and gently. Apply gentle pressure to the puncture site. If the patient is alert and cooperative, tell him to hold the gauze pad in place for several minutes until the bleeding stops to prevent hematoma. If the patient is not alert or cooperative, hold the pad in place or apply a small adhesive bandage.

After collection with a syringe, remove the needle and carefully empty the sample into the appropriate test tube without delay. To prevent foaming and hemolysis, *don't* eject the blood through the needle or force it out of the syringe. Place the appropriate color-coded stoppers on the tubes. Gently invert a tube containing an anticoagulant several times to mix the sample thoroughly. Examine the sample for clots or clumps; if none appear, send the sample to the laboratory. *Don't* shake the tube.

Before leaving the patient, check his condition. If a hematoma develops at the puncture site, apply warm soaks. If the patient has lingering discomfort or excessive bleeding, instruct him to lie down. Watch for anxiety or signs of shock, such as hypotension and tachycardia. Send the sample to the laboratory immediately.

Many laboratories use automated electronic systems that can perform multiple tests on a blood sample.(See *Automatic test series: SMA 12/60 and SMAC.*)

Arterial sample

Arterial blood is rarely required for routine studies. Because arterial puncture carries risks, samples are usually collected by a doctor or a specially trained nurse. Before drawing an arterial blood sample, administer a local anesthetic at the puncture site, if necessary. If available, you may use an arterial blood gas (ABG) kit, which contains all the necessary equipment, including a heparinized syringe. Perform Allen's test to assess radial artery circulation. (See *Performing Allen's test,* page xxiv.) Try to obtain the specimen from the radial artery; use the brachial artery only when necessary. Don't use the arm if the patient has had a vascular graft or has an atrioventricular fistula in situ.

Next, using a circular motion, clean the puncture site with povidone-iodine solution. Then wipe the site with alcohol to remove the povidone-iodine solution, which is sticky and may hinder palpation. Palpate the artery with the forefinger and middle finger of one hand while holding the syringe over the puncture site with the other hand. With the needle bevel up, puncture the skin at a 45-degree angle for the radial artery and at a 60-degree angle for the brachial artery. For a femoral arterial puncture, the needle is inserted at a 90-degree angle.

Advance the needle, but don't pull the plunger back. When you've punctured the artery, blood will pulsate into the syringe. Allow 5 to 10 ml to fill the syringe. If the syringe doesn't fill immediately, you may have pushed the needle through the artery. If so, pull the needle back slightly, but don't pull the plunger back. If the syringe still doesn't

Automatic test series: SMA 12/60 and SMAC

Many laboratories use automated electronic systems, such as the sequential multiple analyzer (SMA) 12/60 and the sequential multiple analyzer with computer (SMAC), to perform chemistry, blood banking, serologic, and bacteriologic tests. (Many laboratories have SMA 6, 12, and 20.)

The *SMA 12/60* can make 12 determinations on 60 serum specimens in 1 hour: glucose, cholesterol, albumin, total protein levels (nutritional status); bilirubin levels (liver function); blood urea nitrogen (BUN) and uric acid levels (kidney function); aspartate aminotransferase (AST) and lactate dehydrogenase (LD) enzyme levels (tissue injury); alkaline phosphatase levels (bone tissue injury); and calcium and phosphate levels (parathyroid function).

The *SMAC* can perform 20 to 40 biochemical determinations on 120 serum specimens in 1 hour. It can analyze selected blood components, singly or in combination, and provide an entire test profile on each specimen. This system also automatically reports special cardiac, renal, hepatic, lipid, bone, enzyme, and electrolyte profiles.

Tests performed on a 450-µl sample include cholesterol, triglycerides, glucose, BUN, calcium, phosphorus, sodium, potassium, chloride, carbon dioxide, total protein, total bilirubin, albumin, creatinine, gamma glutamyl transferase, AST, alanine aminotransferase, LD, uric acid, acid and alkaline phosphatase, and iron.

---

fill, withdraw the needle and start over with a fresh heparinized needle. Never make more than two attempts to draw blood from one site.

After drawing the sample, remove the needle and apply firm pressure to the puncture site with a gauze pad for at least 5 minutes to prevent hematoma (a significant risk after arterial puncture). If the patient is receiving an anticoagulant or has a bleeding disorder, apply pressure for at least 15 minutes. *Do not* ask the patient to apply pressure to the site; he may not apply the continuous, firm pressure that's needed.

Rotate the syringe to mix the heparin with the sample. Try to remove air bubbles by holding the syringe upright and tapping it lightly with your finger. If the bubbles don't disappear, hold the syringe upright and pierce a 2" x 2" gauze pad or alcohol pad with the needle. (Slowly forcing some of the blood out of the syringe eliminates the bubbles,

and the gauze pad catches the ejected blood.) After removing air bubbles, plunge the needle into a rubber stopper to seal it, or remove the needle and apply the syringe stopper from the ABG kit, if available. Transfer the sample to the iced specimen container.

Note on the laboratory request the type and amount of oxygen the patient is receiving. In certain instances (such as hypothermia), you may also be asked to provide the patient's temperature and hemaglobin count. Send the sample to the laboratory immediately.

After releasing pressure on the puncture site, tape a bandage firmly over it. (Don't tape the entire wrist.)

 After arterial puncture, observe the patient closely for signs of circulatory impairment distal to the puncture site, such as swelling or discoloration. Ask if he feels pain, numbness, or tingling in the extremity.

Performing Allen's test

Before obtaining a specimen from an arterial site, assess the blood supply to your patient's hand. If the radial artery is blocked by a blood clot — a common complication — the ulnar artery alone must supply blood to the hand. The Allen's test is a simple, reliable procedure that quickly assesses arterial function.

Just follow these steps:

1. Have the patient rest his arm on the bedside table. Support his wrist with a rolled towel. Ask him to clench his fist.

Use your index and middle fingers to exert pressure over both the radial and the ulnar arteries (as shown).

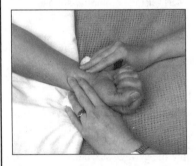

2. Without removing your fingers, ask the patient to unclench his fist (as shown above, right). You'll notice his palm is blanched because you've impaired the normal blood flow with your fingers.

Nursing tip: If your patient is unconscious or unable to clench his fist for some other reason, you can encourage his palm to blanch by oc-cluding both arteries, elevating his hand, and massaging his palm.

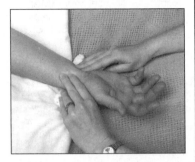

3. Release the pressure on the ulnar artery, and ask the patient to open his fist (as shown).

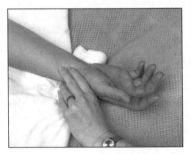

If the ulnar artery is functioning well, his palm will turn pink in about 5 seconds, even though the radial artery is still occluded. But if blood return is slow and his fingers begin to contract, blood supply from the ulnar artery may not be adequate. In that case, try Allen's test on his other wrist; you may get better results. *Note:* Slow blood return may indicate poor cardiac output or poor capillary refill due to shock.

Before drawing an arterial blood sample for ABG analysis, carefully check the patient's oxygen therapy. If ABG levels are being measured to monitor his response to withdrawal of oxygen but the patient continues to receive it, results will be misleading. For the same reason, wait 15 to 30 minutes before drawing an arterial sample after suctioning the patient or placing him on a ventilator to allow circulating blood levels to reflect mechanical ventilation. Blood gases should not be drawn during dialysis.

Capillary sample

Collection of a capillary blood sample requires puncturing the fingertip or earlobe of adults or the great toe or heel of neonates. To facilitate collection of a capillary sample, first dilate the vessels by applying warm, moist compresses to the area for about 10 minutes. Select the puncture site, wipe it with gauze and alcohol pads, and dry it thoroughly with another gauze pad so the blood will well up. Avoid cold, cyanotic, or swollen sites to ensure an adequate blood sample. To draw a sample from the fingertip, use an automatic lancing device and make the puncture perpendicular to the lines of the patient's fingerprints.

After drawing the sample, wipe away the first drop of blood and avoid squeezing the puncture site to reduce the risk of diluting the sample with tissue fluid. After collecting the sample, apply pressure to the puncture site briefly to prevent painful extravasation of blood into the subcutaneous tissues. Ask the adult patient to hold a sterile gauze pad over the puncture site until bleeding has stopped. Then apply a small adhesive bandage.

Interfering factors

Because food and medications can interfere with test methods, be sure to check the patient's diet and medication history before tests, and schedule them after an overnight fast of 12 to 14 hours. Although the concentration of most blood constituents doesn't change significantly after a meal, fasting is customary because blood collected shortly after eating often appears cloudy (turbid) from a temporary increase in triglyceride levels, which can interfere with many chemical reactions. Transient, food-related lipemia usually disappears 4 to

6 hours after a meal, making such short fasts acceptable before blood collection. Baseline studies often depend on the patient's diet. For example, valid glucose tolerance test results require an adequate daily carbohydrate intake (250 mg) for 3 days before testing. Similarly, recent protein and fat consumption influences uric acid, urea, and lipid levels.

Numerous drugs and their metabolites can affect test results by pharmacologic or chemical interference. Pharmacologic interference results from temporary or permanent drug-induced physiologic changes in a blood component. For example, long-term administration of aminoglycosides can damage the kidneys and alter the results of renal function studies. Chemical interference results from a drug's physical characteristic that alters the test reaction. For example, high doses of ascorbic acid may raise blood glucose levels. To identify such interference with test results, all unexpected changes in blood values require a meticulous review of the patient's drug and dietary history and of his clinical status.

Urine

The type of urine specimen required — random, second-voided, clean-catch midstream, first morning, fasting, or timed — depends on the patient's condition and the purpose of the test. Random, second-voided, and clean-catch midstream specimens can be collected at any time; first morning, fasting, and timed specimens require collection at specific times.

To collect a *random specimen* (for such routine tests as urinalysis), the patient simply collects urine from one voiding in a specimen container. Although this method provides quick laboratory results, the information it supplies is less reliable than that from a controlled specimen.

To collect a *second-voided specimen,* the patient voids, discards the urine, and then voids again 30 minutes later into a specimen container.

To collect a *clean-catch specimen,* the patient voids first into either a bedpan or toilet and then collects a sample in midstream. Originally used mainly to test for bacteriuria and pyuria, this type of specimen is now replacing the random specimen because it's aseptic.

First morning and *fasting specimens* must be collected when the patient awakens. Because the first morning specimen is the most concentrated of the day, it's the specimen of choice for nitrate, protein, and urinary sediment analyses. To obtain this specimen, the patient voids and discards the urine just before going to bed, then collects the urine from the first voiding of the morning. For the fasting specimen, which is used for glucose testing, the patient maintains an overnight fast and collects a first morning specimen.

A *timed specimen* determines the urinary concentration of such substances as hormones, proteins, creatinine, and electrolytes over a specified period — usually 2, 12, or 24 hours. The 24-hour collection, the most common duration, provides a measure of average excretion for substances eliminated in variable amounts during the day, such as hormones. A timed specimen may also be collected after administration of a challenge dose of a chemical, to measure physiologic efficiency — for example, ingestion of glucose to test for incipient diabetes mellitus or hypoglycemia. This type of specimen is also preferred for quantitative analysis of urobilinogen, amylase, or dye excretion.

Equipment
For random, second-voided, first morning, or *fasting collection:* clean, dry bedpan or urinal (for nonambulatory patients) ✦ gloves ✦ specimen container ✦ specimen labels ✦ laboratory request.

For clean-catch midstream collection: commercially prepared kit containing necessary equipment and directions for patient in several languages (English, Spanish, French); or antiseptic solution (green soap or povidone-iodine solution) ✦ water ✦ cotton balls ✦ sterile gloves ✦ specimen labels ✦ laboratory request.

For timed collection (24-hour specimen): clean, dry gallon containers or commercial urine collection containers ✦ preservative, as ordered ✦ labels for collection container ✦ display signs.

For pediatric urine collection: gloves ✦ plastic disposable collection bags ✦ specimen containers ✦ laboratory request ✦ cotton swabs ✦ soap and water ✦ diapers.

Random and second-voided collections
For random collection, tell the ambulatory patient to urinate directly into a clean, dry specimen container. Tell the nonambulatory patient to void into a clean bedpan or urinal to minimize bacterial or chemical contamination; then put on gloves, transfer about 30 ml of urine to the specimen container, and secure the cap.

For second-voided collection, instruct the patient to void and discard the urine. Then offer him at least one glass of water to stimulate urine production. Collect urine 30 minutes later, using the random collection technique.

Label the specimen container with the patient's name and room number, and send the labeled container to the laboratory immediately. On the chart, record the procedure and the time the specimen was sent.

First morning and fasting collections

Unless the patient is an infant or is catheterized or unable to urinate, use the following collection techniques.

For fasting specimen collection, instruct the patient to restrict food and fluids after midnight before the test. For both collection procedures, instruct the patient to void and discard the urine before retiring for the night and then collect the first voiding of the next day in a clean, dry specimen container. (If the patient must void during the night, note it on the specimen label — for example, "Urine specimen, 2:15 a.m. to 8:00 a.m.")

Label the container with the patient's name and room number (if applicable), doctor's name, date, and collection time. Send the specimen and a completed request to the laboratory immediately. On the chart, record the procedure and the time the specimen was sent.

Clean-catch midstream collection

This aseptic technique for obtaining a clean-catch midstream urine specimen has become the acceptable procedure for collecting a random urine specimen. It's especially valuable for collecting urine specimens from women because it provides a specimen that's virtually free of bacterial contamination.

Teach the patient how to obtain a clean-catch midstream specimen. Send the specimen to the laboratory immediately or refrigerate it to prevent proliferation of bacteria. On the chart, record the procedure and the time the specimen was sent.

Timed collection

All timed specimens — 2-, 12-, and 24-hour — are collected in virtually the same way. This procedure is used for uncatheterized adults and continent children.

Explain the procedure to the patient, and instruct him to collect all urine during the test period, to notify you after each voiding, and to avoid contaminating the specimen with toilet tissue or stool. Also, provide him with written instructions for home collection. Explain any necessary dietary, drug, or activity restrictions.

Obtain the proper preservative from the laboratory. Write down the test requirements on the nursing-care Kardex. Label a gallon jug or a commercial urine collection container with the patient's name and room number (if applicable); the doctor's name; the date and time the collection begins and ends; a "Do Not Discard" warning; and instructions to keep the container refrigerated. Prominently display signs indicating that a 24-hour urine collection is in progress: one at the head of the patient's bed, a second over the toilet bowl in his bathroom, and a third over the utility room bedpan hopper.

Tell the patient to void and discard the urine; then begin a 24-hour collection with the next voiding. After placing the urine from the first voiding in the container, add the preservative. Add each subsequent urine specimen to the container immediately. If any urine is lost, restart the test, but remember that the test should end at a time that the laboratory is open. Just before the end of the collection period, instruct the patient to void, and add the urine to the gallon jug.

Send the labeled container to the laboratory as soon as the collection period has ended. On the chart, record the time that urine collection ended and when the specimen was sent to the laboratory.

Special timed collections

Some tests require specimen collection at specified times — for example, the glucose tolerance test requires collection of urine at 30 minutes, 1 hour, 2 hours, 3 hours and, occasionally, 4 and 5 hours

Applying a pediatric urine collector

To attach a plastic urine collector to an infant girl (left), stretch the perineum to smooth the skin around the vagina. Working upward from the perineum, press the bag's adhesive ring inside the labia. To attach the collector to an infant boy (right), make sure the adhesive seal attaches firmly to the skin and does not pucker.

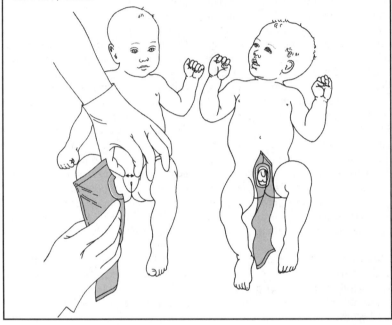

after a test meal. To ensure that the patient can void at the specified times, have him drink water at least every hour. Other tests, including urea clearance, require only 2-hour collection periods. For these tests, give the patient at least 20 oz (600 ml) of water 30 minutes before the test, and instruct him to drink at least one full glass each hour during the test.

Pediatric urine collection

Pediatric urine collection is used to obtain a random, second-voided, first morning, fasting, or timed specimen from infants.

Position the infant on his back, with his hips externally rotated and abducted, and knees flexed. Put on gloves. Clean the perineal area with cotton swabs, soap, and water. Rinse the area with warm water and dry it thoroughly.

For *boys,* apply the collection device over the penis and scrotum with gloved hands, and closely press the flaps of the bag against the perineum to secure it. For *girls,* put on gloves, and tape the pediatric collection device to the perineum, starting between the anus and the vagina and working anteriorly. (See *Applying a pediatric urine collector.*) Place a diaper over the collection bag to discourage the child from tampering with it. Elevate the head of the bed to facilitate drainage.

Remove the bag immediately after

collection is complete to prevent skin excoriation. Transfer the urine to a clean, dry specimen container. Label the container with the patient's name and room number (if applicable), doctor's name, date, and collection time. Send the specimen and the completed request to the laboratory immediately, and note the collection time on the chart.

Catheter collection

Although catheter collection increases the risk of bacterial infection in the lower genitourinary tract, it may be necessary to obtain a random, second-voided, first morning, fasting, or timed specimen in a patient who can't void voluntarily.

Have the following equipment available: sterile catheterization set (sterile gloves, sterile catheter [#16F for adults, #8F for children]) ✦ sterile forceps ✦ soap, water, towelette ✦ sterile water-soluble lubricant ✦ sterile cotton balls ✦ antiseptic solution ✦ sterile drapes ✦ sterile specimen container ✦ labels for specimen container.

Tell the patient you'll collect a urine specimen by inserting a small tube into the bladder through the urethra and that, although this procedure may cause some discomfort, it takes only a few minutes. (See *Inserting a straight catheter*, pages xxx to xxxii.)

Male catheterization: Put on gloves and wash the perineal area with soap and water. Place a sterile drape under the patient's buttocks and around the penis, making sure that you don't contaminate the drape. Remove the contaminated gloves, and put on sterile gloves. Place the antiseptic solution on the cotton balls. Arrange all sterile articles within easy reach on a sterile wrapper. Open the sterile specimen container, and lubricate the sterile catheter. Grasp the shaft of the penis in one hand and elevate it about 90 degrees to the upright position; hold it in this position until the procedure is completed.

Retract the foreskin and, with the forceps, grasp an antiseptic-moistened cotton ball. Clean the urethral meatus, wiping with a circular motion away from the urethral opening toward the glans. Repeat twice, each time with a clean cotton ball. *Gently* insert the lubricated catheter until urine flows. Allow a few milliliters to drain into the basin; then collect 10 to 60 ml in a sterile plastic container, depending on test requirements. After gently removing the catheter, clean and dry the periurethral area.

Send the specimen and the laboratory request to the laboratory within 10 minutes, or refrigerate the specimen. On the chart, record the procedure and the time the specimen is sent.

Female catheterization: Put on gloves. After washing the perineal area with soap and water, place the patient in the supine position, with knees flexed and feet on the bed. Place a sterile drape under her buttocks and around the perineal area, making sure that you don't contaminate the drape. Remove the contaminated gloves, and put on sterile gloves. Place the antiseptic solution on the cotton balls, and lubricate the sterile catheter. Arrange all sterile articles within easy reach on a sterile wrapper, and open the sterile specimen container.

Separate the labia majora and keep them open with one hand. With the forceps, grasp an antiseptic-moistened cotton ball. Make two vertical swipes on the labia minora. (Use a new cotton ball for each swipe, cleaning from the urethral meatus toward the anus.) Position the sterile tray with the lubricated catheter on the sterile field between the patient's legs. *Gently* insert the catheter into the urethra until urine flows. Allow a few milliliters of urine to flow into a basin; then collect 10 to 60 ml in a sterile plastic container, depending on the test re-

Inserting a straight catheter

1. Obtain a prepackaged sterile insertion kit, which contains sterile gloves, drapes (regular and fenestrated), cotton balls, forceps, water-soluble lubricant, a urine collection basin, a sterile urine specimen container with label, and povidone-iodine or another antiseptic solution. If the prepackaged kit does not contain a urinary catheter, obtain one in the proper size. You should also gather a washcloth and towel, gloves, soap and water, a biohazard bag, and a reliable light source.

Explain the procedure to the patient and reassure him.

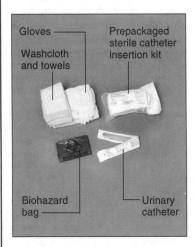

Gloves —

Washcloth and towels

Prepackaged sterile catheter insertion kit

Biohazard bag —

— Urinary catheter

2. Position a female patient flat on her back, with her knees bent and her legs abducted. Place a linen-saver pad under her buttocks, and position her feet about 2' (60 cm) apart

(as shown). Direct the light source toward the perineum.

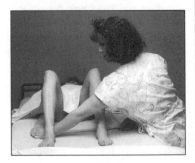

3. Put on gloves and wash the patient's perineum with soap and water; pat it dry with a towel. Then remove your gloves.

Place the sterile catheter insertion kit between the patient's legs (as shown). Open the kit, using aseptic technique. If the catheter is packaged separately, open the package and drop the catheter into the open kit.

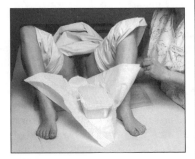

4. Still using aseptic technique, put on sterile gloves and pick up the sterile, fenestrated drape. Ask the patient to raise her pelvis by pushing down on her feet. Slide the drape under her buttocks with your gloved hand. Now tell her to lower her pelvis onto the drape. Position the drape so that the opening is over the perineum (as shown).

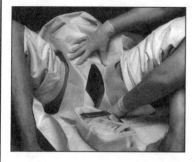

5. To clean the perineal area, use your nondominant hand to spread apart the patient's labia. With the thumb and index finger of the same hand, separate the labia to expose the urethral meatus (as shown).

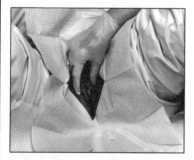

Be careful not to confuse the urethral opening with the vaginal opening. Look for the meatus between the clitoris and the vagina. If you can't see it, it may be hidden in the anterior part of the vagina. If you can't find it there, exert gentle downward pressure when you clean between the labia (see step 6); this should open the meatus briefly.

Caution: The hand used to clean the labia is now considered contaminated. Do *not* use it to insert the catheter.

6. With your uncontaminated hand, use the forceps to pick up a cotton ball saturated with the antiseptic solution. Clean the labia minora with a downward stroke (as shown). Discard the cotton ball in the biohazard bag. Then clean the other side with another saturated cotton ball, and discard the cotton ball. Pick up another cotton ball and wipe directly over the meatus. Discard the cotton ball and the forceps.

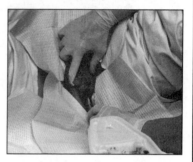

6a. If the patient is male, hold his penis in your nondominant hand. With your uncontaminated hand, use the forceps to pick up a saturated cotton ball (as shown). Clean around the meatus using a circular motion. Then, with another cotton ball, clean in a spiral motion to the corona of the glans penis.

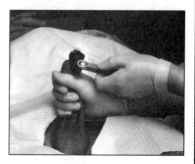

(continued)

7. Now, with your uncontaminated hand, grasp the catheter as you would a pencil (as shown). Making sure that the catheter doesn't touch the unprepped areas of the perineum, gently insert it 2" to 3" (5 to 8 cm) into the meatus. Angle the catheter slightly upward as you advance it.

Caution: Never force the catheter.

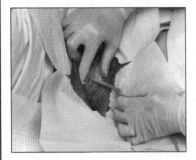

7a. For a male patient, hold the penis at a 90-degree angle to his thighs. Grasp the catheter with your uncontaminated hand, and gently insert it into the meatus (as shown above, right). Advance it 7" to 10" (18 to 25 cm) along the anterior wall of the urethra. A few inches into the urethra (at the internal sphincter, just below the prostate), you'll encounter resistance from most patients. If your patient indicates discomfort, reassure him.

Caution: Never forcibly insert a catheter. If you encounter an obstruction, call the doctor. He'll introduce the catheter using a guide.

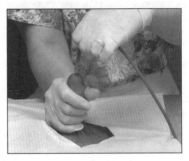

8. As the catheter enters the patient's bladder, urine begins to flow. Release the labia. Using your sterile hand, place the free end of the catheter in the specimen container (as shown). Make sure you grasp the catheter high enough to avoid contaminating the specimen. Let the container fill to the three-quarters mark. When the container has filled, allow the remaining urine to drain.

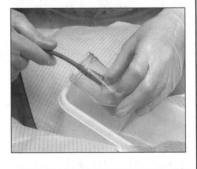

quirements. After gently removing the catheter, clean and dry the urethral area.

Send the specimen and a laboratory request to the laboratory within 10 minutes after collection, or refrigerate the specimen. On the chart, record the procedure and the time that the specimen was sent.

Collection from an indwelling urinary catheter

You can minimize the risk of bacterial contamination by aspirating a urine specimen from an indwelling urinary catheter made of self-sealing rubber or from a collection tube with a special sampling port. (However, *don't* aspirate a Silastic, silicone, or plastic catheter.) This technique can provide a random, second-voided, first morning, fasting, or timed specimen.

Have ready the following equipment: gloves ✦ sterile syringe (10 to 20 ml) ✦ sterile needle (21G to 25G) ✦ alcohol sponge ✦ sterile specimen container ✦ specimen labels ✦ laboratory request.

About 30 minutes before collecting the specimen, clamp the collection tube. (This procedure is contraindicated for patients who've just undergone genitourinary surgery.) Put on gloves. After wiping the sampling port with an alcohol sponge, insert the needle at a 90-degree angle and aspirate the urine into the syringe. If the collection tube has a rubber catheter but not a port, obtain the specimen from the catheter. Wipe the catheter with alcohol just above the connection of the collection tube to the catheter. Insert the needle at a 45-degree angle into the catheter, and withdraw the urine specimen. Never insert the needle into the shaft of the catheter because this may puncture the lumen leading to the balloon.

Failure to unclamp the tube after collecting the specimen can cause bladder distention and may predispose the patient to a bladder infection. If you can't draw any urine, lift the tube a little, but make sure urine doesn't return to the bladder. Aspirate urine, transfer the specimen to a sterile container, and cap the container securely. Send it to the laboratory in a plastic bag.

Interfering factors

A common interfering factor in urine collection, especially in timed collections, is the patient's failure to follow the correct collection procedure. Inaccurate test results may be due to *overcollection,* by failing to discard the last voiding before the test period; *undercollection,* by failing to include all urine voided during the test; *contamination,* by including toilet tissue or stool in the specimen; or, for procedures requiring collection at specified times or for the second-voided collection, the patient's *inability to urinate on demand.* In urine specimens collected from females, vaginal drainage (such as menses, which elevates the RBC count) can alter the results of a urinalysis.

Improper collection or handling of the specimen can also produce unreliable results. For instance, failure to thoroughly clean the urethral meatus and glans before collection can contaminate a clean-catch midstream specimen. Similarly, failure to send a urine specimen to the laboratory immediately allows bacterial proliferation and thus invalidates the colony count on bacterial culture.

Foods and drugs can affect test results by changing the composition of the urine. For example, ingestion of sugar increases urine glucose levels. Drugs can cause chemical or pharmacologic interference with the laboratory analysis. For example, corticosteroids tend to elevate glucose levels.

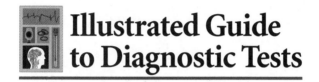

Illustrated Guide to Diagnostic Tests

Second Edition

CHAPTER ONE

Hematology

Learning objectives

After completing this chapter, the reader will be able to:
- describe the formation, components, and functions of red blood cells
- describe the types and functions of white blood cells (WBCs)
- explain how hypoxia stimulates erythropoiesis
- list drugs that decrease the WBC count
- list five disorders that affect serum iron and total iron-binding capacity
- identify the causes of abnormal blood cell production
- discuss the significance of the complete blood count and differential

- state the purpose of each test discussed in the chapter
- prepare the patient physically and psychologically for each test
- describe the procedure for performing each test
- specify appropriate precautions for accurate administration of each test
- implement appropriate post-test care
- state the reference values for each test
- discuss the implications of abnormal test results
- list factors that may interfere with accurate test results.

INTRODUCTION

Blood is a continuously circulating tissue that performs many vital functions as it flows through the body. Most important is its ability to transport oxygen (bound to hemoglobin in red blood cells [RBCs]) from the lungs to the body tissues and to return carbon dioxide from the tissues to the lungs. Blood contains white blood cells (WBCs) called leukocytes, which produce antibodies and consume pathogens by phagocytosis. Blood also contains complement, a group of immunologically significant protein substances.

Other functions performed by blood include maintenance of hemostasis with platelets and with coagulation factors, which repair tissue injuries and prevent bleeding; regulation of body temperature and of acid-base and fluid balances; movement of nutrients and regulatory hormones to body tissues; and disposal of metabolic wastes through the kidneys, lungs, and skin. Abnormalities of either RBCs or WBCs can result in various disorders. (See *Blood cell disorders,* pages 3 and 4.)

Blood is three times as viscous as water, tastes slightly salty, and has an alkaline pH of 7.35 to 7.45. Oxygenated arterial blood is bright red; oxygen-poor venous blood is dark red.

Blood has two major components: plasma, the clear, straw-colored liquid portion; and the formed elements, erythrocytes (red blood cells), leukocytes (white blood cells), and thrombocytes (platelets).

Red cells

Also known as erythrocytes and red corpuscles, RBCs appear in the embryonic yolk sac during the first weeks of fetal development. During the second trimester, the fetal liver and spleen produce most RBCs. Starting just before birth, the marrow of all bones produces RBCs. The total quantity of active marrow decreases as the person grows. By adult-

Blood cell disorders

RED CELL DISORDERS

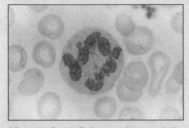

Vitamin B₁₂ deficiency: *characteristically marked by a macrocytic neutrophil cell with increased lobulation, interspersed with macrocytic erythrocytes*

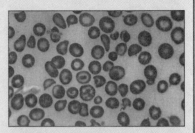

β-thalassemia: *characteristically marked by erythrocytes that vary in size and shape and include target cells (dark centers encircled by pale rings)*

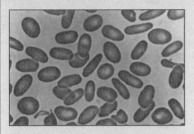

Hereditary ovalocytosis: *characteristically marked by oval erythrocytes with pale centers*

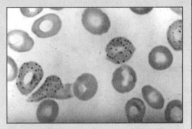

Lead poisoning: *characteristically marked by basophilic stippling of red blood cells*

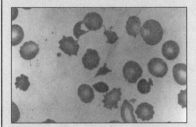

Thrombotic thrombocytopenic purpura: *characteristically marked by helmet, thorn, burr, and fragmented erythrocytes and diffusely basophilic cells*

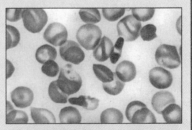

Hemoglobin S-C disease: *characteristically marked by "SC" red cells (dense-staining fingerlike protrusions in center), many target cells (dark centers encircled by pale rings), and several folded and irregular spherical cells*

(continued)

Blood cell disorders (continued)

WHITE CELL DISORDERS

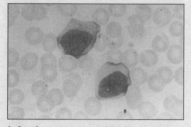

Infectious mononucleosis: *characteristically marked by large, reactive lymphocytes interspersed with normal erythrocytes*

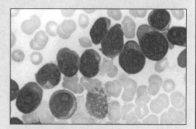

Acute granulocytic leukemia: *characteristically marked by myeloblasts showing early chromatin pattern and nucleoli*

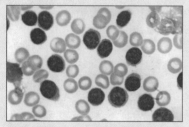

Chronic lymphocytic leukemia: *characteristically marked by increased numbers of mature lymphocytes and thrombocytopenia, shown in the photograph by two disintegrated cells (smudges)*

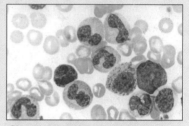

Chronic granulocytic leukemia: *characteristically marked by leukocytosis, shown in the photograph by the presence of a progranulocyte, a neutrophilic myelocyte, a neutrophilic metamyelocyte, neutrophilic bands, and basophils*

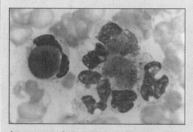

Lupus erythematosus: *characteristically marked by LE cells*

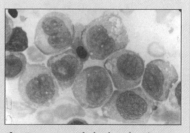

Acute monocytic leukemia: *characteristically marked by monoblasts, promonocytes, prominent nucleoli, nuclear folding, abundant blue cytoplasm, vacuoles, and pseudopods*

hood, the marrow of membranous bones (sternum, ribs, vertebrae, and pelvis) becomes the primary source of red cells. Red cell production declines with advancing age.

Current theory states that hemocytoblasts are the progenitors of red cells. Hemocytoblasts repeatedly change shape and function until they become mature red cells. Most circulating red cells are biconcave and disk-shaped, range in color from pale pink at the center to deep pink at the periphery, and are normally 7 microns in diameter. Abnormal red cells may vary in size (anisocytosis) or in color (anisochromia), or may assume permanent changes in shape (poikilocytosis). In *anisocytosis,* cell diameter ranges from about 6 microns (microcytic) to 9 microns (macrocytic), with slight, moderate, or marked gradations. In *anisochromia,* RBC color ranges from insufficient (hypochromic) to excessive (hyperchromic). In *poikilocytosis,* bizarre shapes, such as teardrop, sickle, or pear, generally reflect abnormal cell formation and development in the bone marrow.

The number of red cells in an adult varies according to sex, age, and geographic location. Men usually have higher counts than women, and the elderly have fewer red cells than young adults. Persons living at high altitudes generally have more red cells than those living at sea level — a compensatory adaptation to the thinner air.

Red cell function

A primary function of red cells is to maintain a high concentration of circulatory hemoglobin. Hemoglobin — the main component of the red cell — is a conjugated protein that enables red cells to carry oxygen from the lungs to the tissues and to carry carbon dioxide from the tissues back to the lungs for excretion. Red cells also transport large quantities of carbon dioxide through the activity of carbonic anhydrase, a red cell enzyme. By accelerating the reaction between carbon dioxide and water, this enzyme promotes absorption into the blood of large quantities of carbon dioxide. Thus, red cells help maintain the body's acid-base balance.

Mature red cells circulate in the blood for about 120 days. As they age, these cells become fragile, finally rupture and decompose, and then are removed by the spleen and the liver.

Hemoglobin

Hemoglobin (Hb), which constitutes about 90% of the mature red cell's dry weight, is composed of 4% heme — an iron and porphyrin complex that colors it — and 96% globin — a simple water-soluble protein. Hemoglobin synthesis depends on the metabolism of the porphyrin complex, globin, and iron.

The body contains about 4 g of iron; more than half this amount is in the hemoglobin of red cells. Iron is absorbed from food in the upper intestine, primarily the duodenum, through the blood; the amount absorbed is normally in response to the amount lost daily. For transport, iron combines with a glycoprotein, transferrin. Some iron is transported to the bone marrow for hemoglobin synthesis; some goes to needy tissues, such as muscle, for myoglobin synthesis; and unused iron is converted to ferritin and is stored in the liver, spleen, bone marrow, and reticuloendothelial system. The iron in the hemoglobin of destroyed red cells is recycled by the spleen, either for inclusion in new red cells or for storage in the liver. Normally, less than 1 mg of iron is lost daily through the skin, feces, and urine.

Three major types of hemoglobin are found in normal blood: Hb A, Hb A_2, and Hb F. Hb A accounts for more than 95% of adult hemoglobin, with Hb A_2 comprising 2% to 3%. Although traces of Hb F appear in adult blood, this type

Abnormal hemoglobins

Abnormal hemoglobins can be classified as homozygous or heterozygous. This chart lists some abnormal hemoglobins and their clinical effects.

CLASSIFICATION	ABNORMAL HEMOGLOBIN	CLINICAL EFFECTS
Homozygous (double complement of genes)	S	Sickle cell anemia
	C	Three variants, two of which cause sickling
	D, E	Mild hemolytic anemia
	M	Methemoglobinemia and cyanosis
Heterozygous (bearing a single gene)	Chesapeake, Hiroshima, Capetown, Bethesda	Increased oxygen affinity and polycythemia
	Kansas, Seattle, Bristol, Yoshizuka	Decreased oxygen affinity, cyanosis, and anemia
	Torino, Ann Arbor, Hasharon	Congenital Heinz body hemolytic anemia
	H, Bart's	Thalassemias

of hemoglobin appears predominately in the fetus and neonate, thereafter decreasing to 2% to 3% of the infant's blood at age 6 months.

Hemoglobin variants

Each heme molecule is attached to a *globin* molecule. Each of these combinations represents a subunit of hemoglobin, and each hemoglobin molecule contains four subunits. One molecule of hemoglobin can carry four molecules of oxygen. The globins are present as two identical pairs. Variations occur, however, creating abnormal hemoglobins. Because the heme portion of all hemoglobins is identical, variations are possible only in these polypeptide globins, resulting from substitutions in any of the amino acid chains. Such substitutions may result in structurally unstable hemoglobin. An identical substitution in both polypeptide pairs produces a *homozygous* variation; a substitution in one pair or nonidentical changes in both pairs result in *heterozygous* variation.

Overall, genetic and acquired variations account for more than 200 abnormal hemoglobins. (See *Abnormal hemoglobins.*)

Abnormal hemoglobins were initially identified using capital letters — for example, Hb S for the abnormal hemoglobin in sickle cell anemia. As the alphabet was nearly exhausted, new abnormal hemoglobins were identified with place names, such as Hb D Punjab. (A letter plus a place name means identical mobility on hemoglobin electrophoresis, but different substitution.) In addition, the Greek letters alpha and beta are used to identify a known abnormal polypeptide chain.

Abnormal red cell production

Erythropoietin, a glycoprotein of low molecular weight originating in the kid-

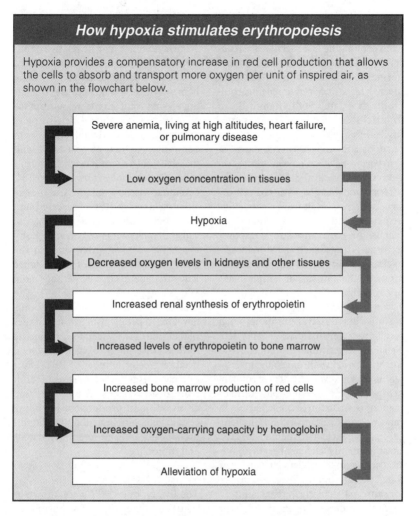

How hypoxia stimulates erythropoiesis

Hypoxia provides a compensatory increase in red cell production that allows the cells to absorb and transport more oxygen per unit of inspired air, as shown in the flowchart below.

> Severe anemia, living at high altitudes, heart failure, or pulmonary disease
>
> Low oxygen concentration in tissues
>
> Hypoxia
>
> Decreased oxygen levels in kidneys and other tissues
>
> Increased renal synthesis of erythropoietin
>
> Increased levels of erythropoietin to bone marrow
>
> Increased bone marrow production of red cells
>
> Increased oxygen-carrying capacity by hemoglobin
>
> Alleviation of hypoxia

neys, stimulates production (erythropoiesis), maturation, and release of red cells from the bone marrow and other blood-forming tissues. Low oxygen levels in the kidneys and in other tissues (hypoxia) cause increased secretion of this glycoprotein, which accelerates red cell production. (See *How hypoxia stimulates erythropoiesis.*) Hypoxia can result from severe anemia, heart failure, pulmonary disease, or living at high altitudes.

Anemias, defined by abnormally low hemoglobin concentration, red cell count, and hematocrit, may reflect acute or chronic blood loss, excessive hemolysis, or deficient blood production. Anemias are classified by their causes or by the structural changes they produce in the red cells — normocytic (normal), microcytic (small), or macrocytic (large) — and by hemoglobin content as normochromic or hypochromic (normal color or pale).

Together these classifications can describe anemia accurately. If the size, shape, and hemoglobin content of RBCs are normal but RBC production is depressed, *normocytic normochromic anemia* is diagnosed. Such anemia results from debilitating disorders, such as cancer and chronic infection. If RBCs have normal color but are abnormally large, *macrocytic normochromic anemia,* commonly associated with vitamin B_{12} or folic acid deficiency, is diagnosed. If RBCs are small and pale from hemoglobin deficiency, the patient has *microcytic hypochromic anemia,* which most often results from iron deficiency.

Hemolytic anemia, with red cell destruction, may result from a congenital defect (such as sickle cell anemia or thalassemia) or as an acquired response to certain drugs (such as methyldopa), to certain disorders (Hodgkin's disease, lupus erythematosus, or lymphomas), or to foreign red cells (transfusion reaction).

Similarly, reduced erythropoiesis may result from various diseases and deficiencies. For example, prolonged X-ray therapy can cause chronic bone marrow hypoplasia and varying degrees of pancytopenia (aplastic anemia). Impairment or destruction of bone marrow by cancer, thymic tumor, or chloramphenicol creates deficiency of hemocytoblasts, causing anemia. Deficient erythropoiesis also results from deficiency of iron, folic acid, or vitamin B_{12}. Another major cause, particularly in renal failure, is impaired secretion of erythropoietin, the hormone that stimulates bone marrow production. Erythropoietin levels drop markedly when the kidneys are removed or damaged, but this condition can now be treated with recombinant erythropoietin.

Polycythemias

The body reacts to hypoxia by a compensatory increase in red cell production. Severe and chronic hypoxia, such as results from congenital heart disease and pulmonary disease, can lead to overcompensation and overproduction of RBCs, a condition called polycythemia.

Polycythemias may be relative or absolute, and either primary or secondary. In *relative* (or *spurious*) *polycythemia,* hematocrit is elevated because circulating plasma volume is decreased, but total red cell mass is normal. Relative polycythemia follows dehydration from vomiting, diarrhea, or heatstroke, and massive fluid loss from extensive burns.

In *absolute polycythemia,* the RBC count may rise to 8 million/μl as the circulating mass of RBCs increases, and hematocrit rises to 70% to 80%. The cause of *primary polycythemia* (polycythemia vera) is unknown, but the bone marrow produces many more RBCs than necessary and perhaps more WBCs and platelets.

Secondary (or *reactive*) *polycythemia* develops in people who live at altitudes higher than 14,000 feet; to compensate for less atmospheric oxygen, the blood needs a greater number of RBCs. Secondary polycythemia may also result from disorders that cause increased erythropoietin production, including certain hemoglobinopathies, cardiopulmonary disease, and certain renal cysts and tumors.

White cells

The five types of WBCs are known as neutrophils, eosinophils, basophils, monocytes, and lymphocytes. *Neutrophils* are so named because they accept both acidic and basic stains. White cells that develop an orange-red cytoplasm when stained with the acid dye eosin are called *eosinophils* (eosin-loving cells), and the cytoplasm of *basophils* readily accepts a basic dye. These three cell types are collectively known as *granulocytes* because they characteristically display irregularly shaped nuclei and granules dispersed in their cytoplasm.

Monocytes and *lymphocytes* are mononuclear cells. Monocytes are phagocytic and develop into macrophages. Most lymphocytes are formed in lymphoid tissue, but some of them, and all neutrophils, basophils, eosinophils, and monocytes, are formed only in bone marrow.

The special function of white cells, particularly neutrophils, is to protect the body against infection. WBCs respond to inflammation by chemotaxis, a process of chemical attraction or repulsion. Inflamed tissue causes positive chemotaxis, a biochemical alarm that draws white cells to the infected area. White cells move about by ameboid motion or diapedesis. In ameboid motion, one end of the cell alternately protrudes and pulls the remainder of the cell along with it. In diapedesis, the cell squeezes itself through pores or interstitial spaces in the capillary endothelium. Once at the infection site, white cells engulf and digest any foreign matter by a process called phagocytosis. (See *Phagocytosis,* page 10.)

Granulocytes

Produced in the bone marrow and stored there until the body needs them, granulocytes normally circulate for about 12 hours, but during severe stress, they survive only 2 or 3 hours. The following abnormal cellular inclusions can appear in granulocytes:

■ *Toxic granules:* Patients with severe bacterial infection or fever associated with extensive tissue damage may have neutrophils with deeply staining granules. These granules may be abnormally activated neutrophilic granules rather than inclusion bodies or phagocytized material.

■ *Döhle's inclusion bodies:* Patients with severe burns, bacterial infection, malignant disease, or extensive cytolysis may have neutrophils with large, round, blue cytoplasmic masses. These bodies reflect a too-rapid proliferation of neutrophils,

but they may also occur in normal pregnancy.

■ *Azurophil granules:* Small, smoothly rounded granules that contain diverse lysosomal enzymes, azurophil granules appear in lymphocytes, monocytes, and immature granulocytes. After such cells mature and specific granulation develops, a few azurophil granules persist in the cells but reflect no pathology.

■ *Auer bodies (Auer rods):* Composed of slender, rodlike masses of pink or purple cytoplasmic material, Auer bodies indicate abnormal cellular development of granulocytes or monocytes. Since these bodies never appear in lymphocytes, their presence makes possible the classification of very immature, undifferentiated leukemic cells as belonging to the myelomonocytic series.

■ *Hypersegmentation and macropolycytes:* Abnormal metabolism of folic acid and vitamin B_{12} may induce production of abnormally large granulocytes and erythrocytes. Hypersegmented neutrophils may have seven or eight lobes in their nuclei, instead of the normal three to five.

Neutrophils

More than half the white cells in the peripheral circulation are neutrophils. Because they quickly phagocytize significant quantities of microorganisms, neutrophils are the body's first line of defense against infection. Each mature neutrophil can inactivate 5 to 20 bacteria.

A small number of slightly immature neutrophils, known as *band cells,* normally appears in peripheral blood. In a differential count, the presence of many band cells and their precursors is known as a shift to the left and indicates infection. A shift to the right describes the presence of mature, hypersegmented neutrophils that have more nuclear segments than normal; this commonly occurs with pernicious anemia and hepat-

Phagocytosis

In response to infection, chemotaxis directs macrophages to the infection site, where phagocytosis — engulfment and destruction of the bacteria or other foreign particles — occurs.

First, bacteria attach to the cell surface, initiating opsonization (figure 1), antibody coating of the bacteria that enables phagocytosis. Then, macrophages surround the bacteria by forming pseudopods — footlike extensions (figure 2). Phagosomes digest the foreign particle and merge with lysosomes, becoming phagolysosomes (figure 3), which release enzymes that help iodine, bromide, and chloride bind to the cell wall to destroy the bacteria. Finally, macrophages release digestive debris (figure 4), so they can continue to fight infection.

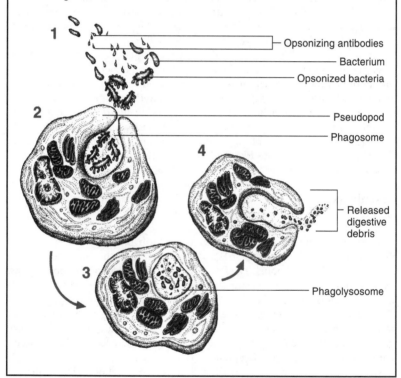

1 — Opsonizing antibodies
— Bacterium
— Opsonized bacteria

2 — Pseudopod
— Phagosome

4 — Released digestive debris

3 — Phagolysosome

ic disease. Increased band cells and a low total WBC count reflect bone marrow depression (as in typhoid fever), known as a degenerative shift. A regenerative shift implies stimulation of the bone marrow (as in pneumonia and appendicitis) and may be noted by increased band cells, metamyelocytes, and myelocytes, together with a high WBC count.

Eosinophils

Although eosinophils are phagocytic, they proliferate in response to allergic conditions rather than to bacterial infection. In allergic reactions, eosinophils pour into the blood and collect at the site of tissue inflammation; they detoxify foreign protein matter and ingest antigen-antibody complexes before these complexes can damage the body. The most common causes of eosinophilia are allergic disorders and parasitic infections.

Basophils

Basophils contain large amounts of histamine. Their most important role is in immediate hypersensitivity reactions. Basophils have specific immunoglobulin E receptors that cause degranulation when the appropriate antigens are present. This reaction may be manifested as anaphylaxis brought on by drugs or insect stings and as some forms of bronchial asthma, hives, or allergic rhinitis.

Monocytes to macrophages

The body's second line of defense, monocytes arrive at infection sites in smaller numbers than do neutrophils. Bone marrow releases immature monocytes into the circulation. Within a few hours, they enter the tissue, where they perform their phagocytic function. As a monocyte matures into a macrophage, it enlarges; its lysosome and hydrolytic enzymes increase, enhancing its bactericidal activity. These macrophages ingest debris; depending on the amount ingested, they may eventually become so engorged that they die. Immature monocytes that become fixed in the tissue are called *tissue macrophages*, or *histiocytes*; they become part of the reticuloendothelial system and establish themselves in the lymph nodes, alveoli of the lungs, the spleen, the bone marrow, and the hepatic sinuses (in the latter, they're known as *Kupffer's cells*).

Lymphocytes

Important in both humoral and cell-mediated immunity, lymphocytes are produced in the lymph nodes, spleen, thymus, tonsils, and lymphoid tissue of the gut. Together with neutrophils, they make up the majority of white cells in

the peripheral blood. In cellular immunity, sensitized T lymphocytes (thymus-derived) attach to and destroy specific foreign antigens. Humoral immunity refers to the production of circulating antibodies by B lymphocytes (bone marrow–derived) that attack invading microorganisms.

Immune reactions to viral infections may cause changes in the appearance of mature lymphocytes, which are then called *variant reactive* (or *atypical*) *lymphocytes*. These cells may appear in infectious mononucleosis, hepatitis, viral pneumonia, and allergic conditions.

Plasma cells

Usually found in the lymphoid tissue and bone marrow, but rarely in the peripheral circulation, plasma cells produce antibodies to help fight disease. Contact with a specific antigen causes certain lymphocytes to become plasma cells and stimulates their immune activity. Plasma cells may appear in the circulation during severe infection to reinforce immunity when sufficient antibodies are not available. The presence of such cells in the blood may also indicate multiple myeloma, plasma cell leukemia, scarlet fever, measles, or chickenpox.

Reticuloendothelial system

The reticuloendothelial system (RES) is made up of tissue histiocytes, macrophages, and lymphatic tissue. Although RES cells are much less mobile than circulating white cells, they're also responsible for removing foreign matter and endogenous debris from the blood, lymph, and interstitial spaces of the body. For example, when hemoglobin is released from ruptured red cells, cells from this system digest it.

Abnormal white cell production

Malignant mutation of the blood-forming tissues can cause unrestrained white cell production, better known as *leukemia.* This condition is marked by a sharp rise in the number of abnormal white cells, first in the tissues of origin and then throughout the body.

Leukemias are classified according to the type of white cell proliferation: lymphocytic, granulocytic, or monocytic. The more immature the blood cell — that is, the more primitive its development — the more severe the disease; the older the cell, the more chronic the disease. For example, abnormal, excessive granulocyte production results in *chronic granulocytic leukemia.* Abnormally high levels of immature lymphocytes and their precursors (lymphoblasts) predominate in *acute lymphoblastic leukemia.*

In *agranulocytosis,* bone marrow stops producing granulocytes, leaving the body virtually defenseless against infection. Acute agranulocytosis, which is fatal if untreated, may result from infection or may be the result of exposure to certain antibodies or certain drugs (such as clindamycin, sulfonamides, melphalan, other chemotherapeutic agents, and barbiturates).

Blood platelets

Derived from megakaryocytes in bone marrow and also known as thrombocytes, platelets protect vascular surfaces and help the blood clot to stop bleeding. Abnormal platelet function (thrombasthenia), increased platelet counts (thrombocythemia), and decreased platelet counts (thrombocytopenia) can interfere with hemostasis. (See Chapter 2 for more information about platelets.)

Complete blood count

This often requested test gives a fairly complete picture of all the blood's formed elements. The complete blood count (CBC) generally is composed of two sections: direct measurement of cellular components, including hemo-globin and erythrocyte indices, and differentiation of WBCs, with an assessment of WBC, RBC, and platelet morphology. The following tests are usually included: hemoglobin concentration, hematocrit, red and white cell counts, differential white cell count, and stained smear for red cell and platelet examination. Besides pointing the way toward further definitive studies, CBC data have proved extremely valuable in themselves.

CBC data can detect anemias, determine their severity, and compare the status of specific blood elements. Thus, the CBC is especially useful for evaluating conditions in which hematocrit does not parallel the RBC count. Normally, as the RBC count rises, so does hematocrit. However, in patients with microcytic or macrocytic anemia, this natural correlation may not hold true. For example, the patient with iron deficiency anemia has undersized red cells that cause his hematocrit to decrease, even though his RBC count may be reported as near-normal. Conversely, the patient with pernicious anemia has many oversized red cells that cause his hematocrit to be higher than his RBC count.

White cell differential

Although the WBC count alone can suggest infection, a white cell differential adds a detailed evaluation of white cell distribution and morphology that can help confirm the possibility of an infection and suggest the type of organism (bacterial or viral). A differential may also indicate that the cause of the WBC count change is something other than infection, such as leukemia.

The stained red cell examination often accompanies the white cell differential as part of the CBC. After the differential, the same stained slide is evaluated for RBC distribution and morphology, including changes in cell contents, color, size, and shape, providing additional information for detecting leukemia, anemia, and thalassemia. Variations in size and shape are reported as occasional, slight, moderate, marked, or very marked; structural variations are reported as the number of immature or nucleated RBCs/100 WBCs, noting cell inclusions.

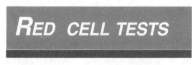

Red blood cell count

This test, also known as an erythrocyte count, reports the number of red blood cells (RBCs) found in a microliter (cubic milliliter) of whole blood, and is included in the complete blood count. Traditionally counted by hand with a hemacytometer, RBCs are now commonly counted with electronic devices such as the Coulter counter, which provide faster, more accurate results. The RBC count itself provides no qualitative information regarding the size, shape, or concentration of hemoglobin within the corpuscles, but it may be used to calculate two erythrocyte indices: mean corpuscular volume (MCV) and mean corpuscular hemoglobin (MCH).

Purpose
- To supply figures for computing the erythrocyte indices, which reveal RBC size and hemoglobin content
- To support other hematologic tests in diagnosis of anemia and polycythemia.

Patient preparation
Explain to the patient that this test evaluates the number of RBCs to detect suspected blood disorders. Inform him that he needn't restrict food or fluids. Tell him this test requires a blood sample, who will perform the venipuncture and when, and that he may experience transient discomfort from the needle puncture and the pressure of the tourniquet. If the patient is an infant or child, explain to the parents (and to the child if he is old enough to understand) that a small amount of blood will be drawn from his finger or earlobe.

Procedure
For adults and older children, draw venous blood into a 7-ml *lavender-top* tube. For younger children, collect capillary blood in a microcollection device.

Precautions
- Completely fill the collection tube, and invert it gently several times to mix the sample and the anticoagulant.
- Handle the sample gently to prevent hemolysis.

Reference values
Normal RBC values vary, depending on age, sex, sample, and geographic location. In adult males, the RBC count ranges from 4.5 to 6.2 million/μl of venous blood; in adult females, from 4.2 to 5.4 million/μl of venous blood; and in children, from 4.6 to 4.8 million/μl of venous blood. In full-term neonates, values range from 4.4 to 5.8 million/μl of capillary blood at birth, fall to 3 to 3.8 million/μl at age 2 months, and increase slowly thereafter. Values are generally higher in persons living at high altitudes.

Implications of results
An elevated RBC count may indicate absolute or relative polycythemia. A depressed count may indicate anemia, fluid overload, or hemorrhage lasting more than 24 hours. Further tests, such as stained cell examination, hematocrit, hemoglobin, red cell indices, and white cell studies, are needed to confirm diagnosis.

Post-test care

If a hematoma develops at the venipuncture site, apply warm soaks to ease discomfort.

Interfering factors

The following factors may alter test results:

- failure to use the proper anticoagulant in the collection tube or to adequately mix the sample and anticoagulant
- hemolysis due to rough handling of the sample
- hemoconcentration due to prolonged tourniquet constriction
- hemodilution caused by drawing the sample from the same arm that is being used for I.V. infusion of fluids
- high WBC count, which falsely elevates the RBC count in semiautomated and automated counters
- diseases that cause RBCs to agglutinate or form rouleaux, leading to a falsely decreased RBC count.

Hematocrit

Hematocrit (HCT), a common, reliable test, may be done by itself or as part of a complete blood count. It measures the percentage by volume of packed red blood cells (RBCs) in a whole blood sample; for example, an HCT of 40% means that a 100-ml sample contains 40 ml of packed RBCs. This packing is achieved by centrifugation of anticoagulated whole blood in a capillary tube, so that red cells are tightly packed without hemolysis.

Most commonly, HCT is measured electronically, producing results 3% lower than when HCT is measured manually. (Manual measurement traps plasma in the column of packed RBCs.) Test results may be used to calculate two erythrocyte indices: mean corpuscular volume (MCV) and mean corpuscular hemoglobin concentration (MCHC).

Purpose

- To aid diagnosis of abnormal states of hydration, polycythemia, and anemia
- To aid in calculating red cell indices.

Patient preparation

Explain to the patient that this test detects anemia and other abnormal conditions of the blood. Inform him that he needn't restrict food or fluids before the test. Tell him the test requires a blood sample, who will perform the venipuncture and when, and that he may experience transient discomfort from the needle puncture and the pressure of the tourniquet. If the patient is an infant or child, explain to the parents (and to the child if he's old enough to understand) that a small amount of blood will be drawn from his finger or earlobe.

Procedure

Perform a fingerstick, using a heparinized capillary tube with a red band on the anticoagulant end.

Precautions

Fill the capillary tube from the red-banded end to about two-thirds capacity, and seal this end with clay. Send the sample to the laboratory immediately. Or, if you perform the test, place the tube in the centrifuge, with the red end pointing outward.

Reference values

Hematocrit values vary, depending on the patient's sex and age, type of sample, and the laboratory performing the test. (See *Normal hematocrit values by age.*)

Implications of results

Low HCT suggests anemia, hemodilution, or massive blood loss; high HCT

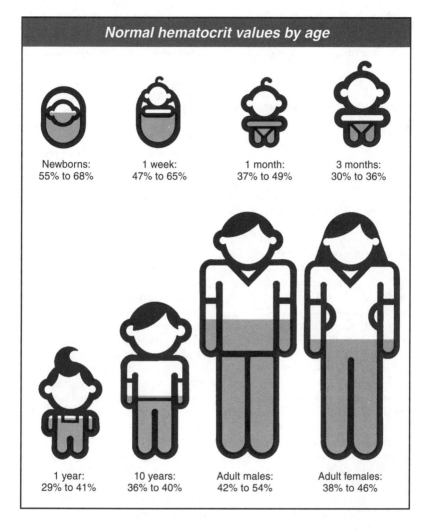

Normal hematocrit values by age

Newborns:
55% to 68%

1 week:
47% to 65%

1 month:
37% to 49%

3 months:
30% to 36%

1 year:
29% to 41%

10 years:
36% to 40%

Adult males:
42% to 54%

Adult females:
38% to 46%

indicates polycythemia or hemoconcentration due to blood loss and dehydration.

Post-test care

If a hematoma develops at the venipuncture site, apply warm soaks to ease discomfort.

Interfering factors

▪ Failure to use the proper anticoagulant in the collection tube, to fill the tube appropriately, or to adequately mix the sample and the anticoagulant may alter test results.

▪ Hemolysis due to rough handling of the sample may affect test results.

▪ Tourniquet constriction for longer than 1 minute causes hemoconcentration and typically raises HCT by 2.5% to 5%.

▪ Taking the blood sample from the same arm that is being used for I.V. infusion causes hemodilution.

■ Failure to adequately mix the sample with the anticoagulant may hinder accurate determination of test results.

Red cell indices

Using the results of the red blood cell (RBC) count, hematocrit, and total hemoglobin tests, the red cell indices (also known as erythrocyte indices) provide important information about the size, hemoglobin concentration, and hemoglobin weight of an average RBC. The indices include mean corpuscular volume (MCV), mean corpuscular hemoglobin (MCH), and mean corpuscular hemoglobin concentration (MCHC).

MCV, the ratio of hematocrit (packed cell volume) to the RBC count, expresses the average size of the erythrocytes and indicates whether they are undersized (microcytic), oversized (macrocytic), or normal (normocytic). MCH, the hemoglobin-RBC ratio, gives the weight of hemoglobin in an average red cell. MCHC, the ratio of hemoglobin weight to hematocrit, defines the concentration of hemoglobin in 100 ml of packed red cells. It helps distinguish normally colored (normochromic) red cells from paler (hypochromic) red cells.

Purpose
■ To aid diagnosis and classification of anemias.

Patient preparation
Explain to the patient that this test helps determine if he has anemia. Tell him the test requires a blood sample, who will perform the venipuncture and when, and that he may experience transient discomfort from the needle puncture and the pressure of the tourniquet.

Procedure
Perform a venipuncture, and collect the sample in a 7-ml *lavender-top* tube.

Precautions
■ Completely fill the collection tube, and invert it gently several times to adequately mix the sample and anticoagulant.
■ Handle the sample gently to prevent hemolysis.

Reference values
The range of normal red cell indices is as follows:
■ *MCV:* 84 to 99 fl
■ *MCH:* 26 to 32 pg
■ *MCHC:* 30 to 36 g/dl.

Implications of results
The red cell indices help to classify anemias. Low MCV and MCHC indicate microcytic, hypochromic anemias caused by iron deficiency anemia, pyridoxine-responsive anemia, or thalassemia. A high MCV suggests macrocytic anemias caused by megaloblastic anemias due to folic acid or vitamin B_{12} deficiency, inherited disorders of DNA synthesis, or reticulocytosis. (See *Comparing red cell indices in anemias.*) Because MCV reflects the average volume of many cells, a value within normal range can encompass RBCs of varying size, from microcytic to macrocytic.

Post-test care
If a hematoma develops at the venipuncture site, apply warm soaks.

Interfering factors
The following factors may interfere with accurate determination of test results:
■ failure to use the proper anticoagulant in the collection tube or to adequately mix the sample and anticoagulant
■ hemolysis due to rough handling of the sample

Comparing red cell indices in anemias

Decreased or increased red cell indices suggest various types of anemia, as shown below.

	NORMAL VALUES (Normocytic, normochromic)	IRON DEFICIENCY ANEMIA (Microcytic, hypochromic)	PERNICIOUS ANEMIA (Macrocytic, normochromic)
MCV	84 to 99 fl	60 to 80 fl	96 to 150 fl
MCH	26 to 32 pg	5 to 25 pg	33 to 53 pg
MCHC	30 to 36 g/dl	20 to 30 g/dl	33 to 38 g/dl

■ hemoconcentration due to prolonged tourniquet constriction
■ high white cell count, which falsely elevates the RBC count in semiautomated and automated counters and thereby invalidates MCV and MCH results
■ falsely elevated hemoglobin values, which invalidate MCH and MCHC results
■ diseases that cause RBCs to agglutinate or form rouleaux, leading to a falsely decreased RBC count and invalid test results.

Erythrocyte sedimentation rate

The erythrocyte sedimentation rate (ESR) measures the degree of erythrocyte settling during a specified time period. As the red blood cells (RBCs) descend in the tube, they displace an equal volume of plasma upward, which retards the downward progress of other settling blood elements. Factors affecting ESR include red cell volume, surface area, density, aggregation, and surface charge. Plasma proteins (notably fibrinogen and globulin) encourage aggregation, increasing the sedimentation rate.

The ESR is a sensitive but nonspecific test that is frequently the earliest indicator of disease when other chemical or physical signs are normal. It often rises significantly in widespread inflammatory disorders due to infection or autoimmune mechanisms; such elevations may be prolonged in localized inflammation and malignancy.

Purpose
■ To monitor inflammatory or malignant disease
■ To aid detection and diagnosis of occult disease, such as tuberculosis, tissue necrosis, or connective tissue disease.

Patient preparation
Explain to the patient that this test evaluates the condition of RBCs. Inform him that he needn't restrict food or fluids. Tell him the test requires a blood

sample, who will perform the venipuncture and when, and that he may experience transient discomfort from the needle puncture and the pressure of the tourniquet.

Procedure
Perform a venipuncture, and collect the sample in a 7-ml *lavender-top* tube or a 4.5-ml *blue-top* tube. (Check with the laboratory to determine its preference.)

Precautions
■ Completely fill the collection tube, and invert it gently several times to adequately mix the sample and the anticoagulant.
■ Since prolonged standing decreases the ESR, send the sample to the laboratory immediately after examining it for clots or clumps. (It must be tested within 2 to 4 hours.)
■ Handle the sample gently to prevent hemolysis.

Reference values
Normal ESR ranges from 0 to 10 mm/hour in males and from 0 to 20 mm/hour in females; rates gradually increase with age.

Implications of results
The ESR rises in pregnancy, acute or chronic inflammation, tuberculosis, paraproteinemias (especially multiple myeloma and Waldenström's macroglobulinemia), rheumatic fever, rheumatoid arthritis, and some cancers. Anemia also tends to raise ESR, since less upward displacement of plasma occurs to retard the relatively few sedimenting RBCs. Polycythemia, sickle cell anemia, hyperviscosity, or low plasma fibrinogen or globulin levels tend to depress ESR.

Post-test care
If a hematoma develops at the venipuncture site, apply warm soaks.

Interfering factors
■ Failure to use the proper anticoagulant in the collection tube, to adequately mix the sample and anticoagulant, or to send the sample to the laboratory immediately may affect test results.
■ Hemolysis due to rough handling or excessive mixing of the sample may affect the sedimentation.
■ Prolonged tourniquet constriction may cause hemoconcentration.

Reticulocyte count

Reticulocytes are nonnucleated, immature red blood cells (RBCs) that remain in the peripheral blood for 24 to 48 hours while they mature. They are generally larger than mature RBCs and contain ribosomes, the centriole, particles of Golgi vesicles, and mitochondria that produce hemoglobin. Because reticulocytes retain remnants of normoblasts (their precursors) that absorb supravital stains, such as new methylene blue or brilliant cresyl blue, they sometimes can be distinguished from other blood cells in a peripheral blood smear.

In this test, reticulocytes in a whole blood sample are counted and expressed as a percentage of the total RBC count. The reticulocyte count is useful for evaluating anemia and is an index of effective erythropoiesis and bone marrow response to anemia. Because the manual method for counting reticulocytes uses a relatively small sample size, values may be imprecise and should be compared with the RBC count or hematocrit.

Purpose
■ To aid in distinguishing between hypoproliferative and hyperproliferative anemias

■ To help assess blood loss, bone marrow response to anemia, and therapy for anemia.

Patient preparation

Tell the patient this test helps detect anemia and monitors its treatment. Advise him that he needn't restrict food or fluids. Tell him that the test requires a blood sample, who will perform the venipuncture and when, and that he may experience transient discomfort from the needle puncture and the pressure of the tourniquet. If the patient is an infant or child, explain to the parents (and to the child if he's old enough to understand) that a small amount of blood will be drawn from his finger or earlobe.

Withhold adrenocorticotropic hormone (ACTH), antimalarials, antipyretics, azathioprine, chloramphenicol, dactinomycin, furazolidone (from infants), levodopa, methotrexate, phenacetin, and sulfonamides, as ordered. If such medications must be continued, note this on the laboratory request.

Procedure

Perform a venipuncture, and collect the sample in a 7-ml *lavender-top* tube.

Precautions

■ Completely fill the collection tube, and invert it gently several times to mix the sample and the anticoagulant.
■ Handle the sample gently.

Reference values

Reticulocytes constitute 0.5% to 2% of the total RBC count. In infants, the percentage is normally higher at birth (2% to 6%) but decreases to adult levels in 1 to 2 weeks.

Implications of results

A low reticulocyte count indicates hypoproliferative bone marrow (hypoplastic anemia) or ineffective erythro-poiesis (pernicious anemia). A high reticulocyte count indicates a bone marrow response to anemia caused by hemolysis or blood loss. The reticulocyte count may also rise after effective therapy for iron deficiency anemia or pernicious anemia.

Post-test care

■ If a hematoma develops at the venipuncture site, ease discomfort by applying warm soaks.
■ As ordered, resume administration of any medications that were withheld before the test.
■ When following a patient with an abnormal reticulocyte count, look for trends in repeated tests or very gross changes in the numerical value.

Interfering factors

■ False-low test results can be caused by azathioprine, chloramphenicol, dactinomycin, and methotrexate. False-high results can be caused by ACTH, antimalarials, antipyretics, furazolidone (in infants), and levodopa. Sulfonamides can cause false-low or false-high results.
■ Failure to use the proper anticoagulant in the collection tube or to adequately mix the sample and anticoagulant may affect the accuracy of test results.
■ Prolonged tourniquet constriction may alter test results.
■ Hemolysis due to rough handling of the sample may affect test results.
■ Recent transfusions may affect results.

Osmotic fragility

Osmotic fragility measures red cell resistance to hemolysis when exposed to a series of increasingly dilute saline solutions. The test is based on osmosis — movement of water across a membrane

Concentration and fluid flow

Isotonic

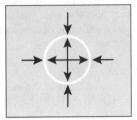

An isotonic fluid has a concentration of dissolved particles, or tonicity, equal to that of intracellular fluid. When isotonic fluids, such as 5% dextrose in water and 0.9% sodium chloride, enter the circulation, they cause no net movement of water across the semipermeable cell membrane. And because the osmotic pressure is the same inside and outside the cells, they neither swell nor shrink.

Hypertonic

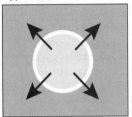

A hypertonic fluid has a concentration greater than that of intracellular fluid. When a hypertonic solution, such as 50% dextrose or 3% sodium chloride, is rapidly infused into the body, water rushes out of the cells to the area of greater concentration, and the cells shrivel. Dehydration can also make extracellular fluid hypertonic, leading to the same kind of cellular shrinking.

Hypotonic

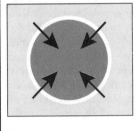

A hypotonic fluid has a concentration less than that of intracellular fluid. When a hypotonic solution, such as 2.5% dextrose or 0.45% sodium chloride, surrounds a cell, water diffuses into the intracellular fluid, causing the cell to swell. Inappropriate use of I.V. fluids or severe electrolyte loss makes body fluids hypotonic.

from a less concentrated solution to a more concentrated one, in a natural tendency to correct the imbalance.

Red cells suspended in an isotonic saline solution — one with the same salt concentration (osmotic pressure) as normal plasma (0.85 g/dl) — keep their shape. If red cells are added to a hypotonic (less concentrated) solution, they take up water until they burst; if placed in a hypertonic solution, they shrink. (See *Concentration and fluid flow*.)

The degree of hypotonicity needed to produce hemolysis varies inversely with the red cell's osmotic fragility; the closer that saline tonicity is to normal physiologic values when hemolysis occurs, the more fragile the cells. In some cases, red cells do not hemolyze immediately, and their incubation in solution for 24 hours improves test sensitivity.

This test offers quantitative confirmation of red cell morphology and should supplement the stained cell examination.

Purpose
- To aid diagnosis of hereditary spherocytosis
- To confirm morphologic red cell abnormalities.

Patient preparation
Explain to the patient that this test helps identify the cause of anemia. Inform him that he needn't restrict food or fluids. Tell the patient the test requires a blood sample, who will perform the venipuncture and when, and that he may experience transient discomfort from the needle puncture and the pressure of the tourniquet.

Procedure
Perform a venipuncture, and collect the sample in a 7-ml *green-top* (heparinized) tube.

Precautions
- Since this is not a routine test, notify the laboratory before drawing the sample if the test is not being performed by the hospital laboratory. Reference laboratories have certain guidelines and testing dates that you'll need to follow.
- Completely fill the tube, and invert it gently several times to mix the sample and anticoagulant adequately.
- Handle the sample gently to prevent hemolysis.

Reference values
Osmotic fragility values (percent of red cells hemolyzed) that have been obtained photometrically are plotted against decreasing saline tonicities to produce an S-shaped curve with a slope characteristic of the disorder.

Implications of results
Low osmotic fragility (increased resistance to hemolysis) is characteristic of thalassemia, iron deficiency anemia, sickle cell anemia, and other red cell disorders in which target cells are found.

Low osmotic fragility also occurs after splenectomy.

High osmotic fragility (increased tendency to hemolysis) is characteristic in patients with hereditary spherocytosis; spherocytosis associated with autoimmune hemolytic anemia, severe burns, or chemical poisoning; or hemolytic disease of the newborn (erythroblastosis fetalis).

Post-test care
If a hematoma develops at the venipuncture site, apply warm soaks.

Interfering factors
The following factors may affect test results:
- failure to use the proper anticoagulant in the collection tube, to fill the tube completely, or to mix the sample and anticoagulant adequately
- hemolysis due to rough handling of the sample
- presence of hemolytic organisms in the sample
- severe anemia or other conditions in which fewer red cells are available for testing
- recent transfusion.

HEMOGLOBIN TESTS

Total hemoglobin

This test measures the grams of hemoglobin (Hb) found in a deciliter (100 ml) of whole blood. Hemoglobin concentration correlates closely with the red blood cell (RBC) count and affects the Hb-RBC ratio (mean corpuscular hemoglobin [MCH] and mean corpuscular hemoglobin concentration

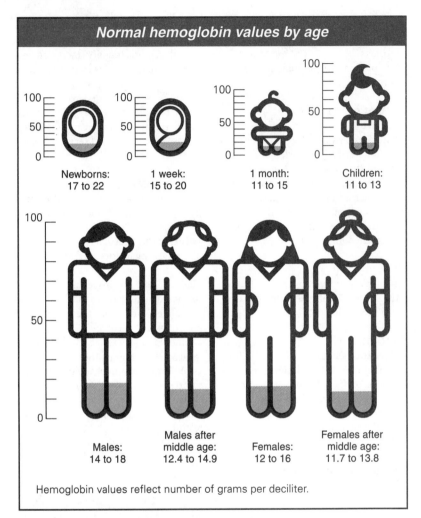

Normal hemoglobin values by age

Newborns:
17 to 22

1 week:
15 to 20

1 month:
11 to 15

Children:
11 to 13

Males:
14 to 18

Males after
middle age:
12.4 to 14.9

Females:
12 to 16

Females after
middle age:
11.7 to 13.8

Hemoglobin values reflect number of grams per deciliter.

[MCHC]). In the laboratory, hemoglobin is chemically converted to pigmented compounds and is measured by either spectrophotometric or colorimetric technique.

The test is usually performed as part of a complete blood count.

Purpose

- To measure the severity of anemia or polycythemia and to monitor response to therapy

- To supply figures for calculating MCH and MCHC.

Patient preparation

Explain to the patient that this test helps determine if he has anemia or polycythemia (or, if appropriate, that it assesses his response to treatment). Inform him that he needn't restrict food or fluids. Tell him the test requires a blood sample, who will perform the venipuncture and when, and that he may experience some discomfort from the needle puncture and the pressure of the tourniquet. If the patient is an infant or child, explain to the parents (and to the child if he's old enough to understand) that a small amount of blood will be drawn from his finger or earlobe.

Procedure

For adults and older children, perform a venipuncture, and collect the sample in a 7-ml *lavender-top* tube. For younger children and infants, collect the sample by fingerstick or heelstick in a microtainer with EDTA.

Precautions

■ Completely fill the collection tube, and invert it gently several times to adequately mix the sample and the anticoagulant.
■ Handle the sample gently to prevent hemolysis.

Reference values

Hemoglobin concentration varies, depending on the patient's age and sex and on the type of blood sample drawn. (See *Normal hemoglobin values by age.*)

Implications of results

Low hemoglobin concentration may indicate anemia, recent hemorrhage, or fluid retention, causing hemodilution; elevated hemoglobin suggests hemoconcentration from polycythemia or dehydration.

Post-test care

If a hematoma develops at the venipuncture site, apply warm soaks.

Interfering factors

■ Failure to use the proper anticoagulant in the collection tube or to adequately mix the sample and anticoagulant may affect test results.
■ Hemolysis due to rough handling may adversely affect the test results.

■ Prolonged tourniquet constriction may cause hemoconcentration.
■ Very high white cell counts, lipemia, or red cells that are resistant to lysis will falsely elevate hemoglobin values.

Hemoglobin electrophoresis

Hemoglobin (Hb) electrophoresis is probably the most useful laboratory method for separating and measuring normal and certain abnormal hemoglobins. Electrophoresis apparatus consists of an anode (+) and a cathode (–), separated by buffered cellulose acetate, on which hemoglobin molecules migrate when an electrical current is passed through the medium. Different types of hemoglobin migrate toward the anode at different speeds, creating a series of distinctively pigmented bands in the medium that are then compared with a normal sample.

The laboratory may change the medium (from cellulose acetate to starch gel) or its pH (from 8.6 to 6.2), depending on the types of hemoglobins being detected. This variation expands the range of this test beyond those hemoglobins routinely checked: Hb A, Hb A_2, Hb S, and Hb C.

Purpose

■ To measure the amount of Hb A and to detect abnormal hemoglobins
■ To aid diagnosis of thalassemias.

Patient preparation

Explain to the patient that this test evaluates hemoglobin. Tell the patient he needn't restrict food or fluids. Inform him that the test requires a blood sample, who will perform the venipuncture and when, and that the puncture and

Hemoglobin types and distribution

This chart shows the distribution pattern and clinical effects associated with some types of hemoglobin.

HEMOGLOBIN	TOTAL HEMOGLOBIN (%)	CLINICAL IMPLICATIONS
Hb A	95% to 100%	Normal
Hb A$_2$	4% to 5.8%	β-thalassemia minor
	2% to 3%	Normal
	Under 2%	Hb H disease
Hb F	Under 1%	Normal
	2% to 5%	β-thalassemia minor
	10% to 90%	β-thalassemia major
	5% to 15%	β-δ-thalassemia minor
	5% to 35%	Heterozygous hereditary persistence of fetal hemoglobin (HPFH)
	100%	Homozygous HPFH
	15%	Homozygous Hb S
Homozygous Hb S	70% to 98%	Sickle cell disease
Homozygous Hb C	90% to 98%	Hb C disease
Heterozygous Hb C	24% to 44%	Hemoglobin C trait

the tourniquet may cause some discomfort. If the patient is a child, explain to the parents (and to the child if he's old enough to understand) that a small amount of blood will be drawn from his finger. Check for a recent blood transfusion (within the past 4 months).

Procedure

Perform a venipuncture, and collect the sample in a 7-ml *lavender-top* tube. For younger children, collect capillary blood in a microcollection device.

Precautions

Completely fill the collection tube, and invert it gently several times to mix the sample and anticoagulant adequately. Don't shake the tube vigorously.

Reference values

In adults, Hb A accounts for over 95% of all hemoglobins; Hb A$_2$, 2% to 3%; and Hb F, less than 1%. In neonates, Hb F normally accounts for half the total; Hb S and Hb C are normally absent.

Implications of results

Hemoglobin electrophoresis allows identification of various types of hemoglobins, many of which may imply the presence of a hemolytic disease. (See *Hemoglobin types and distribution.*)

Post-test care

If a hematoma develops at the venipuncture site, apply warm soaks.

Inheritance patterns in sickle cell anemia

When both parents have sickle cell anemia (left), childbearing — if possible at all — is dangerous for the mother, and all offspring will have sickle cell anemia. When one parent has sickle cell anemia and one is normal (right), all offspring will be carriers of sickle cell anemia.

Sickle cell anemia   Sickle cell trait   Normal

Interfering factors

■ A blood transfusion within the past 4 months may invalidate test results.

■ Failure to use the proper anticoagulant in the collection tube, to fill the tube completely, or to mix the sample and the anticoagulant adequately may alter test results.

■ Hemolysis due to rough handling of the sample may affect the accuracy of test results.

Sickle cells

Sickle cells are severely deformed erythrocytes. The sickling phenomenon is caused by hemoglobinopathy — most commonly, the polymerization of hemoglobin S (Hb S) in the presence of low pH, low oxygen tension, elevated osmolarity, and elevated temperature, to form elongated structures (tactoids) that deform red blood cells (RBCs). Reversing these conditions depolymerizes

Hb S and lets the RBCs resume their normal shape. However, repeated sickling leads to permanent RBC deformity. Sickle cell trait (Hb S) is found almost exclusively in blacks: 0.2% of the blacks born in the United States have sickle cell disease. (See *Inheritance patterns in sickle cell anemia.*)

People who are homozygous for Hb S usually show abundant spontaneously sickled RBCs on a peripheral blood smear. People who are heterozygous for Hb S alone or with another hemoglobinopathy (that is, double heterozygous, sickle cell) may have normal RBCs that can be easily changed to sickled forms by lowering oxygen tension. This sickling tendency can be identified by sealing a drop of blood between a glass slide and coverslip, and adding a reducing agent, such as sodium metabisulfate. The RBC can then be observed under a microscope and compared to a central slide containing blood and saline solution. The concentration of Hb S governs the prevalence and rapidity of the sickling.

Although this test (also known as the hemoglobin S test) is useful as a rapid

Fetal sickle cell test

When both parents of a developing fetus are suspected carriers of sickle cell trait, a reliable test can detect whether the fetus has the sickle cell trait or the disease.

The fetal sickle cell test, developed in 1970 at the University of California at San Francisco, was the first diagnostic tool to result from recombinant DNA research. Many major medical centers throughout the United States currently perform the test. In addition, any doctor can request the test if he suspects that both parents are carriers. He need only mail the appropriate samples to the nearest test center.

The test requires a venous blood sample from both parents and an amniotic fluid specimen. Diagnosis is based on analysis of the genes and DNA in the fetal cell and on the DNA in parental leukocytes. About 1 week is required to complete the test, which is generally performed between the 14th and 18th weeks of pregnancy. This provides a sufficient opportunity for the couple to seek genetic counseling.

screening procedure, it may produce erroneous results; consequently, hemoglobin electrophoresis should be performed if sickle cell trait is strongly suspected.

Fetuses can also be tested for sickle cell disease or trait. (See *Fetal sickle cell test.*)

Purpose

■ To identify sickle cell disease and sickle cell trait. (See *Sickle cell trait.*)

Patient preparation

Explain to the patient that this test helps detect sickle cell disease. Inform him that he needn't restrict food or fluids. Tell him that the test requires a blood sample, who will perform the venipuncture and when, and that he may experience discomfort from the needle puncture and the pressure of the tourniquet. If the patient is an infant or child, explain to the parents (and to the child if he's old enough to understand) that a small amount of blood will be drawn from his finger.

Check the patient history for a blood transfusion within the past 3 months.

Procedure

Perform a venipuncture, and collect the sample in a 7-ml *lavender-top* tube. For younger children, collect capillary blood in a microcollection device.

Precautions

Completely fill the collection tube, and invert it gently several times to adequately mix the sample and the anticoagulant. Don't shake the tube vigorously.

Normal findings

Results of this test are reported as positive or negative. A normal, or negative, test suggests the absence of Hb S.

Implications of results

A positive test may indicate the presence of sickle cells, but hemoglobin electrophoresis is needed to distinguish between homozygous and heterozygous forms. Rarely, other abnormal hemoglobins cause sickling of erythrocytes in the absence of Hb S.

Sickle cell trait

This relatively benign condition results from heterozygous inheritance of the abnormal hemoglobin S–producing gene. Like sickle cell anemia, it's most common in blacks.

In persons with sickle cell trait, 20% to 40% of their total hemoglobin is hemoglobin S; the rest is normal. Such persons, called carriers, usually have no symptoms. They have normal hemoglobin and hematocrit values and can expect a normal life span. Nevertheless, they must avoid situations that provoke hypoxia, which occasionally causes a sickling crisis similar to that in sickle cell anemia.

Genetic counseling is essential for sickle cell carriers. Every child of two sickle cell carriers has a 25% chance of inheriting sickle cell anemia and a 50% chance of being a carrier.

Post-test care
If a hematoma develops at the venipuncture site, apply warm soaks.

Interfering factors
■ Hemoglobin concentration under 10%, elevated Hb S levels in infants under age 6 months, and a blood transfusion within the past 3 months may produce false-negative test results.
■ Failure to use the proper anticoagulant in the collection tube, to completely fill the tube, or to adequately mix the sample and the anticoagulant may affect the accuracy of test results.
■ Hemolysis due to rough handling of the sample may affect test results.

Unstable hemoglobins

Unstable hemoglobins are rare, congenital red cell defects caused by amino acid substitutions in the normally stable structure of hemoglobin. These abnormal replacements produce a molecule that spontaneously denatures into clumps and aggregations called Heinz bodies, which separate from the red cell cytoplasm and accumulate at the cell membrane. Although Heinz bodies are usually efficiently removed by the spleen or liver, they may cause mild to severe hemolysis. (See *Signs and symptoms of unstable hemoglobins,* page 28.)

Unstable hemoglobins are best detected by precipitation tests (heat stability or isopropanol solubility) performed in the laboratory. Although a hemoglobin electrophoresis and the Heinz body test can demonstrate certain unstable hemoglobins, these tests don't always confirm the presence of such hemoglobins. Globin chain analysis identifies them more reliably, but this procedure is time-consuming and technically complex and, therefore, is not performed routinely.

Purpose
■ To detect unstable hemoglobins.

Patient preparation
Explain to the patient that this test detects abnormal hemoglobins in the blood. Inform him that he needn't restrict food or fluids. Tell him the test requires a blood sample, who will perform the venipuncture and when, and that he may experience transient dis-

---

Signs and symptoms of unstable hemoglobins

More than 60 varieties of unstable hemoglobins exist, each named after the city in which it was discovered. Their effects vary according to their number, the degree of instability, the condition of the spleen, and the oxygen-binding abilities of the unstable hemoglobin.

Patients with unstable hemoglobins typically exhibit pallor, jaundice, splenomegaly and, with severely unstable hemoglobins, cyanosis, pigmenturia, and hemoglobinuria. Thalassemia often causes similar signs and symptoms, but the molecular bases of the two diseases differ greatly.

---

comfort from the needle puncture and the pressure of the tourniquet.

As ordered, withhold antimalarials, furazolidone (from infants), nitrofurantoin, phenacetin, procarbazine, and sulfonamides before the test, since these drugs may induce hemolysis. If these medications must be continued, note this on the laboratory request.

Procedure
Perform a venipuncture, and collect the sample in a 7-ml *lavender-top* tube.

Precautions
Completely fill the collection tube, and invert it gently several times to mix the sample and the anticoagulant adequately. Don't shake the tube vigorously because hemolysis may result.

Normal findings
When no unstable hemoglobins appear in the sample, the heat stability test is reported as negative; the isopropanol solubility test, as stable.

Implications of results
A positive heat stability or unstable solubility test, especially with hemolysis, strongly suggests the presence of unstable hemoglobins.

Post-test care
■ If a hematoma develops at the venipuncture site, apply warm soaks.

■ As ordered, resume administration of medications withheld before the test.

Interfering factors
■ Antimalarials, furazolidone (in infants), nitrofurantoin, phenacetin, procarbazine, and sulfonamides can induce Heinz body formation and result in a positive or unstable test.

■ High levels of hemoglobin F may cause a false-positive isopropanol test.

■ Failure to use the proper anticoagulant in the collection tube, to fill the tube completely, or to mix the sample and the anticoagulant adequately may interfere with test results.

■ Hemolysis due to rough handling of the sample or hemoconcentration due to prolonged tourniquet constriction may influence test results.

■ A recent blood transfusion may affect results.

Heinz bodies

Heinz bodies are particles of denatured hemoglobin that have precipitated out of the cytoplasm of red blood cells (RBCs) and have collected in small masses attached to the cell membranes. They form as a result of drug injury to RBCs, the presence of unstable hemoglobins, unbalanced globin chain synthesis due to thalassemia, or a red cell enzyme deficiency (such as glucose-6-phosphate dehydrogenase deficiency). Although Heinz bodies are rapidly removed from RBCs in the spleen, they are a major factor in causing hemolytic anemias. (See *Identifying Heinz bodies.*)

Using a whole blood sample, Heinz bodies can be detected by phase microscopy or with supravital stains, such as crystal violet, brilliant cresyl blue, or new methylene blue. However, when Heinz bodies do not form spontaneously, various oxidant drugs are added to the whole blood sample to induce their formation.

Purpose

■ To help detect the cause of hemolytic anemia.

Patient preparation

Explain to the patient that this test helps determine the cause of anemia. Inform him that he needn't restrict food or fluids before the test. Tell him this test requires a blood sample, who will perform the venipuncture and when, and that he may experience transient discomfort from the needle puncture and the pressure of the tourniquet.

Review the patient's drug history for medications that may alter test results. Withhold antimalarials, furazolidone, nitrofurantoin, phenacetin, procarbazine, and sulfonamides, as ordered. If these medications must be continued, note this on the laboratory request.

Procedure

Perform a venipuncture, and collect the sample in a 7-ml *lavender-top* tube.

Precautions

Completely fill the sample collection tube, and invert it gently several times to adequately mix the sample and the anticoagulant.

Identifying Heinz bodies

After special supravital staining, Heinz bodies (particles of denatured hemoglobin that are usually attached to the cell membrane) appear as small, purple inclusions at cell margins. Heinz bodies are present in certain hemolytic anemias.

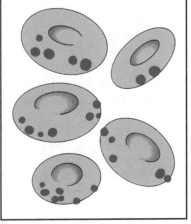

Normal findings

Absence of Heinz bodies is the normal (negative) test result.

Implications of results

The presence of Heinz bodies — a positive test result — may indicate an inherited red cell enzyme deficiency, the presence of unstable hemoglobins, thalassemia, or drug-induced red cell injury. Heinz bodies may also be present after splenectomy.

Post-test care

■ If a hematoma develops at the venipuncture site, ease discomfort by applying warm soaks.
■ As ordered, resume administration of medications withheld before the test.

Interfering factors
- Antimalarials, furazolidone (in infants), nitrofurantoin, phenacetin, procarbazine, and sulfonamides can cause false-positive results.
- Failure to use the appropriate anticoagulant in the collection tube, to fill the collection tube completely, to adequately mix the sample and the anticoagulant, or to send the sample to the laboratory immediately may affect the accuracy of test results.
- A recent transfusion may affect test results.

Serum iron and total iron-binding capacity

Iron is essential to the formation and function of hemoglobin as well as many other heme and nonheme compounds. After iron is absorbed by the intestine, it's distributed to various body compartments for synthesis, storage, and transport. (See *Normal iron metabolism.*) Since iron appears in the plasma, bound to a glycoprotein called transferrin, it is easily sampled and measured. The sample is treated with buffer and color reagents.

Serum iron assay measures the amount of iron bound to transferrin; total iron-binding capacity (TIBC) measures the amount of iron that would appear in plasma if all the transferrin were saturated with iron. The percentage of saturation is obtained by dividing the serum iron result by the TIBC, which reveals the actual amount of saturated transferrin. Normally, transferrin is about 30% saturated.

Serum iron and TIBC are more diagnostically useful when performed with the serum ferritin assay, but these tests may not accurately reflect the state of other iron compartments, such as myoglobin iron and the labile iron pool. Bone marrow or liver biopsy, and iron absorption or excretion studies may yield more information.

Purpose
- To estimate total iron storage
- To aid diagnosis of hemochromatosis (see *Siderocyte stain,* page 32)
- To help distinguish between iron deficiency anemia and anemia of chronic disease
- To provide data for evaluating nutritional status.

Patient preparation
Explain to the patient that this test evaluates his body's capacity to store iron. Inform him that he needn't restrict food or fluids before the test. Tell him that the test requires a blood sample, who will perform the venipuncture and when, and that he may experience transient discomfort from the needle puncture and the pressure of the tourniquet.

Review the patient's drug history for medications that may affect test results. Withhold chloramphenicol, adrenocorticotropic hormone (ACTH), iron supplements, and oral contraceptives, as ordered. If such medications must be continued, note this on the laboratory request.

Procedure
Perform a venipuncture, and collect the sample in a 7-ml *red-top* tube.

Precautions
Handle the sample gently to prevent hemolysis, and send it to the laboratory immediately.

Reference values
- *Serum iron:* 70 to 150 µg/dl for men, 80 to 150 µg/dl for women
- *TIBC:* 300 to 400 µg/dl for men, 300 to 450 µg/dl for women

Normal iron metabolism

Ingested iron, absorbed and oxidated in the bowel, bonds with the protein transferrin for circulation to bone marrow, where hemoglobin synthesis occurs, and to all iron-hungry body cells. In the spleen, hemoglobin breakdown recycles iron back to the bone marrow or into storage. The body conserves iron, losing small amounts through skin, feces, urine, and menses. Storage areas in the liver, spleen, bone marrow, and reticuloendothelial system hold iron as ferritin until the body needs it; the liver alone stores about 60%.

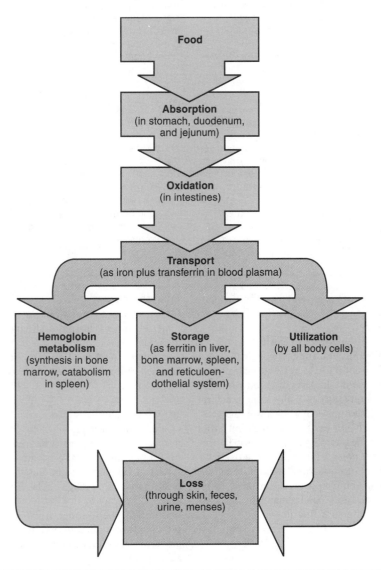

Siderocyte stain

Siderocytes are red blood cells (RBCs) that contain particles of non-hemoglobin iron known as sidero-cytic granules. In newborn infants, siderocytic granules are normally present in normoblasts and reticulo-cytes during hemoglobin synthesis. However, the spleen removes most of these granules from normal RBCs, and they disappear rapidly with age.

In adults, elevated siderocyte levels usually indicate abnormal erythropoiesis, as occurs in congenital spherocytic anemia, chronic hemolytic anemias (such as the thalassemias), pernicious anemia, hemochromatosis, toxicities (such as lead poisoning), infection, and severe burns. Elevated levels may also follow splenectomy because the spleen normally removes siderocytic granules.

The siderocyte stain test measures the number of circulating siderocytes. Venous blood is drawn into a 7-ml *lavender-top* tube or, for infants and children, is collected in a microtainer and smeared directly on a 3" glass slide. When the blood smear is stained, siderocytic granules appear as purple-blue specks clustered around the periphery of mature erythrocytes. Cells containing these granules are counted as a percentage of total RBCs. The results aid differential diagnosis of anemias and hemochromatosis and help detect toxicities.

Normally, siderocyte levels are slightly elevated at birth but reach the normal adult values of 0.5% of total RBCs in 7 to 10 days. In patients with pernicious anemia, the siderocyte level is 8% to 14%; in chronic hemolytic anemia, 20% to 100%; in lead poisoning, 10% to 30%; and in hemochromatosis, 3% to 7%. An elevated siderocyte level requires additional testing — including bone marrow examination — to determine the cause of abnormal erythropoiesis.

■ *Saturation:* 20% to 50% for men and women.

Implications of results

In iron deficiency, serum iron levels drop and TIBC increases to decrease the saturation. In cases of chronic inflammation (such as in rheumatoid arthritis), serum iron may be low in the presence of adequate body stores, but TIBC may be unchanged or may drop to preserve normal saturation. Iron overload may not alter serum levels until relatively late, but in general, serum iron increases and TIBC remains the same to increase the saturation.

Post-test care

■ If a hematoma develops at the venipuncture site, ease discomfort by applying warm soaks.

■ As ordered, resume administration of any medications that were withheld before the test.

Interfering factors

■ Chloramphenicol and oral contraceptives can cause false-positive test results; ACTH can produce false-negative results. Iron supplements can cause false-positive serum iron values but false-negative TIBC.

■ Hemolysis due to rough handling of the sample or failure to send the sample to the laboratory immediately may alter test results.

Serum ferritin

Ferritin, a major iron-storage protein found in reticuloendothelial cells, normally appears in small quantities in serum. In healthy adults, serum ferritin levels are directly related to the amount of available iron stored in the body and can be measured accurately by radioimmunoassay. Unlike many other blood studies, the serum ferritin test isn't affected by moderate hemolysis of the sample or by the patient's use of any known drugs.

Purpose
- To screen for iron deficiency and iron overload
- To measure iron storage
- To distinguish between iron deficiency (a condition of low iron storage) and chronic inflammation (a condition of normal storage).

Precautions
None.

Patient preparation
Explain to the patient that this test assesses the amount of available iron stored in the body. Inform him that he needn't restrict food, fluids, or medications before the test. Tell him that the test requires a blood sample, who will perform the venipuncture and when, and that he may experience transient discomfort from the needle puncture and the pressure of the tourniquet. Review the patient's history for a recent transfusion.

Procedure
Perform a venipuncture, and collect the sample in a 10-ml *red-top* tube.

Reference values
Normal serum ferritin values vary with age, as follows:
- *men:* 20 to 300 ng/ml
- *women:* 20 to 120 ng/ml
- *6 months to 15 years:* 7 to 140 ng/ml
- *2 to 5 months:* 50 to 200 ng/ml
- *1 month:* 200 to 600 ng/ml
- *neonates:* 25 to 200 ng/ml.

Implications of results
High serum ferritin levels may indicate acute or chronic hepatic disease, iron overload, leukemia, acute or chronic infection or inflammation, Hodgkin's disease, or chronic hemolytic anemias; in these disorders, iron stores in the bone marrow may be normal or significantly increased. Serum ferritin levels are characteristically normal or slightly elevated in those patients who have chronic renal disease. Low serum ferritin levels indicate chronic iron deficiency.

Post-test care
If a hematoma develops at the venipuncture site, ease discomfort by applying warm soaks.

Interfering factors
A recent transfusion may cause elevated serum ferritin levels.

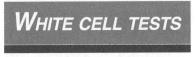

White blood cell count

Part of the complete blood count, the white blood cell (WBC), or leukocyte, count reports the number of WBCs found in a microliter (cubic millimeter) of whole blood by using a hemacytometer or an electronic device, such as the Coulter counter.

On any given day, WBC counts may vary by as much as 2,000 cells/μl. Such variation can be the result of strenuous exercise, stress, or digestion. The WBC count may rise or fall significantly in certain diseases but is diagnostically useful only when interpreted in light of the WBC differential and the patient's current clinical status.

Purpose

- To determine infection or inflammation
- To determine the need for further tests, such as the WBC differential or bone marrow biopsy
- To monitor response to chemotherapy or radiation therapy.

Patient preparation

Explain to the patient that this test helps detect an infection or inflammation. Inform him that he needn't restrict food or fluids but should avoid strenuous exercise for 24 hours before the test. Also tell him that he should avoid ingesting a heavy meal before the test. Explain to him that the test requires a blood sample, who will perform the venipuncture and when, and that he may experience transient discomfort from the needle puncture and the pressure of the tourniquet.

If the patient is being treated for an infection, advise him that this test will be repeated to monitor his progress. Review his drug history for medications that may alter test results. Note the use of such medications on the laboratory request.

Procedure

Perform a venipuncture, and collect the sample in a 7-ml *lavender-top* tube.

Precautions

Completely fill the sample collection tube, and invert it gently several times to adequately mix the sample and the anticoagulant.

Reference values

The WBC count normally ranges from 4,000 to 10,000/μl.

Implications of results

An elevated WBC count (leukocytosis) commonly signals infection, such as an abscess, meningitis, appendicitis, or tonsillitis. A high count may also result from leukemia or tissue necrosis due to burns, myocardial infarction, or gangrene.

A low WBC count (leukopenia) indicates bone marrow depression that may result from viral infections or from toxic reactions, such as those following treatment with antineoplastics, ingestion of mercury or other heavy metals, or exposure to benzene or arsenicals. Leukopenia characteristically accompanies influenza, typhoid fever, measles, infectious hepatitis, mononucleosis, and rubella.

Post-test care

- If a hematoma develops at the venipuncture site, ease discomfort by applying warm soaks.
- As ordered, advise the patient that he may resume normal activities that he discontinued before the test.
- Patients with severe leukopenia may have little or no resistance to infection and, therefore, will require reverse isolation.

Interfering factors

- Hemolysis caused by rough handling of the sample may affect test results.
- Exercise, stress, or digestion raises the WBC count, thus yielding inaccurate results.

LAP stain

Levels of leukocyte alkaline phosphatase (LAP), an enzyme found in neutrophils, may be altered by infection, stress, chronic inflammatory diseases, Hodgkin's disease, and hematologic disorders. Most of these conditions elevate LAP levels; only a few, notably chronic myelogenous leukemia (CML), depress them. Thus, this test is most often used to differentiate CML from other disorders that produce an elevated white blood cell count.

Procedure

To perform this test, a blood sample is obtained by venipuncture or fingerstick. The venous blood sample is collected in a 7-ml *green-top* tube and transported immediately to the laboratory, where a blood smear is prepared; the peripheral blood sample is smeared on a 3" glass slide and fixed in cold formalin-methanol. The blood smear is then stained to show the amount of LAP present in the cytoplasm of the neutrophils. One hundred neutrophils are count-

ed and assessed; each is assigned a score of 0 to 4, according to the degree of LAP staining. Normally, values for LAP range from 40 to 100, depending on the laboratory's standards.

Implications of results

Depressed LAP values typically indicate CML; however, values may also be low in paroxysmal nocturnal hemoglobinuria, aplastic anemia, and infectious mononucleosis. Elevated levels may indicate Hodgkin's disease, polycythemia vera, or a neutrophilic leukemoid reaction — a response to such conditions as infection, chronic inflammation, or pregnancy.

After a diagnosis of CML, the LAP stain may also be used to help detect onset of the blastic phase of the disease, when LAP levels typically rise. However, LAP levels also increase toward normal in response to therapy; because of this, test results must be correlated with the patient's condition.

▪ Some drugs, including most antineoplastic agents; anti-infectives, such as metronidazole and flucytosine; anticonvulsants, such as phenytoin derivatives; thyroid hormone antagonists; and nonsteroidal anti-inflammatory drugs such as indomethacin lower the WBC count, altering results.

White blood cell differential

Because the white blood cell (WBC) differential evaluates the distribution and

morphology of white cells, it provides more specific information about a patient's immune system than the WBC count. In the differential test, the laboratory classifies 100 or more white cells in a stained film of peripheral blood according to five major types of leukocytes — neutrophils, eosinophils, basophils, lymphocytes, and monocytes — and determines the percentage of each type.

The differential count is the relative number of each type of white cell in the blood. By multiplying the percentage value of each type by the total WBC count, the investigator obtains the absolute number of each type of white cell. Abnormally high levels of these cells are

Drugs that influence eosinophil count

Many drugs can affect the accuracy of the eosinophil count, as shown in the chart below.

INCREASE OR DECREASE COUNT:	DECREASE COUNT:	INCREASE COUNT BY PROVOKING AN ALLERGIC REACTION:	
methysergide	indomethacin	anticonvulsants	para-aminosali-cylic acid
desipramine	procainamide	capreomycin	
		cephalosporins	paromomycin
		D-penicillamine	penicillins
		gold compounds	phenothiazines
		isoniazid	rifampin
		nalidixic acid	streptomycin
		novobiocin	sulfonamides
			tetracyclines

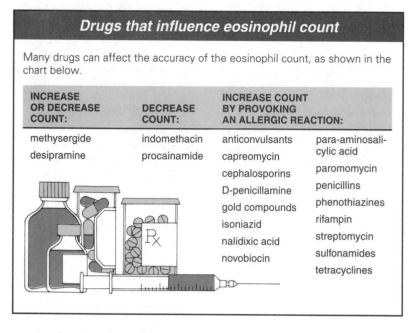

associated with various allergic reactions and parasitic infections. When high levels are reported, an eosinophil count is sometimes ordered as a follow-up to the white cell differential. The eosinophil count is also appropriate if the differential WBC count shows a depressed eosinophil level.

Purpose
■ To evaluate the body's capacity to resist and overcome infection
■ To detect and identify various types of leukemia (see *LAP stain,* page 35, for information on another test used to identify leukemia)
■ To determine the stage and severity of an infection
■ To detect allergic reactions and parasitic infections, and assess their severity (eosinophil count).

Patient preparation
Explain to the patient that this test evaluates how well his immune system is functioning. Inform him that he needn't restrict food or fluids but should refrain from strenuous exercise for 24 hours before the test. Tell him the test requires a blood sample, who will perform the venipuncture and when, and that he may experience transient discomfort from the needle puncture and the pressure of the tourniquet.

Review the patient's history for use of medications that may interfere with test results. (See *Drugs that influence eosinophil count.*)

Procedure
Perform a venipuncture, and collect the sample in a 7-ml *lavender-top* tube.

Precautions
Completely fill the collection tube, and invert it gently several times to mix the sample and the anticoagulant adequately. Handle the tube gently to prevent hemolysis.

Interpreting WBC differential values

The differential count measures the types of white blood cells (WBCs) as a percentage of the total WBC count (the relative value). The absolute value is obtained by multiplying the relative value of each cell type by the total WBC count. Both the relative and absolute values must be considered to obtain an accurate diagnosis.

For example, consider a patient whose WBC count is 6,000/µl and whose differential shows 30% neutrophils and 70% lymphocytes. His relative lymphocyte count seems to be quite high (lymphocytosis), but when this figure is multiplied by his WBC count (6,000 x 70% = 4,200 lymphocytes/µl), it is well within the normal range.

This patient's neutrophil count, however, is low (30%); when this figure is multiplied by the WBC count (6,000 x 30% = 1,800 neutrophils/µl), the result is a low absolute number, which may mean depressed bone marrow.

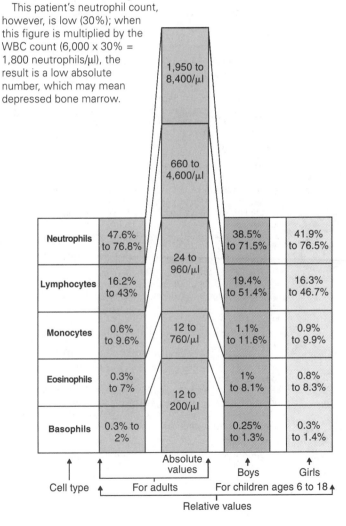

Cell type	For adults (Relative values)	Absolute values	For children ages 6 to 18 Boys	For children ages 6 to 18 Girls
Neutrophils	47.6% to 76.8%	1,950 to 8,400/µl	38.5% to 71.5%	41.9% to 76.5%
Lymphocytes	16.2% to 43%	660 to 4,600/µl	19.4% to 51.4%	16.3% to 46.7%
Monocytes	0.6% to 9.6%	24 to 960/µl / 12 to 760/µl	1.1% to 11.6%	0.9% to 9.9%
Eosinophils	0.3% to 7%	12 to 200/µl	1% to 8.1%	0.8% to 8.3%
Basophils	0.3% to 2%		0.25% to 1.3%	0.3% to 1.4%

How disease affects differential values

CELL TYPE	HOW AFFECTED

Neutrophils

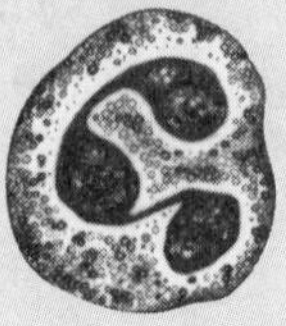

Increased by:
- Infections: osteomyelitis, otitis media, salpingitis, septicemia, gonorrhea, endocarditis, smallpox, chickenpox, herpes, Rocky Mountain spotted fever
- Ischemic necrosis due to myocardial infarction, burns, or cancer
- Metabolic disorders: diabetic acidosis, eclampsia, uremia, thyrotoxicosis
- Stress response due to acute hemorrhage, surgery, excessive exercise, emotional distress, third trimester of pregnancy, or childbirth
- Inflammatory diseases: rheumatic fever, rheumatoid arthritis, acute gout, vasculitis, myositis

Decreased by:
- Bone marrow depression due to radiation or cytotoxic drugs
- Infections: typhoid, tularemia, brucellosis, hepatitis, influenza, measles, mumps, rubella, infectious mononucleosis
- Hypersplenism: hepatic disease and storage diseases
- Collagen vascular diseases, such as systemic lupus erythematosus
- Deficiency of folic acid or vitamin B_{12}

Eosinophils

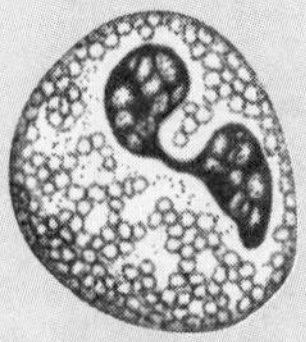

Increased by:
- Allergic disorders: asthma, hay fever, food or drug sensitivity, serum sickness, angioneurotic edema
- Parasitic infections: trichinosis, hookworm, roundworm, amebiasis
- Skin diseases: eczema, pemphigus, psoriasis, dermatitis, herpes
- Neoplastic diseases: chronic myelocytic leukemia, Hodgkin's disease, metastases and necrosis of solid tumors
- Collagen vascular disease, adrenocortical hypofunction, ulcerative colitis, polyarteritis nodosa, scarlet fever, pernicious anemia, excessive exercise, splenectomy

Decreased by:
- Stress response due to trauma, shock, burns, surgery, or mental distress
- Cushing's syndrome

Basophils

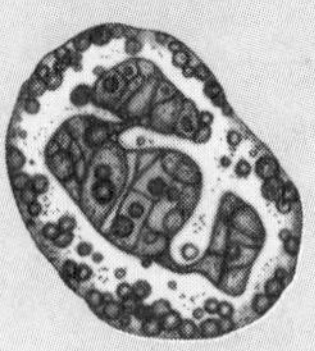

Increased by:
- Chronic myelocytic leukemia, polycythemia vera, some chronic hemolytic anemias, Hodgkin's disease, systemic mastocytosis, myxedema, ulcerative colitis, chronic hypersensitivity states, nephrosis

Decreased by:
- Hyperthyroidism, ovulation, pregnancy, stress

How disease affects differential values (continued)

CELL TYPE	HOW AFFECTED
Lymphocytes	**Increased by:** ■ Infections: pertussis, brucellosis, syphilis, tuberculosis, hepatitis, infectious mononucleosis, mumps, rubella, cytomegalovirus ■ Thyrotoxicosis, hypoadrenalism, ulcerative colitis, immune diseases, lymphocytic leukemia **Decreased by:** ■ Severe debilitating illnesses, such as congestive heart failure, renal failure, and advanced tuberculosis ■ Defective lymphatic circulation, high levels of adrenal corticosteroids, immunodeficiency due to immunosuppressive therapy
Monocytes	**Increased by:** ■ Infections: subacute bacterial endocarditis, tuberculosis, hepatitis, malaria, Rocky Mountain spotted fever ■ Collagen vascular diseases: systemic lupus erythematosus, rheumatoid arthritis, polyarteritis nodosa ■ Carcinomas, monocytic leukemia, lymphomas

Reference values

Normal values for the five types of WBCs classified in the differential — neutrophils, eosinophils, basophils, lymphocytes, and monocytes — are given for adults and children in *Interpreting WBC differential values,* page 37. However, keep in mind that for an accurate diagnosis, differential test results must always be interpreted in relation to the total WBC count.

Implications of results

Abnormal differential patterns suggest a wide range of disease states and other conditions. (See *How disease affects differential values.*)

Post-test care

If a hematoma develops at the venipuncture site, ease discomfort by applying warm soaks.

Interfering factors

■ Hemolysis caused by rough handling of the sample may affect the accuracy of test results.
■ Failure to use the proper anticoagulant, to completely fill the collection tube, or to mix the sample and anticoagulant adequately may affect the accuracy of test results.

SELECTED READINGS

Andrews, C.M., et al. *Color Atlas of Comparative Diagnostic and Experimental Hematology.* St. Louis: Mosby–Year Book, Inc., 1994.

Baer, D.M. "Hematology Testing at the Bedside," *Laboratory Medicine* 26(1):48-53, January 1995.

Diseases, 2nd ed. Springhouse, Pa.: Springhouse Corp., 1997.

Fischbach, F. *A Manual of Laboratory and Diagnostic Tests,* 5th ed. Philadelphia: Lippincott-Raven Pubs., 1996.

Guyton, A.C., and Hall, J.E. *Textbook of Medical Physiology,* 9th ed. Philadelphia: W.B. Saunders Co., 1996.

Harmening, D.M., ed. *Clinical Hematology and Fundamentals of Hemostasis,* 3rd ed. Philadelphia: F.A. Davis Co., 1996.

Henry, J.B., ed.: *Clinical Diagnosis and Management by Laboratory Methods,* 19th ed. Philadelphia: W.B. Saunders Co., 1996.

Kee, J.L. *Laboratory and Diagnostic Tests,* 4th ed. Stamford, Conn.: Appleton & Lange, 1995.

Nursing97 Drug Handbook. Springhouse, Pa.: Springhouse Corp., 1997.

Phipps, W.J., et al. *Medical-Surgical Nursing: Concepts and Clinical Practice,* 5th ed. St. Louis: Mosby–Year Book, Inc., 1995.

Rodak, B.F., ed. *Diagnostic Hematology.* Philadelphia: W.B. Saunders Co., 1995.

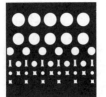

CHAPTER TWO

Hemostasis

Learning objectives

After completing this chapter, the reader will be able to:
- describe how hemostasis protects the body against excessive blood loss
- describe the sequence of physiologic events in blood coagulation
- discuss common coagulation defects, platelet disorders, and vascular defects
- name the defective factor that causes hemophilia A
- state the purpose of each test discussed in the chapter

- prepare the patient physically and psychologically for each test
- describe the procedure for obtaining a specimen for each test
- specify appropriate precautions for accurately obtaining a specimen for each test
- implement appropriate post-test care
- state the reference values for each test
- discuss the implications of abnormal test results
- list factors that may interfere with accurate test results.

INTRODUCTION

The circulatory system protects itself from excessive blood loss or blood clotting by hemostasis. In this process, vascular injury activates a complex chain of events — vasoconstriction, platelet aggregation, and coagulation — that leads to clotting, which stops bleeding. This clotting must be localized to the injury site, and ultimately the clot must be removed.

Vasoconstriction: Primary response

Within seconds of vascular injury, neural reflexes and local smooth-muscle spasms cause the walls of the damaged vessel to contract, aided by secretion of serotonin, epinephrine, and lipoproteins. Constriction lasts about 10 minutes in a small vessel and up to 30 minutes in a larger one. The extent of tissue damage determines the extent of vasospasm; for example, a blood vessel that suffers a clean cut bleeds more than one that is crushed. However, vasoconstric-

tion slows blood flow only briefly in small vessels and is insufficient to prevent blood loss from large ones. Permanent repair requires a hemostatic plug formed of platelet aggregates and a fibrin clot.

Aggregation of platelets

Circulating platelets converge on the wound site, first touching and then adhering to the collagen fibers of the torn vessel lining (endothelium). This contact of platelets with collagen stimulates the platelets to secrete adenosine diphosphate (ADP), which causes them to change shape and aggregate, sticking together in clumps. Additional ADP activates greater numbers of platelets, which also collect at the site. This aggregation loosely plugs the wounds to help prevent further blood loss.

Coagulation (clotting)

When platelet aggregation is underway, blood loses its fluidity and forms a gelatinous clot. More than a score of agents in blood and in tissues influence this process. Some promote coagulation (procoagulants) and others inhibit it (anticoagulants). When vascular injury causes bleeding, procoagulants gather at the injury site and stimulate formation of a stable fibrin clot.

Clotting begins within 60 seconds of injury and proceeds through the interaction of two parallel pathways — extrinsic and intrinsic. The *extrinsic pathway* is activated when tissue thromboplastin is released at the injury site. At the same time, procoagulants in the blood are activated in the *intrinsic pathway* to produce plasma thromboplastin and several other factors. Both systems then interact to continue activating other coagulation factors until a meshwork of fibrin strands is built that traps blood cells, more platelets, and plasma to form a clot.

Three crucial steps

Clotting normally proceeds in three stages:
■ Trauma to blood vessels or tissues triggers thromboplastin activity through intrinsic and extrinsic pathways.
■ Next, these pathways converge to convert prothrombin to thrombin.
■ Thrombin converts fibrinogen in the surrounding plasma to a fibrin plug.

Formation of thromboplastin

When blood contacts injured tissue, the tissue frees factor III (tissue thromboplastin), an ill-defined, clot-promoting substance. Because factor III alone is ineffective, it interacts with factor VII (proconvertin) in the presence of calcium ions. Factor IV (calcium ions [Ca^{++}]) and tissue phospholipids form a complex that initiates the reactions of the extrinsic pathway. This complex then activates factor X (Stuart-Prower factor) at the end of the extrinsic pathway.

In intrinsic clotting, plasma thromboplastin results from progressive activation of several procoagulants. When stimulated by surface contact or vascular injury, factor XII (Hageman factor) activates factor XI (plasma thromboplastin antecedent), which, in the presence of calcium, initiates activity of factor IX (Christmas factor). The activated form of this plasma protein, in the presence of platelet phospholipids, converts factor VIII (antihemophilic factor) to its active state and forms a complex that activates factor X.

Almost simultaneously, factor X reacts with factor V (proaccelerin), in the presence of Ca^{++} and platelet phospholipids, to form a prothrombin-converting complex. Within 15 seconds of its formation, this protein begins to split factor II (prothrombin) to form thrombin. (See *Blood coagulation factors*, page 44.)

Conversion of prothrombin to thrombin

Prothrombin splits into two parts: One is inert and the other is thrombin. Thrombin is a potent enzyme that converts fibrinogen to fibrin, helps stabilize the final clot, and starts clot breakdown (fibrinolysis) after healing.

Conversion of fibrinogen to fibrin

After thrombin is formed in adequate amounts, it hydrolyzes fibrinogen (factor I), splitting two low–molecular-weight peptides from each fibrinogen molecule. The remaining peptides are fibrin monomers, which automatically combine end to end and side by side to form fibrin threads that eventually build a weak, soluble polymer meshwork.

To strengthen this weak fibrin clot, thrombin activates another plasma enzyme called factor XIII (fibrin stabilizing factor). In the presence of Ca^{++}, this enzyme strengthens the fibrin polymer by forming covalent bonds and causing cross-linkage of peptide bonds. This action results in a firm, insoluble clot.

Blood coagulation factors			
FACTOR	**SYNONYM**	**PROFILE**	**SITE OF SYNTHESIS**
I	Fibrinogen	Precursor of fibrin	Liver
II	Prothrombin	Precursor of thrombin	Liver
III	Tissue thromboplastin	Activator of prothrombin	All tissues
IV	Ca⁺⁺	Essential for prothrombin activation and formation of fibrin	From diet
V	Proaccelerin	Accelerates conversion of prothrombin to thrombin	Liver
VII	Serum prothrombin (proconvertin)	Accelerates conversion of prothrombin to thrombin	Liver
VIII	Antihemophilic factor (AHF, hemophilic factor A)	Associated with factors IX, XII, and XI; aids in forming activated factor X via intrinsic system and conversion of prothrombin to thrombin	Reticuloendothelial system
IX	Christmas factor (hemophilic factor B, plasma thromboplastin component [PTC])	Activated by factor XI; essential to formation of activated factor X through intrinsic system; associated with factors XII, XI, and VIII	Liver
X	Stuart-Prower factor	Triggers prothrombin conversion; requires vitamin K	Liver
XI	Plasma thromboplastin antecedent (PTA)	Activated by factor XII; associated with factors XII IX, and VIII in formation of activated factor X through intrinsic system	Unknown
XII	Hageman factor	First factor activated in the intrinsic pathway; activates factor XI	Unknown
XIII	Fibrin stabilizing factor (FSF)	Produces stronger urea-insoluble fibrin clot	Unknown

Coagulation defects and bleeding disorders

Coagulation defects due to *factor I (fibrinogen) deficiency* may be hereditary or acquired. Hereditary errors are classified as quantitative (afibrinogenemia or hypofibrinogenemia) or qualitative (dysfibrinogenemia). Afibrinogenemia causes severe bleeding that may be life-threatening. This disorder, thought to be transmitted as an autosomal recessive trait, first occurs in the newborn as umbilical bleeding. Acquired hypofibrinogenemia can result from conditions such as disseminated intravascular coagulation (DIC), primary fibrinogenolysis, and hepatic disease.

Factor II deficiency, or hypoprothrombinemia, can also be hereditary or acquired. Hereditary transmission, as an autosomal recessive trait, is rare. This defect can be acquired from vitamin K deficiency, warfarin therapy, or hepatic disease. It is frequently associated with deficiencies of factor VII, factor IX, and factor X.

Factor V deficiency can be inherited as an autosomal recessive trait or acquired. Acquired deficiency occurs in severe liver disease or DIC. Severe hereditary deficiency produces effects resembling mild to moderate hemophilia.

Factor VII deficiency can also be inherited as an autosomal recessive trait. Although the clinical effects of this hereditary defect may vary, it commonly causes overt symptoms of abnormal coagulation, such as epistaxis, easy bruising, and bleeding from the gums. An acquired form of factor VII deficiency can result from vitamin K deficiency, warfarin therapy, or hepatic disease.

A *defect of factor VIII* causes two congenital disorders: hemophilia A (classic hemophilia) and von Willebrand's disease. Hemophilia A, a sex-linked recessive disorder transmitted by females that occurs almost exclusively in males, is marked by severe bleeding (hemarthroses, and muscular and gastrointestinal bleeding). Von Willebrand's disease, which causes a milder coagulation dysfunction than hemophilia A, is characterized by abnormal platelet function and a mild-to-moderate deficiency of factor VIII, and is transmitted to both sexes as an autosomal dominant trait. Symptoms of this disorder include epistaxis, ecchymoses, and oozing after tooth extraction. Both DIC and fibrinolysis may induce acquired factor VIII deficiency.

Congenital *deficiency of factor IX* can cause hemophilia B (Christmas disease), a severe bleeding disorder transmitted as a sex-linked recessive trait from mothers to sons. Because factor IX is formed in the liver and depends on the presence of sufficient vitamin K, an acquired deficiency of this factor can result from lack of vitamin K or from warfarin therapy and hepatic disease.

A *factor X deficiency*, inherited as an autosomal recessive trait (rare), is generally associated with depressed levels of vitamin K, hepatic disease, and anticoagulant therapy.

Congenital *deficiency of factor XI* (hemophilia C), transmitted as an autosomal recessive trait, may not produce symptoms unless the patient undergoes trauma or injury. The severity of bleeding may vary from one event to another. A transient form of the deficiency is sometimes detectable in newborns.

Congenital *factor XII deficiency*, also transmitted as an autosomal recessive trait, is similarly unlikely to cause symptoms.

A small number of patients (5% to 10%) with systemic lupus erythematosus (SLE) develop inhibitors known as lupus-like anticoagulants. These inhibitors appear to be directed at the phospholipids that activate the clotting factors. The presence of these anticoagulants is rarely linked to a clinical bleeding tendency unless another abnormality in hemostasis is present. In the case of SLE, this abnormality is a low platelet count (thrombocytopenia).

Various tests are used to help detect coagulation disorders. (See *Common coagulation screening tests,* page 46, and *Collecting specimens for coagulation testing,* page 47.)

Common coagulation screening tests

TEST	IMPLICATIONS OF ABNORMAL FINDINGS
Bleeding time	*Prolonged bleeding time:* thrombocytopenia, disseminated intravascular coagulation, or von Willebrand's disease; *Abnormal bleeding time with normal platelet count:* platelet function disorder
Capillary fragility	*Excessive number of petechiae in 2" (5-cm) circle of skin:* capillary wall weakness or platelet disorder
Activated partial thromboplastin time (APTT)	*Prolonged APTT:* presence of anticoagulant, fibrin split products, fibrinolysins, or antibodies to specific clotting factors; or deficiency of clotting factor other than factor VII or factor XIII
Prothrombin time (PT)	*Prolonged PT:* deficiency of fibrinogen (factor I), prothrombin (factor II), or factors V, VII, or X; hepatic disease; vitamin K deficiency; or ongoing anticoagulant therapy
Plasma thrombin time (TT)	*Prolonged TT:* hepatic disease, fibrin degradation products, effective heparin therapy, hypofibrinogenemia, or dysfibrinogenemia
Fibrin split products (FSP)	*Elevated FSP:* pulmonary embolus, myocardial infarction, deep vein thrombosis, disseminated intravascular coagulation, or primary fibrinogenolysis syndrome.

Platelet disorders

Platelets, oval or discoid cytoplasmic fragments about 2 to 4 microns in diameter, are derived from bone marrow megakaryocytes. Platelet disorders stemming from abnormalities of number (thrombocytopenia and thrombocytosis) or function (thrombasthenia and thrombocytopathia) impair vascular integrity and the coagulation mechanism. However, serious coagulopathy is likely only when large numbers of platelets are dysfunctional or deficient.

In *thrombocytopenia,* the most common platelet deficiency, the number of platelets is abnormally low (less than 150,000/µl); nevertheless, overt bleeding doesn't generally develop until the count drops below 50,000/µl. Thrombocytopenia may result from decreased bone marrow production of platelets related to aplastic anemia, leukemia, and vitamin B_{12} or folic acid deficiency; from

accelerated destruction of platelets by the spleen; from exaggerated destruction of platelets caused by antiplatelet or drug-induced antibodies; from severe blood loss; or from accelerated consumption of platelets, as seen in DIC and idiopathic thrombocytopenic purpura.

Antiplatelet antibodies stimulate the reticuloendothelial system to sequester circulating platelets. Proliferation of antibodies may result from treatment with such medications as quinidine, quinine, and thiazide derivatives. Sulfonamides and phenylbutazone may exert a direct toxic effect on platelets through an unknown mechanism. Drug toxicity is likely to induce bleeding from capillaries rather than from larger vessels. This tendency causes small hemorrhages that appear on the skin as purple discolorations (purpura).

In *thrombocytosis,* which is usually

Collecting specimens for coagulation testing

Proper specimen collection and handling is especially important when collecting blood samples for coagulation testing because damage to the vessel wall during venipuncture can cause coagulation to begin, thus affecting test results. As hospitals expand the role of nurses to include blood collection, you'll need to keep in mind the following guidelines for venipuncture and specimen collection.

Timing
Collect samples for coagulation testing at approximately the same time each day, if possible, to eliminate the circadian variations of the different coagulation proteins.

Venipuncture equipment
Avoid using small-bore (large-gauge [>21G]) needles to collect coagulation test samples because this size needle may mechanically disrupt platelets and activate the coagulation cascade.

Collection technique
A clean venipuncture with a minimum of tissue trauma is essential to obtain a good quality plasma specimen for coagulation testing. Any trauma to the tissue can stimulate the release of tissue thrombo-plastin, which can contaminate the needle. Therefore, when drawing blood for several laboratory tests, don't draw the coagulation test sample first. If no other tests will be performed, first draw a *red-top* discard tube to negate the effect of tissue thromboplastin on test results. If you're drawing from an intermittent access device, discard 20 ml of blood before collecting the coagulation test sample (for a heparinized line, discard 30 ml). Make sure that the coagulation test tube is filled with blood to the appropriate level to achieve a whole blood–anticoagulant ratio of 9:1.

In addition, avoid prolonged application of the tourniquet because this can stimulate the release of tissue thromboplastin and elevate levels of coagulation factor VII, fibrin monomer, and tissue plasminogen activator.

Specimen handling and transport
Coagulation specimens should be kept capped during transport and storage before testing because uncapped specimens lose carbon dioxide. Loss of carbon dioxide would result in a pH increase, which would affect coagulation test results.

secondary to other disorders, the platelet count is abnormally high (more than 400,000/µl) and is associated with inflammatory response, iron deficiency, or splenectomy. Abnormally elevated platelet counts also appear in myeloproliferative disorders, such as polycythemia vera, myelofibrosis, and chronic granulocytic leukemia. Thrombocytosis does not generally cause symptoms but may occasionally lead to bleeding or thrombosis.

Qualitative platelet disorders may be congenital or acquired. Congenital disorders include *thrombasthenia,* a rare autosomal recessive trait; *storage-pool disease,* typified by decreased ADP levels in blood platelets; and *Bernard-Soulier (giant platelet) syndrome,* marked by abnormally large platelets that fail to aggregate with the reagent ristocetin. Acquired defects may result from aspirin ingestion, uremia, dysproteinemias, and chronic hepatic disease.

Vascular defects

Bleeding due to vascular defects results from abnormal vascular permeability (as in vitamin C deficiency) or fragility (as in purpura senilis). Blood vessels can also rupture and bleed after certain abrupt movements because blood vessels are lightly anchored to surrounding tissue. In allergic purpura, increased vascular permeability and tissue hemorrhage result from an inflammatory capillary reaction.

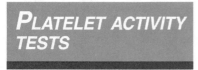

Bleeding time

This test measures the duration of bleeding after a standardized skin incision. Bleeding time depends on the elasticity of the blood vessel wall and on the number and functional capacity of platelets. Although this test is usually performed on patients with a personal or family history of bleeding disorders, it is also useful for preoperative screening, along with a platelet count.

Bleeding time may be measured by one of four methods: Duke, Ivy, template, or modified template. The template methods are the most frequently used and the most accurate, since they standardize the incision size, making test results reproducible.

This test usually isn't recommended for a patient whose platelet count is less than 75,000/µl. However, some patients with altered platelet morphology may have normal bleeding times despite low platelet counts.

Purpose

■ To assess overall hemostatic function (platelet response to injury and functional capacity of vasoconstriction)
■ To detect congenital and acquired platelet function disorders.

Patient preparation

Explain to the patient that this test measures the time required to form a clot and stop bleeding. Tell him who will perform the test and when. Inform him he needn't restrict food or fluids before the test. Advise him that he may feel some discomfort from the incisions, the antiseptic, and the tightness of the blood pressure cuff. Also inform him that the incisions will leave two small, hairline scars that should be barely visible when healed.

Check the patient history for recent ingestion of drugs that prolong bleeding time. If the patient has taken such drugs, check with the laboratory for special instructions. If the test is being used to identify a suspected bleeding disorder, it should be postponed and the drugs discontinued, as ordered; if it's being used preoperatively to assess hemostatic function, it should proceed as scheduled.

Equipment

Blood pressure cuff ✦ disposable lancet ✦ template with 9-mm slits (template method) or 5-mm slits (modified template method) ✦ spring-loaded blade (modified template method) ✦ 70% alcohol or povidone-iodine solution ✦ filter paper ✦ small pressure bandage ✦ stopwatch.

Procedure

For the template and modified template methods: Wrap the pressure cuff around the upper arm and inflate the cuff to 40 mm Hg. Select an area on the forearm free of superficial veins, and clean it with antiseptic. Allow the skin to dry *completely* before making the incision. Apply the appropriate template lengthwise to the forearm. For the template method, use the lancet to make two incisions, 1 mm deep and 9 mm long. For the modified template method, use the spring-loaded blade to make two incisions, 1 mm deep and 5 mm long. Start the stopwatch. Without touching the cuts, gently blot the drops of blood with filter paper every 30 seconds until the bleeding stops in both cuts. Average the time of the two cuts, and record the results.

For the Ivy method: After applying the pressure cuff and preparing the test site, make three small punctures with a disposable lancet. Start the stopwatch immediately. Taking care not to touch the punctures, blot each site with filter paper every 30 seconds until the bleeding stops. Average the bleeding time of the three punctures, and record the result.

For the Duke method: Drape the patient's shoulder with a towel. Clean the earlobe, and let the skin air-dry. Then make a puncture wound 2 to 4 mm deep on the earlobe with a disposable lancet. Start the stopwatch. Being careful not to touch the ear, blot the site with filter paper every 30 seconds until bleeding stops. Record bleeding time.

Precautions
- Maintain a pressure of 40 mm Hg throughout the test.
- If the bleeding doesn't diminish after 15 minutes, discontinue the test.

Reference values
The normal bleeding time is 2 to 8 minutes in the template method, 2 to 10 minutes in the modified template method, 1 to 7 minutes in the Ivy method, and 1 to 3 minutes in the Duke method.

Implications of results
Prolonged bleeding time may indicate the presence of many disorders associated with thrombocytopenia, such as Hodgkin's disease, acute leukemia, disseminated intravascular coagulation, hemolytic disease of the newborn, Schönlein-Henoch purpura, severe hepatic disease (such as cirrhosis), or severe deficiency of factors I, II, V, VII, VIII, IX, and XI. Prolonged bleeding time in a person with a normal platelet count suggests a platelet function disorder (thrombasthenia or thrombocytopathia) and requires further investigation with clot retraction, prothrombin consumption, and platelet aggregation tests.

Post-test care
- For a patient with a bleeding tendency (such as hemophilia), maintain a pressure bandage over the incision for 24 to 48 hours to prevent further bleeding. Keep the edges of the cuts aligned to minimize scarring. Otherwise, a piece of gauze held in place by an adhesive bandage is sufficient. Check the test area frequently.
- As ordered, resume administration of medications discontinued before the test.

Interfering factors
Sulfonamides, thiazide diuretics, antineoplastics, anticoagulants, nonsteroidal anti-inflammatory drugs, aspirin and aspirin compounds, and some nonnarcotic analgesics may prolong bleeding times.

Platelet count

Platelets, or thrombocytes, are the smallest formed elements in the blood. Vital to the formation of the hemostatic plug in vascular injury, they promote coagulation by supplying phospholipids to the intrinsic coagulation pathway.

The platelet count is one of the most important screening tests of platelet function. Accurate counts are vital for monitoring severe thrombocytosis or the thrombocytopenia associated with chemotherapy and radiation therapy. A platelet count that falls below 50,000/µl can cause spontaneous bleeding; when the count drops below 5,000/µl, fatal central nervous system bleeding or massive GI hemorrhage is possible.

Properly prepared and stained, peripheral blood films provide a reliable estimate of platelet number. A more accurate visual method involves use of a hemocytometer counting chamber and a phase microscope. Automated systems use the voltage pulse or electro-optical counting system. Results from such automated systems should always be checked against a visual estimate from a stained blood film.

Purpose

■ To evaluate platelet production
■ To assess effects of chemotherapy or radiation therapy on platelet production
■ To aid diagnosis of thrombocytopenia and thrombocytosis
■ To confirm visual estimate of platelet number and morphology from a stained blood film.

Patient preparation

Explain to the patient that this test helps determine if his blood clots normally. Inform him that he needn't restrict food or fluids before the test. Tell him the test requires a blood sample, who will perform the venipuncture and when, and that he may experience transient discomfort from the needle puncture and the pressure of the tourniquet.

Check the patient history for use of medications that may affect test results. Notify the laboratory if such drugs have been used.

Procedure

Perform a venipuncture, and collect the sample in a 7-ml *lavender-top* tube.

Precautions

■ To prevent hemolysis, handle the sample gently and avoid excessive probing at the venipuncture site.
■ Completely fill the collection tube, and invert it gently several times to mix the sample and anticoagulant adequately.

Reference values

A normal platelet count ranges from 140,000 to 400,000/µl in adults and from 150,000 to 450,000/µl in children.

Implications of results

A decreased platelet count (thrombocytopenia) can result from aplastic or hypoplastic bone marrow; infiltrative bone marrow disease, such as leukemia or disseminated infection; megakaryocytic hypoplasia; ineffective thrombopoiesis due to folic acid or vitamin B_{12} deficiency; pooling of platelets in an enlarged spleen; increased platelet destruction due to drugs or immune disorders; disseminated intravascular coagulation; Bernard-Soulier syndrome; or mechanical injury to platelets.

An increased platelet count (thrombocytosis) can result from hemorrhage, infectious disorders, cancers, iron deficiency anemia, or inflammatory disease, or from recent surgery, pregnancy, or splenectomy. In such cases, the platelet count returns to normal after the patient recovers from the primary disorder. However, the count remains elevated in primary thrombocythemia, myelofibrosis with myeloid metaplasia, polycythemia vera, and chronic myelogenous leukemia.

When the platelet count is abnormal, diagnosis usually requires further studies, such as a complete blood count, bone marrow biopsy, direct antiglobulin test (direct Coombs' test), and serum protein electrophoresis.

Post-test care
If a hematoma develops at the venipuncture site, apply warm soaks.

Interfering factors
- Failure to use the proper anticoagulant or to mix the sample and anticoagulant promptly and adequately may affect test results.
- Hemolysis due to rough handling of the sample or to excessive probing at the venipuncture site may alter test results.
- Medications that may decrease the platelet count include acetazolamide, acetohexamide, antineoplastics, brompheniramine maleate, carbamazepine, chloramphenicol, ethacrynic acid, furosemide, gold salts, hydroxychloroquine, indomethacin, isoniazid, mephenytoin, mefenamic acid, methazolamide, methimazole, methyldopa, oral diazoxide, oxyphenbutazone, penicillamine, penicillin, phenylbutazone, phenytoin, pyrimethamine, quinidine sulfate, quinine, salicylates, streptomycin, sulfonamides, thiazide and thiazide-like diuretics, and tricyclic antidepressants. Heparin causes transient, reversible thrombocytopenia.
- The platelet count normally increases at high altitudes, with persistent cold temperature, and during strenuous exercise and excitement; the count may decrease just before menstruation.

Capillary fragility

A nonspecific method of evaluating bleeding tendencies, the capillary fragility test (also known as the positive-pressure test, tourniquet test, and Rumpel-Leede test) measures the capillaries' ability to remain intact under increased intracapillary pressure. In this test, a blood pressure cuff is placed around the patient's upper arm. The cuff is inflated to 70 to 90 mm Hg or midway between the diastolic and systolic pressures. Pressure is maintained for 5 minutes. This temporary increase in pressure may cause rhexis bleeding of the capillaries and formation of petechiae on the arm, wrist, or hand. The number of petechiae within a given circular space is recorded as the test result.

Purpose
- To assess the fragility of capillary walls
- To identify platelet deficiency (thrombocytopenia).

Patient preparation
Explain to the patient that this test helps identify abnormal bleeding tendencies. Inform him that he needn't restrict food or fluids. Tell him who will perform the procedure and when and that he may feel discomfort from the pressure of the blood pressure cuff.

Procedure
Select and mark a 2" (5-cm) space on the patient's forearm. Ideally, the site should be free of petechiae; otherwise, record the number of petechiae present on the site before starting the test. The patient's skin temperature and the room temperature should be normal to ensure accurate results.

Fasten the cuff around the arm, and raise the pressure to a point midway between the systolic and diastolic blood pressures. Maintain this pressure for 5 minutes; then release the cuff. Count the number of petechiae that appear in the 2" space, and record the results.

Precautions
- Don't repeat this test on the same arm within 1 week.

■ This test is contraindicated in patients with disseminated intravascular coagulation (DIC) or other bleeding disorders and in those who already have significant petechiae.

Reference values

A few petechiae may normally be present before the test. Fewer than 10 petechiae on the forearm 5 minutes after the test is considered normal, or negative; more than 10 petechiae is considered a positive result. The following scale may also be used to report test results:

Number of petechiae/5 cm	Score
0 to 10	1+
10 to 20	2+
20 to 50	3+
50	4+

Implications of results

A positive finding (more than 10 petechiae present or a score of 2+ to 4+) indicates weakness of the capillary walls (vascular purpura) or a platelet defect and occurs in such conditions as thrombocytopenia, thrombasthenia, purpura senilis, scurvy, DIC, von Willebrand's disease, vitamin K deficiency, dysproteinemia, and polycythemia vera, as well as in severe deficiencies of Factor VII, fibrinogen, or prothrombin.

Conditions unrelated to bleeding defects, such as scarlet fever, measles, influenza, chronic renal disease, hypertension, and diabetes with coexistent vascular disease, may also increase capillary fragility. An abnormal number of petechiae sometimes appears before onset of menstruation and at other times in some healthy persons, especially in women over age 40.

Post-test care

Encourage the patient to open and close his hand a few times to hasten return of blood to the forearm.

Interfering factors

■ Decreased estrogen levels in postmenopausal women may increase capillary fragility.

■ Glucocorticoids may increase capillary resistance, even in a patient with thrombocytopenia.

■ Repeating the test on the same arm within 1 week may yield inaccurate results by causing errors in counting the number of petechiae.

Platelet aggregation

After vascular injury, platelets gather at the injury site and clump together to form an aggregate — a plug — that helps maintain hemostasis and promotes healing. The platelet aggregation test, an in vitro procedure, measures the rate at which the platelets in a sample of citrated platelet-rich plasma form a clump after the addition of an aggregating reagent (adenosine diphosphate, epinephrine, thrombin, collagen, or ristocetin).

This test is a major diagnostic tool for detecting von Willebrand's disease; people with this disorder lack the ristocetin cofactor that enables platelets to aggregate in the presence of ristocetin.

Purpose

■ To assess platelet aggregation
■ To detect congenital and acquired platelet bleeding disorders.

Patient preparation

Explain to the patient that this test helps determine if his blood clots properly. Instruct him to fast or to maintain a nonfat diet for 8 hours before the test because lipemia can affect test findings. Tell him that the test requires a blood sample, who will perform the venipunc-

Aspirin and platelet aggregation

Unlike other salicylates, aspirin inhibits platelet aggregation. The inhibition occurs in the second phase of platelet aggregation, when it prevents the release of adenosine diphosphate from platelets. Mean bleeding time may double in healthy individuals after ingestion of aspirin. In children or in patients with bleeding disorders such as hemophilia, bleeding time may be even more prolonged.

Effect on platelets
The effect of aspirin on platelets seems to result from the inhibition of prostaglandin synthesis. A single 325-mg oral dose results in about 90% inhibition of the enzyme cyclooxygenase in circulating platelets, preventing the synthesis of compounds that induce platelet aggregation. The inhibition of cyclooxygenase is irreversible; thus, its effect lasts for 4 to 6 days — the lifespan of platelets. Bleeding time peaks within 12 hours. Altered hemostasis persists about 36 hours after the last dose of aspirin, sometimes longer for patients receiving long-term therapy.

Effect on blood vessels
Aspirin's action on blood vessels may oppose that seen in platelets because cyclooxygenase plays a different role in the vascular endothelium. Here, the enzyme produces prostacyclin, a compound that inhibits platelet aggregation and causes vasodilation. Inhibition of cyclooxygenase in the vascular endothelium, in effect, reverses aspirin's antithrombotic effect on platelets. However, studies suggest that cyclooxygenase in the platelets is more sensitive than that in the vascular endothelium and that, therefore, a low aspirin dosage (for example, 80 mg daily or 325 mg every other day) may prove more effective in preventing thrombosis than higher dosages.

Researchers are continuing to investigate whether antithrombotic therapy with aspirin is beneficial to women.

ture and when, and that he may experience transient discomfort from the needle puncture and the pressure of the tourniquet.

Withhold aspirin and aspirin compounds for 14 days, and phenylbutazone, sulfinpyrazone, phenothiazines, antihistamines, anti-inflammatory drugs, and tricyclic antidepressants for 48 hours, as ordered. If these medications must be continued, note this on the laboratory request. Because the list of medications known to alter the results of this test is long and continually growing, the patient should be as free of drugs as possible before the test. (See *Aspirin and platelet aggregation*.)

Procedure
Perform a venipuncture, and collect the sample in a 7-ml *blue-top* siliconized tube.

Precautions
▪ Be careful to avoid excessive probing at the venipuncture site. Don't leave the tourniquet on too long because it can cause bruising. Apply pressure to the venipuncture site for 5 minutes or until the bleeding stops.
▪ Completely fill the collection tube, and invert it gently several times to mix the sample and anticoagulant adequately.
▪ Handle the sample gently to prevent hemolysis, and keep it between 71.6° F

(22° C) and 98.6° F (37° C) to prevent aggregation.

■ If the patient has taken aspirin within the past 14 days and the test can't be postponed, notify the laboratory. The technician will then use arachidonic acid as the reagent to verify the presence of aspirin in the plasma. If test results are abnormal for such a sample, aspirin use must be discontinued and the test repeated in 2 weeks.

Reference values

Normal aggregation occurs in 3 to 5 minutes, but findings depend on the temperature and vary with the laboratory. Aggregation curves obtained by using different reagents help to distinguish various qualitative platelet defects.

Implications of results

Abnormal findings may indicate von Willebrand's disease, Bernard-Soulier syndrome, storage pool disease, polycythemia vera, or Glanzmann's thrombasthenia.

Post-test care

■ If a hematoma develops at the venipuncture site, apply warm soaks.
■ As ordered, resume diet and administration of medications withheld before the test.

Interfering factors

■ Hemolysis caused by rough handling of the sample or by trauma at the venipuncture site may alter test results.
■ Failure to use the proper anticoagulant or to mix the sample and anticoagulant adequately may alter test results.
■ Failure to observe restrictions of diet and medications may affect test results. Platelet aggregation is inhibited by aspirin and aspirin compounds, phenylbutazone, sulfinpyrazone, phenothiazines, antihistamines, anti-inflammatory drugs, and tricyclic antidepressants.

COAGULATION TESTS

Activated partial thromboplastin time

The activated partial thromboplastin time (APTT) test evaluates all the clotting factors of the intrinsic pathway — except platelets — by measuring the time required for formation of a fibrin clot after the addition of calcium and phospholipid emulsion to a plasma sample. Because most congenital coagulation deficiencies occur in the intrinsic pathway, the APTT test is valuable in preoperative screening for bleeding tendencies. It's also the test of choice for monitoring heparin therapy.

Purpose

■ To screen for deficiencies of the clotting factors in the intrinsic pathways
■ To monitor response to heparin therapy. (For information about another test used to monitor heparin therapy, see *Heparin neutralization assay.*)

Patient preparation

Explain to the patient that this test helps determine if his blood clots normally. Advise him that he needn't restrict food or fluids. Inform him that the test requires a blood sample, who will perform the venipuncture and when, and that he may experience transient discomfort from the needle puncture and the pressure of the tourniquet.

When appropriate, tell the patient receiving heparin therapy that this test may be repeated at regular intervals to assess his response to treatment.

Procedure

Perform a venipuncture, and collect the sample in a 7-ml *blue-top* tube.

Heparin neutralization assay

This complex, quantitative test is sometimes used to monitor heparin therapy. It can also help determine if prolonged thrombin time results from effective heparin therapy or from the presence of other circulating anticoagulants, such as fibrin split products.

To perform this test, a specimen is divided into small plasma samples. Thrombin time is determined on one sample; the other samples are added to various dilutions of protamine sulfate. After a brief incubation, equal amounts of thrombin are added to each solution and thrombin time is measured. Be-

cause protamine sulfate neutralizes heparin, reduced thrombin time in the protamine-treated samples indicates the presence of heparin.

A fibrometer is used to select the sample with the thrombin time closest to the control value. Then, a chart or formula is used to convert the sample's protamine concentration to units of heparin per milliliter, providing an accurate measurement of heparin blood levels. If none of the samples shows a reduced thrombin time, no heparin is present, indicating that prolonged thrombin time is due to other anticoagulants, such as fibrin split products.

Precautions

■ To prevent hemolysis, avoid excessive probing at the venipuncture site, and handle the sample gently.

■ Completely fill the collection tube, invert it gently several times, and send it to the laboratory on ice.

■ For a patient on anticoagulant therapy, additional pressure may be needed at the venipuncture site to control bleeding.

Reference values

Normally, a fibrin clot forms 25 to 36 seconds after addition of reagents. For a patient on anticoagulant therapy, check with the attending doctor to find out the desirable values for the therapy being delivered.

Implications of results

Prolonged APTT may indicate a deficiency of certain plasma clotting factors, the presence of heparin, or the presence of fibrin split products, fibrinolysins, or circulating anticoagulants that are antibodies to specific clotting factors.

Post-test care

If a hematoma develops at the venipuncture site, apply warm soaks.

Interfering factors

■ Failure to use the proper anticoagulant, to fill the collection tube completely, or to mix the sample and the anticoagulant adequately may affect the accuracy of test results.

■ Hemolysis due to rough handling of the sample or to excessive probing at the venipuncture site may alter test results.

■ Failure to send the sample to the laboratory immediately or to place it on ice may cause spurious test results.

Prothrombin time

This test (commonly known as pro time) measures the time required for a fibrin clot to form in a citrated plasma sample after addition of calcium ions and tissue thromboplastin (factor III).

It is an excellent screening procedure for overall evaluation of extrinsic coagulation factors V, VII, and X, and of prothrombin and fibrinogen. Prothrombin time (PT) is the test of choice for monitoring oral anticoagulant therapy.

Purpose
- To evaluate the extrinsic coagulation system
- To monitor response to oral anticoagulant therapy.

Patient preparation
Explain to the patient that this test helps determine if his blood clots normally. Advise him that he needn't restrict food or fluids. Tell him that the test requires a blood sample, who will perform the venipuncture and when, and that he may experience discomfort from the needle puncture and the pressure of the tourniquet. Check the patient history for use of medications that may affect test results.

When appropriate, explain to the patient that this test monitors the effects of medications (oral anticoagulants). Tell him that the test will be performed daily when therapy begins and will be repeated at longer intervals when medication levels stabilize.

Procedure
Perform a venipuncture, and collect the sample in a 7-ml *blue-top* tube.

Precautions
- To prevent hemolysis, avoid excessive probing during venipuncture and handle the sample gently.
- Completely fill the collection tube, and invert it gently several times to mix the sample and the anticoagulant adequately. If the tube isn't filled to the correct volume, an excess of citrate appears in the sample.

Reference values
Normally, PT ranges from 10 to 14 seconds. In a patient receiving warfarin therapy, PT is usually maintained between $1\frac{1}{2}$ and 2 times the normal control value. (See *International Normalized Ratio.*)

Implications of results
Prolonged PT may indicate hepatic disease or deficiencies in fibrinogen; prothrombin; factors V, VII, or X (specific assays can pinpoint such deficiencies); or vitamin K. Or it may result from ongoing oral anticoagulant therapy. Prolonged PT that exceeds $2\frac{1}{2}$ times the control value is commonly associated with abnormal bleeding.

Prolonged PT can result from overuse of alcohol or from the use of adrenocorticotropic hormone, anabolic steroids, cholestyramine resin, I.V. heparin (within 5 hours of collection), indomethacin, mefenamic acid, para-aminosalicylic acid, methimazole, oxyphenbutazone, phenylbutazone, phenytoin, propylthiouracil, quinidine, quinine, thyroid hormones, or vitamin A.

Prolonged or shortened PT can follow ingestion of antibiotics, barbiturates, hydroxyzine, sulfonamides, salicylates (more than 1 g/day prolongs PT), mineral oil, or clofibrate.

Post-test care
If a hematoma develops at the venipuncture site, apply warm soaks.

Interfering factors
- Hemolysis may interfere with the accuracy of test results.
- Failure to mix the sample and anticoagulant adequately or to send the sample to the laboratory promptly may alter test results.
- Fibrin or fibrin split products in the sample or plasma fibrinogen levels less than 100 mg/dl can prolong PT.

International Normalized Ratio

The International Normalized Ratio (INR) system is generally viewed as the best means of standardizing measurement of prothrombin time (PT) to monitor oral anticoagulant therapy. However, the INR should never be used to screen patients for coagulopathies. Since PT testing is performed using different thromboplastin reagents and different instruments, each laboratory may have different "normal values."

Many types of thromboplastin are used in PT testing (rabbit brain, human brain, recombinant). Each type of reagent has a different sensitivity. The greater the reagent's sensitivity, the longer the PT will be. For example, using the same patient plasma, a sensitive thromboplastin will result in a PT of approximately 30 seconds, but a less sensitive thromboplastin will result in a PT of approximately 20 seconds.

The INR helps to standardize oral anticoagulant therapy so that a patient's therapy outcomes can be easily evaluated by various institutions that may use different instruments and thromboplastin reagents. Recent guidelines for patients receiving warfarin therapy recommend an INR of 2.0 to 3.0, except for those with mechanical prosthetic heart valves. For these patients, an INR of 2.5 to 3.5 is suggested.

■ Falsely prolonged results may occur if the collection tube is not filled to capacity with blood; this results in too much anticoagulant for the blood sample.

■ Shortened PT can result from the use of antihistamines, chloral hydrate, corticosteroids, digitalis glycosides, diuretics, glutethimide, griseofulvin, progestin-estrogen combinations, pyrazinamide, vitamin K, or xanthines (caffeine, theophylline).

One-stage factor assay: Extrinsic coagulation system

When prothrombin time (PT) and activated partial thromboplastin time (APTT) are prolonged, a one-stage assay helps detect a deficiency of factor II,

V, or X. If PT is abnormal but APTT is normal, factor VII may be deficient.

In this test, diluted samples of the patient's plasma are added to a substrate plasma deficient in a single factor. The activity of this mixture is compared with normal activity plotted on a predetermined standard curve for each factor. If the clotting time for these patient substrate mixtures is prolonged compared to normal, the patient may be deficient in the factor being tested.

Purpose

■ To identify a specific factor deficiency in persons with prolonged PT or APTT

■ To study patients with congenital or acquired coagulation defects

■ To monitor the effects of blood component therapy in factor-deficient patients.

Patient preparation

Explain that this test assesses the function of the blood coagulation mechanism. Tell the patient that he needn't

Factor XIII assay: The missing link

When a patient shows poor wound healing and other symptoms of a bleeding disorder despite normal coagulation test results, a factor XIII assay is recommended. In this test, a plasma sample is incubated with either chloracetic acid or a urea solution after normal clotting takes place. The clot is observed for 24 hours; if it dissolves, a severe factor XIII deficiency exists.

Factor XIII is responsible for stabilizing the fibrin clot, the final step in the clotting process. If the clot is unstable, it breaks loose, resulting in scarring and poor wound healing. Deficiency of this factor is usually transmitted as an autosomal recessive trait but may result from hepatic disease or from tumors.

Effects of deficiency
The clinical effects of factor XIII deficiency include umbilical bleeding in neonates, prolonged bleeding after trauma, hemarthrosis, spontaneous abortion (rarely), intraovarial bleeding (more common in factor XIII deficiency than in other bleeding disorders), and recurrent ecchymoses, hematomas, and poor wound healing. Bleeding after trauma may begin immediately or may be delayed as long as 12 to 36 hours.

Prognosis improving
Treatment with infusions of plasma or cryoprecipitate has improved the prognosis of patients with factor XIII deficiency; some patients may even live normal lives. However, before appropriate treatment can begin, diagnostic evaluation must rule out other bleeding disorders. Dysfibrinogenemia, hyperfibrinogenemia, and disseminated intravascular coagulation also cause rapid clot dissolution in this assay, but unlike factor XIII deficiency, they also cause an abnormal fibrinogen level and thrombin time.

restrict food or fluids. Inform him that the test requires a blood sample, who will perform the venipuncture and when, and that he may experience discomfort from the puncture and the tourniquet.

Withhold oral anticoagulants before the test, as ordered. If they must be continued, note that on the laboratory request. If the patient is factor-deficient and receiving blood component therapy, tell him that he may need a series of tests. (See *Factor XIII assay: The missing link.*)

Procedure
Perform a venipuncture, and collect the sample in a 7-ml *blue-top* tube.

Precautions
- If the patient has a suspected coagulation defect, avoid excessive probing during venipuncture, don't leave the tourniquet on too long (it will cause bruising), and apply pressure to the puncture site for 5 minutes or until the bleeding stops.
- Completely fill the collection tube, and invert it gently several times to mix the sample and the anticoagulant.
- Handle the sample gently to prevent hemolysis, and send it to the laboratory immediately.

Reference values
The reference range for most factors is approximately 50% to 150% of normal activity.

Implications of results

Deficiency of factor II, VII, or X may indicate hepatic disease or vitamin K deficiency; deficiency of factor X may also indicate disseminated intravascular coagulation (DIC). Factor V deficiency suggests severe hepatic disease, DIC, or fibrinogenolysis. Deficiencies of all four factors may be congenital, although absence of factor II is lethal.

Post-test care

- If a hematoma develops at the venipuncture site, apply warm soaks.
- A patient with a bleeding disorder may require a pressure bandage to stop bleeding at the venipuncture site.

Interfering factors

- Hemolysis caused by rough handling of the sample may affect test results.
- Failure to mix the sample and the anticoagulant adequately or to send the sample to the laboratory immediately may alter test results.
- Oral anticoagulant therapy may increase bleeding time by inhibiting vitamin K–dependent synthesis and activation of clotting factors II, VII, and X, which are formed in the liver.

One-stage factor assay: Intrinsic coagulation system

When prothrombin time is normal but activated partial thromboplastin time is abnormal, a one-stage assay helps identify a deficiency in the intrinsic coagulation system — factor VIII, IX, XI, or XII.

In this test, diluted samples of the patient's plasma are added to a substrate plasma deficient in a single factor. The activity of this mixture is compared with normal activity plotted on a predetermined standard curve for each factor. If the clotting time of these patient substrate mixtures is prolonged compared to normal, the patient may be deficient in the factor being tested.

Purpose

- To identify a specific factor deficiency
- To study patients with congenital or acquired coagulation defects
- To monitor the effects of blood component therapy in factor-deficient patients.

Patient preparation

Explain to the patient that this test assesses the function of the blood coagulation mechanism. Inform him that he needn't restrict food or fluids. Tell him that the test requires a blood sample, who will perform the venipuncture and when, and that he may experience discomfort from the needle puncture and the pressure of the tourniquet.

Withhold oral anticoagulants before the test, as ordered. If such medications must be continued, note this on the laboratory request.

If the patient is factor-deficient and receiving blood component therapy, tell him that a series of tests may be needed to monitor therapeutic progress.

Procedure

Perform a venipuncture, and collect the sample in a 7-ml *blue-top* tube.

Precautions

- If a coagulation defect is suspected, avoid excessive probing during venipuncture, don't leave the tourniquet on too long (it will cause bruising), and apply pressure to the puncture site for 5 minutes or until the bleeding stops.
- Completely fill the collection tube, and invert it gently several times to mix the sample and anticoagulant adequately.

Factor VIII–related antigen test

Bleeding time tests and the patient history can usually distinguish between classic hemophilia and von Willebrand's disease. But when bleeding time tests prove inconclusive and the patient has no family history of bleeding, the factor VIII–related antigen test can provide helpful diagnostic information.

In this test, a sample of the patient's plasma is compared to a control sample after both are placed in an agarose gel impregnated with factor VIII antibody. Electrophoresis is performed; then the gel is examined for rocket-shaped immunoprecipitates indicating a factor VIII antigen response.

People with hemophilia and carriers of hemophilia demonstrate normal activity: 45% to 185% of the control sample. Patients with von Willebrand's disease, however, show absent or deficient levels of factor VIII antigen.

■ Handle the sample gently to prevent hemolysis, and send it to the laboratory immediately.

Reference values
The reference range for most factors is approximately 50% to 150% of normal activity.

Implications of results
Factor VIII deficiency may indicate hemophilia A, von Willebrand's disease, or factor VIII inhibitor. An acquired deficiency of factor VIII may result from disseminated intravascular coagulation or fibrinolysis. The factor VIII antigen and ristocetin cofactor tests distinguish between hemophilia A (and its carrier state) and von Willebrand's disease. (See *Factor VIII-related antigen test.*)

Factor IX deficiency may suggest hemophilia B, or it may be acquired as a result of hepatic disease, factor IX inhibitor, vitamin K deficiency, or coumarin therapy. (Factors VIII and IX inhibitors are antibodies specific to each factor that occur after transfusions in patients deficient in either factor.)

Factor XI deficiency may appear after the stress of trauma or surgery, or transiently in neonates. Factor XII deficiency may be inherited or acquired (as in nephrosis) and may also appear transiently in neonates.

Post-test care
■ If a hematoma develops at the venipuncture site, apply warm soaks.
■ A patient with a bleeding disorder may require a pressure bandage to stop bleeding at the venipuncture site.
■ As ordered, resume administration of medications discontinued before the test.

Interfering factors
■ Hemolysis caused by rough handling of the sample may alter test results.
■ Failure to mix the sample and the anticoagulant adequately or to send the sample to the laboratory immediately may alter test results.
■ Oral anticoagulants decrease factor IX levels; pregnancy elevates factor VIII.

Plasma thrombin time

The plasma thrombin time test measures how quickly a clot forms when a standard amount of bovine thrombin is

Antithrombin III test

This test helps detect the cause of impaired coagulation, especially hypercoagulation, by measuring levels of antithrombin III (AT III). This protein inactivates thrombin and inhibits coagulation. Normally, a balance exists between AT III and thrombin; an AT III deficiency increases coagulation.

AT III may be evaluated by a functional clotting assay or by synthetic substrates. Exogenous heparin is added to a fresh, citrated blood sample to accelerate AT III activity. Then excess thrombin (factor Xa) is added to the plasma. The amount of factor Xa not activated by AT III is quantitated by clotting time or spectrophotometrically and is compared to a normal control. Reference values may vary for each laboratory, but should lie between 80% to 120% of normal activity.

Decreased AT III levels can indicate disseminated intravascular coagulation or thromboembolic, hypercoagulation, or hepatic disorders. Slightly decreased levels can result from use of oral contraceptives. Elevated levels can result from kidney transplantation and use of oral anticoagulants or anabolic steroids.

---

added to a platelet-poor plasma sample from the patient and to a normal plasma control sample. After thrombin is added, the clotting time for each sample is compared and recorded. Because thrombin rapidly converts fibrinogen to a fibrin clot, this test (also known as the thrombin clotting time test) allows a quick but imprecise estimation of plasma fibrinogen levels, which are a function of clotting time. (See *Antithrombin III test* for information about another test that helps determine the cause of coagulation disorders.)

Purpose
■ To detect a fibrinogen deficiency or defect
■ To aid diagnosis of disseminated intravascular coagulation (DIC) and hepatic disease
■ To monitor the effectiveness of treatment with heparin or thrombolytic agents.

Patient preparation
Explain to the patient that this test helps determine if his blood clots normally. Inform him that he needn't restrict food or fluids. Tell him that the test requires a blood sample, who will perform the venipuncture and when, and that he may experience discomfort from the needle puncture and the pressure of the tourniquet.

If possible, withhold heparin therapy before the test, as ordered. If heparin must be continued, note this on the laboratory request.

Procedure
Perform a venipuncture, and collect the sample in a 7-ml *blue-top* tube.

Precautions
■ To prevent hemolysis, avoid excessive probing during venipuncture and rough handling of the sample.
■ Completely fill the collection tube, and invert it gently several times to mix the sample and anticoagulant adequately. If the tube isn't filled to the correct volume, an excess of citrate appears in the sample.
■ Send the sample to the laboratory immediately.

Reference values

Normal thrombin times range from 10 to 15 seconds. Test results are usually reported with a normal control value.

Implications of results

A prolonged thrombin time may indicate heparin therapy, hepatic disease, DIC, hypofibrinogenemia, or dysfibrinogenemia. Patients with prolonged thrombin times may require quantitation of fibrinogen levels; in suspected DIC, the test for fibrin split products is also necessary.

Post-test care

If a hematoma develops at the venipuncture site, apply warm soaks.

Interfering factors

■ Hemolysis caused by excessive probing during venipuncture or rough handling of the sample may affect the accuracy of test results.
■ Failure to use the proper anticoagulant in the collection tube, to mix the sample and the anticoagulant adequately, or to send the sample to the laboratory immediately may affect the accuracy of test results.
■ Administration of heparin may prolong clotting time.

Plasma fibrinogen

Fibrinogen (factor I), a plasma protein originating in the liver, isn't normally present in serum; it's converted to fibrin by thrombin during clotting. Since fibrin is a necessary part of a blood clot, fibrinogen deficiency can produce mild to severe bleeding disorders. When fibrinogen levels drop below 100 mg/dl, accurate interpretation of all coagula-tion tests that have a fibrin clot as an end point becomes difficult.

Purpose

■ To aid the diagnosis of suspected clotting or bleeding disorders caused by fibrinogen abnormalities.

Patient preparation

Explain to the patient that this test helps determine if his blood clots normally. Inform him that he needn't restrict food or fluids before the test. Tell him that a blood sample is required, who will perform the venipuncture and when, and that he may experience discomfort from the needle puncture and the pressure of the tourniquet. Check the patient history for use of heparin and oral contraceptives. Note such drugs on the laboratory request.

Procedure

Perform a venipuncture, and collect the sample in a 7-ml *blue-top* tube.

Precautions

■ This test is contraindicated in patients with active bleeding or acute infection or illness, and in those who have received a blood transfusion within the past 4 weeks.
■ If the patient is receiving heparin therapy, notify the laboratory; such therapy requires use of a different reagent.
■ Completely fill the collection tube, invert it gently several times, and send it to the laboratory immediately.
■ Avoid excessive probing during the venipuncture, and handle the sample gently.

Reference values

Fibrinogen levels normally range from 195 to 365 mg/dl.

Implications of results

Depressed fibrinogen levels may indicate congenital afibrinogenemia, hypofibrinogenemia or dysfibrinogenemia, disseminated intravascular coagulation, fibrinolysis, severe hepatic disease, bone marrow lesions, or cancer of the prostate, pancreas, or lung. Obstetric complications or trauma may also cause low levels.

Elevated levels may indicate cancer of the stomach, breast, or kidney, or inflammatory disorders, such as pneumonia or membranoproliferative glomerulonephritis.

Prolonged activated partial thromboplastin time, prothrombin time, and thrombin time may also indicate a fibrinogen deficiency.

Post-test care
If a hematoma develops at the venipuncture site, apply warm soaks.

Interfering factors
■ Fibrinogen levels may be elevated during the third trimester of pregnancy and in postoperative patients.
■ Hemolysis caused by traumatic venipuncture or rough handling of the sample may affect test results.
■ Failure to fill the collection tube completely, to mix the sample and anticoagulant adequately, or to send the sample to the laboratory promptly may affect the accuracy of test results.

Fibrin split products

After a fibrin clot forms in response to vascular injury, the fibrinolytic system acts to degrade the clot by converting plasminogen into the fibrin-dissolving enzyme plasmin. Plasmin breaks down fibrin and fibrinogen into fragments (known as fibrin split products or fibrin degradation products) labeled X, Y, D, and E, in order of decreasing molecular weight. An excess of these products in the circulation may combine with fibrin monomers to prevent polymerization; that is, the fragments cause anticoagulant activity. This excess may lead to coagulation disorders, which may be due to fibrinogenolysis or clotting excesses such as disseminated intravascular coagulation (DIC).

Fibrin split products (FSP) are detected by an immunoprecipitation reaction, in which diluted serum left in a blood sample after clotting is mixed on a slide with latex particles that carry antibodies to D and E split products. Clumping of the latex particles occurs if FSP are present in the serum dilution.

Purpose
■ To detect FSP in the circulation
■ To help determine the presence and approximate severity of a hyperfibrinolytic state that may be associated with primary fibrinogenolysis or hypercoagulability such as DIC. (See *Causes of disseminated intravascular coagulation,* page 64.)

Patient preparation
Explain to the patient that this test helps determine if his blood clots normally. Tell him that he needn't restrict food or fluids before the test. Inform him that the test requires a blood sample, who will perform the venipuncture and when, and that he may experience transient discomfort from the needle puncture and the pressure of the tourniquet.

Check the patient history for use of any medications (especially heparin) that may affect the accuracy of test results.

Procedure
Perform a venipuncture, and draw 2 ml of blood into a plastic syringe. Transfer the sample to the tube provided by the laboratory, which contains a soybean trypsin inhibitor and bovine thrombin.

Causes of disseminated intravascular coagulation

Obstetric: Amniotic fluid embolism, eclampsia, retained dead fetus, retained placenta, abruptio placentae, and toxemia

Neoplastic: Sarcoma, metastatic carcinoma, acute leukemia, prostate cancer, and giant hemangioma

Infectious: Acute bacteremia, septicemia, and rickettsemia; viral, fungal, or protozoal infection

Necrotic: Trauma, destruction of brain tissue, extensive burns, heat stroke, rejection of transplant, and hepatic necrosis

Cardiovascular: Fat embolism, acute venous thrombosis, cardiopulmonary bypass surgery, hypovolemic shock, cardiac arrest, and hypotension

Other: Snakebite, cirrhosis, transfusion of incompatible blood, purpura, and glomerulonephritis

(Evacuated tubes are available in kits designed to provide a rapid semi-quantitative analysis of FSP. Follow the manufacturer's directions for specimen collection and handling.)

Precautions

■ Drawing the sample before administering heparin will help avoid false-positive test results.

■ Gently invert the collection tube several times to mix the contents adequately. The blood clots within 2 seconds and must then be sent to the laboratory immediately to be incubated at 98.6° F (37° C) for 30 minutes before testing proceeds.

Reference values

Serum contains less than 10 μg/ml of FSP. A quantitative assay shows levels of less than 3 μg/ml.

Implications of results

FSP levels rise in primary fibrinolytic states because of increased levels of circulating profibrinolysin; in secondary states, because of DIC and subsequent fibrinolysis. Levels also increase in alcoholic cirrhosis, preeclampsia, abruptio placentae, congenital heart disease, sunstroke, burns, intrauterine death, pulmonary embolus, deep vein thrombosis (transient increase), and myocardial infarction (after 1 or 2 days). FSP levels usually exceed 100 μg/ml in active renal disease or kidney transplant rejection.

Post-test care

If a hematoma develops at the venipuncture site, apply warm soaks.

Interfering factors

■ Pretest administration of heparin causes false-positive results.

■ Fibrinolytic drugs, such as urokinase and streptokinase, and large doses of barbiturates increase FSP levels.

■ Failure to fill the collection tube completely, to mix the sample and additive adequately, or to send the sample to the laboratory immediately may affect the accuracy of test results.

■ Hemolysis caused by rough handling of the sample may alter test results.

Plasma plasminogen

Measurement of plasminogen, the precursor of plasmin, is one way to evaluate the fibrinolytic system. During fibrinolysis, plasmin dissolves fibrin clots to prevent excessive coagulation and resultant impairment of blood flow. However, because plasmin doesn't circulate in active form, it can't be measured directly; instead, measurement of its circulation precursor, plasminogen, provides a parameter to evaluate this system.

In this test, streptokinase, a plasminogen activator, is added to a plasma sample. Streptokinase converts plasminogen to active plasmin; the plasmin then converts a substrate, a colored substance that's measured spectrophotometrically or fluorometrically. The colored amount is proportional to the functional plasminogen in the sample. Plasminogen may also be measured immunologically.

Purpose
■ To assess fibrinolysis
■ To detect congenital and acquired fibrinolytic disorders.

Patient preparation
Explain to the patient that this test evaluates blood clotting. Inform him that he needn't restrict food or fluids. Tell him that the test requires a blood sample, who will perform the venipuncture and when, and that he may experience minor discomfort from the needle puncture and the pressure of the tourniquet. Check the patient history for use of streptokinase or other drugs that may cause inaccurate test results. If these drugs must be continued, note this on the laboratory request.

Procedure
Perform a venipuncture, and collect the sample in a 7-ml *blue-top* tube.

Precautions
■ Collect the sample as quickly as possible to prevent stasis, which can slow blood flow, causing coagulation and plasminogen activation.
■ To prevent hemolysis, avoid excessive probing during venipuncture and rough handling of the specimen.
■ Invert the tube gently several times, and send the sample to the laboratory immediately. If testing must be delayed, plasma must be separated and frozen at −94° F (−70° C).

Reference values
Normal plasminogen levels range from 10 to 20 mg/dl by immunologic methods and from 80 to 120 U/dl by functional methods.

Implications of results
Diminished plasminogen levels can result from disseminated intravascular coagulation, tumors, preeclampsia, and eclampsia, which accelerate plasminogen conversion to plasmin and increase fibrinolysis. Some liver diseases prevent formation of sufficient plasminogen, decreasing fibrinolysis.

Post-test care
■ If a hematoma develops at the venipuncture site, apply warm soaks.
■ Resume medications withheld before the test, as ordered.

Interfering factors
■ Failure to use the proper tube, to mix the sample and citrate adequately, to send the sample to the laboratory immediately, or to have it separated and frozen may alter results.
■ Hemolysis due to excessive probing during venipuncture or rough handling of the sample may alter results.

- Prolonged tourniquet use before venipuncture may cause stasis, falsely decreasing plasminogen levels.
- Oral contraceptives may slightly increase plasminogen levels. Thrombolytic drugs, such as streptokinase or urokinase, may decrease levels also.

Protein C

A vitamin K–dependent protein, protein C is produced in the liver and circulates in the plasma. After activation by thrombin in the presence of a capillary endothelial cofactor, it acts as a potent anticoagulant that suppresses the procoagulation activity of activated factors V and VIII. Both acquired and congenital deficiencies of protein C have been identified.

Homozygous deficiency of protein C, which is rare, is characterized by rapidly fatal thrombosis in the perinatal period, a syndrome known as purpura fulminans. The more common heterozygous deficiency is associated with familial susceptibility to venous thromboembolism before age 30 and continuing throughout life.

Measurement of protein C should include a functional assay and an immunologic approach to determine the type of deficiency. Protein C values are used to investigate the cause of otherwise unexplained thrombosis and to establish patterns of inheritance. A positive finding for heterozygous deficiency suggests the possible need for long-term treatment with warfarin therapy or protein C supplements from plasma fractions.

Purpose
- To investigate the mechanism of idiopathic venous thrombosis.

Patient preparation
Explain to the patient that this test evaluates the blood clotting mechanism. Tell him that the test requires a blood sample, who will perform the venipuncture and when, and that he may have some discomfort from the needle puncture and the tourniquet pressure. If the patient is receiving anticoagulant therapy, note this on the laboratory request.

Procedure
Perform a venipuncture. Collect a 3-ml sample in a *blue-top* vacuum specimen tube or in a special syringe with anticoagulant provided by the laboratory.

Precautions
- Avoid excessive probing during venipuncture; handle the sample gently.
- Completely fill the collection tube, and invert it several times to mix the sample and anticoagulant adequately.
- Send the sample to the laboratory immediately.

Reference values
The normal range is 70% to 140% of the population mean, depending on the test method.

Implications of results
Identifying the role of protein C deficiency in idiopathic venous thrombosis may help prevent thromboembolism.

Post-test care
If a hematoma develops at the venipuncture site, apply warm soaks.

Interfering factors
- Hemolysis due to excessive probing during venipuncture or to rough handling of the sample may alter test results.
- Anticoagulant therapy may alter test results.

Euglobulin lysis time

This test measures the interval between clot formation and dissolution in the euglobulin fraction of plasma. In the laboratory, a precipitated plasma extract is clotted with thrombin. The time required for this clot to lyse is then recorded.

Purpose
■ To assess the fibrinolytic system
■ To help detect abnormal fibrinolytic states.

Patient preparation
Explain to the patient that this test evaluates the clotting mechanism. Tell him that the test requires a blood sample, who will perform the venipuncture and when, and that he may have some discomfort from the needle puncture and the tourniquet pressure.

Procedure
Perform a venipuncture. Collect a 4.5-ml sample in a *blue-top* tube or in a chilled tube with 0.5 ml sodium oxalate.

Precautions
■ When drawing the sample, be careful not to rub the area over the vein too vigorously, not to pump the fist excessively, and not to leave the tourniquet in place too long. Avoid excessive probing during venipuncture, and handle the sample gently.
■ If a blue-top tube is used, mix the sample and anticoagulant thoroughly. If a chilled tube containing 0.5 ml sodium oxalate is used, mix the sample and preservative adequately, pack the sample in ice, and send it to the laboratory immediately.

Normal findings
Lysis normally occurs in 2 to 4 hours.

Implications of results
Clot lysis within 1 hour indicates increased plasminogen activator activity. In pathologic fibrinolysis, lysis time may be as brief as 5 to 10 minutes.

Post-test care
If a hematoma develops at the venipuncture site, ease discomfort by applying warm soaks.

Interfering factors
■ Prolonged tourniquet constriction, vigorous vein preparation, or excessive pumping of the fist shortens lysis time.
■ Hemolysis resulting from excessive probing during venipuncture or from rough handling of the sample may alter test results.
■ Failure to follow appropriate precautions for the type of collection tube used may affect the accuracy of test results.
■ Depressed fibrinogen levels (less than 100 mg/dl) can shorten lysis time.

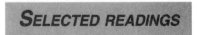

SELECTED READINGS

Diseases, 2nd ed. Springhouse, Pa.: Springhouse Corp., 1996.

Ebert, R.F. "PTs, PRs, ISIs, and INRs: A Primer on Prothrombin Time Reporting, Part I: Calibration of Thromboplastin Reagents and Principles of Prothrombin Time Reporting," *Clinical Hemostasis Review* 7(11):1–9, 1993.

Ebert, R.F. "PTs, PRs, ISIs, and INRs: A Primer on Prothrombin Time Reporting, Part II: Limitations of INR Reporting," *Clinical Hemostasis Review* 7(12):1–9, 1993.

Fischbach, F. *A Manual of Laboratory and Diagnostic Tests,* 5th ed. Philadelphia: Lippincott-Raven Pubs., 1996.

Guyton, A.C., and Hall, J.E. *Textbook of Medical Physiology*, 9th ed. Philadelphia: W.B. Saunders Co., 1996.

Harmening, D.M., ed. *Clinical Hematology and Fundamentals of Hemostasis*, 3rd ed. Philadelphia: F.A. Davis Co., 1996.

Henry, J.B., ed. *Clinical Diagnosis and Management by Laboratory Methods*, 19th ed. Philadelphia: W.B. Saunders Co., 1996.

Jensen, R. "Pre-Analytical Variables in Hemostasis Testing," *Clinical Hemostasis Review* 9(10):1–7, 1995.

Nursing97 Drug Handbook. Springhouse, Pa.: Springhouse Corp., 1997.

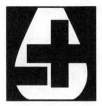

CHAPTER THREE

Blood gases and electrolytes

Learning objectives

After completing this chapter, the reader will be able to:
- identify the three major fluid compartments
- state the arterial blood gas results commonly associated with respiratory acidosis and alkalosis and with metabolic acidosis and alkalosis
- identify the functions of the major serum electrolytes
- explain the physiology of calcium absorption
- state the causes, signs, and symptoms of hypovolemia and hypervolemia
- explain how the sodium pump works
- state the purpose of each test discussed in this chapter
- prepare the patient physically and psychologically for each test
- describe the procedure for obtaining a specimen for each test
- specify appropriate precautions for accurately obtaining a specimen for each test
- recognize signs of abnormal serum levels of the major electrolytes and respond appropriately
- implement appropriate post-test care
- state the reference values for each test
- discuss the implications of abnormal test results
- list factors that may interfere with accurate test results.

INTRODUCTION

Laboratory analysis of blood gases and electrolytes helps evaluate the body's respiratory and metabolic status. Arterial blood gas (ABG) values provide important information about the adequacy of gas exchange in the lungs, the integrity of the ventilatory control system, and blood pH and acid-base balance. Serum electrolyte levels also supply valuable data about the body's acid-base balance and fluid balance.

Metabolic processes continually form acids, which must be eliminated to maintain acid-base balance. To maintain this balance, the lungs and kidneys interact to maintain pH within an acceptable range. Blood gas studies measure the lungs' capacity to regulate carbon dioxide concentration in the blood; serum electrolyte assays determine the kidneys' capacity to retain or excrete metabolic acids and bases. Because these functions are so closely interwoven, accurate assessment of homeostasis requires simultaneous interpretation of blood gas and electrolyte studies.

Arterial blood gases

Blood gas studies are usually performed on arterial blood, which contains oxygen (O_2) and carbon dioxide (CO_2). ABGs are measurements of the partial pressure that oxygen (Pao_2) and carbon dioxide ($Paco_2$) exert in the blood. As the concentration of the gas rises, so does its partial pressure. To understand the clinical significance of ABG values, one must first understand the phenomenon of gas exchange in the lungs.

Environmental oxygen, about 21% of inspired air, travels through the airways into the lungs; the waste product, carbon dioxide, travels from the lungs to the surrounding air. Consequently, the alveoli in the lungs contain a mixture of inspired oxygen moving through the capillaries and into circulation, and car-

Important definitions

Partial pressure	A measure of the force that a gas exerts on the fluid in which it is dissolved
Pao_2	Partial pressure of oxygen in arterial blood
$Paco_2$	Partial pressure of carbon dioxide in arterial blood
pH	A measure of acid-base balance, or the concentration of free hydrogen ions in the blood
O_2CT	Oxygen content, or the volume of oxygen combined with hemoglobin in arterial blood
Sao_2	Arterial oxygen saturation, a measure of the percentage of oxygen combined with hemoglobin compared to the total amount of oxygen with which hemoglobin could combine
Electrolytes	Substances that dissociate into ions when fused or in solution and that thus conduct electricity
Cations	Positively charged ions
Anions	Negatively charged ions
Acidosis	Metabolic or respiratory changes that result in a loss of base or an accumulation of acid
Alkalosis	Metabolic or respiratory changes that result in a loss of acid or an accumulation of base

bon dioxide (waste product of metabolism) moving through the capillaries for exhalation.

Oxygen taken up in the lungs is transported to the tissues through the circulatory system. Only a small amount of inspired oxygen can dissolve in arterial blood; how much dissolves depends on the partial pressure of the oxygen. The remainder combines chemically with hemoglobin. *Oxygen content* (O_2CT) measures the amount of oxygen combined with hemoglobin; this value is used infrequently. *Oxygen saturation* (Sao_2) is the ratio of the amount of oxygen in the blood that is combined with hemoglobin to the total amount of oxygen that the hemoglobin could carry. (See *Important definitions.*)

Carbon dioxide is produced by cellular metabolism and is released into the bloodstream. Because it's more soluble than oxygen, it dissolves in the blood, mostly forming bicarbonate (HCO_3-) and lesser amounts of carbonic acid (H_2CO_3) and carbamino compounds (bound to hemoglobin).

Acid-base balance

Enzymes that control vital cellular functions perform most efficiently when the body's pH ranges between 7.35 and 7.45. The carbonic acid–bicarbonate buffer system helps maintain body pH at this desirable level. The system may be represented by these equations:

$$CO_2 + H_2O \rightarrow H_2CO_3$$

(carbon dioxide + water $\rightarrow$ carbonic acid).

In turn, carbonic acid can undergo the following change:

$$H_2CO_3 \rightarrow H^+ + HCO_3-$$

(carbonic acid $\rightarrow$ hydrogen ion + bicarbonate).

Bicarbonate and carbonic acid normally exist in a 20:1 ratio. Any change in this ratio causes a blood pH that is abnormally acid or alkaline.

The lungs control carbonic acid levels by converting carbonic acid to carbon dioxide and water for excretion. By changing the rate and depth of respiration, the lungs can adjust the amount of carbon dioxide lost to maintain the normal ratio. This compensatory mechanism is rapidly effective. For example, in metabolic acidosis, the lungs increase their rate and depth in order to "blow off" excess carbon dioxide (carbonic acid), thus raising the pH to acceptable levels.

When the lungs are functioning inadequately, they can actually produce an acid-base imbalance. For example, they cause *respiratory acidosis* by hypoventilation and excessive retention of carbon dioxide (carbonic acid excess); they cause *respiratory alkalosis* by hyperventilation and excessive exhalation of carbon dioxide (carbonic acid deficit).

The kidneys — primary regulators of bicarbonate — excrete, reabsorb, or regenerate the amount of bicarbonate needed to maintain the normal carbonic acid–bicarbonate ratio. This can effectively compensate for an imbalance that results from pulmonary dysfunction. However, this compensatory response is notably slower than pulmonary compensation and usually occurs over a 3- to 4-day period.

The kidneys have another important role to play: Because the acids resulting from metabolic processes — with the exception of carbonic acid — can't be converted to gases for exhalation by the lungs, they must be excreted by the kidneys. Thus, renal dysfunction can cause metabolic acid-base imbalance. Summarized briefly, metabolic acidosis results when the body loses too much base (bicarbonate) or retains excessive acid; metabolic alkalosis results when the body retains too much base (bicarbonate) or loses too much acid.

Clinical significance of ABGs

Abnormal variations in ABG levels may result from respiratory or metabolic causes. Compensatory mechanisms, such as those in the lungs and kidneys, automatically attempt to correct an imbalance. But compensation is not correction, and compensatory mechanisms are limited.

Although valuable in assessing overall respiratory and metabolic status, ABG measurements are not diagnostically specific. For example, taken alone, ABG values do not distinguish between pulmonary and cardiac disorders. These values are most useful when considered with other factors, such as cardiac output, regional blood flow, and tissue oxygen consumption.

The significance of ABG studies is also limited by the fact that these studies don't necessarily detect disease. For example, the lungs may continue to function properly, with unchanged ABG values, despite the presence of pulmonary disease. Therefore, other diagnostic screening tests, such as spirometry or chest X-ray, must be performed. When dealing with ABG values, make sure you check the accepted values for your hospital. Normal ranges may vary according to the laboratory method used.

Serum electrolytes

Electrolytes are substances that dissociate into ions when dissolved in the blood. Electrolytes that carry a positive charge are called cations; those that carry a negative charge are called anions. Sodium, calcium, chloride, and bicarbonate are the major extracellular electrolytes. Sodium is the most abundant extracellular cation; chloride, the most abundant anion. Potassium, magnesium, and phosphate are the major intracellular electrolytes. Potassium is the

Functions of serum electrolytes		
CATIONS	Sodium (Na+)	■ Maintains osmotic pressure of extracellular fluid
		■ Helps regulate neuromuscular activity
		■ Influences acid-base balance, and chloride and potassium levels
		■ Helps regulate water excretion
	Potassium (K+)	■ Maintains cellular osmotic equilibrium
		■ Helps regulate neuromuscular and enzymatic activity, and acid-base balance
		■ Influences kidney function
	Calcium (Ca++)	■ Helps regulate and promote neuromuscular activity, skeletal development, and blood coagulation
	Magnesium (Mg++)	■ Helps regulate intracellular activity, and sodium, potassium, calcium, and phosphorus levels
ANIONS	Chloride (Cl–)	■ Influences acid-base balance
		■ Helps maintain blood osmotic pressure and arterial pressure
	Bicarbonate (HCO$_3$–)	■ Acts with carbonic acid in buffer system that regulates blood pH
	Phosphate (HPO$_4$–)	■ Helps regulate calcium levels, energy metabolism, and acid-base balance

most abundant intracellular cation; phosphate, the most abundant anion. Note that hemolyzed blood samples will show a false increase in potassium levels because of the way potassium is release from red blood cells.

Serum concentrations of electrolytes influence movement of fluid within and between body compartments. (See *Functions of serum electrolytes.*) Such movement depends on osmolality — the concentration of electrolytes in the respective fluid compartments. Total electrolyte concentration (usually expressed in milliequivalents [mEq] per liter of serum) plus other dissolved substances, such as glucose, determine the osmolality of a given compartment. During osmosis, water flows from a compartment of lower osmolality to one of higher osmolality, until the osmotic pressure in the two compartments is equal. (See *Body fluids,* page 74.)

Electrolytes and homeostasis
The body can function properly only if the kidneys and lungs (with the aid of endocrine hormones) maintain electrolyte balance between intracellular and extracellular compartments. The hypothalamus and the pituitary control osmolality by regulating antidiuretic hor-

---

Body fluids

Fluids — mainly water — account for 60% of an adult's total body weight. Body fluids contain substances that dissociate in solutions and conduct a weak electric current (electrolytes), as well as substances that don't break down into smaller substances. Electrolytes with a positive charge are called *cations;* those carrying a negative charge are called *anions.* A cation-anion balance results in electric neutrality.

Two main compartments house the body's fluids. With its 100 trillion cells, the *intracellular compartment* accounts for 40% of the total body weight (approximately 25 liters of fluid). In the spaces between the cells, the *extracellular compartment* constitutes 15% of the total body weight (approximately 15 liters of interstitial fluid). Intravascular fluid, or plasma, accounts for the final 5%. A change in the amount or composition of these compartments can be fatal.

Electrolytes play a crucial role in the body's water distribution, osmolality, acid-base balance, and neuromuscular irritability. Potassium (K^+) is the principal cation, and phosphate (HPO_4-) is the dominant anion in the intracellular compartment. Like plasma, the interstitial fluid contains high concentrations of sodium (Na^+) and chloride ($Cl-$). Together, fluids and electrolytes nourish and maintain the body.

---

mone, which promotes water reabsorption by the kidneys. The kidneys govern fluid and electrolytes through filtration, reabsorption, and excretion.

Electrolytes also help maintain acid-base balance. The kidneys may exchange potassium or sodium for hydrogen and absorb or excrete bicarbonate or chloride ions to maintain a proper pH. Serum electrolyte concentrations affect all metabolic activity in some way. Also, electrolyte concentration differences between intracellular fluid and extracellular fluid regulate neuromuscular function. Consequently, serum electrolyte studies are essential to routine medical evaluation in all hospitalized patients. Abnormal electrolyte values may reflect fluid or acid-base imbalance or kidney, neuromuscular, endocrine, or skeletal dysfunction.

BLOOD GAS ANALYSIS

Arterial blood gas analysis

Arterial blood gas (ABG) analysis evaluates gas exchange in the lungs by measuring the partial pressures of oxygen (Pao_2) and carbon dioxide ($Paco_2$) as well as the pH of an arterial sample. Pao_2 indicates how much oxygen the lungs are delivering to the blood. $Paco_2$ indicates how efficiently the lungs eliminate carbon dioxide. The pH indicates the acid-base level of the blood, or the hydrogen ion (H^+) concentration. Acidity indicates H^+ excess; alkalinity, H^+ deficit. (See *Balancing pH.*) Oxygen content (O_2CT), oxygen saturation (Sao_2), and

Balancing pH

To measure the acidity or alkalinity of a solution, chemists use a pH scale of 1 to 15 that measures hydrogen ion concentrations. As hydrogen ions and acidity increase, pH falls below 7.0, which is neutral. Conversely, when hydrogen ions decrease, pH and alkalinity increase. Acid-base balance, or homeostasis of hydrogen ions, is necessary if the body's enzyme systems are to work properly.

The slightest change in ionic hydrogen concentration alters the rate of cellular chemical reactions; a sufficiently severe change can be fatal. To maintain a normal blood pH — generally between 7.35 and 7.45 — the body relies on the following three mechanisms.

Buffers

Chemically composed of two substances, buffers prevent radical pH changes by replacing strong acids added to a solution (such as blood) with weaker ones. For example, strong acids capable of yielding many hydrogen ions are replaced by weaker ones that yield fewer hydrogen ions. Because of the principal buffer coupling of bicarbonate and carbonic acid — normally in a ratio of 20:1 — the plasma acid-base level rarely fluctuates. Increased bicarbonate, however, indicates alkalosis, whereas decreased bicarbonate points to acidosis. Increased carbonic acid indicates acidosis, and decreased carbonic acid indicates alkalosis.

Respiration

Respiration is important in maintaining blood pH. The lungs convert carbonic acid to carbon dioxide and water. With every expiration, carbon dioxide and water leave the body, decreasing the carbonic acid content of the blood. Consequently, fewer hydrogen ions are formed, and blood pH increases. When the blood's hydrogen ion or carbonic acid content increases, neurons in the respiratory center stimulate respiration.

Hyperventilation eliminates carbon dioxide and hence carbonic acid from the body, reduces hydrogen ion formation, and increases pH. Conversely, increased blood pH from alkalosis — decreased hydrogen ion concentration — causes hypoventilation, which restores blood pH to its normal level by retaining carbon dioxide and thus increasing hydrogen ion formation.

Urinary excretion

The third factor in acid-base balance is urine excretion. Because the kidneys excrete varying amounts of acids and bases, they control urine pH, which in turn affects blood pH. For example, when blood pH is decreased, the distal and collecting tubules remove excessive hydrogen ions (carbonic acid forms in the tubular cells and dissociates into hydrogen and bicarbonate) and displaces them in urine, thereby eliminating hydrogen from the body. In exchange, basic ions in the urine — most often sodium — diffuse into the tubular cells, where they combine with bicarbonate. This sodium bicarbonate is then reabsorbed in the blood, resulting in decreased urine pH and, more important, increased blood pH.

bicarbonate (HCO_3-) values also aid diagnosis. A blood sample for ABG analysis may be drawn by percutaneous arterial puncture or from an arterial line.

Purpose

- To evaluate the efficiency of pulmonary gas exchange
- To assess integrity of the ventilatory control system
- To determine the acid-base level of the blood
- To monitor respiratory therapy.

Patient preparation

Explain to the patient that this test evaluates how well the lungs are delivering oxygen to blood and eliminating carbon dioxide. Inform him he needn't restrict food or fluids. Tell him the test requires a blood sample, who will perform the arterial puncture and when, and which site — radial, brachial, or femoral artery — has been selected for the puncture. Instruct the patient to breathe normally during the test, and warn him that he may experience brief cramping or throbbing pain at the puncture site.

Procedure

Perform an arterial puncture.

Precautions

- Wait at least 20 minutes before drawing arterial blood if a change in oxygen therapy has been made or when starting or discontinuing oxygen therapy.
- Before sending the sample to the laboratory, make sure the following information is included on the laboratory request:
  –whether the patient was breathing room air or receiving oxygen therapy when the sample was drawn (if he was receiving oxygen therapy, give the flow rate)
  –if the patient is on a ventilator, the fraction of inspired oxygen and tidal volume

–the patient's rectal temperature and respiratory rate.

Reference values

Normal ABG values fall within the following ranges:

- Pao_2: 75 to 100 mm Hg
- $Paco_2$: 35 to 45 mm Hg
- pH: 7.35 to 7.45
- O_2CT: 15% to 23%
- Sao_2: 94% to 100%
- HCO_3-: 22 to 26 mEq/L.

Implications of results

Low Pao_2, O_2CT, and Sao_2 levels, in combination with a high $Paco_2$, may be due to conditions that impair respiratory function, such as respiratory muscle weakness or paralysis (as in Guillain-Barré syndrome or myasthenia gravis), respiratory center inhibition (from head injury, brain tumor, or drug abuse, for example), and airway obstruction (possibly from mucus plugs or a tumor). Low readings also may result from bronchiole obstruction due to asthma or emphysema, from an abnormal ventilation-perfusion ratio due to partially blocked alveoli or pulmonary capillaries, or from alveoli that are damaged or filled with fluid because of disease, hemorrhage, or near-drowning.

When inspired air contains insufficient oxygen, Pao_2, O_2CT, and Sao_2 also decrease but $Paco_2$ may be normal. Such findings are common in pneumothorax, impaired diffusion between alveoli and blood (due to interstitial fibrosis, for example), or in an arteriovenous shunt that permits blood to bypass the lungs.

Low O_2CT — with normal Pao_2, Sao_2, and possibly $Paco_2$ — may result from severe anemia, decreased blood volume, and reduced oxygen-carrying capacity of hemoglobin.

In addition to clarifying blood oxygen disorders, ABG values can provide considerable information about acid-base disorders. (See *Acid-base disorders.*)

Acid-base disorders

This chart lists the arterial blood gase (ABG) values, possible causes, and clinical effects associated with acid-base disorders.

DISORDERS AND A.B.G. FINDINGS	POSSIBLE CAUSES	SIGNS AND SYMPTOMS
Respiratory acidosis (excess CO_2 retention) pH < 7.35 HCO_3- > 26 mEq/L (if compensating) $Paco_2$ > 45 mm Hg	▪ Central nervous system depression from drugs, injury, or disease ▪ Asphyxia ▪ Hypoventilation due to pulmonary, cardiac, musculoskeletal, or neuromuscular disease	▪ Diaphoresis, headache, tachycardia, confusion, restlessness, apprehension
Respiratory alkalosis (excess CO_2 excretion) pH > 7.42 HCO_3- < 22 mEq/L (if compensating) $Paco_2$ < 35 mm Hg	▪ Hyperventilation due to anxiety, pain, or improper ventilator settings ▪ Respiratory stimulation due to drugs, disease, hypoxia, fever, or high room temperature ▪ Gram-negative bacteremia	▪ Rapid, deep respirations; paresthesias; light-headedness; twitching; anxiety; fear
Metabolic acidosis (HCO_3- loss, acid retention) pH < 7.35 HCO_3- < 22 mEq/L $Paco_2$ < 35 mm Hg (if compensating)	▪ HCO_3- depletion due to renal disease, diarrhea, or small-bowel fistulas ▪ Excessive production of organic acids due to hepatic disease, endocrine disorders (including diabetes mellitus), hypoxia, shock, or drug intoxication ▪ Inadequate excretion of acids due to renal disease	▪ Rapid, deep breathing; fruity breath; fatigue; headache; lethargy; drowsiness; nausea; vomiting; coma (if severe)
Metabolic alkalosis (HCO_3- retention, acid loss) pH > 7.42 HCO_3- > 26 mEq/L $Paco_2$ > 45 mm Hg (if compensating)	▪ Loss of hydrochloric acid from prolonged vomiting or gastric suctioning ▪ Loss of potassium due to increased renal excretion (as in diuretic therapy) or steroid overdose ▪ Excessive alkali ingestion	▪ Slow, shallow breathing; hypertonic muscles; restlessness; twitching; confusion; irritability; apathy; tetany; seizures; coma (if severe)

Post-test care

▪ After applying pressure for 3 to 5 minutes to the puncture site, tape a gauze pad firmly over it. (If the puncture site is on the arm, don't tape the entire circumference; this may restrict circulation.) If the patient is receiving anticoagulants or has a coagulopathy, hold the puncture site longer than 5 minutes if necessary.

 ■ Monitor vital signs, and observe for signs of circulatory impairment, such as swelling, discoloration, pain, numbness, or tingling in the bandaged arm or leg. Watch for bleeding from the puncture site.

Interfering factors
■ Exposing the sample to air affects Pao_2 and $Paco_2$ and interferes with accurate determination of results.
■ Failure to comply with correct specimen handling procedures (heparinize the syringe, place the sample in an iced bag, and transport the sample to the laboratory immediately) will adversely affect the test results.
■ Venous blood in the sample may lower Pao_2 and elevate $Paco_2$.
■ Bicarbonate, ethacrynic acid, hydrocortisone, metolazone, prednisone, and thiazides may elevate $Paco_2$. Acetazolamide, methicillin, nitrofurantoin, and tetracycline may decrease $Paco_2$.

Total carbon dioxide content

Carbon dioxide (CO_2) is present in small amounts in the air, and in the body as an end product of food metabolism. When the pressure of CO_2 in the red cells exceeds 40 mm Hg, CO_2 spills out of the cells and dissolves in plasma. There it may combine with water (H_2O) to form carbonic acid (H_2CO_3), which in turn can dissociate into hydrogen (H^+) and bicarbonate ions (HCO_3^-).

This test measures the total concentration of all such forms of CO_2 in se-rum, plasma, or whole blood samples. Since about 90% of CO_2 in serum is in the form of bicarbonate, this test closely assesses bicarbonate levels. Total CO_2 content reflects the adequacy of gas exchange in the lungs and the efficiency of the carbonic acid–bicarbonate buffer system, which maintains acid-base balance and normal pH. Consequently, this test is commonly ordered for patients with respiratory insufficiency and is usually included in any assessment of electrolyte balance. For maximum clinical significance, test results must be considered with both pH and arterial blood gas values.

Purpose
■ To help evaluate acid-base balance.

Patient preparation
Explain to the patient that this test measures the amount of CO_2 in the blood. Inform him that he needn't restrict food or fluids. Tell him this test requires a blood sample, who will perform the venipuncture and when, and that he may feel some transient discomfort from the needle puncture and the pressure of the tourniquet. Check the patient history for use of medications that may influence CO_2 blood levels.

Procedure
Perform a venipuncture. Because CO_2 content is usually measured along with electrolytes, a 7-ml *red-marble-top* tube may be used. When this test is performed alone, a *green-top* (heparinized) tube is appropriate.

Precautions
Fill the tube completely to prevent diffusion of CO_2 into the vacuum.

Reference values
Normally, total CO_2 levels range from 22 to 34 mEq/L.

Implications of results

High CO_2 levels may occur in metabolic alkalosis (due to excessive ingestion or retention of base bicarbonate), respiratory acidosis (from hypoventilation, for example, as in emphysema or pneumonia), primary aldosteronism, and Cushing's syndrome. CO_2 levels may also be elevated after excessive loss of acids, as in severe vomiting and continuous gastric drainage.

Decreased CO_2 levels are common in metabolic acidosis (as in diabetic acidosis or renal tubular acidosis due to renal failure). Decreased total CO_2 levels in metabolic acidosis also result from loss of bicarbonate (as in severe diarrhea or intestinal drainage). Levels also may fall below normal in respiratory alkalosis (for example, from hyperventilation after trauma).

Post-test care

If a hematoma develops at the venipuncture site, apply warm soaks.

Interfering factors

■ CO_2 levels rise with excessive use of adrenocorticotropic hormone, cortisone, or thiazide diuretics or with excessive ingestion of alkalis or licorice.
■ CO_2 levels decrease with use of salicylates, paraldehyde, methicillin, dimercaprol, ammonium chloride, or acetazolamide and after accidental ingestion of ethylene glycol or methyl alcohol.

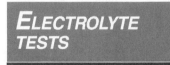

Serum calcium

This test measures serum levels of calcium, a predominantly extracellular cation that helps regulate and promote neuromuscular and enzyme activity, skeletal development, and blood coagulation. The body absorbs calcium from the GI tract, provided sufficient vitamin D is present, and excretes it in the urine and feces. Over 98% of the body's calcium is found in the bones and teeth. However, calcium can shift in and out of these structures. For example, when calcium concentrations in the blood fall below normal, calcium ions can move out of the bones and teeth to help restore blood levels.

Parathyroid hormone, vitamin D, and to a lesser extent, calcitonin and adrenal steroids control calcium blood levels. Calcium and phosphorus are closely related, usually reacting together to form insoluble calcium phosphate. To prevent formation of a precipitate in the blood, calcium levels vary inversely with phosphorus; as serum calcium levels rise, phosphorus levels should decrease through renal excretion. Because the body excretes calcium daily, regular ingestion of calcium in food (at least 1 g/day) is necessary for normal calcium balance.

Purpose

■ To aid diagnosis of neuromuscular, skeletal, and endocrine disorders; arrhythmias; blood-clotting deficiencies; and acid-base imbalance.

Patient preparation

Explain to the patient that this test determines blood calcium level. Inform him that he needn't restrict food or fluids. Tell him that the test requires a blood sample, who will perform the venipuncture and when, and that he may feel some discomfort from the puncture.

Procedure

Perform a venipuncture without using a tourniquet if possible, and collect the sample in a 7-ml *red-top* or *red-marble-top* tube.

Precautions

None.

Reference values

Normally, serum calcium levels should range from 8.9 to 10.1 mg/dl in adults (as measured by atomic absorption). Serum calcium levels are higher in children than in adults; they can rise as high as 10.6 mg/dl during periods of rapid bone growth.

Implications of results

Abnormally high serum calcium levels (hypercalcemia) may occur in hyperparathyroidism and parathyroid tumors (due to oversecretion of parathyroid hormone), Paget's disease of the bone, multiple myeloma, metastatic carcinoma, multiple fractures, or prolonged immobilization. Elevated serum calcium levels may also result from inadequate excretion of calcium, as in adrenal insufficiency and renal disease; from excessive calcium ingestion; or from overuse of antacids such as calcium carbonate.

 Observe the patient with hypercalcemia for deep bone pain, flank pain due to renal calculi, and muscle hypotonicity. Hypercalcemic crisis begins with nausea, vomiting, and dehydration and may lead to stupor, coma, and possibly cardiac arrest.

Low calcium levels (hypocalcemia) may result from hypoparathyroidism, total parathyroidectomy, or malabsorption. Decreased serum levels of calcium may follow calcium loss in Cushing's syndrome, renal failure, acute pancreatitis, or peritonitis.

 In a patient with hypocalcemia, be alert for circumoral and peripheral numbness and tingling, muscle twitching, Chvostek's sign (facial muscle spasm), tetany, muscle cramping, Trousseau's sign (carpopedal spasm), seizure activity, and arrhythmias. (See *Checking for Trousseau's and Chvostek's signs.*)

Post-test care

If a hematoma develops at the venipuncture site, ease discomfort by applying warm soaks.

Interfering factors

▪ Prolonged application of a tourniquet causes venous stasis and may falsely increase calcium results.

▪ Excessive ingestion of vitamin D or its derivatives (dihydrotachysterol, calcitriol) or the use of androgens, calciferol-activated calcium salts, progestins-estrogens, or thiazide diuretics can elevate serum calcium levels.

▪ Chronic laxative use, excessive transfusions of citrated blood, and administration of acetazolamide, corticosteroids, or mithramycin can alter test results.

Serum chloride

This test, a quantitative analysis, measures serum levels of chloride, the major extracellular fluid anion. Interacting with sodium, chloride helps maintain the osmotic pressure of blood and therefore helps regulate blood volume and arterial pressure. Chloride levels also affect acid-base balance. Serum concentrations of this electrolyte are regulated by aldosterone secondarily to regulation of sodium. Chloride is absorbed from the intestines and is excreted primarily by the kidneys.

Checking for Trousseau's and Chvostek's signs

Hypocalcemia causes nerve fiber membranes to become partially charged. This increased neuromuscular irritability characterizes tetany, a condition distinguished by carpopedal spasms, muscle twitchings, cramps, and seizures. Testing for Trousseau's and Chvostek's signs aids diagnosis of tetany.

To check for Trousseau's sign, occlude the arterial blood flow of the patient's arm with a blood pressure cuff. After 1 to 5 minutes, a carpopedal spasm — an adducted thumb and extended phalangeal joints — indicates tetany.

Trousseau's sign

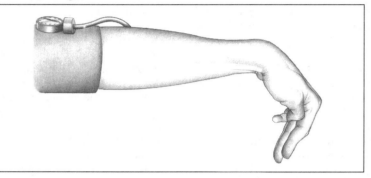

You can induce Chvostek's sign by tapping the patient's facial nerve adjacent to the ear. A brief contraction of the upper lip, nose, or side of the face is a positive sign.

Chvostek's sign

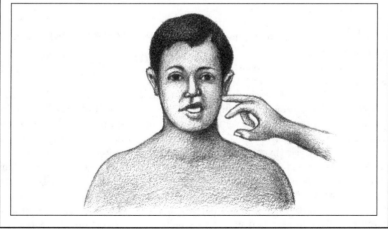

Purpose

■ To detect acid-base imbalance (acidosis and alkalosis) and to aid evaluation of fluid status and extracellular cation-anion balance.

Patient preparation

Explain to the patient that this test evaluates the chloride content of blood. Tell him this test requires a blood sample, who will perform the venipuncture and when, and that he may feel some transient discomfort from the needle puncture and the pressure of the tourniquet.

Check the patient history for use of drugs that influence chloride levels.

Procedure

Perform a venipuncture, and collect the sample in a 7-ml *red-top* or *red-marble-top* tube.

Precautions

Handle the sample gently to prevent hemolysis.

Reference values

Normally, serum chloride levels range from 100 to 108 mEq/L.

Implications of results

Chloride levels relate inversely to those of bicarbonate and thus reflect acid-base balance. Excessive loss of gastric juices or of other secretions containing chloride may cause hypochloremic metabolic alkalosis; excessive chloride retention or ingestion may lead to hyperchloremic metabolic acidosis.

Elevated serum chloride levels (hyperchloremia) may result from HCO_3^- loss due to diarrhea, severe dehydration, complete renal shutdown, head injury (producing neurogenic hyperventilation), or primary aldosteronism.

Low chloride levels (hypochloremia) are usually associated with low sodium and potassium levels. Possible underlying causes include prolonged vomiting, gastric suctioning, intestinal fistula, chronic renal failure, and Addison's disease. Congestive heart failure or edema resulting in excess extracellular fluid can cause dilutional hypochloremia.

Observe a patient with hypochloremia for hypertonicity of muscles, tetany, and depressed respirations. In a patient with hyperchloremia, be alert for signs of developing stupor, rapid deep breathing, and weakness that may lead to coma.

Post-test care

If a hematoma develops at the venipuncture site, ease discomfort by applying warm soaks.

Interfering factors

■ Elevated serum chloride levels may result from administration of ammonium chloride, cholestyramine, boric acid, oxyphenbutazone, or phenylbutazone or from excessive I.V. infusion of sodium chloride.

■ Serum chloride levels are decreased by thiazide diuretics, ethacrynic acid, furosemide, bicarbonates, or prolonged I.V. infusion of dextrose 5% in water.

■ Hemolysis due to rough handling of the sample may interfere with accurate determination of test results.

Serum magnesium

This test, a quantitative analysis, measures serum levels of magnesium, the most abundant intracellular cation after potassium. Vital to neuromuscular function, this often overlooked electrolyte helps regulate intracellular metabolism, activates many essential enzymes, and affects the metabolism of nucleic acids and proteins. Magnesium also helps transport sodium and potassium across cell membranes and, through its effect on the secretion of parathyroid hormone, influences intracellular calcium levels. Most magnesium is found in bone and in intracellular fluid; a small amount is found in extracellular fluid. Magnesium is absorbed by the small intestine and is excreted in the urine and feces.

Purpose
- To evaluate electrolyte status
- To assess neuromuscular or renal function.

Patient preparation
Explain to the patient that this test determines the magnesium content of the blood. Instruct him not to use magnesium salts (such as milk of magnesia or Epsom salts) for at least 3 days before the test, but tell him that he needn't restrict food or fluids. Tell him that the test requires a blood sample, who will perform the venipuncture and when, and that he may feel transient discomfort from the needle puncture.

Procedure
Perform a venipuncture, without a tourniquet if possible, and collect the sample in a 7-ml *red-top* or *red-marble-top* tube.

Precautions
Handle the sample gently to prevent hemolysis. This is crucial since 75% of the blood's magnesium is present in red blood cells.

Reference values
Normally, serum magnesium levels range from 1.7 to 2.1 mg/dl (atomic absorption) or from 1.5 to 2.5 mEq/L.

Implications of results
Elevated serum magnesium levels (hypermagnesemia) that are not due to magnesium administration or ingestion most commonly occur in renal failure, when the kidneys excrete inadequate

amounts of magnesium. Adrenal insufficiency (Addison's disease) can also elevate serum magnesium levels.

 In suspected or confirmed hypermagnesemia, observe the patient for lethargy; flushing; diaphoresis; decreased blood pressure; slow, weak pulse; diminished deep tendon reflexes; muscle weakness; and slow, shallow respirations.

Decreased serum magnesium levels (hypomagnesemia) most commonly result from chronic alcoholism. Other causes include malabsorption syndrome, diarrhea, faulty absorption following bowel resection, prolonged bowel or gastric aspiration, acute pancreatitis, primary aldosteronism, severe burns, hypercalcemic conditions (including hyperparathyroidism), and use of certain diuretics.

 In hypomagnesemia, watch for leg and foot cramps, hyperactive deep tendon reflexes, cardiac arrhythmias, muscle weakness, seizures, twitching, tetany, and tremors.

Post-test care
If a hematoma develops at the venipuncture site, ease discomfort by applying warm soaks.

Interfering factors
- Using a tourniquet causes venous stasis and may alter magnesium results.
- Obtaining a specimen above an I.V. site that's receiving a solution containing magnesium may alter results.
- Excessive use of antacids or cathartics, or excessive infusion of magnesium sulfate raises magnesium levels.
- Prolonged I.V. infusions without magnesium suppress levels. Excessive use of diuretics decreases magnesium levels.
- I.V. administration of calcium gluconate may falsely decrease serum magne-

sium levels if measured by the Titan yellow method.
- Hemolysis causes falsely elevated serum magnesium levels.

Serum phosphates

This test measures serum levels of phosphates, the dominant cellular anions. Phosphates help store and utilize body energy and help regulate calcium levels, carbohydrate and lipid metabolism, and acid-base balance. Phosphates are essential to bone formation; about 85% of the body's phosphates are found in bone.

The intestine absorbs a considerable amount of phosphates from dietary sources, but adequate levels of vitamin D are necessary for their absorption. The kidneys excrete phosphates and serve as a regulatory mechanism. Because calcium and phosphates interact in a reciprocal relationship, urinary excretion of phosphates increases or decreases in inverse proportion to serum calcium levels.

Abnormal phosphate levels result more often from improper excretion than from abnormal ingestion or absorption from dietary sources.

Purpose
- To aid diagnosis of renal disorders and acid-base imbalance
- To detect endocrine, skeletal, and calcium disorders.

Patient preparation
Explain to the patient that this test measures the blood levels of phosphate. Inform him that he needn't restrict food or fluids. Tell him that this test requires a blood sample, who will perform the venipuncture and when, and that he may feel discomfort from the needle puncture. Check the patient history for use of drugs that alter phosphate levels.

Procedure
Perform a venipuncture, without using a tourniquet if possible, and collect the sample in a 7-ml *red-top* or *red-marble-top* tube.

Precautions
Handle the sample gently to prevent hemolysis.

Reference values
Normally, serum phosphate levels in adults range from 2.5 to 4.5 mg/dl (atomic absorption) or from 1.8 to 2.6 mEq/L. Children have higher serum phosphate levels than adults; their levels can rise as high as 7 mg/dl or 4.1 mEq/L during periods of increased bone growth.

Implications of results
Because serum phosphate values alone are of limited use diagnostically (only a few rare conditions directly affect phosphate metabolism), they should be interpreted in light of serum calcium results.

Depressed phosphate levels (hypophosphatemia) may result from malnutrition, malabsorption syndromes, hyperparathyroidism, renal tubular acidosis, or treatment of diabetic acidosis. In children, hypophosphatemia can suppress normal growth.

Elevated levels (hyperphosphatemia) may result from skeletal disease, healing fractures, hypoparathyroidism, acromegaly, diabetic acidosis, high intestinal obstruction, and renal failure. Hyperphosphatemia is rarely clinically significant; however, if prolonged, it can alter bone metabolism by causing abnormal calcium phosphate deposits.

Post-test care
If a hematoma develops at the venipuncture site, apply warm soaks.

Interfering factors

- Using a tourniquet causes venous stasis and may alter phosphate results.
- Obtaining a specimen above an I.V. site receiving a solution containing phosphate may alter results.
- Excessive vitamin D intake and therapy with anabolic steroids or androgens may elevate serum phosphate levels.
- Hemolysis of the sample falsely increases serum phosphate levels.
- Suppressed phosphate levels may result from excessive excretion due to prolonged vomiting and diarrhea, vitamin D deficiency, extended I.V. infusion of dextrose 5% in water, use of phosphate-binding antacids, and use of acetazolamide, insulin, and epinephrine.

Serum potassium

This test, a quantitative analysis, measures serum levels of potassium, the major intracellular cation. Small amounts of potassium may also be found in extracellular fluid. Vital to homeostasis, potassium maintains cellular osmotic equilibrium and helps regulate muscle activity. (It's essential for maintaining electrical conduction within the cardiac and skeletal muscles.) Potassium also helps regulate enzyme activity and acid-base balance, and influences kidney function.

Potassium levels are affected by variations in the secretion of adrenal steroid hormones and by fluctuations in pH, serum glucose levels, and serum sodium levels. A reciprocal relationship appears to exist between potassium and sodium; a substantial intake of one element causes a corresponding decrease in the other. Although it readily conserves sodium, the body has no efficient method for conserving potassium. Even in potassium depletion, the kidneys continue to excrete potassium; therefore, potassium deficiency can develop rapidly and is quite common.

Since the kidneys excrete nearly all ingested potassium daily, a dietary intake of at least 40 mEq/day is essential. A normal diet usually includes 60 to 100 mEq of potassium. (See *Dietary sources of potassium*, page 86, and *Treating potassium imbalance*, page 87.)

Purpose

- To evaluate clinical signs of potassium excess (hyperkalemia) or potassium depletion (hypokalemia)
- To monitor renal function, acid-base balance, and glucose metabolism
- To evaluate neuromuscular and endocrine disorders
- To detect the origin of arrhythmias.

Patient preparation

Explain to the patient that this test determines the potassium content of blood. Inform him he needn't restrict food or fluids. Tell him the test requires a blood sample, who will perform the venipuncture and when, and that he may feel some transient discomfort from the needle puncture and the pressure of the tourniquet.

Check the patient history for use of drugs that may influence test results. If these medications must be continued, note this on the laboratory request.

Procedure

Perform a venipuncture, and collect the sample in a 7-ml *red-top* or *red-marble-top* tube.

Precautions

- Draw the sample immediately after applying the tourniquet because a delay may elevate the potassium level by allowing intracellular potassium to leak into the serum.

Dietary sources of potassium

A healthy person needs to consume at least 40 mEq of potassium daily.

FOODS AND BEVERAGES	SERVING SIZE	AMOUNT OF POTASSIUM (mEq)
Meats		
Beef	4 oz (112 g)	11.2
Chicken	4 oz	12.0
Scallops	5 large	30.0
Veal	4 oz	15.2
Vegetables		
Artichokes	1 large bud	7.7
Asparagus, fresh, frozen, cooked	½ cup	5.5
raw	6 spears	7.7
Beans, dried, cooked	½ cup	10.0
lima	½ cup	9.5
Broccoli, cooked	½ cup	7.0
Carrots, cooked	½ cup	5.7
raw	1 large	8.8
Mushrooms, raw	4 large	10.6
Potato, baked	1 small	15.4
Spinach, fresh, cooked	½ cup	8.5
Squash, winter, baked	½ cup	12.0
Tomato, raw	1 medium	10.4
Fruits		
Apricots, dried	4 halves	5.0
fresh	3 small	8.0
Banana	1 medium	12.8
Cantaloupe	small	13.0
Figs, dried	7 small	17.5
Peach, fresh	1 medium	6.2
Pear, fresh	1 medium	6.2
Beverages		
Apricot nectar	1 cup (240 ml)	9.0
Grapefruit juice	1 cup	8.2
Orange juice	1 cup	11.4
Pineapple juice	1 cup	9.0
Prune juice	1 cup	14.4
Tomato juice	1 cup	11.6
Milk, whole, skim	1 cup	8.8

Treating potassium imbalance

Both hypokalemia and hyperkalemia can cause serious problems if not treated promptly.

Hypokalemia

Most patients with potassium deficiency can be treated with oral potassium chloride replacement and increased dietary intake. In severe cases, potassium can be replaced by I.V. infusion at a rate not exceeding 20 mEq/hour and at a concentration of no more than 80 mEq/L of I.V. fluid. Mix the potassium well in the I.V. solution because it can settle near the neck of the bottle or plastic bag. Failure to mix the solution adequately or to infuse it properly can cause a burning sensation at the I.V. site and possibly even fatal hyperkalemia.

Monitor the electrocardiogram, urine output, and serum potassium levels frequently during the infusion. Never administer I.V. potassium replacement to a patient with inadequate urine flow because diminished excretion can rapidly lead to hyperkalemia.

Hyperkalemia

Dangerously high potassium levels may be reduced with sodium polystyrene sulfonate — a potassium-removing resin — administered orally, rectally, or through a nasogastric tube. Hyperkalemia may also be treated with an I.V. infusion of sodium bicarbonate or of glucose and insulin, which lowers blood potassium by causing potassium to move into cells.

A calcium I.V. infusion provides fast but transient relief from the cardiotoxic effects of hyperkalemia; however, it does not directly lower serum potassium levels. In renal failure, dialysis may help remove excess potassium, but this corrects the imbalance much more slowly.

■ Handle the sample gently to avoid hemolysis.

Reference values

Normally, serum potassium levels range from 3.8 to 5.5 mEq/L.

Implications of results

Hyperkalemia is common in patients with burns, crushing injuries, diabetic ketoacidosis, or myocardial infarction — conditions in which excessive cellular potassium enters the blood. Hyperkalemia may also indicate reduced sodium excretion, possibly due to renal failure (preventing normal sodium-potassium exchange) or Addison's disease (because of the absence of aldosterone, which results in potassium buildup and sodium depletion).

 Observe a patient with hyperkalemia for weakness, malaise, nausea, diarrhea, colicky pain, muscle irritability progressing to flaccid paralysis, oliguria, and bradycardia.

In hyperkalemia, an electrocardiogram (ECG) reveals a prolonged PR interval, wide QRS complex, ST-segment depression, and tall, tented T waves.

Hypokalemia often results from aldosteronism or Cushing's syndrome (marked by hypersecretion of adrenal steroid hormones), loss of body fluids (as in long-term diuretic therapy), or excessive licorice ingestion (due to the aldosterone-like effect of glycyrrhizic acid). Although serum values and clinical symptoms can indicate a potassium imbalance, an ECG provides the definitive diagnosis.

Observe a patient with hypokalemia for decreased reflexes; rapid, weak, irregular pulse; mental confusion; hypotension; anorexia; muscle weakness; and paresthesia.

In hypokalemia, an ECG shows a flattened T wave, ST-segment depression, and U wave elevation. In severe cases, ventricular fibrillation, respiratory paralysis, and cardiac arrest can develop.

Post-test care
If a hematoma develops at the venipuncture site, apply warm soaks.

Interfering factors
■ Excessive or rapid potassium infusion, spironolactone or penicillin G potassium therapy, or renal toxicity from administration of amphotericin B, methicillin, or tetracycline elevates serum potassium levels.
■ Insulin and glucose administration, diuretic therapy (especially with thiazides, but not with triamterene, amiloride, or spironolactone), or I.V. infusions without potassium suppress serum potassium levels.
■ Excessive hemolysis of the sample or delay in drawing blood following the application of a tourniquet elevates potassium levels.
■ Repeated clenching of the fist prior to venipuncture may cause elevated potassium levels.

Serum sodium

This test measures serum levels of sodium, the major extracellular cation. Sodium affects body water distribution, maintains osmotic pressure of extracellular fluid, and helps promote neuromuscular function; it also helps maintain acid-base balance and influences chloride and potassium levels. Sodium is absorbed by the kidneys; a small amount is lost through the skin.

Since extracellular sodium concentration helps the kidneys to regulate body water (decreased sodium levels promote water excretion and increased levels promote retention), serum levels of sodium are evaluated in relation to the amount of water in the body. For example, a sodium deficit (hyponatremia) refers to a decreased level of sodium in relation to the body's water level. (See *Fluid imbalances.*) The body normally regulates this sodium-water balance through aldosterone, which inhibits sodium excretion and promotes its resorption (with water) by the renal tubules, to maintain balance. Low sodium levels stimulate aldosterone secretion; elevated sodium levels depress aldosterone secretion.

Purpose
■ To evaluate fluid-electrolyte and acid-base balance and related neuromuscular, renal, and adrenal functions.

Patient preparation
Explain to the patient that this test determines the sodium content of blood. Inform him that he needn't restrict food or fluids. Tell him this test requires a blood sample, who will perform the venipuncture and when, and that he may feel some discomfort from the needle puncture and the pressure of the tourniquet.

Check the patient's medication history for use of drugs that influence sodium levels. If these medications must be continued, note this on the laboratory request.

Procedure
Perform a venipuncture, and collect the sample in a 7-ml *red-top* or *red-marble-top* tube.

Fluid imbalances

This chart lists the causes, signs and symptoms, and diagnostic test findings associated with hypervolemia (increased fluid volume) and hypovolemia (decreased fluid volume).

CAUSES	SIGNS AND SYMPTOMS	LABORATORY FINDINGS
Hypervolemia		
■ Increased water intake ■ Decreased water output due to renal disease ■ Congestive heart failure ■ Excessive ingestion or infusion of sodium chloride ■ Long-term administration of adrenocortical hormones ■ Excessive infusion of isotonic solutions	■ Increased blood pressure, pulse rate, body weight, and respiratory rate ■ Bounding peripheral pulses ■ Moist pulmonary crackles ■ Moist mucous membranes ■ Moist respiratory secretions ■ Edema ■ Weakness ■ Seizures and coma due to swelling of brain cells	■ Decreased red blood cell (RBC) count, hemoglobin concentration, packed cell volume, serum sodium concentration (dilutional decrease), and urine specific gravity
Hypovolemia		
■ Decreased water intake ■ Fluid loss due to fever, diarrhea, vomiting ■ Systemic infection ■ Impaired renal concentrating ability ■ Fistulous drainage ■ Severe burns ■ Hidden fluid in body cavities	■ Increased pulse and respiratory rates ■ Decreased blood pressure and body weight ■ Weak and thready peripheral pulses ■ Thick, slurred speech ■ Thirst ■ Oliguria ■ Anuria ■ Dry skin	■ Increased RBC count, hemoglobin concentration, packed cell volume, serum sodium concentration, and urine specific gravity

Precautions
Handle the sample gently to prevent hemolysis.

Reference values
Normally, serum sodium levels range from 135 to 145 mEq/L.

Implications of results
Sodium imbalance can result from a loss or gain of sodium or from a change in water volume. Remember, serum sodium results must be interpreted in light of the patient's state of hydration.

Elevated serum sodium levels (hypernatremia) may be due to inadequate water intake, water loss that exceeds sodium loss (as in diabetes insipidus, impaired renal function, prolonged hyperventilation, and occasionally, severe vomiting or diarrhea), and sodium retention (as in aldosteronism). Hypernatremia can also result from excessive sodium intake.

 In a patient with hypernatremia and associated loss of water, observe for signs of thirst, restlessness, dry and sticky mucous membranes, flushed skin, oliguria, and diminished reflexes.

However, if increased total body sodium causes water retention, observe for hypertension, dyspnea, and edema.

Abnormally low serum sodium levels (hyponatremia) may result from inadequate sodium intake or excessive sodium loss due to profuse sweating, GI suctioning, diuretic therapy, diarrhea, vomiting, adrenal insufficiency, burns, or chronic renal insufficiency with acidosis. Urine sodium determinations are frequently more sensitive to early changes in sodium balance and should always be evaluated simultaneously with serum sodium findings.

 In a patient with hyponatremia, watch for apprehension, lassitude, headache, decreased skin turgor, abdominal cramps, and tremors that may progress to seizures.

Post-test care
If a hematoma develops at the venipuncture site, apply warm soaks.

Interfering factors
▪ Most diuretics suppress serum sodium levels by promoting sodium excretion; lithium, chlorpropamide, and vasopressin suppress sodium levels by inhibiting water excretion.

▪ Corticosteroids elevate serum sodium levels by promoting sodium retention. Antihypertensives, such as methyldopa, hydralazine, and reserpine, may cause sodium and water retention.

▪ Hemolysis due to rough handling of the sample may interfere with accurate determination of test results.

Anion gap

The anion gap reflects anion-cation balance in the serum and helps distinguish types of metabolic acidosis without expensive, time-consuming measurement of all serum electrolytes. This test uses serum levels of routinely measured electrolytes — sodium (Na^+), chloride (Cl^-), and bicarbonate (HCO_3^-) — for a quick calculation based on a simple physical principle: Total concentrations of cations and anions are normally equal, thereby maintaining electrical neutrality in serum.

Because sodium accounts for more than 90% of circulating cations, whereas chloride and bicarbonate together account for 85% of the counterbalancing anions, the "gap" between measured cation and anion levels represents those anions not routinely measured (sulfate, phosphates, organic acids such as ketone bodies and lactic acid, and proteins).

An increased anion gap indicates an increase in one or more of these unmeasured anions, which may occur with acidosis characterized by excessive organic or inorganic acids, such as lactic acidosis or ketoacidosis.

A normal anion gap occurs in hyperchloremic acidoses, renal tubular acidosis, and severe bicarbonate-wasting conditions, such as biliary or pancreatic fistulas and poorly functioning ileal loops.

Purpose
▪ To distinguish types of metabolic acidosis
▪ To monitor renal function and total parenteral nutrition.

Patient preparation
Explain to the patient that this test helps determine the cause of metabolic acidosis. Inform him that he needn't re-

Anion gap and metabolic acidosis

Metabolic acidosis with a *normal anion gap* (8 to 14 mEq/L) occurs in conditions characterized by loss of bicarbonate, such as:
- hypokalemic acidosis due to renal tubular acidosis, diarrhea, or ureteral diversions
- hyperkalemic acidosis due to acidifying agents (for example, ammonium chloride, hydrochloric acid), hydronephrosis, or sickle cell nephropathy.

Metabolic acidosis with an *increased anion gap* (>14 mEq/L) occurs in conditions characterized by accumulation of organic acids, sulfates, or phosphates, such as:
- renal failure
- ketoacidosis due to starvation, diabetes mellitus, or alcohol abuse
- lactic acidosis
- ingestion of toxins, such as salicylates, methanol, ethylene glycol (antifreeze), and paraldehyde.

strict food or fluids before the test. Tell the patient that the test requires a blood sample, who will perform the venipuncture and when, and that he may feel some transient discomfort from the needle puncture and the pressure of the tourniquet.

Check the patient history for use of drugs that may influence sodium, chloride, or bicarbonate blood levels (such as diuretics, corticosteroids, and antihypertensives). If these drugs must be continued, note this on the laboratory request.

Procedure
Perform a venipuncture, and collect the sample in a 7-ml *red-top* or *red-marble-top* tube.

Precautions
Handle the sample gently to prevent hemolysis, which can interfere with accurate determination of test results.

Reference values
Normally, the anion gap ranges from 8 to 14 mEq/L.

Implications of results
A normal anion gap doesn't rule out metabolic acidosis. When acidosis re-

sults from loss of bicarbonate in the urine or other body fluids, renal reabsorption of sodium promotes retention of chloride, and the anion gap remains unchanged. Thus, metabolic acidosis due to excessive chloride levels is known as *normal anion gap acidosis*.

When acidosis results from accumulation of metabolic acids — as occurs in lactic acidosis, for example — the anion gap increases (above 14 mEq/L) with the increase in unmeasured anions. Metabolic acidosis caused by such accumulation is known as a *high anion gap acidosis*. (See *Anion gap and metabolic acidosis*.)

Because the anion gap only determines total anion-cation balance, it doesn't necessarily reflect abnormal values for individual electrolytes. Further investigation and diagnostic tests are usually necessary to determine the specific cause of metabolic acidosis.

A decreased anion gap (less than 8 mEq/L) is rare but may occur in hypermagnesemia and in paraproteinemic states, such as multiple myeloma and Waldenström's macroglobulinemia.

Post-test care
- If a hematoma develops at the veni-

puncture site, ease discomfort by applying warm soaks.

▪ As ordered, instruct the patient to resume use of any drugs discontinued before the test.

Interfering factors

▪ Diuretics, lithium, chlorpropamide, and vasopressin suppress serum sodium levels, possibly decreasing the anion gap; corticosteroids and antihypertensives elevate serum sodium levels, possibly increasing the anion gap.

▪ Salicylates, paraldehyde, methicillin, dimercaprol, ammonium chloride, acetazolamide, ethylene glycol, and methyl alcohol decrease serum bicarbonate levels, which may increase the anion gap; adrenocorticotropic hormone, cortisone, mercurial or chlorthiazide diuretics, and excessive ingestion of alkalis or licorice elevate serum bicarbonate levels, which may decrease the anion gap.

▪ Ammonium chloride, cholestyramine, boric acid, oxyphenbutazone, phenylbutazone, and excessive I.V. infusion of sodium chloride may elevate serum chloride levels, possibly decreasing the anion gap.

▪ Thiazide diuretics, ethacrynic acid, furosemide, bicarbonates, and prolonged I.V. infusion of dextrose 5% in water can lower serum chloride levels, possibly increasing the anion gap.

▪ Iodine absorption from wounds packed with povidone-iodine or excessive use of magnesium-containing antacids (especially by patients with renal failure) may cause a falsely low anion gap.

▪ Hemolysis due to rough handling of the sample may interfere with accurate determination of test results.

SELECTED READINGS

Black, J.M., and Matassarin-Jacobs, E., eds. *Luckmann and Sorensen's Medical-Surgical Nursing: A Psychophysiologic Approach,* 4th ed. Philadelphia: W.B. Saunders Co., 1993.

Diseases, 2nd ed. Springhouse, Pa.: Springhouse Corp., 1996.

Fischbach, F. *A Manual of Laboratory and Diagnostic Tests,* 5th ed. Philadelphia: Lippincott-Raven Pubs., 1996.

Guyton, A.C., and Hall, J.E. *Textbook of Medical Physiology,* 9th ed. Philadelphia: W.B. Saunders Co., 1996.

Henry, J.B., ed. *Clinical Diagnosis and Management by Laboratory Methods,* 19th ed. Philadelphia: W.B. Saunders Co., 1996.

Kee, J.L. *Laboratory and Diagnostic Tests,* 4th ed. Stamford, Conn.: Appleton & Lange, 1995.

Nursing97 Drug Handbook. Springhouse, Pa.: Springhouse Corp., 1997.

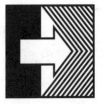

CHAPTER FOUR

Enzymes

INTRODUCTION

Enzymes are reusable proteins that catalyze the thousands of chemical reactions needed to keep a single cell alive and functioning. They accelerate and control reaction rates without being destroyed themselves in the process.

Different kinds of cells produce different enzymes, and most tissues contain many different enzymes. When tissue cells are damaged by disease or some other defect, they release enzymes specific to that area into the bloodstream, where they can be readily detected. For example, leakage from dying cells is the source of elevated serum enzyme levels in myocardial infarction (MI), infectious hepatitis, and other disease states.

Although serum levels of any one enzyme may not identify its tissue of origin, comparing serum levels of several enzymes may provide important diagnostic information because individual enzymes are present in different tissues

in different ratios. Such analysis may reveal the extent of pathology and monitor the progress of healing. (See *How enzymes work.*)

Sensitivity and specificity

Because certain diseases that produce similar symptoms cause distinctively different enzyme abnormalities, enzyme tests can be used to separate them. The diagnostic value of these tests depends on their sensitivity and specificity. Sensitivity indicates how reliably the test gives a positive result when a particular disease is present; specificity indicates how often the test is "normal" when the disease is absent. Thus, enzymes tests with low sensitivity produce negative readings when the disease is present; tests with low specificity show positive readings when the disease is absent.

Some enzymes, such as *creatine kinase* (CK) and *lactate dehydrogenase* (LD), occur in multiple forms — isoenzymes — that differ in molecular details while retaining their basic identities. CK also appears in isoenzyme subunits

How enzymes work

According to current theory, enzymes work as catalysts because of their surface activity. Because each reactant has its own unique three-dimensional surface, an enzyme combines with reactants whose molecular surfaces fit its own (top left). To initiate a reaction, the reactants and an enzyme specific to them combine briefly (bottom left). At the end of the reaction, the enzyme and the reactants separate, leaving the enzyme unchanged (right).

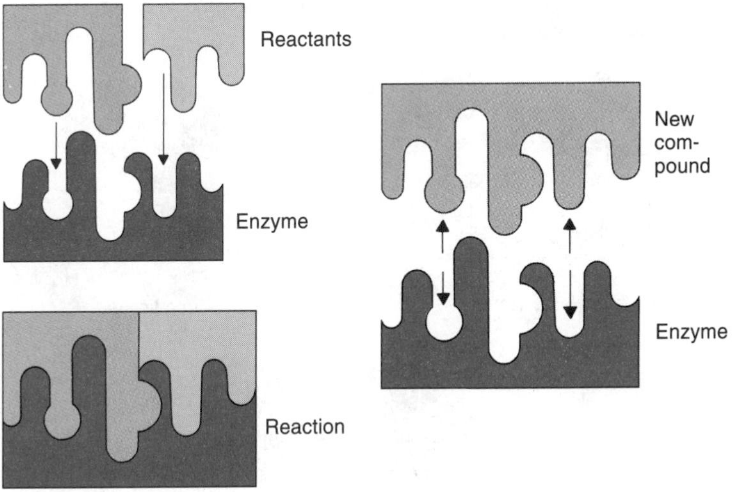

Reactants

New compound

Enzyme

Enzyme

Reaction

called isoforms. Certain organs or tissues contain more or less of one isoenzyme than another; therefore, testing for isoenzymes may provide better sensitivity or specificity than measuring an entire enzyme group.

CK is present in heart muscle, skeletal muscle, and brain tissue. CK isoenzymes are combinations of the subunits M (muscle) and B (brain). For example, CK-BB is found primarily in brain and nerve tissue, CK-MB in heart muscle, and CK-MM in skeletal muscle. Therefore, in a suspected acute MI, elevated CK-MB levels reliably indicate cardiac damage.

LD has five isoenzymes that are formed from different combinations of two subunits: M (muscle) and H (heart).

The patterns of LD_1 and LD_2 levels are monitored — along with other serum enzyme levels — to trace the progress of an MI. LD_3 levels are elevated primarily in patients with pulmonary infarction, whereas LD_4 and LD_5 elevations are characteristic of skeletal muscle and hepatic disorders. (See *Isoenzymes of lactate dehydrogenase,* page 96.)

Enzyme test batteries
Isoenzymes may be separated and assayed by several laboratory methods, including electrophoresis, column chromatography, difference in heat stability, substrate alterations, and the use of chemical inhibitors. These techniques take advantage of physical or chemical properties of the isoenzyme molecule.

Isoenzymes of lactate dehydrogenase

Individual monomers of the five lactate dehydrogenase (LD) isoenzymes carry the letter H, for those subunits that appear most consistently in heart tissue, or the letter M, for those predominant in skeletal muscle tissue. Injury to almost any tissue stimulates the release of isoenzymes with a tetrametric pattern peculiar to the injured tissue and roughly parallel to the degree of damage. For instance, in myocardial infarction, blood levels of LD_1 (HHHH) and LD_2 (HHHM) are elevated. Damage to pulmonary tissue causes the release of LD_3 (HHMM); injury to the liver and skeletal muscle causes the release of LD_4 (HMMM) and LD_5 (MMMM).

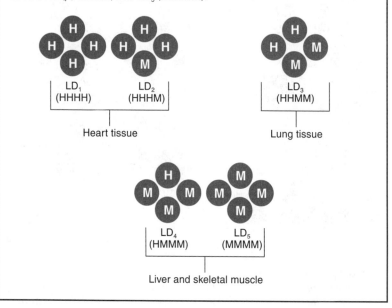

LD_1 (HHHH) LD_2 (HHHM)

Heart tissue

LD_3 (HHMM)

Lung tissue

LD_4 (HMMM) LD_5 (MMMM)

Liver and skeletal muscle

Some enzymes and isoenzymes are routinely tested in groups to aid identification of disorders such as MI and hepatic and pancreatic disease. Nevertheless, because some enzymes are present in many organs and disease states, positive test results are meaningful only in light of the patient's overall clinical status.

Cardiac enzymes and isoenzymes

CK-MB levels rise 4 to 8 hours after onset of infarction, peak at 12 to 24 hours, and may remain elevated for as long as 72 hours. LD_1 and LD_2 levels usually rise within 24 hours after an episode, tapering off 72 to 96 hours later.

Some laboratories also measure hydroxybutyric dehydrogenase (HBD) in suspected acute MI when electrophoresis equipment is not available or when the total LD is not sufficient to confirm diagnosis. Serum HBD levels rise 8 to 10 hours after MI, peak in 48 to 96 hours, and return to normal in 16 to 18 days. (See *Hydroxybutyric dehydrogenase.*)

Aspartate aminotransferase (AST) also rises during acute MI, increasing 6 to 8

Hydroxybutyric dehydrogenase

Hydroxybutyric dehydrogenase (HBD), or alpha-hydroxybutyric dehydrogenase, is actually total lactate dehydrogenase (LD) that's tested using a hydroxybutyric acid substrate instead of lactic or pyruvic acid. With this substrate, the electrophoretically fast-moving LD_1 and LD_2 (cardiac) isoenzymes exhibit more activity than the slow-moving LD_5 (liver) fraction, so that HBD activity roughly parallels LD_1 and LD_2 activity. Measurement of serum HBD is sometimes used as a substitute for LD isoenzyme fractionation because this analysis is easier to perform and less expensive than LD electrophoresis.

Although HBD concentration primarily reflects LD_1 and LD_2 activity, it may also show LD_5 activity if enough of this isoenzyme is present (as it is in some forms of hepatic disease). Therefore, this test isn't consistently reliable in distinguishing between myocardial and hepatic cellular damage and is used infrequently.

hours after the infarction and peaking in 18 to 24 hours. The AST level may increase to 4 to 10 times normal but returns to normal in 4 to 5 days. Because AST is also found in other tissues, such as liver and muscle, an increase is not sufficient to diagnose MI. Thus, correct interpretation of enzyme analyses always requires careful comparison with the patient's clinical status and correlation to other enzyme assays.

Because the diagnostic value of some enzyme tests depends on the comparison of sequential test results, *each* blood sample must be labeled with both the date and hour it was collected. For example, in acute MI, the first set of tests is ordered to obtain a baseline. Subsequent sets of tests are ordered serially (perhaps at 6, 12, and 24 hours after the episode and daily thereafter) to monitor changes in enzyme concentrations, particularly elevations. However, decreases can also be important in evaluating the patient's prognosis. Adding "Rule out MI" to the laboratory request will aid the diagnostician, but it's also essential to record the time that the sample was drawn.

Liver enzymes and isoenzymes
The liver is the site of many biochemical reactions that are controlled by numerous enzymes. Many of these reactions occur at diagnostically significant levels in the serum in a spectrum of hepatobiliary disorders ranging from minute changes within hepatic cells (hepatitis) to extrahepatic disorders, such as biliary obstruction.

Although neither AST nor *alanine aminotransferase* (ALT) is confined to the liver, both can reliably identify hepatic disease. In severe necrosis (as in viral hepatitis), AST levels may rise as high as 100 times the reference range because of massive tissue destruction. ALT levels may rise even higher and remain elevated longer than AST. These enzymes changes become detectable early in the disease and persist longer than changes in other liver function studies.

Gamma glutamyl transferase (GGT) is a sensitive indicator of early hepatocellular damage, obstruction, or alcohol-induced hepatic disease; it's usually measured with other enzymes to confirm hepatic disease. Elevated levels rise in patterns similar to those of serum alkaline phosphatase.

The enzyme *alkaline phosphatase* (ALP) can be separated into several isoenzymes, each of which is found in different tissues. Isoenzyme type 1 is specific to hepatic disorders; serum levels rise dramatically in biliary cirrhosis and in bile duct obstruction that impedes phosphatase excretion.

When ALP levels are elevated, measuring another phosphatase enzyme — *5'-nucleotidase* (5'NT), which is formed mostly in the liver — can determine whether ALP elevations are liver- or bone-related. Usually, both 5'NT and ALP levels are elevated in hepatic disease, whereas only ALP levels rise in skeletal disease.

Two isoenzymes of LD — LD_4 and LD_5 — occur predominantly in the liver. Their serum levels are commonly elevated even before jaundice appears and return to normal while clinical symptoms are still evident.

Pancreatic enzymes

Amylase and *lipase* are produced by the pancreas and secreted into the small intestine, where they break down starches and fats, respectively. Both appear in serum after acute pancreatitis. Serum amylase levels rise rapidly in acute pancreatitis, reaching twice the normal values just 4 hours after onset of symptoms; however, levels also drop quickly, returning to normal 48 to 72 hours later. Serum lipase levels rise similarly but remain elevated for as long as 14 days.

Prostatic and other enzymes

Acid phosphatase is found mainly in the adult prostate gland. Elevated levels of this enzyme usually indicate prostatic cancer that has penetrated the prostatic capsule.

Miscellaneous enzyme tests

Special enzyme tests that aren't part of specific organ test profiles include plasma renin activity, cholinesterase, glucose-6-phosphate dehydrogenase (G6PD), pyruvate kinase (PK), hexosaminidase A and B, uroporphyrinogen I synthase, galactose-1-phosphate uridyltransferase, and angiotensin-converting enzyme (ACE).

Plasma renin testing helps identify primary aldosteronism. Pseudocholinesterase may aid diagnosis of pesticide poisonings and succinyldicholine hypersensitivity. Assays for G6PD, PK, uroporphyrinogen I synthase, and galactose-1-phosphate uridyltransferase can help detect inherited enzyme deficiencies. Hexosaminidase A and B testing is used to diagnose Tay-Sachs disease. The ACE test is used mainly to detect sarcoidosis.

CARDIAC ENZYME TESTS

Creatine kinase

Creatine kinase (CK) is an enzyme that catalyzes the creatine-creatinine metabolic pathway in muscle cells and brain tissue. Because of its important role in energy production, CK levels reflect normal tissue catabolism; above-normal serum levels indicate trauma to cells with high CK content. CK may be separated into three isoenzymes with distinct molecular structures: CK-BB (CK_1), found primarily in brain tissue; CK-MB (CK_2), found primarily in cardiac muscle (a small amount also appears in skeletal muscle); and CK-MM (CK_3), found mainly in skeletal muscle.

Total serum CK levels were once widely used to detect acute myocardial infarction (MI), but elevated levels caused by skeletal muscle damage reduce the test's specificity for this disorder. Fractionation and measurement of CK isoenzymes has replaced total CK assay to accurately localize the site of increased tissue destruction. In addition, subunits of CK-MM and CK-MB, called *isoforms*, can be assayed to increase the sensitivity of the test.

Purpose
■ To detect and diagnose acute MI and reinfarction (CK-MB primarily used)
■ To evaluate possible causes of chest pain and to monitor the severity of myocardial ischemia after cardiac surgery, cardiac catheterization, or cardioversion (CK-MB primarily used)
■ To detect early dermatomyositis and skeletal muscle disorders that are not neurogenic in origin, such as Duchenne's muscular dystrophy (total CK primarily used).

Patient preparation
Explain to the patient that this test helps assess myocardial and skeletal muscle function and that multiple blood samples are required to detect fluctuations in serum levels. Inform him that he need not restrict food or most fluids before the test. If the patient is being evaluated for skeletal muscle disorders, advise him to avoid exercising for 24 hours before the test. Tell him who will perform the venipuncture and when and that he may feel some discomfort from the needle or the tourniquet.

Before the test, withhold alcohol, aminocaproic acid, and lithium, as ordered. If these substances must be continued, note this on the laboratory request.

Procedure
Perform a venipuncture, and collect the sample in a 7-ml *red-top* tube.

Precautions
■ Draw the sample before giving an I.M. injection, or wait at least 1 hour after the injection, because muscle trauma raises total CK levels.
■ Obtain the sample as scheduled. Since timing is important to the diagnosis, recording the date and time the sample was drawn and the number of hours that elapsed since the onset of chest pain is critical.
■ Handle the collection tube gently to prevent hemolysis.
■ Send the sample to the laboratory immediately because CK activity diminishes significantly after 2 hours at room temperature.

Reference values
Total CK values determined by ultraviolet or kinetic measurement normally range from 52 to 336 U/L for men and from 38 to 176 U/L for women. CK levels may be significantly higher in very muscular people. Infants up to age 1 have levels two to four times higher than adults, possibly reflecting birth trauma and striated muscle development.

Normal ranges for isoenzyme levels are as follows: CK-BB, undetectable; CK-MB, undetectable to 7 U/L; CK-MM, 5 to 70 U/L.

Implications of results
CK-MM constitutes over 99% of total CK normally present in serum. Detectable CK-BB levels may indicate brain tissue injury, certain widespread malignant tumors, severe shock, or renal failure. However, such elevations don't confirm a specific diagnosis.

CK-MB levels greater than 5% of total CK (or more than 10 U/L) indicate MI, especially if the LD_1/LD_2 isoenzyme ratio is greater than 1 (flipped LD). In acute MI and after cardiac surgery, CK-MB levels begin to rise in 2 to 4 hours, peak in 12 to 24 hours, and usually return to normal in 24 to 48 hours; per-

Enzyme and isoenzyme changes after MI

Because they're released by damaged tissue, serum enzymes and isoenzymes — catalytic proteins that vary in concentration in specific organs — can help identify the compromised organ and assess the extent of damage. The graph below shows how serum levels of the enzymes and isoenzymes that are most significant in myocardial infarction (MI) fluctuate in the days following an MI.

Enzymes
■ Hydroxybutyric dehydrogenase (HBD): an indirect measurement of Lactate dehydrogenase 1 and 2 (LD_1, LD_2)
■ Aspartate aminotransferase (AST): found primarily in heart muscle and liver; less extensively in skeletal muscles, kidneys, pancreas, and red blood cells (RBCs)

Isoenzymes
■ Creatine kinase-MB (CK-MB): found primarily in heart muscle; a small amount in skeletal muscle
■ LD_1 and LD_2 found in the heart, brain, kidneys, liver, skeletal muscles, and RBCs

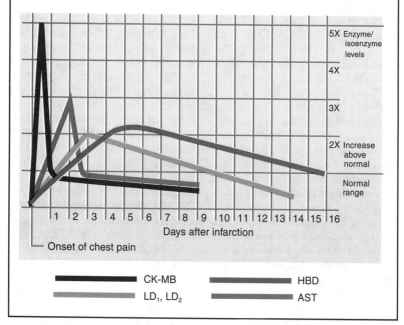

sistent elevations or increasing levels indicate ongoing myocardial damage. (See *Enzyme and isoenzyme changes after MI*.) Total CK follows roughly the same pattern but rises slightly later. CK-MB levels don't rise in congestive heart failure or during angina pectoris not accompanied by myocardial cell necrosis. (Not all researchers agree about this, however.)

Serious skeletal muscle injury that occurs in certain muscular dystrophies, polymyositis, and severe myoglobinuria may produce mildly elevated CK-MB levels because a small amount of this isoenzyme is present in some skeletal muscles.

Rising CK-MM values follow skeletal muscle damage from trauma, such as surgery and I.M. injections, or from diseases, such as dermatomyositis and muscular dystrophy (values may be 50 to 100 times normal). A moderate rise in CK-MM levels develops in patients with hypothyroidism; sharp elevations occur with muscular activity caused by agitation, such as an acute psychotic episode.

Total CK levels may be elevated in patients with severe hypokalemia, carbon monoxide poisoning, malignant hyperthermia, or alcoholic cardiomyopathy; in those who have recently had a seizure; and occasionally in those who have suffered pulmonary or cerebral infarctions.

Post-test care
▪ If a hematoma develops at the venipuncture site, apply warm soaks.
▪ Resume medications discontinued before the test, as ordered.

Interfering factors
▪ Hemolysis may alter test results.
▪ Failure to send the sample to the laboratory immediately or to refrigerate the serum if testing will be delayed for more than 2 hours may decrease the concentration and affect test results.
▪ Failure to draw the samples at the scheduled time may miss peak levels.
▪ Halothane and succinylcholine, alcohol, lithium, and large doses of aminocaproic acid as well as I.M. injections, cardioversion, invasive diagnostic procedures, recent vigorous exercise or muscle massage, and severe coughing and trauma raise total CK values.

▪ Surgery through skeletal muscle will raise total CK levels.

Creatine kinase isoforms

An enzyme found in muscle tissue, creatine kinase has three isoenzymes: CK-MM (CK_3), CK-MB (CK_2), and CK-BB (CK_1). CK-MM and CK-MB are found primarily in skeletal and heart muscle. CK-BB, most prevalent in brain tissue, is not usually seen in serum. Isoforms, or subforms, of CK-MM and CK-MB are called $CK-MM_1$, $CK-MM_2$, $CK-MB_1$, and $CK-MB_2$. Isoforms are determined by high-voltage electrophoresis or isoelectric focusing.

Cardiac muscle damage releases CK-MM, CK-MB, and lactate dehydrogenase isoenzymes into serum. An increase in CK-MB levels indicates myocardial infarction (MI). Serum levels begin to rise 6 to 8 hours after myocardial damage; isoform levels, 4 to 6 hours after. Evaluating these increases speeds diagnosis and treatment of MI.

Purpose
▪ To detect or provide early confirmation of MI
▪ To evaluate reperfusion therapy.

Patient preparation
Explain that the test will help to confirm or rule out MI. Tell the patient that it will require a blood test, with specimens drawn at timed intervals. Tell him who will perform the venipuncture and when and that he may feel discomfort from the tourniquet and the needle.

Procedure
Perform a venipuncture and collect blood in a 7-ml *lavender-top* tube.

Record the time the specimen was drawn. Obtain another specimen every 2 hours, as indicated, and note the time on each. Place each specimen on ice, and deliver it to the laboratory at once.

Precautions
- Obtain each specimen on schedule, and note the collection time and date on each.
- Handle the specimens gently.

Reference values
Normally, CK-MB$_2$ concentrations are less than 1 U/L. The CK-MB$_2$/CK-MB$_1$ ratio is less than 1.5.

Implications of results
Within 2 to 4 hours after MI, more than 50% of patients will have a CK-MB$_2$/CK-MB$_1$ ratio greater than 1.5. By 6 hours after MI, more than 90% of patients will have a ratio of 1.5 or greater. Giving thrombolytic drugs may restore coronary perfusion. The increased blood flow through the damaged area removes accumulated CK isoenzymes and causes the CK-MB$_2$/CK-MB$_1$ ratio to peak sooner.

Post-test care
If a hematoma develops at the venipuncture site, apply warm soaks.

Interfering factors
- Hemolysis may alter test results.
- Failure to draw the samples at the scheduled times may result in missing peak levels.

Lactate dehydrogenase

Lactate dehydrogenase (LD) catalyzes the reversible conversion of muscle lactic acid into pyruvic acid. This essential final step in the Embden-Meyerhof glycolytic pathway provides the metabolic bridge to the Krebs cycle (citric acid or tricarboxylic acid cycle), ultimately producing cellular energy.

Because LD is present in almost all body tissues, cellular damage causes an elevation of total serum LD, thus limiting its diagnostic usefulness. However, five tissue-specific isoenzymes can be identified and measured, using immunochemical separation and quantitation or electrophoresis. Two of these isoenzymes, LD$_1$ and LD$_2$, appear primarily in the heart, red blood cells (RBCs), and kidneys; LD$_3$, primarily in the lungs; and LD$_4$ and LD$_5$, in the liver and the skeletal muscles. Also, the midzone fractions (LD$_2$, LD$_3$, LD$_4$) can be elevated in granulocytic leukemia, lymphomas, and platelet disorders.

The specificity of LD isoenzymes and their distribution pattern is useful in diagnosing hepatic, pulmonary, and erythrocytic damage. But their widest clinical application is in aiding diagnosis of acute myocardial infarction (MI). An LD isoenzyme assay is useful when creatine kinase (CK) hasn't been measured within 24 hours of an acute MI. The myocardial LD level rises later than CK (12 to 48 hours after infarction begins), peaks in 2 to 5 days, and drops to normal in 7 to 10 days if tissue necrosis doesn't persist. (See *LD isoenzyme variations in disease.*)

Purpose
- To aid differential diagnosis of MI, pulmonary infarction, anemias, and hepatic disease
- To support CK isoenzyme test results in diagnosing MI or to provide diagnosis when CK-MB samples are drawn too late to display elevation
- To monitor patient response to some forms of chemotherapy.

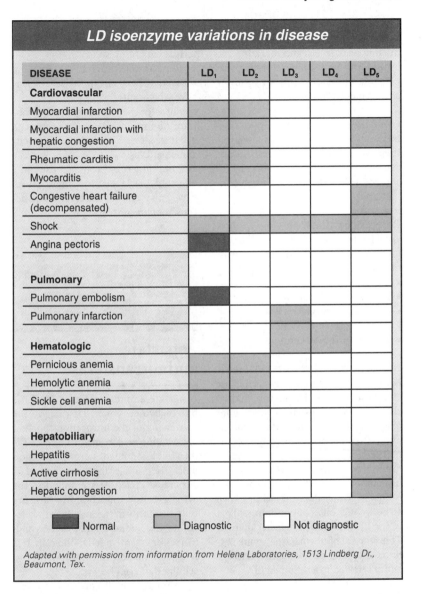

LD isoenzyme variations in disease

DISEASE	LD_1	LD_2	LD_3	LD_4	LD_5
Cardiovascular					
Myocardial infarction	Diagnostic	Diagnostic	Not diagnostic	Not diagnostic	Not diagnostic
Myocardial infarction with hepatic congestion	Diagnostic	Diagnostic	Not diagnostic	Not diagnostic	Diagnostic
Rheumatic carditis	Diagnostic	Diagnostic	Not diagnostic	Not diagnostic	Not diagnostic
Myocarditis	Diagnostic	Diagnostic	Not diagnostic	Not diagnostic	Not diagnostic
Congestive heart failure (decompensated)	Not diagnostic	Not diagnostic	Not diagnostic	Not diagnostic	Diagnostic
Shock	Diagnostic	Diagnostic	Diagnostic	Diagnostic	Diagnostic
Angina pectoris	Normal	Not diagnostic	Not diagnostic	Not diagnostic	Not diagnostic
Pulmonary					
Pulmonary embolism	Normal	Not diagnostic	Not diagnostic	Not diagnostic	Not diagnostic
Pulmonary infarction	Not diagnostic	Not diagnostic	Diagnostic	Not diagnostic	Not diagnostic
Hematologic			Diagnostic	Diagnostic	
Pernicious anemia	Diagnostic	Diagnostic	Not diagnostic	Not diagnostic	Not diagnostic
Hemolytic anemia	Diagnostic	Diagnostic	Not diagnostic	Not diagnostic	Not diagnostic
Sickle cell anemia	Diagnostic	Diagnostic	Not diagnostic	Not diagnostic	Not diagnostic
Hepatobiliary					
Hepatitis	Not diagnostic	Not diagnostic	Not diagnostic	Not diagnostic	Diagnostic
Active cirrhosis	Not diagnostic	Not diagnostic	Not diagnostic	Not diagnostic	Diagnostic
Hepatic congestion	Not diagnostic	Not diagnostic	Not diagnostic	Not diagnostic	Diagnostic

Normal | Diagnostic | Not diagnostic

Adapted with permission from information from Helena Laboratories, 1513 Lindberg Dr., Beaumont, Tex.

Patient preparation

Explain that this test is used primarily to detect tissue alterations. Inform the patient he needn't restrict food or fluids before the test. Tell him that the test requires a blood sample, who will perform the venipuncture and when, and that he may experience discomfort from the needle and the tourniquet. If an MI is suspected, tell him that the test is likely to be repeated for the next few mornings to monitor progressive changes.

Procedure

Perform a venipuncture, and collect the sample in a 7-ml *red-top* tube.

Precautions

- Draw the samples on schedule to avoid missing peak levels, and mark the collection time on the laboratory request.
- Handle the sample gently to prevent artifact blood sample hemolysis because RBCs contain LD_1.
- Send the sample to the laboratory immediately or, if transport is delayed, keep the sample at room temperature. Changes in temperature reportedly inactivate LD_5, thus altering isoenzyme patterns.

Reference values

Total LD levels normally range from 48 to 115 U/L. Normal isoenzyme distribution is as follows:

- LD_1: 14% to 26% of total
- LD_2: 29% to 39% of total
- LD_3: 20% to 26% of total
- LD_4: 8% to 16% of total
- LD_5: 6% to 16% of total.

Implications of results

Because many common diseases cause elevations in total LD levels, isoenzyme electrophoresis is usually necessary for diagnosis. In some disorders, total LD may be within normal limits, but abnormal proportions of each isoenzyme indicate specific organ tissue damage. For instance, in acute MI, the concentration of LD_1 is greater than LD_2 within 12 to 48 hours after onset of symptoms. (That is, the LD_1/LD_2 ratio is greater than 1.) This reversal of normal isoenzyme patterns is typical of myocardial damage and is referred to as "flipped LD."

Post-test care

If a hematoma develops at the venipuncture site, apply warm soaks.

Interfering factors

- Hemolysis due to rough handling of the sample may affect results.

- For diagnosis of acute MI, failure to draw the sample on schedule may interfere with test results.
- Failure to centrifuge the sample and separate the cells from the serum may affect the results.
- Failure to send the sample to the laboratory immediately may interfere with accurate determination of LD isoenzyme patterns.
- Recent surgery or pregnancy can cause elevated LD levels. Prosthetic heart valves may also increase LD levels because of chronic hemolysis.

HEPATIC ENZYME TESTS

Aspartate aminotransferase

Aspartate aminotransferase (AST) is one of two enzymes that catalyze the conversion of the nitrogenous portion of an amino acid to an amino acid residue. It is essential to energy production in the Krebs cycle (tricarboxylic acid or citric acid cycle). AST is found in the cytoplasm and mitochondria of many cells, primarily in the liver, heart, skeletal muscles, kidneys, and pancreas and, to a lesser extent, in red blood cells. It is released into serum in proportion to cellular damage.

Although a high correlation exists between myocardial infarction (MI) and elevated AST levels, this test is sometimes considered superfluous for diagnosing MI because of its relatively low organ specificity; it doesn't allow differentiation between acute MI and the effects of hepatic congestion due to heart failure.

Purpose
- To aid detection and differential diagnosis of acute hepatic disease
- To monitor patient progress and prognosis in cardiac and hepatic diseases
- To aid in diagnosing MI in correlation with creatine kinase and lactate dehydrogenase levels.

Patient preparation
Explain to the patient that this test helps assess heart and liver function. Tell him that he needn't restrict food or fluids. Inform him that the test usually requires three venipunctures: one at admission and one each day for the next 2 days. Reassure him that any discomfort from the needle and the tourniquet will be temporary.

Before the test, withhold morphine, codeine, meperidine, chlorpropamide, methyldopa, phenazopyridine, and antitubercular drugs (isoniazid, para-aminosalicylic acid, and pyrazinamide), as ordered. If any of these medications must be continued, note this on the laboratory request.

Procedure
Perform a venipuncture, and collect the sample in a 7-ml *red-top* tube.

Precautions
- To avoid missing peak AST levels, draw serum samples at the same time each day.
- Handle the collection tube gently to prevent hemolysis, and send the sample to the laboratory immediately.

Reference values
AST levels range from 8 to 20 U/L in males and from 5 to 40 U/L in females. Children's values are typically higher.

Implications of results
AST levels fluctuate in response to the extent of cellular necrosis and therefore may be transiently and minimally elevated early in the disease process and extremely elevated during the most acute phase. Depending on when during the course of the disease the initial sample was drawn, AST levels can rise — indicating increasing disease severity and tissue damage — or fall — indicating disease resolution and tissue repair. Thus, the relative change in AST values serves as a reliable monitoring mechanism.

Very high AST levels (more than 20 times normal) may indicate acute viral hepatitis, severe skeletal muscle trauma, extensive surgery, drug-induced hepatic injury, or severe passive liver congestion.

High levels (ranging from 10 to 20 times normal) may indicate severe MI, severe infectious mononucleosis, or alcoholic cirrhosis. They also occur during the prodromal or resolving stages of conditions that cause very high elevations.

Moderate to high levels (ranging from 5 to 10 times normal) may indicate Duchenne muscular dystrophy, dermatomyositis, or chronic hepatitis. They also occur during prodromal and resolving stages of diseases that cause high elevations.

Low to moderate levels (ranging from 2 to 5 times normal) may indicate hemolytic anemia, metastatic hepatic tumors, acute pancreatitis, pulmonary emboli, delirium tremens, or fatty liver. AST levels also rise slightly after the first few days of biliary duct obstruction.

Post-test care
- If a hematoma develops at the venipuncture site, apply warm soaks.
- Resume medications discontinued before the test, as ordered.

Interfering factors
- Chlorpropamide, opiates, methyldopa, erythromycin, sulfonamides, pyridoxine, dicumarol, and antitubercular

agents; large doses of acetaminophen, salicylates, or vitamin A; and many other drugs known to affect the liver cause elevated AST levels. Strenuous exercise and muscle trauma due to I.M. injections also raise AST levels.

■ Hemolysis due to rough handling of the sample may affect test results.

■ Failure to draw the sample as scheduled, thus missing peak AST levels, may interfere with accurate determination of test results.

Alanine aminotransferase

Alanine aminotransferase (ALT) is one of two enzymes that catalyze a reversible amino group transfer reaction in the Krebs cycle (citric acid or tricarboxylic acid cycle) and is necessary for tissue energy production. Unlike aspartate aminotransferase (AST), the other aminotransferase, ALT primarily appears in hepatocellular cytoplasm — with lesser amounts in the kidneys, heart, and skeletal muscles — and is a relatively specific indicator of acute hepatocellular damage. When such damage occurs, ALT is released from the cytoplasm into the bloodstream, often before jaundice appears, resulting in abnormally high serum levels that may not return to normal for days or weeks. This test measures serum ALT levels using the spectrophotometric method.

Purpose

■ To help detect and evaluate treatment of acute hepatic disease — especially hepatitis and cirrhosis without jaundice
■ To help distinguish between myocardial and hepatic tissue damage (used with AST)
■ To assess hepatotoxicity of some drugs.

Patient preparation

Explain to the patient that this test helps assess liver function. Inform him that he need not restrict food or fluids. Tell him that the test requires a blood sample, who will perform the venipuncture and when, and that he may experience transient discomfort from the needle puncture and the pressure of the tourniquet.

Withhold hepatotoxic or cholestatic drugs, such as methotrexate, chlorpromazine, salicylates, and narcotics, before the test. If they must be continued, note this on the laboratory request.

Procedure

Perform a venipuncture, and collect the sample in a 7-ml *red-top* tube.

Precautions

Handle the sample gently to prevent hemolysis. ALT activity is stable in serum for up to 3 days at room temperature.

Reference values

Normally, serum ALT levels range from 10 to 35 U/L in males and from 9 to 24 U/L in females.

Implications of results

Very high ALT levels (up to 50 times normal) suggest viral or severe drug-induced hepatitis or another hepatic disease with extensive necrosis. (AST levels are also elevated but usually to a lesser degree.) Moderate to high levels may indicate infectious mononucleosis, chronic hepatitis, intrahepatic cholestasis or cholecystitis, early or improving acute viral hepatitis, or severe hepatic congestion due to heart failure.

Slight to moderate ALT elevations (usually with higher increases in AST levels) may appear in any condition that produces acute hepatocellular injury, such as active cirrhosis and drug-induced or alcoholic hepatitis. Marginal elevations occasionally occur in acute myocardial infarction, reflecting secondary hepatic congestion or the release of small amounts of ALT from myocardial tissue.

Post-test care
■ If a hematoma develops at the venipuncture site, apply warm soaks.
■ As ordered, resume administration of drugs that were withheld before the test.

Interfering factors
■ Many medications produce hepatic injury by competitively interfering with cellular metabolism. Falsely elevated ALT levels can follow use of barbiturates, griseofulvin, isoniazid, nitrofurantoin, methyldopa, phenothiazines, phenytoin, salicylates, tetracycline, chlorpromazine, para-aminosalicylic acid, and other drugs that affect the liver. Narcotic analgesics (morphine, codeine, meperidine) may also falsely elevate ALT levels by increasing intrabiliary pressure.
■ Ingestion of lead or exposure to carbon tetrachloride causes direct injury to hepatic cells and sharp elevations of ALT.
■ Hemolysis due to rough handling of the sample may affect test results.

Alkaline phosphatase

An enzyme that is most active at about pH 10.0, alkaline phosphatase (ALP) influences bone calcification and lipid and metabolite transport. Total serum levels reflect the combined activity of several ALP isoenzymes found in the liver, bones, kidneys, intestinal lining, and placenta. (See *ALP isoenzymes,* page 108.) Bone and liver ALP are always present in adult serum, with liver ALP most prominent — except during the third trimester of pregnancy (when the placenta originates about half of all ALP). The intestinal variant of this enzyme can be a normal component (in less than 10% of normal patterns; a genetically controlled characteristic found almost exclusively in the sera of blood groups B and O), or it can be an abnormal finding associated with hepatic disease.

The ALP test is particularly sensitive to mild biliary obstruction and is a primary indicator of space-occupying hepatic lesions. Although both skeletal and hepatic diseases can raise ALP levels, this test is most useful for diagnosing metabolic bone disease. Additional liver function studies are usually required to identify hepatobiliary disorders.

Purpose
■ To detect and identify skeletal diseases, primarily those characterized by marked osteoblastic activity
■ To detect focal hepatic lesions causing biliary obstruction, such as tumor or abscess
■ To supplement information from other liver function studies and GI enzyme tests
■ To assess response to vitamin D treatment of deficiency-induced rickets.

Patient preparation
Explain to the patient that this test assesses liver or bone function. Instruct him to fast for at least 8 hours before the test because fat intake stimulates intestinal ALP secretion. Tell him that this test requires a blood sample, who will perform the venipuncture and when, and that he may experience discomfort from the needle puncture and the pressure of the tourniquet.

Procedure
Perform a venipuncture, and collect the sample in a 7-ml *red-top* tube.

ALP isoenzymes

Separation of alkaline phosphatase (ALP) isoenzymes in the laboratory, using heat inactivation, electrophoresis, or chemical means, is sometimes used in place of serum gamma glutamyl transferase, leucine aminopeptidase, or 5'-nucleotidase to differentiate hepatic and skeletal disease.

Sixteen molecularly distinct isoenzyme fractions have been identified electrophoretically in human serum, stimulating continuing controversy about the origins, proportions, and methods of isoenzyme determination. Although the number and concentration of ALP isoenzymes in total serum levels vary with the laboratory separation method used, the five isoenzyrnes of greatest clinical significance originate in the liver (includes kidney and bile fractions), bone (may also include bile fraction), intestine, and placenta.

Reference values

On electrophoresis, liver isoenzyme levels usually range from 20 to 130 U/L; bone isoenzyme levels, from 20 to 120 U/L; and intestinal isoenzyme levels (which occur almost exclusively in individuals with blood group B or O and are markedly elevated 8 hours after a fatty meal), from undetectable to 18 U/L.

The placental isoenzyme first appears in the second trimester of pregnancy, accounts for roughly half of all ALP during the third trimester, and drops to normal levels the first month postpartum. Another isoenzyme, Regan, resembles the placental isoenzyme and appears in a small percentage of patients with cancer; it may be used as a tumor marker.

Precautions

Handle the collection tube gently to prevent hemolysis, and send the sample to the laboratory immediately because ALP activity increases at room temperature due to a rise in pH.

Reference values

When measured by chemical inhibition, total ALP levels normally range from 98 to 251 U/L for males and from 81 to 312 U/L for females (depending on age).

Implications of results

Although significant ALP elevations are possible with diseases that affect many organs, they usually indicate skeletal disease or extrahepatic or intrahepatic biliary obstruction causing cholestasis. Many acute hepatic diseases cause ALP elevations before they result in any change in serum bilirubin levels. A moderate rise in ALP levels may reflect acute biliary obstruction from hepatocellular inflammation, inactive cirrhosis, mononucleosis, or viral hepatitis. Moderate increases are also seen in osteomalacia and deficiency-induced rickets.

Sharp elevations of ALP levels may result from complete biliary obstruction by malignant or infectious infiltrations or fibrosis. Such markedly high levels are most common in Paget's disease and, occasionally, in biliary obstruction, extensive bone metastases, or hyperparathyroidism. Metastatic bone tumors resulting from pancreatic cancer raise ALP levels without a concomitant rise in serum alanine aminotransferase levels.

Isoenzyme fractionation and additional enzyme tests — gamma glutamyl transferase, lactate dehydrogenase, 5'-nucleotidase, and leucine aminopeptidase — are sometimes performed when the cause of ALP elevations (skeletal or hepatic disease) is in doubt. However, hepatic scans are taking the place of these tests as a diagnostic tool and sometimes are used to follow disease progression. Rarely, low ALP levels are associated with hypophosphatasia or with protein or magnesium deficiency.

Post-test care
■ If a hematoma develops at the venipuncture site, apply warm soaks.
■ Tell the patient that he may resume his usual diet.

Interfering factors
■ Recent ingestion of vitamin D may increase ALP levels because of vitamin D's effect on osteoblastic activity.
■ Recent infusion of albumin prepared from placental venous blood causes a marked increase in serum ALP levels.
■ Drugs that influence liver function or cause cholestasis, such as barbiturates, chlorpropamide, oral contraceptives, isoniazid, methyldopa, phenothiazines, phenytoin, and rifampin, can mildly elevate ALP levels; halothane sensitivity may increase levels drastically. Clofibrate decreases ALP levels.
■ Healing long-bone fractures and pregnancy (third trimester) can increase ALP levels. Levels are also typically elevated in infants, children, adolescents, and women over age 45.
■ Hemolysis due to rough handling of the sample may alter test results.
■ The specimen should be analyzed within 4 hours.

Gamma glutamyl transferase

Gamma glutamyl transferase (GGT), also known as gamma glutamyl transpeptidase, participates in the transfer of amino acids across cellular membranes and, possibly, in glutathione metabolism. Highest concentrations of GGT exist in the renal tubules, where amino acids are reabsorbed from glomerular filtrate, but this enzyme also appears in the liver, biliary tract epithelium, pancreas, lymphocytes, brain, and testes. At least four isoenzymes exist, but fractionation is not clinically useful or practical.

Because GGT is not elevated in bone growth or pregnancy, this test is a somewhat more sensitive indicator of hepatic necrosis than the aspartate aminotransferase assay and is as sensitive as or more sensitive than the alkaline phosphatase (ALP) assay. However, the test is nonspecific, providing little data about the type of hepatic disease, because increased levels also occur in renal, cardiac, and prostatic disease and with use of certain medications. GGT is particularly sensitive to the effects of alcohol in the liver, and levels may be elevated after moderate alcohol intake and in chronic alcoholism, even without clinical evidence of hepatic injury. (See *Bilirubin and enzyme changes in hepatobiliary disease,* page 110.)

Purpose
■ To provide information about hepatobiliary disease, to assess liver function, and to detect alcohol ingestion
■ To distinguish between skeletal disease and hepatic disease when serum ALP levels are elevated. (Normal GGT levels suggest that ALP elevation stems from skeletal disease.)

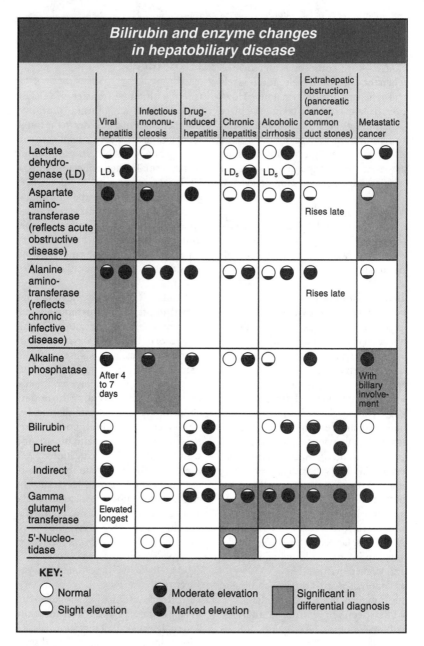

Bilirubin and enzyme changes in hepatobiliary disease

Patient preparation

Explain to the patient that this test evaluates liver function. Tell him who will perform the venipuncture and when and that he may experience discomfort from the needle puncture and the pressure of the tourniquet.

Procedure

Perform a venipuncture, and collect the sample in a 7-ml *red-top* tube.

Precautions

■ Handle the collection tube gently to prevent hemolysis.
■ GGT activity is stable in serum at room temperature for 2 days.

Reference values

Serum GGT values vary with the assay method used (kinetic or end-point method). Normal levels range from 8 to 37 U/L in males, from 5 to 27 U/L in females < 45 years, and from 6 to 37 U/L in females ≥ 45 years.

Implications of results

Serum GGT levels rise in any acute hepatic disease as enzyme production increases in response to hepatocellular injury. Moderate increases occur in acute pancreatitis, renal disease, prostatic metastases, in some patients with epilepsy or brain tumors, and postoperatively. Levels also increase after alcohol ingestion. The sharpest elevations occur in patients with obstructive jaundice or hepatic metastatic infiltrations. GGT may increase 5 to 10 days after acute myocardial infarction, either as a result of tissue granulation and healing or as an indication of the effects of cardiac insufficiency on the liver.

Post-test care

If a hematoma develops at the venipuncture site, apply warm soaks to ease discomfort.

Interfering factors

■ Clofibrate and oral contraceptives decrease serum GGT levels. Aminoglycosides, barbiturates, and phenytoin produce elevated values.
■ Moderate intake of alcohol causes increased serum GGT levels that may persist for at least 60 hours.

■ Hemolysis due to rough handling of the sample may alter test results.

5'-Nucleotidase

The enzyme 5'-nucleotidase (5'NT) is a phosphatase formed almost entirely in the hepatobiliary tract. Unlike alkaline phosphatase (ALP), an enzyme that is nonspecific, this enzyme hydrolyzes nucleoside 5'-phosphate groups only. Although serum 5'NT, ALP, and leucine aminopeptidase (LAP) levels all rise in hepatic metastases, hepatocarcinoma, and biliary tract obstruction, only 5'NT remains normal in skeletal disease and pregnancy; thus, 5'NT is more specific for hepatic dysfunction than ALP or LAP.

This test, which measures serum 5'NT levels, is technically more difficult than the ALP assay. It hasn't been widely used as a liver function study, although some authorities consider it more sensitive than ALP to cholangitis, biliary cirrhosis, and malignant infiltrations of the liver. However, 5'NT is used most often to determine whether ALP elevation is due to skeletal or hepatic disease.

Purpose

■ To distinguish between hepatobiliary and skeletal disease when the source of elevated ALP levels is uncertain
■ To help differentiate biliary obstruction from acute hepatocellular damage
■ To detect hepatic metastasis in the absence of jaundice.

Patient preparation

Explain to the patient that this test evaluates liver function. Inform him that he need not restrict food or fluids. Tell him that the test requires a blood sample, who will perform the venipuncture and when, and that he may experience discomfort from the needle puncture and the pressure of the tourniquet.

Procedure
Perform a venipuncture, and collect the sample in a 7-ml *red-top* tube.

Precautions
Handle the sample gently.

Reference values
Serum 5'NT values for adults range from 2 to 17 U/L; values for children may be lower.

Implications of results
Marked 5'NT elevations occur in common bile duct obstruction due to calculi or tumors in diseases that cause severe intrahepatic cholestasis, such as neoplastic infiltrations of the liver. Slight to moderate increases may reflect acute hepatocellular damage or active cirrhosis.

Post-test care
If a hematoma develops at the venipuncture site, apply warm soaks.

Interfering factors
- Hemolysis may interfere with results.
- Ingestion of cholestatic drugs, such as phenothiazines, morphine, meperidine, and codeine, elevates 5'NT levels.

PANCREATIC ENZYME TESTS

Serum amylase

Alpha-amylase (amylase or AML) is synthesized primarily in the pancreas and the salivary glands and secreted into the GI tract. This enzyme helps digest starch and glycogen in the mouth, stomach, and intestine. In cases of suspected acute pancreatic disease, measurement of serum or urine amylase is the most important laboratory test.

More than 20 methods of measuring serum amylase exist, with different ranges of normal values. Unfortunately, test values can't always be converted to a standard measurement.

Purpose
- To diagnose acute pancreatitis
- To distinguish between acute pancreatitis and other causes of abdominal pain that require immediate surgery
- To evaluate possible pancreatic injury caused by abdominal trauma or surgery.

Patient preparation
Explain to the patient that this test helps assess pancreatic function. Inform him that he needn't fast before the test but must abstain from alcohol, as ordered. Tell him that this test requires a blood sample, who will perform the venipuncture and when, and that he may experience transient discomfort from the needle puncture and the pressure of the tourniquet.

Withhold drugs that may elevate serum amylase levels, as ordered. If these drugs must be continued, note this on the laboratory request.

Procedure
Perform a venipuncture, and collect the sample in a 7-ml *red-top* tube.

Precautions
- If the patient has severe abdominal pain, draw the sample before diagnostic or therapeutic intervention. For accurate results, it's important to obtain an early sample.
- Handle the sample gently to prevent hemolysis.

Macroamylasemia

An uncommon, benign condition, macroamylasemia doesn't cause any symptoms, but it occasionally causes elevated serum amylase levels. This condition occurs when macroamylase — a complex of amylase and an immunoglobulin or other protein — is present in a patient's serum.

A typical patient with macroamylasemia has an elevated serum amylase level and a normal or slightly decreased urine amylase level. This characteristic pattern helps differentiate macroamylasemia from conditions in which both serum and urine amylase levels rise such as pancreatitis. But it doesn't differentiate macroamylasemia from hyperamylasemia due to impaired renal function, which may raise serum amylase levels and lower urine amylase levels. Chromatographic, ultracentrifugation, or precipitation tests are necessary to detect macroamylase in serum and definitively confirm macroamylasemia.

Reference values

Serum amylase levels for adults ≥ 18 years normally range from 35 to 115 U/L.

Implications of results

After the onset of acute pancreatitis, serum amylase levels begin to rise in 2 hours, peak at 12 to 48 hours, and return to normal in 3 to 4 days. Determination of urine levels should follow normal serum amylase results to rule out pancreatitis.

Moderate serum elevations may accompany pancreatic injury from perforated peptic ulcer, pancreatic cancer, acute salivary gland disease, impaired renal function, or obstruction of the common bile duct, the pancreatic duct, or the ampulla of Vater. Levels may be slightly elevated in a patient who is asymptomatic or who is responding unusually to therapy.

Depressed amylase levels can occur in chronic pancreatitis, pancreatic cancer, cirrhosis, hepatitis, and toxemia of pregnancy.

Post-test care

∎ If a hematoma develops at the venipuncture site, apply warm soaks.

∎ As ordered, resume administration of drugs discontinued before the test.

Interfering factors

∎ Hemolysis may alter test results.

∎ The following conditions may produce false-positive test results: ingestion of ethyl alcohol in large amounts; use of certain drugs, such as aminosalicylic acid, asparaginase, azathioprine, corticosteroids, cyproheptadine, narcotic analgesics, oral contraceptives, rifampin, sulfasalazine, and thiazide or loop diuretics; recent peripancreatic surgery, perforated ulcer or intestine, or abscess; spasm of the sphincter of Oddi; or, rarely, macroamylasemia. (See *Macroamylasemia.*)

Serum lipase

Lipase is produced in the pancreas and secreted into the duodenum, where it converts triglycerides and other fats into fatty acids and glycerol. Destruction of pancreatic cells, which occurs in acute pancreatitis, releases large amounts of

Blocked enzyme pathway

The pancreas secretes lipase, amylase, and other enzymes that pass through the pancreatic duct into the duodenum. In pancreatitis and obstruction of the pancreatic duct by a tumor or calculus (shown below), these enzymes can't reach their intended destination. Instead, they're diverted into the bloodstream by a mechanism that's not fully understood.

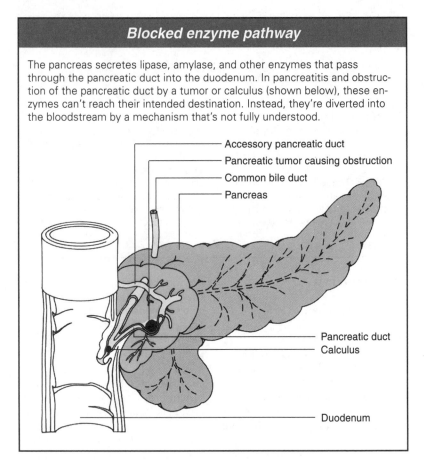

lipase into the blood. (See *Blocked enzyme pathway.*)

This test measures serum lipase levels by the kinetic turbidimetric technique; it's most useful when performed with a serum or urine amylase test.

Purpose
- To aid diagnosis of acute pancreatitis.

Patient preparation
Explain that this test evaluates pancreatic function. Instruct the patient to fast overnight before the test. Tell him that the test requires a blood sample, who will perform the venipuncture and when, and that he may feel some transient discomfort.

Withhold cholinergics, codeine, meperidine, and morphine before the test, as ordered. If any of these drugs must be continued, note this on the laboratory request.

Procedure
Perform a venipuncture, and collect the sample in a 7-ml *red-top* tube.

Precautions
Handle the collection tube gently.

Reference values

Serum levels are method-dependent and are generally less than 300 U/L.

Implications of results

High lipase levels lasting up to 14 days suggest acute pancreatitis or pancreatic duct obstruction. Lipase levels may also increase in other pancreatic injuries, such as perforated peptic ulcer with chemical pancreatitis due to gastric juices, and in patients with a high intestinal obstruction, pancreatic cancer, or renal disease with impaired excretion.

Post-test care

- If a hematoma develops at the venipuncture site, apply warm soaks.
- As ordered, resume administration of drugs discontinued before the test.

Interfering factors

- Cholinergics, codeine, meperidine, and morphine cause spasm of the sphincter of Oddi, producing false-positive results.
- Hemolysis may alter test results.

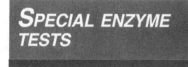

SPECIAL ENZYME TESTS

Acid phosphatase

Acid phosphatase, a group of phosphatase enzymes most active at a pH of about 5.0, appears in the prostate gland and semen and, to a lesser extent, in the liver, spleen, red blood cells, bone marrow, and platelets. Prostatic and erythrocytic enzymes are this group's two major isoenzymes, which can be separated in the laboratory; the prostatic isoenzyme is more specific for prostate cancer.

This test measures total acid phosphatase and the prostatic fraction in serum by radioimmunoassay or biochemical enzyme assay. It's usually restricted to adult males to detect prostate cancer. The more widespread the cancer, the more likely that serum acid phosphatase levels will be increased.

Purpose

- To detect prostate cancer
- To monitor response to therapy for prostate cancer (successful treatment decreases acid phosphatase levels).

Patient preparation

Explain to the patient that this test helps evaluate prostate function. Inform him that he needn't restrict food or fluids before the test. Tell him that the test requires a blood sample, who will perform the venipuncture and when, and that he may experience discomfort from the needle puncture and the tourniquet.

Withhold fluorides, phosphates, and clofibrate before the test, as ordered. If any of these drugs must be continued, be sure to note this on the laboratory request.

Procedure

Perform a venipuncture, and collect the sample in a 7-ml *red-top* tube, which should be iced for delivery to the laboratory. Some laboratories ask for a *green-top* (heparinized) tube so they won't have to wait for the sample to clot. If the sample can't be analyzed in less than 30 minutes, it should be frozen.

Precautions

- Don't draw the sample within 48 hours of prostate manipulation (rectal examination).
- Handle the collection tube gently.
- Send the sample to the laboratory immediately. Acid phosphatase levels drop by 50% within 1 hour if the sample re-

mains at room temperature without a preservative or if it's not packed in ice.

Reference values
Total serum acid phosphatase levels depend on the assay method; they generally range from 0.5 to 1.9 U/L.

Implications of results
High levels of acid phosphatase in the prostate usually indicate a tumor that has spread beyond the prostatic capsule. If the tumor has metastasized to bone, high acid phosphatase levels are accompanied by high alkaline phosphatase (ALP) levels, reflecting increased osteoblastic activity.

Misleading results may occur if ALP levels are high, because acid phosphatase and ALP enzymes are very similar and differ mainly in the optimum pH ranges. Some ALP isoenzymes may react at a lower pH and thus be detected as acid phosphatase.

Acid phosphatase levels rise moderately in prostatic infarction, Paget's disease (some patients), Gaucher's disease, and occasionally in other conditions such as multiple myeloma.

Post-test care
- If a hematoma develops at the venipuncture site, apply warm soaks to ease discomfort.
- As ordered, resume administration of any medications discontinued before the test.

Interfering factors
- Fluorides, phosphates, and oxalates can cause false-negative test results; clofibrate can cause false-positive results.
- Prostate massage, catheterization, or rectal examination within 48 hours of the test may interfere with interpretation of the test results.
- Hemolysis due to rough handling of the sample or improper sample storage may interfere with test results.

- Delayed delivery of specimen to the laboratory may cause false-low results or results in the reference range.

Prostate-specific antigen

Until recently, digital rectal examination and measurement of prostatic acid phosphatase were the primary methods of monitoring the progression of prostate cancer. Now measurement of prostate-specific antigen (PSA) helps track the course of this disease and evaluate response to treatment.

Biochemically and immunologically distinct from prostatic acid phosphatase, PSA appears in varying concentrations in normal, benign hyperplastic, and malignant prostatic tissue as well as in metastatic prostate cancer. For this reason, measurement of serum PSA levels along with a digital rectal examination is now recommended as a screening test for prostate cancer in men over age 50. (See *Controversy over PSA screening.*) It's also useful in assessing response to treatment in patients with stage B3 to D1 prostate cancer and in detecting tumor spread or recurrence.

Purpose
- To screen for prostate cancer in men over age 50
- To monitor the course of prostate cancer and help evaluate the effectiveness of treatment.

Patient preparation
Explain to the patient that this test is used to screen for prostate cancer or, if appropriate, to monitor the course of treatment. Inform him that he needn't restrict food or fluids. Tell him that this test requires a blood sample, who will

Controversy over PSA screening

Measurement of prostate-specific antigen (PSA) allows earlier detection of prostate cancer than digital rectal examination (DRE) alone. Accordingly, the American Cancer Society and the American Urological Association currently recommend that PSA screening begin at age 40 (in combination with DRE) in black men and any man who has a father or brother with prostate cancer, and at age 50 in all other men.

But does this test actually reduce mortality from prostate cancer? The answer to that question remains unknown. Some specialists question the value of all prostate cancer screening tests because of the costs involved, the uncertain benefits, and the known risks associated with current treatments.

Before undergoing a PSA test, the patient should understand that controversy surrounds nearly every aspect of prostate cancer screening and treatment. Among the issues he'll face are the following:

■ Even if cancer is detected, treatment may not be advisable, either because of the patient's advanced age or because the doctor believes the tumor is so slow-growing that it will not result in death.

■ The current treatments for prostate cancer — surgery and radiation therapy — may not be as effective as experts formerly believed, and no effective chemotherapy protocol is currently available.

■ Surgery and radiation therapy carry a high risk of impotence, incontinence, and other problems, which the patient must weigh against the uncertain benefits of therapy.

■ Screening tests sometimes yield false-positive results, requiring transrectal ultrasonography or a biopsy to confirm the diagnosis.

■ A mildly elevated PSA level may be the result of normal age-related increases. (Data from a study of more than 9,000 men showed that PSA levels increase about 30% a year in men under age 70 and more than 40% a year in men over age 70.)

In summary, the value of prostate cancer screening in general and PSA testing in particular won't be clearly established until studies show a definitive link between early treatment and reduced mortality.

---

perform the venipuncture and when, and that he may experience discomfort from the needle puncture.

Procedure
Perform a venipuncture, and collect the sample in a 7-ml *red-top* tube.

Precautions
■ Collect the sample either before a digital rectal examination or at least 48 hours after it to avoid falsely elevated PSA levels.
■ Send the sample, on ice, to the laboratory immediately.

■ Handle the sample gently to prevent hemolysis.

Reference values
■ *40 to 50 years:* 2 to 2.8 ng/ml
■ *51 to 60 years:* 2.9 to 3.8 ng/ml
■ *61 to 70 years:* 4 to 5.3 ng/ml
■ *≥ 71 years:* 5.6 to 7.2 ng/ml

Implications of results
About 80% of patients with prostate cancer have pretreatment PSA values greater than 4 ng/ml. This percentage is higher in advanced stages and lower in early stages.

However, PSA results alone should not be considered diagnostic for prostate cancer because approximately 20% of patients with benign prostatic hypertrophy also have levels over 4 ng/ml. Further testing, including tissue biopsy and digital rectal examination, is needed to confirm a diagnosis of cancer.

Post-test care
If a hematoma develops at the venipuncture site, apply warm soaks.

Interfering factors
■ Hemolysis caused by rough handling of the sample may alter test results.
■ Excessive doses of chemotherapeutic drugs, such as cyclophosphamide, diethylstilbestrol, and methotrexate, may alter test results.

Plasma renin activity

Renin secretion is the first stage of the renin-angiotensin-aldosterone cycle, which controls the body's sodium-potassium balance, fluid volume, and blood pressure. Renin is released by the juxtaglomerular cells of the kidneys into the renal veins in response to sodium depletion and blood loss. It catalyzes the conversion of angiotensinogen, an alpha$_2$-globulin plasma protein, to angiotensin I, which in turn is converted by hydrolysis into angiotensin II, a vasoconstrictor that stimulates aldosterone production in the adrenal cortex. (See *Renin-angiotensin feedback system.*) When present in excessive amounts, angiotensin II causes renal hypertension.

The plasma renin activity (PRA) test is a screening procedure for renovascular hypertension but does not unequivocally confirm it. When supplemented by other special tests, the PRA test can help establish the cause of hypertension. For instance, sampling blood obtained from both renal veins by renal vein catheterization and analyzing the renal venous renin ratio can identify renovascular disorders. Indexing renin levels against urinary sodium excretion can help identify primary aldosteronism. A sodium-depleted PRA test can then confirm this.

Some experts believe that the type of treatment chosen for essential hypertension should depend on whether renin levels are low, normal, or high; the PRA test can categorize the disease to allow for appropriate therapy.

PRA is measured by radioimmunoassay of a peripheral or renal blood sample; results are expressed as the rate of angiotensin I formation per unit of time. Patient preparation is crucial and may take up to 1 month.

Purpose
■ To screen for renal origin of hypertension
■ To help plan treatment of essential hypertension, a genetic disease often aggravated by excessive sodium intake
■ To help identify hypertension linked to unilateral (sometimes bilateral) renovascular disease by renal vein catheterization
■ To help identify primary aldosteronism (Conn's syndrome) resulting from aldosterone-secreting adrenal adenoma
■ To confirm primary aldosteronism (sodium-depleted PRA test).

Patient preparation
Explain to the patient that this test helps determine the cause of hypertension. As ordered, tell him to stop using diuretics, antihypertensives, vasodilators, oral contraceptives, and licorice for 2 to 4 weeks before the test and to maintain a normal-sodium diet (3 g/day) during this period.

Renin-angiotensin feedback system

The renin-angiotensin-aldosterone system, sometimes known as the juxta-glomerular apparatus, is an important homeostatic device for regulating the body's sodium and water levels, and blood pressure. It works this way:

   Juxtaglomerular cells (1) in each of the kidney's glomeruli secrete the enzyme renin into the blood. The rate of renin secretion depends on the rate of perfusion in the afferent renal arterioles (2) and on the amount of sodium in the serum. A low sodium load and low perfusion pressure (as in hypovolemia) increase renin secretion; high sodium and high perfusion pressure decrease it.

   Renin circulates throughout the body. In the liver, renin converts angiotensinogen to angiotensin I (3), which passes to the lungs. There it is converted by hydrolysis to angiotensin II (4), a potent vasoconstrictor that acts on the adrenal cortex to stimulate production of the hormone aldosterone (5). Aldosterone acts on the juxtaglomerular cells to stimulate or depress renin secretion, completing the feedback cycle that automatically readjusts homeostasis.

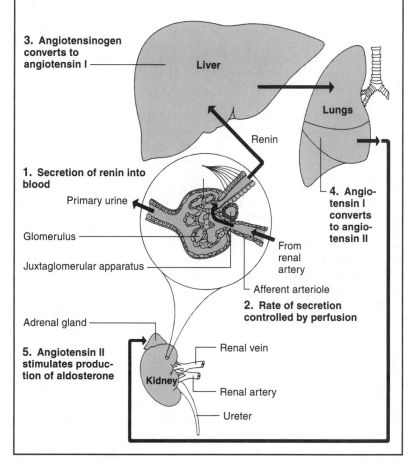

3. Angiotensinogen converts to angiotensin I

Liver

Lungs

Renin

1. Secretion of renin into blood

Primary urine

4. Angiotensin I converts to angiotensin II

Glomerulus

From renal artery

Juxtaglomerular apparatus

Afferent arteriole

2. Rate of secretion controlled by perfusion

Adrenal gland

5. Angiotensin II stimulates production of aldosterone

Renal vein

Kidney

Renal artery

Ureter

For the sodium-depleted PRA test, tell the patient that he'll receive furosemide or, if he has angina or cerebrovascular insufficiency, that he'll receive chlorothiazide and follow a specific low-sodium diet for 3 days. The patient shouldn't receive radioactive treatments for several days prior to the test.

Inform the patient that the test requires a blood sample, who will perform the venipuncture and when, and that he may experience transient discomfort from the needle puncture and the pressure of the tourniquet. Collect a morning sample if possible.

If a recumbent sample is ordered, instruct the patient to remain in bed at least 2 hours before the sample is obtained. (Posture influences renin secretion.) If an upright sample is ordered, instruct him to stand or sit upright for 2 hours before the test is performed.

If renal vein catheterization is ordered, make sure the patient has signed an informed consent form. Tell him that the procedure will be done in the X-ray department and that he'll receive a local anesthetic.

Procedure

For peripheral vein sample: Perform a venipuncture, and collect the sample in a chilled 7-ml *lavender-top* tube. Note on the laboratory request if the patient was fasting and whether he was upright or supine during sample collection.

For renal vein catheterization: A catheter is advanced to the kidneys through the femoral vein, under fluoroscopic control, and samples are obtained from both renal veins and the vena cava.

Precautions

■ Because renin is very unstable, the sample must be drawn into a chilled syringe and collection tube, placed on ice, and sent to the laboratory immediately.

■ Completely fill the collection tube, and invert it gently several times to mix the sample and the anticoagulant.

Reference values

Plasma renin activity and aldosterone levels decrease with age.

■ *Sodium-depleted, upright, peripheral vein:* For ages 18 to 39, the range is 2.9 to 24 ng/ml/hour; mean, 10.8 ng/ml/hour. For age 40 and over, the range is 2.9 to 10.8 ng/ml/hour; mean, 5.9 ng/ml/hour.

■ *Sodium-replete, upright, peripheral vein:* For ages 18 to 39, the range is less than or equal to 0.6 to 4.3 ng/ml/hour; mean, 1.9 ng/ml/hour. For age 40 and over, the range is less than or equal to 0.6 to 3.0 ng/ml/hour; mean, 1 ng/ml/hour.

■ *Renal vein catheterization:* The renal venous renin ratio (the renin level in the renal vein compared to the level in the inferior vena cava) is less than 1.5 to 1.

Implications of results

Elevated renin levels may occur in essential hypertension (uncommon), malignant and renovascular hypertension, cirrhosis, hypokalemia, hypovolemia due to hemorrhage, renin-producing renal tumors (Bartter's syndrome), and adrenal hypofunction (Addison's disease). High renin levels may also be found in chronic renal failure with parenchymal disease, end-stage renal disease, and kidney transplant rejection.

Decreased renin levels may indicate hypervolemia due to a high-sodium diet, salt-retaining steroids, primary aldosteronism, Cushing's syndrome, licorice ingestion syndrome, or essential hypertension with low renin levels.

High serum and urine aldosterone levels, with low PRA, help identify primary aldosteronism: In the sodium-depleted test, low PRA confirms this and differentiates it from secondary aldosteronism (characterized by increased renin levels).

Post-test care

■ If a hematoma develops at the venipuncture site, apply warm soaks.
■ After renal vein catheterization, apply pressure to the catheterization site for 10 to 20 minutes to prevent extravasation. Monitor vital signs, and check the catheterization site every half hour for 2 hours, then every hour for 4 hours, to ensure that the bleeding has stopped. Check distal pulse for signs of thrombus formation and arterial occlusion (cyanosis, loss of pulse, cool skin).
■ Resume diet and administration of any medications that were discontinued, as ordered.

Interfering factors

■ Failure to use the proper anticoagulant in the collection tube, to completely fill it, or to adequately mix the sample and the anticoagulant may influence renin levels. (EDTA helps preserve angiotensin I; heparin does not.)
■ Failure to chill the collection tube, syringe, and sample or to send the sample to the laboratory immediately promotes breakdown of renin.
■ Renin levels may be affected by failure to observe diet restrictions and by improper patient positioning during tests.
■ Levels are increased by salt intake, severe blood loss, licorice use, and therapy with diuretics, antihypertensives, or vasodilators.
■ Pregnancy or use of oral contraceptives also raises levels.
■ Salt-retaining steroid therapy and antidiuretic therapy decrease levels.

Cholinesterase

The cholinesterase test measures the amounts of two similar enzymes that hydrolyze acetylcholine: acetylcholinesterase (or true cholinesterase) and pseudocholinesterase (also known as serum cholinesterase). Acetylcholinesterase is present in nerve tissue, red cells of the spleen, and the gray matter of the brain. It inactivates acetylcholine at nerve junctions and helps transmit impulses across nerve endings to muscle fibers. (See *Role of acetylcholinesterase in nerve impulse transmission,* page 122.)

Pseudocholinesterase is produced primarily in the liver and appears in small amounts in the pancreas, intestine, heart, and white matter of the brain. Although pseudocholinesterase has no known function, its measurement is significant because certain chemicals that inactivate acetylcholinesterase also affect pseudocholinesterase.

Two groups of anticholinesterase chemicals — organophosphates and muscle relaxants — are important. Organophosphates, which are used by the military as nerve gases and are common ingredients in many insecticides, inactivate acetylcholinesterase directly. Muscle relaxants (such as succinylcholine), which interfere with acetylcholine-mediated transmission across nerve endings, are normally destroyed by pseudocholinesterase.

When poisoning by an organophosphate (such as parathion) is suspected, either cholinesterase may be measured. For technical reasons, pseudocholinesterase is generally tested (although this analysis is less sensitive than the one for acetylcholinesterase).

In muscle relaxant poisoning, prolonged apnea develops not from the drug itself, but because the patient lacks

Role of acetylcholinesterase in nerve impulse transmission

Each time a nerve impulse arrives at the neuromuscular junction (between a myelinated nerve fiber and a skeletal muscle fiber), the nerve terminals release about 300 vesicles (bubbles) of acetylcholine into the synaptic clefts. Then acetylcholinesterase (one component of cholinesterase) inactivates acetylcholine by hydrolyzing it to acetate and choline. This action is necessary to allow the muscle fiber to recover between excitation by acetylcholine. Without acetylcholinesterase, muscle excitation would be continuous.

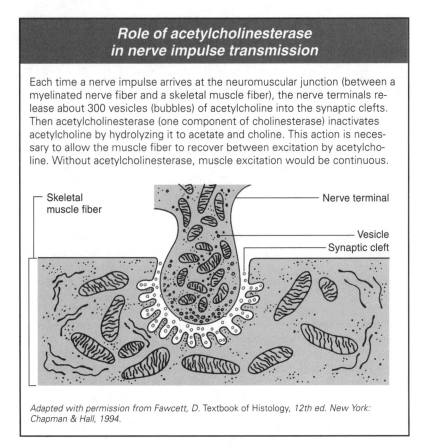

Adapted with permission from Fawcett, D. Textbook of Histology, *12th ed. New York: Chapman & Hall, 1994.*

adequate pseudocholinesterase, which normally inactivates the muscle relaxant. In this case, measurement of pseudocholinesterase is required.

Purpose
- To evaluate, preoperatively or before electroconvulsive therapy, the patient's potential response to succinylcholine, which is hydrolyzed by cholinesterase
- To identify atypical forms of pseudocholinesterase to detect those patients who may have reactions to muscle relaxants
- To assess overexposure to insecticides containing organophosphates
- To assess liver function and aid diagnosis of liver disease (a rare purpose).

Patient preparation
Explain to the patient that this test assesses muscle function or the extent of exposure to poisoning. Inform him that he needn't restrict food or fluids. Tell him the test requires a blood sample, who will perform the venipuncture and when, and that he may experience transient discomfort from the needle puncture and the pressure of the tourniquet.

Withhold substances that affect serum cholinesterase levels, as ordered. If such substances must be continued, note this on the laboratory request.

Procedure
Perform a venipuncture, and collect the sample in a 7-ml *red-top* tube.

Precautions
- Handle the collection tube gently to prevent hemolysis.
- If the sample can't be sent to the laboratory within 6 hours after being drawn, refrigerate it.

Reference values
Pseudocholinesterase levels range from 8 to 18 U/ml (when determined by kinetic colorimetric technique).

Implications of results
Very low pseudocholines-terase levels suggest a congenital deficiency or organophosphate insecticide poisoning; levels near zero necessitate emergency treatment.

Pseudocholinesterase levels are usually normal in early extrahepatic obstruction and decreased in hepatocellular damage, such as hepatitis or cirrhosis. Levels also decline in acute infections, chronic malnutrition, anemia, myocardial infarction, obstructive jaundice, and metastasis.

Post-test care
- If a hematoma develops at the venipuncture site, apply warm soaks.
- As ordered, resume administration of medications that were discontinued before the test.

Interfering factors
- Hemolysis due to rough handling of the sample may alter test results.
- Pregnancy or recent surgery may affect test results.
- Serum cholinesterase levels can be falsely depressed by cyclophosphamide, echothiophate iodide, monoamine oxidase inhibitors, succinylcholine, neostigmine, quinine, quinidine, chloroquine, caffeine, theophylline, epinephrine, ether, barbiturates, atropine, morphine, codeine, phenothiazines, vitamin K, and folic acid.

Glucose-6-phosphate dehydrogenase

Glucose-6-phosphate dehydrogenase (G6PD), an enzyme found in most body cells, is part of the pentose phosphate pathway (hexose monophosphate shunt) that metabolizes glucose. This test, which measures serum G6PD levels, detects deficiency of this enzyme. Such deficiency is a hereditary, sex-linked condition carried on the female X chromosome (with clinical disease found mostly in males) that impairs the stability of the red cell membrane and makes red cells susceptible to destruction by strong oxidizing agents.

Red cell enzyme levels normally decrease as cells age, but G6PD deficiency accelerates this process, making older red cells more prone to destruction than younger ones. In mild deficiency, young red cells retain enough G6PD to survive; in severe deficiency, all red cells are destroyed.

About 10% of all black males in the United States inherit a mild G6PD deficiency; some people of Mediterranean origin inherit a severe deficiency. In some whites, fava beans may produce hemolytic episodes. Although deficiency of G6PD provides partial immunity to falciparum malaria, it precipitates an adverse reaction to antimalarials.

Purpose
- To detect hemolytic anemia caused by G6PD deficiency
- To aid differential diagnosis of hemolytic anemia.

Patient preparation
Explain to the patient that this test detects an inherited enzyme deficiency that may affect the life span of red blood cells. Inform him that he needn't restrict food or fluids. Tell him that the test re-

quires a blood sample, who will perform the venipuncture and when, and that he may experience some transient discomfort from the needle puncture and the pressure of the tourniquet.

Check the patient history, and report a recent blood transfusion or ingestion of aspirin, sulfonamides, phenacetin, nitrofurantoin, vitamin K derivatives, antimalarials, or fava beans, which cause hemolysis in G6PD–deficient persons.

Procedure

Perform a venipuncture, and collect the sample in a 7-ml *lavender-top* tube.

Precautions

- Completely fill the collection tube, and invert it gently several times to mix the sample and the anticoagulant.
- Handle the sample gently to prevent hemolysis.
- If you can't send the sample to the laboratory immediately, refrigerate it.

Normal findings

Serum G6PD values vary with the measurement method used but usually range from 8.6 to 18.6 U/g of hemoglobin. They may also be reported simply as normal or abnormal.

Implications of results

Fluorescent spot testing or staining for Heinz bodies or erythrocytes can test for G6PD deficiency. If results are positive, the kinetic quantitative assay for G6PD may be performed. Electrophoretic techniques assess genetic variants of deficiencies (which may cause lifelong, mild, or asymptomatic anemia). Some variants are symptomatic only when the patient experiences stress or illness or is exposed to drugs or agents that elicit hemolytic episodes.

Post-test care

If a hematoma develops at the venipuncture site, apply warm soaks .

Interfering factors

- Performing the test after a hemolytic episode or a blood transfusion can cause false-negative results.
- Failure to use a collection tube containing the proper anticoagulant or to adequately mix the sample and anticoagulant may alter test results.
- Hemolysis caused by rough handling of the sample may affect test results.
- The following substances decrease G6PD enzyme activity and precipitate hemolytic episodes: aspirin, sulfonamides, nitrofurantoin, vitamin K derivatives, primaquine, and fava beans.

Pyruvate kinase

The erythrocyte enzyme pyruvate kinase (PK) takes part in the anaerobic metabolism of glucose (Embden-Meyerhof pathway). Abnormally low PK levels, revealed by erythrocyte enzyme assay using a serum sample, are inherited as an autosomal recessive trait and may result in a nonspherocytic red cell membrane defect associated with congenital hemolytic anemia.

Although PK deficiency is fairly uncommon, it's the most prevalent congenital nonspherocytic hemolytic anemia after glucose-6-phosphate dehydrogenase (G6PD) deficiency. PK assay confirms PK deficiency when red cell enzyme deficiency is the suspected cause of anemia.

Purpose

- To differentiate PK-deficient hemolytic anemia from other congenital hemolytic anemias (such as G6PD deficiency) and from acquired hemolytic anemia (when the patient history or laboratory tests fail to indicate a genetic red cell defect)

■ To detect PK deficiency in asymptomatic, heterozygous inheritance.

Patient preparation

Explain to the patient that this test is used to detect inherited enzyme deficiencies. Inform him that he need not restrict food or fluids. Tell him that this test requires a blood sample, who will perform the venipuncture and when, and that he may experience transient discomfort from the needle puncture and the pressure of the tourniquet.

Check the patient history for a recent blood transfusion, and note it on the laboratory request.

Procedure

Perform a venipuncture, and collect the sample in a 7-ml *lavender-top* tube.

Precautions

■ Completely fill the collection tube, and invert it gently several times to mix the sample and the anticoagulant.
■ Handle the sample gently.
■ Refrigerate the sample if you can't send it to the laboratory immediately.

Reference values

In a routine assay (ultraviolet), serum PK levels range from 9 to 22 U/g of hemoglobin; in the low substrate assay, from 1.7 to 6.8 U/g of hemoglobin.

Implications of results

Low serum PK levels confirm a diagnosis of PK deficiency and allow differentiation between PK-deficient hemolytic anemia and other inherited disorders.

Post-test care

If a hematoma develops at the venipuncture site, apply warm soaks.

Interfering factors

■ Failure to use a collection tube with the proper anticoagulant or to adequately mix the sample and anticoagulant may affect test results.
■ Hemolysis caused by rough handling of the sample may affect test results.
■ Because PK levels in white blood cells remain normal in hemolytic anemia, the laboratory removes white cells from the sample to prevent false results.
■ Failure to notify the laboratory of a recent blood transfusion may alter test results.

Serum hexosaminidase A and B

This fluorometric test measures the hexosaminidase A and B content of serum samples drawn by venipuncture or collected from a neonate's umbilical cord, or of amniotic fluid obtained by amniocentesis. Hexosaminidase deficiency can also be identified by testing cultured skin fibroblasts; however, this procedure is costly and technically complex. A reference center for congenital disease should be consulted for the preferred screening method and specimen.

Hexosaminidase is a group of enzymes necessary for the metabolism of gangliosides — water-soluble glycolipids found primarily in brain tissue. A deficiency of hexosaminidase A (one of the two hexosaminidase isoenzymes) causes Tay-Sachs disease. In this autosomal recessive disorder, GM_2 ganglioside builds up in brain tissue, resulting in progressive destruction and demyelination of central nervous system cells and, usually, death before age 5.

In the United States each year, fewer than 100 infants are born with Tay-Sachs disease. However, the disorder strikes people of Eastern European Jewish ancestry about 100 times more often than the general population; about 1 in 30 such persons in New York City carries this defective gene. If two such carriers have a child, this child and subsequent offspring have a 25% chance of inheriting Tay-Sachs disease. Sandhoff's disease, which results from total hexosaminidase deficiency (both A and B), is uncommon and not prevalent in any ethnic group.

Purpose

- To confirm or rule out Tay-Sachs disease in neonates
- To screen for Tay-Sachs carriers
- To establish a prenatal diagnosis of hexosaminidase A deficiency.

Patient preparation

When testing an adult, explain that this test identifies carriers of Tay-Sachs disease. Emphasize the test's importance to a Jewish couple of Eastern European ancestry who plan to have children, and explain that both must carry the defective gene to transmit Tay-Sachs disease to their offspring. Tell the patient the test requires a blood sample, who will perform the venipuncture and when, and that he may feel some discomfort from the needle and the tourniquet.

When testing a neonate, explain to the parents that this test detects Tay-Sachs disease. Tell them blood will be drawn from the neonate's arm, neck, or umbilical cord, and explain that the procedure is safe and quickly performed. Tell them the infant will have a small bandage on the site of the venipuncture.

Inform the patient or parents that no pretest restrictions of food or fluid are necessary. If the test is being performed prenatally, teach the patient how to prepare for amniocentesis.

Procedure

Perform a venipuncture, collect cord blood, or assist with amniocentesis, as appropriate. Collect the sample in a 7-ml *red-top* tube. When testing a neonate, find out the laboratory's preferred method for collecting serum samples. Take the sample from the neonate's arm, neck, or umbilical cord, as appropriate.

Precautions

- Handle the collection tube gently.
- This test can't be done on a pregnant woman's serum, but the father's blood may be tested. If it's negative, the child won't get Tay-Sachs. The mother's leukocytes or amniotic fluid may be tested if necessary.
- If the test can't be performed immediately, freeze the sample.

Reference values

Total serum hexosaminidase levels range from 5 to 12.9 U/L; hexosaminidase A makes up 55% to 76% of the total.

Implications of results

Absence of hexosaminidase A indicates Tay-Sachs disease (total hexosaminidase levels can be normal). Absence of both hexosaminidase A and hexosaminidase B indicates Sandhoff's disease, an uncommon, virulent variant of Tay-Sachs disease that causes faster deterioration.

Post-test care

- If a hematoma develops at the venipuncture site, apply warm soaks.
- If both partners are Tay-Sachs carriers, refer them for genetic counseling. Stress the importance of having amniocentesis as early as possible during pregnancy. If only one partner is a carrier, reassure the couple that their offspring cannot inherit the disease, since both parents must be carriers in order to transmit Tay-Sachs disease.

Interfering factors

- Hemolysis may alter test results.
- Oral contraceptives may falsely increase test results.

Uroporphyrinogen I synthase

This test measures blood levels of uroporphyrinogen I synthase, an enzyme that converts porphobilinogen to uroporphyrinogen during heme biosynthesis. This enzyme (also known as uroporphyrinogen I synthetase and porphobilinogen deaminase) is normally present in erythrocytes, fibroblasts, lymphocytes, liver cells, and amniotic fluid cells. However, a hereditary deficiency can reduce uroporphyrinogen I synthase levels by 50% or more, resulting in acute intermittent porphyria (AIP). An autosomal dominant disorder of heme biosynthesis, AIP can be latent indefinitely, until certain factors (some sex hormones and drugs, a low-carbohydrate diet, or an infection) precipitate active disease.

An improvement over traditional urine tests that can detect AIP only during an acute episode, the uroporphyrinogen I synthase test can detect AIP even during its latent phase. Thus, it can identify affected individuals before their first acute episode. Because it's specific for AIP, this test can also differentiate AIP from other types of porphyria.

Enzyme activity is determined by fluorometrically measuring the conversion rate of porphobilinogen to uroporphyrinogen. If levels are indeterminate, urine and stool tests for aminolevulinic acid (ALA) and porphobilinogen may be ordered to support the diagnosis, since excretion of these porphyrin precursors increases substantially during an acute episode of AIP and may increase slightly during the latent phase.

Purpose
■ To aid diagnosis of latent or active AIP.

Patient preparation
Explain to the patient that this test helps detect a red blood cell disorder. Inform him that he'll need to fast for 12 to 14 hours before the test and to abstain from alcohol for 24 hours, but that he may drink water. Tell him that the test requires a blood sample, who will perform the venipuncture and when, and that he may experience slight discomfort from the needle puncture and the pressure of the tourniquet.

If the patient's hematocrit is available, record this on the laboratory request. Check the patient's history for any medications that may decrease enzyme levels, and withhold them as ordered. If they must be continued, note this on the laboratory request.

Procedure
Perform a venipuncture, and collect the sample in a 10-ml *green-top* tube.

Precautions
■ Handle the sample gently.
■ Send the specimen, on ice, to the laboratory immediately.

Reference values
Normal values for this enzyme are greater than or equal to 7 nmol/sec/L.

Implications of results
Decreased levels usually indicate latent or active AIP; symptoms differentiate these phases. Levels below 6 nmol/sec/L confirm AIP; levels from 6 to 6.9 nmol/sec/L are indeterminate. When levels are indeterminate, urine and stool tests for the porphyrin precursors ALA and porphobilinogen may be ordered.

Post-test care
■ If a hematoma develops at the venipuncture site, apply warm soaks.
■ As ordered, instruct the patient to resume his usual diet and medications.

■ If the patient has AIP, provide nutritional and genetic counseling. Teach him to avoid low-carbohydrate diets, alcohol, and drugs that may trigger an acute episode, such as steroid hormones, estrogens, barbiturates, sulfonamides, phenytoin, griseofulvin, chlordiazepoxide, meprobamate, glutethimide, methyprylon, and ergot. Remind him to seek medical care promptly for all infections to avoid precipitating an acute episode.

Interfering factors
■ Hemolytic and hepatic diseases may elevate uroporphyrinogen I synthase levels.
■ Hemolysis caused by rough handling of the sample may alter test results.
■ Failure to freeze the sample will cause false-positive results.
■ Failure to fast before the test may increase enzyme levels.
■ A low-carbohydrate diet, alcohol, infection, and use of the drugs listed above may decrease enzyme levels.

Galactose-1-phosphate uridyltransferase

This enzyme (commonly known as GPUT), with galactokinase and uridine diphosphate glucose 4-epimerase, converts galactose to glucose during lactose metabolism. Deficiency of these enzymes causes galactosemia, an autosomal recessive disorder marked by elevated serum galactose and decreased serum glucose. Unless detected and treated soon after birth, galactosemia can impair eye, brain, and liver development, causing irreversible cataracts, mental retardation, and cirrhosis.

A deficiency of GPUT causes the most common and severe form of galac-

tosemia, detected by both qualitative and quantitative tests. The qualitative method, a simple screening test performed at birth, is required in some hospitals for all neonates. Blood collected on specially treated filter paper is checked for fluorescence after 1- and 2-hour exposures under an ultraviolet light. Normal blood fluoresces; GPUT-deficient blood does not.

The quantitative test requires a blood sample and measures the amount of a fluorescent substance generated during a coupled enzyme reaction. This is generally ordered as soon as possible after a positive screening test and may occasionally be ordered for an adult to detect a carrier state.

Prenatal testing of amniotic fluid can also detect GPUT deficiency, but it's rarely performed because neonatal screening can detect the deficiency in time to prevent irreversible damage.

Purpose
■ To screen infants for galactosemia
■ To detect heterozygous carriers of galactosemia.

Patient preparation
When testing a neonate, explain to the parents that the test screens for galactosemia, a potentially dangerous enzyme deficiency. If a blood sample was not taken from the umbilical cord at birth, tell the parents that a small amount of blood will be drawn from the infant's heel. Explain that the procedure is safe and quickly performed.

When testing an adult, explain that the test identifies carriers of galactosemia, a genetic disorder that may be transmitted to his offspring. Tell the patient that the test requires a blood sample, who will perform the venipuncture and when, and that he may feel discomfort from the needle puncture and the tourniquet.

Procedure

For a qualitative (screening) test, collect cord blood or blood from a heelstick on special filter paper, saturating all three circles.

For a quantitative test, perform a venipuncture and collect a 4-ml sample in a *green-top* or *lavender-top* tube, depending on the laboratory method used.

Indicate the patient's age on the laboratory request. Check his history for a recent exchange transfusion. Note this on the laboratory request or postpone the test, as ordered.

Precautions

■ Handle the collection tube gently to prevent hemolysis.

■ Send the collection tube to the laboratory on wet ice.

Reference values

Normally, the qualitative test is negative (fluorescence is strong 1 and 2 hours after the test begins).

The normal range for the quantitative test is 18.5 to 28.5 U/g of hemoglobin. Check the normal range for your laboratory if it uses a different method.

Implications of results

A positive qualitative test, in which no fluorescence is observed, may indicate GPUT deficiency. A follow-up quantitative test should be performed as soon as possible.

Quantitative test results less than 5 U/g of hemoglobin indicate galactosemia; levels between 5 and 18.5 U/g may indicate a carrier state.

Post-test care

■ If a hematoma develops at the venipuncture site, apply warm soaks.

■ If test results indicate galactosemia, provide nutritional counseling for the parents and a galactose- and lactose-free diet for their infant. A soybean- or meat-based formula may replace milk.

■ If one or both parents are carriers, stress the importance of having a screening test performed on their infant at birth.

Interfering factors

■ Failure to use the proper tube or to send the sample on wet ice may cause a false-positive result because heat inactivates the transferase.

■ A total exchange transfusion causes a transient false-negative result because normal transfused blood contains the transferase.

■ Hemolysis caused by rough handling of the sample may affect test results.

Angiotensin-converting enzyme

This test measures serum levels of angiotensin-converting enzyme (ACE), an enzyme found in high concentrations in lung capillaries and in lesser concentrations in blood vessels and kidney tissue. Its primary function is to help regulate arterial pressure by converting angiotensin I to angiotensin II, a powerful vasoconstrictor.

Despite ACE's role in blood pressure regulation, this test is of little use in diagnosing hypertension. Instead, it's primarily used to diagnose sarcoidosis because of the high correlation between elevated serum ACE levels and this disease. Presumably, elevated serum levels reflect macrophage activity. This test also monitors response to treatment in sarcoidosis and helps confirm a diagnosis of Gaucher's disease or leprosy.

Purpose

■ To aid diagnosis of sarcoidosis, especially pulmonary sarcoidosis

- To monitor response to therapy in sarcoidosis
- To help confirm Gaucher's disease or leprosy.

Patient preparation

Explain to the patient that this test helps diagnose sarcoidosis, Gaucher's disease, or leprosy or, if appropriate, that it checks his response to treatment for sarcoidosis. Inform him that he must fast for 12 hours before the test. Tell him that the test requires a blood sample, who will perform the venipuncture and when, and that he may experience slight discomfort from the needle puncture and the pressure of the tourniquet.

Note the patient's age on the laboratory request. If the patient is under age 20, ask the doctor about postponing the test; ACE levels vary under age 20.

Procedure

Perform a venipuncture, and collect the sample in a 7-ml *red-top* tube.

Precautions

- Avoid using a *lavender-top* tube or contaminating the sample with EDTA because this can decrease ACE levels, altering test results.
- Handle the collection tube gently to prevent hemolysis, which may interfere with determination of ACE levels.
- Send the sample to the laboratory immediately, or freeze it and place it on dry ice until the test can be done.

Reference values

In the colorimetric assay, normal serum ACE values for patients age 20 and over range from 6.1 to 21.1 U/L.

Implications of results

Elevated serum ACE levels may indicate sarcoidosis, Gaucher's disease, or leprosy, but results must be correlated with the patient's clinical condition. In some patients, elevated ACE levels may result from hyperthyroidism, diabetic retinopathy, or liver disease.

Serum ACE levels decline as the patient responds to steroid or prednisone therapy for sarcoidosis.

Post-test care

If a hematoma develops at the venipuncture site, apply warm soaks.

Interfering factors

- Use of a *lavender-top* collection tube or other EDTA contamination can decrease ACE levels.
- Hemolysis caused by excessive agitation of the sample may alter test results.
- Failure to fast before the test may cause significant lipemia of the sample, interfering with accurate test results.
- Failure to send the sample to the laboratory at once or to freeze it and place it on dry ice may cause enzyme degradation and artificially low ACE levels.

SELECTED READINGS

Fischbach, F. *A Manual of Laboratory and Diagnostic Tests,* 5th ed. Philadelphia: Lippincott-Raven Pubs., 1996.

Guyton, A.C., and Hall, J.E. *Textbook of Medical Physiology,* 9th ed. Philadelphia: W.B. Saunders Co., 1996.

Henry, J.B., ed. *Clinical Diagnosis and Management by Laboratory Methods,* 19th ed. Philadelphia: W.B. Saunders Co., 1996.

Isselbacher, K.J., et al., eds. *Harrison's Principles of Internal Medicine,* 13th ed. New York: McGraw-Hill Book Co., 1994.

Leavelle, D., ed. *Mayo Medical Laboratories Interpretive Handbook.* Rochester, Minn.: Mayo Medical Laboratories, 1994.

Mayo Medical Laboratories 1996 Test Catalog. Rochester, Minn.: Mayo Medical Laboratories, 1996.

Tietz, N.W. *Clinical Guide to Laboratory Tests,* 3rd ed. Philadelphia: W.B. Saunders Co., 1995.

Hormones

Learning objectives

After completing this chapter, the reader will be able to:
- identify the major hormones, their secretion sites, and principal actions
- tell the patient the purpose of each test and prepare him for the test
- describe the procedure for obtaining a specimen for each test
- state the reference values for each test and list factors that may affect results.

INTRODUCTION

Hormones are powerful, complex chemicals that are normally produced by the endocrine system and transported through the bloodstream to stimulate or inhibit the metabolic activity of target glands or organs. Some hormones, such as epinephrine, have profound and widespread effects on body tissues; others regulate the production and release of another hormone by the target cell and are referred to as trophic hormones — thyroid-stimulating hormone is an example. Hormones continuously interact in complicated feedback systems, both negative and positive, to maintain hormonal homeostasis. Thus, a change in the circulating blood level of any one hormone eventually changes the secretion of others. Consequent-

ly, the circulating blood levels of hormones have enormous diagnostic significance, and numerous tests have been devised to detect and evaluate abnormal secretion.

In chemical terms, hormones can be divided into three classes of compounds: polypeptides, amines, and steroids. The polypeptides include hormones such as antidiuretic hormone and gastrin; the amines include hormones such as thyroxine and the catecholamines; and the steroids include the gonadal hormones — estrogen and testosterone.

Chemical transmitters

Basically, hormones are chemical transmitters, or messengers. Most hormones attach to specific receptor sites on cell membranes, activating adenyl cyclase, an enzyme responsible for production of cyclic adenosine monophosphate (cAMP) within the cell. Just as the hormone travels through the blood with a chemical message for its target gland, cAMP acts as the third messenger within the cell itself. Prostaglandins have been implicated as the second messenger in the response system. The end result of this delicate and intricate communications network is a change in cellular function — increased protein synthesis, for example, or the release of more metabolic fuel, such as glycogen. Hormones are thus indispensable to the maintenance of homeostasis and to the growth or repair of body tissues.

Sites of secretion
Most hormones are secreted by the ductless glands or organs of the endocrine system: the pituitary, thyroid, parathyroid, and adrenal glands, and the pancreas, gonads (ovaries and testes), and placenta. (See *Sites of hormonal secretion,* page 134.) Most of these glands and organs are controlled — directly or indirectly — by the hypothalamus, the clearinghouse or message coordinator for both the endocrine and autonomic nervous systems. Some hormones are secreted by nonendocrine organs; gastrin, for example, is secreted by the stomach.

The *pituitary gland* (or hypophysis) is situated within the sella turcica of the sphenoid bone, inside the skull. This small gland dominates and regulates most of the secretory activity of the endocrine system. It has an anterior lobe (adenohypophysis) and a posterior lobe (neurohypophysis).

The *anterior pituitary* consists of glandular tissue connected to the hypothalamus by a vascular network called the hypothalamic-pituitary portal venous system. It secretes many hormones whose bloodstream levels have diagnostic significance. The basophilic cells of the anterior pituitary secrete four

polypeptide hormones that affect other endocrine glands: adrenocorticotropic hormone, follicle-stimulating hormone, luteinizing hormone, and thyroid-stimulating hormone. The acidophilic cells secrete two hormones that directly affect peripheral tissues: prolactin and growth hormone. Hyposecretion or hypersecretion of these hormones leads to serious disorders, such as Cushing's syndrome, sterility, and dwarfism.

The *posterior pituitary* comprises neural tissue or neuroepithelial cells and is continuous with the hypothalamus. It releases stored antidiuretic hormone (ADH) on neural stimulation by the hypothalamus, where ADH is formed.

The *thyroid gland* consists of two lobes, straddling the trachea and connected by an isthmus, that lie just below the cricoid cartilage. A primary regulator of body metabolism, the thyroid secretes two vital hormones — thyroxine (T_4) and triiodothyronine (T_3) — to maintain the proper metabolic rate for cellular function. The thyroid hormones have a stimulatory effect on calorigenesis (increased oxygen consumption in body tissues) and affect the growth and development of the nervous and musculoskeletal systems. They also regulate the synthesis, storage, and use of carbohydrates, fats, proteins, vitamins, and body fluids.

Serum T_4 and T_3 — probably the most often evaluated hormones — are measured to detect hyperthyroidism or hypothyroidism. If confirming tests are needed, free forms of T_4 and T_3 (FT_4 and FT_3) — unbound to thyroxine-binding globulin (TBG) — can be measured. Tests of protein binding, such as serum TBG electrophoresis, also help assess thyroid function.

The *parathyroids* — four small glands usually located behind the thyroid — release parathyroid hormone, which maintains calcium and phosphorus homeostasis. PTH, with vitamin D, stim-

Sites of hormonal secretion

Powerful, complex chemicals, hormones circulate through the bloodstream to stimulate or inhibit the activity of target glands or organs. In coordination with the nervous system, these target glands secrete the hormones that maintain homeostasis.

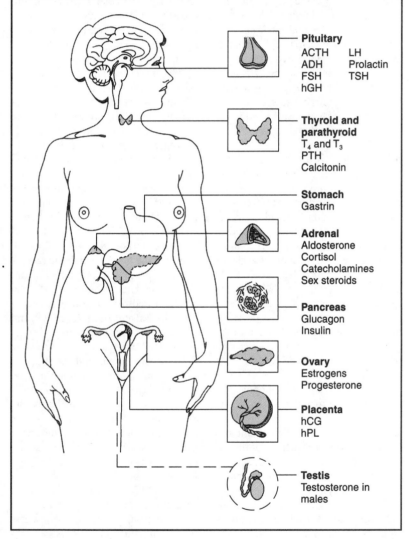

Pituitary
ACTH   LH
ADH   Prolactin
FSH   TSH
hGH

Thyroid and parathyroid
T_4 and T_3
PTH
Calcitonin

Stomach
Gastrin

Adrenal
Aldosterone
Cortisol
Catecholamines
Sex steroids

Pancreas
Glucagon
Insulin

Ovary
Estrogens
Progesterone

Placenta
hCG
hPL

Testis
Testosterone in males

ulates the osteocytes to release calcium from the bones in order to raise the serum calcium level. In contrast, calcitonin — a polypeptide hormone secreted by the parafollicular cells of the thyroid gland — and high levels of phosphate stimulate absorption of calcium ions into the bones to lower the calcium level.

The *adrenal glands* secrete mineralocorticoids (primarily aldosterone) to maintain sodium and water balance; glucocorticoids (primarily cortisol) to regulate carbohydrate, fat, and protein metabolism; sex steroids (androgens and estrogens); and catecholamines (mainly epinephrine, norepinephrine, and dopamine) to regulate reaction to stress. The adrenal cortex secretes mineralocorticoids, glucocorticoids, and sex steroids. The adrenal medulla secretes catecholamines — this is part of the body's fight-or-flight response to stress.

In the *pancreas,* the islets of Langerhans (beta cells) secrete insulin and the alpha cells secrete glucagon; both hormones have a marked effect on total body metabolism but especially on carbohydrate metabolism. The *stomach* secretes gastrin, a hormone that plays an indispensable role in facilitating digestion.

The *ovaries* and *testes* secrete the gonadal hormones estrogen and testosterone, respectively, which govern development of secondary sex characteristics and reproductive function. The ovaries also secrete progesterone, which serves primarily to prepare the endometrium for the implantation of a fertilized ovum. During pregnancy, the *placenta* serves as a temporary endocrine organ, secreting the hormones human chorionic gonadotropin and human placental lactogen.

Hormonal "watchdog" mechanisms

Because hormones are so powerful, despite the minute quantities in which they appear in the blood, the body monitors their activities closely to prevent unwanted physiologic effects. Two important "watchdog" mechanisms to control hormonal levels are *neurohumoral regulation* and a closed-loop *feedback system*. In neurohumoral regulation, certain releasing or inhibiting factors produced in the supraoptic hypothalamic nuclei travel to the pituitary, where they regulate secretion of hormones.

The positive loop of the feedback system, which is constantly at work within the endocrine system, encompasses the initial stimulus, such as an elevated blood glucose level, that results in the secretion of the controlling hormone — in this case, insulin. The negative loop goes into action when the desired secretory response or hormonal concentration is achieved. For example, decreased blood glucose levels cause the pancreas to curtail its secretion of insulin.

Hormone assay methods

Radioimmunoassay and enzyme immunoassay are two testing methods used by laboratories to measure hormone levels. But the assay method is just one consideration that affects the reliability of test results. For example, diurnal variations in hormone secretion require careful scheduling of the sample collection to coincide with or avoid times of peak secretion.

Other important considerations in evaluating hormone levels are age, gender, exercise, emotional stress, nutritional status, and medication use, all of which may affect the level of the hormone to be tested.

Assessment crucial

Remember to assess your patients accurately for endocrine disorders, such as hypothyroidism or diabetes. In children, watch especially for indications of abnormal growth patterns, such as absent or delayed puberty, irregular bone structure, muscular atrophy, or weight changes. (See *Clinical indications for hormone tests,* page 136.)

Remember, careful observation, accurate history taking, and patient teaching are essential to the care of patients scheduled for hormone tests.

Clinical indications for hormone tests

DISEASE OR DISORDER	HORMONES TESTED
Acromegaly, gigantism	ACTH, hGH, FSH, LH, TSH
Addison's disease	ACTH, cortisol
Aldosteronism	Aldosterone
Anemia	Erythropoietin
Congenital adrenal hyperplasia	ACTH, cortisol, androgens, estrogens, hCG, androstenedione
Cushing's syndrome	ACTH, cortisol, androstenedione, DHEA
Diabetes insipidus	ADH
Diabetes mellitus	Insulin, cortisol, glucagon
Dwarfism	ACTH, hGH, FSH, LH, TSH
Gigantism	hGH
Hyperparathyroidism and hypoparathyroidism	PTH
Hyperthyroidism and hypothyroidism	T_4 and T_3, FT_4 and FT_3, TSH, TBG
Hypogonadism	Estrogens, testosterone, FSH, LH, androstenedione
Hypopituitarism	ACTH, hGH, FSH, LH, TSH, T_4, T_3, alpha PGH
Medullary thyroid carcinoma	Calcitonin
Performance enhancers, suspected use of	Erythropoietin, anabolic steroids, androgens
Pituitary tumors	ACTH, hGH, prolactin, FSH, LH
Polycythemia	Erythropoietin
Precocious puberty	FSH, LH, estrogens, androgens, androstenedione
Specific tumors	Erythropoietin, hCG
Zollinger-Ellison syndrome	Gastrin

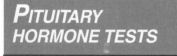

PITUITARY HORMONE TESTS

Plasma ACTH

This test measures the plasma levels of adrenocorticotropic hormone (ACTH) — also known as corticotropin — by radioimmunoassay. ACTH, a polypeptide hormone released by the basophilic cells of the anterior pituitary, stimulates the adrenal cortex to secrete cortisol and, to a lesser degree, androgens and aldosterone. ACTH also has some melanocyte-stimulating activity and increases the uptake of amino acids by muscle cells, promotes lipolysis by fat cells, stimulates pancreatic beta cells to secrete insulin, and may contribute to the release of growth hormone. ACTH levels vary diurnally, peaking between 6 a.m. and 8 a.m. and ebbing between 6 p.m. and 11 p.m.

Through a negative feedback mechanism, plasma cortisol levels control ACTH secretion — for example, high cortisol levels suppress ACTH secretion. Emotional and physical stress (pain, surgery, insulin-induced hypoglycemia) stimulate secretion and can override the effects of plasma cortisol levels.

The plasma ACTH test may be ordered for patients with signs of adrenal hypofunction (insufficiency) or hyperfunction (Cushing's syndrome). However, ACTH suppression or stimulation testing is usually necessary to confirm diagnosis. The instability and unavailability of plasma ACTH greatly limit its diagnostic significance and reliability.

Purpose

■ To facilitate differential diagnosis of primary and secondary adrenal hypofunction
■ To aid differential diagnosis of Cushing's syndrome.

Patient preparation

Explain to the patient that this test helps to determine if his hormonal secretion is normal. Advise him to fast and limit his physical activity for 10 to 12 hours before the test. Tell him that the test requires a blood sample, who will perform the venipuncture and when, and that he may experience some transient discomfort from the needle puncture and the pressure of the tourniquet. Advise him that the laboratory requires up to 4 days to complete the analysis.

Check the patient's drug history for the use of any medications that may affect accurate determination of test results, such as corticosteroids and drugs that affect cortisol levels — estrogens,

amphetamines, spironolactone, calcium gluconate, and alcohol (ethanol). Withhold these drugs, as ordered, for 48 hours or longer before the test. If these medications must be continued, note this on the laboratory request. Arrange with the dietary department to provide a low-carbohydrate diet for 2 days before the test. This requirement may vary, depending on the laboratory.

Procedure

For a patient with suspected adrenal hypofunction, perform the venipuncture for a baseline level between 6 a.m. and 8 a.m. (peak secretion); for a patient with suspected Cushing's syndrome, perform the venipuncture between 6 p.m. and 11 p.m. (low secretion). Collect the sample in a *plastic* tube because ACTH may adhere to glass, or in a *lavender-top* (EDTA) tube. The tube must be full because excess anticoagulant will affect results. Pack the sample in ice, and send it to the laboratory immediately. The collection technique may vary, depending on the laboratory.

Precautions

Because proteolytic enzymes in the plasma degrade ACTH, a temperature of 39.2° F (4° C) is necessary to retard enzyme activity. Immediate transfer of the sample, packed in ice, to the laboratory is essential for reliable test results.

Reference values

Normal baseline values are usually less than 60 pg/ml, but they may vary, depending on the laboratory.

Implications of results

A higher-than-normal plasma ACTH level may indicate primary adrenal hypofunction (Addison's disease), in which the pituitary gland attempts to compensate for the unresponsiveness of the target organ by releasing excessive ACTH. The underlying cause of adrenocortical hypofunction may be idiopathic atrophy of the adrenal cortex, or partial destruction of the gland by granuloma, neoplasm, amyloidosis, or inflammatory necrosis.

A low-normal plasma ACTH level suggests secondary adrenal hypofunction resulting from pituitary or hypothalamic dysfunction. The primary determinant may be panhypopituitarism, absence of corticotropin-releasing hormone in the hypothalamus, or chronic blunting of ACTH levels by long-term corticosteroid therapy.

In suspected Cushing's syndrome, an elevated plasma ACTH level suggests *Cushing's disease,* in which pituitary dysfunction (due to adenoma) causes continuous hypersecretion of ACTH and, consequently, continuously elevated plasma cortisol levels, without diurnal variations. Moderately elevated ACTH levels suggest pituitary-dependent adrenal hyperplasia as well as nonadrenal tumors, such as oat cell carcinoma of the lungs.

A low-normal ACTH level implies adrenal hyperfunction due to adrenocortical tumor or hyperplasia as the source of high cortisol levels; in such hyperfunction, ACTH levels are low-normal (or undetectable) because the high plasma cortisol levels suppress ACTH secretion through negative feedback.

Post-test care

■ If a hematoma develops at the puncture site, apply warm soaks.
■ Resume diet and administration of medications that were discontinued before the test, as ordered.

Interfering factors

■ Failure to observe restrictions of diet, medications, or physical activity may interfere with accurate determination of test results. ACTH levels are depressed by corticosteroids, including cortisone and its analogues, and by drugs that increase endogenous cortisol secretion (estrogens, calcium gluconate, amphetamines, spironolactone, and ethanol). Lithium carbonate decreases cortisol levels and may interfere with ACTH secretion. ACTH levels are also affected by the menstrual cycle and pregnancy.
■ A radioactive scan performed within 1 week before the test may influence test results.

Rapid ACTH

The rapid adrenocorticotropic hormone (ACTH) test (also known as the cosyntropin test) is gradually replacing the 8-hour ACTH stimulation test as the most effective test for evaluating adrenal hypofunction (insufficiency). Using cosyntropin, a synthetic analogue of the biologically active part of ACTH, the rapid ACTH test provides faster results and causes fewer allergic reactions than the 8-hour test, which uses natural ACTH from animal sources. This test requires prior determination of baseline plasma cortisol levels to evaluate the effect of cosyntropin administration on cortisol secretion. An equivocally high morning cortisol level rules out adrenal hypofunction and makes further testing unnecessary.

Purpose

■ To aid in identification of primary and secondary adrenal hypofunction.

Patient preparation

Explain to the patient that this test helps determine if his condition is due to a hormonal deficiency. Inform him that he may be required to fast for 10 to 12 hours before the test and that he must be relaxed and rest quietly for 30 minutes before the test. Tell him the test, which takes at least 1 hour to perform, requires three venipunctures and an injection.

This test may be given on an outpatient basis. If so, instruct the patient to withhold ACTH and all steroid medications before the test, as ordered. If the patient is hospitalized, withhold these medications. If they must be continued, note this on the laboratory request.

Procedure

Draw 5 ml of blood for a baseline value. Collect the sample in a 5-ml *green-top* (heparinized) tube. Label this sample "preinjection" and send it to the laboratory. Inject 250 mcg (0.25 mg) of cosyntropin I.V. (preferably) or I.M. (I.V. administration yields more accurate test results because ineffective absorption after I.M. administration may cause wide variations in response.) Direct I.V. injection should take 2 minutes.

Draw another 5 ml of blood 30 and 60 minutes after the cosyntropin injection. Collect the samples in 5-ml *green-top* (heparinized) tubes. Label the samples "30 minutes postinjection" and "60 minutes postinjection"; then send them to the laboratory. Also include the actual collection times on the laboratory request.

Precautions

Handle the samples gently to prevent hemolysis. These samples require no special precautions other than avoiding stasis.

Reference values

Normally, plasma cortisol levels rise 7 or more µg/dl above the baseline value to a peak of 18 µg/dl (or more) 60 minutes after the cosyntropin injection. Generally, a doubling of the baseline value indicates a normal response.

Implications of results

A normal result excludes adrenal hypofunction. In patients with primary adrenal hypofunction (Addison's disease), cortisol levels remain low. Thus, the rapid ACTH test provides an effective method of screening for adrenal hypofunction. However, if test results show subnormal increases in plasma cortisol levels, prolonged stimulation of the adrenal cortex may be required to differentiate between primary and secondary adrenal hypofunction.

Post-test care

- If a hematoma develops at the venipuncture sites, apply warm soaks.
- Observe the patient for signs of an allergic reaction to cosyntropin (rare), such as hives, itching, or tachycardia.
- As ordered, resume diet and administration of medications that were discontinued before the test.

Interfering factors

- Failure to observe restrictions of diet, medications, and physical activity may hinder accurate determination of test results. Drugs that increase plasma cortisol levels — including estrogens (which increase plasma cortisol-binding proteins) and amphetamines — may interfere with test results. Smoking and obesity may also increase plasma cortisol levels. Lithium carbonate decreases plasma cortisol levels.
- A radioactive scan performed within 1 week before the test may influence test results, since plasma cortisol levels are determined by radioimmunoassay.
- Hemolysis due to rough handling of the sample may interfere with accurate determination of test results.

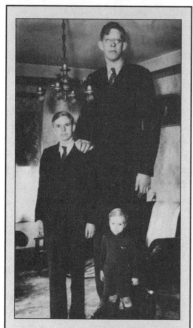

Robert Pershing Wadlow, the tallest person on record, is pictured here at age 14, at which point he was already much taller than his brothers. At his death in 1940 at age 22, he measured 8'11" (267.5 cm).

Serum human growth hormone

Human growth hormone (hGH), also known as growth hormone and somatotrophic hormone, is a protein secreted by acidophils of the anterior pituitary and is the primary regulator of human growth. Unlike other pituitary hormones, hGH has no easily defined feedback mechanism or single target gland — it affects many body tissues. Like insulin, hGH promotes protein synthesis and stimulates amino acid uptake by cells. It also raises plasma glucose levels by inhibiting glucose up-take and utilization by cells, and increases free fatty acid concentrations by enhancing lipolysis.

Secretion of hGH appears to be regulated by the hypothalamus by means of a growth hormone–releasing factor and a growth hormone release–inhibiting factor (somatostatin). Secretion of hGH is diurnal and varies with such factors as exercise, sleep, stress, and nutritional status. Hyposecretion or hypersecretion of this hormone may induce pathologic states (such as dwarfism or gigantism). Altered hGH levels are common in patients with pituitary dysfunction.

This test, a quantitative analysis of plasma hGH levels, is usually performed as part of an anterior pituitary stimulation or suppression test. Such testing is crucial because clinical manifestations of an hGH deficiency can rarely be reversed by therapy.

Purpose
- To aid differential diagnosis of dwarfism because retarded growth in children can result from pituitary or thyroid hypofunction
- To confirm a diagnosis of acromegaly and gigantism
- To aid diagnosis of pituitary or hypothalamic tumors
- To help evaluate hGH therapy.

Patient preparation
Explain to the patient or his parents (if the patient is a child) that this test measures hormone levels and helps determine the cause of abnormal growth. Instruct him to fast and limit physical activity for 10 to 12 hours before the test. Tell him the test requires a blood sample, who will perform the venipuncture and when, and that he may feel some discomfort from the needle puncture. Advise him that another sample may have to be drawn the following day for comparison and that the laboratory requires at least 2 days for analysis.

Withhold all medications that affect hGH levels, such as pituitary-based steroids, as ordered. If these medications must be continued, note this on the laboratory request. Make sure the patient is relaxed and recumbent for 30 minutes before the test, since stress and physical activity elevate hGH levels.

Procedure

Between 6 a.m. and 8 a.m. on 2 consecutive days, or as ordered, draw venous blood into a 7-ml *red-top* collection tube.

Precautions

■ Handle the sample gently to prevent hemolysis.
■ Send it to the laboratory immediately because hGH has a half-life of only 20 to 25 minutes.

Reference values

Normal hGH levels for men range from undetectable to 5 ng/ml; for women, from undetectable to 10 ng/ml. Higher values in women are due to estrogen effects. Children generally have higher hGH levels; nevertheless, they may range from undetectable to 16 ng/ml.

Implications of results

Increased hGH levels may indicate a pituitary or hypothalamic tumor (frequently an adenoma), which causes gigantism in children and acromegaly in adults and adolescents. Patients with diabetes mellitus sometimes have elevated hGH levels without acromegaly. Suppression testing is necessary to confirm the diagnosis.

Pituitary infarction, metastatic disease, and tumors may reduce hGH levels. Dwarfism may be due to low hGH levels, although only 15% of all cases of growth failure relate to endocrine dysfunction. Confirmation of the diagnosis requires stimulation testing with arginine or insulin.

Post-test care

■ If a hematoma develops at the venipuncture site, apply warm soaks to ease discomfort.
■ As ordered, resume diet and any medications that were discontinued before the test.

Interfering factors

■ Failure to follow restrictions of diet, medications, or physical activity may alter test results.
■ Arginine, beta blockers (propranolol), and estrogens increase hGH secretion and may affect test results.
■ Amphetamines, bromocriptine, levodopa, dopamine, methyldopa, and histamine also increase hGH secretion.
■ Insulin (induced hypoglycemia), glucagon, and nicotinic acid also raise hGH levels.
■ Phenothiazines (chlorpromazine) and corticosteroids reduce hGH secretion.
■ A radioactive scan performed within 1 week before the test may affect results.
■ Hemolysis due to rough handling of the sample may interfere with accurate determination of test results.

Growth hormone suppression

This test (also known as the glucose loading test) evaluates excessive baseline levels of growth hormone (hGH) from the anterior pituitary by measuring the secretory response to a loading dose of glucose. Normally, hGH raises plasma glucose and fatty acid concentrations; in response, insulin secretion increases to counteract these effects. Consequently, a glucose load should suppress hGH secretion. In a patient with excessive hGH levels, failure of suppression indicates anterior pituitary dysfunction and

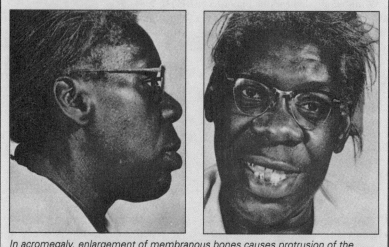

In acromegaly, enlargement of membranous bones causes protrusion of the jaw, forward slanting of the forehead, and enlargement of the nose to twice normal size.

confirms a diagnosis of acromegaly or gigantism.

Purpose
- To assess elevated baseline hGH levels
- To confirm a diagnosis of gigantism in children and acromegaly in adults.

Patient preparation
Explain to the patient and to his family (if the patient is a child) that this test helps determine the cause of his abnormal growth. Instruct him to fast and limit physical activity for 10 to 12 hours before the test. Tell him two blood samples will be drawn, and warn that he may experience nausea after drinking the glucose solution and feel some discomfort from the needle punctures. Inform him that the test takes about 1 hour but that the laboratory requires at least 2 days to complete the analysis.

Before the test, as ordered, withhold all steroids — including estrogens and progestogens — and other pituitary-based hormones. If these or other medications must be continued, note this on the laboratory request.

Because hGH levels rise after exercise or excitement, make sure the patient is relaxed and recumbent for 30 minutes before the test.

Procedure
Between 6 a.m. and 8 a.m., draw 6 ml of venous blood (basal sample) into a 7-ml *red-top* collection tube. Administer 100 g of glucose solution P.O. To prevent nausea, advise the patient to drink the glucose slowly. About an hour later, draw venous blood into a second 7-ml *red-top* collection tube. Label the tubes appropriately, and send them to the laboratory.

Precautions
- Handle the samples gently to prevent hemolysis.
- Send each sample to the laboratory immediately because hGH has a half-life of only 20 to 25 minutes.

Reference values

Normally, glucose suppresses hGH to levels ranging from undetectable to 3 ng/ml in 30 minutes to 2 hours. In children, rebound stimulation may occur after 2 to 5 hours.

Implications of results

In a patient with active acromegaly, basal hGH levels are elevated (75 ng/ml) and are not suppressed to less than 5 ng/ml during the test. Unchanged or increased hGH levels in response to glucose loading indicate hGH hypersecretion and may confirm suspected acromegaly or gigantism. This response may be verified by repeating the test after a 1-day rest.

Post-test care

■ If a hematoma develops at the puncture sites, apply warm soaks.
■ As ordered, resume diet and medications that were discontinued before the test.

Interfering factors

■ Failure to observe restrictions of diet, medications, and physical activity may interfere with accurate determination of test results. Release of hGH may be impaired by corticosteroids and phenothiazines (chlorpromazine), and may be increased by arginine, levodopa, amphetamines, glucagon, niacin, or estrogens.
■ A radioactive scan performed within 1 week before the test may affect results, since hGH levels are determined by radioimmunoassay.
■ Hemolysis due to rough handling of the sample may interfere with accurate determination of test results.

Insulin tolerance

This test measures serum levels of human growth hormone (hGH) and adrenocorticotropic hormone (ACTH) after administration of a loading dose of insulin. It's more reliable than direct measurement of hGH and ACTH because many healthy people have undetectable fasting levels of these hormones. Insulin-induced hypoglycemia stimulates hGH and ACTH secretion in persons with an intact hypothalamic-pituitary-adrenal axis. Failure of stimulation indicates anterior pituitary or adrenal hypofunction, and helps confirm an hGH or ACTH insufficiency.

Because the insulin tolerance test stimulates an adrenergic response, it's not recommended for patients with cardiovascular or cerebrovascular disorders, epilepsy, or low basal plasma cortisol levels.

Purpose

■ To aid diagnosis of hGH or ACTH deficiency
■ To identify pituitary dysfunction
■ To aid differential diagnosis of primary and secondary adrenal hypofunction.

Patient preparation

Explain to the patient or to his family that this test evaluates hormonal secretion. Instruct him to fast and to restrict physical activity for 10 to 12 hours before the test. Explain that the test involves I.V. infusion of insulin and the collection of multiple blood samples. Warn him that he may experience an increased heart rate, diaphoresis, hunger, and anxiety after administration of insulin. Reassure him that these symptoms are transient but that if they become severe, the test will be discontinued. Inform him that the test takes about 2 hours and that results are usually available in 2 days.

Because physical activity and excitement increase hGH and ACTH levels, make sure the patient is relaxed and recumbent for 90 minutes before the test.

Procedure

Between 6 a.m. and 8 a.m., collect three 5-ml samples of venous blood for basal levels — one in a *gray-top* tube for blood glucose (laboratory requirements may vary) and two in *green-top* tubes for hGH and ACTH. Then administer an I.V. bolus of U-100 regular insulin (0.15 U/kg or as ordered) over a 1- to 2-minute period. Draw additional blood samples 15, 30, 45, 60, 90, and 120 minutes after administration of insulin. Use an indwelling venous catheter to avoid repeated venipunctures. At each interval, collect three samples: one in a *gray-top* tube and two in *green-top* tubes. Label the tubes appropriately and send them to the laboratory immediately.

Precautions

 ■ Be sure to have concentrated glucose solution readily available in case the patient has a severe hypoglycemic reaction to insulin.
■ Label the tubes appropriately, including the time of collection, on the laboratory request, and send all samples to the laboratory immediately.
■ Handle the samples gently to prevent hemolysis.

Reference values

Normally, blood glucose falls to 50% of the fasting level 20 to 30 minutes after insulin administration. This stimulates a 10- to 20-ng/dl increase over baseline values in both hGH and ACTH, with peak levels occurring 60 to 90 minutes after insulin administration.

Implications of results

Failure of stimulation or a blunted response suggests dysfunction of the hypothalamic-pituitary-adrenal axis. An increase in hGH levels of less than 10 ng/dl above basal suggests hGH deficiency. However, a definitive diagnosis requires a supplementary stimulation test, such as the arginine test. Additional testing is necessary to determine the site of the abnormality.

An increase in ACTH levels of less than 10 ng/dl above basal suggests adrenal insufficiency. The metyrapone or ACTH stimulation test then confirms the diagnosis and determines whether insufficiency is primary or secondary.

Post-test care

■ If a hematoma develops at the I.V. or venipuncture site, apply warm soaks.
■ As ordered, instruct the patient to resume diet, activity, and medications.

Interfering factors

■ Failure to follow restrictions of diet, physical activity, and medications can prevent reliable test results.
■ Steroids, such as progestogen and estrogen, and pituitary-based drugs elevate hGH levels; glucocorticoids and beta blockers depress hGH levels.
■ Glucocorticoids, estrogens, calcium gluconate, amphetamines, methamphetamines, spironolactone, and ethanol depress ACTH levels.
■ Hemolysis caused by rough handling of the sample may affect test results.

Arginine

This test (also known as the growth hormone stimulation test) measures plasma growth hormone (hGH) levels after I.V. administration of arginine, an amino acid that normally stimulates hGH secretion. It's commonly used to identify pituitary dysfunction in infants and children with growth retardation and to confirm hGH deficiency. This test may be performed concomitantly with an insulin tolerance test or after administration of other hGH stimulants, such as glucagon, vasopressin, and L-dopa.

Purpose
- To aid diagnosis of pituitary tumors
- To confirm hGH deficiency in infants and children with low baseline levels.

Patient preparation
Explain to the patient or his parents that this test identifies hGH deficiency. Instruct him to fast and limit physical activity for 10 to 12 hours before the test. Explain that this test requires venous infusion of a drug and collection of several blood samples. The test takes at least 2 hours to perform; results are available in 2 days.

Before the test, withhold all steroid medications — including pituitary-based hormones — as ordered. If these medications must be continued, record this on the laboratory request. Because hGH levels may rise after exercise or excitement, make sure the patient is relaxed and recumbent for at least 90 minutes before the test.

Procedure
Between 6 a.m. and 8 a.m., draw 6 ml of venous blood (basal sample) into a *red-top* tube. Start I.V. infusion of arginine (0.5 g/kg of body weight) in normal saline solution, and continue for 30 minutes. Use of an indwelling venous catheter avoids repeated venipunctures and minimizes stress and anxiety. After discontinuing the I.V. infusion, draw a total of three 6-ml samples at 30-minute intervals. Collect each sample in a *red-top* collection tube, and label it appropriately.

Precautions
- Draw each sample at the scheduled time, and specify the collection time on the laboratory request.
- Send each sample to the laboratory immediately because hGH has a half-life of 20 to 25 minutes.
- Handle the samples gently to prevent hemolysis.

Reference values
Arginine should raise hGH levels to more than 10 ng/ml in men, to more than 15 ng/ml in women, and to 48 ng/ml in children. Such an increase may appear in the first sample drawn 30 minutes after arginine infusion is discontinued or in the samples drawn 60 and 90 minutes afterward.

Implications of results
Elevated fasting levels and increases during sleep help to rule out hGH deficiency. Failure of hGH levels to rise after arginine infusion indicates decreased anterior pituitary hGH reserve. In children, this deficiency causes dwarfism; in adults, it can indicate panhypopituitarism. When hGH levels fail to reach 10 ng/ml, retesting is required at the same time of day as the original test.

Post-test care
- If a hematoma develops at the venipuncture site, apply warm soaks.
- As ordered, resume diet and medications discontinued before the test.

Interfering factors
- Failure to observe restrictions of diet, medications, and physical activity may affect test results.
- A radioactive scan performed within 1 week before the test may affect results.
- Hemolysis due to rough handling of the sample may affect test results.

Serum follicle-stimulating hormone

This test of gonadal function, performed more often on females than on males, measures follicle-stimulating hormone (FSH) levels by radioimmunoassay and is vital to infertility studies. Its overall diagnostic significance often depends on the results of related hormone tests (for luteinizing hormone, estrogen, or progesterone, for example).

A glycoprotein secreted by the anterior pituitary, FSH stimulates gonadal activity in both sexes. In females, it spurs development of primary ovarian follicles into graafian follicles for ovulation. Secretion varies diurnally and fluctuates during the menstrual cycle, peaking at ovulation. In males, continuous secretion of FSH (and testosterone) stimulates and maintains spermatogenesis. Plasma levels fluctuate widely in females; to obtain a true baseline level, daily testing may be necessary (for 3 to 5 days), or multiple samples may be drawn on the same day.

Purpose

- To aid in the diagnosis of infertility and disorders of menstruation, such as amenorrhea
- To aid in the diagnosis of precocious puberty in girls (before age 9) and in boys (before age 10)
- To aid in the differential diagnosis of hypogonadism.

Patient preparation

Explain to the patient that this test helps determine if her hormonal secretion is normal. Inform her that she needn't fast or limit physical activity before the test. Tell her a blood sample will be drawn and that she may feel some discomfort from the needle puncture. Advise her

that the laboratory requires at least 3 days to complete the analysis.

As ordered, withhold medications that may interfere with accurate determination of test results, such as estrogens and progestogen, for 48 hours before the test. If these medications must be continued, note this on the laboratory request.

Make sure the patient is relaxed and recumbent for 30 minutes before the test.

Procedure

Perform a venipuncture, preferably between 6 a.m. and 8 a.m., using a 7-ml *red-top* collection tube, and send the sample to the laboratory immediately.

Precautions

- Handle the sample gently to prevent hemolysis.
- If the patient is a female, indicate the phase of her menstrual cycle on the laboratory request. If she is menopausal, note this as well.

Reference values

Reference values vary greatly, depending on the patient's age and stage of sexual development, and — for a female — the phase of her menstrual cycle. For menstruating females, approximate values are as follows:

- *follicular phase:* 5 to 20 mIU/ml
- *ovulatory phase:* 15 to 30 mIU/ml
- *luteal phase:* 5 to 15 mIU/ml.

Approximate values for adult males are 5 to 20 mIU/ml; for menopausal females, 50 to 100 mIU/ml.

Implications of results

Decreased FSH levels may cause male or female infertility: aspermatogenesis in males and anovulation in females. Low FSH levels may indicate secondary hypogonadotropic states, which can result from anorexia nervosa, panhypopituitarism, or hypothalamic lesions.

High FSH levels in females may indicate ovarian failure associated with Turner's syndrome (primary hypogonadism) or Stein-Leventhal syndrome (polycystic ovary syndrome). Elevated levels may occur in patients with precocious puberty (idiopathic or with CNS lesions) and in postmenopausal women. In males, abnormally high FSH levels may indicate destruction of the testes (from mumps orchitis or X-ray exposure), testicular failure, seminoma, or male climacteric. Congenital absence of the gonads and early-stage acromegaly may cause FSH levels to rise in both sexes.

Post-test care
■ If a hematoma develops at the venipuncture site, apply warm soaks.
■ As ordered, resume medications that were discontinued before the test.

Interfering factors
■ Failure to observe restriction of medications may hinder accurate determination of test results. Ovarian steroid hormones, such as estrogen or progesterone, and related compounds may, through negative feedback, inhibit the flow of releasing hormones from the hypothalamus and pituitary; phenothiazines (such as chlorpromazine) may exert a similar effect.
■ Radioactive scan performed within 1 week before the test may affect results.
■ Hemolysis due to rough handling of the sample may interfere with accurate determination of test results.

Serum luteinizing hormone

This test (also known as the interstitial-cell–stimulating hormone test) is a quantitative analysis of serum luteinizing hormone (LH) levels. Performed most often on females, it's usually ordered for anovulation and infertility studies. For accurate diagnosis, results must be evaluated in light of findings obtained from related hormone tests (follicle-stimulating hormone [FSH], estrogen, and testosterone, for example).

LH is a glycoprotein secreted by basophilic cells of the anterior pituitary. In females, cyclic LH secretion (with FSH) causes ovulation and transforms the ovarian follicle into the corpus luteum, which, in turn, secretes progesterone. (See *LH secretion cycle,* page 148.) In males, continuous LH secretion stimulates the interstitial (Leydig) cells of the testes to release testosterone, which stimulates and maintains spermatogenesis (with FSH).

Purpose
■ To detect ovulation
■ To assess male or female infertility
■ To evaluate amenorrhea
■ To monitor therapy designed to induce ovulation.

Patient preparation
Explain to the patient that this test helps determine if her secretion of female hormones is normal. Since there is no evidence that LH levels are affected by fasting, eating, or exercise, such pretest restrictions may be unnecessary. Tell the patient that this test requires a blood sample, who will perform the venipuncture and when, and that she may feel some discomfort from the needle puncture. Inform her that the laboratory requires at least 3 days to complete the analysis.

As ordered, withhold drugs that may interfere with plasma LH levels, such as steroids (including estrogens or progesterone), for 48 hours before the test. If these medications must be continued, note this on the laboratory request.

LH secretion cycle

The menstrual cycle is divided into three distinct phases: the menstrual phase (days 1 to 5); the proliferative, or follicular, phase (days 6 to 13); and after ovulation on day 14, the secretory, or luteal, phase (days 15 to 28). In a normal cycle, the menstrual phase is characterized by endometrial sloughing, corpus luteum degeneration, and new follicle growth. During this stage, estrogen and progesterone levels are low, triggering increased secretion of follicle-stimulating hormone (FSH) and luteinizing hormone (LH).

During the follicular phase, the follicle stimulated by FSH reaches full size and increases its secretion of estrogen. Simultaneously, FSH decreases while LH increases slowly but steadily. During the late follicular phase, LH rises sharply and FSH rises slightly. At about the 14th day, within hours of this abrupt surge in LH, estrogen levels in the plasma drop and ovulation occurs. After ovulation, the concentration of both LH and FSH falls rapidly.

During the final, or luteal, phase, the follicle reorganizes as the corpus luteum secretes progesterone and estrogen. Within 7 or 8 days following ovulation, if fertilization has not occurred, the corpus luteum regresses while progesterone and estrogen levels decrease. The endometrium sloughs, and the menstrual cycle begins again.

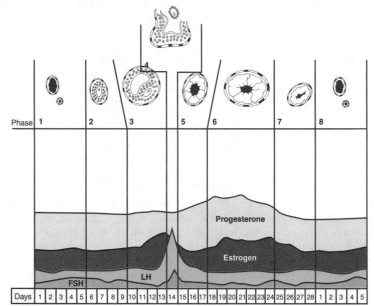

1. Menstrual phase (degeneration of corpus luteum)
2. Early follicular phase (development of follicle)
3. Late follicular phase (development of follicle)
4. Ovulation at midcycle (rupture of follicle)
5. Early luteal phase (development of corpus luteum)
6. Midluteal phase (development of corpus luteum)
7. Late luteal phase (development of corpus luteum)
8. Menstrual phase (degeneration of corpus luteum)

Procedure

Perform a venipuncture, and collect the sample in a 7-ml *red-top* tube.

Precautions

- Handle the sample gently to prevent hemolysis.
- If the patient is a female, indicate the phase of her menstrual cycle on the laboratory request. If the patient is menopausal, note this on the laboratory request.

Reference values

Normal values vary widely:

- *adult females:* values vary, depending on the phase of the patient's menstrual cycle; follicular phase — 5 to 15 mIU/ml; ovulatory phase — 30 to 60 mIU/ml; luteal phase — 5 to 15 mIU/ml
- *postmenopausal females:* 50 to 100 mIU/ml
- *adult males:* 5 to 20 mIU/ml
- *children:* 4 to 20 mIU/ml.

Implications of results

In females, absence of a midcycle peak in LH secretion may indicate anovulation. Decreased or low-normal levels may indicate hypogonadotropism; these findings are commonly associated with amenorrhea. High LH levels may indicate congenital absence of ovaries or ovarian failure associated with Stein-Leventhal syndrome (polycystic ovary syndrome), Turner's syndrome (ovarian dysgenesis), menopause, or early-stage acromegaly. Infertility can result from either primary or secondary gonadal dysfunction.

In males, low values may indicate secondary gonadal dysfunction (of hypothalamic or pituitary origin); high values may indicate testicular failure (primary hypogonadism) or destruction or congenital absence of testes.

Post-test care

- If a hematoma develops at the venipuncture site, apply warm soaks.
- As ordered, resume administration of medications that were discontinued before the test.

Interfering factors

- Failure to observe restrictions of medications may interfere with accurate determination of test results. Steroids (including estrogens, progesterone, and testosterone) may decrease plasma LH levels.
- A radioactive scan performed within 1 week before the test may influence test results because plasma LH levels are determined by radioimmunoassay.
- Hemolysis due to rough handling of the sample may interfere with accurate determination of test results.

Serum prolactin

Similar in molecular structure and biological activity to growth hormone (hGH), prolactin is a polypeptide hormone secreted by the anterior pituitary. It's essential for the development of the mammary glands for lactation during pregnancy and for stimulating and maintaining lactation postpartum. (See *Physiology of lactation,* page 150.) Prolactin (also known as lactogenic hormone or lactogen) is also secreted in males and nonpregnant females, but its function in these groups is unknown. Like hGH, prolactin acts directly on tissues, and its levels rise in response to sleep and to physical or emotional stress.

This radioimmunoassay is a quantitative analysis of serum prolactin levels, which normally rise ten- to twentyfold during pregnancy, corresponding to concomitant elevations in human

Physiology of lactation

During pregnancy, progesterone and estrogen normally interact to suppress milk secretion while developing the breasts for lactation. Estrogen causes the breasts to grow by increasing their fat content; progesterone causes lobule growth and develops the alveolar cells' secretory capacity.

After childbirth, the mother's anterior pituitary gland secretes prolactin (suppressed during pregnancy), which helps the alveolar epithelium produce and release colostrum. Usually, within 3 days of prolactin release, the breasts secrete large amounts of milk rather than colostrum. The infant's sucking stimulates nerve ending at the nipple, initiating the let-down reflex that allows the expression of milk from the mother's breasts. Sucking also stimulates the release of another pituitary hormone, oxytocin, into the mother's bloodstream. This hormone causes alveolar contraction, which forces milk into the ducts and the lactiferous sinuses beneath the alveolar surface, making milk available to the infant. (It also promotes normal involution of the uterus.) Because the infant's suckling stimulates both milk production and milk expression, the more the infant breast-feeds, the more milk the breast produces.

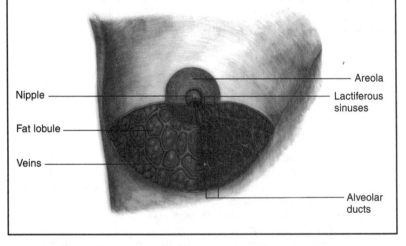

Nipple

Fat lobule

Veins

Areola

Lactiferous sinuses

Alveolar ducts

placental lactogen levels. After delivery, prolactin secretion falls to basal levels in mothers who don't breast-feed. However, prolactin secretion increases during breast-feeding, apparently as a result of a stimulus triggered by suckling that curtails the release of prolactin-inhibiting factor by the hypothalamus. This, in turn, allows transient elevations of prolactin secretion by the pituitary. This test is considered useful in patients suspected of having pituitary tumors, which are known to secrete prolactin in excessive amounts.

Another test used to evaluate hypothalamic dysfunction is the thyrotropin-releasing hormone (TRH) stimulation test. (See *TRH stimulation test.*)

Purpose

- To facilitate diagnosis of pituitary dysfunction that may be due to pituitary adenoma
- To aid in the diagnosis of hypothalamic dysfunction regardless of cause

TRH stimulation test

This test evaluates hypothalamic dysfunction and pituitary tumors by stimulating the release of prolactin. The procedure is as follows: perform a venipuncture to obtain a baseline prolactin level; then place the patient supine. Administer an I.V. bolus of synthetic thyrotropin-releasing hormone (TRH) in a dose of 500 µg/ml over 15 to 30 seconds. Blood samples are taken at 15- and 30-minute intervals to measure prolactin.

A baseline prolactin reading greater than 200 ng/ml indicates a pituitary tumor, yet levels between 30 and 200 ng/ml are also consistent with this condition. Normally, patients show at least a twofold increase in prolactin after injection of TRH. If the prolactin level fails to rise, hypothalamic dysfunction or adenoma of the pituitary gland is likely.

■ To evaluate secondary amenorrhea and galactorrhea.

Patient preparation
Tell the patient that this test helps evaluate hormonal secretion. Advise her to restrict food and fluids and limit physical activity for 12 hours before the test. Encourage her to relax for about 30 minutes before the test. Tell her who will draw the blood sample and when and that she may experience some discomfort from the needle puncture. Advise her that the laboratory requires at least 4 days to complete the analysis. As ordered, withhold drugs that may influence serum prolactin levels, such as chlorpromazine and methyldopa. If they must be continued, note this on the laboratory request.

Procedure
Perform a venipuncture at least 3 hours after the patient wakes; samples drawn earlier are likely to show sleep-induced peak levels. Collect the sample in a 7-ml *red-top* tube.

Precautions
■ Handle the sample gently to prevent hemolysis.

■ Confirm slight elevations with repeat measurements on two other occasions.

Reference values
Normal values range from undetectable to 23 ng/ml in nonlactating females.

Implications of results
Abnormally high prolactin levels (100 to 300 ng/ml) suggest autonomous prolactin production by a pituitary adenoma, especially when amenorrhea or galactorrhea is present (Forbes-Albright syndrome). Rarely, hyperprolactinemia may also result from severe endocrine disorders, such as hypothyroidism. Idiopathic hyperprolactinemia may be associated with anovulatory infertility.

Decreased prolactin levels in a lactating mother cause failure of lactation and may be associated with postpartum pituitary infarction (Sheehan's syndrome). Abnormally low prolactin levels have also been found in a few patients with empty-sella syndrome. In these patients, a flattened pituitary gland makes the pituitary fossa look empty.

Post-test care
■ If a hematoma develops at the venipuncture site, apply warm soaks.

- As ordered, resume administration of discontinued medications.

Interfering factors

- Failure to take into account physiologic variations related to sleep or stress may invalidate test results.
- Pretest use of drugs that raise prolactin levels (such as ethanol, morphine, methyldopa, and estrogens) may interfere with test results.
- Pretest use of apomorphine, ergot alkaloids, and levodopa — which lower prolactin levels — may also affect results.
- Radioactive scan performed within 1 week before the test or recent surgery may interfere with test results.
- Breast stimulation may alter results.
- Hemolysis due to rough handling of the sample may affect test results.

Serum thyroid-stimulating hormone

Thyroid-stimulating hormone (TSH) is a glycoprotein secreted by the anterior pituitary after stimulation by thyrotropin-releasing hormone (TRH) from the hypothalamus. TSH stimulates an increase in the size, number, and secretory activity of thyroid cells; heightens "iodine pump activity," often raising the ratio of intracellular to extracellular iodine as much as 350:1; and stimulates the release of triiodothyronine (T_3) and thyroxine (T_4). These hormones affect total body metabolism and are essential for normal growth and development.

This test (also known as the serum thyrotropin test) measures serum TSH levels by radioimmunoassay. It can detect primary hypothyroidism and can determine whether it results from thyroid gland failure or from pituitary or hypothalamic dysfunction. Normal serum TSH levels rule out primary hypothyroidism. This test may not distinguish between low-normal and subnormal levels, especially in secondary hypothyroidism.

The TRH challenge test evaluates thyroid function and can be performed after a baseline TSH reading has been obtained. (See *TRH challenge test.*)

Purpose

- To confirm or rule out primary hypothyroidism and distinguish it from secondary hypothyroidism
- To monitor drug therapy in patients with primary hypothyroidism.

Patient preparation

Explain to the patient that this test helps assess thyroid gland function. Tell him that the test requires a blood sample, who will perform the venipuncture and when, and that he may feel discomfort from the needle puncture. Advise him that the laboratory requires up to 2 days to complete the analysis. As ordered, withhold steroids, thyroid hormones, aspirin, and other drugs that may influence test results. If these medications must be continued, note this on the laboratory request. Keep the patient relaxed and recumbent for 30 minutes before the test.

Procedure

Between 6 a.m. and 8 a.m., perform a venipuncture. Collect the sample in a 5-ml *red-top* tube.

Precautions

Handle the sample gently to prevent hemolysis.

Reference values

Normal values for adults and children range from undetectable to 15 µIU/ml.

TRH challenge test

This test, which evaluates thyroid function and is the first direct test of pituitary reserve, is a reliable tool for diagnosing thyrotoxicosis (Graves' disease). The challenge test requires an injection of thyrotropin-releasing hormone (TRH).

One commonly accepted procedure is the following: After a venipuncture is performed to obtain a baseline thyroid-stimulating hormone (TSH) reading, synthetic TRH (protirelin) is administered by I.V. bolus in a dose of 200 to 500 µg. As many as five samples (5 ml each) are then drawn at 5-, 10-, 15-, 20-, and 60-minute intervals to assess thyroid response. To facilitate blood collection, an indwelling catheter can be used to obtain the required samples.

A sudden spike above the baseline TSH reading indicates a normally functioning pituitary but suggests hypothalamic dysfunction. If the TSH level fails to rise or remains undetectable, pituitary failure is likely. In thyrotoxicosis or thyroiditis, TSH levels fail to rise when challenged by TRH.

Implications of results

TSH levels that exceed 20 µIU/ml suggest primary hypothyroidism or, possibly, an endemic goiter (due to dietary iodine deficiency). TSH levels may be slightly elevated in euthyroid patients with thyroid cancer.

Low or undetectable TSH levels may be normal but may occasionally indicate secondary hypothyroidism (with inadequate secretion of TSH or TRH). Low TSH levels may also result from hyperthyroidism (Graves' disease) or thyroiditis; both are marked by hypersecretion of thyroid hormones, which suppresses TSH release. Provocative testing with TRH is necessary to confirm the diagnosis.

Post-test care

- If a hematoma develops at the venipuncture site, apply warm soaks.
- As ordered, resume administration of drugs discontinued before the test.

Interfering factors

- Failure to observe restrictions of medications may cause spurious test results.
- Hemolysis due to rough handling of the sample may affect test results.

Neonatal thyroid-stimulating hormone

This immunoassay (also known as the neonatal thyrotropin test) confirms congenital hypothyroidism after an initial screening test detects low thyroxine (T_4) levels. Normally, thyroid-stimulating hormone (TSH) levels surge after birth, triggering a rise in thyroid hormone levels that's essential for neurologic development. In primary congenital hypothyroidism, the thyroid gland doesn't respond to TSH stimulation, resulting in diminished thyroid hormone levels and elevated TSH levels. Early detection and treatment of congenital hypothyroidism is critical to prevent mental retardation and cretinism.

Purpose

- To confirm a diagnosis of congenital hypothyroidism.

Patient preparation

Explain to the infant's parents that this test helps confirm a diagnosis of congenital hypothyroidism. Emphasize the test's importance in detecting the disorder early so that prompt therapy can prevent irreversible brain damage.

Equipment

For a filter paper sample: alcohol or povidone-iodine swabs ✦ sterile lancet ✦ specially marked filter paper ✦ sterile 2" x 2" gauze pads ✦ adhesive bandage ✦ labels ✦ gloves.
For a serum sample: venipuncture equipment.

Procedure

For a filter paper sample: Assemble the necessary equipment, wash your hands thoroughly, and put on gloves. Wipe the infant's heel with an alcohol or povidone-iodine swab; then dry it thoroughly with a gauze pad. Perform a heelstick. Squeezing the infant's heel gently, fill the circles on the filter paper with blood. Make sure the blood saturates the paper. Gently apply pressure with a gauze pad to ensure hemostasis at the puncture site. Allow the filter paper to dry, label it appropriately, and send it to the laboratory.
For a serum sample: Perform a venipuncture and collect the sample in a 5-ml *red-top* tube. Label the sample and send it to the laboratory immediately.

Precautions

Handle the samples carefully.

Reference values

At age 1 to 2 days, TSH levels are normally 25 to 30 µIU/ml. Thereafter, levels are normally less than 25 µIU/ml.

Implications of results

Neonatal TSH levels must be interpreted in light of T_4 concentrations. Elevated TSH accompanied by decreased T_4 indicates primary congenital hypothyroidism (thyroid gland dysfunction). Depressed TSH and T_4 may be present in secondary congenital hypothyroidism (pituitary or hypothalamic dysfunction). Normal TSH accompanied by depressed T_4 may indicate hypothyroidism due to a congenital defect in thyroxine-binding globulin, or it may indicate transient congenital hypothyroidism due to prematurity or prenatal hypoxia. A complete thyroid workup must be done to confirm the cause of hypothyroidism before treatment can begin.

Post-test care

If a hematoma develops at the venipuncture site, apply warm soaks. Heelsticks require no special care.

Interfering factors

■ Corticosteroids, T_3, and T_4 lower TSH levels; lithium carbonate, potassium iodide, excessive topical resorcinol, and TSH injection raise TSH levels.
■ Failure to let a filter paper sample dry completely may alter test results.
■ Rough handling of a serum sample may cause hemolysis and may interfere with accurate testing.

Serum antidiuretic hormone

Antidiuretic hormone (ADH), also known as vasopressin, is a polypeptide produced by the hypothalamus and released from storage sites in the posterior pituitary on neural stimulation. The primary function of ADH is to promote water reabsorption in response to *increased* osmolality (water deficiency with high concentration of sodium and other solutes). In response to *decreased* osmolality (water excess), reduced secretion of ADH allows increased excretion of water to maintain fluid balance.

(See *ADH release and regulation,* page 156.) In an interlocking feedback mechanism with aldosterone, ADH helps regulate sodium, potassium, and fluid balance. It also stimulates vascular smooth-muscle contraction, causing an increase in arterial blood pressure.

This relatively rare test, a quantitative analysis of serum ADH level, may identify diabetes insipidus and other causes of severe homeostatic imbalance. It may be ordered as part of dehydration or hypertonic saline infusion testing, which determines the body's response to states of hyperosmolality.

Purpose
■ To aid in the differential diagnosis of pituitary diabetes insipidus, nephrogenic diabetes insipidus (congenital or familial), and syndrome of inappropriate antidiuretic hormone (SIADH).

Patient preparation
Explain to the patient that this test to measure hormonal secretion may aid in identifying the cause of his symptoms. Instruct him to fast and limit physical activity for 10 to 12 hours before the test. Tell him a blood sample will be drawn and that he may feel some discomfort from the needle puncture. Advise him that the laboratory requires at least 5 days to complete the analysis.

As ordered, withhold conjugated estrogens, morphine, tranquilizers, hypnotics, oxytocin, anesthetics (such as ether), lithium carbonate, vincristine, carbamazepine, cyclophosphamide, and chlorothiazide before the test; these drugs and others may cause SIADH. If these medications must be continued, note this on the laboratory request.

Make sure the patient is relaxed and recumbent for 30 minutes before the test.

Procedure
Perform a venipuncture, and collect the sample in a *red-top,* plastic collection tube or a chilled *lavender-top* (EDTA) tube. Immediately send the sample to the laboratory, where serum or plasma must be separated from the red blood cells within 10 minutes. Do a serum osmolality test at the same time to facilitate interpretation of results.

Precautions
The syringe and the collection tube *must* be plastic because the fragile ADH degrades on contact with glass.

Reference values
ADH values range from 1 to 5 pg/ml, but they can be evaluate in light of serum osmolality. If serum osmolality is less than 285 mOsm/kg, ADH is normally less than 2 pg/ml. If it's greater than 290 mOsm/kg, ADH may range from 2 to 12 pg/ml.

Implications of results
Absent or below-normal ADH levels indicate pituitary diabetes insipidus resulting from a neurohypophysial or hypothalamic tumor, a viral infection, metastatic disease, sarcoidosis, tuberculosis, Hand-Schüller-Christian disease, syphilis, neurosurgical procedures, or head trauma.

Normal ADH levels in the presence of signs of diabetes insipidus (such as polydipsia, polyuria, and hypotonic urine) may indicate the nephrogenic form of the disease, marked by renal tubular resistance to ADH; however, levels may rise if the pituitary tries to compensate.

Elevated ADH levels may also indicate SIADH, possibly as a result of bronchogenic carcinoma, acute porphyria, hypothyroidism, Addison's disease, cirrhosis of the liver, infectious hepatitis, severe hemorrhage, or circulatory shock.

ADH release and regulation

Neural impulses signal the supraoptic nuclei of the hypothalamus to produce antidiuretic hormone (ADH). After it is formed, ADH moves along the hypothalamicohypophysial tract to the posterior pituitary, where it is stored until needed by the kidneys to maintain fluid balance. In the kidneys, ADH acts on the collecting tubules to retain water.

Homeostasis is maintained by a negative feedback mechanism: Ample water or water excess inhibits further ADH secretion by the supraoptic nuclei of the hypothalamus or ADH release from the posterior pituitary. A similar negative feedback mechanism that is vital to hormonal homeostasis prevents oversecretion of other hormones.

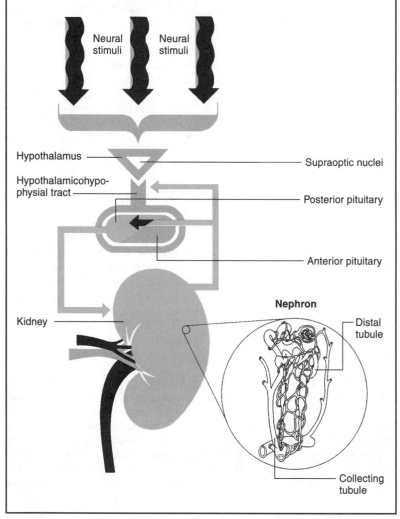

Post-test care
■ If a hematoma develops at the venipuncture site, apply warm soaks.
■ As ordered, resume diet and medications discontinued before the test.

Interfering factors
■ Failure to restrict diet, medications, or activity may affect test results. Morphine, anesthetics, estrogen, oxytocin, chlorpropamide, vincristine, carbamazepine, cyclophosphamide, and chlorothiazide elevate ADH levels, as do stress, pain, and positive-pressure ventilation. Alcohol and negative-pressure ventilation inhibit ADH secretion.
■ A radioactive scan performed within 1 week before the test may influence test results.

Alpha-subunit of pituitary glycoprotein hormones

Using radioimmunoassay, this test measures the alpha-subunit of the pituitary glycoprotein hormones (alpha-PGH). These hormones — follicle-stimulating hormone (FSH), luteinizing hormone (LH), and thyroid-stimulating hormone (TSH) — comprise similar alpha-subunits but differ in their beta-subunits. Alpha-PGH measurement assesses total pituitary production of these hormones.

Purpose
■ To aid in the diagnosis of pituitary hypofunction related to reduced production of FSH, LH, and TSH
■ To aid in the diagnosis of recurrent pituitary tumors.

Patient preparation
Explain to the patient that this test helps assess pituitary function. Inform him that he needn't fast. Tell him that this test requires a blood sample, who will perform the venipuncture and when, and that he may feel discomfort from the needle puncture. Advise him that the laboratory needs up to 4 days to do the analysis.

Procedure
Perform a venipuncture, and collect the sample in a 5-ml *red-top* tube. Send the sample to the laboratory immediately.

Precautions
■ Handle the specimen gently.
■ Indicate the sex of the patient on the laboratory request.

Reference values
Normal alpha-PGH values can range up to 1.2 ng/ml.

Implications of results
Low levels of alpha-PGH appear in patients with inadequate pituitary hormone production. Hypopituitarism results in reduced FSH, LH, and TSH levels.

Elevated levels indicate recurrent pituitary tumors or ineffective treatment.

Post-test care
If a hematoma develops at the venipuncture site, apply warm soaks.

Interfering factors
Hemolysis due to rough handling of the sample may affect the accuracy of test results.

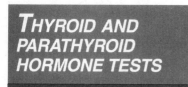

THYROID AND PARATHYROID HORMONE TESTS

Serum thyroxine

Thyroxine (T_4) is an amine secreted by the thyroid gland in response to thyroid-stimulating hormone (TSH) from the pituitary and, indirectly, to thyrotropin-releasing hormone (TRH) from the hypothalamus. The rate of secretion is normally regulated by a complex system of negative and positive feedback involving the thyroid, anterior pituitary, and hypothalamus. The suspected precursor, or prohormone, of triiodothyronine (T_3), T_4 is believed to convert to T_3 by monodeiodination, which occurs mainly in the liver and kidneys.

Only a fraction of T_4 (about 0.3%) circulates freely in the blood; the rest binds strongly to plasma proteins, primarily to thyroxine-binding globulin (TBG). This minute fraction is responsible for the clinical effects of thyroid hormone. TBG binds so tenaciously that T_4 survives in the plasma for a relatively long time, with a half-life of about 6 days. This immunoassay, one of the most common thyroid diagnostic tools, measures the total circulating T_4 level when TBG is normal. An alternative test is the Murphy-Pattee or T_4(D) test, based on competitive protein binding.

Purpose

■ To evaluate thyroid function
■ To aid diagnosis of hyperthyroidism and hypothyroidism
■ To monitor response to antithyroid medication in hyperthyroidism or to thyroid replacement therapy in hypothyroidism. (Confirmation of hypothyroidism requires TSH estimates.)

Patient preparation

Explain that this test helps evaluate thyroid gland function. Inform the patient that he needn't fast or restrict physical activity. Tell him a blood sample is needed, who will perform the venipuncture and when, and that he may feel some discomfort from the needle puncture.

As ordered, withhold any medications that may interfere with test results. If these medications must be continued, note this on the laboratory request. (If this test is being performed to monitor thyroid therapy, the patient continues to receive daily thyroid supplements.)

Procedure

Perform a venipuncture, and collect the sample in a 7-ml *red-top* tube. Send the sample to the laboratory immediately so the serum can be separated.

Precautions

Handle the sample gently to prevent hemolysis.

Reference values

Normally, total T_4 levels range from 5 to 13.5 µg/dl.

Implications of results

Abnormally elevated levels of T_4 are consistent with primary and secondary hyperthyroidism, including excessive T_4 (levothyroxine) replacement therapy (factitious or iatrogenic hyperthyroidism). Subnormal levels of T_4 suggest primary or secondary hypothyroidism or T_4 suppression by normal, elevated, or replacement levels of T_3. In doubtful cases of hypothyroidism, the TSH or TRH test may be indicated. Normal T_4 levels don't guarantee euthyroidism; for example, normal readings occur in T_3 thyrotoxicosis. Overt signs of hyperthyroidism require further testing.

Post-test care
- If a hematoma develops at the venipuncture site, apply warm soaks.
- As ordered, resume administration of medications discontinued before the test.

Interfering factors
- Hemolysis may alter test results.
- Hereditary factors and hepatic disease can change TBG concentration; protein-wasting disease (nephrotic syndrome) and androgens may reduce TBG.
- Estrogens, progestins, levothyroxine, and methadone increase T_4 levels. Free fatty acids, heparin, iodides, liothyronine sodium, lithium, methylthiouracil, phenylbutazone, phenytoin, propylthiouracil, salicylates (high doses), steroids, sulfonamides, and sulfonylureas all decrease T_4. Clofibrate can do either.

Serum triiodothyronine

This highly specific radioimmunoassay measures total (bound and free) serum content of triiodothyronine (T_3) to investigate clinical indications of thyroid dysfunction. T_3, the more potent thyroid hormone, is an amine derived primarily from thyroxine (T_4) through the process of monodeiodination. At least 50% and as much as 90% of T_3 is thought to be derived from T_4 as a result of this pivotal transformation, during which T_4 loses one of its iodine atoms to become T_3. The remaining 10% or more is secreted directly by the thyroid gland.

Like T_4 secretion, T_3 secretion occurs in response to thyroid-stimulating hormone (TSH) released by the pituitary and, secondarily, to thyrotropin-releasing hormone from the hypothalamus through a complex negative feedback mechanism.

Although T_3 is present in the bloodstream in minute quantities and is metabolically active for only a short time, its impact on body metabolism dominates that of T_4. Another significant difference between the two major thyroid hormones is that T_3 binds less firmly to thyroxine-binding globulin (TBG). Consequently, T_3 persists in the bloodstream for a short time — half of it disappears in about 1 day — whereas half of T_4 disappears in 6 days.

Purpose
- To aid diagnosis of T_3 toxicosis
- To aid diagnosis of hypothyroidism or hyperthyroidism
- To monitor clinical response to thyroid replacement therapy in hypothyroidism.

Patient preparation
Explain to the patient that this test helps to evaluate thyroid gland function and to determine the cause of his symptoms. Tell him that the test requires a blood sample, who will perform the venipuncture and when, and that he may experience some transient discomfort from the needle puncture.

As ordered, withhold medications that may influence thyroid function, such as steroids, propranolol, and cholestyramine. If such medications must be continued, record this information on the laboratory request.

Procedure
Draw venous blood into a 7-ml *red-top* tube. Send the sample to the laboratory as soon as possible to avoid stasis and to allow early separation of serum from the clotted blood.

Precautions
Handle the sample gently to prevent hemolysis. If a patient must receive thy-

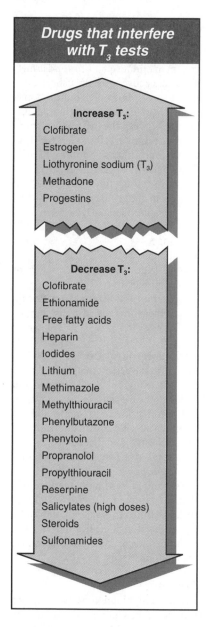

Drugs that interfere with T₃ tests

Increase T₃:
Clofibrate
Estrogen
Liothyronine sodium (T₃)
Methadone
Progestins

Decrease T₃:
Clofibrate
Ethionamide
Free fatty acids
Heparin
Iodides
Lithium
Methimazole
Methylthiouracil
Phenylbutazone
Phenytoin
Propranolol
Propylthiouracil
Reserpine
Salicylates (high doses)
Steroids
Sulfonamides

roid preparations such as T_3 (liothyronine), note the time of drug administration on the laboratory request. Otherwise, T_3 levels are not reliable.

Reference values

Serum T_3 levels normally range from 90 to 230 ng/dl. These values may vary with the laboratory performing this test.

Implications of results

Serum T_3 and T_4 levels usually rise and fall in tandem. However, in T_3 toxicosis, only T_3 levels rise, while total and free T_4 levels remain normal. T_3 toxicosis occurs in patients with Graves' disease, toxic adenoma, or toxic nodular goiter. T_3 levels also surpass T_4 levels in patients receiving thyroid replacement containing more T_3 than T_4. In iodine-deficient areas, the thyroid may produce larger amounts of the more cellularly active T_3 than of T_4 in an effort to maintain the euthyroid state.

Generally, T_3 levels appear to be a more accurate diagnostic indicator of hyperthyroidism than T_4 levels. Although hyperthyroidism increases both T_3 and T_4 levels in about 90% of patients, it causes a disproportionate increase in T_3. In some patients with hypothyroidism, T_3 levels may fall within the normal range and may not be diagnostically significant.

A rise in serum T_3 levels normally occurs during pregnancy. Low T_3 levels may appear in euthyroid patients with systemic illness (especially hepatic or renal disease), during severe acute illness, or following trauma or major surgery; in such patients, however, TSH levels are within normal limits. Low serum T_3 levels are sometimes found in euthyroid patients with malnutrition.

Post-test care

▪ If a hematoma develops at the venipuncture site, apply warm soaks.
▪ As ordered, resume administration of drugs discontinued before the test.

Interfering factors

▪ Markedly increased or decreased TBG levels, regardless of cause, may affect the accuracy of test results.

■ Hemolysis due to rough handling of the sample may influence test results.

■ Failure to take into account medications that affect T_3 levels, such as steroids, clofibrate, and propranolol, may influence test results. (See *Drugs that interfere with T_3 tests.*)

Serum thyroxine-binding globulin

This test measures the serum level of thyroxine-binding globulin (TBG), the predominant protein carrier for circulating thyroxine (T_4) and triiodothyronine (T_3). TBG values may be identified by saturating the sample for TBG determination with radioactive T_4, then subjecting this to electrophoresis and quantitating the amount of TBG by the amount of radioactive T_4 bound or by radioimmunoassay.

Any condition that affects TBG levels and subsequent binding capacity also affects the amount of free T_4 (FT_4) and free T_3 (FT_3) in circulation. This can be clinically significant because only FT_4 and FT_3 are metabolically active. An underlying TBG abnormality renders tests for total T_3 and T_4 inaccurate but does not alter tests for FT_3 and FT_4.

Purpose

■ To evaluate abnormal thyrometabolic states that do not correlate with thyroid hormone (T_3 or T_4) values (for example, a patient with overt signs of hypothyroidism and a low FT_4 level with a high total T_4 level due to a marked increase of TBG secondary to use of oral contraceptives)

■ To identify TBG abnormalities.

Patient preparation

Explain to the patient that this test helps evaluate thyroid function. Tell him the test requires a blood sample, who will perform the venipuncture and when, and that he may feel transient discomfort from the needle puncture.

As ordered, withhold medications that may interfere with accurate testing, such as estrogens, anabolic steroids, phenytoin, salicylates, and thyroid preparations. If these medications must be continued, note this on the laboratory request. (They may be continued to determine if prescribed drugs are affecting TBG levels.)

Procedure

Draw venous blood into a 10-ml *red-top* tube.

Precautions

Be sure to handle the sample gently because excessive agitation may cause hemolysis.

Reference values

Normal values for serum TBG by electrophoresis range from 10 to 26 µg T_4 (binding capacity) per deciliter. Values by immunoassay range from 12 to 25 mg/L for males and from 14 to 30 mg/L for females.

Implications of results

Elevated TBG levels may indicate hypothyroidism and congenital (genetic) excess, some forms of hepatic disease, or acute intermittent porphyria. TBG levels normally rise during pregnancy and are high in neonates. Suppressed levels may indicate hyperthyroidism or congenital deficiency, and can occur in active acromegaly, nephrotic syndrome and malnutrition with hypoproteinemia, acute illness, or surgical stress.

Patients with TBG abnormalities require additional testing, such as the serum FT$_3$ and serum FT$_4$ tests, to evaluate thyroid function more precisely.

Post-test care
- If a hematoma develops at the venipuncture site, apply warm soaks.
- As ordered, resume administration of medications that were discontinued before the test.

Interfering factors
- Estrogens (including oral contraceptives) and phenothiazines (perphenazine) elevate TBG levels.
- Androgens, prednisone, phenytoin, and high doses of salicylates depress TBG levels.
- Hemolysis due to rough handling of the sample may interfere with accurate determination of test results.

Serum free thyroxine and serum free triiodothyronine

These tests measure serum levels of free thyroxine (FT$_4$) and free triiodothyronine (FT$_3$), the minute portions of T$_4$ and T$_3$ not bound to thyroxine-binding globulin (TBG) and other serum proteins. As the active components of T$_4$ and T$_3$, these unbound hormones enter target cells and are responsible for the thyroid's effects on cellular metabolism. Since levels of circulating FT$_4$ and FT$_3$ are regulated by a feedback mechanism that compensates for changes in binding protein concentrations by adjusting total hormone levels, measurement of free hormone levels is the best indicator of thyroid function. Of the two tests, FT$_3$ is the better indicator. This test may be useful in the 5% of patients in whom

the standard T$_3$ or T$_4$ tests fail to produce diagnostic results.

Purpose
- To measure the metabolically active form of the thyroid hormones
- To aid diagnosis of hypothyroidism or hyperthyroidism when TBG levels are abnormal.

Patient preparation
Explain to the patient that this special test helps evaluate thyroid function. Tell him the test requires a blood sample, who will perform the venipuncture and when, and that he may feel transient discomfort from the needle puncture.

Procedure
Draw venous blood into a 7-ml *red-top* tube.

Precautions
Handle the sample gently to prevent hemolysis.

Reference values
Normal range for FT$_4$ is 0.8 to 3.3 ng/dl; for FT$_3$, 0.2 to 0.6 ng/dl. Values vary, depending on the laboratory. (See *Measuring FT$_3$*.)

Implications of results
Elevated FT$_4$ and FT$_3$ levels indicate hyperthyroidism, unless peripheral resistance to thyroid hormone is present. T$_3$ toxicosis, a distinct form of hyperthyroidism, yields high FT$_3$ levels, with normal or low FT$_4$ values. Low FT$_4$ levels usually indicate hypothyroidism, except in patients receiving replacement therapy with T$_3$. Patients receiving thyroid hormone replacement therapy may have varying levels of FT$_4$ and FT$_3$, depending on the preparation used and the time of sample collection.

Measuring FT₃

Free triiodothyronine (FT$_3$) levels can be determined by procedures using monoclonal antibodies. These engineered antibodies are highly specific and sensitive and permit rapid testing. Basically, FT$_3$ reacts with the antibody, which is coupled to a chromogenic (color-producing) enzyme or a fluorescent marker. Under test conditions, a color is produced or fluorescence is detected in proportion to the FT$_3$ concentration.

Post-test care

If a hematoma develops at the venipuncture site, apply warm soaks.

Interfering factors

Except for hemolysis due to rough handling of the sample, this test is virtually free of interfering factors. Agents that compete with T$_4$ and T$_3$ binding to TBG increase FT$_4$ fraction; this does not affect in vitro TBG studies due to serum dilution. Depending on the dosage, thyroid therapy may increase FT$_4$ or FT$_3$ levels. However, these medications should not be withheld; serial tests may be performed to evaluate thyroid function.

Serum long-acting thyroid stimulator

This test is used to determine whether a patient's serum contains long-acting thyroid stimulator (LATS), an abnormal immunoglobulin (called 75 IgG) that mimics the action of thyroid-stimulating hormone (TSH), although its effects are more prolonged. LATS (also known as thyroid-stimulating immunoglobulin) stimulates the thyroid gland to produce and secrete thyroid hormones in excessive amounts. Thus, through the normal negative feedback mechanism, it inhibits TSH secretion. LATS is often found in patients with Graves' disease (about 80%) and in neonates whose mothers have Graves' disease because LATS crosses the placenta.

Some authorities believe that the thyroid gland hyperplasia seen in Graves' disease may be due to LATS or other circulating antibodies. Some consider the clinical significance of this test questionable.

Purpose

- To confirm diagnosis of Graves' disease. (This test is not done routinely to diagnose thyroid disorders.)

Patient preparation

Explain to the patient (or the infant's parents) that this test helps evaluate thyroid function. Tell him this test requires a blood sample, who will perform the venipuncture and when, and that he may feel transient discomfort from the needle puncture. Advise him that the laboratory requires several days to complete the analysis.

Procedure

Draw venous blood into a 5-ml *red-top* tube. (See *Measuring LATS,* page 164.)

Precautions

- Handle the sample gently to prevent hemolysis.

Measuring LATS

In this test, samples of the patient's serum are mixed with cultured rat thyroid cells. The activation of the enzyme adenylate cyclase in the cells is a measure of long-acting thyroid stimulator (LATS).

- Note on the laboratory request if the patient had a radioactive scan within 48 hours before the test.

Normal findings

LATS should not appear in serum.

Implications of results

LATS in serum indicates Graves' disease, whether or not overt signs of hyperthyroidism are present. About 80% of patients with Graves' disease have detectable LATS in their sera.

Post-test care

If a hematoma develops at the venipuncture site, apply warm soaks.

Interfering factors

- Radioactive iodine in the serum may affect test results.
- Hemolysis due to rough handling of the sample may interfere with accurate determination of test results.

Screening test for congenital hypothyroidism

This test measures serum thyroxine (T_4) levels in neonates to detect congenital hypothyroidism. Characterized by low or absent levels of T_4, congenital hypothyroidism affects roughly 1 in 5,000 neonates, occurring in girls three times more often than in boys. This disorder can result from thyroid dysgenesis or hypoplasia, congenital goiter, or maternal use of thyroid inhibitors during pregnancy. If untreated, it can lead to irreversible brain damage by age 3 months.

Because clinical signs are few, in the past, most cases of congenital hypothyroidism went undetected until cretinism became apparent or death followed respiratory distress. Recently, however, radioimmunoassays of T_4 and thyroid-stimulating hormone (TSH) have been used effectively to screen neonates for congenital hypothyroidism. This test is now mandatory in some states.

Purpose

- To screen neonates for congenital hypothyroidism.

Patient preparation

Explain to the parents that although hypothyroidism is uncommon in infants, this screening test detects the disorder early enough to begin therapy before irreversible brain damage occurs. Tell them the test will be performed before the infant is discharged from the hospital and again 4 to 6 weeks later. Emphasize the importance of the screening and the need for following the test protocol.

Because false-positive findings can result from variations in the test procedure or from a congenital thyroxine-binding globulin (TBG) defect, inform the parents that a second test may be done before the infant is discharged.

Equipment

Gloves ✦ alcohol or povidone-iodine swabs ✦ sterile lance ✦ specially marked filter paper ✦ sterile 2" x 2" gauze pads ✦ small adhesive bandage strip ✦ labels for infant's and mother's names, doctor's name, room number, and date.

Procedure
After assembling the necessary equipment and washing your hands, put on gloves. Wipe the infant's heel with an alcohol or povidone-iodine swab, and then dry it thoroughly with a gauze pad.

Perform a heelstick. Squeezing the heel gently, fill the circles on the filter paper with blood. Make sure the blood saturates the paper. Apply gentle pressure with a gauze pad to ensure hemostasis at the puncture site. When the filter paper is dry, label it appropriately and send it to the laboratory.

Precautions
None.

Reference values
Immediately after birth, neonatal T_4 levels are considerably higher than normal adult levels. By the end of the first week, however, they decrease markedly, as follows:
- *1 to 5 days:* ≤ 4.9 µg/dl
- *6 to 8 days:* ≤ 4.0 µg/dl
- *9 to 11 days:* ≤ 3.5 µg/dl
- *12 to 120 days:* ≤ 3.0 µg/dl.

Implications of results
Low serum T_4 levels in the neonate require TSH testing to clarify the diagnosis. Decreased T_4 levels accompanied by elevated TSH readings (more than 25 µIU/ml) indicate primary congenital hypothyroidism (thyroid gland dysfunction). Decreased T_4 and TSH levels suggest secondary congenital hypothyroidism (resulting from pituitary or hypothalamic dysfunction).

If T_4 levels are subnormal but TSH readings are normal, further testing is required. Serum TBG levels must be analyzed to identify infants with hypothyroidism resulting from congenital defects in TBG. This low T_4–normal

TSH pattern also occurs in a transient form of congenital hypothyroidism that may accompany prematurity or prenatal hypoxia.

A complete thyroid workup — including serum triiodothyronine (T_3), TBG, and free T_4 levels — is necessary for an unequivocal diagnosis of congenital hypothyroidism before treatment begins.

Post-test care
- Heelsticks heal readily and require no special care.
- If results of the screening test indicate congenital hypothyroidism, tell the parents additional testing is necessary to determine the cause of the disorder.
- If the diagnosis is confirmed, inform the parents that replacement therapy can restore normal thyroid gland function. Also tell them that such therapy is lifelong and that the dosage will increase until the adult requirement is reached.
- If the sample is not processed in the hospital laboratory, make sure the parents are notified when test results are available.

Interfering factors
- Failure to allow the filter paper to dry completely may affect test results.
- Failure to follow special directions for obtaining the sample may affect the accuracy of test results.

Plasma calcitonin

This radioimmunoassay measures plasma levels of calcitonin (also known as thyrocalcitonin), a polypeptide hormone secreted by interstitial or parafollicular cells called specialized C cells of the thyroid gland in response to rising plasma calcium levels. The exact role of

Calcitonin stimulation tests

Stimulation testing is often necessary in patients with medullary thyroid carcinoma when baseline calcitonin levels fail to rise high enough to confirm the diagnosis. The most common test is a 4-hour I.V. calcium infusion (15 mg/kg) to provoke calcitonin secretion. Samples are taken just before the infusion and at 3 and 4 hours postinfusion. Calcitonin levels rise rapidly after the infusion in patients with medullary thyroid carcinoma.

Another test involves I.V. infusion of pentagastrin (0.5 mcg/kg over 5 to 10 seconds). A blood sample is drawn just before the I.V. infusion and at 90 seconds, 5 minutes, and 10 minutes postinfusion. In patients with medullary thyroid carcinoma, calcitonin levels rise markedly over the baseline reading.

calcitonin in normal human physiology has not been fully determined. However, calcitonin is known to inhibit bone resorption by osteoclasts and osteocytes and to increase calcium excretion by the kidneys; therefore, calcitonin acts as an antagonist to parathyroid hormone and lowers serum calcium levels.

The usual clinical indication for this test is suspected medullary carcinoma of the thyroid, which causes hypersecretion of calcitonin (without associated hypocalcemia). Equivocal results require provocative testing with I.V. pentagastrin or calcium to rule out this disease. (See *Calcitonin stimulation tests.*)

Purpose
■ To aid diagnosis of thyroid medullary carcinoma or ectopic calcitonin-producing tumors (rare).

Patient preparation
Explain to the patient that this test helps evaluate thyroid function. Instruct him to observe an overnight fast, since eating may interfere with calcium homeostasis and, subsequently, calcitonin levels. Tell him this test requires a blood sample, who will perform the venipuncture and when, and that he may feel transient discomfort from the needle puncture. Advise him that the laboratory requires several days to complete the analysis.

Procedure
Draw venous blood into a 10-ml *green-top* (heparinized) tube.

Precautions
Handle the sample gently to prevent hemolysis, and send it to the laboratory immediately.

Reference values
Normal plasma calcitonin levels (basal) are:
■ *males:* ≤ 40 pg/ml
■ *females:* ≤ 20 pg/ml.
Values after provocative testing with 4-hour calcium infusion are:
■ *males:* ≤ 190 pg/ml
■ *females:* ≤ 130 pg/ml.
Values after provocative testing with pentagastrin infusion are:
■ *males:* ≤ 110 pg/ml
■ *females:* ≤ 30 pg/ml.

Implications of results
Elevated plasma calcitonin levels in the absence of hypocalcemia usually indicate medullary carcinoma of the thyroid. Transmitted as an autosomal dominant trait, this disease may occur as part

of multiple endocrine neoplasia. Occasionally, increased calcitonin levels may be due to ectopic calcitonin production resulting from oat cell carcinoma of the lung or from breast carcinoma.

Post-test care
If a hematoma develops at the venipuncture site, apply warm soaks.

Interfering factors
■ Failure to observe an overnight fast before the test may interfere with accurate determination of test results.
■ Hemolysis due to rough handling of the sample may interfere with accurate determination of test results.

Serum parathyroid hormone

Parathyroid hormone (PTH), also known as parathormone, is a polypeptide secreted by the parathyroid glands that regulates plasma concentration of calcium and phosphorus. Normally, PTH release is regulated by a negative feedback mechanism involving serum calcium. Normal or elevated circulating calcium levels (especially the ionized form) inhibit PTH release; decreased levels stimulate PTH release. The overall effect of PTH is to raise plasma levels of calcium while lowering phosphorus levels by stimulating osteoclasts and osteocytes to mobilize both calcium and phosphorus from bone, acting on renal tubular cells to promote calcium reabsorption and phosphorus excretion (phosphaturia), and (with biological vitamin D [1,25-dihydroxycholecalciferol]) promoting intestinal absorption of calcium.

Circulating PTH exists in three distinct molecular forms: the intact PTH molecule, which originates in the parathyroids, and two smaller circulating forms — N-terminal fragments and C-terminal fragments — that are cleaved from the intact molecule by the kidneys, liver and, to a lesser extent for the C-fragment, the parathyroids.

Currently, two radioimmunoassays are available to detect intact PTH and the N- and C-terminal fragments. Both tests can be used to confirm a diagnosis of hyperparathyroidism and hypoparathyroidism, but they have other specific applications as well. The C-terminal PTH assay is more useful for diagnosing chronic disturbances in PTH metabolism, such as secondary and tertiary hyperparathyroidism; it's also better for differentiating ectopic from primary hyperparathyroidism. The assay for intact PTH and the N-terminal fragment (both forms are measured concomitantly) more accurately reflects acute changes in PTH metabolism and thus is useful in monitoring a patient's response to PTH therapy.

An inappropriate deficiency or excess of PTH has clinical and diagnostic consequences directly related to the effects of PTH on bone and the renal tubules and to the interaction of PTH with ionized calcium and biologically active vitamin D. Consequently, measuring serum calcium, phosphorus, and creatinine levels with serum PTH is useful in identifying states of pathologic parathyroid function. Suppression or stimulation tests may be of confirming value.

Purpose
■ To aid in the differential diagnosis of parathyroid disorders.

Patient preparation
Explain to the patient that this test helps evaluate parathyroid function. Instruct him to observe an overnight fast because food may affect PTH levels and interfere with the test results. Tell him that

Clinical implications of abnormal parathyroid secretion

CONDITIONS	CAUSES	P.T.H. LEVELS	CALCIUM (IONIZED) LEVELS
Primary hyperparathyroidism	■ Parathyroid adenoma or carcinoma ■ Parathyroid hyperplasia	High	High to Normal
Secondary hyperparathyroidism	■ Chronic renal disease ■ Severe vitamin D deficiency ■ Calcium malabsorption ■ Pregnancy and lactation	High	Low
Tertiary hyperparathyroidism	■ Progressive secondary hyperparathyroidism leading to autonomous hyperparathyroidism	High	High to Normal
Hypoparathyroidism	■ Usually, accidental removal of the parathyroid glands during surgery ■ Occasionally associated with autoimmune disease	Low	Low
Malignant tumors	■ Squamous cell carcinoma of the lung ■ Renal, pancreatic, or ovarian carcinoma	High to Normal	High

KEY: High ● (dark)   Normal ● (gray)   Low ○ (open)

this test requires a blood sample, who will perform the venipuncture and when, and that he may experience transient discomfort from the needle puncture. Advise him that the laboratory will need several days to complete the analysis.

Procedure

Draw 3 ml of venous blood into two separate 7-ml *red-top* tubes.

Precautions

Handle the sample gently to prevent hemolysis. Send it to the laboratory immediately so the serum can be separated and frozen for assay.

Reference values

Normal serum PTH levels vary, depending on the laboratory, and must be interpreted in relation to serum calcium levels. Typical values are as follows:
- *intact PTH:* 210 to 310 pg/ml
- *N-terminal fraction:* 230 to 630 pg/ml
- *C-terminal fraction:* 410 to 1760 pg/ml.

Implications of results

Measured concomitantly with serum calcium levels, abnormally elevated PTH values may indicate primary, secondary, or tertiary hyperparathyroidism. Abnormally low PTH levels may result from hypoparathyroidism and from certain malignant diseases. (See

Clinical implications of abnormal parathyroid secretion.)

Post-test care
- If a hematoma develops at the venipuncture site, apply warm soaks.
- As ordered, resume the patient's normal diet after the test.

Interfering factors
- Failure to observe an overnight fast may interfere with accurate determination of test results.
- Hemolysis due to rough handling of the sample may interfere with accurate determination of test results.

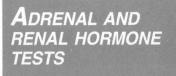

ADRENAL AND RENAL HORMONE TESTS

Serum aldosterone

This test measures serum aldosterone levels by quantitative analysis and radioimmunoassay. Aldosterone, the principal mineralocorticoid secreted by the zona glomerulosa of the adrenal cortex, regulates ion transport across cell membranes in the renal tubules to promote reabsorption of sodium and chloride in exchange for potassium and hydrogen ions. (See *Sites of adrenal hormone production,* page 170.) Consequently, aldosterone helps to maintain blood pressure and blood volume and to regulate fluid and electrolyte balance.

Aldosterone secretion is controlled primarily by the renin-angiotensin system and by the circulating concentration of potassium. Thus, high serum potassium levels elicit secretion of aldosterone through a potent feedback system; similarly, hyponatremia, hypo-

volemia, and other disorders that provoke the release of renin stimulate aldosterone secretion.

This test identifies aldosteronism and, when supported by plasma renin levels, distinguishes between the primary and secondary forms of this disorder. Thus, it's helpful in identifying adrenal adenoma and adrenal hyperplasia, causes of primary aldosteronism. Secondary aldosteronism is commonly associated with salt depletion, potassium excess, congestive heart failure with ascites, or other conditions that increase activity of the renin-angiotensin system.

Purpose
- To aid diagnosis of primary and secondary aldosteronism, adrenal hyperplasia, hypoaldosteronism, and salt-losing syndrome.

Patient preparation
Explain to the patient that this test helps determine whether his symptoms are due to improper hormonal secretion. Instruct him to maintain a low-carbohydrate, normal-sodium diet for at least 2 weeks or, preferably, for 30 days before the test. Tell him that the test requires a blood sample and that he may feel some discomfort from the needle puncture. Advise him that the laboratory requires up to 5 days to complete the multistage analysis.

As ordered, withhold all drugs that alter fluid, sodium, and potassium balance — especially diuretics, antihypertensives, steroids, cyclic progestational agents, and estrogens — for at least 2 weeks or, preferably, for 30 days before the test. Also withhold all renin inhibitors (such as propranolol) for 1 week before the test. If these medications must be continued, note this on the laboratory request. Licorice produces an aldosterone-like effect and should be avoided for at least 2 weeks before the test.

Sites of adrenal hormone production

The adrenal glands are paired structures located retroperitoneally, one atop each kidney. Each gland consists of the cortex, composed of three layers, and the medulla. The outer layer of the cortex, the zona glomerulosa, produces aldosterone; the first inner layer, the zona fasciculata, produces cortisol; the next inner layer, the zona reticularis, secretes sex hormones (primarily androgens); and the medulla stores catecholamines (epinephrine and norepinephrine).

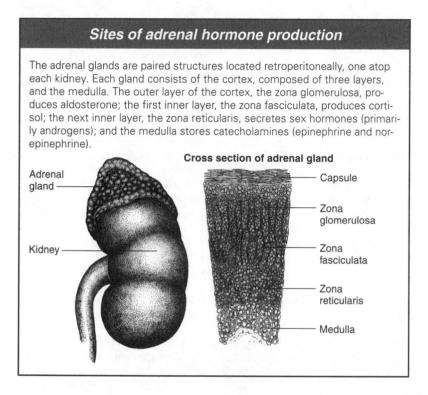

Cross section of adrenal gland

Adrenal gland

Kidney

Capsule

Zona glomerulosa

Zona fasciculata

Zona reticularis

Medulla

Procedure

While the patient is still supine after a night's rest, perform a venipuncture. Collect the sample in a 7-ml *red-top* collection tube, and send it to the laboratory. To evaluate the effect of postural change, draw another sample 4 hours later, after the patient has been up and about and while he is standing. Collect the second sample in a 7-ml *red-top* collection tube, and send it to the laboratory. Alternatively, a 24-hour urine collection may be used.

Precautions

■ Handle the sample gently to prevent hemolysis.

■ Record on the laboratory request whether the patient was supine or standing during the venipuncture. If the patient is a premenopausal female, specify the phase of her menstrual cycle be-

cause aldosterone levels may fluctuate during the menstrual cycle.

■ Send the specimen to the laboratory immediately.

Reference values

Normal serum aldosterone levels vary with age, as follows:

■ *0 to 3 weeks:* 16.5 to 154 ng/dl
■ *1 to 11 months:* 6.5 to 86 ng/dl
■ *1 to 10 years:* 3 to 39.5 ng/dl (supine); 3.5 to 124 ng/dl (upright)
■ *11 years and older:* 1 to 21 ng/dl.

Implications of results

Excessive aldosterone secretion may indicate a primary or secondary disease. Primary aldosteronism (Conn's syndrome) may result from adrenocortical adenoma or carcinoma or from bilateral adrenal hyperplasia. Secondary aldosteronism can result from renovascular hypertension, congestive heart failure, cirrhosis of the liver, nephrotic syndrome, idiopathic cyclic edema, or the third trimester of pregnancy.

Depressed serum aldosterone levels may indicate primary hypoaldosteronism, salt-losing syndrome, toxemia of pregnancy, or Addison's disease.

Post-test care
■ If a hematoma develops at the venipuncture site, apply warm soaks.
■ As ordered, resume diet and medications discontinued before the test.

Interfering factors
■ Hemolysis due to rough handling of the sample may interfere with accurate determination of test results.
■ Failure to observe restrictions of diet, medications, or posture may interfere with accurate determination of test results. Some antihypertensives, such as methyldopa, promote sodium and water retention and therefore may reduce aldosterone levels. Diuretics promote sodium excretion and may raise aldosterone levels. Some corticosteroids, such as fludrocortisone, mimic mineralocorticoid activity and therefore may lower aldosterone levels.
■ A radioactive scan performed within 1 week before the test may influence test results.

Plasma cortisol

Cortisol — the principal glucocorticoid secreted by the zona fasciculata of the adrenal cortex, primarily in response to adrenocorticotropic hormone (ACTH) stimulation — helps metabolize nutrients, mediate physiologic stress, and regulate the immune system. Cortisol secretion normally follows a diurnal pattern: Levels rise during the early morning hours and peak around 8 a.m., then decline to very low levels in the evening and during the early phase of sleep. (See *Diurnal variations in cortisol secretion,* page 172.) Production of this hormone is influenced by physical or emotional stress, which activates ACTH. Thus, intense heat or cold, infection, trauma, exercise, obesity, and debilitating disease influence cortisol secretion.

This radioimmunoassay, a quantitative analysis of plasma cortisol levels, is usually ordered for patients with signs of adrenal dysfunction, but dynamic tests, suppression tests for hyperfunction, and stimulation tests for hypofunction are generally required to confirm the diagnosis.

Purpose
■ To aid in the diagnosis of Cushing's disease, Cushing's syndrome, Addison's disease, and secondary adrenal insufficiency.

Patient preparation
Explain to the patient that this test helps determine if his symptoms are due to improper hormonal secretion. Instruct him to maintain a normal-sodium diet for 3 days before the test and to fast and limit physical activity for 10 to 12 hours before the test. Tell him a blood sample is required, who will perform the venipuncture and when, and that he may experience some discomfort from the needle puncture. Advise him that the laboratory requires at least 2 days to complete the analysis.

As ordered, withhold all medications that may interfere with plasma cortisol levels, such as estrogens, androgens, and phenytoin, for 48 hours before the test. If the patient is receiving replacement therapy and is dependent on exogenous steroids for survival, note this on the laboratory request as well as any other medications that must be continued.

Diurnal variations in cortisol secretion

Cortisol secretion rises in the early morning, peaking after the patient awakens. Levels decline sharply in the evening and during the early phase of sleep. They rise again during the night and peak by the next morning.

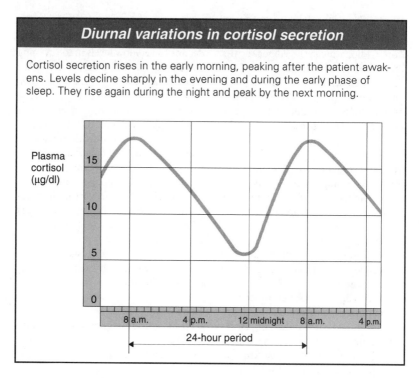

Plasma cortisol (µg/dl)

15 — 10 — 5 — 0

8 a.m.　　4 p.m.　　12 midnight　　8 a.m.　　4 p.m.

24-hour period

Make sure the patient is relaxed and recumbent for at least 30 minutes before the test.

Procedure

Between 6 and 8 a.m., perform a venipuncture. Collect the sample in a 7-ml *green-top* tube, label it appropriately, and send it to the laboratory immediately. For diurnal variation testing, draw another sample between 4 and 6 p.m. Collect it in a *green-top* tube, label it appropriately, and send it to the laboratory immediately.

Precautions
- Handle the sample gently to prevent hemolysis.
- Record the collection time on the laboratory request.

Reference values

Normally, plasma cortisol levels range from 7 to 28 µg/dl in the morning, and from 2 to 18 µg/dl in the afternoon. (The afternoon level is usually half the morning level.)

Implications of results

Increased plasma cortisol levels may indicate adrenocortical hyperfunction in Cushing's disease (a rare disease due to basophilic adenoma of the pituitary gland) or in Cushing's syndrome (glucocorticoid excess from any cause). In most patients with Cushing's syndrome, the adrenal cortex tends to secrete independently of any natural rhythm. Thus, absence of diurnal variations in cortisol secretion is a significant finding in almost all patients with Cushing's syndrome; in these patients, little difference in values, if any, is found between morning samples and those taken in the afternoon. Diurnal variations may also be absent in otherwise healthy persons who are under considerable emotional or physical stress.

Decreased cortisol levels may indicate primary adrenal hypofunction (Addison's disease), usually due to idiopathic glandular atrophy (a presumed autoimmune process). Tuberculosis, fungal invasion, and hemorrhage can cause adrenocortical destruction. Low cortisol levels resulting from secondary adrenal insufficiency may occur in conditions of impaired ACTH secretion, such as hypophysectomy, postpartum pituitary necrosis, craniopharyngioma, or chromophobe adenoma.

Post-test care

■ If a hematoma develops at the venipuncture site, apply warm soaks.

■ As ordered, resume diet and administration of medications that were discontinued before the test.

Interfering factors

■ Failure to observe restrictions of diet, medications, or physical activity may interfere with accurate determination of test results. Plasma cortisol levels are falsely elevated by estrogens (during pregnancy or in oral contraceptives), which increase plasma proteins that bind with cortisol. Obesity, stress, or severe hepatic or renal disease may also increase these levels. Plasma cortisol levels may be decreased by androgens and phenytoin, which decrease cortisol-binding proteins.

■ A radioactive scan performed within 1 week before the test may influence the results.

■ Hemolysis due to rough handling of the sample may interfere with accurate determination of test results.

Plasma catecholamines

This test, a quantitative (total or fractionated) analysis of plasma catecholamines, is clinically significant in patients with hypertension and signs of adrenal medullary tumor and in patients with neural tumors that affect endocrine function. Elevated plasma catecholamine levels necessitate supportive confirmation by urinalysis that shows catecholamine degradation products, such as vanillylmandelic acid and metanephrine.

Major catecholamines include the hormones epinephrine, norepinephrine, and dopamine (produced almost entirely in the brain, sympathetic nerve endings, and adrenal medulla). When secreted into the bloodstream, adrenal medullary catecholamines prepare the body for the fight-or-flight reaction: They increase heart rate and contractility, constrict blood vessels, redistribute circulating blood toward the skeletal and coronary muscles, mobilize carbohydrate and lipid reserves, and sharpen alertness. (See *Fight-or-flight reaction*, page 174.) These effects resemble those produced by direct stimulation of the sympathetic nervous system, but they're intensified and prolonged. Excessive catecholamine secretion by tumors causes hypertension, weight loss, episodic sweating, headache, palpitations, and anxiety.

Plasma levels commonly fluctuate in response to temperature, stress, postural change, diet, smoking, anoxia, volume depletion, renal failure, obesity, and use of certain drugs.

Purpose

■ To rule out pheochromocytoma (adrenal medullary or extra-adrenal) in patients with hypertension

Fight-or-flight reaction

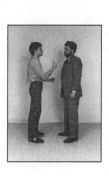 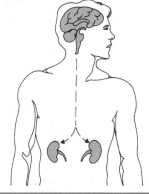

Stress — emotional or physical — initiates the transmission of nerve impulses by way of the sympathetic nervous system to the adrenal medullae.

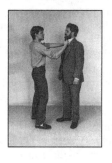 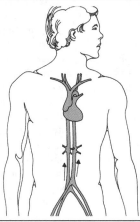

Nerve impulses cause the adrenal medullae to release catecholamines (primarily epinephrine and norepinephrine) into the bloodstream to prepare the body to react to stress (fight or flight).

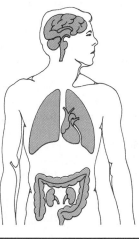

The fight-or-flight reaction is characterized by the following signs and symptoms:
- increased respiratory rate
- increased blood pressure, pulse rate, and cardiac output
- increased muscle strength
- increased blood supply to major organs (brain, heart, kidneys)
- decreased blood supply to periphery (skin) and intestines.

■ To identify neuroblastoma, ganglio-neuroblastoma, and ganglioneuroma

■ To aid diagnosis of autonomic nervous system dysfunction, such as idiopathic orthostatic hypotension

■ To distinguish between adrenal medullary tumors and other catecholamine-producing tumors through fractional analysis. (Urinalysis for catecholamine degradation products is recommended to support the diagnosis.)

Patient preparation

Explain that this test helps determine if hypertension or other symptoms are related to improper hormonal secretion. Advise the patient to strictly follow pretest instructions to ensure a reliable test result. Instruct him to refrain from using self-prescribed medications (especially cold or allergy remedies that may contain sympathomimetics) for 2 weeks, to exclude amine-rich foods and beverages (such as bananas, avocados, cheese, coffee, tea, cocoa, beer, and Chianti) from his diet for 48 hours, to maintain vitamin C intake (necessary for formation of catecholamines), to abstain from smoking for 24 hours, and to fast for 10 to 12 hours.

Tell the patient that this test requires one or two blood samples, who will perform the venipunctures and when, and that he may feel some discomfort from the needle punctures. Advise the patient that the laboratory requires up to 1 week to complete the analysis.

If the patient is hospitalized, withhold medications that affect catecholamine levels, such as amphetamines, phenothiazines, sympathomimetics, and tricyclic antidepressants, as ordered.

Also, insert an indwelling venous catheter (heparin lock) 24 hours before the test, as ordered. This may be needed because the stress of the venipuncture itself may significantly raise catecholamine levels. Make sure the patient is relaxed and recumbent for 45 to 60 minutes before the test. If necessary, provide blankets to keep him warm; low temperatures stimulate catecholamine secretion.

Procedure

Perform a venipuncture between 6 a.m. and 8 a.m. Collect the sample in a 10-ml chilled tube containing EDTA (sodium metabisulfite solution), which can be obtained from the laboratory on request. If a second sample is requested, have the patient stand for 10 minutes, and draw the sample into another tube exactly like the first. If a heparin lock is used, you may need to discard the first 1 or 2 ml of blood. Check with the laboratory for the preferred procedure.

Precautions

After collecting each sample, roll the tube slowly between your palms to distribute the EDTA without agitating the blood. Then pack the tube in crushed ice to minimize deactivation of catecholamines, and send it to the laboratory immediately. Indicate on the laboratory request whether the patient was supine or standing and the time the sample was drawn.

Reference values

In fractional analysis, catecholamine levels range as follows:

■ *supine:* epinephrine, undetectable to 110 pg/ml; norepinephrine, 70 to 750 pg/ml; dopamine, undetectable to 30 pg/ml

■ *standing:* epinephrine, undetectable to 140 pg/ml; norepinephrine, 200 to 1,700 pg/ml; dopamine, undetectable to 30 pg/ml.

Implications of results

High catecholamine levels may indicate pheochromocytoma, neuroblastoma, ganglioneuroblastoma, or ganglioneu-

---

Clonidine suppression test

This test aids in the differential diagnosis of pheochromocytoma and essential hypertension. It requires the administration of clonidine.

To perform the test, first place the patient in the supine position. Collect a blood sample to obtain baseline catecholamine levels, and then administer 0.3 mg of oral clonidine. Collect a blood sample after 3 hours to measure catecholamine levels again and to allow comparison of findings.

Patients with pheochromocytoma show no decrease in catecholamine levels after clonidine administration. In contrast, patients with essential hypertension have catecholamine levels in the normal range.

---

roma. (See *Clonidine suppression test.*) Elevations are possible with — but do not directly confirm — thyroid disorders, hypoglycemia, or cardiac disease. Electroconvulsive therapy or shock resulting from hemorrhage, endotoxins, or anaphylaxis also raises catecholamine levels.

In the patient with normal or low baseline catecholamine levels, failure to show an increase in the sample taken after standing suggests autonomic nervous system dysfunction.

Fractional analysis helps identify the cause of elevated catecholamine levels. For example, adrenal medullary tumors secrete epinephrine, whereas ganglioneuromas, ganglioblastomas, and neuroblastomas secrete norepinephrine.

Post-test care
■ If a hematoma develops at the venipuncture site, apply warm soaks to ease discomfort.
■ As ordered, resume normal diet and any medications discontinued before the test.

Interfering factors
■ Failure to observe pretest restrictions may interfere with test results.
■ Epinephrine, levodopa, amphetamines, phenothiazines, sympathomimetics, decongestants, and tricyclic antidepressants raise plasma catecholamine levels. Reserpine lowers them.
■ A radioactive scan performed within 1 week before the test may affect results.

Androstenedione

This test identifies the causes of disorders related to altered estrogen levels. Androstenedione, secreted by the adrenal cortex and the gonads, is converted to estrone (an estrogen of relatively low biological activity) by adipose tissue and the liver. In premenopausal women, the amount of estrogen derived from androstenedione is relatively small compared to the amount of estradiol, a more potent estrogen secreted by the ovaries. Usually, estrogen derived from androstenedione doesn't interfere with gonadotropin feedback during the menstrual cycle. But in obese patients, increased levels of estrone may interfere with normal feedback, causing menstrual irregularities.

In children and postmenopausal women, estrone is a major source of estrogen. Increased androstenedione production may induce premature sexual development in children. It may produce renewed ovarian stimulation, endometriosis, bleeding, and polycystic ovaries in postmenopausal women. In men, overproduction of androstenedione may cause feminizing signs, such as gynecomastia.

Purpose
■ To aid in determining the cause of gonadal dysfunction, menstrual or menopausal irregularities, and premature sexual development.

Patient preparation
Explain that this test determines the cause of symptoms. Tell the patient that the test requires a blood sample, who will perform the venipuncture and when, and that she may experience transient discomfort from the needle puncture. If appropriate, explain that the test should be done 1 week before or after her menstrual period and that it may be repeated. As ordered, withhold steroid and pituitary-based hormones before the test. If they must be continued, note this on the laboratory request.

Procedure
Perform a venipuncture, and collect a serum sample in a 10-ml *red-top* tube. (Collect a plasma sample in a *green-top* tube.) Label it appropriately and send it to the laboratory immediately.

Precautions
■ Handle the sample gently to prevent hemolysis. Refrigerate plasma samples or place them on ice.
■ Record the patient's age, sex, and (if appropriate) phase of menstrual cycle on the laboratory request.

Reference values
Normal values by radioimmunoassay for females ≥ 18 years are 0.2 to 3.1 ng/

ml; for males ≥ 18 years, 0.3 to 3.1 ng/ml. Children's values vary by age.

Implications of results
Elevated androstenedione levels are associated with Stein-Leventhal syndrome, Cushing's syndrome, ectopic tumors that produce adrenocorticotropic hormone, late-onset congenital adrenal hyperplasia, ovarian stromal hyperplasia, and ovarian, testicular, or adrenocortical tumors. Elevated levels result in increased estrone levels, causing premature sexual development in children; menstrual irregularities in premenopausal women; bleeding, endometriosis, or polycystic ovaries in postmenopausal women; and feminizing signs, such as gynecomastia, in men. Decreased levels occur in hypogonadism.

Post-test care
■ If a hematoma develops at the venipuncture site, apply warm soaks to ease discomfort.
■ As ordered, resume medications discontinued before the test.

Interfering factors
■ Hemolysis caused by rough handling of the sample may interfere with accurate determination of test results.
■ Ingestion of steroids or pituitary hormones may alter test results.

Erythropoietin

This test of renal hormone production measures erythropoietin by immunoassay. It's used to evaluate anemia, polycythemia, and kidney tumors. It's also used to evaluate abuse of commercially prepared erythropoietin by athletes who believe the drug enhances performance.

A glycoprotein hormone, erythropoietin is secreted by the liver of fetuses but by the kidneys in adults. The hormone acts on stem cells in the bone marrow to stimulate production of red blood cells. It's regulated by a feedback loop involving red cell volume and oxygen saturation of the blood, especially in the brain.

Purpose

■ To aid diagnosis of anemia and polycythemia
■ To aid diagnosis of kidney tumors
■ To detect abuse of erythropoietin by athletes.

Patient preparation

Explain to the patient that this test determines whether hormonal secretion is causing changes in his red blood cells. Instruct him to fast for 8 to 10 hours before the test. Tell him that this test requires a blood sample, who will perform the venipuncture and when, and that he may feel transient discomfort from the puncture. Advise him that the laboratory requires up to 4 days to complete the analysis. Keep the patient relaxed and recumbent for 30 minutes before the test.

Procedure

Perform a venipuncture, and collect the sample in a 5-ml *red-top* tube. If requested, a hematocrit may be performed at the same time by collecting an additional sample in a 2-ml *lavender-top* tube.

Precautions

Handle the specimen gently to prevent hemolysis.

Reference values

The normal range is up to 24 mU/ml.

Implications of results

Low levels of erythropoietin appear in anemic patients with inadequate or absent hormone production and may occur in severe renal disease. Congenital absence of erythropoietin also can occur.

Elevated levels occur in anemias as a compensatory mechanism in the reestablishment of homeostasis. Inappropriate elevations (when the hematocrit level is normal to high) are seen in polycythemia and erythropoietin-secreting tumors.

Erythropoietin can be produced for sale by recombinant gene technology and is used by some athletes as a performance enhancer. The increased red cell volume conveys additional oxygen-carrying capacity to the blood. Adverse reactions from such use may include clotting abnormalities, headache, seizures, hypertension, nausea, vomiting, diarrhea, and rash.

Post-test care

If a hematoma develops at the venipuncture site, apply warm soaks.

Interfering factors

■ Failure to collect a sample in the fasting state will affect test results.
■ Hemolysis may affect results.

Plasma atrial natriuretic factor

This radioimmunoassay measures the plasma level of atrial natriuretic factor (ANF), a vasoactive and natriuretic hormone that's secreted from the heart when expansion of blood volume stretches atrial tissue. An extremely potent natriuretic agent and vasodilator, ANF (also known as atrial natriuretic hormone, atrionatriuretic peptides, and atriopeptins) rapidly produces diuresis and increases the glomerular filtration rate.

ANF's role in regulating extracellular fluid volume, blood pressure, and sodium metabolism appears critical. It promotes sodium excretion, inhibits the renin-angiotensin system's effect on aldosterone secretion, and decreases atrial pressure by decreasing venous return, thereby reducing blood pressure and volume.

Researchers have found that patients with overt congestive heart failure (CHF) have highly elevated ANF levels. Patients with cardiovascular disease and elevated cardiac filling pressure, but without CHF, also have markedly elevated ANF levels. Recent findings support ANF as a possible marker for early asymptomatic left ventricular dysfunction and increased cardiac volume.

Purpose
▪ To confirm CHF
▪ To identify asymptomatic cardiac volume overload.

Patient preparation
As appropriate, explain the purpose of the test to the patient. Inform him that he must fast before the test. Tell him that this test requires a blood sample, who will perform the venipuncture and when, and that he may feel transient discomfort from the needle puncture. Advise him that the laboratory needs up to 4 days for analysis.

Check the patient history for use of medications that can influence test results. Withhold beta blockers, calcium antagonists, diuretics, vasodilators, and digitalis glycosides for 24 hours before sample collection.

Procedure
Perform a venipuncture, and collect the sample in a prechilled potassium-EDTA tube. After chilled centrifugation, the EDTA plasma should be promptly frozen and sent to the laboratory to be analyzed.

Precautions
▪ Handle the specimen gently to prevent hemolysis.
▪ Place the specimen on ice, and send it to the laboratory immediately.

Reference values
ANF levels normally range from 20 to 77 pg/ml.

Implications of results
Markedly elevated ANF levels are found in patients with frank CHF and significantly elevated cardiac filling pressure.

Post-test care
▪ If a hematoma develops at the venipuncture site, apply warm soaks.
▪ The patient may resume his normal diet and any medications discontinued before the test.

Interfering factors
Cardiovascular drugs, including beta blockers, calcium antagonists, diuretics, vasodilators, and digitalis glycosides, interfere with test results.

*P*ANCREATIC AND *G*ASTRIC *H*ORMONE *T*ESTS

Serum insulin

This radioimmunoassay is a quantitative analysis of serum insulin levels, which are usually measured concomitantly with glucose levels, since glucose

How the pancreas produces insulin

The pancreas is composed of an exocrine portion — acinar cells, which secrete digestive enzymes — and an endocrine portion — the islets of Langerhans, which secrete insulin and glucagon into the bloodstream in response to changes in blood glucose levels. The islets of Langerhans contain two principal types of cells — beta cells, which produce insulin when blood glucose increases, and alpha cells, which produce glucagon when blood glucose decreases. Splenic arteries transport oxygenated blood to the pancreas; mesenteric veins transport insulin and glucagon, contained in deoxygenated blood, from the pancreas.

Insulin lowers blood glucose levels by facilitating transport of glucose into cells and by increasing the conversion of glucose into liver and muscle glycogen; it also prevents breakdown of liver glycogen to yield glucose. Glucagon exerts the opposite effect.

Cross section of pancreas

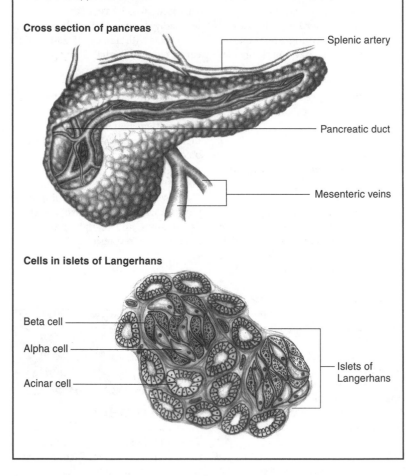

Splenic artery

Pancreatic duct

Mesenteric veins

Cells in islets of Langerhans

Beta cell

Alpha cell

Acinar cell

Islets of Langerhans

C-peptide assay

Connecting peptide (C-peptide) is a biologically inactive peptide chain formed during the proteolytic conversion of proinsulin to insulin in the pancreatic beta cells. It has no insulin effect, either biologically or immunologically. This is important because circulating insulin is measured by immunologic assay. As insulin is released into the bloodstream, the C-peptide chain splits off from the hormone. Except in patients with islet cell tumors and, possibly, in obese patients, serum C-peptide levels generally parallel those of insulin (normal vales range between 0.9 and 4.2 ng/ml).

A C-peptide assay may help to:
- determine the cause of hypoglycemia by distinguishing between endogenous hyperinsulinism or insulinoma (elevated C-peptide levels) and surreptitious insulin injection (decreased C-peptide levels)
- indirectly measure insulin secretion in the presence of circulating insulin antibodies, which interfere with insulin assays but not with C-peptide assays
- detect residual tissue (some C-peptide present) after total pancreatectomy for carcinoma
- indicate the remission phase (some C-peptide present) of diabetes mellitus
- determine beta-cell function in patients with diabetes mellitus. (Absence of C-peptide indicates no beta-cell function; presence indicates residual beta-cell function.)

is the primary stimulus for insulin release from pancreatic islet cells. (See *How the pancreas produces insulin.*) The test helps evaluate patients suspected of having hyperinsulinemia due to pancreatic tumor or hyperplasia.

Insulin, a hormone secreted by beta cells of the islets of Langerhans, regulates the metabolism and transport or mobilization of carbohydrates, amino acids, proteins, and lipids. Stimulated by increased plasma levels of glucose, insulin secretion reaches peak levels after meals, when metabolism and food storage are greatest. Insulin insufficiency or resistance is the primary abnormality in diabetes mellitus.

Purpose
- To aid diagnosis of hypoglycemia resulting from tumor or hyperplasia of pancreatic islet cells, glucocorticoid deficiency, or severe hepatic disease
- To aid diagnosis of diabetes mellitus

and insulin-resistant states. (For information on a related test, see *C-peptide assay.*)

Patient preparation
Explain that this test helps determine if the pancreas is functioning normally. Instruct the patient to fast for 10 to 12 hours before the test. (Questionable results may require a repeat test or, frequently, a simultaneous glucose tolerance test, which requires the patient to drink glucose solution.) Tell him that the test requires blood samples, who will perform the venipunctures and when, and that he may feel discomfort from the needle.

As ordered, withhold adrenocorticotropic hormone (ACTH), steroids (including oral contraceptives), thyroid supplements, epinephrine, and other medications that may interfere with test results. If they must be continued, note this on the laboratory request.

Make sure the patient is relaxed and recumbent for 30 minutes before the test.

Procedure

Perform a venipuncture; collect one sample for insulin testing in a 7-ml *lavender-top* tube; then collect a sample for glucose testing in a *gray-top* tube, if requested.

Precautions

■ Make sure that the patient is relaxed before sample collection because agitation or stress may affect insulin levels.
■ Pack the sample for insulin testing in ice, and immediately send it, along with the glucose sample, to the laboratory.

 ■ In the patient with an insulinoma, fasting for this test may precipitate dangerously severe hypoglycemia. Keep glucose I.V. (50%) available to combat this reaction.
■ Handle the sample gently.

Reference values

Serum insulin levels normally range from 0 to 25 µU/ml.

Implications of results

Insulin levels are interpreted in light of the glucose concentration. A normal insulin level may be inappropriate for the glucose results. High insulin and low glucose levels after a significant fast suggest an insulinoma. Prolonged fasting or stimulation testing may be required to confirm the diagnosis. In insulin-resistant diabetic states, insulin levels are elevated; in non-insulin-resistant diabetes, they are low.

Post-test care

■ If a hematoma develops at the venipuncture site, apply warm soaks.
■ Resume diet and medications discontinued before the test, as ordered.

Interfering factors

■ Failure to observe restrictions of diet and activity may affect test results.
■ Use of ACTH, steroids (including oral contraceptives), thyroid hormones, or epinephrine may raise serum insulin levels.
■ Use of insulin by non-insulin-dependent patients may lower levels.
■ In patients with insulin-dependent diabetes mellitus, high levels of insulin antibodies may interfere with the test.
■ Failure to pack the insulin sample in ice and send it to the laboratory promptly may affect test results.
■ Hemolysis due to rough handling of the sample may alter test results.

Plasma glucagon

Glucagon, a polypeptide hormone secreted by the alpha cells of the islets of Langerhans in the pancreas, acts primarily on the liver to promote glucose production and control glucose storage. Glucagon is secreted in response to hypoglycemia; secretion is inhibited by the other pancreatic hormones, insulin and somatostatin. Normally, the coordinated release of glucagon, insulin, and somatostatin ensures an adequate and constant fuel supply while maintaining blood glucose levels within relatively stable limits.

This test, a quantitative analysis of plasma glucagon by radioimmunoassay, evaluates patients suspected of having glucagonoma (alpha cell tumor) or hypoglycemia due to idiopathic glucagon deficiency or pancreatic dysfunction. Glucagon is usually measured concomitantly with serum glucose and insulin because glucose and insulin levels influence glucagon secretion.

Purpose
- To aid diagnosis of glucagonoma and hypoglycemia due to chronic pancreatitis or idiopathic glucagon deficiency.

Patient preparation
Explain to the patient that this test helps evaluate pancreatic function. Instruct him to fast for 10 to 12 hours before the test. Tell him that the test requires a blood sample, who will perform the venipuncture and when, and that he may feel transient discomfort from the needle puncture.

As ordered, withhold insulin, catecholamines, and other drugs that could influence test results. If these drugs must be continued, note this on the laboratory request.

Since exercise and stress elevate serum glucagon levels, make sure the patient is relaxed and recumbent for 30 minutes before the test.

Procedure
Perform a venipuncture, and collect a blood sample in a chilled 10-ml *lavender-top* tube.

Precautions
- Make sure the patient is relaxed before sample collection because stress may elevate glucagon levels.
- Place the sample on ice and send it to the laboratory immediately.
- Handle the sample gently to prevent hemolysis.

Reference values
Fasting glucagon levels are normally less than 250 pg/ml.

Implications of results
Markedly elevated fasting glucagon levels (900 to 7,800 pg/ml) occur in glucagonoma. Elevated levels also occur in diabetes mellitus, acute pancreatitis, and pheochromocytoma.

Abnormally low glucagon levels are associated with idiopathic glucagon deficiency and hypoglycemia due to chronic pancreatitis. Stimulation or suppression tests may be necessary to confirm the diagnosis.

Post-test care
- If a hematoma develops at the venipuncture site, apply warm soaks.
- As ordered, resume diet and medications discontinued before the test.

Interfering factors
- Prolonged fasting, undue stress, or use of catecholamines or insulin before sample collection may elevate glucagon levels.
- Failure to pack the sample in ice and send it to the laboratory immediately may affect test results.
- Hemolysis due to rough handling of the sample may alter test results.

Serum gastrin

Gastrin is a polypeptide hormone produced and stored primarily by specialized G cells in the antrum of the stomach and, to a lesser degree, by the islets of Langerhans in the pancreas. The main function of gastrin is to facilitate digestion of food by triggering gastric acid secretion in the parietal area of the stomach in response to food (especially proteins), vagal stimulation, or decreased stomach acidity. Secondarily, gastrin stimulates the release of pancreatic enzymes and the gastric enzyme pepsin, increases gastric and intestinal motility, and stimulates bile flow from the liver.

Through a strong negative feedback control mechanism, acid in the gastric antrum inhibits gastrin release in re-

Gastrin stimulation tests

Since some patients with duodenal or gastric ulcers have normal fasting gastrin levels, provocative testing is necessary to identify them; a protein-rich test meal serves this purpose. In a patient with duodenal or gastric ulcers, gastrin levels increase markedly after such a meal; in a healthy person, they rise only moderately.

Provocative testing is also necessary to distinguish a patient with duodenal or gastric ulcers from one suspected of having Zollinger-Ellison syndrome, since both may show similar baseline gastrin levels. One effective test involves I.V. infusion of calcium gluconate in a dosage of 5 mg/kg of body weight over 3 hours. After the infusion, 10 ml of venous blood is drawn and sent to the laboratory. In a patient with Zollinger-Ellison syndrome, gastrin levels double, rising to about 500 pg/ml; in a patient with duodenal or gastric ulcers, levels rise only moderately or don't change at all.

A third indication for provocative testing is an abnormally — but not strikingly — high fasting serum gastrin level. This is possible in both Zollinger-Ellison syndrome and in pernicious anemia. To distinguish between the two, hydrochloric acid may be infused into the stomach through a nasogastric tube. Such infusion causes a sharp drop in gastrin levels in patients with pernicious anemia but not in patients with Zollinger-Ellison syndrome.

sponse to all stimuli. However, abnormal secretion of gastrin can result from tumors (gastrinomas) and from pathologic disorders affecting the stomach, pancreas and, less commonly, the esophagus and small bowel.

This radioimmunoassay, a quantitative analysis of gastrin levels, is diagnostically significant in patients suspected of having gastrinomas (Zollinger-Ellison syndrome). In doubtful situations, provocative testing may be necessary. However, gastrin estimation has limited value in persons with duodenal ulcer because the role of gastrin in peptic ulcers is unclear.

Purpose

■ To confirm diagnosis of gastrinoma, the gastrin-secreting tumor in Zollinger-Ellison syndrome
■ To aid differential diagnosis of gastric and duodenal ulcers and pernicious anemia. (See *Gastrin stimulation tests*.)

Patient preparation

Explain to the patient that this test helps determine the cause of his GI symptoms. Instruct him to abstain from alcohol for at least 24 hours before the test and to fast for 12 hours before it (water is permitted). Tell him the test requires a blood sample, who will perform the venipuncture and when, and that he may feel some transient discomfort from the needle puncture.

As ordered, withhold all medications that may interfere with test results, especially anticholinergics (such as atropine and belladonna) and insulin. If these medications must be continued, note this on the laboratory request.

Because stress can increase gastrin levels, make sure the patient is relaxed and recumbent for at least 30 minutes before the test.

Procedure

Perform a venipuncture, and collect the sample in a 10- to 15-ml *red-top* tube.

Precautions

■ Handle the sample gently to avoid hemolysis.

■ To prevent destruction of serum gastrin by proteolytic enzymes, send the sample to the laboratory immediately to have the serum separated and frozen.

Reference values

Normal serum gastrin levels are less than 300 pg/ml.

Implications of results

Strikingly high serum gastrin levels (over 1,000 pg/ml) confirm Zollinger-Ellison syndrome. (Levels as high as 450,000 pg/ml have been reported.)

Gastrin levels may be high in various conditions, but the concomitant findings of very low gastric juice pH and a very high serum gastrin level indicate autonomous hormone secretion not governed by a negative feedback mechanism. Increased serum levels of gastrin may occur in a few patients with duodenal ulceration (less than 1%) and in patients with achlorhydria (with or without pernicious anemia) or with extensive stomach carcinoma (because of hyposecretion of gastric juices and hydrochloric acid).

Post-test care

■ If a hematoma develops at the venipuncture site, apply warm soaks.

■ As ordered, resume diet and medications that were discontinued before the test.

Interfering factors

■ Failure to observe restrictions of diet, medications, or physical activity may interfere with accurate determination of test results.

■ Gastrin secretion is increased by amino acids (especially glycine), calcium carbonate, acetylcholine, calcium chloride, and ethanol; gastrin secretion is decreased by anticholinergics (atropine), hydrochloric acid, and secretin (a strongly basic polypeptide).

■ Insulin-induced hypoglycemia increases gastrin secretion.

■ Hemolysis caused by rough handling of the sample may interfere with accurate determination of test results.

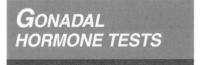

GONADAL HORMONE TESTS

Serum estrogens

Estrogens (and progesterone) are secreted by the ovaries under the influence of the pituitary gonadotropins, follicle-stimulating hormone (FSH) and luteinizing hormone (LH). Estrogens — in particular, estradiol, the most potent estrogen — interact with the hypothalamic-pituitary axis through both negative and positive feedback mechanisms. Slowly rising or sustained high levels inhibit secretion of FSH and LH (negative feedback), but a rapid rise in estrogen just before ovulation seems to stimulate LH secretion (positive feedback).

Estrogens are responsible for the development of secondary female sexual characteristics and for normal menstruation; levels are usually undetectable in children. These hormones are secreted by ovarian follicular cells during the first half of the menstrual cycle and by the corpus luteum during the luteal phase and during pregnancy. In menopause, estrogen secretion drops to a constantly low level.

Estriol: Clue to fetal well-being

Estriol represents about 90% of the estrogen produced during pregnancy after 20 weeks' gestation. The placenta converts fetal adrenal precursors into estriol, which is then conjugated by the maternal liver and excreted in maternal urine. Because estriol production depends on the fetus and placenta, levels serve as an index of fetal well-being and placental adequacy.

Disagreement exists as to the merits of measuring total plasma estriol, plasma unconjugated estriol (about 10% to 15% of total plasma estriol), or urine estriol. However, plasma estriol has several advantages over urine estriol: Samples don't have to be collected at specific times, and they're less affected by medications. Of the plasma samples, unconjugated estriol appears to be preferred because it's easier to analyze in the laboratory. Despite these differences, all three types of samples are used to assess placental function and fetal well-being.

This radioimmunoassay, which measures serum levels of estradiol, estrone, and estriol (the only estrogens that appear in serum in measurable amounts) has diagnostic significance in evaluating female gonadal dysfunction. (See *Estriol: Clue to fetal well-being.*) Tests of hypothalamic-pituitary function may be required to confirm the diagnosis.

Purpose
■ To determine sexual maturation and fertility
■ To aid diagnosis of gonadal dysfunction, such as precocious or delayed puberty, menstrual disorders (especially amenorrhea), or infertility
■ To determine fetal well-being
■ To aid diagnosis of tumors known to secrete estrogen.

Patient preparation
Explain to the patient that this test helps determine if secretion of female hormones is normal and may be repeated during various phases of the menstrual cycle. Tell her she needn't restrict food or fluids. Inform her that the test requires a blood sample, who will perform the venipuncture and when, and that she may experience transient discomfort from the needle puncture.

Withhold all steroid and pituitary-based hormones (including estrogens and progestogen), as ordered. If these medications must be continued, note this on the laboratory request.

Procedure
Perform a venipuncture, and collect the sample in a 10-ml *red-top* tube. If the patient is premenopausal, indicate the phase of her menstrual cycle on the laboratory request.

Precautions
To prevent hemolysis, handle the sample gently. Send it to the laboratory immediately for centrifugation.

Reference values
Normal serum estrogen levels for premenopausal females vary widely during the menstrual cycle, as follows:
■ *1 to 10 days:* 24 to 68 pg/ml
■ *11 to 20 days:* 50 to 186 pg/ml
■ *21 to 30 days:* 73 to 149 pg/ml.

Serum estrogen levels in males range from 12 to 34 pg/ml. In girls age 6 and older, levels rise gradually to adult female values. In children under age 6, the normal range is 3 to 10 pg/ml.

Implications of results

Decreased estrogen levels may indicate primary hypogonadism or ovarian failure, as in Turner's syndrome or ovarian agenesis; secondary hypogonadism, as in hypopituitarism; or menopause. Abnormally high levels can occur with estrogen-producing tumors, in precocious puberty, or in severe hepatic disease, such as cirrhosis, that prevents clearance of plasma estrogens. High levels may also result from congenital adrenal hyperplasia (increased conversion of androgens to estrogen).

Post-test care

■ If a hematoma develops at the venipuncture site, apply warm soaks.
■ As ordered, resume administration of medications discontinued before the test.

Interfering factors

■ Pregnancy and pretest use of estrogens (oral contraceptives) can increase serum estrogen levels. Clomiphene, an estrogen antagonist, can decrease serum estrogen levels. Ingestion of steroids or pituitary-based hormones can alter test results. For example, dexamethasone may suppress adrenal androgen secretion.
■ Hemolysis caused by rough handling of the sample may interfere with accurate determination of test results.

Plasma progesterone

Progesterone, an ovarian steroid hormone secreted by the corpus luteum, causes thickening and secretory development of the endometrium in preparation for implantation of the fertilized ovum. Progesterone levels, therefore, peak during the midluteal phase of the menstrual cycle. Progesterone may prolong the surge of luteinizing hormone after ovulation. If implantation doesn't occur, progesterone (and estrogen) levels drop sharply and menstruation begins about 2 days later. (See *The endometrial cycle,* page 188.)

During pregnancy, the placenta releases about 10 times the normal monthly amount of progesterone to maintain the pregnancy. Increased secretion begins toward the end of the first trimester and continues until delivery. Progesterone causes thickening of the endometrium, which contains large amounts of stored nutrients for the developing ovum (blastocyst). In addition, progesterone prevents abortion by decreasing uterine contractions and, with estrogen, prepares the breasts for lactation.

This radioimmunoassay is a quantitative analysis of plasma progesterone levels. It provides reliable information about corpus luteum function in fertility studies or placental function in pregnancy. Serial determinations are recommended. Although plasma levels provide accurate information, progesterone can also be monitored by measuring urine pregnanediol, a catabolite of progesterone.

Purpose

■ To assess corpus luteum function as part of infertility studies
■ To evaluate placental function during pregnancy
■ To aid in confirming ovulation. Test results support basal body temperature readings.

Patient preparation

Explain to the patient that this test helps determine if her female sex hormone secretion is normal. Inform her that she

The endometrial cycle

Each month progesterone, released by the corpus luteum, stimulates endometrial thickening in preparation for implantation of a fertilized ovum. The endometrial layer contains nutrients necessary for growth of the blastocyst. Immediately after menstruation, in the proliferative phase, the endometrium is thin and relatively homogenous. It continuously thickens until the end of the secretory phase, just before the menstrual phase begins again.

Menstrual	Proliferative	Secretory	Menstrual

Days 1 2 3 4 5 6 7 8 9 10 11 12 13 14 15 16 17 18 19 20 21 22 23 24 25 26 27 28 1 2 3 4 5 →

needn't restrict food or fluids. Tell her the test requires a blood sample, who will perform the venipuncture and when, and that she may experience transient discomfort from the needle puncture. Inform her that the test may be repeated at specific times coinciding with phases of her menstrual cycle or at each prenatal visit.

Procedure
Perform a venipuncture, and collect the sample in a 7-ml *green-top* (heparinized) tube.

Precautions
■ Handle the sample gently to prevent hemolysis.
■ Completely fill the collection tube; then invert it gently at least 10 times to mix sample and anticoagulant adequately.
■ Indicate the date of the patient's last menstrual period and the phase of her cycle on the laboratory request. If the patient is pregnant, indicate the month of gestation.
■ Send the sample to the laboratory immediately.

Reference values
Normal values during menstruation are:
■ *follicular phase:* less than 150 ng/dl
■ *luteal phase:* about 300 ng/dl (rises daily during periovulation)
■ *midluteal phase:* 2,000 ng/dl.
  Normal values during pregnancy are:
■ *first trimester:* 1,500 to 5,000 ng/dl
■ *second and third trimesters:* 8,000 to 20,000 ng/dl.

Implications of results

Elevated progesterone levels may indicate ovulation, luteinizing tumors, ovarian cysts that produce progesterone, or adrenocortical hyperplasias and tumors that produce progesterone along with other steroidal hormones.

Low progesterone levels are associated with amenorrhea due to several causes (such as panhypopituitarism or gonadal dysfunction), toxemia of pregnancy, threatened abortion, and fetal death.

Post-test care

If a hematoma develops at the venipuncture site, apply warm soaks.

Interfering factors

■ Hemolysis caused by rough handling of the sample may affect test results.
■ Progesterone or estrogen therapy may interfere with test results.
■ Use of radioisotopes or scans within 1 week of the test may affect test results.

Testosterone

The principal androgen secreted by the interstitial cells of the testes (Leydig cells), testosterone induces puberty in the male and maintains male secondary sex characteristics. (See *Sites of testosterone secretion*, page 190.) Prepubertal levels of testosterone are low. Increased testosterone secretion during puberty stimulates growth of the seminiferous tubules and the production of sperm; it also contributes to the enlargement of external genitalia, accessory sex organs (such as prostate glands), and voluntary muscles as well as to the growth of facial, pubic, and axillary hair.

Testosterone production begins to increase at the onset of puberty, under the influence of luteinizing hormone (LH)

from the anterior pituitary, and continues to rise during adulthood. Testosterone inhibits gonadotropin secretion by a negative feedback mechanism similar to that of ovarian hormones in females. Production begins to taper off at about age 40, eventually dropping to approximately one fifth the peak level by age 80. In females, the adrenal glands and the ovaries secrete small amounts of testosterone.

This competitive protein-binding test measures plasma or serum testosterone levels. When combined with plasma gonadotropin levels (follicle-stimulating hormone and LH), it reliably aids evaluation of gonadal dysfunction in males and females.

Purpose

■ To evaluate male infertility or other sexual dysfunction
■ To facilitate differential diagnosis of male sexual precocity (before age 10). True precocious puberty must be distinguished from pseudoprecocious puberty.
■ To aid differential diagnosis of hypogonadism. Primary hypogonadism must be distinguished from secondary hypogonadism.
■ To evaluate hirsutism and virilization in females.

Patient preparation

Explain to the patient that this test helps determine if male sex hormone production is adequate. Inform him that he needn't restrict food or fluids. Tell him this test requires a blood sample, who will perform the venipuncture and when, and that he may experience some discomfort from the needle puncture.

Procedure

Perform a venipuncture, and collect the sample in a 7-ml *red-top* tube. Use a *green-top* (heparinized) tube if plasma is to be collected. Indicate the patient's

Sites of testosterone secretion

In the testis, several hundred pyramid-shaped lobules contain one or several seminiferous tubules. Within the tissue connecting the tubules, large polygonal Leydig cells secrete testosterone, the most potent androgenic hormone.

Cross section of a testis

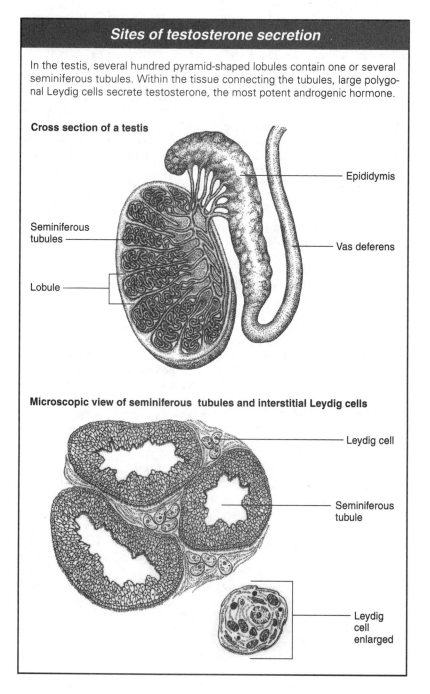

Seminiferous tubules

Lobule

Epididymis

Vas deferens

Microscopic view of seminiferous tubules and interstitial Leydig cells

Leydig cell

Seminiferous tubule

Leydig cell enlarged

Sex hormone–binding globulin

This radioimmunoassay measures levels of sex hormone–binding globulin (SHBG), also known as testosterone-binding globulin. It helps to evaluate conditions related to sex hormone levels and requires no special procedure. Note the patient's sex on the laboratory request.

Normal SHBG values are 8 to 49 mmol/L for males and 20 to 106 mmol/L for females. Androgenizing disorders and adrenal problems can cause decreased SHBG values. Increased levels occur in women with hyperthyroidism and in those receiving estrogen.

age, sex, and history of hormone therapy on the laboratory request.

Precautions

Handle the sample gently to prevent hemolysis, and send it to the laboratory. The sample is stable and requires no refrigeration or preservative for up to 1 week. Frozen samples are stable for at least 6 months.

Reference values

Normal levels of testosterone are as follows (laboratory values vary slightly):
- *males:* 300 to 1,200 ng/dl
- *females:* 30 to 95 ng/dl
- *prepubertal children:* in boys, less than 100 ng/dl; in girls, less than 40 ng/dl.

Implications of results

Elevated testosterone levels in prepubertal males may indicate true sexual precocity due to excessive gonadotropin secretion or pseudoprecocious puberty due to male hormone production by a testicular tumor. They can also indicate congenital adrenal hyperplasia, which results in precocious puberty in males (from ages 2 to 3) and pseudohermaphroditism and milder virilization of females. Increased levels can occur with a benign or malignant adrenal tumor, hyperthyroidism, or incipient puberty. In females with ovarian tumors or poly-

cystic ovarian syndrome, testosterone levels may rise, leading to hirsutism.

Depressed testosterone levels can indicate primary hypogonadism (as in Klinefelter's syndrome) or secondary hypogonadism (hypogonadotropic eunuchoidism) from hypothalamic-pituitary dysfunction. Depressed testosterone levels can also follow orchiectomy, testicular or prostatic cancer, delayed male puberty, estrogen therapy, or cirrhosis.

Post-test care

If a hematoma develops at the venipuncture site, apply warm soaks.

Interfering factors

- Exogenous sources of estrogens or androgens, thyroid and growth hormones, and other pituitary-based hormones may interfere with test results. Estrogens decrease free testosterone levels by increasing sex hormone–binding globulin, which binds testosterone; androgens can elevate these levels. (See *Sex hormone–binding globulin.*)
- Hemolysis may affect test results.

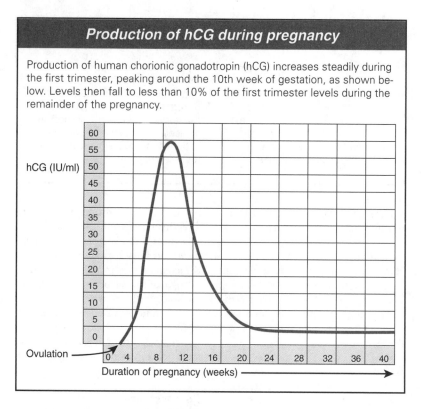

Production of hCG during pregnancy

Production of human chorionic gonadotropin (hCG) increases steadily during the first trimester, peaking around the 10th week of gestation, as shown below. Levels then fall to less than 10% of the first trimester levels during the remainder of the pregnancy.

hCG (IU/ml)

Ovulation

Duration of pregnancy (weeks)

PLACENTAL HORMONE TESTS

Serum human chorionic gonadotropin

Human chorionic gonadotropin (hCG) is a glycoprotein hormone produced by the trophoblastic cells (probably the syncytiotrophoblasts) of the placenta. If conception occurs, a specific assay for hCG — commonly known as the beta-subunit assay — may detect this hormone in the blood 9 days after ovulation. This interval coincides with the implantation of the fertilized ovum into the uterine wall. Although the precise function of this hormone is still unclear, it appears that hCG, with progesterone, maintains the corpus luteum during early pregnancy. Production of hCG increases steadily during the first trimester, peaking around the 10th week of gestation. Levels then fall to less than 10% of first trimester peak levels during the remainder of the pregnancy. At approximately 2 weeks after delivery, the hormone may no longer be detectable. (See *Production of hCG during pregnancy* and *Site of hCG secretion.*)

This serum immunoassay, a quantitative analysis of the hCG beta-subunit level, is more sensitive (and costly) than the routine pregnancy test using a urine specimen.

Site of hCG secretion

Nine days after ovulation, the trophoblastic cells of the blastocyst begin secreting human chorionic gonadotropin (hCG). Under the influence of hCG, the corpus luteum secretes increasing amounts of estrogen and progesterone—vital for a successful pregnancy. The trophoblastic cells develop into the chorionic villi of the placenta and continue secreting hCG. Levels of hCG peak during the 10th week of gestation.

Female reproductive system

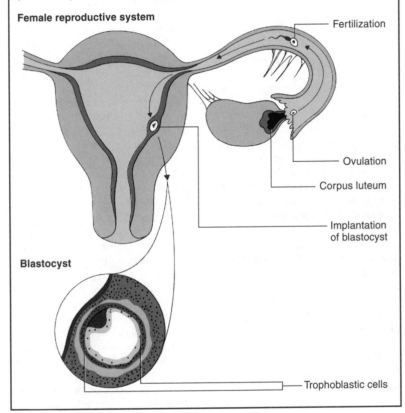

Fertilization

Ovulation

Corpus luteum

Implantation of blastocyst

Blastocyst

Trophoblastic cells

Purpose
■ To detect early pregnancy
■ To determine the adequacy of hormone production in high-risk pregnancies (for example, habitual abortion)
■ To aid diagnosis of trophoplastic tumors, such as hydatidiform mole or choriocarcinoma, and of tumors that ectopically secrete hCG
■ To monitor treatment for induction of ovulation and conception.

Patient preparation
Explain to the patient that this test determines if she is pregnant. (If detection of pregnancy isn't the diagnostic objective, offer the appropriate explanation.) Inform her she needn't restrict food or fluids. Tell her the test requires a blood sample, who will perform the venipuncture and when, and that she may feel transient discomfort from the needle puncture.

Procedure

Perform a venipuncture, and collect the sample in a 7-ml *red-top* tube.

Precautions

Handle the sample gently to prevent hemolysis, and send it to the laboratory immediately.

Reference values

Normal values for hCG are less than 4 IU/L. During pregnancy, hCG levels are quite variable and depend partially on the number of days after the last normal menstrual period.

Implications of results

Elevated hCG beta-subunit levels indicate pregnancy; significantly higher concentrations are present in a multiple pregnancy. Increased levels may also suggest hydatidiform mole, trophoblastic neoplasm of the placenta, or nontrophoblastic carcinomas that secrete hCG (including gastric, pancreatic, and ovarian adenocarcinomas). Beta-subunit levels cannot differentiate between pregnancy and tumor recurrence because levels are high in both conditions.

Low hCG beta-subunit levels can occur in ectopic pregnancy or pregnancy of less than 9 days.

Post-test care

If a hematoma develops at the venipuncture site, apply warm soaks.

Interfering factors

▪ Heparin anticoagulants and EDTA depress plasma hCG levels and may alter test results. Check with the laboratory to find out if the test is to be performed on plasma or serum.

▪ Hemolysis due to rough handling of the sample may affect test results.

Serum human placental lactogen

A polypeptide hormone secreted by placental syncytial trophoblasts, human placental lactogen (hPL) displays lactogenic and somatotropic (growth hormone) properties in the pregnant female. In combination with prolactin, hPL (also known as human chorionic somatomammotropin) prepares the breasts for lactation. It also promotes lipolysis, liberating free fatty acids to provide energy for maternal metabolism and fetal nutrition.

By exerting an anti-insulin effect, hPL causes the pancreas to secrete more insulin in response to rising blood sugar levels, thus facilitating protein synthesis and mobilization essential to fetal growth. Secretion is autonomous, beginning about the fifth week of gestation and declining rapidly after delivery. According to some evidence, this hormone may not be essential for a successful pregnancy.

This radioimmunoassay measures serum hPL levels, which are roughly proportional to placental mass, as evidenced by higher levels in a multiple pregnancy. Such assays may be required in high-risk pregnancies (patients with diabetes mellitus, hypertension, or toxemia) or in suspected placental tissue dysfunction. Because values vary widely during the last half of pregnancy, serial determinations over several days provide the most reliable test results. This test, when combined with measurement of estriol levels, is a reliable indicator of placental function and fetal well-being. It may also be useful as a tumor marker in certain malignant states, such as ectopic tumors that secrete hPL.

Purpose

- To assess placental function
- To aid diagnosis and monitor treatment of nontrophoblastic tumors that ectopically secrete hPL
- To aid diagnosis of hydatidiform mole and choriocarcinoma. (However, human chorionic gonadotropin levels are more diagnostic in these conditions.)

Patient preparation

Explain to the patient that this test helps assess placental function and fetal well-being. (If assessing fetal well-being isn't the diagnostic objective, offer an appropriate explanation.) Tell her the test requires a blood sample, who will perform the venipuncture and when, and that she may experience transient discomfort from the needle puncture. Inform the pregnant patient that this test may be repeated during her pregnancy.

Procedure

Perform a venipuncture, and collect the sample in a 7-ml *red-top* tube.

Precautions

Handle the sample gently to prevent hemolysis, and send it to the laboratory without delay.

Reference values

For pregnant females, normal hPL values vary with gestational age:
- *5 to 27 weeks:* < 4.6 µg/ml
- *28 to 31 weeks:* 2.4 to 6.1 µg/ml
- *32 to 35 weeks:* 3.7 to 7.7 µg/ml
- *36 weeks to term:* 5.0 to 8.6 µg/ml.

At term, diabetic patients may have mean levels of 9 to 11 µg/ml.

Normal levels for nonpregnant females are < 0.5 µg/ml; for males, < 0.5 µg/ml.

Implications of results

For reliable interpretation, hPL levels must be correlated with gestational age;

for example, after 30 weeks' gestation, levels below 4 µg/ml may indicate placental dysfunction. Subnormal hPL levels are also associated with trophoblastic neoplastic disease, such as hydatidiform mole or choriocarcinoma, and with postmaturity syndrome, intrauterine growth retardation, and toxemia of pregnancy. Although low hPL concentrations don't confirm fetal distress, they may help differentiate incomplete abortion from threatened abortion.

Conversely, hPL levels over 4 µg/ml after 30 weeks' gestation don't guarantee fetal well-being, since elevated levels have been reported after fetal death. An hPL value above 6 µg/ml after 30 weeks' gestation may suggest an unusually large placenta, which commonly occurs in patients with diabetes mellitus, multiple pregnancy, or Rh isoimmunization. Nevertheless, this test has limited use in predicting fetal death in a patient with diabetes or in managing Rh isoimmunization during pregnancy.

Abnormal concentrations of hPL have been found in the sera of patients with various types of cancer, including bronchogenic carcinoma, hepatoma, lymphoma, and pheochromocytoma. In these patients, hPL levels are used as tumor markers to evaluate chemotherapy, to monitor tumor growth and recurrence, and to detect residual tissue after excision.

Post-test care

If a hematoma develops at the venipuncture site, ease discomfort by applying warm soaks.

Interfering factors

Hemolysis caused by rough handling of the sample may alter test results.

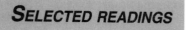

Behrman, R.E., et al., eds. *Nelson Textbook of Pediatrics,* 15th ed. Philadelphia: W.B. Saunders Co., 1996.

Bennett, J.C., and Plum, F., eds. *Cecil Textbook of Medicine,* 20th ed. Philadelphia: W.B. Saunders Co., 1996.

Cunningham, F.G., et al. *Williams Obstetrics,* 19th ed. Stamford, Conn.: Appleton & Lange, 1993.

Fischbach, F. *A Manual of Laboratory and Diagnostic Tests,* 5th ed. Philadelphia: Lippincott-Raven Pubs., 1996.

Guyton, A.C., and Hall, J.E. *Textbook of Medical Physiology,* 9th ed. Philadelphia: W.B. Saunders Co., 1996.

Henry, J.B., ed. *Clinical Diagnosis and Management by Laboratory Methods,* 19th ed. Philadelphia: W.B. Saunders Co., 1996.

Isselbacher, K.J., et al., eds. *Harrison's Principles of Internal Medicine,* 13th ed. New York: McGraw-Hill Book Co., 1994.

Mayo Medical Laboratories 1996 Test Catalog. Rochester, Minn.: Mayo Medical Laboratories, 1996.

Nursing97 Drug Handbook. Springhouse, Pa.: Springhouse Corp., 1997.

Ravel, R.A. *Clinical Laboratory Medicine: Clinical Application of Laboratory Data,* 6th ed. St. Louis: Mosby–Year Book, Inc., 1995.

Treseler, K.M. *Clinical Laboratory and Diagnostic Tests: Significance and Nursing Implications,* 3rd ed. Stamford, Conn.: Appleton & Lange, 1995.

CHAPTER SIX

Lipids and lipoproteins

INTRODUCTION

Lipids, also called fats, are organic substances with a hydrophobic side chain or a steroid nucleus (or with both of these molecular features) that causes them to be insoluble in water. The major lipids are the triglycerides, free cholesterol, cholesteryl esters, and phospholipids. For transportation through the body, lipids must combine with plasma proteins into a lipid-protein molecular complex called lipoproteins: nonesterified fatty acids (free fatty acids) bind to albumin; other blood lipids (free and esterified cholesterol, triglycerides, and phospholipids) bind to globulin.

Lipid differences

Lipoproteins can be described as an inner core of hydrophobic lipids (triglycerides and cholesteryl esters) within a membrane of proteins (apoproteins), associated with free cholesterol and phospholipids. Lipoproteins differ based on the relative amount of the four lipids each apoprotein contains and the specific apoprotein associated with each specific lipoprotein.

Lipoproteins are classified by ultracentrifugation density and electrophoretic mobility as follows:

- *Chylomicrons,* the lowest density lipoproteins, consist mostly of triglycerides and are the form in which long-chain fats and cholesterol are transported from the intestine to the blood. Eventually, chylomicrons break down into other lipids and nonesterified fatty acids.

- *Very-low-density (prebeta) lipoproteins* (VLDLs) consist mostly of triglycerides and smaller amounts of phospholipids, cholesterol, and protein.

- *Intermediate-density lipoproteins* (IDLs) are short-lived and contain almost equal amounts of cholesterol and triglycerides, and smaller amounts of phospholipids and protein. They're converted to LDLs by lipase.

- *Low-density (beta) lipoproteins* (LDLs) are about half cholesterol and half protein, phospholipids, and triglycerides.

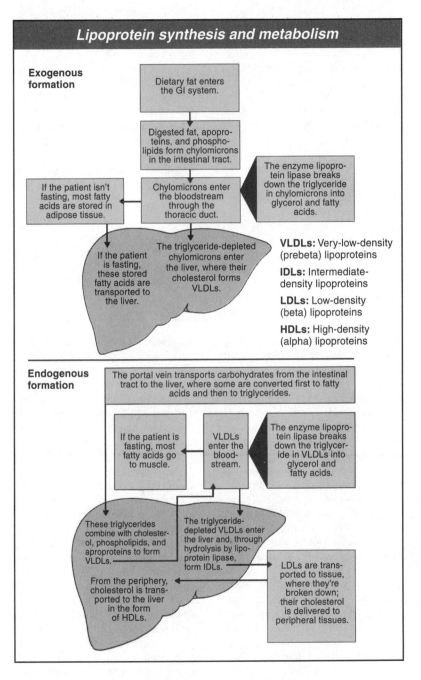

Lipoprotein synthesis and metabolism

Exogenous formation

Dietary fat enters the GI system.

Digested fat, apoproteins, and phospholipids form chylomicrons in the intestinal tract.

Chylomicrons enter the bloodstream through the thoracic duct.

The enzyme lipoprotein lipase breaks down the triglyceride in chylomicrons into glycerol and fatty acids.

If the patient isn't fasting, most fatty acids are stored in adipose tissue.

If the patient is fasting, these stored fatty acids are transported to the liver.

The triglyceride-depleted chylomicrons enter the liver, where their cholesterol forms VLDLs.

VLDLs: Very-low-density (prebeta) lipoproteins

IDLs: Intermediate-density lipoproteins

LDLs: Low-density (beta) lipoproteins

HDLs: High-density (alpha) lipoproteins

Endogenous formation

The portal vein transports carbohydrates from the intestinal tract to the liver, where some are converted first to fatty acids and then to triglycerides.

If the patient is fasting, most fatty acids go to muscle.

VLDLs enter the bloodstream.

The enzyme lipoprotein lipase breaks down the triglyceride in VLDLs into glycerol and fatty acids.

These triglycerides combine with cholesterol, phospholipids, and aproproteins to form VLDLs.

The triglyceride-depleted VLDLs enter the liver and, through hydrolysis by lipoprotein lipase, form IDLs.

From the periphery, cholesterol is transported to the liver in the form of HDLs.

LDLs are transported to tissue, where they're broken down; their cholesterol is delivered to peripheral tissues.

■ *High-density (alpha) lipoproteins* (HDLs) are about half protein and half phospholipids, cholesterol, and triglyc-erides. (See *Lipoprotein synthesis and metabolism*.)

Clinical implications

Lipoprotein phenotyping — classifying patients by the pattern of their lipoprotein levels — is an important procedure for diagnosing and treating hyperlipoproteinemias and hypolipoproteinemias. These disorders produce a variety of symptoms ranging from mild (such as xanthomas) to severe (such as pancreatitis).

Lipoprotein determinations are also useful in evaluating the risk of coronary artery disease (CAD). At one time, total blood cholesterol — the amount of cholesterol in all lipoproteins — was considered the major indicator of CAD for patients under age 50. However, the Framingham Heart Study found that high levels of HDL actually help prevent CAD, whereas high levels of LDL increase the risk. Apparently, HDLs help the enzyme lecithin cholesterol acyltransferase remove cholesterol from arterial walls. Further studies have shown that patients with angina pectoris or myocardial infarction generally have lower HDL levels than healthy persons and that low HDL levels — which can be hereditary — are not just associated with CAD but precede it. Low HDL levels are also connected with diabetes mellitus, hypertension, cigarette smoking, obesity, and lack of exercise.

The higher incidence of heart disease among men and postmenopausal women, compared with premenopausal women, may result from low levels of estrogen, a hormone that helps regulate synthesis of HDLs. Paradoxically, oral contraceptives and pregnancy elevate HDL levels. However, since HDL levels are only 5% to 8% lower in premenopausal women than in men of the same age, the potentially protective action of estrogens against atherosclerosis remains controversial.

Although HDL and LDL levels are good indicators of potential CAD, a full lipoprotein profile is a more useful measure. This battery of tests includes total cholesterol, total triglycerides, and lipoprotein phenotyping.

Antilipemic regimen

Care for patients with elevated LDL levels consists of teaching diet and lifestyle changes to reduce the risk of heart disease. For example, exercise (especially running), a low-fat diet, and reducing high blood pressure may raise levels of beneficial HDLs.

LIPID TESTS

Triglycerides

This test provides quantitative analysis of triglycerides, the main storage form of lipids, which constitute about 95% of fatty tissue. Although not in itself diagnostic, serum triglyceride analysis permits early identification of hyperlipidemia (characteristic in nephrotic syndrome and other conditions) and risk of coronary artery disease (CAD).

Triglyceride consists of one molecule of glycerol bonded to three molecules of fatty acids (usually some combination of stearic, oleic, and palmitic). Thus, the degradation of triglyceride leads directly to the production of fatty acid. Together with carbohydrates, these compounds furnish energy for metabolism. Serum triglycerides are associated with several lipid aggregates, primarily chylomicrons, whose major function is transport of dietary triglycerides. When present in serum, chylomicrons appear milky, which interferes with many laboratory tests. Very-low-density lipoproteins are also rich in triglycerides, though less so than chylomicrons. When present in excess amounts, they may cause plasma to become turbid, which also interferes with many laboratory tests.

Purpose
- To screen for hyperlipidemia
- To help identify nephrotic syndrome
- To determine the risk of CAD.

Patient preparation
Explain triglycerides to the patient, and tell him that this test helps detect disorders of fat metabolism. Advise him to abstain from food for 10 to 14 hours before the test and to abstain from alcohol for 24 hours. Tell him that he may drink water.

Inform the patient that the test requires a blood sample, who will perform the venipuncture and when, and that he may experience transient discomfort from the needle puncture and the pressure of the tourniquet.

As ordered, withhold medications that may interfere with the accuracy of test results. These include antilipemics, corticosteroids, estrogen, and some diuretics, which can raise or lower triglyceride levels.

Procedure
Perform a venipuncture, and collect a serum or plasma sample in a 7-ml *lavender-top* tube. (If plasma is used, use a tube that contains the anticoagulant EDTA.)

Precautions
Send the sample to the laboratory immediately.

Reference values
Triglyceride values are age- and sex-related. Some controversy exists over the most appropriate normal ranges. Nonetheless, serum values of 40 to 160 mg/dl for adult men and 35 to 135 mg/dl for adult women are widely accepted.

Implications of results
Increased or decreased serum triglyceride levels merely suggest a clinical abnormality; additional tests are required for a definitive diagnosis. For example, measurement of cholesterol may also be necessary, since cholesterol and triglyceride levels vary independently. High levels of triglyceride and cholesterol reflect an increased risk of CAD.

A mild to moderate increase in serum triglyceride levels may indicate biliary obstruction, diabetes, nephrotic syndrome, endocrinopathies, or overconsumption of alcohol. Markedly increased levels without an identifiable cause reflect congenital hyperlipoproteinemia and necessitate lipoprotein phenotyping to confirm the diagnosis.

Decreased serum levels are rare, occurring mainly in malnutrition or abetalipoproteinemia. In the latter, serum is virtually devoid of beta-lipoproteins and triglycerides because the body lacks the capacity to transport preformed triglycerides from the epithelial cells of the intestinal mucosa or from the liver.

Post-test care
- If a hematoma develops at the venipuncture site, apply warm soaks.
- As ordered, resume medications and diet discontinued before the test.

Interfering factors
- Failure to comply with dietary restrictions may alter test results.
- Ingestion of alcohol within 24 hours of the test may cause elevated triglyceride levels. In fact, excessive consumption of alcohol is a common cause of high triglyceride levels. That's because alcohol is heavily hydrogenated. As a result, this hydrogen has to be disposed of during alcohol metabolism; most of it ultimately ends up in triglyceride. Fatty liver is an early manifestation of this metabolic phenomenon.

■ Certain drugs lower cholesterol levels but raise or may have no effect on triglyceride levels. All antilipemics lower serum lipid concentration in the bloodstream, although their mechanism of action may differ. Cholestyramine and colestipol lower cholesterol; they raise or have no effect on triglycerides.

■ Long-term use of corticosteroids increases triglyceride levels, as does use of oral contraceptives, estrogen, ethyl alcohol, furosemide, and miconazole.

■ Don't use glycol-lubricated collection tubes because they may alter test results.

■ Clofibrate, dextrothyroxine, gemfibrozil, and niacin lower cholesterol and triglyceride levels.

■ Certain drugs have a variable effect: Probucol inhibits transport of cholesterol from the intestine and may also affect cholesterol synthesis. It lowers cholesterol but has a variable effect on triglycerides.

Total cholesterol

This test, the quantitative analysis of serum cholesterol, measures the circulating levels of free cholesterol and cholesterol esters; it reflects the level of the two forms in which this biochemical compound appears in the body.

Cholesterol, a structural component in cell membranes and plasma lipoproteins, is absorbed from the diet and synthesized in the liver and other body tissues. It's then metabolized to steroid hormones, glucocorticoids, and bile acids.

A diet high in saturated fat raises cholesterol levels by stimulating absorption of lipids, including cholesterol, from the intestine; a diet low in saturated fats lowers them. High serum cholesterol levels may be associated with an increased risk of coronary artery disease (CAD).

Purpose

■ To assess the risk of CAD
■ To evaluate fat metabolism
■ To aid diagnosis of nephrotic syndrome, pancreatitis, hepatic disease, and hypothyroidism and hyperthyroidism.

Patient preparation

Explain that this test determines the body's fat metabolism. Advise the patient to abstain from food and drink for 12 hours before the test. Tell him the test requires a blood sample, who will perform the venipuncture and when, and that he may experience discomfort from the needle puncture and the pressure of the tourniquet. As ordered, withhold drugs that may affect test results.

Procedure

Perform a venipuncture, and collect the sample in a 7-ml *lavender-top* tube containing EDTA.

Precautions

Send the sample to the laboratory immediately.

Reference values

Total cholesterol concentrations vary with age and sex. The normal range is 170 to 240 mg/dl. Levels of 280 to 320 mg/dl are considered elevated.

Implications of results

An elevated serum cholesterol level (hypercholesterolemia) may indicate risk of CAD as well as incipient hepatitis, lipid disorders, bile duct blockage, nephrotic syndrome, obstructive jaundice, pancreatitis, and hypothyroidism. Hypercholesterolemia due to increased intake of fats and cholesterol-rich foods requires dietary changes and, possibly, medication to retard absorption of cholesterol.

A low serum cholesterol level (hypocholesterolemia) is commonly associated with malnutrition, cellular necrosis of the liver, or hyperthyroidism.

Abnormal cholesterol levels commonly require further testing to pinpoint the causative disorder, depending on the type of abnormality and the presence of overt signs. Abnormal levels associated with cardiovascular diseases, for example, may require lipoprotein phenotyping.

Post-test care
■ If a hematoma develops at the venipuncture site, apply warm soaks.
■ As ordered, resume diet and medications discontinued before the test.

Interfering factors
■ Cholesterol levels are lowered by cholestyramine, clofibrate, colestipol, dextrothyroxine, haloperidol, neomycin, niacin, and chlortetracycline. Levels are raised by epinephrine, chlorpromazine, trifluoperazine, oral contraceptives, and trimethadione. Androgens may have a variable effect on cholesterol levels.
■ Failure to follow dietary restrictions may interfere with test results.

Phospholipids

The phospholipid assay was formerly an important test because of the lack of more specific tests and the relative unreliability of other lipid assays. Today, however, this quantitative analysis of phospholipid levels adds minimal information to that provided by cholesterol levels. Phospholipids are not associated with coronary artery disease and are seldom included in routine lipid evaluation.

Phospholipids, the largest and most soluble of the lipid elements, are molecules composed of glycerol, fatty acids, and phosphate. In human plasma, the main phospholipids are lecithins, cephalins, and sphingomyelins. Dietary phospholipids are partially broken down by pancreatic enzymes before absorption by the mucosal cells.

Phospholipids fulfill a variety of body functions, including cellular membrane composition and permeability, and some control of enzyme activity within the membrane. They have a tendency to concentrate at cell membranes and aid the transport of fatty acids and lipids across the intestinal barrier, and from the liver and other fat depots to other body tissues. Phospholipids, especially saturated lecithin, are also essential for pulmonary gas exchange, as evidenced by neonatal respiratory distress syndrome in premature infants who lack them.

Purpose
■ To aid in the evaluation of fat metabolism
■ To aid diagnosis of hypothyroidism, diabetes mellitus, nephrotic syndrome, chronic pancreatitis, obstructive jaundice, and hypolipoproteinemia.

Patient preparation
Explain to the patient that this test helps determine how the body metabolizes fats. Instruct him to abstain from ingestion of alcohol for 24 hours before the test and from food and fluids after midnight before the test. Tell him the test requires a blood sample, who will perform the venipuncture and when, and that he may experience transient discomfort from the needle puncture and the pressure of the tourniquet. Withhold antilipemic drugs, as ordered.

Procedure
Perform a venipuncture, and collect the sample in a 10- to 15-ml *red-top* tube.

Precautions
Send the sample to the laboratory immediately because spontaneous redistribution may occur among plasma lipids.

Reference values

Normal phospholipid levels range from 180 to 320 mg/dl. Although males usually have higher levels than females, values in pregnant females exceed those of males.

Implications of results

Elevated levels may indicate hypothyroidism, diabetes mellitus, nephrotic syndrome, chronic pancreatitis, or obstructive jaundice. Decreased levels may indicate primary hypolipoproteinemia.

Post-test care

■ If a hematoma develops at the venipuncture site, apply warm soaks.
■ Resume diet and administration of medications that were discontinued before the test, as ordered.

Interfering factors

■ Clofibrate and other antilipemics may lower phospholipid levels; estrogens, epinephrine, and some phenothiazines increase them.
■ Failure to follow dietary restrictions may interfere with test results.

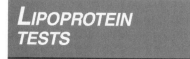

LIPOPROTEIN TESTS

Lipoprotein-cholesterol fractionation

Cholesterol fractionation tests isolate and measure the cholesterol in serum — low-density lipoproteins (LDLs) and high-density lipoproteins (HDLs) — by ultracentrifugation or electrophoresis. The amount of LDL and HDL fractions in serum is significant because the Framingham Heart Study has shown that the HDL level is inversely related to the incidence of coronary artery disease (CAD) — the higher the HDL level, the lower the incidence of CAD; conversely, the higher the LDL level, the higher the incidence of CAD.

Measurement of apolipoproteins may also be clinically important in determining an individual's risk of CAD. (See *Apolipoproteins and CAD.*)

Purpose

■ To assess the risk of CAD.

Patient preparation

Tell the patient that this test helps determine the risk of CAD. Instruct him to maintain his normal diet for 2 weeks before the test, to abstain from alcohol for 24 hours before the test, and to fast and avoid exercise for 12 to 14 hours before the test. Tell the patient the test requires a blood sample, who will perform the venipuncture and when, and that he may experience transient discomfort from the needle puncture and the pressure of the tourniquet.

As ordered, withhold thyroid hormones, oral contraceptives, and antilipemics, which alter test results.

Procedure

Perform a venipuncture, and collect the sample in a 7-ml *red-top* or *red-marble-top* tube.

Precautions

Send the sample to the laboratory immediately to avoid spontaneous redistribution among the lipoproteins. If the sample can't be transported immediately, refrigerate, but don't freeze, it.

Reference values

Since normal cholesterol values vary according to age, sex, geographic region, and ethnic group, check the laboratory for the normal values in your hospital. An alternative method (measuring cholesterol and triglyceride levels, separat-

Apolipoproteins and CAD

Although measurement of apolipoproteins — the protein fractions of lipoprotein molecules — is primarily a research procedure, mounting evidence suggests that it may have important clinical applications as well. Because apolipoprotein levels can be measured directly in serum, they may indicate an individual's risk of coronary artery disease (CAD) more accurately than high-density lipoprotein (HDL) or low-density lipoprotein (LDL) levels, which must be measured indirectly.

Currently, eight apolipoproteins have been identified. Of these, apolipoprotein A (ApoA) — the major protein component of HDL — and apolipoprotein B (ApoB) — the major protein component of LDL — are the most clinically significant. Reduced ApoA levels (below 140 mg/dl) occur in ischemic heart disease, whereas elevated ApoB levels (above 135 mg/dl) occur in hyperlipidemia, angina pectoris, and myocardial infarction.

ing out HDL by selective precipitation, and using these values to calculate LDL) provides normal HDL levels that range from 29 to 77 mg/dl and normal LDL levels that range from 62 to 185 mg/dl.

Implications of results

High LDL levels increase the risk of CAD. Elevated HDL levels generally reflect a healthy state, but they can also indicate chronic hepatitis, early-stage primary biliary cirrhosis, or alcohol consumption. Rarely, a sharp rise (to as high as 100 mg/dl) in a second type of HDL (alpha$_2$-HDL) may signal CAD.

Although cholesterol fractionation provides valuable information about the risk of heart disease, other risk factors (diabetes mellitus, hypertension, cigarette smoking) are at least as important.

Post-test care

■ If a hematoma develops at the venipuncture site, apply warm soaks.
■ Resume diet and medications withheld before the test, as ordered.

Interfering factors

■ Values are lowered by antilipemic medications, such as clofibrate, cholestyramine, colestipol, dextrothyroxine, niacin, probucol, and gemfibrozil.

■ Oral contraceptives, disulfiram, alcohol, miconazole, and high doses of phenothiazines may increase values.
■ Estrogens usually increase but may decrease values.
■ Failure to send the sample to the laboratory immediately may allow spontaneous redistribution of the lipoproteins and alter test results.
■ Collecting the sample in a heparinized tube may produce false elevations of values through activation of the enzyme lipase, which, in turn, causes the release of fatty acids from triglycerides.
■ The presence of bilirubin, hemoglobin, salicylates, iodine, vitamins A and D, and some other substances may affect test results.
■ Concurrent illness, especially if accompanied by fever, recent surgery, or myocardial infarction, may interfere with test results.

Lipoprotein phenotyping

In lipoprotein phenotyping, ultracentrifugation and electrophoresis of a blood sample determine lipoprotein levels. The density of the four major lipoproteins varies, depending on their relative percentages of triglyceride and protein: chylomicrons, which are very light lipid aggregates, consist of 85% to 95% triglycerides, 5% to 10% phospholipids, 3% to 5% cholesterol, and 1% to 2% protein; very-low-density (prebeta) lipoproteins consist of 45% to 65% triglycerides, 7% to 14% phospholipids, 7% to 14% cholesterol, and 2% to 13% protein; low-density (beta) lipoproteins consist of 7% to 10% triglycerides, 20% to 30% phospholipids, 35% to 45% cholesterol, and 15% to 38% protein; and high-density (alpha) lipoproteins consist of about 1% to 7% triglycerides, 28% to 30% phospholipids, 17% to 20% cholesterol, and 49% to 50% protein.

For transport through the blood, most lipids must combine with water-soluble proteins (apoproteins) to form lipoproteins. Several types of lipoproteins normally exist in the body, but in certain familial disorders, the blood levels of these types change. Classification of patients by the pattern of their lipoprotein levels identifies hyperlipoproteinemias and hypolipoproteinemias.

Purpose

▪ To determine classification of hyperlipoproteinemia or hypolipoproteinemia.

Patient preparation

Explain to the patient that this test helps determine how his body metabolizes fats. Instruct him to abstain from alcohol for 24 hours before the test, to eat a low-fat meal the night before the test, and to fast after midnight before the test. Tell him that this test requires a blood sample, who will perform the venipuncture and when, and that he may experience transient discomfort from the needle puncture and the pressure of the tourniquet.

Check the patient's drug history for use of heparin. As ordered, withhold antilipemics, such as cholestyramine, for about 2 weeks before the test.

Notify the laboratory if the patient is hospitalized for any other condition that might significantly alter lipoprotein metabolism, such as diabetes mellitus, nephrosis, or hypothyroidism.

Procedure

Perform a venipuncture, and collect the sample in a 7-ml *lavender-top* tube.

Precautions

 ▪ When drawing multiple samples, collect the sample for lipoprotein phenotyping first, if possible, because venous obstruction by the tourniquet for 2 minutes (while other blood samples are being drawn) can affect test results.

▪ Fill the collection tube completely, and invert it gently several times to mix the sample and the anticoagulant.

▪ Handle the sample gently to prevent hemolysis, which can alter test results.

Normal findings

The types of hyperlipoproteinemias or hypolipoproteinemias are identified by their characteristic electrophoretic patterns. The laboratory reports the type of lipoproteinemia present.

Implications of results

Familial lipoprotein disorders are classified as either hyperlipoproteinemias or hypolipoproteinemias. (See *Familial hyperlipoproteinemias*.)

The hyperlipoproteinemias break down into six types — I, IIa, IIb, III, IV, and V. Types IIa, IIb, and IV are relatively common. In contrast, all hypolipoproteinemias are rare; they include hypobetalipoproteinemia, abetalipoproteinemia (Bassen-Kornzweig syn-

Familial hyperlipoproteinemias

TYPE	CAUSES AND INCIDENCE	SIGNS AND SYMPTOMS	LABORATORY FINDINGS
I	■ Deficient lipoprotein lipase, resulting in increased chylomicrons ■ May be induced by alcoholism ■ Incidence: rare	■ Eruptive xanthomas ■ Lipemia retinalis ■ Abdominal pain	■ Increased chylomicron, total cholesterol, and triglyceride levels ■ Normal or slightly increased very-high-density lipoprotein (VLDL) levels ■ Normal or decreased low-density lipoprotein (LDL) levels and high-density lipoprotein (HDL) levels ■ Cholesterol-triglyceride ratio under 0.2
IIa	■ Deficient cell receptor, resulting in increased LDL levels and excessive cholesterol synthesis ■ May be induced by hypothyroidism ■ Incidence: common	■ Premature coronary artery disease (CAD) ■ Arcus cornea ■ Xanthelasma ■ Tendinous and tuberous xanthomas	■ Increased LDL levels ■ Normal VLDL levels ■ Cholesterol-triglyceride ratio over 2.0
IIb	■ Deficient cell receptor, resulting in increased LDL levels and excessive cholesterol synthesis ■ May be induced by dysgammaglobulinemia, hypothyroidism, uncontrolled diabetes mellitus, or nephrotic syndrome ■ Incidence: common	■ Premature CAD ■ Obesity ■ Possible xanthelasmas	■ Increased LDL, VLDL, total cholesterol, and triglyceride levels
III	■ Unknown cause, resulting in deficient VLDL-to-LDL conversion ■ May be induced by hypothyroidism, uncontrolled diabetes mellitus, or paraproteinemia ■ Incidence: rare	■ Premature CAD ■ Arcus cornea ■ Eruptive tuberous xanthomas	■ Increased total cholesterol, VLDL, and triglyceride levels ■ Normal or decreased LDL levels ■ Cholesterol-triglyceride ratio of VLDL over 0.4 ■ Broad beta band observed on electrophoresis

(continued)

Familial hyperlipoproteinemias (continued)

TYPE	CAUSES AND INCIDENCE	SIGNS AND SYMPTOMS	LABORATORY FINDINGS
IV	■ Unknown cause, resulting in decreased levels of lipoprotein lipase ■ May be induced by uncontrolled diabetes mellitus, alcoholism, pregnancy, steroid or estrogen therapy, dysgammaglobulinemia, or hyperthyroidism ■ Incidence: common	■ Possible premature CAD ■ Obesity ■ Hypertension ■ Peripheral neuropathy	■ Increased VLDL and triglyceride levels ■ Normal LDL ■ Cholesterol-triglyceride ratio of VLDL under 0.25
V	■ Unknown cause, resulting in defective triglyceride clearance ■ May be induced by alcoholism, dysgammaglobulinemia, uncontrolled diabetes mellitus, nephrotic syndrome, pancreatitis, or steroid therapy ■ Incidence: rare	■ Premature CAD ■ Abdominal pain ■ Lipemia retinalis ■ Eruptive xanthomas ■ Hepatosplenomegaly	■ Increased VLDL, total cholesterol, and triglyceride levels ■ Chylomicrons present ■ Cholesterol-triglyceride ratio under 0.6

drome), and alpha-lipoprotein deficiency (Tangier disease).

Post-test care
■ If a hematoma develops at the venipuncture site, apply warm soaks.
■ Instruct the patient to resume his normal diet.
■ As ordered, resume administration of medications withheld before the test.

Interfering factors
■ Hemolysis due to rough handling of the sample may affect test results.
■ Failure to observe dietary and alcohol restrictions or recent use of antilipemics, which lower lipid levels, may affect the accuracy of test results.
■ Administration of heparin (which activates the enzyme lipase, producing fatty acids from triglycerides) or collection of the sample in a heparinized tube may falsely elevate values.

SELECTED READINGS

Guyton, A.C., and Hall, J.E. *Textbook of Medical Physiology,* 9th ed. Philadelphia: W.B. Saunders Co., 1996.

Henry, J.B., ed. *Clinical Diagnosis and Management by Laboratory Methods,* 19th ed. Philadelphia: W.B. Saunders Co., 1996.

Kaplan, L.A., and Pesce, A.J. *Clinical Chemistry: Theory, Analysis, and Correlation,* 3rd ed. St. Louis: Mosby–Year Book, Inc., 1995.

Ravel, R.A. *Clinical Laboratory Medicine: Clinical Application of Laboratory Data,* 6th ed. St. Louis: Mosby–Year Book, Inc., 1995.

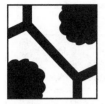

CHAPTER SEVEN

Proteins, protein metabolites, and pigments

Learning objectives

After completing this chapter, the reader will be able to:
- describe the formation and metabolism of serum proteins
- identify the five major steps in the formation of bile pigments
- identify the four stages of hepatic coma
- explain bilirubin metabolism
- recognize the signs of hemolysis in patients with low serum haptoglobin levels
- state the purpose of each test discussed in the chapter
- prepare the patient physically and psychologically for each test
- describe the procedure for obtaining a specimen for each test
- specify appropriate precautions for accurately obtaining a specimen for each test
- implement appropriate post-test care
- state the reference values for each test
- discuss the implications of abnormal test results
- list factors that may interfere with accurate test results.

INTRODUCTION

Serum proteins, the most abundant compounds in serum, function quite differently from tissue proteins. They have great diagnostic significance because of their vital functions: binding and detoxifying drugs and other potentially toxic substances; performing as antibodies, enzymes, and hormones; sustaining the oncotic pressure of blood; maintaining acid-base balance through their buffering action; and serving as a reserve source of nutrition for tissues.

One protein — *albumin* — makes up more than 50% of the total proteins in serum; a group of proteins, collectively called *globulins*, accounts for the remainder. Fibrinogen, a major plasma protein, does not appear in serum because it is converted to fibrin during coagulation. But it does appear in anticoagulated blood (or plasma).

Serum protein formation

The major serum proteins are albumin and the globulins (alpha$_1$, alpha$_2$, beta, and gamma). The liver forms most of the albumin as well as the alpha and beta globulins. The reticuloendothelial system and immature plasma cells in the spleen, lymph nodes, and bone marrow produce gamma globulin.

Albumin is primarily responsible for maintaining the oncotic pressure of plasma, which in turn maintains normal distribution of water in the various body compartments. Albumin also helps transport many drugs, dyes, and fatty acids by combining with them in the plasma.

Reflecting their heterogeneous composition, globulins have many diverse functions, including binding free hemoglobin and certain hormones, transporting metals, and forming antibodies. For example, ceruloplasmin, an alpha$_2$-globulin, binds most of the circulating copper in the body (Wilson's disease is characterized by defective formation of ceruloplasmin); haptoglobin, another alpha$_2$-globulin, binds free plasma hemoglobin; and transferrin, a beta globulin, binds and transports dietary iron.

Poor nutrition inhibits formation of

plasma proteins. Declining plasma protein levels, in turn, can have serious clinical consequences. For example, a sharp decline in albumin leads to edema, and low levels of gamma globulin weaken the host's defense to infection.

Protein metabolism

Unlike carbohydrates and fats, proteins are not stored by the body. Instead, they're continuously broken down into amino acids in the intestinal mucosa and other sites. These amino acids form a common reserve for the synthesis of new proteins, hormones, enzymes, and nonprotein nitrogenous compounds such as creatine. Certain genetic disorders, such as phenylketonuria, can result from lack of a specific enzyme or inadequate transport activity, which alters the metabolic function of one or more amino acids.

The major end product of protein metabolism is *urea,* which is formed in the liver by deamination of amino acids. Urea is excreted in urine and is the primary method of nitrogen elimination. Blood levels of urea, measured as blood urea nitrogen, begin to rise with impaired glomerular excretion and are an important index of renal function.

Another important protein metabolite is *ammonia,* most of which is ultimately metabolized to urea in the liver and then excreted. Because impaired hepatic function inhibits such conversion of ammonia, serum ammonia levels rise in severe hepatic disease and can lead to hepatic coma.

Creatine is a nonprotein nitrogenous compound that combines with phosphate to form phosphocreatine, an important storage form of high-energy phosphate. This compound is particularly prevalent in muscles. *Creatinine,* the end product of creatine metabolism, is excreted in urine and, like blood urea nitrogen levels, reflects the efficiency of renal excretory function.

Uric acid is the end product of purine metabolism and is excreted in urine. Serum uric acid levels and urate crystal deposits in synovial fluid are significant in the diagnosis of gout.

Bile pigments

Bile pigments are waste products of heme degradation, initiated by the breakdown of erythrocytes at the end of their life cycle. The five major steps in bile pigment metabolism include formation, plasma transport, hepatic uptake, conjugation, and biliary excretion. In humans, the bone marrow and spleen are the main sites of normal red cell destruction and heme degradation.

Although bile pigments have no known function, abnormalities in their overall transformation are significant in diagnosing hepatobiliary disease and conditions marked by excessive hemolysis. Conjugated bilirubin is converted into pigments responsible for the characteristic color of bile and feces; unconjugated bilirubin migrates in normal plasma, largely combined with albumin. Serum bilirubin levels may rise in hemolytic anemia, hepatocellular injury, and biliary duct occlusion.

PROTEIN TESTS

Serum protein electrophoresis

This test separates serum albumin and globulins by using an electric field to differentiate the proteins according to their size, shape, and electric charge at pH 8.6 into five distinct fractions: albumin, $alpha_1$, $alpha_2$, beta, and gamma proteins. Because each moves at a dif-

How hepatic diseases affect protein fractions

Because the liver synthesizes albumin as well as alpha and beta globulins, changes in the concentration of these major plasma proteins can indicate hepatic malfunction or hepatocellular damage. Although total protein levels — the sum of albumin and globulin fractions — may remain normal, hepatic disease will alter one, several, or all of the protein fractions.

	NORMAL	HEPATITIS	CIRRHOSIS	OBSTRUC-TIVE JAUNDICE	METASTATIC LIVER CANCER
Total protein	100%	0	–	0	0
Albumin	53%	0	–	0/–	–
Alpha$_1$-globulin	14%	–	0	0	+
Alpha$_2$-globulin	14%	–	0	0/+	+
Beta globulin	12%	+	+	0/+	0/+
Gamma globulin	20%	+	+	0	0/+

KEY: 0 = normal   + = increased   – = decreased

ferent rate, the fractions have recognizable, measurable patterns.

Albumin, which constitutes more than 50% of total serum protein, maintains oncotic pressure (preventing leakage of capillary plasma) and transports substances that are insoluble in water alone, such as bilirubin, fatty acids, hormones, and drugs. Four types of globulins exist — alpha$_1$, alpha$_2$, beta, and gamma. The first three types act primarily as carrier proteins that transport lipids, hormones, and metals through the blood. The fourth type, gamma globulin, is an important component in the body's immune system.

Chemical analysis of total and individual proteins is a common laboratory procedure, and electrophoresis yields meaningful data about the five major fractions. When the relative percentage of each component protein fraction is multiplied by the total protein concentration, the proportions can be converted into absolute values. Regardless of test method used, however, a single protein fraction value is rarely significant by itself. The usual clinical indication for this test is suspected hepatic disease or protein deficiency. (See *How hepatic diseases affect protein fractions*.)

Purpose

■ To aid diagnosis of hepatic disease, protein deficiency, and renal disorders, as well as GI and neoplastic diseases.

Patient preparation

Explain to the patient that this test determines the protein content of blood. Inform him that he needn't restrict food or fluids. Tell him that the test requires

Alpha₁-antitrypsin test

Using radioimmunoassay or isoelectric focusing, this test measures fasting serum levels of alpha₁-antitrypsin (AAT), a major component of alpha₁-globulin. AAT is believed to inhibit release of protease into body fluids by dying cells.

Congenital absence or deficiency of AAT increases susceptibility to emphysema. As a result, the serum AAT test provides a useful screening tool for high-risk patients. Such patients must be instructed to avoid smoking because irritants in tobacco stimulate leukocytes in the lungs to release protease.

The AAT test also is a nonspecific method of detecting inflammation, severe infection, and necrosis.

a blood sample, who will perform the venipuncture and when, and that he may feel some discomfort from the needle puncture and the pressure of the tourniquet.

Review the patient's medication history for drugs that may influence serum protein levels. If they must be continued, note this on the laboratory request.

Procedure

Perform a venipuncture, and collect the sample in a 7-ml *red-top* or *red-marble-top* tube.

Precautions

This test must be performed on a serum sample to avoid measuring the fibrinogen fraction. (The fibrinogen fraction, if present, would be indistinguishable from certain monoclonal gammopathies.)

Reference values

- *total serum protein:* 6.6 to 7.9 g/dl
- *albumin:* 3.3 to 4.5 g/dl
- *alpha₁-globulin:* 0.1 to 0.4 g/dl
- *alpha₂-globulin:* 0.5 to 1.0 g/dl
- *beta globulin:* 0.7 to 1.2 g/dl
- *gamma globulin:* 0.5 to 1.6 g/dl.

For information on another test involving alpha₁-globulin, see *Alpha₁-antitrypsin test.*

Implications of results

See *Clinical implications of abnormal protein levels,* page 214.

Post-test care

If a hematoma develops at the venipuncture site, apply warm soaks.

Interfering factors

- Pretest administration of a contrast agent (such as sulfobromophthalein) falsely elevates total protein test results.
- Pregnancy or cytotoxic drug use may lower serum albumin levels.
- Use of plasma instead of serum alters test results.

Serum ceruloplasmin

This test measures serum levels of ceruloplasmin, an alpha₂-globulin that binds about 95% of serum copper, usually in the liver. (Little copper exists in a free state.) Because ceruloplasmin catalyzes oxidation of ferrous compounds to ferric ions, it is thought to regulate iron uptake by transferrin, making iron available to reticulocytes for heme syn-

Clinical implications of abnormal protein levels

Abnormal levels of albumin or globulins are characteristic in many pathologic states, such as those listed below.

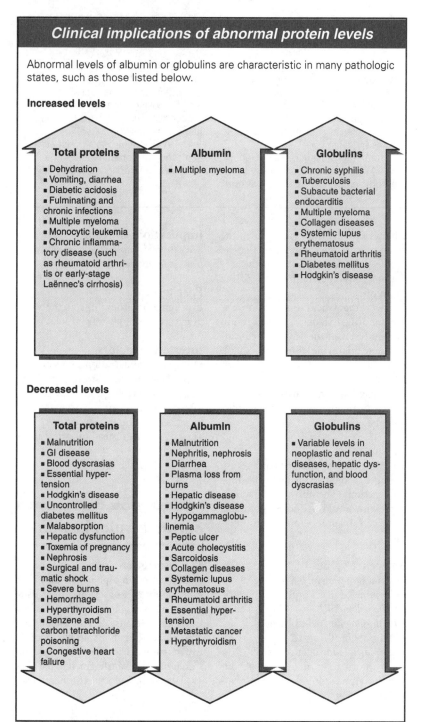

Increased levels

Total proteins
- Dehydration
- Vomiting, diarrhea
- Diabetic acidosis
- Fulminating and chronic infections
- Multiple myeloma
- Monocytic leukemia
- Chronic inflammatory disease (such as rheumatoid arthritis or early-stage Laënnec's cirrhosis)

Albumin
- Multiple myeloma

Globulins
- Chronic syphilis
- Tuberculosis
- Subacute bacterial endocarditis
- Multiple myeloma
- Collagen diseases
- Systemic lupus erythematosus
- Rheumatoid arthritis
- Diabetes mellitus
- Hodgkin's disease

Decreased levels

Total proteins
- Malnutrition
- GI disease
- Blood dyscrasias
- Essential hypertension
- Hodgkin's disease
- Uncontrolled diabetes mellitus
- Malabsorption
- Hepatic dysfunction
- Toxemia of pregnancy
- Nephrosis
- Surgical and traumatic shock
- Severe burns
- Hemorrhage
- Hyperthyroidism
- Benzene and carbon tetrachloride poisoning
- Congestive heart failure

Albumin
- Malnutrition
- Nephritis, nephrosis
- Diarrhea
- Plasma loss from burns
- Hepatic disease
- Hodgkin's disease
- Hypogammaglobulinemia
- Peptic ulcer
- Acute cholecystitis
- Sarcoidosis
- Collagen diseases
- Systemic lupus erythematosus
- Rheumatoid arthritis
- Essential hypertension
- Metastatic cancer
- Hyperthyroidism

Globulins
- Variable levels in neoplastic and renal diseases, hepatic dysfunction, and blood dyscrasias

thesis. The usual clinical indications for this assay are Menkes' kinky hair syndrome, suspected copper deficiency from total parenteral nutrition, and suspected Wilson's disease.

Purpose
■ To aid diagnosis of Wilson's disease, Menkes' kinky hair syndrome, and copper deficiency.

Patient preparation
Explain to the patient that this test helps determine the copper content of the blood. Tell him the test requires a blood sample, who will perform the venipuncture and when, and that he may feel discomfort from the needle puncture and the tourniquet. Check his medication history for drugs that may influence ceruloplasmin levels.

Procedure
Perform a venipuncture, and collect the sample in a 7-ml *red-top* or *red-marble-top* tube.

Precautions
Send the sample to the laboratory immediately.

Reference values
Serum ceruloplasmin concentrations for adults normally range from 22.9 to 43.1 mg/dl.

Implications of results
Low ceruloplasmin levels usually indicate Wilson's disease; this is confirmed by Kayser-Fleischer rings (copper deposits in the corneas that form green-gold rings) or by liver biopsy results that show 250 µg of copper per gram of dry weight. Low ceruloplasmin levels may also occur in Menkes' kinky hair syndrome, nephrotic syndrome, and hypocupremia caused by total parenteral nutrition. Elevated levels may indicate certain hepatic diseases and infections.

Post-test care
If a hematoma develops at the venipuncture site, apply warm soaks.

Interfering factors
Estrogen, methadone, phenytoin, and pregnancy may elevate serum ceruloplasmin levels.

Serum haptoglobin

Using radial immunodiffusion or nephelometry, this test measures serum levels of haptoglobin, a glycoprotein produced in the liver. Haptoglobin binds with free hemoglobin and prevents its accumulation in plasma, permitting clearance by reticuloendothelial cells and conserving body iron. Hemoglobin circulates inside erythrocytes; when aged erythrocytes die, they release free hemoglobin into plasma. Certain anemias, bacterial toxins, mechanical disruption (from a prosthetic heart valve, for example), or antibodies can increase intravascular hemolysis. In acute intravascular hemolysis, haptoglobin levels fall rapidly; low levels may last for 5 to 7 days, until the liver synthesizes more glycoprotein.

Purpose
■ To serve as an index of hemolysis
■ To distinguish between hemoglobin and myoglobin in plasma because haptoglobin doesn't bind with myoglobin
■ To investigate hemolytic transfusion reactions
■ To establish proof of paternity, using genetic (phenotypic) variations in haptoglobin structure.

Patient preparation
Explain to the patient that this test helps determine the condition of red blood

cells. Inform him that he needn't restrict food or fluids. Tell him the test requires a blood sample, who will perform the venipuncture and when, and that he may feel some discomfort from the needle puncture and the pressure of the tourniquet. Check the patient's medication history for drugs that may influence haptoglobin levels.

Procedure
Draw a venous blood sample into a 7-ml *red-top* or *red-marble-top* tube.

Precautions
Handle the sample gently.

Reference values
Serum haptoglobin concentrations, measured in terms of the protein's hemoglobin-binding capacity, normally range from 38 to 270 mg/dl. Nephelometric procedures yield lower results.

Implications of results
Markedly depressed serum haptoglobin levels are characteristic in acute and chronic hemolysis, severe hepatocellular disease, infectious mononucleosis, and transfusion reactions. Hepatocellular disease inhibits the synthesis of haptoglobin. In hemolytic transfusion reactions, haptoglobin levels begin falling after 6 to 8 hours and drop to 40% of pretransfusion levels after 24 hours.

 If serum haptoglobin values are very low, watch for symptoms of hemolysis: chills, fever, back pain, flushing, distended neck veins, tachycardia, tachypnea, and hypotension.

Although haptoglobin is absent in 90% of neonates, levels usually rise to normal by age 4 months. However, in about 1% of the population — including 4% of blacks — haptoglobin is permanently absent; this disorder is known as congenital ahaptoglobinemia.

Markedly elevated serum haptoglobin levels occur in diseases marked by chronic inflammatory reactions or tissue destruction, such as rheumatoid arthritis and malignant neoplasms.

Post-test care
If a hematoma develops at the venipuncture site, apply warm soaks.

Interfering factors
- Steroids and androgens can elevate haptoglobin levels and mask hemolysis in patients with inflammatory disease.
- Hemolysis caused by rough handling of the sample can alter test results.

Serum transferrin

Using radial immunodiffusion or nephelometry, this test measures serum transferrin levels to evaluate iron metabolism. Transferrin (also known as siderophilin), a glycoprotein formed in the liver, transports circulating iron obtained from dietary sources and from the breakdown of red blood cells by reticuloendothelial cells. Most of this iron is transported to bone marrow for use in hemoglobin synthesis; some is converted to hemosiderin and ferritin and stored in the liver, spleen, and bone marrow. Inadequate transferrin levels may therefore lead to impaired hemoglobin synthesis and, possibly, anemia. Transferrin is normally about 30% saturated with iron. Serum iron levels are usually obtained simultaneously.

Purpose
- To determine the iron-transporting capacity of the blood
- To evaluate iron metabolism in iron deficiency anemia.

Patient preparation

Explain to the patient that this test helps determine the cause of anemia. Inform him that he needn't restrict food or fluids. Tell him the test requires a blood sample, who will perform the venipuncture and when, and that he may feel some discomfort from the needle puncture and the pressure of the tourniquet. Check his medication history for drugs that may affect transferrin levels.

Procedure

Perform a venipuncture, and collect the sample in a 7-ml *red-top* or *red-marble-top* tube.

Precautions

Handle the sample gently, and send it to the laboratory immediately.

Reference values

Normal serum transferrin values range from 200 to 400 mg/dl, of which 65 to 170 mg/dl are usually bound to iron.

Implications of results

Depressed serum transferrin levels may indicate inadequate production due to hepatic damage or excessive protein loss from renal disease. They may also result from acute or chronic infection or from cancer. Elevated serum transferrin levels may indicate severe iron deficiency.

Post-test care

If a hematoma develops at the venipuncture site, apply warm soaks.

Interfering factors

■ Late pregnancy or the use of oral contraceptives may raise transferrin levels.
■ Hemolysis due to rough handling of the sample may affect test results.

PROTEIN METABOLITE TESTS

Plasma amino acids

This is a qualitative but effective test performed on neonates to detect inborn errors of amino acid metabolism. The test uses thin-layer chromatography, which can profile many amino acids simultaneously.

Amino acids are the chief components of all proteins and polypeptides. The body contains at least 20 amino acids; 10 are considered "essential" — that is, they must be acquired through diet because the body doesn't form them. Certain congenital enzymatic deficiencies interfere with normal metabolism of one or more amino acids, causing them to accumulate or become deficient.

Excessive accumulation of amino acids typically produces overflow aminoacidurias. Congenital abnormalities of the amino acid transport system in the kidneys produce a second group of disorders called renal aminoacidurias.

Purpose

■ To screen for inborn errors of amino acid metabolism.

Patient preparation

Explain to the parents that this test determines how well their infant metabolizes amino acids. Tell the parents the infant must fast for 4 hours before the test and that a small amount of blood will be drawn from his heel.

Procedure

Perform a heelstick, and collect 0.1 ml of blood in a heparinized capillary tube.

Precautions

Handle the sample gently.

Normal findings

Chromatography shows a normal plasma amino acid pattern.

Implications of results

The plasma amino acid pattern is normal in renal aminoacidurias and abnormal in overflow aminoacidurias. Comparisons of blood and urine chromatography can help distinguish between the two types of aminoacidurias.

Post-test care

- If a hematoma develops at the heelstick site, apply warm soaks.
- The infant can resume feeding, as ordered.

Interfering factors

- Failure to observe dietary restrictions may influence amino acid levels.
- Hemolysis may alter results.

Serum phenylalanine

This test (also known as the Guthrie screening test) is a screening method used to detect elevated levels of serum phenylalanine, a naturally occurring amino acid essential to growth and nitrogen balance. Such an elevation may indicate phenylketonuria (PKU), a metabolic disorder inherited as an autosomal recessive trait. An infant with PKU usually has normal phenylalanine levels at birth, but after he begins feeding with milk or formula (both contain phenylalanine), levels gradually rise because of a deficiency of the liver enzyme that converts phenylalanine to tyrosine. The resulting accumulation of phenylalanine, phenylpyruvic acid, and other metabolites hinders normal development of central nervous system cells, causing mental retardation.

Dietary restriction of foods that contain phenylalanine prevents accumulation of toxic compounds and hence prevents mental retardation. As the child matures, other metabolic pathways develop to metabolize phenylalanine.

The serum phenylalanine screening test detects abnormal phenylalanine levels through the growth rate of *Bacillus subtilis*, an organism that needs phenylalanine to thrive. To ensure accurate results, the test must be performed after 3 full days (preferably 4 days) of milk or formula feeding.

Purpose

- To screen infants for PKU.

Patient preparation

Explain to the parents of the infant that the test is a routine screening measure for PKU and is required in many states. Tell them that a small amount of blood will be drawn from the infant's heel.

Procedure

Perform a heelstick, and collect three drops of blood — one in each circle — on the filter paper.

Precautions

Note the infant's name and birth date and the date of the first milk or formula feeding on the laboratory request, and send the sample to the laboratory immediately.

Normal findings

In the laboratory, the sample is added to a culture medium containing a phenylalanine-dependent strain of *B. subtilis* and an antagonist to phenylalanine. A negative test, in which the presence of the phenylalanine antagonist inhibits growth of *B. subtilis* around the blood on the filter paper, indicates normal phenylalanine levels (less than 2 mg/dl) and no appreciable danger of PKU.

Confirming PKU

After the Guthrie screening test detects the possible presence of phenylketonuria (PKU), serum phenylalanine and tyrosine levels are measured to confirm the diagnosis. Phenylalanine hydroxylase is the enzyme that converts phenylalanine to tyrosine. If this enzyme is absent, increasing phenylalanine levels and falling tyrosine levels indicate PKU.

Samples are obtained by venipuncture (femoral or external jugular) and measured by fluorometry. Serum phenylalanine levels greater than 4 mg/dl and tyrosine levels less than 0.6 mg/dl — with urinary excretion of phenylpyruvic acid — confirm PKU.

Implications of results

Growth of B. *subtilis* on the filter paper indicates that serum phenylalanine levels are high enough to overcome the antagonist. Such a positive test suggests the *possibility* of PKU. Diagnosis requires exact serum phenylalanine measurement and urine testing. (See *Confirming PKU.*) A positive test may also result from hepatic disease, galactosemia, or delayed development of certain enzyme systems.

Post-test care

Reassure the parents of a child who may have PKU that early detection and continuous treatment with a low-phenylalanine diet can prevent permanent mental retardation.

Interfering factors

Performing the test before the infant has received at least 3 full days of milk or formula feeding yields a false-negative finding.

Plasma ammonia

This test measures plasma levels of ammonia, a nonprotein nitrogen compound that helps maintain acid-base balance. Most ammonia is absorbed from the intestinal tract, where it is produced by bacterial action on protein; a smaller amount of ammonia is produced in the kidneys from hydrolysis of glutamine. Normally, the body uses the nitrogen fraction of ammonia to rebuild amino acids, then converts the ammonia to urea in the liver for excretion by the kidneys. In such diseases as cirrhosis of the liver, however, ammonia can bypass the liver and accumulate in the blood. Therefore, plasma ammonia levels may help indicate the severity of hepatocellular damage.

Purpose

- To help monitor the progression of severe hepatic disease and the effectiveness of therapy
- To recognize impending or established hepatic coma. (See *Recognizing hepatic coma,* page 220.)

Patient preparation

Explain to the patient that this test evaluates liver function. (If the patient is comatose, explain the procedure to a family member.) Inform the patient who is conscious that he must observe an overnight fast before the test because plasma ammonia levels may vary with protein intake. Tell him that the test requires a blood sample, who will perform the venipuncture and when, and that he may feel transient discomfort from the needle puncture. Check the patient's

Recognizing hepatic coma

Patients in hepatic coma progress through the following four stages, with accompanying clinical features:
- *Prodromal:* mild confusion, euphoria or depression, vacant stare, inappropriate laughter, forgetfulness, inability to concentrate, slow mentation, slurred speech, untidiness, lethargy, belligerence, minimal asterixis (flapping tremor). Watch carefully for these subtle symptoms. They are not necessarily all present at the same time.
- *Impending:* obvious obtundation, aberrant behavior, asterixis, constructional apraxia. To test for asterixis (flapping tremor), have the patient raise both arms, with forearms flexed and fingers extended. To test for constructional apraxia, keep a serial record of the patient's handwriting and figure construction, and check it for progressive deterioration.
- *Stuporous* (patient can still be aroused): marked confusion, incoherent speech, asterixis, noisiness, abusiveness, violence, abnormal EEG. Restraints may be necessary at this stage. *Do not sedate the patient; sedation could be fatal.*
- *Comatose* (patient cannot be aroused, responds only to painful stimuli): no asterixis but positive Babinski's sign, hepatic fetor (musty, sweet breath odor), elevated serum ammonia level. The degree of hepatic fetor correlates with the degree of somnolence and confusion.

medication history for drugs that may influence plasma ammonia levels.

Procedure
Perform a venipuncture, and collect the sample in a 10-ml *green-marble-top* (heparinized) tube.

Precautions
- Notify the laboratory before performing the venipuncture so that preliminary preparations can begin.
- Handle the sample gently, pack it in ice, and send it to the laboratory immediately. *Don't* use a chilled container.

Reference values
Normally, plasma ammonia levels are less than 50 µg/dl.

Implications of results
Elevated plasma ammonia levels are common in severe hepatic disease, such as cirrhosis and acute hepatic necrosis, and may lead to hepatic coma. Elevated levels are also possible in Reye's syndrome, severe congestive heart failure, GI hemorrhage, and erythroblastosis fetalis.

Post-test care
- Make sure bleeding has stopped before removing pressure from the venipuncture site. If a hematoma develops, apply warm soaks.
- Watch for signs of impending or established hepatic coma if plasma ammonia levels are high.

Interfering factors
- Acetazolamide, thiazides, ammonium salts, and furosemide raise ammonia levels, as can total parenteral nutrition or a portacaval shunt. Lactulose, neomycin, and kanamycin depress ammonia levels.
- Hemolysis caused by rough handling of the sample may alter test results.
- Smoking, poor venipuncture tech-

nique, and exposure to ammonia cleaners in the laboratory may elevate results.
■ Delay in testing may alter results.

Blood urea nitrogen

This test measures the nitrogen fraction of urea, the chief end product of protein metabolism. Formed in the liver from ammonia and excreted by the kidneys, urea constitutes 40% to 50% of the blood's nonprotein nitrogen. The blood urea nitrogen (BUN) level reflects protein intake and renal excretory capacity, but it's a less reliable indicator of uremia than the serum creatinine level. Photometry is a commonly used test method.

Purpose
■ To evaluate renal function and aid diagnosis of renal disease
■ To aid assessment of hydration.

Patient preparation
Tell the patient that this test evaluates kidney function. Inform him that he needn't restrict food or fluids but should avoid a diet high in meat. Tell him the test requires a blood sample, who will perform the venipuncture and when, and that he may feel some discomfort from the needle puncture and the pressure of the tourniquet. Check the patient's medication history for drugs that may influence BUN levels.

Procedure
Perform a venipuncture, and collect the sample in a 7-ml *red-top* or *red-marble-top* tube.

Precautions
Handle the sample gently to prevent hemolysis.

Reference values
BUN values normally range from 8 to 20 mg/dl, with slightly higher values in elderly patients.

Implications of results
Elevated BUN levels occur in renal disease, reduced renal blood flow (due to dehydration, for example), urinary tract obstruction, and increased protein catabolism (as occurs in burns).

Depressed BUN levels occur in severe hepatic damage, malnutrition, and overhydration.

Post-test care
If a hematoma develops at the venipuncture site, apply warm soaks.

Interfering factors
■ Chloramphenicol can depress BUN levels.
■ Nephrotoxic drugs, such as aminoglycosides, amphotericin B, and methicillin, can elevate BUN levels.
■ Hemolysis caused by rough handling of the sample may affect test results.

Serum creatinine

A quantitative analysis of serum creatinine levels, this test provides a more sensitive measure of renal damage than BUN levels because renal impairment is virtually the only cause of creatinine elevation. Creatinine is a nonprotein end product of creatine metabolism. Similar to creatine, creatinine appears in serum in amounts proportional to the body's muscle mass; unlike creatine it is easily excreted by the kidneys, with minimal or no tubular reabsorption. Creatinine levels, therefore, are directly related to the glomerular filtration rate.

Because creatinine levels normally remain constant, elevated levels usually indicate diminished renal function. Determination of serum creatinine is commonly based on the Jaffé reaction or on coupled enzymatic reactions.

Purpose
- To assess renal glomerular filtration
- To screen for renal damage.

Patient preparation
Explain to the patient that this test evaluates kidney function. Tell him that the test requires a blood sample, who will perform the venipuncture and when, and that he may feel some discomfort from the needle puncture and the pressure of the tourniquet. Check the patient's medication history for drugs that may interfere with test results.

Procedure
Perform a venipuncture, and collect the sample in a 7-ml *red-top* or *red-marble-top* tube.

Precautions
Handle the specimen gently, and send it to the laboratory immediately.

Reference values
Serum creatinine levels in males normally range from 0.8 to 1.2 mg/dl; in females, from 0.6 to 0.9 mg/dl.

Implications of results
Elevated serum creatinine levels generally indicate renal disease that has seriously damaged 50% or more of the nephrons. They may also be associated with gigantism and acromegaly.

Post-test care
If a hematoma develops at the venipuncture site, apply warm soaks.

Interfering factors
- Ascorbic acid, barbiturates, and diuretics may raise serum creatinine levels.
- Sulfobromophthalein or phenolsulfonphthalein given within the previous 24 hours can elevate creatinine levels if the test is based on the Jaffé reaction.
- Patients with exceptionally large muscle mass, such as athletes, may have above-average creatinine levels, even with normal renal function.
- Hemolysis may elevate results.

Serum uric acid

Used primarily to detect gout, this test measures serum levels of uric acid, the major end metabolite of purine. Large amounts of purines are present in nucleic acids and derive from dietary and endogenous sources. Uric acid clears the body by glomerular filtration and tubular secretion. However, uric acid is not very soluble at a pH of 7.4 or lower. Disorders of purine metabolism, rapid destruction of nucleic acids, and conditions marked by impaired renal excretion characteristically raise serum uric acid levels.

Purpose
- To confirm diagnosis of gout
- To help detect kidney dysfunction.

Patient preparation
Explain to the patient that this test helps detect gout or kidney dysfunction. Inform him that he must fast for 8 hours before the test. Tell him that the test requires a blood sample, who will perform the venipuncture and when, and that he may feel some discomfort from the needle puncture and the pressure of the tourniquet. Check the patient's medica-

tion history for any drugs that may influence uric acid levels.

Procedure
Perform a venipuncture, and collect the sample in a 7-ml *red-top* or *red-marble-top* tube.

Precautions
Handle the sample gently to prevent hemolysis.

Reference values
Uric acid concentrations in men normally range from 4.3 to 8.0 mg/dl; in women, from 2.3 to 6.0 mg/dl.

Implications of results
Increased serum uric acid levels may indicate gout or impaired renal function (levels don't correlate with severity of disease). Levels may also rise in congestive heart failure, glycogen storage disease (type I, von Gierke's disease), infections, hemolytic or sickle cell anemia, polycythemia, neoplasms, and psoriasis.

Depressed uric acid levels may indicate defective tubular absorption (as in Fanconi's syndrome and Wilson's disease) or acute hepatic atrophy.

Post-test care
If a hematoma develops at the venipuncture site, apply warm soaks.

Interfering factors
■ Loop diuretics, ethambutol, vincristine, pyrazinamide, thiazides, and low doses of aspirin may raise uric acid levels. When using the colorimetric method, false elevations may be caused by acetaminophen, ascorbic acid, levodopa, and phenacetin. Aspirin in high doses may decrease uric acid levels.
■ Starvation, a high-purine diet, stress, and abuse of alcohol may raise uric acid levels.

PIGMENT TESTS

Serum bilirubin

This test measures serum levels of bilirubin, the main pigment in bile. Bilirubin is the major product of hemoglobin catabolism. After being formed in the reticuloendothelial cells, bilirubin is bound to albumin and transported to the liver, where it is conjugated with glucuronide by the enzymatic action of glucuronyl transferase. The resulting compound — bilirubin diglucuronide — is then excreted in bile. (See *Bilirubin metabolism,* page 224.)

Effective bilirubin conjugation and excretion depend on a properly functioning hepatobiliary system and a normal red blood cell (RBC) turnover rate. Therefore, measurement of unconjugated (indirect or prehepatic) bilirubin and conjugated (direct or posthepatic) bilirubin can help evaluate hepatobiliary and erythropoietic function. Serum bilirubin values are especially significant in neonates because excessive unconjugated bilirubin can accumulate in the brain, causing irreparable damage.

Purpose
■ To evaluate liver function
■ To aid differential diagnosis of jaundice and to monitor its progression
■ To aid diagnosis of biliary obstruction and hemolytic anemia
■ To determine whether a neonate requires an exchange transfusion or phototherapy because of dangerously high unconjugated bilirubin levels.

Patient preparation
Explain that this test evaluates liver function and the condition of RBCs. If the patient is a neonate, tell his parents why the test is important. Inform the

Bilirubin metabolism

After formation in the reticuloendothelial cells, bilirubin is bound to albumin and transported to the liver, where it is conjugated with glucuronic acid to form bilirubin diglucuronide, and is excreted into the bile. A small portion of conjugated bilirubin recycles into the reticuloendothelial system.

In the intestine, bacteria convert the remaining bilirubin diglucuronide into urobilinogen, a portion of which is reabsorbed into the portal blood and carried back to the liver. Most urobilinogen eventually travels back through bile into the intestine, but a small amount reaches the kidneys and is excreted in urine. The urobilinogen that escaped portal reabsorption is excreted in feces. With exposure to air, urobilinogen in urine oxidizes to urobilin, and urobilinogen in feces oxidizes to stercobilin.

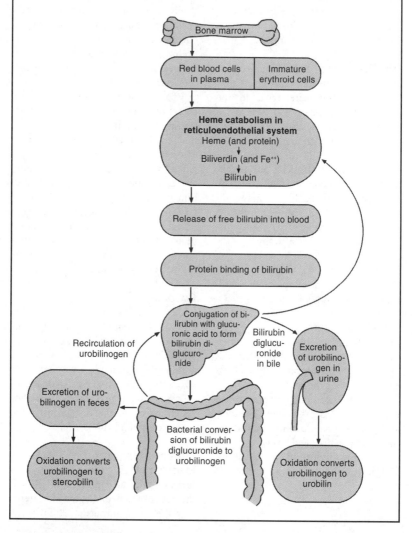

adult patient that he needn't restrict fluids but should fast for at least 4 hours before the test. (Fasting isn't necessary for neonates.) Tell the patient that this test requires a blood sample, who will perform the venipuncture and when, and that he may feel discomfort from the needle puncture and the tourniquet. Tell the parents of an infant that a small amount of blood will be drawn from the infant's heel as well as who will perform the heelstick and when. Check the patient's medication history for use of drugs that are known to interfere with serum bilirubin levels.

Procedure

If the patient is an adult, perform a venipuncture, and collect the sample in a 7-ml *red-top* or *red-marble-top* tube.

If the patient is an infant, perform a heelstick, and fill the microcapillary tube to the designated level with blood.

Precautions

- Protect the sample from strong sunlight and ultraviolet light because bilirubin breaks down when exposed to light.
- Handle the sample gently, and send it to the laboratory immediately.

Reference values

In adults, indirect serum bilirubin measures 1.1 mg/dl or less; direct serum bilirubin, less than 0.5 mg/dl. In neonates, total serum bilirubin measures 1 to 12 mg/dl.

Implications of results

Elevated indirect serum bilirubin levels often indicate hepatic damage in which the parenchymal cells can no longer conjugate bilirubin with glucuronide. Consequently, indirect bilirubin reenters the bloodstream. High levels of indirect bilirubin are also common in severe hemolytic anemia, when excessive indirect bilirubin overwhelms the liver's conjugating mechanism. If

hemolysis continues, both direct and indirect bilirubin may rise. Other causes of elevated indirect bilirubin levels include congenital enzyme deficiency, such as Gilbert's disease and Crigler-Najjar syndrome.

Elevated direct serum bilirubin levels usually indicate biliary obstruction, in which direct bilirubin, blocked from its normal pathway from the liver into the biliary tree, overflows into the bloodstream. If the obstruction continues, both direct and indirect bilirubin eventually may be elevated because of hepatic damage. In severe chronic hepatic damage, direct bilirubin concentrations may return to normal or near-normal levels, but elevated indirect bilirubin levels persist.

In neonates, total bilirubin levels that reach or exceed 18 mg/dl indicate the need for an exchange transfusion.

Post-test care

If a hematoma develops at the venipuncture or heelstick site, apply warm soaks.

Interfering factors

- Exposure of the sample to direct sunlight or ultraviolet light may depress bilirubin levels.
- Hemolysis due to rough handling of the sample may alter test results.

Fractionated erythrocyte porphyrins

This test measures erythrocyte porphyrins (also known as erythropoietic porphyrins) — specifically, protoporphyrin, coproporphyrin, and uroporphyrin. Porphyrins, pigments that are present in all protoplasm, have a significant role in energy storage and use. Protoporphyrin, coproporphyrin, and uroporphyrin are produced during heme biosynthesis. Small amounts of these porphyrins or their precursors normally appear in blood, urine, and feces. Production and excretion of porphyrins or their precursors increase in porphyrias, which are separated into erythropoietic and hepatic types. This test detects erythropoietic porphyrias.

Total porphyrins can be quantitated and separated by high-performance liquid chromatography into uroporphyrin, coproporphyrin, and protoporphyrin. Elevated levels suggest the need for further enzyme testing, which can identify the specific porphyria present.

Purpose
- To aid diagnosis of congenital or acquired erythropoietic porphyrias
- To help confirm diagnosis of disorders affecting red blood cell (RBC) activity.

Patient preparation
Explain to the patient that this test helps detect RBC disorders. Tell him that the test requires a blood sample, who will perform the venipuncture and when, and that he may feel some transient discomfort from the needle puncture and from the pressure of the tourniquet.

Procedure
Perform a venipuncture, and collect the sample in a 5-ml or larger *green-top* tube. Label the sample, place it on ice, and send it to the laboratory at once.

Precautions
- Handle the sample gently to prevent hemolysis.
- Send the sample to the laboratory promptly.

Reference values
Total porphyrin levels range from 16 to 60 µg/dl of packed RBCs. Protoporphyrin levels range from 16 to 60 µg/dl.

Coproporphyrin and uroporphyrin levels are less than 2 µg/dl.

Implications of results
Elevated protoporphyrin levels may indicate erythropoietic protoporphyria, infection, increased erythropoiesis, thalassemia, sideroblastic anemia, iron deficiency anemia, or lead poisoning.

Increased coproporphyrin levels may indicate congenital erythropoietic porphyria, erythropoietic protoporphyria or coproporphyria, or sideroblastic anemia.

Post-test care
If a hematoma develops at the venipuncture site, apply warm soaks.

Interfering factors
Hemolysis due to rough handling of the sample may interfere with test results.

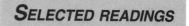

SELECTED READINGS

Henry, J.B., ed. *Clinical Diagnosis and Management by Laboratory Methods,* 19th ed. Philadelphia: W.B. Saunders Co., 1996.

Marshall, W.J. *Clinical Chemistry,* 3rd ed. St. Louis: Mosby–Year Book, Inc., 1995.

Mayo Medical Laboratories 1996 Test Catalog. Rochester, Minn.: Mayo Medical Laboratories, 1996.

Ravel, R.A. *Clinical Laboratory Medicine: Clinical Application of Laboratory Data,* 6th ed. St. Louis: Mosby–Year Book, Inc., 1995.

Tilkian, S.M., et al. *Clinical and Nursing Implications of Laboratory Tests,* 5th ed. St. Louis: Mosby–Year Book, Inc., 1995.

Weinstein, R.S., et al. *Advances in Pathology and Laboratory Medicine,* vol. 9. St. Louis: Mosby–Year Book, Inc., 1996.

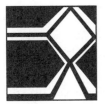

CHAPTER EIGHT

Carbohydrates

Learning objectives

After completing this chapter, the reader will be able to:
- explain carbohydrate metabolism after food intake and after fasting
- state the effects of abnormal insulin secretion
- list the signs and symptoms of diabetes mellitus
- describe how the pancreas functions
- explain how to administer oral glucose solutions
- describe the body's response to hypoglycemia and hyperglycemia
- state the purpose of each test discussed in the chapter
- prepare the patient physically and psychologically for each test
- describe the procedure for obtaining a specimen for each test
- specify appropriate precautions for safe administration of each test
- recognize signs of hypoglycemia and respond appropriately
- implement appropriate post-test care
- state the reference values for each test
- discuss the implications of abnormal test results
- list factors that may interfere with accurate test results.

INTRODUCTION

Tests that measure the body's tolerance for carbohydrates — that is, the capacity to metabolize carbohydrates — have great clinical significance and rank among the most commonly performed laboratory tests. Blood glucose determinations are also useful for evaluating the function of hormone-secreting organs that help regulate blood glucose, for assessing intestinal absorption of glucose, and for evaluating liver function.

Such tests actually measure the capacity for conversion of carbohydrates by insulin. Because direct assay of insulin is technically difficult and costly, the most useful tests measure insulin activity indirectly — by measuring blood concentrations of glucose.

These tests encompass many techniques for measuring blood glucose and differ greatly in specificity and sensitivity. The type of sample used also varies; normal values given in many common reference sources represent values derived from analysis of whole blood, which includes all reducing substances present in blood, such as fructose and other sugars, and some drugs. However, most current automated laboratory equipment is specific for true glucose. (Reference values listed in this book are for plasma and for true glucose, unless otherwise specified.)

Why measure glucose?

Glucose, a 6-carbon monosaccharide, is the body's major source of energy. Blood glucose derives from the conversion of ingested carbohydrates to glucose and to other simple sugars by enzymatic activity in the digestive tract; from the metabolic conversion of noncarbohydrate sources in the liver and kidneys; and from the breakdown of hepatic glycogen (a major storage form of glucose).

Insulin and glucagon are the two chief regulators of glucose levels, but several other hormones also influence glucose levels and are vital to normal carbohydrate metabolism. Growth hormone and adrenocorticotropic hormone, secreted by the anterior pituitary, raise glucose levels by promoting glucose formation from fat and protein. Cortisol and similar 11-oxysteroids, secreted by the adrenal cortex, produce the same effect. Epinephrine and thyroxine raise blood levels by stimulating the conversion of glycogen to glucose.

Metabolism after eating and fasting

Carbohydrate metabolism is most easily explained by examining the body's response to food ingestion and to fasting. Ingestion of food causes a modest rise in blood glucose levels, triggering secretion of the hormone insulin by the beta cells of the islets of Langerhans, located in the pancreas.

Insulin, a simple protein, acts as a hypoglycemic by stimulating cellular absorption of glucose and promoting its conversion to storage forms. In the liver, insulin increases the synthesis of glucose to glycogen (glycogenesis) and thus inhibits the breakdown of hepatic glycogen to glucose. Normally, the liver stores 60% or more of ingested glucose as glycogen; peripheral tissues receive the remainder. In the muscles, insulin enhances protein synthesis and the storage of amino acids, and promotes the conversion of glucose to glycogen or fat. In adipose tissue, most of the absorbed glucose acts to synthesize triglycerides, inhibiting their breakdown to free fatty acids and glycerol. The two major determinants of hepatic and peripheral glucose uptake are prompt secretion of insulin and the normal responsiveness of the tissues to insulin.

In the fasting state, the body derives energy from stored sources. In response to diminishing levels of circulating carbohydrates, insulin secretion decreases and the glucagon concentration rises. *Glucagon* is a hyperglycemic, a small protein secreted by the alpha cells of the islets of Langerhans. (See *Functions of the pancreas,* pages 230 and 231.) When dietary carbohydrates, the body's preferred source of energy, are in short supply, glucagon stimulates the formation of glucose from protein and fat catabolized in the liver and kidneys (glyconeogenesis) and from the breakdown of hepatic glycogen stores (glycogenolysis). In adipose tissue, glucagon stimulates the breakdown of triglycerides to free fatty acids and glycerol (lipolysis); in the muscles, glucagon breaks down protein into amino acids (proteolysis).

Effects of abnormal insulin secretion

Insulin deficiency, as occurs in diabetes mellitus, causes profound abnormalities in carbohydrate, lipid, and protein metabolism that ultimately affect all body tissues, especially skeletal muscle, adipose tissue, and the liver. Without adequate insulin, the body is unable to use ingested carbohydrates efficiently. The resulting deficiency of carbohydrate energy sources causes the body to metabolize fat. Consequently, ketone bodies — intermediate products of fat metabolism — accumulate in the blood. The end result of this abnormal metabolic pattern is marked hyperglycemia, osmotic diuresis, severe dehydration, electrolyte imbalance, metabolic acidosis, and severe weight loss.

Excessive insulin secretion, as occurs in insulinoma, causes similarly disruptive metabolic effects. Insulin excess produces *hypoglycemia* (low blood glucose levels), characterized by diaphoresis, nervousness, weakness, nausea, and tachycardia. In patients without diabetes, insulinoma is one cause of severe episodes of hypoglycemia. Unlike other causes of hypoglycemia, in which excessive insulin secretion follows immediately after eating (functional or reactive hypoglycemia), insulin secretion in insulinoma follows no distinct pattern.

Functions of the pancreas

The pancreas, a 3" to 4" (7.5- to 10-cm) triangularly shaped gland, lies behind the stomach. Two major tissue types perform its dual functions: the *acini* secrete digestive juices into the duodenum, and the *islets of Langerhans* secrete insulin and glucagon into the bloodstream. The three major islet cells are *alpha, beta,* and *delta.*

Beta cells secrete insulin
The polygonal beta cells contain insulin-bearing capsules. After a carbohydrate meal (and in response to other stimuli, including amino acids, as well as GI and pituitary hormones), these cells rapidly secrete insulin.

Insulin is a metabolic hormone that regulates the body's carbohydrate metabolism. One of insulin's primary functions is glycogenesis, whereby the liver stores 60% of the ingested glucose for later use. Insulin also influences synthesis and storage of muscle glycogen, triglycerides, and protein. An insulin deficiency, as in diabetes mellitus, inhibits the body's normal metabolism of glucose, resulting in glucose accumulation in the blood. In turn, the unavailability of glucose for energy needs causes the increased conversion of stored fats and protein for energy and eventually leads to ketosis and acidosis. At the same time, hyperglycemia increases osmotic pressure and causes dehydration and loss of glucose in the urine. Insulin deficiency also promotes lipid deposits in the vascular cells and leads to atherosclerosis.

Alpha cells secret glucagon
The alpha cells are larger than the beta cells and contain dark granules that secrete the hormone glucagon. Unlike insulin, glucagon has a hyperglycemic effect. When blood glucose levels are low (during periods of fasting) and insulin secretion falls, the alpha cells secrete glucagon to maintain body glucose levels (insulin's hypoglycemic role suppresses glucagon secretion). Glucagon breaks down stored liver glycogen and combats hypoglycemia. Because glucose is the brain's only nutrient, maintaining normal glucose levels is essential.

Delta cells secret somatostatin
The delta cells secrete somatostatin, a hormone whose metabolic role isn't completely understood. Because somatostatin can inhibit insulin and gluca-

Hypoglycemia may develop long after eating (fasting hypoglycemia).

Although *hyper*glycemia is usually characteristic of diabetes, *hypo*glycemia may result from kidney failure, hepatic disease, alcoholism, decreased food intake, or excessive administration of insulin. Brain tissue is most vulnerable to hypoglycemia, because it doesn't synthesize glucose or store it in significant amounts. Thus, hypoglycemia is likely to impair cerebral function.

Glucagon imbalance rare
Primary glucagon imbalance is rare. Primary causes of elevated glucagon levels include familial hyperglucagonemia (an autosomal dominant disorder) and glucagonoma (islet alpha-cell tumor). Because abnormal islet alpha cells and abnormal beta cells may appear simultaneously, glucagonoma is characteristically associated with mild diabetes.

gon secretion, it might someday be used to control the secretion of one or both of these hormones. Somatostatin is also secreted by the hypothalamus (where it's known as growth hormone inhibitory factor) and by the mucosa of the upper GI tract, where its function is unknown.

GI tract

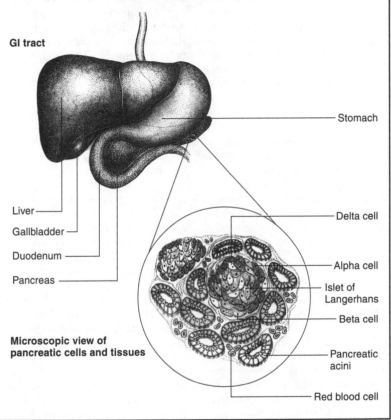

Stomach

Liver

Gallbladder

Duodenum

Pancreas

Delta cell

Alpha cell

Islet of Langerhans

Beta cell

Microscopic view of pancreatic cells and tissues

Pancreatic acini

Red blood cell

Elevated glucagon levels are usually linked to diabetes and to insulin deficiency. Because insulin inhibits glucagon secretion, its absence or deficiency allows secretion of glucagon to continue, even in the presence of hyperglycemia. Another factor that enhances the activity of glucagon is unresponsiveness to insulin of the hepatic cells. Thus, glucagon may contribute to hyperglycemia, especially in hypoinsulinemia diabetes.

Carbohydrate metabolism tests
Various tests screen for diabetes mellitus by measuring the body's response to fasting and to carbohydrate ingestion. The *fasting plasma glucose test* measures plasma glucose levels after a 12- to 14-hour fast. A patient with diabetes will have consistently high glucose levels because of insufficient insulin levels.

The *2-hour postprandial plasma glucose test,* performed 2 hours after the patient has eaten a high-carbohydrate meal, measures immediate insulin response to carbohydrate ingestion.

The *oral glucose tolerance test* (OGTT), the most sensitive method of evaluating borderline diabetes in selected patients, measures carbohydrate metabolism after ingestion of a challenge dose of glucose. This test is used to confirm diabetes and to aid diagnosis of hypoglycemia. It has significant limitations, however. Because no universal agreement exists regarding what values indicate an abnormal OGTT curve, the test allows no absolute distinction between a healthy person and one with mild diabetes. Moreover, this test has been known to suggest diabetes in a significant percentage of healthy people. (This overdiagnosis of diabetes may be related to the release of epinephrine in response to stress resulting from the numerous venipunctures required in the OGTT. Epinephrine stimulates the conversion of glycogen to glucose.) Thus, an OGTT-confirmed diagnosis of latent or asymptomatic diabetes is not necessarily significant.

Another limitation of this test is that different test methods provide different sets of values. Moreover, even when the same values are used for repeated testing, test results aren't consistently reproducible. Because of these limitations, the trend in laboratory testing is away from the OGTT and toward the fasting plasma glucose test for diagnosing diabetes mellitus.

Variations of the OGTT

The *I.V. glucose tolerance test,* an infrequently used variation of the OGTT, is more specific than the OGTT but less sensitive. The clinical significance of the test is under investigation, and the American Diabetes Association has yet to suggest a standardized procedure.

Another variation of the OGTT is the *cortisone glucose tolerance test.* In this test, the patient is given an oral dose of cortisone acetate $8\frac{1}{2}$ hours and 2 hours before an OGTT is performed. Because cortisone elevates plasma glucose by promoting glyconeogenesis, it is useful in detecting probable diabetes in patients with borderline deficiencies in carbohydrate tolerance or with a family history of diabetes. However, because the test's sensitivity and specificity have been challenged, it isn't considered a primary tool in diagnosing diabetes.

Other useful tests

The *beta-hydroxybutyrate assay* helps detect carbohydrate deprivation resulting from dietary imbalances, digestive disturbances, frequent vomiting, or starvation. This test, which measures one of the three ketone bodies, is especially helpful in monitoring the effect of insulin therapy during treatment of diabetic ketoacidosis. It's also helpful during emergency care of hypoglycemia, acidosis, and alcohol ingestion.

The *glycosylated hemoglobin test* measures the reactive amount of glucose in hemoglobin and evaluates carbohydrate status for up to 120 days. This test is useful because patients with diabetes are known to have abnormal concentrations of hemoglobins A_{1a}, A_{1b}, and A_{1c} in the red blood cells — about twice the level in people without diabetes. In patients with poorly controlled diabetes, the abnormal concentrations of these hemoglobins may rise to three times the normal levels.

The *oral lactose tolerance test,* which measures plasma glucose levels after a challenge dose of lactose, helps diagnose lactose intolerance due to lactase deficiency.

Levels of *blood lactate,* the reduction product of pyruvate, are measured by enzymatic methods using lactate dehydrogenase. These methods are recommended for evaluating patients with symptoms of lactic acidosis, such as

Kussmaul's respirations. Either arterial or venous blood can be used for this test, but venous samples are easily obtained and so are more commonly used. However, unless the patient rests for 1 hour before testing, venous blood may yield higher values than arterial blood. Comparison of pyruvate and lactate levels reliably indicates tissue oxidation, but measurement of pyruvate is technically difficult and infrequently performed.

Home blood glucose monitoring
The long-term goal of diabetes therapy is to maintain blood glucose levels at normal or near-normal levels, because persistent hyperglycemia leads to serious complications, such as retinopathy, vascular insufficiency, urinary tract infection, and peripheral neuropathy. Self-testing of blood glucose at home can help the diabetic patient improve blood glucose control by allowing him to record and monitor daily fluctuations. It also helps promote the patient's independence.

The home monitoring systems now available allow rapid, reliable blood glucose measurement. These systems use a reagent test strip either alone or in combination with a reflectance meter. After applying a drop of capillary blood to the test strip, the patient compares the color on the strip to a color-coded key (for an approximate measurement) or inserts the test strip into a reflectance meter (for a precise measurement).

Home monitoring of blood glucose levels is becoming more widely accepted because findings closely approximate laboratory results if the patient follows directions carefully. However, improper timing of the test or overzealous washing of the reagent strip can alter test results.

CARBOHYDRATE METABOLISM TESTS

Fasting plasma glucose

Commonly used to screen for diabetes mellitus, the fasting plasma glucose test (also known as the fasting blood sugar test) measures plasma glucose levels following a 12- to 14-hour fast.

In the fasting state, plasma glucose levels decrease, stimulating release of the hormone glucagon. Glucagon then acts to raise plasma glucose by accelerating glycogenolysis, stimulating glyconeogenesis, and inhibiting glycogen synthesis. Normally, secretion of insulin checks this rise in glucose levels. In diabetes, however, absence or deficiency of insulin allows persistently high glucose levels. (See *Recognizing symptoms of diabetes,* page 234.)

Purpose
▪ To screen for diabetes mellitus
▪ To monitor drug or dietary therapy in patients with diabetes mellitus.

Patient preparation
Explain to the patient that this test detects disorders of glucose metabolism and aids diagnosis of diabetes. Advise him to fast for 12 to 14 hours before the test. Tell him that this test requires a blood sample, who will perform the venipuncture and when and that he may experience transient discomfort from the needle puncture and the pressure of the tourniquet.

Withhold drugs that affect test results, as ordered. If these medications must be continued, note this on the laboratory request. Advise the patient with diabetes that he will receive his medication after the test.

Recognizing symptoms of diabetes

When you suspect diabetes, observe the patient carefully for the following classic symptoms:
- *Polyuria:* Excessive plasma glucose overflows into the urine and exerts an osmotic pressure because of its concentration. This inhibits normal reabsorption of water by the renal tubules and leads to osmotic diuresis and dehydration.

- *Polydipsia:* Frequent urination leads to dehydration and severe thirst.
- *Weight loss:* Depletion of fat and protein stores to satisfy energy requirements causes severe, unexplained weight loss.
- *Polyphagia:* In some patients, tissue destruction raises metabolic requirements and produces severe hunger.

Alert the patient to the symptoms of hypoglycemia — weakness, restlessness, nervousness, hunger, and sweating — and tell him to report such symptoms immediately.

Procedure
Perform a venipuncture, and collect the sample in a 5-ml *gray-top* tube.

Precautions
- Send the sample to the laboratory immediately because blood glucose levels decrease when the sample is left at room temperature. If transport is delayed, refrigerate the sample.
- Specify on the laboratory request the time that the patient last ate, the sample collection time, and the time that he received the last pretest dose of insulin or oral antidiabetic drug (if applicable).

Reference values
The normal range for fasting plasma glucose varies according to the laboratory procedure. Generally, normal values after a 12- to 14-hour fast are 70 to 100 mg of "true glucose"/dl of blood when measured by the glucose oxidase and hexokinase methods.

Implications of results
A fasting plasma glucose level of 140 mg/dl or more obtained on two or more occasions confirms diabetes mellitus;

however, a borderline or transiently elevated level requires the 2-hour postprandial plasma glucose test or the oral glucose tolerance test to confirm the diagnosis.

Although increased fasting plasma glucose levels most commonly occur with diabetes, they can also result from pancreatitis, recent acute illness (such as myocardial infarction), Cushing's syndrome, acromegaly, and pheochromocytoma. Hyperglycemia may also stem from hyperlipoproteinemia (especially type III, IV, or V), chronic hepatic disease, nephrotic syndrome, brain tumor, sepsis, or gastrectomy with dumping syndrome, and is typical in eclampsia, anoxia, and seizure disorders.

Depressed plasma glucose levels can result from hyperinsulinism, insulinoma, von Gierke's disease, functional or reactive hypoglycemia, myxedema, adrenal insufficiency, congenital adrenal hyperplasia, hypopituitarism, malabsorption syndrome, and some cases of hepatic insufficiency.

Post-test care
- If a hematoma develops at the venipuncture site, apply warm soaks.
- Provide a balanced meal or a snack. As ordered, resume administration of medications withheld before the test.

Interfering factors

■ False-positive findings may be caused by acetaminophen when the glucose oxidase or hexokinase method is used. Other drugs known to elevate plasma glucose levels are chlorthalidone, thiazide diuretics, furosemide, triamterene, oral contraceptives (estrogen-progestogen combination), benzodiazepines, phenytoin, phenothiazines, lithium, epinephrine, arginine, phenolphthalein, dextrothyroxine, diazoxide, large doses of nicotinic acid, corticosteroids, and recent I.V. glucose infusions. Ethacrynic acid may also cause hyperglycemia, but large doses can produce hypoglycemia in patients with uremia.

■ Decreased plasma glucose levels may be caused by beta-adrenergic blockers, ethanol, clofibrate, insulin, oral antidiabetic agents, and monoamine oxidase inhibitors.

■ Failure to observe dietary restrictions may elevate plasma glucose levels.

■ Recent illness, infection, or pregnancy can elevate plasma glucose levels; strenuous exercise can depress them.

■ Glycolysis due to failure to refrigerate the sample or to send it to the laboratory immediately can result in false-negative results.

Two-hour postprandial plasma glucose

The 2-hour postprandial test is a valuable screening tool for detecting diabetes mellitus. This procedure is performed on patients who have symptoms of diabetes (polydipsia and polyuria) or on patients whose fasting plasma glucose test results suggest diabetes.

The 2-hour postprandial test reliably indicates the body's insulin response to carbohydrate ingestion. It relies solely

---

Preferred screening test

Because the 2-hour postprandial test is a simpler procedure than the oral glucose tolerance test or the fasting plasma glucose test, it's often the preferred test for diabetes screening in patients with any of the following conditions:
■ obesity
■ family history of diabetes
■ transient glycosuria or hyperglycemia (especially during pregnancy, surgery, or use of adrenal steroids) or after trauma, emotional stress, myocardial infarction, or cerebrovascular accident
■ unexplained hypoglycemia, neuropathy, retinopathy, nephropathy, or peripheral vascular disease
■ pregnancy resulting in abortion, premature labor, stillbirth, neonatal death, or a very large infant
■ recurrent infection, especially boils and abscesses.

---

on the 2-hour glucose level, avoiding the multiple venipunctures required for the oral glucose tolerance test (OGTT). If postprandial test results are borderline, the OGTT may confirm the diagnosis. (See *Preferred screening test.*)

Purpose

■ To aid diagnosis of diabetes mellitus
■ To monitor drug or diet therapy in patients with diabetes mellitus.

Patient preparation

Explain to the patient that this test evaluates glucose metabolism and helps detect diabetes. Tell him to eat a balanced meal or one containing 100 g of carbohydrate (recommended by the American Diabetes Association) before the test and then to fast for 2 hours. Instruct him to avoid smoking and strenuous exercise after the meal. Tell him this test requires a blood sample, who will per-

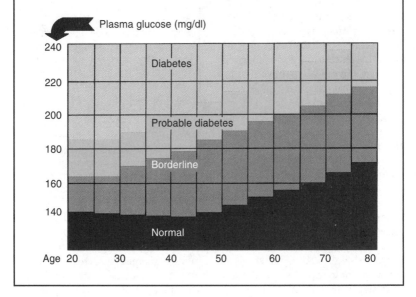

Two-hour postprandial glucose levels by age

The greatest difference in normal and diabetic insulin responses and, thus, in plasma glucose concentration, occurs about 2 hours after a glucose challenge. However, normal glucose values can fluctuate according to the patient's age (as shown below). After age 50, for example, normal levels rise markedly and steadily, sometimes reaching 160 mg/dl or higher. In younger patients, glucose levels over 145 mg/dl suggest incipient diabetes and require further evaluation.

Plasma glucose (mg/dl)

Diabetes

Probable diabetes

Borderline

Normal

Age 20 30 40 50 60 70 80

form the venipuncture and when, and that he may experience transient discomfort from the needle puncture and the pressure of the tourniquet.

Procedure
Perform a venipuncture, and collect the sample in a 5-ml *gray-top* tube. Many laboratories will accept other color top tubes as long as the sample is processed in a reasonable amount of time.

Precautions
▪ Send the sample to the laboratory immediately or refrigerate it.
▪ Specify on the laboratory request the time that the patient last ate, the sample collection time, and the time that he

received the last pretest dose of insulin or oral antidiabetic drug (if applicable). If the sample is to be drawn by a technician, tell him the exact time the venipuncture must be performed.

Reference values
In a person without diabetes, postprandial glucose values are less than 145 mg/dl by the glucose oxidase or hexokinase method; levels are slightly elevated in people over age 50. (See *Two-hour postprandial glucose levels by age.*)

Implications of results
Two-hour postprandial plasma glucose values of 200 mg/dl or more indicate diabetes mellitus. High levels may also

result from pancreatitis, Cushing's syndrome, acromegaly, or pheochromocytoma. Hyperglycemia may also be caused by hyperlipoproteinemia (especially type III, IV, or V), chronic hepatic disease, nephrotic syndrome, brain tumor, sepsis, gastrectomy with dumping syndrome, eclampsia, anoxia, or convulsive disorders.

Depressed glucose levels can result from hyperinsulinism, insulinoma, von Gierke's disease, functional or reactive hypoglycemia, myxedema, adrenal insufficiency, congenital adrenal hyperplasia, hypopituitarism, malabsorption syndrome, and some cases of hepatic insufficiency.

Post-test care

■ If a hematoma develops at the venipuncture site, ease discomfort by applying warm soaks.

■ As ordered, resume diet, normal activity, and administration of medications that were discontinued before the test.

Interfering factors

■ False-positive results may be caused by acetaminophen when the glucose oxidase or hexokinase method is used. Other drugs known to elevate plasma glucose levels are chlorthalidone, thiazide diuretics, furosemide, triamterene, oral contraceptives (estrogen-progestogen combination), benzodiazepines, phenytoin, phenothiazines, lithium, epinephrine, arginine, phenolphthalein, dextrothyroxine, diazoxide, large doses of nicotinic acid, corticosteroids, and recent I.V. glucose infusions. Ethacrynic acid may also cause hyperglycemia, but large doses can produce hypoglycemia in patients with uremia.

■ Depressed glucose levels may result from the use of beta-adrenergic blockers, amphetamines, ethanol, clofibrate, insulin, oral antidiabetic drugs, and monoamine oxidase inhibitors.

■ Recent illness, infection, or pregnancy may raise glucose levels; strenuous exercise or stress may depress them.

■ Glycolysis caused by failure to refrigerate the sample or to send it to the laboratory immediately can depress glucose levels.

Oral glucose tolerance

The oral glucose tolerance test (OGTT), the most sensitive method of evaluating borderline cases of diabetes mellitus in selected patients, measures carbohydrate metabolism after ingestion of a challenge dose of glucose. (See *Administering oral glucose solutions,* page 238.) The body absorbs this dose rapidly, causing plasma glucose levels to rise and peak within 30 minutes to 1 hour. The pancreas responds by secreting more insulin, causing glucose levels to return to normal after 2 to 3 hours.

During this period, plasma and urine glucose levels are monitored to assess insulin secretion and the body's ability to metabolize glucose. Occasionally, glucose levels are monitored an additional 2 to 3 hours to aid diagnosis of hypoglycemia and malabsorption syndrome. However, such extended testing is contraindicated when insulinoma is strongly suspected because prolonged fasting in such a patient can lead to fainting and coma.

In a patient with mild or diet-controlled diabetes, fasting plasma glucose levels may be in the normal range; however, insufficient secretion of insulin after ingestion of carbohydrates causes plasma glucose levels to rise sharply and return to normal slowly. This decreased tolerance for glucose helps to confirm mild diabetes.

The OGTT is not usually used in patients with fasting plasma glucose val-

Administering oral glucose solutions

The oral glucose load in a glucose tolerance test usually varies from 50 to 100 g. The American Diabetes Association, however, recommends a glucose dose of 40 g/m^2 of body surface area, as calculated by a nomogram based on height and weight. Others advocate a glucose load of 1.75 g/kg of body weight, which is especially useful in testing pediatric patients.

Many patients become nauseated after drinking the overly sweet glucose solution. One way to make the solution more palatable is to dissolve it in water, flavor it with lemon juice, and chill it. Another is to substitute Glucola, a carbonated drink, or Gel-a-dex, a cherry-flavored gelatin, for the appropriate amount of glucose.

ues above 140 mg/dl or postprandial plasma glucose above 200 mg/dl. Two other tests are also used to confirm or sensitize OGTT findings. (See *Supplementary glucose tolerance tests.*)

Purpose
▪ To confirm diabetes mellitus in selected patients
▪ To aid diagnosis of hypoglycemia and malabsorption syndrome.

Patient preparation
Explain to the patient that this test evaluates glucose metabolism. Instruct him to maintain a high-carbohydrate diet for 3 days and then to fast for 10 to 16 hours before the test. Advise him not to smoke, drink coffee or alcohol, or exercise strenuously for 8 hours before or during the test. Tell him this test usually requires five blood samples and five urine specimen, who will perform the venipunctures and when, and that he may expe-

rience transient discomfort from the needle punctures and the pressure of the tourniquet. Suggest that he bring a book or other quiet diversions with him to the test because the procedure usually takes 3 hours but can last as long as 6 hours.

Withhold drugs that may affect test results, as ordered. If these drugs must be continued, note this on the laboratory request. Alert the patient to the symptoms of hypoglycemia — weakness, restlessness, nervousness, hunger, and sweating — and tell him to report such symptoms immediately.

Procedure
Between 7 a.m. and 9 a.m., draw a fasting blood sample in a 7-ml *gray-top* tube. Collect a urine specimen at the same time, if your institution includes this as part of the test. After collecting these samples, administer the test load of oral glucose, and record the time of ingestion. Encourage the patient to drink the entire glucose solution within 5 minutes.

Draw blood samples 30 minutes, 1 hour, 2 hours, and 3 hours after giving the loading dose, using 7-ml *gray-top* tubes. Collect urine specimens at the same intervals. Tell the patient to lie down if he feels faint from the numerous venipunctures. Encourage him to drink water throughout the test to promote adequate urine excretion.

Precautions
▪ Send blood and urine samples to the laboratory immediately, or refrigerate them. Specify when the patient last ate and the blood and urine collection times. As appropriate, record the time that the patient received his last pretest dose of insulin or oral antidiabetic drug.

 ▪ If the patient develops severe hypoglycemia, notify the doctor. Draw a blood sample, record the time on the laboratory request, and discontinue

Supplementary glucose tolerance tests

Although the oral glucose tolerance test (OGTT) is the most effective test for detecting diabetes, two other tests are sometimes used as research tools to sensitize or confirm OGTT findings.

I.V. glucose tolerance test
This test measures blood glucose after the patient receives an I.V. infusion of 50% glucose over 3 or 4 minutes. Blood samples are then drawn at $\frac{1}{2}$-, 1-, 2-, and 3-hour intervals. After an immediate glucose peak of 300 to 400 mg/dl (accompanied by glycosuria), the normal glucose curve falls steadily, reaching fasting levels within 1 to $1\frac{1}{4}$ hours.

Failure to achieve fasting glucose levels within 2 to 3 hours generally confirms diabetes. A similarly delayed return to fasting glucose levels may result from fever, stress, old age, inactivity, carbohydrate deprivation, neoplasms, cirrhosis, or steroid-producing endocrine diseases. Nevertheless, the I.V. glucose tolerance test (IVGTT) has the following advantages over the OGTT:
- GI hormones that cause insulin secretion won't affect IVGTT glucose tolerance curves.
- Patients with intestinal absorption syndromes won't present abnormal curves.
- The IVGTT provides an alternative to flat OGTT curves resulting from hypopituitarism, hypoparathyroidism, or Addison's disease.
- This test does not require the patient to ingest an unpalatable oral glucose load.

Cortisone glucose tolerance test
This test is occasionally used for patients with borderline carbohydrate-tolerance deficiencies or a strong familial predisposition to diabetes who produce a normal OGTT curve. After a 3-day high-carbohydrate diet, oral cortisone acetate is administered $8\frac{1}{2}$ and 2 hours before the standard OGTT. (Cortisone promotes glyconeogenesis and may accentuate carbohydrate intolerance in latent or mild diabetes.)

Although this test is used primarily for research, values that rise approximately 20 mg/dl above those of the standard OGTT after 2 hours indicate probable diabetes in some people with only minimally decreased carbohydrate intolerance.

---

the test. Have the patient drink a glass of orange juice with sugar added, or administer glucose I.V. to reverse the reaction.

Reference values
Normal plasma glucose levels peak at 160 to 180 mg/dl 30 minutes to 1 hour after administration of an oral glucose test dose and return to fasting levels or lower in 2 to 3 hours. (See *Interpreting results of the OGTT,* page 240.) Urine glucose tests remain negative throughout.

Implications of results
Depressed glucose tolerance, in which levels peak sharply before falling slowly to fasting levels, may confirm diabetes or may result from Cushing's disease, hemochromatosis, pheochromocytomas, or central nervous system lesions.

Increased glucose tolerance, in which levels may peak at less than normal, may indicate insulinoma, malabsorption syndrome, adrenocortical insufficiency (Addison's disease), hypothyroidism, or hypopituitarism.

Interpreting results of the OGTT

Because plasma glucose levels in the oral glucose tolerance test (OGTT) can be measured various ways, inconsistent results and misinterpretation are common. Age, race, inactivity, and obesity may also affect established OGTT criteria. The American Diabetes Association recommends using the reference values obtained by the Wilkerson point system, the Fajans-Conn system, or the NIH system, depending on whether the patient is a child or is pregnant.

METHOD	HOUR	WHOLE BLOOD	PLASMA	POINTS
Wilkerson point system	Fasting	≥110 mg/dl	≥130 mg/dl	1
	1	≥170 mg/dl	≥195 mg/dl	½
	2	≥120 mg/dl	≥140 mg/dl	½
	3	≥110 mg/dl	≥130 mg/dl	1

Two or more total points confirm the diagnosis of diabetes.

Fajans-Conn	1	≥160 mg/dl	≥185 mg/dl	
	1½	≥140 mg/dl	≥165 mg/dl	
	2	≥120 mg/dl	≥140 mg/dl	

If all levels equal or exceed established values, the diagnosis of diabetes is confirmed.

National Institutes of Health (NIH)	Fasting		>140 mg/dl	
	2		>200 mg/dl	

If all levels exceed established values, the diagnosis of diabetes is confirmed.

Post-test care

- If a hematoma develops at the venipuncture site, apply warm soaks.
- Provide a balanced meal or a snack, but observe for a hypoglycemic reaction.
- As ordered, resume administration of medications withheld before the test.

Interfering factors

- Elevated plasma glucose levels may result from chlorthalidone, thiazide diuretics, furosemide, triamterene, oral contraceptives (estrogen-progestogen combination), benzodiazepines, phenytoin, phenothiazines, lithium, epinephrine, phenolphthalein, caffeine, arginine, dextrothyroxine, diazoxide, large doses of nicotinic acid, corticosteroids, and recent I.V. glucose infusions.
- Depressed glucose levels may be caused by ingestion of beta-adrenergic blockers, amphetamines, ethanol, clofibrate, insulin, oral antidiabetic drugs, and monoamine oxidase inhibitors.
- Failure to adhere to dietary and exercise restrictions may alter test results.
- Carbohydrate deprivation before the test can produce a diabetic response (abnormal increase in plasma glucose with a delayed decrease) because the pancreas is unaccustomed to responding to high-carbohydrate load.
- A recent infection, fever, pregnancy, or acute illness such as myocardial infarction may elevate glucose levels.
- People over age 50 tend to exhibit decreasing carbohydrate tolerance, which causes an increase in glucose tolerance to upper limits of about 1 mg/dl for every year over age 50.

Serum beta-hydroxybutyrate

A quantitative colorimetric assay, this test measures levels of beta-hydroxybutyrate, which is one of three ketone bodies. (The other two are acetoacetate and acetone.) At 78%, its relative proportion in the blood is greater than acetoacetate (20%) or acetone (2%).

A small amount of acetoacetate and beta-hydroxybutyrate is formed during the normal hepatic metabolism of free fatty acids and is then metabolized in the peripheral tissues. In some conditions, increased acetoacetate production may exceed the metabolic capacity of the peripheral tissues. As acetoacetate accumulates in the blood, a small portion is converted to acetone by spontaneous decarboxylation. The remaining and greater portion of acetoacetate is converted to beta-hydroxybutyrate. This accumulation of all three ketone bodies is referred to as ketosis: excessive formation of ketone bodies in the blood is called ketonemia.

Purpose

■ To diagnose carbohydrate deprivation, which may result from starvation, digestive disturbances, dietary imbalances, or frequent vomiting
■ To aid diagnosis of diabetes mellitus resulting from decreased utilization of carbohydrates
■ To aid diagnosis of glycogen storage diseases, specifically Von Gierke's disease (see *Glycogen storage diseases,* page 242)
■ To diagnose or monitor the treatment of metabolic acidosis, such as diabetic ketoacidosis or lactic acidosis.

Patient preparation

Explain to the patient that this test evaluates ketones in the blood and doesn't require him to fast. Tell him that the test requires a blood sample, who will perform the venipuncture and when, and that he may experience transient discomfort from the needle puncture and the pressure of the tourniquet.

Procedure

Perform a venipuncture, and collect the sample in a 5-ml *red-top* tube. Let the specimen clot. Centrifuge and remove the serum. If an acetone level is requested, have this analysis performed first.

Serum beta-hydroxybutyrate remains stable for at least 1 week at 25.6° to 46.4° F (2° to 8° C). Plasma may also be used for analysis of beta-hydroxybutyrate.

Precautions

Send the specimen to the laboratory immediately.

Reference values

The normal value for serum or plasma beta-hydroxybutyrate levels is less than 0.4 mmol/L.

Implications of results

The determination of ketone bodies in the blood, more so than in the urine, is extremely helpful in treating ketosis associated with diabetes and other conditions. Because it possesses greater concentration and stability than acetoacetate and acetone, beta-hydroxybutyrate has become an extremely reliable guide in monitoring the effect of insulin therapy during treatment of diabetic ketoacidosis. This test is also helpful during emergency management of hypoglycemia, acidosis, alcohol ingestion, or an unexplained increase in the anion gap.

Notify the patient's doctor at once if values exceed 2 mmol/L.

Post-test care

If a hematoma develops at the venipuncture site, applying warm soaks relieves discomfort.

Glycogen storage diseases

Glycogen storage diseases alter the synthesis or degradation of glycogen, the form in which glucose is stored in the body.

Von Gierke's disease, a Type I glycogen storage disease, is caused by a deficiency of glucose-6-phosphate dehydrogenase. It affects the liver and kidneys, causing hepatomegaly, hypoglycemia, hyperuricemia, xanthomas, bleeding, and adiposity.

Von Gierke's disease is transmitted as an autosomal recessive trait.

Two types, Types Ia and Ib, exist. Type Ib (pseudo Type I) is similar to, but more severe than, Type Ia. However, patients with this disease may live well into adulthood.

Laboratory studies of plasma demonstrate low glucose levels but high levels of free fatty acids, triglycerides, cholesterol, and uric acid in Type Ia disease. Serum analysis reveals elevated pyruvic acid and lactic acid levels.

Interfering factors

- Hemolysis, jaundice, or lipemia have little or no effect on results.
- Heparin doesn't appear to interfere with the reaction.
- The presence of both lactate dehydrogenase (at high concentrations) and lactic acid (at concentrations greater than 10 mmol/L) may elevate beta-hydroxybutyrate levels by at least 0.2 mmol/L, thereby altering test results.
- Sodium fluoride, at concentrations greater than 2.5 nmol/L, appears to lower the levels of beta-hydroxybutyrate by at least 0.1 mmol/L.
- If the patient has fasted, values will increase with increased fasting time.

Glycosylated hemoglobin

The glycosylated hemoglobin test (also known as the total fasting hemoglobin or glycohemoglobin test) is a diagnostic tool that helps to monitor the effectiveness of diabetes therapy. The three minor hemoglobins measured in this test — hemoglobins (Hb) A_{1a}, A_{1b}, and A_{1c} — are variants of Hb A formed by glycosylation, a nearly irreversible molecular process in which glucose becomes chemically incorporated in Hb A. Because glycosylation occurs at a constant rate during the 120-day life span of an erythrocyte, glycosylated hemoglobin levels reflect the average blood glucose level during the preceding 2 to 3 months and thus are useful in evaluating the long-term effectiveness of diabetes therapy.

The glycosylated hemoglobin test has distinct advantages over traditional blood and urine glucose tests. Blood glucose testing requires repeated venipunctures; each measurement reflects glucose control only at the moment the sample was taken. Measuring urinary glucose excretion also reflects glucose control only at the time of collection. In contrast, the glycosylated hemoglobin test requires only one venipuncture every 6 to 8 weeks and reflects diabetes control over several months. In addition, because this test measures glucose within an erythrocyte, levels are more stable than with plasma glucose, which is affected by metabolic processes.

Glycosylated hemoglobin is measured by processing red cell hemolysates through a cation exchange chromatog-

Avoiding complications of diabetes

Because the glycosylated hemoglobin test measures glucose levels over a 120-day period — the life span of erythrocytes — this test helps assess average daily glucose levels over a long period in patients with diabetes. In doing so, it may also help prevent serious complications even in patients whose insulin regimen, antidiabetic drug use, and diet are strictly controlled.

Without proper management, patients with diabetes are at risk for the following chronic complications, which can affect all body systems:
■ cardiovascular diseases such as atherosclerosis, resulting in strokes and myocardial infarction
■ peripheral vascular disorders, such as gangrene, intermittent claudication, and microangiopathy
■ renal failure, specifically intercapillary glomerulosclerosis (Kimmelstiel-Wilson syndrome)
■ urinary tract infections
■ neuropathies, ranging from extraocular muscle palsies to more common peripheral nerve problems
■ neuropathies of the bladder, GI tract, and reproductive system
■ skin lesions and infections, such as candidiasis
■ tooth loss due to periodontal disease
■ cataracts and retinopathy, leading to impaired vision and blindness
■ diabetic acidosis, possibly resulting in coma.

raphy column to separate glycosylated hemoglobins from Hb A.

Purpose
■ To assess control of diabetes mellitus. (See *Avoiding complications of diabetes*.)

Patient preparation
Explain to the patient that this test evaluates the effectiveness of diabetes therapy. Advise him that he need not restrict food or fluids, and instruct him to maintain his prescribed medication or diet regimen. Tell him the test requires a blood sample, who will perform the venipuncture and when, and that he may experience transient discomfort from the needle puncture and the pressure of the tourniquet.

Procedure
Perform a venipuncture, and collect the sample in a 5-ml *lavender-top* tube.

Precautions
Fill the collection tube completely, and invert it gently several times to mix the sample and anticoagulant adequately.

Reference values
Glycosylated hemoglobin values are reported as a percentage of the total hemoglobin within an erythrocyte. Because Hb A_{1c} is present in a larger quantity than the other minor hemoglobins, it's commonly measured and reported separately. Hb A_{1a} and Hb A_{1b} account for about 1.6% and 0.8%, respectively; Hb A_{1c} accounts for approximately 5%; and total glycosylated hemoglobin accounts for 5.5% to 9.0%.

Implications of results
In diabetes, Hbs A_{1a} and A_{1b} constitute approximately 2.5% to 3.9% of total hemoglobin; Hb A_{1c} constitutes 8.0% to 11.9%; and total glycosylated hemoglobin, 10.9% to 15.5%. Glycosylated hemoglobin levels approach normal range as therapy begins to control diabetes.

Post-test care

■ If a hematoma develops at the venipuncture site, ease discomfort by applying warm soaks.

■ Schedule the patient for an appointment in 6 to 8 weeks for appropriate follow-up testing.

Interfering factors

Failure to mix the sample and the anticoagulant adequately may affect the accuracy of test results.

Oral lactose tolerance

This test measures plasma glucose levels after ingestion of a challenge dose of lactose. It's used to screen for lactose intolerance due to lactase deficiency.

Lactose, a disaccharide, is found in milk and other dairy products. The intestinal enzyme lactase splits lactose into the monosaccharides glucose and galactose for absorption by the intestinal epithelium. Absence or deficiency of lactase causes undigested lactose to remain in the intestinal lumen, producing abdominal cramps and watery diarrhea. Congenital lactase deficiency is rare; lactose intolerance is usually acquired as lactase levels decline with age.

Purpose

■ To detect lactose intolerance.

Patient preparation

Explain to the patient that this test determines if his symptoms are due to an inability to digest lactose. Instruct him to fast and to avoid strenuous activity for 8 hours before the test. Tell him this test requires four blood samples, who will perform the venipunctures and when, and that he may feel transient discomfort from the needle punctures

and the pressure of the tourniquet. Explain that the entire procedure may take as long as 2 hours.

As ordered, withhold drugs that may affect plasma glucose levels. If these drugs must be continued, note this on the laboratory request.

Procedure

After the patient has fasted for 8 hours, perform a venipuncture and collect a blood sample in a 7-ml *gray-top* tube. Then administer the test load of lactose — for an adult, 50 g of lactose dissolved in 400 ml of water; for a child, 50 g/m² of body surface area. Record the time of ingestion.

Draw a blood sample 30, 60, and 120 minutes after giving the loading dose, using 7-ml *gray-top* tubes. Collect a stool sample 5 hours after the loading dose, if ordered.

Precautions

■ Send blood and stool samples to the laboratory immediately, or refrigerate them if transport is delayed. Note the collection time on the laboratory request.

■ Watch for symptoms of lactose intolerance — abdominal cramps, nausea, bloating, flatulence, and watery diarrhea — caused by the loading dose.

Reference values

Normally, plasma glucose levels rise more than 20 mg/dl over fasting levels within 15 to 60 minutes after ingestion of the lactose loading dose. Stool sample analysis shows normal pH (7 to 8) and low glucose content (less than 1+ on a glucose-indicating dipstick).

Implications of results

A rise in plasma glucose of less than 20 mg/dl indicates lactose intolerance, as does stool acidity (pH of 5.5 or less) and high glucose content (greater than 1+ on the dipstick). Accompanying signs and symptoms provoked by the test also suggest but do not confirm the diagnosis because such symptoms may develop for patients with normal lactase activity after a loading dose of lactose. Small-bowel biopsy with lactase assay may be done to confirm the diagnosis.

Post-test care
■ If a hematoma develops at the venipuncture site, apply warm soaks.
■ As ordered, instruct the patient to resume diet, activity, and medications withheld before the test.

Interfering factors
■ Drugs that affect plasma glucose levels — such as thiazide diuretics, oral contraceptives, benzodiazepines, propranolol, and insulin — may alter test results.
■ Delayed emptying of stomach contents can cause depressed glucose levels.
■ Failure to follow diet and exercise restrictions may alter test results.
■ Glycolysis may cause false-negative results.

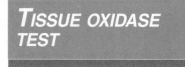

TISSUE OXIDASE TEST

Lactic acid and pyruvic acid

Lactic acid, present in blood as lactate ion, is derived primarily from muscle cells and erythrocytes. It is an intermediate product of carbohydrate metabolism and is normally metabolized by the liver. Blood lactate concentration depends on the rate of production and on the rate of metabolism; lactate levels may rise significantly during exercise.

Lactate is the reduction product of pyruvate, a by-product of carbohydrate metabolism. Together these compounds form a reversible reaction that's regulated by oxygen supply. When oxygen levels are deficient, pyruvate converts to lactate; when they're adequate, lactate converts to pyruvate.

When the hepatic system fails to metabolize lactate sufficiently, or when excess pyruvate converts to lactate due to tissue hypoxia and circulatory collapse, lactic acidosis (lactate levels more than 2 mEq/L, with a pH lower than 7.35) may result. Measurement of blood lactate levels by enzymatic methods, using lactic dehydrogenase, is recommended for all patients with symptoms of lactic acidosis, such as Kussmaul's respiration.

Although arterial or venous blood can be used for lactate analysis, a venous sample is more convenient to obtain. However, unless the patient rests for 1 hour before the test, venous blood may yield higher values than arterial blood. Comparison of pyruvate and lactate levels reliably mirrors tissue oxidation, but measurement of pyruvate is technically difficult and performed infrequently.

Purpose
■ To assess tissue oxidation
■ To help determine the cause of lactic acidosis.

Patient preparation
The patient with acidosis is likely to be comatose or extremely lethargic. Nevertheless, explain to him that this blood test evaluates the oxygen level in tissues. Tell him the test requires a blood sample, who will perform the venipuncture and when, and that he may experience transient discomfort from the needle puncture and the tourniquet pressure. Withhold food overnight, and make sure the patient rests for at least 1 hour before the test.

Procedure

Perform a venipuncture, and collect the sample in a 5-ml *gray-top* tube.

Precautions

■ Because venostasis may raise blood lactate levels, it's best to avoid using a tourniquet; if you do use one, release it at least 2 minutes before collecting the sample so the blood can circulate. Tell the patient he must not clench his fist during the venipuncture.

■ Because lactate and pyruvate are extremely unstable, place the sample container in an ice-filled cup, and send it to the laboratory immediately.

Reference values

Blood lactate values range from 0.93 to 1.65 mEq/L; pyruvate levels, from 0.08 to 0.16 mEq/L. Normally, the lactate-pyruvate ratio is less than 10:1.

Implications of results

Elevated blood lactate levels associated with hypoxia may result from strenuous muscle exercise, shock, hemorrhage, septicemia, myocardial infarction, pulmonary embolism, or cardiac arrest. When no reason for diminished tissue perfusion is apparent, increased lactate levels may result from systemic disorders (such as diabetes mellitus, leukemias, lymphomas, hepatic disease, and renal failure) or from enzymatic defects (as in von Gierke's disease and fructose 1,6-diphosphatase deficiency).

Lactic acidosis can follow ingestion of large doses of acetaminophen or ethanol as well as I.V. infusion of epinephrine, glucagon, fructose, or sorbitol. Because phenformin causes severe lactic acidosis, the Food and Drug Administration has removed it from clinical use as an antidiabetic agent.

Post-test care

■ If a hematoma develops at the venipuncture site, apply warm soaks.

■ As ordered, instruct the patient to resume his normal diet.

Interfering factors

■ Failure to adhere to restrictions of diet and activity may affect test results.

■ Failure to pack the sample in ice and to transport it to the laboratory immediately may elevate blood lactate levels.

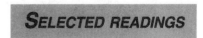

SELECTED READINGS

Fischbach, F. *A Manual of Laboratory and Diagnostic Tests,* 5th ed. Philadelphia: Lippincott-Raven Pubs., 1996.

Gaedeke, M.K. *Laboratory and Diagnostic Tests.* Reading, Mass.: Addison-Wesley Publishing Co., 1996.

Higgins, C. "Pathology Testing of Blood Glucose Levels," *Nursing Times* 9(3):42-44, January 18-24, 1995.

Tietz, N.W. *Clinical Guide to Laboratory Tests,* 3rd ed. Philadelphia: W.B. Saunders Co., 1995.

Watson, J., et al. *Nurse's Manual of Laboratory and Diagnostic Tests,* 2nd ed. Philadelphia: F.A. Davis Co., 1995.

CHAPTER NINE

Vitamins and trace elements

Learning objectives

After completing this chapter, the reader will be able to:

- explain why proper intake of vitamins and trace elements is necessary to maintain health
- identify food sources of major vitamins and minerals
- name and define the two classes of vitamins
- describe physical manifestations of vitamin or mineral imbalances
- list the principal properties and actions of vitamins and trace elements
- state the purpose of each test discussed in the chapter
- prepare the patient physically and psychologically for each test
- describe the procedure for obtaining a specimen for each test
- specify appropriate precautions for accurately obtaining a specimen for each test
- implement appropriate post-test care
- state the reference values for each test
- discuss the implications of abnormal test results
- list factors that may interfere with accurate test results.

INTRODUCTION

Vitamins and trace elements — organic and inorganic nutrients, respectively — are indispensable to normal metabolism and proper nutrition. Because the body can't synthesize most of these compounds, an adequate intake from nutritional sources is essential to maintain normal concentrations in the body. This is rarely a problem, except in people with very inadequate diets, because generous amounts of vitamins and trace elements are found in the basic food groups. Although food processing and cooking can reduce or destroy some of the nutrients in food, a balanced diet usually provides sufficient amounts to maintain health. Supplements are recommended only for severely inadequate diet or a known deficiency.

Today, a far greater danger than trace element deficiency is toxic excess — through industrial exposure to potentially toxic levels of trace elements. Fortunately, sophisticated diagnostic techniques have been developed to detect minute concentrations of trace elements in serum. One such technique is atomic absorption spectroscopy. Equally sensitive bioassays and chemical assays are available to investigate vitamin toxicity or deficiency. For example, radioisotopes have been used to measure minute amounts of a specific vitamin such as vitamin B_{12} in serum.

Vitamins: Vital to support life

Originally classified as "vital amines," vitamins differ in chemical composition and are not, in fact, all amines. However, they are vital for body maintenance, growth, and reproduction. Laboratory animals fed vitamin-depleted diets of carbohydrates, fats, minerals, and proteins failed to survive; only the animals fed diets containing adequate vitamins survived.

Because vitamins are generously prevalent in so many foods, absence of a vitamin, or *avitaminosis*, is rare indeed. A more common condition is *hypovitaminosis*, in which serum levels of a particular vitamin are below normal and may produce adverse clinical reactions. (See

Signs and symptoms of nutritional imbalances, pages 250 and 251.)

Classification

Vitamins are classified as fat soluble or water soluble. *Fat-soluble vitamins,* which include vitamins A, D, E, and K, are associated with lipids in food sources and are similarly absorbed. Although these vitamins are necessary for survival, excessive or prolonged ingestion of most fat-soluble vitamins — especially in doses that exceed the recommended daily allowance — can have toxic effects, because the body stores them in varying amounts and does not readily excrete them.

Fat-soluble vitamins have different functions that are only partially understood. Vitamin A maintains night vision and the integrity of epithelial cells: vitamin D regulates calcium and phosphorus metabolism and is thus primarily associated with bone maintenance; vitamin E, an antioxidant of polyunsaturated fatty acids, is associated with various synthetic processes in the body; and vitamin K is necessary for formation of certain blood-clotting factors.

Unlike fat-soluble vitamins, which tend to be stored and accumulate in the body, *water-soluble vitamins,* including vitamin C and the B complex vitamins, are readily excreted in the urine. Consequently, excessive dietary ingestion doesn't produce toxicity, and deficiency of these vitamins is more common.

Water-soluble vitamins have many important functions. The B complex vitamins prevent certain diseases (vitamin B_1 [thiamine], for example, is an anti-beriberi factor), serve as coenzymes in energy metabolism (vitamin B_6 [pyridoxine], for example, is essential to protein metabolism), and contribute to cell growth and the development of blood-forming factors (vitamin B_{12} is essential for normal hematopoiesis, as is folic acid). Vitamin C is necessary for collagen synthesis and for maintaining healthy bone and cartilage.

The vitamins and trace elements that will be discussed in detail in this chapter are vitamins A (and carotene), B_2, B_{12}, C, D_3, and folic acid, and the trace elements manganese and zinc.

Trace elements

Trace elements are minerals found in the body in minute quantities. Vital to health, many trace elements are an integral part of intracellular enzyme systems necessary for energy metabolism and other important biological processes. Although more than 20 trace elements have been identified, only a few (including manganese, cobalt, chromium, and zinc) are known to be essential to body functions. Manganese and zinc, for example, figure prominently in enzyme activation; cobalt is a critical factor in hematopoiesis; and chromium is essential in amino acid transport. (Copper, another essential trace element, is often measured indirectly [see "Serum ceruloplasmin" in Chapter 7] or in urine [see "Urine copper" in Chapter 17].)

Trace elements are found throughout nature in water, plants, and soil. Their concentrations in plant and animal food sources can lead to deficiencies or toxicity. However, because amounts required are so small and available from so many food sources, trace element deficiencies are rare. They're most likely to develop during long-term total parenteral nutrition unless the feeding solution contains trace element supplements.

Excessive accumulations and toxicity are becoming a more common problem. For example, heavy industrial use of such minerals as chromium and zinc can result in overexposure through inhalation, skin contact, or accidental ingestion. Similarly, contamination of drinking water and of edible plants by industrial wastes dispersed in the soil

(Text continues on page 252.)

Signs and symptoms of nutritional imbalances

VITAMIN/ TRACE ELEMENT	DEFICIENCY	TOXICITY
Vitamin A and carotene	■ Night blindness ■ Xerophthalmia ■ Bitot's spots ■ Skin and mucous membrane infections ■ Follicular hyperkeratosis	■ Hyperirritability ■ Yellow skin ■ Alopecia ■ Bone and joint pain ■ Headaches, vertigo ■ Hepatosplenomegaly ■ Malaise ■ Abdominal pain, anorexia ■ Transient hydrocephalus and vomiting (in infants)
Vitamin B$_{12}$	*Megaloblastic anemia with:* ■ Yellow skin ■ Anorexia and weight loss ■ Dyspnea ■ Prolonged bleeding time ■ Abdominal pain, constipation, anorexia, and weight loss ■ Glossitis ■ Peripheral neuropathy ■ Ataxia ■ Weakness	Nontoxic (even in high doses)
Vitamin C	■ Bleeding gums, loose teeth ■ Joint pain ■ Irritability ■ Retarded growth ■ Dyspnea ■ Poor wound healing ■ Increased susceptibility to infection ■ Weight loss ■ Fever ■ Vomiting and diarrhea	*Only after prolonged ingestion of massive doses (5,000 to 15,000 mg daily):* ■ Nausea and vomiting ■ Possible formation of urinary tract calculi, especially uric acid calculi
Folic acid	*Megaloblastic anemia with:* ■ Yellow skin ■ Dyspnea ■ Prolonged bleeding ■ Abdominal pain, anorexia, and weight loss ■ Peripheral neuropathy ■ Ataxia ■ Weakness	Nontoxic (even in high doses)

Signs and symptoms of nutritional imbalances (continued)

VITAMIN/ TRACE ELEMENT	DEFICIENCY	TOXICITY
Vitamin D₃	*Rickets in infants and children, characterized by:* ■ In early stages, profuse sweating, restlessness and irritability ■ In late stages, bony malformations due to bone softening, delayed closing of fontanelles, poorly developed muscles, and tetany *Osteomalacia in adults, characterized by:* ■ Bone malformation due to softening of bones in pelvis, spine, legs, and thorax ■ Rheumatic pain in lower back and legs ■ Spontaneous fractures	*Early:* ■ Anorexia ■ Nausea ■ Vomiting ■ Diarrhea ■ Headache *Late:* ■ Hypercalcemia leading to metastatic calcification and renal failure ■ Osteoporosis due to increased mobilization from bone
Chromium	■ Possible impaired glucose tolerance	■ Dermatitis ■ Vertigo ■ Abdominal pain ■ Anuria ■ Shock, seizures, coma
Manganese	■ Retarded growth ■ Bone abnormalities ■ Reproductive dysfunction ■ Ataxia	■ Pulmonary dysfunction ■ Early-stage encephalitis-like syndrome: anorexia, weakness, headache, impotence ■ Late-stage parkinsonian syndrome: mask-like facies, monotone voice, tremor, muscle rigidity, spastic gait, clonus
Zinc	■ Sparse hair growth ■ Hepatosplenomegaly ■ Severe anemia ■ Impaired taste and smell acuity ■ Foul odor in nasopharynx ■ Anorexia ■ Pica (in children) ■ Retarded growth ■ Testicular atrophy ■ Hyperpigmentation ■ Impaired wound healing ■ Diarrhea ■ Increased susceptibility to infection	*From ingestion:* ■ GI irritation with fever, cramps, diarrhea, nausea and vomiting ■ Metallic taste in mouth *From inhalation:* ■ Metal fume fever ■ Dry throat, cough, chest discomfort ■ Tachycardia, hypertension ■ Pulmonary edema due to inhalation

Radioimmunoassays

Radioimmunoassays, a collection of laboratory procedures based on displacement reactions, allow sensitive and specific measurement of vitamins, hormones, and other compounds.

In this procedure, the laboratory technician radioactively tags a specific quantity of the subject substance, or antigen (Ag* in diagram), and then combines it with an equal amount of its specific antibody (Ab). This forms the bound complex (Ag*-Ab). When the technician introduces a patient's serum sample containing the subject substance, this new and untagged antigen (Ag) displaces the tagged antigen in the complex and itself combines with the antibody until all the untagged antigen is bound. Because the amount of the freed radioactive antigen equals the amount of bound antigen, measurement of the tagged substance gives a clear accounting of the amount of nonradioactive antigen present in the serum sample.

Although antibodies are the most widely used binding reagents, certain naturally occurring binding proteins and receptors are also used. Binding proteins need little preparation and are stable, inexpensive, and of uniform consistency. However, they are available for only a limited number of compounds, have lower affinity constants, and don't always have good specificity. Receptors measure biologic rather than immunologic activity. They're uniformly consistent, but unstable and difficult to isolate.

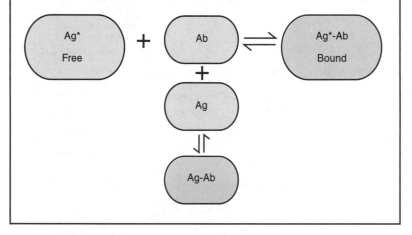

can also cause overexposure to trace elements.

Managing imbalances

A patient suspected of having a vitamin or trace element imbalance requires close observation for characteristic clinical features that may aid diagnosis. Accurate assessment of the patient's nutritional status is essential to identify dietary needs and appropriate intervention. One of the most effective methods of measuring nutrients in the body is radioimmunoassay. (See *Radioimmunoassays*.)

The hospitalized patient with a nutritional imbalance requires careful monitoring of his diet to replace deficient nutrients; he may also need dietary supplements, as appropriate. To maintain the proper balance after he leaves the hospital, the patient needs thorough teaching about good nutrition to make it an integral part of his life.

VITAMIN ASSAYS

Serum vitamin A and carotene

This test measures serum levels of vitamin A (retinol) and its precursor, carotene. A fat-soluble vitamin normally supplied by diet, vitamin A is important for reproduction, vision (especially night vision), and epithelial tissue and bone growth. It also maintains cellular and subcellular membranes and synthesis of mucopolysaccharides (the ground substance of collagenous tissue). Vitamin A is found mostly in fruits, vegetables, eggs, poultry, meat, and fish. Carotene is present in leafy green vegetables and in yellow fruits and vegetables.

The body absorbs vitamin A from the intestines as a fatty acid ester; chylomicrons in the lymphatic system then transport it to the liver, where nearly 90% is stored. Absorption of vitamin A requires the presence of adequate amounts of dietary fat and bile salts. Thus, impaired fat absorption or biliary obstruction inhibits vitamin A absorption, causing a deficiency of this vitamin. Serum levels of vitamin A can remain normal as long as the liver retains even a low reserve of vitamin A.

In this serum test, the color reactions produced by vitamin A and related compounds with various reagents provide both quantitative and qualitative determinations.

Purpose
- To investigate suspected vitamin A deficiency or toxicity
- To aid diagnosis of visual disturbances, especially night blindness and xerophthalmia
- To aid diagnosis of skin diseases, such as keratosis follicularis or ichthyosis
- To screen for malabsorption.

Patient preparation
Explain to the patient that this test measures the level of vitamin A in the blood. Instruct him to fast overnight, but advise him that he need not restrict water before the test. Tell him the test requires a blood sample, who will perform the venipuncture and when, and that he may feel some discomfort from the needle puncture and the pressure of the tourniquet.

Procedure
Perform a venipuncture, and collect the sample in a chilled, 7-ml *red-top* or *blue-top* tube.

Precautions
- Protect the sample from light, because vitamin A characteristically absorbs light.
- Handle the sample gently, and send it to the laboratory immediately.
- Keep the specimen on ice.

Reference values
Values differ according to age and gender. For adults, the range is 30 to 95 µg/dl, with values for men usually 20% higher than for women. For children ages 1 to 6, the range is 20 to 43 µg/dl; for ages 7 to 12, 26 to 50 µg/dl; and for ages 13 to 19, 26 to 72 µg/dl.

Implications of results
Low serum levels of vitamin A (hypovitaminosis A) may indicate impaired fat absorption, as in celiac disease, infectious hepatitis, cystic fibrosis of the

pancreas, or obstructive jaundice. These disorders interfere with intestinal absorption of vitamin A and thus slower serum levels. Low levels are also associated with protein-calorie malnutrition (marasmic kwashiorkor), a rare condition in the United States but a major nutritional disorder worldwide, especially among children. Similar decreases in vitamin A levels may also result from excessive loss of vitamin A in urine due to chronic nephritis.

Elevated vitamin A levels (hypervitaminosis A) usually indicate chronic excessive intake of vitamin A supplements or of foods high in vitamin A. Increased levels are also associated with hyperlipemia and hypercholesterolemia due to uncontrolled diabetes mellitus.

Decreased serum carotene levels may indicate impaired fat absorption or, rarely, insufficient dietary intake of carotene. Carotene levels may also be suppressed during pregnancy because of the body's increased metabolic demand for carotene. Elevated carotene levels indicate grossly excessive dietary intake.

Post-test care

■ If a hematoma develops at the venipuncture site, apply warm soaks.
■ As ordered, allow the patient to resume his normal diet.

Interfering factors

■ Patient failure to observe overnight fast may influence test results.
■ Mineral oil, neomycin, and cholestyramine may decrease vitamin A and carotene levels. Glucocorticoids and oral contraceptives may increase levels.
■ Hemolysis caused by rough handling of the sample may alter test results.

Serum vitamin B_2

This test evaluates the nutritive status and metabolism of vitamin B_2 (riboflavin) and thus helps to detect vitamin B_2 deficiency. Absorbed from the intestinal tract and excreted in urine, vitamin B_2 is essential for growth and tissue function. In the tissues, it combines with phosphate to produce the coenzymes flavin mononucleotide and flavin adenine dinucleotide (FAD); these coenzymes then participate in oxidation-reduction reactions with oxidative enzymes, such as glutathione reductase.

In this test, glutathione reductase activity is measured before and after administration of exogenous FAD. Normally, glutathione reductase binds with FAD. If vitamin B_2 supply is inadequate, glutathione reductase activity and the degree of FAD unsaturation will markedly increase, inversely proportional to vitamin B_2 concentration.

This serum test is considered more reliable than the urine vitamin B_2 test, which can produce artificially high values in patients after surgery or prolonged fasting.

Purpose

■ To detect vitamin B_2 deficiency.

Patient preparation

Explain to the patient that this test evaluates vitamin B_2 levels. Instruct him to maintain a normal diet before the test. Inform him that the test requires a blood sample, who will perform the venipuncture and when, and that he may experience some discomfort from the needle puncture and the pressure of the tourniquet.

Procedure

Perform a venipuncture, and collect the sample in a 7-ml *blue-top* tube.

Precautions

- Handle the sample gently to prevent hemolysis.
- Send the sample to the laboratory immediately.
- Do not refrigerate or freeze the sample.

Reference values

Normally, glutathione reductase has an activity index of 0.9 to 1.3.

Implications of results

An index of 1.4 or greater indicates vitamin B$_2$ deficiency, which can result from insufficient dietary intake of vitamin B$_2$, malabsorption syndrome, or conditions that increase metabolic demands, such as stress.

Post-test care

- If a hematoma develops at the venipuncture site, ease discomfort by applying warm soaks.
- Inform the patient with vitamin B$_2$ deficiency that good dietary sources of vitamin B$_2$ are milk products, organ meats (liver and kidneys), fish, green leafy vegetables, and legumes.

Interfering factors

Hemolysis caused by rough handling of the sample may alter test results.

Serum vitamin B$_{12}$

This radioisotopic assay of competitive binding is a quantitative analysis of serum levels of vitamin B$_{12}$ (also known as cyanocobalamin, antipernicious anemia factor, and extrinsic factor). This

Cobalt: Critical trace element

A trace element found mainly in the liver, cobalt is an essential component of vitamin B$_{12}$ and therefore is a critical factor in hematopoiesis.

A balanced diet supplies sufficient cobalt to maintain hematopoiesis, primarily through foods containing vitamin B$_{12}$. However, excessive ingestion of cobalt may have toxic effects. For example, people who consumed large quantities of beer containing cobalt as a stabilizer suffered toxicity, resulting in congestive heart failure from cardiomyopathy.

Because quantitative analysis of cobalt alone is difficult owing to the minute amount found in the body, cobalt is often measured by bioassay as part of vitamin B$_{12}$ tests. The normal cobalt concentration in human plasma is about 60 to 80 pg/ml.

test is usually performed concurrently with measurement of serum folic acid levels, because deficiencies of vitamin B$_{12}$ and folic acid are the two most common causes of megaloblastic anemia.

A water-soluble vitamin containing cobalt, vitamin B$_{12}$ is essential to hematopoiesis, synthesis and growth of deoxyribonucleic acid, and myelin synthesis and nervous system integrity. (See *Cobalt: Critical trace element.*) Ingested almost exclusively in animal products, such as meat, shellfish, milk, and eggs, vitamin B$_{12}$ is absorbed from the ileum after forming a complex with intrinsic factor and is stored in the liver. (See *Vitamin B$_{12}$ absorption,* page 256.)

A clinical vitamin B$_{12}$ deficiency takes years to develop, because almost total conservation is provided by a cyclic

Vitamin B₁₂ absorption

This illustration shows the route vitamin B_{12} takes as it passes through the GI system and bloodstream.

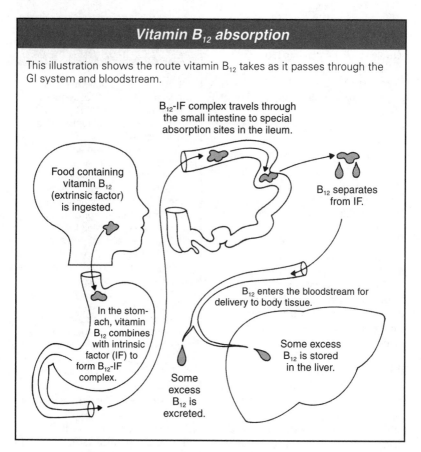

B_{12}-IF complex travels through the small intestine to special absorption sites in the ileum.

Food containing vitamin B_{12} (extrinsic factor) is ingested.

B_{12} separates from IF.

B_{12} enters the bloodstream for delivery to body tissue.

In the stomach, vitamin B_{12} combines with intrinsic factor (IF) to form B_{12}-IF complex.

Some excess B_{12} is excreted.

Some excess B_{12} is stored in the liver.

pathway (enterohepatic circulation) that allows reabsorption of the vitamin B_{12} normally excreted in bile. Deficiency of intrinsic factor, however, causes malabsorption of vitamin B_{12} and may result in pernicious anemia.

Purpose

■ To aid differential diagnosis of megaloblastic anemia, which may be due to a deficiency of vitamin B_{12} or folic acid
■ To aid differential diagnosis of central nervous system (CNS) disorders affecting peripheral and spinal myelinated nerves.

Patient preparation

Explain that this test determines the amount of vitamin B_{12} in the blood. If folic acid is also being measured, instruct the patient to observe an overnight fast before the test. Tell him this test requires a blood sample, who will perform the venipuncture and when, and that he may feel some discomfort from the needle puncture and pressure of the tourniquet.

Check the patient history for use of drugs that may alter test results, such as para-aminosalicylic acid, phenytoin, neomycin, and colchicine.

Procedure

Perform the venipuncture, and collect the sample in a 7-ml *blue-top* tube.

Precautions

Handle the sample gently to prevent hemolysis, and send it to the laboratory immediately.

Reference values

Normally, serum vitamin B_{12} values range from 200 to 900 pg/ml. For newborns, the range is 160 to 1,200 pg/ml.

Implications of results

Decreased serum levels may indicate inadequate dietary intake of vitamin B_{12}, especially if the patient is a strict vegetarian. Low levels are also associated with malabsorption syndromes (such as celiac disease), isolated malabsorption of vitamin B_{12}, hypermetabolic states (such as hyperthyroidism), pregnancy, and CNS damage (such as posterolateral sclerosis or funicular degeneration).

Elevated levels of serum vitamin B_{12} may result from excessive dietary intake, hepatic disease such as cirrhosis or acute or chronic hepatitis, and myeloproliferative disorders such as myelocytic leukemia. These conditions raise levels of serum vitamin B_{12}-binding proteins, causing high serum levels of vitamin B_{12}.

Post-test care

- If a hematoma develops at the venipuncture site, apply warm soaks.
- As ordered, resume diet.

Interfering factors

- Drugs such as neomycin, metformin, anticonvulsants, and ethanol may decrease vitamin B_{12} levels. Use of oral contraceptives may decrease levels.
- Failure to fast overnight and administration of substances that decrease absorption of vitamin B_{12} may alter test results.

Plasma vitamin C

This chemical assay measures plasma levels of vitamin C, a water-soluble vitamin required for collagen synthesis and cartilage and bone maintenance. Vitamin C (also known as ascorbic acid) also promotes iron absorption, influences folic acid metabolism, and may be necessary for withstanding the stresses of injury and infection.

After vitamin C is absorbed from the small intestine, it's transported in the blood to the kidneys and oxidized to dehydroascorbic acid. Then it's stored in the adrenal and salivary glands, pancreas, spleen, testes, and brain. However, because the adrenal glands contain high concentrations of vitamin C, stimulation of these glands by adrenocorticotropic hormone may deplete stores of vitamin C.

This vitamin is present in generous amounts in citrus fruits, berries, tomatoes, raw cabbage, green peppers, and green leafy vegetables. Severe vitamin C deficiency, or scurvy, causes capillary fragility, joint abnormalities, and numerous systemic symptoms.

Purpose

- To aid diagnosis of scurvy, scurvylike conditions, and metabolic disorders, such as malnutrition and malabsorption syndromes.

Patient preparation

Explain to the patient that this test detects the amount of vitamin C in the blood. Instruct him to observe an overnight fast before the test. Tell him that this test requires a blood sample, who will perform the venipuncture and when, and that he may feel some discomfort from the needle puncture and the pressure of the tourniquet.

Risks of ingesting high-dose vitamin C

In the early 1970s, Nobel Laureate Linus Pauling sparked interest in vitamin C when he suggested that megadoses of this vitamin might increase resistance to viral and bacterial infection, increase resistance to cancer, and lower serum cholesterol levels. Pauling recommended daily doses of vitamin C at two to five times the recommended dietary allowance (60 mg daily for adults) and much higher doses during times of stress or illness. In particular, he advocated very high doses to treat cancer and to relieve common cold symptoms.

To date, clinical studies have not supported Pauling's theories. In fact, a recent study has proved definitively that high-dose vitamin C is no more effective than a placebo in the treatment of cancer. Other studies have shown that high-dose vitamin C has little or no effect on the severity of colds. But despite this, many people supplement their diets

with high doses of vitamin C. In addition to delaying proper treatment, such high doses can cause severe adverse effects.

The most common adverse effects of vitamin C are diarrhea and vomiting. However, in some people, high-dose vitamin C promotes formation of uric acid crystals, which may trigger or intensify gout, and causes oxalic acid accumulation in the kidneys, which may lead to formation of calculi. Vitamin C also promotes iron absorption, which may lead to iron toxicity.

Additional risks include interference with drug metabolism and diagnostic tests. For example, high-dose vitamin C impairs the effectiveness of warfarin and other anticoagulants and can cause rapid excretion of other drugs by acidifying urine pH. And it interferes with fecal occult blood testing and produces false-positive test results for glycosuria.

Procedure

Perform the venipuncture, and collect the sample in a 7-ml *green-top* tube.

Precautions

■ Avoid rough handling or excessive agitation of the sample in order to prevent hemolysis.

■ Send the sample to the laboratory immediately.

Reference values

Plasma vitamin C values of 0.3 mg/dl or more are considered acceptable.

Implications of results

Vitamin C values of 0.2 to 0.29 mg/dl are considered borderline; values under

0.2 mg/dl indicate deficiency. Vitamin C levels diminish during pregnancy and reach a low point immediately postpartum. Depressed levels occur with infection, fever, anemia, and burns. Severe deficiencies result in scurvy.

High plasma levels can indicate increased ingestion of vitamin C in amounts exceeding the recommended dietary allowance. Excess vitamin C is converted to oxalate, which is excreted in the urine. Excessive oxalate can produce urinary calculi. (See *Risks of ingesting high-dose vitamin C.*)

Post-test care

■ If a hematoma develops at the venipuncture site, apply warm soaks.

- As ordered, resume diet that was discontinued before the test.

Interfering factors
- Failure to follow dietary restrictions or to transport the sample to the laboratory promptly may alter test results.
- Hemolysis due to rough handling of the sample may affect test results.

Serum vitamin D₃

Vitamin D₃ (cholecalciferol), the major form of vitamin D, is endogenously produced in the skin by the sun's ultraviolet rays and occurs naturally in fish oils, egg yolks, liver, and butter. Like other fat-soluble vitamins, vitamin D₃ is absorbed from the intestine in the presence of bile salts and is stored in the liver. To become active, this vitamin must undergo conversion to 25-hydroxycholecalciferol, its circulating metabolite, and then to 1,25-dihydroxycholecalciferol, a potent compound — often called a hormone — that controls bone mineralization.

The hormonal function of vitamin D₃ closely parallels that of parathyroid hormone in maintaining calcium and phosphorus homeostasis. Low serum calcium and phosphorus levels stimulate production of parathyroid hormone, which then stimulates renal secretion of 1,25-dihydroxycholecalciferol to promote intestinal absorption of calcium and phosphate. Together the two hormones stimulate renal absorption of calcium and mobilization of calcium from bone.

This test, a competitive protein-binding assay, determines serum levels of 25-hydroxycholecalciferol after chromatography has separated it from other vitamin D metabolites and contaminants.

Clinically useful in evaluating nutritional status and the biological activity of vitamin D₃, this test is commonly combined with measurement of serum calcium and alkaline phosphatase levels.

Purpose
- To evaluate skeletal diseases, such as rickets and osteomalacia
- To aid diagnosis of hypercalcemia
- To detect vitamin D toxicity
- To monitor therapy with vitamin D₃.

Patient preparation
Explain to the patient that this test measures vitamin D in the body. Tell him that he shouldn't eat or drink anything for 8 to 12 hours before the test, that the test requires a blood sample, who will perform the venipuncture and when, and that he may feel discomfort from the needle puncture and the tourniquet. Check for drugs that may alter test results, such as corticosteroids and anticonvulsants. If these drugs must be continued, note this on the laboratory request.

Procedure
Perform a venipuncture, and collect the sample in a 7-ml *blue-top* tube.

Precautions
Handle the sample carefully to prevent hemolysis.

Reference values
Serum vitamin D₃ levels normally range from 10 to 55 ng/ml; values are typically higher in summer.

Implications of results
Low or undetectable levels may result from vitamin D deficiency, which can cause rickets or osteomalacia. Such deficiency may stem from poor diet, decreased exposure to the sun, or impaired absorption of vitamin D (secondary to hepatobiliary disease, pancreatitis, celi-

ac disease, cystic fibrosis, or gastric or small-bowel resection). Low levels may also be related to various hepatic diseases that directly affect vitamin D metabolism.

Elevated levels (over 100 ng/ml) may indicate toxicity due to excessive self-medication or prolonged therapy. Elevated levels associated with hypercalcemia may be due to hypersensitivity to vitamin D, as in sarcoidosis.

Post-test care
- If a hematoma develops at the venipuncture site, apply warm soaks.
- Tell the patient that he may resume his normal diet.

Interfering factors
- Drugs that may decrease vitamin D_3 levels include anticonvulsants, isoniazid, mineral oil, glucocorticoids, aluminum hydroxide, cholestyramine, and colestipol.
- Anticonvulsants and corticosteroids may lower serum levels by inhibiting formation of vitamin D_3 metabolites.
- Hemolysis may alter test results.

Serum folic acid

A quantitative analysis of serum folic acid levels by radioisotopic assay of competitive binding, this test is often performed concomitantly with serum vitamin B_{12} determinations. Like vitamin B_{12}, folic acid (also known as pteroylglutamic acid, folacin, and folate) is a water-soluble vitamin that influences hematopoiesis, DNA synthesis, and overall body growth. The parent compound of folate vitamins, folic acid is biologically inactive and requires enzymatic breakdown in the small intestine for absorption into the bloodstream.

Once in the bloodstream, folic acid is rapidly absorbed into the tissues.

Normally, diet supplies folic acid in liver, kidney, yeast, fruits, leafy vegetables, eggs, and milk. Because the body stores only small amounts of folic acid (mostly in the liver), inadequate dietary intake causes a deficiency, especially during pregnancy, when the metabolic demand for folic acid rises. Because of folic acid's vital role in hematopoiesis, the usual indication for this test is a suspected hematologic abnormality.

Purpose
- To aid differential diagnosis of megaloblastic anemia, which may result from deficiency of folic acid or vitamin B_{12}
- To assess folate stores in pregnancy.

Patient preparation
Explain to the patient that this test determines the folic acid level in the blood. Instruct him to observe an overnight fast before the test. Tell him the test requires a blood sample, who will perform the venipuncture and when, and that he may experience some discomfort from the needle puncture and the pressure of the tourniquet.

Check the patient's medication history for drugs that may affect test results.

Procedure
Perform a venipuncture, and collect the sample in a 7-ml *red-top* tube.

Precautions
Handle the sample gently to prevent hemolysis. Protect it from light, and send it to the laboratory immediately.

Reference values
Normally, serum folic acid values range from 3 to 16 ng/ml.

Implications of results
Low serum levels (less than 2 ng/ml) may indicate hematologic abnormali-

ties, such as anemia (especially megaloblastic anemia), leukopenia, or thrombocytopenia. The Schilling test is often performed to rule out vitamin B_{12} deficiency, which also causes megaloblastic anemia (pernicious anemia). Decreased folic acid levels can also result from hypermetabolic states (such as hyperthyroidism), inadequate dietary intake, chronic alcoholism, small-bowel malabsorption syndrome, or pregnancy.

High serum levels (more than 20 ng/ml) may indicate excessive dietary intake of folic acid or folic acid supplements. This vitamin is nontoxic in humans, even when taken in large doses.

Post-test care
■ If a hematoma develops at the venipuncture site, apply warm soaks.
■ Tell the patient that he may resume his normal diet.

Interfering factors
■ Alcohol and phenytoin interfere with folic acid absorption and lower serum folic acid. Pyrimethamine can induce folate deficiency, thus lowering folic acid levels. Other drugs that may decrease levels include anticonvulsants such as primidone; antineoplastics; antimalarials; and oral contraceptives.
■ Hemolysis may alter test results.
■ Folate deterioration may occur if the specimen is not protected from light.

TRACE ELEMENT ASSAYS

Serum manganese

This test, an analysis by atomic absorption spectroscopy, measures serum levels of manganese, a trace element. Manganese is found throughout the body but concentrates mainly in the pituitary, pineal, and lactating mammary glands, as well as in the liver and bones. Although the function of this element in humans is only partially understood, manganese is known to activate several enzymes — including cholinesterase and arginase — that are essential to metabolism. Arginase, for example, is necessary for the formation of urea during protein catabolism.

Because of poor intestinal absorption, the body retains only a fraction of the manganese supplied by such foods as unrefined cereals, green leafy vegetables, and nuts.

Industrial workers exposed to potentially dangerous levels of manganese may require testing for toxicity. Such toxicity can follow inhalation of manganese dust or fumes — a constant hazard in the steel and dry-cell battery industries — or ingestion of contaminated water.

Purpose
■ To detect manganese toxicity.

Patient preparation
Explain to the patient that this test determines the level of manganese in the blood. Inform him that he needn't restrict food or fluids. Tell him this test requires a blood sample, who will perform the venipuncture and when, and that he may feel some discomfort from the needle puncture and the pressure of the tourniquet.

Check the patient's medication history for use of drugs that may influence serum manganese levels.

Procedure
Perform a venipuncture, and collect the sample in a metal-free collection tube. Laboratories will supply a special kit for this test on request.

Precautions
Handle the sample gently to prevent hemolysis, and send it to the laboratory immediately.

Reference values
Normally, serum manganese values range from 0.04 to 1.4 µg/dl.

Implications of results
Significantly elevated serum levels indicate manganese toxicity, which requires prompt medical attention to prevent central nervous system deterioration. Depressed serum manganese levels may indicate deficient dietary intake, although deficiency hasn't been linked to human disease.

Post-test care
If a hematoma develops at the venipuncture site, apply warm soaks.

Interfering factors
■ High dietary intake of calcium and phosphorus can interfere with intestinal absorption of manganese and thus decrease serum levels.
■ Serum manganese levels are influenced by estrogen, which increases the circulating level. Glucocorticoids affect levels by altering the distribution of manganese in the body.
■ Hemolysis caused by rough handling of the sample may alter test results.
■ Failure to use a metal-free collection tube can affect test results.

Serum zinc

This test, an analysis by atomic absorption spectroscopy, measures serum levels of zinc, an important trace element. Zinc is found throughout the body but concentrates primarily in the blood cells, especially in the leukocytes. This element is an integral component of more than 80 enzymes and proteins, and plays a critical role in enzyme catalytic reactions. For example, zinc is closely linked to the activity of carbonic anhydrase, the enzyme that catalyzes the elimination of carbon dioxide.

Zinc occurs naturally in water and in most foods; high concentrations are found in meat, seafood, dairy products, whole grains, nuts, and legumes. Zinc deficiency can seriously impair body metabolism, growth, and development. This defect is most apt to develop in patients with certain diseases that tend to deplete its body stores, such as chronic alcoholism and renal disease. Zinc toxicity is rare but can occur after inhalation of zinc oxide during industrial exposure. (See *Industrial exposure to zinc oxide.*)

Purpose
■ To detect zinc deficiency or toxicity.

Patient preparation
Explain to the patient that this test determines the concentration of zinc in the blood. Inform him that he needn't restrict food or fluids. Tell him the test requires a blood sample, who will perform the venipuncture and when, and that he may feel some discomfort from the needle puncture and the pressure of the tourniquet.

Ask the patient's recent drug history for use of zinc-chelating agents and other medications that may interfere with the test results.

Procedure
Perform a venipuncture, and collect a 7- to 10-ml sample in a zinc-free collection tube.

Precautions
Handle the sample gently to prevent hemolysis, which can invalidate the test

Industrial exposure to zinc oxide

Approximately 50,000 industrial workers risk toxic exposure to zinc oxide. Such overexposure can result from inhalation of dust or fumes in the following industries and occupations:

- alloy manufacturing
- brass foundry work
- bronze foundry work
- electric fuse manufacturing
- gas welding
- electroplating
- galvanizing
- junk metal refining
- paint manufacturing
- metal cutting
- metal spraying
- rubber manufacturing
- roof making
- zinc manufacturing.

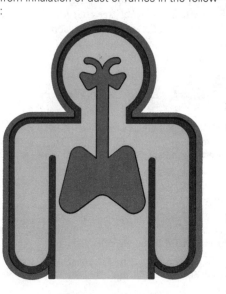

results. Send the sample to the laboratory immediately. Analysis must begin before platelet disintegration can alter test results.

Reference values
Normally, serum zinc values range from 60 to 150 µg/dl.

Implications of results
Fasting values below 70 µg/dl indicate zinc deficiency. Decreased serum zinc levels may indicate an acquired deficiency (due to insufficient dietary intake or to an underlying disease) or a hereditary deficiency. Markedly depressed levels are common in leukemia and may be related to impaired zinc-dependent enzyme systems. Low serum zinc levels are commonly associated with alcoholic cirrhosis of the liver, myocardial infarction, ileitis, chronic renal failure,

rheumatoid arthritis, anemia (such as hemolytic or sickle cell anemia), and severe diarrhea.

Elevated and potentially toxic serum zinc levels may result from accidental ingestion or industrial exposure.

Post-test care
If a hematoma develops at the venipuncture site, applying warm soaks can ease discomfort.

Interfering factors
- Zinc levels may be affected by time of day specimen is drawn and by time of last meal.
- Zinc-chelating agents (such as penicillinase) and corticosteroids decrease serum zinc levels and may interfere with determination of results. Other drugs that may decrease levels include estrogens, penicillamine, antineoplastic

drugs (such as cisplatin), antimetabolites, and diuretics.
- Hemolysis caused by rough handling of the sample may interfere with accurate determination of test results.
- Failure to use a metal-free collection tube, or to send the sample to the laboratory immediately can alter results.

SELECTED READINGS

Fischbach, F. *A Manual of Laboratory and Diagnostic Tests*, 5th ed. Philadelphia: Lippincott-Raven Pubs., 1996.

Guyton, A.C., and Hall, J.E. *Textbook of Medical Physiology*, 9th ed. Philadelphia: W.B. Saunders Co., 1996.

Henry, J.B., ed. *Clinical Diagnosis and Management by Laboratory Methods*, 19th ed. Philadelphia: W.B. Saunders Co., 1996.

Jacobs, D., et al. *Laboratory Test Handbook*, 3rd ed. Baltimore: Williams & Wilkins Co., 1994.

Kee, J.L. *Laboratory and Diagnostic Tests*, 4th ed. Stamford, Conn.: Appleton & Lange, 1995.

Mayo Medical Laboratories 1996 Test Catalog. Rochester, Minn.: Mayo Medical Laboratories, 1996.

Ravel, R.A. *Clinical Laboratory Medicine: Clinical Application of Laboratory Data*, 6th ed. St. Louis: Mosby–Year Book, Inc., 1995.

Tilkian, S.M., et al. *Clinical and Nursing Implications of Laboratory Tests*, 5th ed. St. Louis: Mosby–Year Book, Inc., 1995.

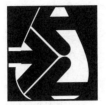

CHAPTER TEN

Immunohematology

Learning objectives

After completing this chapter, the reader will be able to:

- explain the ABO and Rh blood group systems
- list the health standards required of prospective blood donors
- name the compatibility tests commonly performed on donor blood
- state the causes and major characteristics of nine transfusion reactions and complications
- discuss safety precautions for transfusing blood
- state the purpose of each test discussed in the chapter
- prepare the patient physically and psychologically for each test
- describe the procedure for obtaining a specimen for each test
- specify appropriate precautions for safe administration of each test
- implement appropriate post-test care
- state the normal findings for each test
- discuss the implications of abnormal test results
- list factors that may interfere with accurate test results.

INTRODUCTION

Immunohematology is the study of antigen-antibody reactions and their effects on blood. An *antigen* is a substance that can initiate an immune response and induce the formation of a corresponding antibody. The established major antigens found in blood are inherited, such as those in the ABO system and the Rh-Hr system; others can be introduced into the body from exogenous sources, such as blood transfusions or drugs. An *antibody* is an immunoglobulin molecule synthesized in response to a specific antigen.

Successful blood transfusions require tests that identify these naturally occurring or acquired antigens and antibodies to make possible correct matching of donor and recipient blood. Among the most important of these tests are ABO blood typing, Rh typing, crossmatching, direct antiglobulin test, and antibody screening test. If a transfusion reaction occurs despite correct transfusion of compatible blood, tests for oth-

er antibodies (such as leukoagglutinins) help identify the cause and prevent further reactions.

ABO blood group system

All blood group classifications are based on the types of antigens present or absent on the surfaces of red blood cells (RBCs). Austrian immunologist Karl Landsteiner, winner of the 1930 Nobel prize for his work in physiology, created the most important of these classifications — the ABO blood group system. Landsteiner classified human RBCs as type A, B, AB, or O, depending on the presence or absence of these antigens on the surface of RBCs. Persons with group A blood have RBCs with A antigens; those with group B blood have B antigens. AB blood contains both A and B antigens; group O blood contains neither.

In the ABO system, one or both of two naturally occurring antibodies, anti-A and anti-B, are found in the serum. Thus, a person with group A blood has anti-B antibodies, rather than anti-A antibodies, because the latter would destroy his RBCs. Similarly, a person with group B blood has anti-A antibodies. A person with group O blood, has both anti-A and anti-B antibodies; a person with AB blood has neither type of antibody.

Because group O blood lacks both A and B antigens, it can be transfused in limited amounts to any recipient in an emergency, regardless of his blood type, with little risk of agglutination. For this reason, a person with group O blood is called a *universal donor*. However, transfusions of universal donor blood should be given as packed RBCs, from which the plasma has been removed. A person with AB blood, who has neither anti-A nor anti-B antibodies, can receive A, B, or O blood (packed cells) and is called a *universal recipient*.

Typing and crossmatching of donor and recipient blood are required before a transfusion to establish compatibility. These tests minimize the risk of a hemolytic reaction — the greatest danger with blood transfusions. A hemolytic reaction is an immune reaction that occurs when the donor's and recipient's blood types are mismatched — that is, when blood containing anti-A antibodies is mixed with blood containing A antigens or when blood containing anti-B antibodies is mixed with blood containing B antigens.

When mismatching happens, the antibodies attach to the surface of the foreign RBCs, causing the cells to clump together. This clumping can eventually plug small blood vessels and arterioles. Such an antibody-antigen reaction activates the body's complement system — a group of enzymatic proteins — which promotes and accelerates RBC hemolysis and phagocytosis by the reticuloendothelial cells. RBC hemolysis releases free hemoglobin into the blood-stream, which can damage the renal tubules and lead to renal failure and death.

Rh blood group system

In 1940, Landsteiner and immunoserologist Alexander S. Wiener developed the Rh blood group system after discovering a certain antigen on the surface of RBCs in virtually all rhesus monkeys. Among humans, about 85% of whites and an even higher percentage of blacks, Native Americans, and Asians carry this Rh antigen — known as $Rh_o(D)$ factor — on their RBCs. Such blood is therefore classified as *Rh-positive*. The remaining 15% or less of the population lack this factor, and their blood is typed *Rh-negative*. The Rh antigen is highly immunogenic — that is, it is more likely to stimulate formation of an antibody than other known antigens.

Consequently, a person with Rh-positive blood does not carry anti-Rh antibodies in his serum because they would destroy his RBCs. However, a person with Rh-negative blood develops anti-Rh antibodies following exposure to Rh-positive blood (by transfusion or pregnancy). A transfusion reaction usually does not occur after the initial exposure to Rh-positive blood. Rather, anti-Rh antibodies generally develop slowly, over several weeks, causing the transfusion recipient to become sensitized to the Rh antigen. Subsequent exposure to Rh-positive blood then provokes a transfusion reaction and hemolysis, as in hemolytic disease of the newborn.

An important variation in the Rh system is the D^u antigen. This antigen, considered Rh-positive, is somewhat less immunogenic than $Rh_o(D)$ and may not provoke antibody production in persons who lack it. Thus, all prospective donors must be screened for the D^u antigen, which is more common in blacks than in whites. Persons whose blood contains this antigen are considered Rh-positive donors but are generally transfused as Rh-negative recipients. This precaution is taken to protect persons with a D^u variant whose blood may not be distinguished serologically from that of D^u blood.

Other clinically significant Rh antigens have been discovered since Landsteiner's and Wiener's work; these additional antigens, such as rh' (C), rh" (E), hr' (c), and hr" (e) are much less immunogenic and not as likely to provoke an antibody reaction as $Rh_o(D)$. Tests for these antigens are done only in special cases, as for establishing paternity, determining family studies, or distinguishing between heterozygous and homozygous Rh-positive factors.

Screening blood donors

To qualify for selection, prospective blood donors must meet strict criteria established by the Scientific Committee of the Joint Blood Council and the Standards Committee of the American Association of Blood Banks. The purpose of these guidelines is to protect the donor and the recipient and to ensure a safe, therapeutic blood transfusion.

Before donation, a detailed medical history must be obtained from the prospective donor to detect disorders or conditions that could exclude or defer the donation. Such conditions include any disease that can be transmitted by blood transfusion (such as viral hepatitis, malaria, Creutzfeldt-Jakob disease, babesiosis, Chagas' disease, or acquired immunodeficiency syndrome [AIDS]), active tuberculosis, alcoholism, drug addiction or drug therapy, pregnancy, and recent immunizations or dental surgery.

A physical examination and laboratory tests must then be done to determine if the prospective donor meets the following minimum health standards:
- *age:* should be at least 17
- *weight:* should weigh at least 110 lb (50 kg)
- *blood pressure:* systolic pressure no higher than 180 mm Hg; diastolic pressure no higher than 100 mm Hg

- *pulse:* between 50 and 100 beats/minute and regular
- *oral temperature:* should not exceed 99.5% (37.5% C)
- *skin:* should be free of all lesions at the venipuncture site; should show no evidence of intravenous drug abuse
- *hemoglobin:* no less than 12.5 g/dl
- *hematocrit:* no less than 38%.

Testing donor blood

Except in the case of identical twins or autologous transfusion (in which a person receives his own blood), testing for blood compatibility between donor and recipient can never be foolproof. However, the following tests on donor blood can improve selection for the recipient:
- determining ABO and Rh blood groups
- detecting unexpected antibodies that can coat, hemolyze, or agglutinate RBCs
- crossmatching of donor blood and recipient blood (prior to transfusion)
- detecting hepatitis B surface antigen (HBsAg) as well as antibodies to hepatitis B core antigen (anti-HB$_c$); to hepatitis C virus (anti-HCV); to human T-cell lymphotropic virus, type I (anti-HTLV-I); to human immunodeficiency viruses (anti-HIV-1 and anti-HIV-2); and to syphilis.

Nursing considerations

After the compatibility of donor and recipient blood has been established, the most important nursing consideration is to make sure you match the *right* blood with the *right* patient. Hemolytic reactions are most often caused by giving blood to the wrong person and mislabeling the sample.

Double-check the patient's name, medical record number, and ABO and Rh status, preferably with another nurse or a doctor. If there is a discrepancy — no matter how slight — *don't* administer the blood. Instead, notify the blood bank immediately so a substitution can be made without delay. Preventing potentially fatal hemolytic reactions from mismatched blood transfusions ranks among the most critical of nursing responsibilities. Uncompromising thoroughness and strict adherence to protocol ensures your patients' safety.

After blood is administered, watch for signs and symptoms of a transfusion reaction. Check the patient's vital signs before and during the blood transfusion. For the first 15 minutes, transfuse the blood slowly to lessen the severity of any reaction that may occur, and stay with the patient. Notify the doctor immediately at the first signs of a transfusion reaction.

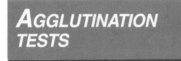

AGGLUTINATION TESTS

ABO blood typing

This test classifies blood according to the presence of major antigens A and B on red blood cell (RBC) surfaces and according to serum antibodies anti-A and anti-B. ABO blood typing is required before transfusions to prevent a lethal reaction — even if the patient is carrying an ABO blood group identification card.

In forward typing, the patient's RBCs are mixed with anti-A serum, then with anti-B serum; the presence or absence of agglutination determines the blood group. In reverse typing, the results of the forward method are verified by mixing the patient's serum with known group A and group B cells. Blood group determination is confirmed when the results of forward and reverse typing match perfectly. (See *ABO blood types*, page 270.)

Purpose
■ To establish blood group according to the ABO system
■ To check compatibility of donor and recipient blood before a transfusion.

Patient preparation
Tell the patient that this test determines his blood group. If he's scheduled for a transfusion, explain that once his blood group is known, it can be matched with the right donor blood. Inform him that he needn't fast. Tell him the test requires a blood sample, who will perform the venipuncture and when, and that he may feel transient discomfort from the needle puncture and the pressure of the tourniquet. Check his history for recent administration of blood, dextran, or I.V. contrast media.

Before the transfusion, compare current and past ABO typing and crossmatching to detect mistaken identification and prevent transfusion reaction.

Procedure
Perform the venipuncture, and collect the sample in a 10-ml *red-top* tube, as ordered.

Precautions
■ Label the sample with the patient's name, the hospital or blood bank number, the date, and the initials of the phlebotomist.
■ Handle the sample gently, and send it to the laboratory immediately with a properly completed laboratory request.

Normal findings and implications of results
In forward typing, if agglutination occurs when the patient's RBCs are mixed with anti-A serum, the A antigen is present and the blood is typed A. If agglutination occurs when the patient's RBCs are mixed with anti-B serum, the B antigen is present and the blood is typed B. If agglutination occurs in both

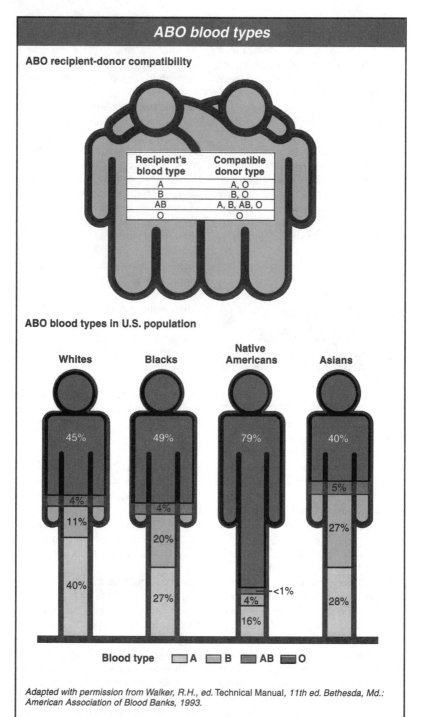

ABO blood types

ABO recipient-donor compatibility

Recipient's blood type	Compatible donor type
A	A, O
B	B, O
AB	A, B, AB, O
O	O

ABO blood types in U.S. population

Whites
45%
4%
11%
40%

Blacks
49%
4%
20%
27%

Native Americans
79%
<1%
4%
16%

Asians
40%
5%
27%
28%

Blood type ☐ A ☐ B ■ AB ■ O

Adapted with permission from Walker, R.H., ed. Technical Manual, *11th ed. Bethesda, Md.: American Association of Blood Banks, 1993.*

mixes, both A and B antigens are present and the blood is typed AB. If it does not occur in either mix, no antigens are present and the blood is typed O.

In reverse typing, if agglutination occurs when B cells are mixed with the patient's serum, anti-B is present and the blood is typed A. If agglutination occurs when A cells are mixed, anti-A is present and the blood is typed B. If agglutination occurs when both A and B cells are mixed, anti-A and anti-B are present and the blood is typed O. If agglutination does not occur when both A and B cells are mixed, neither anti-A nor anti-B is present and the blood is typed AB.

Post-test care
If a hematoma develops at the venipuncture site, apply warm soaks.

Interfering factors
- Recent administration of dextran or I.V. contrast media causes cellular aggregation that resembles agglutination.
- Hemolysis due to rough handling of the sample may affect test results.
- If the patient has received blood or been pregnant in the past 3 months, new antibodies may interfere with compatibility testing.

Rh typing

The Rh system classifies blood by the presence or absence of the $Rh_o(D)$ antigen on the surface of RBCs. In this test, a patient's RBCs are mixed with serum containing anti $Rh_o(D)$ antibodies and are observed for agglutination. If agglutination occurs, the $Rh_o(D)$ antigen is present, and the patient's blood is typed Rh-positive; if agglutination doesn't occur, the antigen is absent, and the patient's blood is typed Rh-negative.

Rh typing is performed routinely on prospective blood donors and on blood recipients before a transfusion. Only prospective blood donors are fully tested to exclude the D^u variant of the $Rh_o(D)$ antigen before being classified as having Rh-negative blood. Persons who have this antigen are considered Rh-positive donors but are generally transfused as Rh-negative recipients.

Purpose
- To establish blood type according to the Rh system
- To help determine the compatibility of the donor before transfusion
- To determine if the patient will require an $Rh_o(D)$ immune globulin injection.

Patient preparation
Explain to the patient that this test determines or verifies his blood group — an important step in ensuring a safe transfusion. Inform him that he needn't fast before the test. Tell him the test requires a blood sample, who will perform the venipuncture and when, and that he may experience transient discomfort from the needle puncture and the pressure of the tourniquet.

Check the patient history for recent administration of dextran, I.V. contrast media, or drugs that may alter results.

Procedure
Perform a venipuncture, and collect the sample in a 10-ml *red-top* tube, as ordered.

Precautions
- Label the sample with the patient's name, the hospital or blood bank number, the date, and the initials of the phlebotomist.
- Handle the sample gently, and send it to the laboratory immediately.

Implications of $Rh_o(D)$ typing test results

Classified as $Rh_o(D)$-positive, $Rh_o(D)$-negative, or $Rh(D^u)$-positive, donor blood may be transfused only if it's compatible with the recipient's blood, as shown below.

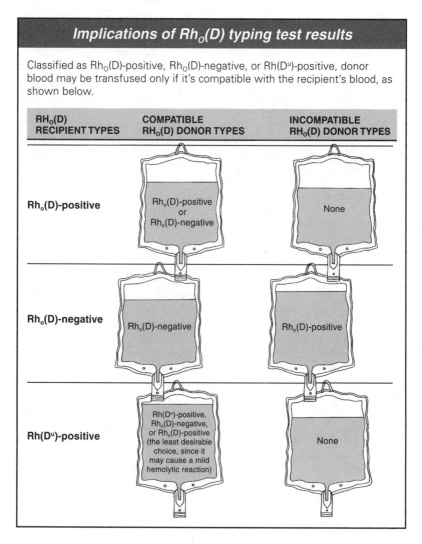

$RH_o(D)$ RECIPIENT TYPES	COMPATIBLE $RH_o(D)$ DONOR TYPES	INCOMPATIBLE $RH_o(D)$ DONOR TYPES
$Rh_o(D)$-positive	$Rh_o(D)$-positive or $Rh_o(D)$-negative	None
$Rh_o(D)$-negative	$Rh_o(D)$-negative	$Rh_o(D)$-positive
$Rh(D^u)$-positive	$Rh(D^u)$-positive, $Rh_o(D)$-negative, or $Rh_o(D)$-positive (the least desirable choice, since it may cause a mild hemolytic reaction)	None

■ If a transfusion is ordered, a transfusion request form must accompany the sample to the laboratory.

Normal findings and implications of results

Classified as Rh-positive, Rh-negative, or Rh-positive D^u, donor blood may be transfused only if it's compatible with the recipient's blood. (See *Implications of $Rh_o(D)$ typing test results.*)

If an Rh-negative woman delivers an Rh-positive baby or aborts a fetus whose Rh-type is unknown, she should receive an injection of $Rh_o(D)$ immune globulin within 72 hours to prevent hemolytic disease of the newborn in future births.

Post-test care

■ If a hematoma develops at the venipuncture site, apply warm soaks to ease discomfort.

- If available, give the pregnant patient a card identifying that she may need to receive $Rh_o(D)$ immune globulin.

Interfering factors

- Recent administration of dextran or I.V. contrast media results in cellular aggregation, which resembles antibody-mediated agglutination.
- If the patient has received blood or been pregnant in the past 3 months, antibodies may develop and linger, thus interfering with compatibility testing.
- Methyldopa, cephalosporins, and levodopa may cause a false-positive result for the D^u antigen because these drugs may produce a positive direct antiglobulin (Coombs') test.

Fetal-maternal erythrocyte distribution

Some transfer of red blood cells (RBCs) from fetal to maternal circulation occurs during most spontaneous or elective abortions and most normal deliveries. Usually, the amount of blood transferred is minimal and has no clinical significance. But transfer of significant amounts of blood from an Rh-positive fetus to an Rh-negative mother can result in maternal immunization to the $Rh_o(D)$ antigen and the development of anti-Rh-positive antibodies in maternal circulation. During a subsequent pregnancy, the maternal immunization subjects an Rh-positive fetus to potentially fatal hemolysis and erythroblastosis.

To prevent maternal $Rh_o(D)$ immunization, $Rh_o(D)$ immune globulin is given to an unsensitized Rh-negative mother shortly after the birth of an Rh-positive infant or after an abortion. The amount needed depends on the volume of fetal blood transferred; this test measures the number of fetal RBCs in maternal circulation to allow calculation of the $Rh_o(D)$ immune globulin dosage needed for protection.

This test usually employs a modification of the Kleihauer-Betke technique, using a maternal blood smear fixed with ethanol. The adult hemoglobin is eluted from the RBCs by a buffer at an acid pH of 3.2. Removal of hemoglobin doesn't destroy the RBCs and therefore permits the counting of these adults cells and the normally stained fetal RBCs. (A counterstain, such as aniline blue, may aid visualization of the eluted adult RBCs by giving them a light gray-blue color.) After counting, the percentage of fetal RBCs is used to calculate the approximate fetal-maternal erythrocyte volume, based on average total RBC volume.

Purpose

- To detect and measure fetal-maternal blood transfer
- To determine the amount of $Rh_o(D)$ immune globulin needed to prevent maternal immunization to the $Rh_o(D)$ antigen.

Patient preparation

Explain that this test determines or verifies blood group — an important step in ensuring a safe transfusion. Inform the patient that she needn't fast before the test. Tell her that the test requires a blood sample, who will perform the venipuncture and when, and that she may feel transient discomfort from the needle puncture and the pressure of the tourniquet.

Check the patient's history for recent administration of dextran, I.V. contrast media, or drugs that may alter results.

Procedure

Perform the venipuncture, and collect the sample in a 10-ml *lavender-top* tube, as ordered.

Precautions

▪ Label the sample with the patient's name, the hospital or blood bank number, the date, and the initials of the phlebotomist.

▪ Send the sample to the laboratory immediately with a properly completed laboratory request.

Normal findings

Fetal maternal whole blood should contain no fetal RBCs.

Implications of results

An elevated fetal RBC volume in maternal circulation necessitates administration of more than one dose of $Rh_o(D)$ immune globulin. The number of vials needed is determined by dividing the calculated fetomaternal hemorrhage by 30 (a single vial of $Rh_o(D)$ immune globulin will provide protection against a 30-ml fetomaternal hemorrhage).

Administration of $Rh_o(D)$ immune globulin to an unsensitized Rh-negative mother as soon as possible (no later than 72 hours) after the birth of an Rh-positive infant or after a spontaneous or elective abortion prevents complications in subsequent pregnancies. Most clinicians now administer $Rh_o(D)$ immune globulin prophylactically at 28 weeks' gestation to women who are Rh-negative but have no detectable Rh antibodies.

The following patients should be screened for Rh isoimmunization or irregular antibodies: all Rh-negative mothers during their first prenatal visit and at 28 weeks' gestation; and all Rh-positive mothers with a history of transfusion, a jaundiced infant, stillbirth, cesarean delivery, or induced or spontaneous abortion.

Post-test care

If a hematoma develops at the venipuncture site, apply warm soaks to ease discomfort.

Interfering factors

▪ Hemolysis caused by improper temperature or rough handling may alter test results.

▪ Delays of more than 72 hours after collection may yield inaccurate results and will prevent timely administration of $Rh_o(D)$ immune globulin.

▪ An improper test request, such as ordering a "Kleihauer test," may result in performance of the wrong test. (The Kleihauer method is also used to detect abnormal hemoglobin with hereditary persistence of high fetal hemoglobin levels.)

Crossmatching

Crossmatching establishes the compatibility or incompatibility of a donor's and a recipient's blood. It's the best antibody detection test available for avoiding lethal transfusion reactions.

After the donor's and the recipient's ABO blood type and Rh factor type are determined, *major crossmatching* tests for compatibility between the donor's red blood cells (RBCs) and the recipient's serum. They're compatible if the recipient's serum has no antibodies that would destroy transfused cells and possibly cause an acute hemolytic reaction. *Minor crossmatching* tests for compatibility between the donor's serum and the recipient's RBCs. This crossmatch is less important, however, because the donor's antibodies are greatly diluted in the recipient's plasma. Indeed, because the antibody-screening test is routinely performed on all blood donors, minor crossmatching is often omitted.

Blood is always crossmatched before a transfusion, except in emergencies. Because a complete crossmatch may take from 45 minutes to 2 hours, an incomplete (10-minute) crossmatch may be acceptable in some emergencies, such as severe blood loss due to trauma. In such cases, transfusion can begin with limited amounts of group O packed RBCs while crossmatching is completed. An emergency transfusion must proceed with special awareness of the complications that may arise because of incomplete typing and crossmatching. After crossmatching, compatible units of blood are labeled, and a compatibility record is completed.

Purpose

- To serve as the final check for compatibility between the donor's blood and the recipient's blood.

Patient preparation

Explain to the patient that this test ensures that the blood he receives correctly matches his own to prevent a transfusion reaction. Inform him that he needn't fast before the test. Tell him the test requires a blood sample, who will perform the venipuncture and when, and that he may experience some transient discomfort from the needle puncture and the pressure of the tourniquet.

Check the patient's history for recent administration of blood, dextran, or I.V. contrast media.

Procedure

Perform the venipuncture, and collect the sample in a 10-ml *red-top* tube. ABO typing, Rh typing, and crossmatching are all done together.

Precautions

- Handle the sample gently to prevent hemolysis, which can mask hemolysis of

the donor RBCs.

- Label the sample with the patient's name, the hospital or blood bank number, the date, and the initials of the phlebotomist.

- Indicate on the laboratory request the amount and type of blood component needed.

- Send the sample to the laboratory immediately. Crossmatching must be performed on the sample within 72 hours.

- If more than 72 hours have elapsed since a previous transfusion, previously crossmatched donor blood must be recrossmatched with a new recipient serum sample to detect newly acquired incompatibilities before the transfusion.

- If the patient is scheduled for surgery and has received a transfusion or been pregnant within the past 3 months, antibodies may develop and linger. The patient's blood will need to be crossmatched again if his surgery is rescheduled to detect recently acquired incompatibilities.

Normal findings

Absence of agglutination indicates compatibility between the donor's and the recipient's blood, which means that the transfusion of donor blood can proceed.

Implications of results

A *positive* crossmatch indicates incompatibility between the donor's blood and the recipient's blood, which means the donor's blood can't be transfused to the recipient. The sign of a positive crossmatch is agglutination, or clumping, when the donor's RBCs and the recipient's serum are correctly mixed and incubated. Agglutination indicates an undesirable antigen-antibody reaction. The donor's blood must be withheld and the crossmatch continued to determine the cause of the incompatibility and to identify the antibody.

A *negative* crossmatch — the absence of agglutination — indicates probable compatibility between the donor's blood and the recipient's blood, which means the transfusion of donor blood can proceed. It doesn't guarantee a safe transfusion, but it's the best method available to prevent an acute hemolytic reaction.

Post-test care

If a hematoma develops at the venipuncture site, apply warm soaks.

Interfering factors

- Previous administration of dextran or I.V. contrast media causes aggregation resembling agglutination. A previous blood transfusion may produce antibodies to the donor blood that could interfere with compatibility testing.
- Hemolysis may affect results.
- The administration of certain drugs may produce antibodies that could interfere with testing.

Direct antiglobulin

Also known as the direct Coombs' test, the direct antiglobulin test detects immunoglobulins (antibodies) on the surfaces of red blood cells (RBCs). These immunoglobulins coat RBCs when they become sensitized to an antigen, such as Rh factor.

In this test, antiglobulin (Coombs') serum added to saline-washed RBCs results in agglutination if immunoglobulins or complement is present. This test is "direct" because it requires only one step — the addition of Coombs' serum to washed cells.

Purpose

- To diagnose hemolytic disease of the newborn (HDN)

- To investigate hemolytic transfusion reactions
- To aid differential diagnosis of hemolytic anemias, which may be congenital or may result from an autoimmune reaction or use of certain drugs.

Patient preparation

If the patient is a neonate, explain to the parents that this test helps diagnose HDN. If the patient is suspected of having hemolytic anemia, explain that this test determines whether the condition results from an abnormality in the body's immune system, from the use of certain drugs, or from some unknown cause.

Inform the adult patient that he needn't fast. Tell the patient (or the infant's parents) that the test requires a blood sample, who will perform the venipuncture and when, and that he may experience transient discomfort.

As ordered, withhold medications that may induce autoimmune hemolytic anemia.

Procedure

For an adult, perform a venipuncture and collect the sample in two 5-ml *lavender-top* tubes. For a neonate, draw 5 ml of cord blood into a *red-top* or *lavender-top* tube, as ordered, after the cord is clamped and cut.

Precautions

- Handle the sample gently to prevent hemolysis.
- Send it to the laboratory immediately. The test must be performed within 24 hours.
- Label the sample with the patient's full name, the hospital or blood bank number, the date, and the initials of the phlebotomist.

Normal findings

A negative test, in which neither antibodies nor complement appears on the RBCs, is normal.

Implications of results

A positive test on umbilical cord blood indicates that maternal antibodies have crossed the placenta and have coated fetal RBCs, causing HDN. Transfusion of compatible blood lacking the antigens to these maternal antibodies may be necessary to prevent anemia.

In other patients, a positive test result may indicate hemolytic anemia and may help differentiate between autoimmune and secondary hemolytic anemia, which can be drug-induced or associated with an underlying disease such as lymphoma. A positive test result can also indicate sepsis.

A weakly positive test result may suggest a transfusion reaction in which the patient's antibodies react with transfused RBCs containing the corresponding antigen.

Post-test care

■ If a hematoma develops at the venipuncture site, apply warm soaks.
■ As ordered, resume administration of medications withheld before the test.
■ Tell the patient or the parents of an infant with HDN that further testing will be necessary to monitor anemia.

Interfering factors

■ Hemolysis caused by rough handling of the sample may alter test results.
■ Positive results may follow use of quinidine, methyldopa, cephalosporins, sulfonamides, chlorpromazine, diphenylhydantoin, dipyrone, ethosuximide, hydralazine, levodopa, mefenamic acid, melphalan, penicillin, procainamide, rifampin, streptomycin, tetracyclines, or isoniazid. A positive test caused by these drugs may or may not be associated with immune hemolysis.

Antibody screening

This test (also known as the indirect Coombs' test and the indirect antiglobulin test) detects unexpected circulating antibodies in the patient's serum. After incubating the serum with group O red blood cells (RBCs), which are unaffected by anti-A or anti-B antibodies, an antiglobulin (Coombs') serum is added. Agglutination occurs if the patient's serum contains an antibody to one or more antigens on the RBCs.

The antibody screening test detects 95% to 99% of the circulating antibodies. After this screening procedure detects them, the antibody identification test can determine the specific identity of the antibodies present. (See *Antibody identification test,* page 278.)

Purpose

■ To detect unexpected circulating antibodies to RBC antigens in the recipient's or donor's serum before a transfusion
■ To determine the presence of anti-$Rh_o(D)$ (Rh-positive) antibody in maternal blood
■ To evaluate the need for administration of $Rh_o(D)$ immune globulin
■ To aid diagnosis of acquired hemolytic anemia.

Patient preparation

Explain to the prospective blood recipient that the antibody screening test helps evaluate the possibility of a transfusion reaction. If the test is being performed because the patient is anemic, explain to him that it helps identify the specific type of anemia.

Inform the patient that he needn't fast before the test. Tell him that this test requires a blood sample, who will perform the venipuncture and when, and that he may experience transient dis-

Antibody identification test

This test identifies unexpected circulating antibodies detected by the antibody screening test (indirect Coombs' test). In this test, group O red blood cells (RBCs) — at least three with and three without a specific antigen — are combined with serum containing unknown antibodies and are observed for agglutination. If the serum contains the corresponding antibody to the RBC antigen, a positive reaction occurs with RBCs that have the antigen but not with those that lack the antigen. Serum that reacts with Rh-positive cells, for example, but not with Rh-negative cells, probably contains the anti-$Rh_O(D)$ antibody.

At least three RBCs containing the antigen and three without it are used in each test to reduce error. Serum that contains rare or multiple antibodies requires more complicated procedures.

comfort from the needle puncture and the pressure of the tourniquet.

Check the patient history for recent administration of blood, dextran, or I.V. contrast media. Be sure to note any such administration on the laboratory request to prevent spurious interpretation of test results.

Procedure
Perform a venipuncture, and collect the sample in two 10-ml *red-top* tubes. Some laboratories require 20 ml of clotted blood to perform this test.

Precautions
■ Handle the sample gently to prevent hemolysis.
■ Label the sample with the patient's name, the hospital or blood bank number, the date, and the initials of the phlebotomist. Be sure to include the patient's diagnosis and any history of transfusions, pregnancy, or drug therapy on the laboratory request.
■ Send the sample to the laboratory immediately. The antibody screening must be done within 72 hours after the sample is drawn.

Normal findings
A negative test result is normal. That is, agglutination does not occur, indicating that the patient's serum contains no circulating antibodies (other than anti-A and anti-B).

Implications of results
A positive result indicates the presence of unexpected circulating antibodies to RBC antigens. Such a reaction demonstrates donor and recipient incompatibility.

A positive result in a pregnant patient with Rh-negative blood may indicate the presence of antibodies to the Rh factor from previous a transfusion with incompatible blood or from a previous pregnancy with an Rh-positive fetus.

A positive result above a titer of 1:8 indicates that the fetus may develop hemolytic disease of the newborn. As a result, repeated testing throughout the patient's pregnancy is necessary to evaluate progressive development of circulating antibody levels.

Post-test care
If a hematoma develops at the venipuncture site, apply warm soaks.

Interfering factors
- Previous administration of blood, dextran, or I.V. contrast media causes aggregation that resembles agglutination.
- Hemolysis caused by rough handling of the sample may affect the accuracy of test results.
- If the patient has received a transfusion or been pregnant within the past 3 months, antibodies may develop and linger, thereby interfering with the patient's compatibility testing.
- The administration of certain drugs can produce antibodies that may alter test results.

Leukoagglutinins

This test detects leukoagglutinins (also known as white cell antibodies or HLA antibodies) — antibodies that react with white blood cells (WBCs) and may cause a transfusions reaction. These antibodies usually develop after exposure to foreign WBCs through transfusions, pregnancies, or allografts.

If a blood recipient has these antibodies, a febrile nonhemolytic reaction may occur 1 to 4 hours after the start of whole blood, red blood cell, platelet, or granulocyte transfusion. (All these blood products contain some granulocytes, which react with the antibodies.) This nonhemolytic reaction (marked by fever and severe chills, sometimes with nausea, headache, and transient hypertension) must be distinguished from a true hemolytic reaction before the transfusion can proceed. The presence of these antibodies in a recipient can also cause immune-mediated platelet refractoriness, a condition that is characterized by the failure of the platelet count to increase after the transfusion of suitably preserved platelets.

The standard technique used to detect leukoagglutinins is the microlymphocytotoxicity test, in which recipient serum is tested against donor lymphocytes or against a panel of lymphocytes of known HLA phenotype. The antibodies in the recipient serum will bind to the corresponding antigen present on the lymphocytes and will cause cell membrane injury when complement is added to the test system. Cell injury is detected by examination of the lymphocytes using a phase contrast microscope to observe dye exclusion (negative test) or dye uptake (positive test).

Purpose
- To detect leukoagglutinins in blood recipients who develop a transfusion reaction, thus differentiating between hemolytic and febrile nonhemolytic transfusion reactions
- To detect leukoagglutinins in recipients who develop platelet refractoriness after multiple transfusions of blood products.

Patient preparation
Explain to the patient that this test helps determine the cause of his transfusion reaction. Tell him that the test requires a blood sample, who will perform the venipuncture and when, and that he may feel transient discomfort from the needle puncture and the pressure of the tourniquet.

Note recent administration of blood or dextran or testing with I.V. contrast media on the laboratory request.

Procedure
Perform a venipuncture and collect the sample in a 10-ml *red-top* tube. The laboratory will require 3 to 4 ml of serum for testing.

Precautions
Label the sample with the patient's name, the hospital or blood bank num-

ber, the date, and the initials of the phlebotomist. Be sure to include on the laboratory request the patient's suspected diagnosis and any history of blood transfusions, pregnancies, and drug therapy.

Normal findings

A negative test result is normal. That is, agglutination does not occur, indicating that the patient's serum contains no antibodies.

Implications of results

A positive result in a blood recipient indicates the presence of agglutinins, identifying his transfusion reaction as a febrile nonhemolytic reaction to these antibodies. Recipients who test positive for HLA antibodies may need HLA-matched platelets to control bleeding episodes caused by thrombocytopenia.

Post-test care

■ If a hematoma develops at the venipuncture site, ease discomfort by applying warm soaks.

 ■ If a transfusion recipient has a positive leukoagglutinin test, continued transfusions require premedication with acetaminophen 1 to 2 hours before the transfusion, specially prepared leukocyte-poor blood, or use of leukocyte removal blood filters to prevent further reactions.

■ Tests for these antibodies are not useful in deciding which patients should receive leukocyte-poor blood components; the decision must be based on clinical experience.

■ The use of leukocyte-poor blood components is becoming routine for patients who require long-term platelet and red blood cell transfusions and is especially important for patients who are likely to become transplant candidates.

Interfering factors

Previous administration of dextran or I.V. contrast media causes aggregation resembling agglutination.

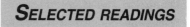

Bennett, J.C., and Plum, F., eds. *Cecil Textbook of Medicine*, 20th ed. Philadelphia: W.B. Saunders Co., 1996.

Beutler, E., et al. *Williams Hematology*, 5th ed. New York: McGraw-Hill Book Co., 1995.

Diseases. 2nd ed. Springhouse, Pa.: Springhouse Corp., 1996.

Fischbach, F. *A Manual of Laboratory and Diagnostic Tests*, 5th ed. Philadelphia: Lippincott-Raven Pubs., 1996.

Guyton, A.C., and Hall, J.E. *Textbook of Medical Physiology*, 9th ed. Philadelphia: W.B. Saunders Co., 1996.

Henry, J.B., ed. *Clinical Diagnosis and Management by Laboratory Methods*, 19th ed. Philadelphia: W.B. Saunders Co., 1996.

Klein, H.G., ed. *Standards for Blood Banks and Transfusion Services*, 17th ed. Bethesda, Md.: American Association of Blood Banks, 1996.

Mayo Medical Laboratories 1996 Test Catalog. Rochester, Minn.: Mayo Medical Laboratories, 1996.

Nursing97 Drug Handbook. Springhouse, Pa.: Springhouse Corp., 1997.

Ravel, R.A. *Clinical Laboratory Medicine: Clinical Application of Laboratory Data*, 6th ed. St. Louis: Mosby–Year Book, Inc., 1995.

Reeder, S.J., et al. *Maternity Nursing: Family, Newborn and Women's Health Care*, 18th ed. Philadelphia: Lippincott-Raven Pubs., 1996.

Walker, R.H., ed. *Technical Manual*, 11th ed. Bethesda, Md.: American Association of Blood Banks, 1993.

Immune response

Learning objectives

After completing this chapter, the reader will be able to:
- explain how the immune system protects the body
- describe seven common techniques used in immunologic tests
- define the term autoimmunity
- explain the purpose and procedure of each test discussed in this chapter
- prepare the patient physically and psychologically for each test
- state the reference values or normal findings for each test
- discuss the implications of normal test results
- list factors that may interfere with accurate test results.

INTRODUCTION

A normally functioning immune system provides continuous physiologic surveillance. It protects the body from the effects of invasion by microorganisms and maintains homeostasis by governing the degradation and removal of damaged cells. It also discovers and disposes of abnormal cells that continually arise within the body. Abnormal immune function causes serious physiologic disruptions. For example, immune hyperreactivity leads to allergic symptoms; immunodeficiency may lead to exaggerated vulnerability to infection; a misdirected immune response leads to autoimmune disorders; failure of surveillance may allow uncontrolled growth of tumor cells. Thus, tests for immune dysfunction have great clinical significance.

The range of immunologic tests to study antigen-antibody reactions has expanded rapidly since the mid-1970s. Existing tests have been modified or replaced to reflect new data and technology. New tests of the cell-mediated immune response and of its components have been developed from the application of immunopotentiation, immunosuppression, and immunomodulation to clinical therapeutic medicine. New tests of the autoimmune response and of tumors have been developed using cell sorter technology and monoclonal antibodies.

Both nonspecific and specific defense mechanisms protect the body against "nonself" attack. Nonspecific mechanisms — such as skin, mucous membranes and their secretions, and various enzymes, secretions, and cellular activities — protect the body from foreign invasion. However, when a foreign agent penetrates the body, a specific immune mechanism takes over, destroying the invading organism through the specialized activity of lymphocytes and macrophages. This response is the focus of the tests described in this chapter.

Lymphoreticular system
The lymphoreticular system — which consists of primary and secondary lymphoid organs (thymus, spleen, and lymph nodes and related areas in the liver, bone marrow, and respiratory and GI tracts) — is responsible for specific immune reactions to foreign substances. This system includes macrophages and T and B lymphocytes. To become properly differentiated, *T lymphocytes* need an intact, functioning thymus during their development. *B lymphocytes* mature through action of an unknown primary lymphoid organ, thought to be the bone marrow.

Macrophages recognize and phagocytize an antigen that enters the body, making it recognizable to lymphocytes as foreign. The lymphocytes then divide rapidly, forming a clone of cells that attempt (sometimes with the aid of complement) to destroy the antigen.

Antigenicity
Antigenicity is the very root of the immune response. A molecule or substance must be recognized as foreign and must provoke a specific immune response to be considered an *antigen*. Generally, antigens are proteins, polysaccharides, or lipoproteins of high molecular weight (10,000 daltons or more). The more complex the molecular configuration of the immunogenic substance, the more antigenic determinants it contains. The amount of antigen that penetrates the body and the route of invasion are also significant. An antigen must be presented in a unique manner to be optimally antigenic.

A *hapten* — a substance of lower molecular weight than an antigen — isn't antigenic by itself but can combine with a carrier protein to form a complete antigen that is recognized as such and is dealt with by antibodies specific for the hapten alone, the carrier protein, or the hapten-protein complex. Certain drugs may be haptens and can cause an allergic response if they combine with body proteins.

Immune response
Three sequentially dependent mechanisms, referred to as limbs, make up the immune response:
- The *afferent limb* recognizes and processes antigens and involves macrophages as well as T and B lymphocytes. (See *T and B cells: Their origin and role in the immune response,* pages 284 and 285.)
- The *central limb* makes possible an efferent immune response and includes cell cooperation, clonal expansion, and production of effectors and memory cells.
- The *efferent limb* involves destruction of specific antigens by sensitized T and B lymphocytes and their products. This destruction results from a system of

(Text continues on page 286.)

T and B cells: Their origin and role in the immune response

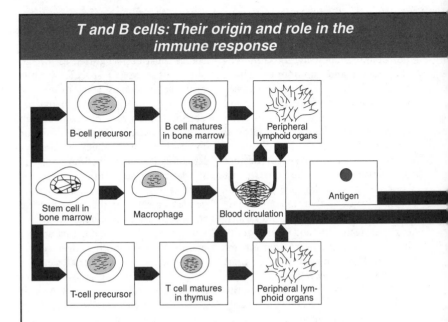

When the immune system recognizes an antigen as nonself, two distinct types of immune responses cooperate to protect the body. Both involve lymphocytes that share a common origin in stem cells. However, these lymphocytes differentiate and mature in different microenvironments, producing two populations: B cells and T cells.

In humoral immunity, antigen-stimulated B cells produce immunoglobulins (antibodies) to destroy antigens before they reach host cells. In cell-mediated immunity, antigen-activated T cells destroy antigens by direct cell-to-cell interaction. Macrophages, phagocytic cells of the reticuloendothelial system, affect both types of immune response by presenting antigens in the proper orientation to B cells and T cells for recognition and destruction.

Two groups of activated T cells trigger overlapping humoral and cell-mediated immune responses. T-regulatory cells (consisting of T-helper and T-suppressor cells) are influenced by interleukin-1 (IL-1), a monokine produce by antigen-stimulated macrophages. IL-1 activates T-helper cells and induces them to produce interleukin-2 (IL-2), B-cell growth factor (BCGF), and B-cell differentiating factor (BCDF); activated B cells then respond to these lymphokines by proliferating into clones of B cells, which differentiate into antibody-secreting plasma cells. The antibodies circulate through the body, find the antigen and bind to it, and assist in its destruction. IL-2 also stimulates effector-T-cell (natural killer and cytotoxic-T-cell) function and induces the production of immune interferon by T cells. Interferon suppresses B cells and enhances the cell-mediated immune response by effector T cells, which destroy antigenic substances. These effector T cells also play a role in graft tissue rejection, delayed hypersensitivity, and graft-versus-host disease.

Macrophages activated by macrophage activating factor (MAF), a T-helper lymphokine, regulate the response by producing prostaglandin E2, which suppresses T-helper lymphokine activity and activates T-suppressor function.

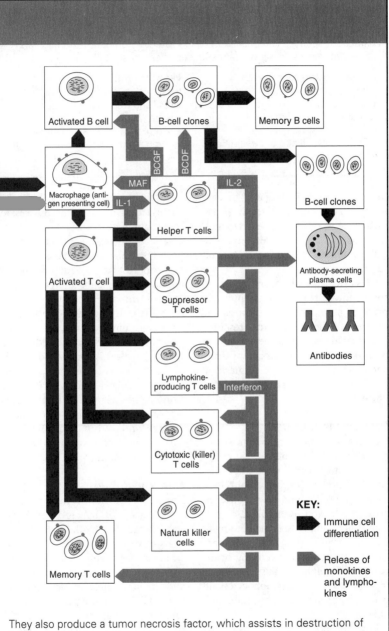

They also produce a tumor necrosis factor, which assists in destruction of foreign antigens.

Both humoral and cell-mediated immune responses record the battle by producing B- and T-memory cells. These memory cells can respond again to the same antigen, providing long-term immunity.

Types of immune response

Immune responses can be either cell-mediated or humoral. This chart lists some of the common immune responses of each type.

Cell-mediated responses
- Transplant rejection
- Delayed hypersensitivity-tuberculin reaction, contact dermatitis
- Graft-vs-host reactions
- Tumor surveillance or destruction
- Intracellular infections

Humoral responses
- Bacterial phagocytosis and lysis
- Viral and toxin neutralization
- Anaphylaxis
- Allergic hay fever and asthma
- Immune complex disease

humoral and cell-mediated mechanisms; although both humoral and cell-mediated responses are present in most immune reactions, one response typically dominates. (See *Types of immune response.*)

Classification of the immune response into three functional limbs has practical application in diagnosis and treatment. When the immune response is evaluated, testing for defects in one or more limbs is common. Many drugs and therapies are directed primarily at particular activities or cell types within one limb.

Humoral immunity

Humoral immunity results from a clone of activated B lymphocytes that differentiates into plasma cells and synthesizes antibodies (immunoglobulins). These antibodies bind to specific antigens on cell surfaces or circulate unattached body fluids. Specific binding of an antibody to an antigen typically leads to the destruction and removal of the complex. B lymphocytes usually require the cooperation of T lymphocytes and macrophages to initiate the production of antibodies.

Immunoglobulins, secreted by plasma cells as the effector agents of humoral immunity, circulate in the vascular system and in the intercellular fluids. Each immunoglobulin molecule is made up of two light and two heavy polypeptide chains attached by disulfide bridges. All four chains have a constant portion and a variable portion. The constant (Fc) portions of the heavy chains have certain regions that are of an unchanging amino acid sequence and can bind to any cell with an Fc receptor. The variable antibody portion (Fab) has a changing amino acid sequence and can lock onto the specific antigen that originally provoked its production. Thus, the Fab portion of immunoglobulin includes the antigen-binding variable portions of the heavy and light chains, whereas the Fc portion is associated with secondary biological activities, such as complement fixation and the release of histamine from mast cells.

Immunoglobulins

The known classes of immunoglobulins — IgG, IgM, IgA, IgE, and IgD — are distinguished by the constant portions of their heavy chains. However, each class has a kappa or a lambda light chain, which gives rise to many subtypes and provides almost limitless combinations of light and heavy chains that give immunoglobulins their specificity. The five classes of immunoglobulins are described below:

- *IgG*, the smallest immunoglobulin, appears in all body fluids because of its ability to move across membranes as a

Four types of hypersensitivity

Hypersensitivity states have been grouped into four major types:

■ *Type I* (immediate hypersensitivity): Antigen reacts with an antibody (IgE) fixed on the surfaces of mast cells or basophils, causing release of vasoactive amines and histamine. These amines produce allergic symptoms, such as hives, secretions, erythema, itching, smooth-muscle contraction, and possibly, shock.

■ *Type II* (cytotoxic): Antibody reacts with an antigenic component of a cell, or with an antigen or a hapten associated with a cell. Complement or mononuclear cells (lymphocytes and macrophages) cause actual cellular destruction, resulting in lysis of the target cell. Thus, if erythrocytes are the target, such destruction causes hemolytic anemia; if platelets are the target, thrombocytope-

nia; and if white cells are the target, leukopenia.

■ *Type III* (immune-complex mediated): Complexes of antigen-antibody and complement, forming in the blood, may precipitate onto "innocent bystander" cells and tissues, which are damaged by local inflammation. Type III hypersensitivity reactions include glomerulonephritis, arteritis, and rheumatoid arthritis.

■ *Type IV* (delayed hypersensitivity): Sensitized T cells respond to antigens by excessive release of lymphokines or by direct cytotoxic injury. Type IV reactions are a delayed type of sensitivity, requiring 48 to 72 hours to occur. This form of hypersensitivity includes allergic contact dermatitis due to exposure to poison ivy as well as skin reactions to cosmetics, drugs, and industrial chemicals.

single structural unit (a monomer). It accounts for 75% of total immunoglobulins and is the major antibacterial and antiviral antibody.

■ *IgM*, the largest immunoglobulin, appears as a pentamer (five monomers joined by a J-chain). Unlike IgG — which is produced mainly in the secondary, or recall, immune response — IgM dominates in the primary, or initial immune response. But like IgG, IgM is involved in classic antibody reactions, including precipitation, agglutination, neutralization, and complement fixation. Because of its size, IgM cannot readily cross membrane barriers and is usually present only in the vascular system. IgM constitutes 5% of total serum immunoglobulins.

■ *IgA* exists in serum primarily as a monomer; in secretory form, IgA exists

almost exclusively as a dimer (two monomer molecules joined by a J-chain and a secretory component chain). As a secretory immunoglobin, IgA defends external body surfaces and is present in colostrum, saliva, tears, nasal fluids, and respiratory, GI, and genitourinary secretions. This antibody is considered important in preventing antigenic agents from attaching to epithelial surfaces. IgA makes up 20% of total immunoglobulins.

■ *IgE*, present in trace amounts in serum, is involved in the release of vasoactive amines stored in basophils and tissue mast cell granules. When released, these bioamines cause the allergic effects characteristic of this type of hypersensitivity (erythema, itching, smooth-muscle contraction, secretions, and swelling). (See *Four types of hypersensitivity*.)

■ *IgD*, present as a monomer in serum in minute amounts, is the predominant antibody found on the surface of B lymphocytes and serves mainly as an antigen receptor. It may also help control lymphocyte activation or suppression.

Complement system

Complement is the collective term for a system of plasma proteins — labeled C1 through C9 — circulating in the blood as inactive precursors of enzymes. The complement system is activated by the coupling of antigen and antibody on the surface of a cell, with a subsequent bonding of C1 to the Fc portion of the immunoglobulin heavy chain. The complement cascade that follows this activation causes cell membranes to undergo lysis. Activated complement fragments also cause chemotaxis of neutrophils and macrophages, initiate release of histamine from mast cells, neutralize viruses, and enhance phagocytosis and other nonspecific inflammatory effects. Alternately, the complement system can be activated by foreign polysaccharides and bacterial endotoxins.

Cell-mediated immune response

In the cell-mediated immune response, macrophages present antigens to T lymphocytes and activate them. Once activated, these T lymphocytes destroy the presenting antigen, either directly by cytotoxicity or indirectly by secreting lymphokines — soluble substances that stimulate proliferation of lymphocytes and cytotoxic macrophages. Thus, T lymphocytes respond differently than B lymphocytes. For example, B lymphocytes are not required to be present at the antigen site, whereas T lymphocytes must be present and must actively participate in destroying the offending antigen.

Two subsets of regulatory T lymphocytes — *T-helper cells* and *T-suppressor cells* — function in both humoral and cell-mediated immune responses and regulate the magnitude, intensity, and duration of the immune response. An equal number of helper and suppressor lymphocytes is required for a normally functioning immune response. An excess of either type can change the intensity and outcome of the immune response. T-helper cells appear to enhance the immune response, whereas T-suppressor cells seem to prevent an excessive immune response.

Activated by interleukin-1 (a soluble monokine produced by macrophages), T-helper cells secrete the lymphokine interleukin-2, which induces the growth and differentiation of B lymphocytes into antibody-secreting plasma cells and potentiates T-cell proliferation with subsequent cytotoxicity of effector cells. T-suppressor cells are also activated by interleukin-1 to produce interferon, a soluble protein that suppresses the growth and differentiation of B lymphocytes.

T-cell interferon enhances cell-mediated immune destruction by activating effector T cells — cytotoxic T lymphocytes and natural killer (NK) cells. Interferon can also promote the production of natural killer cells. These cells have the capacity to respond to an antigen immediately and without differentiation when they're targeting tumor cells, certain microbially infected cells, and perhaps other cells.

Misdirected response

Autoimmunity is the one form of hypersensitivity in which the immune response is misdirected against the body's own tissues. Disorders thought to result from autoimmunity include rheumatoid arthritis, systemic lupus erythematosus, scleroderma, Sjögren's syndrome, and hemolytic anemia. Autoantibodies usually attack intracellular "self-antigens" that are normally not exposed to the lymphoreticular system, including inner layers of cell membranes, nucleoprotein, nucleic acids, and cytoplasmic structures such as mitochondria.

Viruses or haptens attached to the body's own cells also provoke autoimmune cell and tissue destruction. In many instances, tissue destruction results when intracellular antigens escape to form immune complexes, which are then deposited in the kidneys or blood vessels, activating complement and causing cytotoxic damage (type III hypersensitivity). Depletion of T-suppressor cells is believed to cause autoimmune disease by allowing unregulated function of T-helper cells.

In other hypersensitivity states, excessive amounts of immunoglobulins, T-helper cells, T-suppressor cells, B lymphocytes, or complement — or a combination of any of these — are present. In such conditions, overproduction of one immune response component retards the production of others. In multiple myeloma, for example, the excessive production of a single clone of plasma cells can result in a single type of immunoglobulin that completely inhibits the production of other types. In this respect, hypersensitivity reactions can lead to immunodeficiency.

Immunodeficiency is a congenital or acquired deficiency of the immune response. Congenital deficiencies include Bruton's agammaglobulinemia (B-cell deficiency) and DiGeorge's syndrome (thymic parathyroid aplasia). Acquired immunodeficiency disorders can result from chemotherapy or from radiation or corticosteroid therapy. They're related to a change in the ratio of T-helper to T-suppressor cells or macrophages. An imbalance of these regulatory cells may also result from infection, stress, drug use, old age, malnutrition, and cancer.

Immunologic test methods

Most immunologic tests use a combination of techniques to evaluate humoral and cell-mediated immune responses or their individual components. The most commonly used laboratory methods include precipitation, immunodiffusion, agglutination, histochemical techniques (such as immunofluorescence), radioimmunoassay, enzyme-linked immunosorbent assay (ELISA), complement fixation and, most recently, monoclonal antibody assays. The ELISA test is used to screen blood for contamination with HIV antibodies. (See *Screening blood for HIV antibodies,* page 290.)

Precipitation

When a soluble antibody reacts with a soluble antigen, cross-linking occurs between the antibody and the antigen. This phenomenon, known as the *lattice hypothesis,* results from the presence of multiple receptor sites on the surfaces of the antibody and the antigen, allowing cross-linkage between them. As more antigens and antibodies cross-link, they create an insoluble lattice structure and precipitate out of solution.

The quantity of antibody and antigen in solution determines the precipitation reaction. When a small amount of antigen is added to a large amount of antibody, all antigen sites are satisfied, and the resultant complexes contain much antibody and little antigen. Optimal cross-linking occurs when antigen and antibody are present in equal proportions; this point of optimal proportion is called the *zone of equivalence.* An excess of antigen or antibody may produce false-negative test results.

Screening blood for HIV antibodies

Currently, the most common method of screening blood for human immunodeficiency virus (HIV) involves the detection of HIV antibodies. These screening tests are most commonly used to determine whether an individual has been exposed to HIV. In order to ensure a safe supply of banked blood, donations at all blood banks are screened for HIV antibodies to prevent contamination of the blood supply.

Test methods
Many different test methods are commercially available to screen blood for the presence of HIV antibodies. Among the most common are enzyme immunoassay, fluorescence immunoassay, and enzyme-linked immunosorbent assay (ELISA). However, these screening tests are not 100% sensitive and specific and may give false results. For instance, because test sensitivity varies among laboratories, a negative result does not necessarily mean that HIV antibodies are absent. A false-positive result may reflect a lack of specificity in that particular method. As a result, various government health agencies all recommend confirmation of any positive result using the Western blot test. The Western blot test detects the presence of specific viral proteins. The presence of the virus particle confirms the presence of HIV

and thus the possibility of transmitting the virus.

Your role
Encourage the patient with positive screening tests to seek medical follow-up care, even if he is asymptomatic. Signs and symptoms of AIDS vary widely. Nonspecific ones often precede complications and may include fatigue, afternoon fevers, night sweats, weight loss, diarrhea, and a cough. A child with AIDS may exhibit dysmorphic features. Patients may be otherwise asymptomatic until abrupt onset of complications, such as opportunistic infections, Kaposi's sarcoma, and HIV encephalopathy (dementia), which is marked by confusion, apathy, paranoia, and loss of coordination.

Assume that a person with positive test results can transmit HIV to others. To prevent possible contagion, instruct him not to share razors, toothbrushes, or utensils (which may be contaminated with blood) and to clean such items with household bleach diluted 1:10 in water. Advise him to avoid donating blood, tissues, or an organ. If you suspect I.V. drug abuse, warn the patient not to share needles.

Encourage the patient to inform his doctor and dentist about his condition so they can take proper precautions.

Immunodiffusion
Immunodiffusion relies on the tendency of antigen and antibody particles to diffuse in an agar matrix and to form a precipitin line where they meet. This test may be performed using one of three methods:

■ *Single diffusion* (radial immunodiffusion) uses an agar slide containing antibody specific to a certain antigen. A well is punched in the agar and is filled with the specific antigen. After 24 hours, a precipitation ring forms around the well. The distance between the precipitation line and the well is proportional to the antigen concentration. Clinically, single diffusion is used to measure serum immunoglobulin concentrations. However, interference with diffusion (molecular size or weight) or precipitation (excess antigen or antibody) affects accurate determination of findings.

■ *Double diffusion*, a similar method, uses an agar-filled slide or a Petri dish with small wells. After the addition of antigen to one well and antibody to the other, precipitin lines form where optimal proportions of antigen and antibody meet. The number of precipitin lines indicates the number of different antigen-antibody complexes present. Formation of a single precipitin line provides a rough quantitative estimate of antigen or antibody purity. Although double diffusion is a simple, useful method for detecting unknown antigens or antibodies, it lacks sensitivity and thus has limited practical application.

■ *Immunoelectrophoresis* combines electrophoresis and immunodiffusion to identify and measure serum immunoglobulins and other proteins. A direct electric current is applied to an agar slide, causing each protein to migrate at a different speed, according to its size and net electrical charge. After the proteins are separated, addition of antigen to each one results in diffusion and the formation of precipitin lines; these lines may be photographed or stained for a permanent record. Clinically, immunoelectrophoresis aids diagnosis of monoclonal and polyclonal gammopathies as well as immunodeficiency diseases.

Agglutination
Agglutination occurs when large, insoluble particles, such as bacteria or red blood cells (RBCs), are clumped together by antibodies to the particles or to the antigens attached to the particles. Unlike precipitation, agglutination uses high-molecular-weight antigens for rough quantitation of antibody levels.

Direct agglutination results from the addition of antibody to a cell or to insoluble particulate native antigen. If the antigen is added to increasing dilutions of antiserum in tubes or wells with rounded bottoms, the reciprocal of the dilution of antiserum in the last tube to show visible agglutination is the titer (relative concentration) of antibody.

Indirect or passive agglutination refers to the agglutination of soluble antigen attached to blood cells, bacteria, or latex particles, which are inert carrier particles.

Agglutination is clinically useful to detect specific antibodies, such as those that cause rheumatoid arthritis, syphilis, or salmonella infections.

Immunofluorescence
In this histochemical technique, fluorescent dyes are attached to antibody molecules. When complexed with antigen and viewed under an ultraviolet microscope, the antibody appears as a colored fluorescence. Both direct and indirect immunofluorescence allow precise detection and demonstration of human tissue antigens and of bacterial, viral, and protozoan antigens. In the *direct* method, the fluorescein-labeled antibody reacts with an antigen specific to it. In the *indirect* method, a fluorescein-labeled antiglobulin reacts with an unlabeled antigen-antibody complex; the antiglobulin then binds to the unlabeled antibody.

Both methods are widely used to detect autoantibodies, immunoglobulins of cell surfaces, components of complement, T and B lymphocytes, tumor-specific antigens, and microorganisms.

Radioimmunoassay
This technique measures small quantities of a substance by combining a radiolabeled antigen with a particular antibody. Radiolabeled antigen is added to the sample, and binds with about 70%

of antibody. Various amounts of unlabeled antibody are then added to the mixture, and the radiolabeled and unlabeled antigens compete for binding sites on the antibody. A curve is then constructed from the amount of radiolabeled antigen at various unlabeled antigen concentrations to determine the amount of antigen already present in the serum sample.

Enzyme-linked immunosorbent assay

Commonly known as the ELISA test, this technique can identify antibodies or antigens, and is replacing or supplementing radioimmunoassay and immunofluorescence. The ELISA test is safe, sensitive, and simple to perform, and provides reproducible results at a low cost. To measure a specific antibody, antigen is fixed to a solid-phase medium, incubated with a serum sample, and then incubated with an anti-immunoglobulin-tagged enzyme. Excess unbound enzyme is washed from the system and a substrate is added. To measure a specific antigen, antibody instead of antigen is fixed to a solid-phase medium. Hydrolysis of the substrate produces a color change that's quantified by a spectrophotometer. The amount of substrate hydrolyzed is directly proportional to the amount of antigen or antibody in the serum sample.

Complement fixation

Used to determine the presence and extent of an antigen-antibody reaction, complement fixation is performed by adding a known antigen or antibody, directed against an unknown antibody or antigen, to a patient's serum and incubating the sample. Then, RBCs coated with the same known antigen or antibody are added. If hemolysis doesn't occur, complement must have been depleted in the original reaction; that is, the unknown antibody or antigen was present in the sample. The unknown antibody or antigen is then assayed.

Monoclonal antibody assays

B lymphocytes respond to antigen stimulation by rapidly proliferating and producing antibodies against the antigen. Laboratory production of monoclonal antibodies takes advantage of the B-lymphocyte reaction to an antigen to create unlimited numbers of completely homogenous antibodies.

Typically, a selected antigen is injected into a mouse, stimulating its immune response to develop antibody-secreting plasma cells. These cells are then harvested from the mouse's spleen and fused with myeloma cells — malignant cells that secrete an infinite amount of the single antibody specific to the antigen that's been injected. The resulting hybridomas are grown in culture, cloned, and tested for the desired antibody. Finally, selected hybridomas are grown in culture or injected into a mouse to produce monoclonal antibodies, which are purified for future use.

Monoclonal antibodies have been used extensively for typing cells and cell subsets, detecting specific antigens, and differentiating malignant from nonmalignant cells.

GENERAL CELLULAR TESTS

T- and B-lymphocyte assays

Lymphocytes — key cells in the immune system — have the capacity to recognize antigens through special receptors found on their surfaces. The two primary kinds of lymphocytes, T and

B cells, originate in the bone marrow. T cells mature under the influence of the thymus gland; B cells evolve without thymic influence.

Cell separation is used to isolate lymphocytes from other cellular blood elements. In this method, a whole blood sample is layered on Ficoll-Hypaque in a narrow tube, which is then centrifuged. Granulocytes and erythrocytes form a sediment at the bottom of the tube, and lymphocytes, monocytes, and platelets form a distinct band at the Ficoll-Hypaque-plasma interface.

This procedure recovers approximately 80% of the lymphocytes but doesn't differentiate between T and B cells. The percentage of T and B cells is determined by attaching a label or marker and by using different identification techniques. The E rosette test identifies T cells, which tend to form unstable clusterlike shapes (or rosettes) after exposure to sheep red blood cells (RBCs) at 39.2° F (4° C). Direct immunofluorescence detects B cells, which have monoclonal immunoglobulin on their surfaces; unlike T cells, B cells present receptors for complement as well as for Fc portions of immunoglobulin.

Null cells, which make up the remainder of the lymphocytes, possess Fc receptors but no other detectable surface markers, and presently have no diagnostic significance. Null cells are usually determined by subtracting the sum of T and B cells from total lymphocytes.

Purpose
- To aid diagnosis of primary and secondary immunodeficiency diseases
- To distinguish benign from malignant lymphocytic proliferative diseases
- To monitor response to therapy.

Patient preparation
Explain to the patient that this test measures certain white blood cells (WBCs). Tell him that this test requires a blood sample, who will perform the venipuncture and when, and that he may experience transient discomfort from the needle puncture and the pressure of the tourniquet.

Procedure
Perform a venipuncture, and collect the sample in a 7 ml *green-top* tube.

Precautions
- Fill the collection tube completely, and invert it gently several times to mix the sample and anticoagulant adequately.
- Send the sample to the laboratory immediately to ensure viable lymphocytes.
- If antilymphocyte antibodies are suspected, as in autoimmune disease, notify the laboratory.

Reference values
T-cell and B-cell values may differ from one laboratory to another, depending on test technique. Generally, T cells constitute 68% to 75% of total lymphocytes; B cells, 10% to 20%; and null cells, 5% to 20%. The total lymphocyte count ranges from 1,500 to 3,000/µl; the T-cell count varies from 1,400 to 2,700/µl; and the B-cell count ranges from 270 to 640/µl. These counts are higher in children.

Implications of results
An abnormal T-cell or B-cell count suggests but doesn't confirm specific diseases. The B-cell count is elevated in chronic lymphocytic leukemia (thought to be a B-cell malignancy), multiple myeloma, Waldenström's macroglobulinemia, and DiGeorge's syndrome (a congenital T-cell deficiency). The B-cell count decreases in acute lymphocytic leukemia and in certain congenital or acquired immunoglobulin deficiency diseases. In other immunoglobulin deficiency diseases, especially if only one immunoglobulin class is deficient, the B-cell count remains normal.

The T-cell count rises occasionally in infectious mononucleosis; it rises more often in multiple myeloma and acute lymphocytic leukemia. T cells decrease in congenital T-cell deficiency diseases, such as DiGeorge's, Nezelof's, and Wiskott-Aldrich syndromes, and in certain B-cell proliferative disorders, such as chronic lymphocytic leukemia, Waldenström's macroglobulinemia, and acquired immunodeficiency syndrome.

Normal T-cell and B-cell counts don't necessarily ensure a competent immune system. In autoimmune diseases, such as systemic lupus erythematosus and rheumatoid arthritis, T and B cells may be present in normal numbers but may not be functionally competent.

Post-test care

Because many patients with T- and B-cell changes have a compromised immune system, keep the venipuncture site clean and dry. If a hematoma develops at the site, apply warm soaks.

Interfering factors

■ Failure to use the proper collection tube, to mix the sample and anticoagulant adequately, or to send the sample to the laboratory immediately can interfere with accurate testing.
■ T- and B-cell counts can change rapidly with changes in health status, from the effects of stress, or after surgery, chemotherapy, steroid or immunosuppressive therapy, and X-rays.
■ The presence of immunoglobulins, such as autologous antilymphocyte antibodies that sometimes occur in autoimmune disease, can alter test results.

Lymphocyte transformation

Transformation tests evaluate lymphocyte competence without injection of antigens into the patient's skin. These in vitro tests eliminate the risk of adverse effects but can still accurately assess the ability of lymphocytes to proliferate and to recognize and respond to antigens.

The *mitogen assay,* performed using nonspecific plant lectins, evaluates the miotic response of T and B lymphocytes to a foreign antigen. The mitogens phytohemagglutinin (PHA) and concanavalin A (Con-A) stimulate T lymphocytes preferentially, whereas pokeweed stimulates B lymphocytes primarily and T lymphocytes to a lesser extent.

In the mitogen assay, a purified culture of lymphocytes from the patient's blood is incubated with a nonspecific mitogen for 72 hours — the interval during which the greatest effect on deoxyribonucleic acid (DNA) synthesis usually occurs. The culture is then pulse-labeled with tritiated thymidine, which is incorporated in the newly formed DNA of dividing cells.

The uptake of radioactive thymidine can be measured by a liquid scintillation spectrophotometer in counts per minute (cpm), which parallels the rate of mitosis. Lymphocyte responsiveness, or the extent of mitosis, is then reported as a stimulation index, determined by dividing the cpm of the stimulated culture by the cpm of a control culture. The antigen assay uses specific antigens, such as purified protein derivative (PPD), *Candida,* mumps, tetanus toxoid, and streptokinase, to stimulate lymphocyte transformation. After incubation of 4½ to 7 days, transformation is measured by the same method used in the mitogen assay.

The *mixed lymphocyte culture (MLC) assay* tests the response of lymphocytes to histocompatibility antigens determined by the D locus of the sixth chromosome. The MLC assay is useful in matching transplant recipients and donors and in testing immunocompetence. In this assay, lymphocytes from a recipient and potential donor are cultured together for 5 days to test compatibility. Recipient and potential donor lymphocytes (if viable and unaltered) will recognize any genetic differences and undergo transformation, demonstrating incompatibility. In the one-way MLC, one group of lymphocytes is pretreated with radiation or mitomycin C so that it can't divide but can still stimulate the other group of lymphocytes.

Lymphocyte transformation is identified by an increased incorporation of radioactive thymidine labeling and reported as the stimulation index. After the culture is labeled with radioactive thymidine, the MLC stimulation index is determined. Various lymphocyte marker assays can be performed to analyze malignant and normal cell populations. (See *Lymphocyte marker assays,* page 296.)

The neutrophils' ability to engulf and destroy bacteria and foreign particles can also be determined. (See *Neutrophil function tests,* page 297.)

Purpose
■ To assess and monitor genetic and acquired immunodeficiency states
■ To provide histocompatibility typing of both tissue transplant recipients and donors
■ To detect if a patient has been exposed to various pathogens, such as those that cause malaria, hepatitis, and mycoplasmal pneumonia.

Patient preparation
Explain to the patient that this test evaluates lymphocyte function, which is the keystone of the immune system. If appropriate, inform him that the test monitors his response to therapy. For histocompatibility typing, explain that this test helps determine the best match for a transplant.

Advise the patient that he needn't restrict food or fluids. Tell him that this test requires a blood sample, who will perform the venipuncture and when, and that he may feel transient discomfort from the needle puncture and the pressure of the tourniquet. If a radioisotope scan is scheduled, make sure the serum sample for this test is drawn first.

Procedure
Perform a venipuncture. If the patient is an adult, collect the sample in a 7-ml *green-top* (heparinized) tube; for a child, use a 5-ml *green-top* tube.

Precautions
Fill the collection tube completely, and invert it gently several times to mix the sample and anticoagulant. Send the sample to the laboratory immediately.

Reference values
Results depend on the mitogens used. Reference ranges accompany test results.

Implications of results
In the mitogen and antigen assays, a low stimulation index or unresponsiveness indicates a depressed or defective immune system. Serial testing can be performed to monitor the effectiveness of therapy in a patient with an immunodeficiency disease.

In the MLC test, the stimulation index is a measure of compatibility. A high index indicates poor compatibility; conversely, a low stimulation index indicates good compatibility.

Lymphocyte marker assays

A normal immune response requires a balance between the regulatory activities of several interacting cell types — primarily T-helper and T-suppressor cells. By using highly specific monoclonal antibodies, levels of lymphocyte differentiation can be defined, and both normal and malignant cell populations can be analyzed.

Direct and indirect immunofluorescence, microcytotoxicity, and immunoperoxidase immunoassay techniques are used most frequently: these tests use an anticoagulated blood sample combined with monoclonal antibodies that react with specific T- and B-cell markers. The chart below lists some commonly ordered lymphocyte marker assays and their indications.

LYMPHOCYTE MARKER ASSAY	INDICATIONS
CD3	▪ To measure mature T cells in immune dysfunction
CD4	▪ To identify and characterize the proportion of T-helper cells in autoimmune or immunoregulatory disorders ▪ To detect immunodeficiency disorders, such as AIDS ▪ To differentiate T-cell acute lymphoblastic leukemia from T-cell lymphomas and other lymphoproliferative disorders
CD8	▪ To identify and characterize the proportion of T-suppressor cells in autoimmune and immunoregulatory disorders ▪ To characterize lymphoproliferative disorders
CD2	▪ To differentiate lymphoproliferative disorders of T-cell origin, such as T-cell lymphocytic leukemia and lymphoblastic lymphoma, from those of non–T-cell origin
CD20	▪ To differentiate lymphoproliferative disorders of B-cell origin, such as B-cell chronic lymphocytic leukemia, from those of T-cell origin
CD19	▪ To identify B-cell lymphoproliferative disorders, such as B-cell chronic lymphocytic leukemia
CALLA (common acute lymphocytic leukemia antigen) marker, CD10	▪ To identify bone marrow regeneration ▪ To identify non–T-cell acute lymphocytic leukemia
Lymphocyte subset panel (CD3/CD4/ CD8/CD19)	▪ To evaluate immunodeficiencies ▪ To identify immunoregulation associated with autoimmune disorders ▪ To characterize lymphoid malignancies
Lymphocytic leukemia marker panel (CD3/ CD4/CD8/CD19/CD10)	▪ To characterize lymphocytic leukemias as T, B, non-T, or non-B, regardless of the stage of differentiation of the malignant cells

Neutrophil function tests

Normal neutrophils — the body's primary defense against bacterial invasion — engulf and destroy bacteria and foreign particles by a process known as phagocytosis. In patients who suffer from repeated bacterial infections, neutrophil function tests may reveal the inability of neutrophils to kill a target bacteria or to migrate to the bacterial site (chemotaxis).

Neutrophil killing ability can be evaluated by the *nitroblue tetrazolium (NBT) test,* which relies on neutrophil generation of bactericidal enzymes and toxins during killing. This action results in increased oxygen consumption and glucose metabolism, which reduces colorless NBT to blue formazan. The reduced dye is then extracted with pyridine and measured photometrically; the level of reduction indicates phagocytic activity.

Neutrophil killing activity can also be evaluated by noting the neutrophils' *chemiluminescence* — ability to emit light. After a neutrophil phagocytizes a microorganism, oxygen-containing substances form within phagocytic vacuoles. As the cell is stimulated, it emits light in proportion to the amount of oxygen-containing substances that are formed, providing an indirect measurement of phagocytosis.

Chemotaxis can be assessed in vitro by placing bacteria in the lower half of a two-part chamber and phagocytic neutrophils in the upper half. After incubation, migrating cells are counted microscopically and compared to standard values.

A high stimulation index, in response to the relevant pathogen, can also demonstrate exposure to malaria, hepatitis, mycoplasmal pneumonia, periodontal disease, and certain viral infections in patients who no longer have detectable serum antibodies.

Post-test care
Because many of these patients may have a compromised immune system, take special care to keep the venipuncture site clean and dry. If a hematoma develops at the venipuncture site, apply warm soaks.

Interfering factors
■ Pregnancy or the use of oral contraceptives depresses lymphocyte response to PHA and thus causes a low stimulation index.

■ Chemotherapy may affect the accuracy of test results unless pretherapy baseline values are available for comparison.
■ A radioisotope scan performed within 1 week before the test or failure to send the sample to the laboratory immediately can affect the accuracy of test results.

Terminal deoxynucleotidyl transferase

Using indirect immunofluorescence, this test measures levels of terminal deoxynucleotidyl transferase (TdT), an intranuclear enzyme found in certain primitive lymphocytes in the normal thymus and bone marrow. Because TdT acts as a biochemical marker for these lymphocytes, it can help classify the origin of a particular tissue. Thus, the TdT test is useful in differentiating certain types of leukemias and lymphomas marked by primitive cells that can't be identified by histology alone. Measurement of TdT may also help determine the prognosis for these diseases and may provide early diagnosis of a relapse.

Purpose

- To help differentiate acute lymphocytic leukemia (ALL) from acute nonlymphocytic leukemia
- To help differentiate lymphoblastic lymphomas from non-Hodgkin's lymphomas
- To monitor response to therapy.

Patient preparation

Explain to the patient that this test detects an enzyme that can help classify tissue origin and that it may require either a blood or bone marrow sample. If the patient is scheduled for a blood test, tell him to fast for 12 to 14 hours before the test. Tell him the test requires a blood sample, who will perform the venipuncture and when, and that he may experience transient discomfort from the needle puncture and the pressure of the tourniquet.

If the patient is scheduled for a bone marrow aspiration, describe the procedure to him and answer any questions. Inform him that he needn't restrict food or fluids before the test. Tell him who will perform the biopsy and where and that it usually takes only 5 to 10 minutes to perform. Make sure the patient or a responsible family member has signed a consent form.

Check the patient's history for hypersensitivity to the local anesthetic. After checking with the doctor, tell the patient which bone will be the biopsy site. Inform him that he will receive a local anesthetic but will feel pressure on insertion of the biopsy needle and a brief, pulling pain when the marrow is withdrawn. As ordered, administer a mild sedative 1 hour before the test.

Procedure

If a blood test is scheduled, perform a venipuncture and collect the sample in one 10-ml heparinized blood tube and one *lavender-top* EDTA tube. Send the sample to the laboratory immediately.

If you're assisting with a bone marrow aspiration, inject 1 ml of bone marrow into a 7-ml *green-top* tube, and dilute it with 5 ml of sterile saline or submit four air-dried marrow smears. Send the sample to the laboratory immediately.

Precautions

- Contact the laboratory before performing the venipuncture to ensure that they are able to process the sample and to find out how much blood to draw.
- Because patients with leukemia are more susceptible to infection, clean the skin thoroughly before performing the venipuncture.
- Send the sample to the laboratory immediately.

Reference values

TdT is present in less than 2% of marrow cells and is undetectable in normal peripheral blood.

Implications of results

Positive cells are present in over 90% of patients with acute lymphocytic leukemia, in one-third of patients with chronic myelogenous leukemia in blast crisis, and in 5% of patients with nonlymphocytic leukemias. TdT-positive cells are absent in patients with ALL who are in remission.

Post-test care
■ Because patients with leukemia may bleed excessively, apply pressure to the venipuncture site until bleeding stops completely.
■ If a hematoma develops at the venipuncture site, applying warm soaks will ease discomfort.
■ Check the bone marrow aspiration site for bleeding and inflammation, and observe the patient for signs of hemorrhage and infection.

Interfering factors
■ Failure to obtain a representative sample may affect the accuracy of bone marrow aspiration results.
■ Performing a bone marrow aspiration on a child may produce false-positive results because TdT is normally present in bone marrow during proliferation of prelymphocytes.
■ Bone marrow regeneration, idiopathic thrombocytopenic purpura, and neuroblastoma may produce false-positive bone marrow aspiration results because these conditions cause TdT-positive bone marrow.

GENERAL HUMORAL TESTS

Immunoglobulins G, A, and M

Immunoglobulins, proteins that can function as specific antibodies in response to antigen stimulation, are responsible for the humoral aspects of immunity. They are classified into five groups — IgG, IgA, IgM, IgD, and IgE — that are normally present in serum in predictable percentages.

IgG constitutes about 75% of serum immunoglobulins and includes the warm-temperature type; IgA, about 15% of the total; IgM, 5% to 7% and includes cold agglutinins, rheumatoid factor, and ABO blood groups isoagglutinins; IgD and allergen-specific IgE, less than 2%. Deviations from these normal percentages are characteristic in many immune disorders, such as cancer, hepatic disorders, rheumatoid arthritis, and systemic lupus erythematosus.

Immunoelectrophoresis identifies IgG, IgA, and IgM in a serum sample; the level of each is measured by radial immunodiffusion or nephelometry. Some laboratories detect immunoglobulin by indirect immunofluorescence and radioimmunoassay.

In immunoelectrophoresis, serum is placed in a well on a slide containing agar gel, and an electric current is passed through the gel. Immunoglobulins (and other serum proteins) separate according to their different electric charges. Then antiserum is deposited in a shallow trough alongside the separated proteins, from which it diffuses into the agar. Distinct precipitin arcs form wherever the antiserum reacts with specific serum proteins, allowing identification of the immunoglobulins and other proteins.

In radial immunodiffusion, addition of a class-specific antiserum diffuses the serum to form a precipitation ring that is proportional to the immunoglobulin concentration. In nephelometry, photometric measurement of the degree of light scattering caused by the immunoprecipitation reaction provides the relative immunoglobulin concentration.

Purpose
■ To diagnose paraproteinemias, such as multiple myeloma and Waldenström's macroglobulinemia
■ To detect hypogammaglobulinemia and hypergammaglobulinemia, as well

as nonimmunologic diseases that are associated with abnormally high immunoglobulin levels, such as cirrhosis and hepatitis
- To assess the effectiveness of chemotherapy or radiation therapy.

Patient preparation
Explain to the patient that this test measures antibody levels. If appropriate, tell him that the test evaluates the effectiveness of treatment. Instruct him to restrict food and fluids, except for water, for 12 to 14 hours before the test. Tell him the test requires a blood sample, who will perform the venipuncture and when, and that he may experience transient discomfort from the needle puncture and the pressure of the tourniquet.

Check the patient's medication history for drugs that may affect test results. If these medications must be continued, note this on the laboratory request.

Procedure
Perform a venipuncture, and collect the sample in a 7-ml *red-top* tube.

Precautions
Send the sample to the laboratory immediately to prevent deterioration of immunoglobulins.

Reference values
When using nephelometry, serum immunoglobulin levels for adults range as follows:
- *IgG:* 700 to 1,500 mg/dl
- *IgA:* 60 to 400 mg/dl
- *IgM:* 60 to 300 mg/dl.

Implications of results
IgG, IgA, and IgM levels change in various disorders. (See *Immunoglobulin incidence in various disorders.*) In congenital and acquired hypogammaglobulinemias, myelomas, and macroglobulinemia, the findings confirm the diagnosis. In hepatic and autoimmune diseases, leukemias, and lymphomas, such findings are less important but can support the diagnosis based on other tests, such as biopsies and white blood cell differential, and on physical examination findings.

Post-test care
- Advise the patient with abnormally low immunoglobulin levels (especially of IgG or IgM) to protect himself against bacterial infection. When caring for such a patient, watch for signs of infection, such as fever, chills, rash, or skin ulcers.
- Instruct the patient with abnormally high immunoglobulin levels and symptoms of monoclonal gammopathies to report bone pain and tenderness. Such a patient has numerous antibody-producing malignant plasma cells in bone marrow, which hamper production of other blood components. When caring for such a patient, watch for signs of hypercalcemia, renal failure, and spontaneous pathologic fractures.
- If a hematoma develops at the venipuncture site, apply warm soaks.
- As ordered, allow the patient to resume his normal diet and any medications withheld before the test.

Interfering factors
- Radiation therapy or chemotherapy — for example, with methotrexate — may reduce immunoglobulin levels because of the suppressive effects of these treatments on bone marrow.
- Aminophenazone, anticonvulsants, asparaginase, hydralazine, hydantoin derivatives, oral contraceptives, and phenylbutazone may raise all immunoglobulin levels. Methotrexate and severe hypersensitivity to bacille Calmette-Guérin vaccine may lower all levels. Dextrans, phenytoin, and high doses of methylprednisolone lower IgG and IgA levels; dextrans and methylprednisolone lower IgM levels. Methadone

Immunoglobulin incidence in various disorders

The chart below shows the changes in serum levels of immunoglobulins (IgG, IgA, and IgM) that are associated with certain diseases.

DISORDER	IgG	IgA	IgM
Immunoglobulin disorders			
Lymphoid aplasia	D	D	D
Agammaglobulinemia	D	D	D
Type I dysgammaglobulinemia (selective IgG and IgA deficiency)	D	D	N or I
Type II dysgammaglobulinemia (absent IgA and IgM)	N	D	D
IgA globulinemia	N	D	N
Ataxia-telangiectasia	N	D	N
Multiple myeloma, macroglobulinemia, lymphomas			
Heavy chain disease (Franklin's disease)	D	D	D
IgG myeloma	I	D	D
IgA myeloma	D	I	D
Macroglobulinemia	D	D	I
Acute lymphocytic leukemia	N	D	N
Chronic lymphocytic leukemia	D	D	D
Acute myelocytic leukemia	N	N	N
Chronic myelocytic leukemia	N	D	N
Hodgkin's disease	N	N	N
Hepatic disorders			
Hepatitis	I	I	I
Laënnec's cirrhosis	I	I	N
Biliary cirrhosis	N	N	I
Hepatoma	N	N	D
Other disorders			
Rheumatoid arthritis	I	I	I
Systemic lupus erythematosus	I	I	I
Nephrotic syndrome	D	D	N
Trypanosomiasis	N	N	I
Pulmonary tuberculosis	I	N	N

KEY: N = normal; I = increased; D = decreased

raises IgA levels; addiction to narcotics may raise IgM levels.

Serum immune complex

When immune complexes are produced faster than they can be cleared by the lymphoreticular system, immune complex disease may occur — for example, postinfectious syndromes, serum sickness, drug sensitivity, rheumatoid arthritis, and systemic lupus erythematosus (SLE). Immune complexes can develop when a certain ratio of antigen reacts with antibody of isotopes IgG 1, 2, 3, or IgM in tissues. These complexes can fix the first component of complement (C1) and activate the complement cascade. Subsequent complement-mediated activity leads to inflammation and local tissue necrosis. In the blood, soluble circulating immune complexes may also activate complement and eventually cause damage, usually in the renal glomeruli, the aorta, and other large blood vessels.

Histologic examination of tissue obtained by biopsy and the use of fluorescence or peroxidase staining with antibodies specific for immunologic types generally detect immune complexes. However, because tissue biopsies cannot provide information about titers of complexes still in circulation, serum assays, which detect circulating immune complexes indirectly, may be required. Because of the inherent variability of these complexes, several serum test methods may be appropriate, using C1, rheumatoid factor (RF), or cellular substrates, such as Raji cells, as reagents.

Purpose
- To demonstrate circulating immune complexes in serum
- To monitor response to therapy
- To estimate severity of disease.

Patient preparation
Explain to the patient that these tests help evaluate his immune system. If appropriate, inform him that the test will be repeated to monitor his response to therapy. Advise him that he needn't restrict food or fluids before the test. Tell him that this test requires a blood sample, who will perform the venipuncture and when, and that he may experience transient discomfort from the needle puncture and the pressure of the tourniquet.

If the patient is scheduled for a C1q (a component of C1) assay, check his history for recent heparin therapy. Report such therapy to the laboratory because it may affect test results.

Procedure
Perform a venipuncture, and collect the sample in a 7-ml *red-top* tube.

Precautions
Send the sample to the laboratory immediately to prevent deterioration of immune complexes.

Normal findings
Normally, immune complexes are not detectable in serum.

Implications of results
The presence of detectable immune complexes in serum has etiologic importance in many autoimmune diseases, such as SLE and rheumatoid arthritis. However, for a definitive diagnosis, the presence of these complexes must be considered in light of other test results. For example, in SLE, immune complexes are associated with high ti-

ters of antinuclear antibodies and circulating antinative deoxyribonucleic acid antibodies.

Because of their filtering function, renal glomeruli seem most vulnerable to immune complex deposition, although blood vessel walls and choroid plexuses (vascular folds in the ventricles of the brain) can be affected. A renal biopsy to detect immune complexes can provide conclusive evidence for immune complex (Type III) glomerulonephritis, differentiating it from other types of glomerulonephritis.

Post-test care
Because many patients with immune complexes have compromised immune systems, take special care to keep the venipuncture site clean and dry. If a hematoma develops at the site, ease discomfort by applying warm soaks.

Interfering factors
■ Failure to send the serum sample to the laboratory immediately can result in the deterioration of immune complexes and thus alter test results.
■ The presence of cryoglobulins in the patient's serum can affect test results.
■ Inability to standardize RF inhibition tests and platelet aggregation assays can affect the accuracy of test results.

Raji cells

This assay, which is performed to detect the presence of circulating immune complexes, studies the Raji lymphoblastoid cell line. Identifying these cells, which have receptors for IgG complement, is helpful in evaluating autoimmune disease.

Purpose
■ To detect circulating immune complexes
■ To aid the study of autoimmune disease.

Patient preparation
Explain the purpose of the test and tell the patient that it requires a blood sample, who will perform the venipuncture and when, and that he may experience transient discomfort from the needle puncture and the pressure of the tourniquet.

Procedure
Perform a venipuncture, and collect the sample in a *red-top* or *red-marble-top* tube. Send the sample to the laboratory promptly.

Precautions
Handle the specimen gently to avoid hemolysis.

Normal findings
No Raji cells should be present.

Implications of results
The Raji cell assay can detect immune complexes found in viral, microbial, and parasitic infections, metastasis, autoimmune disorders, and drug reactions. This test may also detect immune complexes associated with celiac disease, cirrhosis, Crohn's disease, cryoglobulinemia, dermatitis herpetiformis, sickle cell anemia, and ulcerative colitis.

Post-test care
If a hematoma develops at the venipuncture site, apply warm soaks.

Interfering factors
Hemolysis of the sample can cause misinterpretation of results.

Complement

Complement is a collective term for a system of at least 20 serum proteins designed to destroy foreign cells and to help remove foreign materials. The system may be triggered by contact with antigen-antibody complexes or by clotting factor XIIa. A cascade of events follows, resulting in the formation of a complex that ruptures cell membranes.

Complement components are numerically designated as C1 through C9, with C1 having three subcomponents: C1q, C1r, and C1s. These components constitute 3% to 4% of total serum globulins and play a key role in antibody-mediated immune reactions.

Complement can function as a defense by promoting removal of infectious agents or as a threat by triggering destructive reactions in host tissues. Therefore, complement deficiency can increase susceptibility to infection and can predispose a person to other diseases. Complement assays are thus indicated in patients with known or suspected immunomediated disease or repeatedly abnormal response to infection.

Normally, complement is present in serum in an inactive state until "fixed," or activated, in the classic pathway by binding to an antibody-coated surface. In the classic pathway, a specific antibody identifies and coats an antigen that enters the body. C1 then recognizes and binds with this specific antibody, activating the complement cascade — a series of enzymatic reactions involving all complement components — and producing a coordinated inflammatory response, which usually results in cell lysis or some other damaging outcome.

In the alternate pathway, substances such as polysaccharides, bacterial endotoxins, and aggregated immunoglobulins react with properdin and factors B, D, H, and I, producing an enzyme that activates C3. In turn, C3 activates the remainder of the complement cascade.

In both pathways, specific inhibitors regulate the sequential activation of complement components. The C1 esterase inhibitor, the most commonly studied inhibitor, regulates the classic pathway; the C3b inhibitor can regulate either pathway because C3 is a pivotal component of both.

Although various laboratory methods are used to evaluate and measure total complement and its components, hemolytic assay, laser nephelometry, and radial immunodiffusion are the most common. Hemolytic assay evaluates the lytic capacity of complement and is expressed as hemolytic units per millimeter (the dilution of serum needed to lyse 50% of the erythrocytes in the assay). In this test, sheep red blood cells (RBCs) are mixed with a specific antiserum that lacks complement. Antibody-antigen complexes form, but because complement is absent, lysis can't occur. After the patient's serum sample is serially diluted, equal volumes of these sensitized sheep RBCs are added to each dilution. Complement activity, reported in CH_{50} units, is the dilution capable of lysing 50% of available RBCs.

Laser nephelometry measures C1 esterase inhibitor; immunodiffusion measures C3, C4, C5, properdin, factor B, and C1 inhibitor. In laser nephelometry, the serum sample is mixed with mono-specific antiserum for C1 esterase inhibitor. It reacts to form a precipitate that scatters light from a laser beam directed through it. The amount of light scattered reflects the amount of C1 esterase inhibitor in the serum.

In radial immunodiffusion, an agar slide is impregnated with monospecific antibody for the factor to be studied. Known standards of complement and the patient's serum are placed in appropriate wells punched in the agar. Within 24 hours, a precipitation ring forms around the well where antigen and antibody react; its diameter is proportional to the concentration of complement component.

Although complement assays provide valuable information about the patient's immune system, the results must be considered in light of serum immunoglobulin and autoantibody tests for a definitive diagnosis of immunomediated disease or abnormal response to infection.

Purpose
- To help detect immunomediated disease or genetic complement deficiency
- To monitor effectiveness of therapy.

Patient preparation
Explain to the patient that this test measures a group of proteins that fight infection. Advise him that he needn't restrict food or fluids. Tell him the test requires a blood sample, who will perform the venipuncture and when, and that he may experience transient discomfort from the needle puncture and the pressure of the tourniquet.

If the patient is scheduled for C1q assay, check his history for recent heparin therapy. Report such therapy to the laboratory because it may affect test results.

Procedure
Perform a venipuncture, and collect the sample in a 7-ml *red-top* tube.

Precautions
- Handle the sample gently to prevent hemolysis.
- Send it to the laboratory immediately, because complement is heat labile and deteriorates rapidly.

Reference values
Normal values for complement range as follows:
- *Total complement:* 25 to 110 U

- *C1 esterase inhibitor:* 8 to 24 mg/dl
- *C3:* 70 to 150 mg/dl
- *C4:* 14 to 40 mg/dl.

Implications of results
Complement abnormalities may be genetic or acquired; acquired abnormalities are most common. Depressed total complement levels (which are clinically more significant than elevations) may result from excessive formation of antigen-antibody complexes, insufficient synthesis of complement, inhibitor formation, or increased complement catabolism; decreased levels are characteristic in such conditions as systemic lupus erythematosus (SLE), acute poststreptococcal glomerulonephritis, and acute serum sickness. Low levels may also occur in some patients with advanced cirrhosis of the liver, multiple myeloma, hypogammaglobulinemia, and rapidly rejecting allografts.

Elevated total complement may occur in obstructive jaundice, thyroiditis, acute rheumatic fever, rheumatoid arthritis, acute myocardial infarction, ulcerative colitis, and diabetes.

C1 esterase inhibitor deficiency is characteristic in hereditary angioedema, the most common genetic abnormality associated with complement; C3 deficiency is characteristic in recurrent pyogenic infection; C4 deficiency is characteristic in SLE.

Post-test care
Because many patients with complement defects have a compromised immune system, keep the venipuncture site clean and dry. If a hematoma develops at the venipuncture site, apply warm soaks.

Interfering factors
- Hemolysis caused by rough handling of the sample or failure to send the sample to the laboratory immediately may affect the accuracy of test results.

■ Recent heparin therapy can affect test results.

Radioallergosorbent test

The radioallergosorbent test (RAST) measures IgE antibodies in serum by radioimmunoassay and identifies specific allergens that cause rashes, asthma, hay fever, drug reactions, or other atopic complaints. Before RAST was developed, skin testing was the only reliable method of identifying allergens. RAST is easier to perform and more specific than skin testing; it is also less painful for and less dangerous to the patient. However, careful selection of specific allergens, based on the patient's clinical history, is crucial for effective testing.

Although skin testing is still the preferred means of diagnosing IgE-mediated hypersensitivities, RAST may be more useful when a skin disorder makes accurate reading of skin tests difficult, when a patient requires continual antihistamine therapy, or when skin tests are negative but the patient's clinical history supports IgE-mediated hypersensitivity.

In RAST, a sample of the patient's serum is exposed to a panel of allergen particle complexes (APCs) on cellulose disks. The patient's IgE complexes with those APCs to which it is sensitive. Radio-labeled anti-IgE antibody is then added, and this binds to the IgE-APC complexes. After centrifugation, the amount of radioactivity in the particulate material is directly proportional to the amount of IgE antibodies present. Test results are compared with control values and represent the patient's reactivity to a specific allergen.

Purpose
■ To identify allergens to which the patient has an immediate (IgE-mediated) hypersensitivity
■ To monitor response to therapy.

Patient preparation
Explain to the patient that this test may detect the cause of an allergy or, as appropriate, that it monitors the effectiveness of treatment. Inform him that he needn't restrict food or fluids. Tell him that the test requires a blood sample, who will perform the venipuncture and when, and that he may experience transient discomfort from the needle puncture and the pressure of the tourniquet. If the patient is scheduled for a radioactive scan, make sure the sample is collected before the scan.

Procedure
Perform a venipuncture, and collect the sample in a 7-ml *red-top* tube. Generally, 1 ml of serum is sufficient for five allergen assays. Be sure to note on the laboratory request the specific allergens tested.

Precautions
None.

Normal findings
RAST results are interpreted in relation to a control or reference serum, which differs among laboratories.

Implications of results
Elevated serum IgE levels suggest hypersensitivity to the specific allergen or allergens used.

Post-test care
If a hematoma develops at the venipuncture site, apply warm soaks.

Interfering factors

A radioactive scan within 1 week before sample collection may affect the accuracy of test results.

Ham test

The Ham test (also known as the acidified serum lysis test) is performed to determine the cause of undiagnosed hemolytic anemia, hemoglobinuria, or bone marrow aplasia. It helps establish a diagnosis of paroxysmal nocturnal hemoglobinuria (PNH), a rare hematologic disease.

The Ham test relies on the susceptibility of red blood cells (RBCs) to lysis: RBCs from patients with PNH are unusually susceptible to lysis by complement. To perform the test, washed RBCs are mixed with ABO-compatible normal serum and acid. After incubation at 98.6% F (37% C), the cells are examined for hemolysis. In the presence of acidified human serum, a substantial portion of PNH cells are lysed, whereas normal RBCs show no hemolysis.

Purpose

- To help establish a diagnosis of PNH.

Patient preparation

Explain to the patient that this test helps determine the cause of his anemia or other signs. Advise him that he needn't restrict food or fluids. Tell him that this test requires a blood sample, who will perform the venipuncture and when, and that he may experience transient discomfort from the needle puncture and the pressure of the tourniquet.

Procedure

Because the blood sample must be defibrinated immediately, laboratory personnel will perform the venipuncture and collect the sample.

Precautions

None.

Normal findings

RBCs do not normally undergo hemolysis.

Implications of results

Hemolysis of RBCs indicates PNH.

Post-test care

If a hematoma develops at the venipuncture site, apply warm soaks.

Interfering factors

- Blood containing large numbers of spherocytes may produce false-positive results.
- Blood from patients with congenital dyserythropoietic anemia or HEM-PAS (a rare hematologic disorder) will produce false-positive results.

Human leukocyte antigen

The human leukocyte antigen (HLA) test identifies a group of antigens that are present on the surfaces of all nucleated cells but most easily detected on lymphocytes. These antigens are essential to immunity and determine the degree of histocompatibility between transplant recipients and donors. Numerous antigenic determinants (over 60, for instance, at the HLA-B locus) are present for each site; one set of each antigen is inherited from each parent.

Three types of HLA (HLA-A, HLA-B, and HLA-C) are measured with a lymphocyte microcytotoxicity assay. A lymphocyte sample is mixed with known antisera to these antigens and complement. Lymphocytes that react with a specific antiserum lyse and allow a dye to enter; they may then be detected by phase microscopy.

A fourth type of HLA, HLA-D, is measured by a mixed leukocyte reaction. Leukocytes from the recipient and the donor are combined in culture to determine HLA-D compatibility. If the leukocytes are incompatible, the culture will demonstrate blast formation, DNA synthesis, and proliferation.

A high incidence of specific HLA types has been linked to specific diseases, such as rheumatoid arthritis and multiple sclerosis, but these findings have little diagnostic significance. Thus, HLA testing is best used as an adjunct to diagnosis. It is also useful in genetic counseling and paternity testing.

Purpose

- To provide histocompatibility typing of tissue recipients and donors
- To aid genetic counseling
- To aid paternity testing.

Patient preparation

Explain to the patient that this test detects antigens on white blood cells. Advise him that he needn't restrict food or fluids before the test.

Tell the patient that this test requires a blood sample, who will perform the venipuncture and when, and that he may experience transient discomfort from the needle puncture and the pressure of the tourniquet.

Check the patient's history for recent blood transfusions, and report such transfusions to the doctor. He may want to postpone HLA testing.

Procedure

Perform a venipuncture, and collect the sample in an ACD collection tube.

Precautions

Handle the sample gently to avoid hemolysis.

Normal findings

In HLA-A, HLA-B, and HLA-C testing, lymphocytes that react with the test antiserum undergo lysis; they're detected by phase microscopy. In HLA-D testing, leukocyte incompatibility is marked by blast formation, DNA synthesis, and proliferation.

Implications of results

Incompatible HLA-A, HLA-B, HLA-C, or HLA-D groups may cause unsuccessful tissue transplantation.

Many diseases have a strong association with certain types of HLAs. For example, HLA-DR5 is associated with Hashimoto's thyroiditis. HLA-B8 and HLA-Dw3 are associated with Graves' disease, whereas HLA-B8 alone is associated with chronic autoimmune hepatitis, celiac disease, and myasthenia gravis. Dw3 alone is associated with Addison's disease, Sjögren's syndrome, dermatitis herpetiformis, and systemic lupus erythematosus.

In paternity testing, a putative father who presents a phenotype (two haplotypes: one from the father and one from the mother) with no haplotype or antigen pair identical to one of the child's is excluded as the father. A putative father with one haplotype identical to one of the child's *may* be the father; the probability varies with the incidence of the haplotype in the population.

Post-test care

If a hematoma develops at the venipuncture site, ease discomfort by applying warm soaks.

Interfering factors

- Hemolysis caused by rough handling of the sample may affect the accuracy of test results.

- HLA from blood transfused within 72 hours before collection of a blood sample may affect the accuracy of test results.

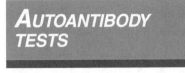

Antinuclear antibodies

In conditions such as systemic lupus erythematosus (SLE), scleroderma, and certain infections, the body's immune system may perceive portions of its own cell nuclei as foreign and may produce antinuclear antibodies (ANA). Specific types of ANA include antibodies to deoxyribonucleic acid (DNA), nucleoprotein, histones, nuclear ribonucleoprotein, and other nuclear constituents. Although ANA are harmless in themselves because they don't penetrate living cells, they sometimes form antigen-antibody complexes that cause damage (as in SLE). Because of multiorgan involvement, test results are not diagnostic and can only partially confirm clinical evidence.

This test measures the relative concentration of ANA in a serum sample through indirect immunofluorescence. Serial dilutions of serum are mixed with either Hep-2 or mouse kidney substrate. If the serum contains ANA, it forms antigen-antibody complexes with the substrate. After the preparation is mixed with fluorescein-labeled antihuman serum, it's examined under an ultraviolet microscope. If ANA are present, the complex fluoresces. Titer is taken as the greatest dilution that shows the reaction.

About 99% of patients with SLE exhibit ANA; a large percentage of these patients do so at high titers. (See *ANA incidence in various disorders,* page 310.) Although this test is not specific for SLE, it is a useful screening tool. Failure to detect ANA essentially rules out active SLE.

Purpose
- To screen for SLE
- To monitor the effectiveness of immunosuppressive therapy for SLE.

Patient preparation
Explain that this test evaluates the immune system and that further testing is usually required for diagnosis. If appropriate, inform the patient that the test will be repeated to monitor his response to therapy. Advise him that he needn't restrict food or fluids. Tell him that this test requires a blood sample, who will perform the venipuncture and when, and that he may experience discomfort from the needle puncture and the pressure of the tourniquet.

Check the patient's history for drugs that may affect test results, such as isoniazid, hydralazine, and procainamide. Note such drug use on the laboratory request.

Procedure
Perform a venipuncture, and collect the sample in a 7-ml *red-top* tube.

Precautions
None.

Reference values
Using Hep-2 cells, the test for ANA is negative at a titer of 1:40 or below. If mouse kidney substrate is being used, the test is negative at a titer of less than 1:20.

Implications of results
Although this test is a sensitive indicator of ANA, it is not specific for SLE. Low titers may occur in patients with viral diseases, chronic hepatic disease,

ANA incidence in various disorders

The chart below indicates the percentage of patients with certain disorders whose serum contains antinuclear antibodies (ANA). About 40% of elderly people and 5% of the general population also show ANA.

DISORDER	POSITIVE A.N.A.
Systemic lupus erythematosus (SLE)	95% to 100%
Lupoid hepatitis	95% to 100%
Felty's syndrome	95% to 100%
Progressive systemic sclerosis (scleroderma)	75% to 80%
Drug-associated SLE-like syndrome: (hydralazine, procainamide, isoniazid)	Approximately 50%
Sjögren's syndrome	40% to 75%
Rheumatoid arthritis	25% to 60%
Healthy family member of SLE patient	Approximately 25%
Chronic discoid lupus erythematosus	15% to 50%
Juvenile arthritis	15% to 30%
Polyarteritis nodosa	15% to 25%
Miscellaneous diseases	10% to 50%
Dermatomyositis, polymyositis	10% to 30%
Rheumatic fever	Approximately 5%

collagen vascular disease, or autoimmune diseases as well as in some healthy adults; incidence increases with age. The higher the titer, the more specific the test is for SLE (titer often exceeds 1:256).

The pattern of nuclear fluorescence helps identify the type of immune disease present. A peripheral pattern is almost exclusively associated with SLE because it indicates the presence of anti-DNA antibodies; anti-DNA antibodies are sometimes measured by radioimmunoassay if ANA titers are high or a peripheral pattern is observed. A homogeneous, or diffuse, pattern is also associated with SLE as well as with related connective tissue disorders; a nucleolar pattern, with scleroderma; and a speckled, irregular pattern, with infectious mononucleosis and mixed connective tissue disorders (such as SLE and scleroderma).

A single serum sample, especially one collected from a patient with collagen vascular disease, may contain antibodies to several parts of the cell's nucleus. In addition, as serum dilution increases, the fluorescent pattern may change, because different antibodies are reactive at different titers.

Post-test care

■ Because a patient with an autoimmune disease has a compromised immune system, observe the venipuncture site for signs of infection, and report any changes to the doctor immediately. Keep a clean, dry bandage over the site for at least 24 hours.
■ If a hematoma develops at the venipuncture site, apply warm soaks.

Interfering factors

Certain drugs — most commonly isoniazid, hydralazine, and procainamide — can produce a syndrome resembling SLE; other such drugs include para-aminosalicylic acid, chlorpromazine, clofibrate, phenytoin, griseofulvin, ethosuximide, gold salts, methyldopa, oral contraceptives, penicillin, propylthiouracil, phenylbutazone, methysergide, streptomycin, sulfonamides, tetracyclines, mephenytoin, quinidine, primidone, reserpine, and trimethadione.

Anti-deoxyribonucleic acid antibodies

This test measures antinative deoxyribonucleic acid (DNA) antibody levels in a serum sample, using radioimmunoassay or a less sensitive technique, such as agglutination, complement fixation, or immunoelectrophoresis. For radioimmunoassay, the sample is mixed with radio-labeled native DNA. If antinative DNA antibodies are in the serum sample, they combine with the native DNA, forming complexes that are too large to pass through a membrane filter. If such antibodies are not present, the radiolabeled DNA is able to pass through the filter. The DNA that does not pass through the membrane filter is then counted.

In autoimmune diseases such as systemic lupus erythematosus (SLE), native DNA is thought to be the antigen that complexes with antibody and complement, causing local tissue damage where these complexes are deposited. Serum antinative DNA levels are directly related to the extent of renal or vascular damage caused by the disease.

Two different types of anti-DNA antibodies are present in patients with SLE: anti-single-stranded (denatured) DNA and anti-double-stranded (native) DNA. Antibodies to native DNA, however, are more specific for SLE. Determination of these antibodies, with serum complement, is also useful in monitoring immunosuppressive therapy.

Purpose

- To confirm SLE after a positive antinuclear antibody test
- To monitor response to therapy.

Patient preparation

Explain to the patient that this test detects certain antibodies and that test results help determine the diagnosis and appropriate therapy. Or, when indicated, tell him that the test assesses the effectiveness of present treatment. Advise him that he needn't restrict food or fluids. Tell him the test requires a blood sample, who will perform the venipuncture and when, and that he may experience transient discomfort from the needle puncture and the pressure of the tourniquet.

If the patient is scheduled for a radionuclide scan, make sure the sample is collected before the scan.

Procedure

Perform a venipuncture and collect the sample in a 7-ml *red-top* tube. (Some laboratories may specify a *lavender-top* or *gray-top* tube.)

Precautions

Handle the sample gently.

Reference values

Normal values are less than 7 IU of native DNA bound per milliliter of serum.

Implications of results

Elevated antinative DNA levels may indicate SLE. A value of 1 to 2.5 mg/ml suggests a remission phase of SLE or the presence of other autoimmune disorders. A value of 10 to 15 mg/ml indicates active SLE. Depressed levels following immunosuppressive therapy demonstrate effective treatment of SLE.

Post-test care

If a hematoma develops at the venipuncture site, ease discomfort by applying warm soaks.

Interfering factors

■ Hemolysis caused by rough handling of the sample may alter test results.

■ A radioactive scan performed within 1 week of collecting the sample may alter test results.

Extractable nuclear antigen antibodies

Extractable nuclear antigen (ENA) is a complex of at least two and possibly three antigens. One of these — ribonucleoprotein (RNP) — is susceptible to degradation by ribonuclease. The second — Smith(Sm) antigen — is an acidic nuclear protein that resists ribonuclease degradation. The third antigen sometimes included in this group — Sjögren's (SS-B) antigen — forms a precipitate when antibody is present. Antibodies to these antigens are associated with certain autoimmune disorders.

Tests to determine ENA antibodies (also known as ribonucleoprotein antibodies, anti-Smith antibodies, and Sjögren's antibodies) help differentiate autoimmune disorders with similar signs and symptoms. The *RNP antibody test* detects RNP autoantibodies, which are associated with systemic lupus erythematosus (SLE), progressive systemic sclerosis, and other rheumatic disorders. This test aids in the differential diagnosis of systemic rheumatic disease and is a useful follow-up test for collagen vascular autoimmune disease.

The *anti-Sm antibody test* detects Sm autoantibodies, which are a specific marker for SLE; positive results thus strongly suggest a diagnosis of SLE. This test, too, helps monitor collagen vascular autoimmune disease. The *Sjögren's antibody test* detects the SS-B autoantibodies produced in Sjögren's syndrome, an immunologic abnormality sometimes associated with rheumatic arthritis and SLE. However, this test does not confirm a diagnosis of Sjögren's syndrome.

To perform these tests, sheep red blood cells are sensitized with ENA extracted from rabbit thymus and then incubated with serum samples; ENA antibodies present in the serum will agglutinate the cells. If the serum sample shows agglutination, differential double immunoassays are performed to determine which of the antibodies are present. Anti-ENA tests are most useful in tandem with anti-DNA, serum complement, and antinuclear antibody tests.

Purpose

■ To aid differential diagnosis of autoimmune disease

■ To distinguish between anti-RNP and anti-Sm antibodies

■ To screen for anti-RNP antibodies (common in mixed connective tissue disease)

■ To screen for anti-Sm antibodies (common in SLE)

■ To support diagnosis of collagen vascular autoimmune diseases

■ To monitor response to therapy.

Patient preparation

Explain to the patient that this test detects certain antibodies and that test results help determine diagnosis and treatment. Or, when indicated, explain that the test assesses the effectiveness of treatment. Advise him that he needn't restrict food or fluids. Tell him the test requires a blood sample, who will perform the venipuncture and when, and that he may experience transient discomfort from the needle puncture and the pressure of the tourniquet.

Procedure
Perform a venipuncture, and collect the sample in a 7-ml *red-top* tube.

Precautions
Send the sample to the laboratory immediately.

Normal findings
Serum should be negative for anti-RNP, anti-Sm, and SS-B antibodies.

Implications of results
The presence of anti-Sm antibodies strongly suggests a diagnosis of SLE. A high level of anti-RNP antibodies with a low titer of anti-Sm antibodies suggests mixed connective tissue disease. Although SS-B antibodies are associated with primary Sjögren's disease, their presence does not confirm a diagnosis of this disorder; however, a positive test for SS-B antibodies mandates further testing.

Post-test care
■ Because a patient with an autoimmune disease has a compromised immune system, check the venipuncture site for infection, and report any change promptly. Keep a clean, dry bandage over the site for at least 24 hours.
■ If a hematoma develops at the venipuncture site, ease discomfort by applying warm soaks.

Interfering factors
Failure to send the sample to the laboratory immediately may affect the accuracy of test results.

Antimitochondrial antibodies

Usually performed with the test for anti–smooth-muscle antibodies, this test detects antimitochondrial antibodies in serum by indirect immunofluorescence. Antimitochondrial antibodies react with mitochondria in the renal tubules, gastric mucosa, and other organs in which cells expend large amounts of energy.

These autoantibodies are present in several hepatic diseases, although their etiology is unknown and there's no evidence they cause hepatic damage. They're most commonly associated with primary biliary cirrhosis and sometimes with chronic active hepatitis and drug-induced jaundice. Antimitochondrial antibodies are also associated with autoimmune diseases, such as systemic lupus erythematosus, rheumatoid arthritis, pernicious anemia, and idiopathic Addison's disease.

Purpose
■ To aid diagnosis of primary biliary cirrhosis
■ To distinguish between extrahepatic jaundice and biliary cirrhosis.

Patient preparation
Explain that this test evaluates liver function. Advise the patient that he need not restrict food or fluids. Tell him that this test requires a blood sample, who will perform the venipuncture and when, and that he may feel some dis-

Incidence of serum antibodies in various disorders

The chart below shows the percentage of patients with certain disorders who have antimitochondrial or anti–smooth-muscle antibodies in the serum. The presence of these antibodies requires further testing to confirm the diagnosis. (Up to 1% of healthy people also show antimitochondrial antibodies.)

DISORDER	ANTIMITOCHONDRIAL ANTIBODIES	ANTI–SMOOTH-MUSCLE ANTIBODIES
Primary biliary cirrhosis	75% to 95%	0% to 50%[a]
Chronic active hepatitis	0% to 30%	50% to 80%
Extrahepatic biliary obstruction	0% to 5%	0%
Cryptogenic cirrhosis	0% to 25%	0% to 1%
Viral (infectious) hepatitis	0%	1% to 2%[b]
Drug-induced jaundice	50% to 80%	
Intrinsic asthma		20%
Rheumatoid arthritis and other collagen diseases	1% to 2%	
Systemic lupus erythematosus	3% to 5%[c]	0%

[a] In chronic disease values fall at upper end of range.

[b] Much higher incidence occurs with hepatic damage.

[c] Much higher incidence occurs with renal involvement.

comfort from the needle puncture and the pressure of the tourniquet.

Check the patient's medication history for oxyphenisatin use, and report such use to the laboratory because this drug may produce antimitochondrial antibodies.

Procedure

Perform a venipuncture, and collect the sample in a 7-ml *red-top* tube.

Precautions

None.

Normal findings

Serum is negative for antimitochondrial antibodies at a titer below 20.

Implications of results

Although antimitochondrial antibodies appear in 75% to 95% of patients with primary biliary cirrhosis, this test alone does not confirm the diagnosis. Further tests, such as serum alkaline phosphatase, serum bilirubin, alanine aminotransferase, aspartate aminotransferase, and possibly liver biopsy or cholangiography, may also be necessary.

Antimitochondrial autoantibodies also appear in some patients with chronic active hepatitis, drug-induced jaundice, or cryptogenic cirrhosis. (See *Incidence of serum antibodies in various disorders.*) However, they rarely appear in patients with extrahepatic biliary obstruction, and a positive test helps rule out this condition.

Post-test care
Because patients with hepatic disease may bleed excessively, apply pressure to the venipuncture site until bleeding stops. If a hematoma develops at the venipuncture site, apply warm soaks.

Interfering factors
■ Confusion of antimitochondrial antibodies with heterophil antibodies, cardiolipin antibodies to syphilis, ribosomal antibodies, or microsomal hepatic or renal autoantibodies may affect the accuracy of test results.
■ Oxyphenisatin can produce antimitochondrial antibodies in patients taking this drug.

Anti–smooth-muscle antibodies

Using indirect immunofluorescence, this test measures the relative concentration of anti–smooth-muscle antibodies in serum and is usually performed with the test for antimitochondrial antibodies. The serum sample is exposed to a thin section of smooth muscle and incubated; then a fluorescent-labeled antiglobulin is added. This antiglobulin binds only to antibodies that have complexed with smooth muscle and appears fluorescent when viewed through the microscope under ultraviolet light.

Anti–smooth-muscle antibodies appear in several hepatic diseases, especially chronic active hepatitis and, less often, primary biliary cirrhosis. Although these antibodies are most commonly associated with hepatic diseases, their etiology is unknown, and there's no evidence that they cause hepatic damage.

Purpose
■ To aid diagnosis of chronic active hepatitis and primary biliary cirrhosis.

Patient preparation
Explain to the patient that this test helps evaluate liver function. Inform him that he needn't restrict food or fluids. Tell him the test requires a blood sample, who will perform the venipuncture and when, and that he may experience transient discomfort from the needle puncture and the pressure of the tourniquet.

Procedure
Perform a venipuncture, and collect the sample in a 7-ml *red-top* tube.

Precautions
None.

Reference values
Normal titer of anti–smooth-muscle antibodies is less than 1:20.

Implications of results
The test for anti–smooth-muscle antibodies is not very specific; these antibodies appear in about 66% of patients with chronic active hepatitis and 30% to 40% of patients with primary biliary cirrhosis. Anti–smooth-muscle antibodies may also be present in patients with infectious mononucleosis, acute viral hepatitis, malignant tumor of the liver, and intrinsic asthma.

Post-test care
Because patients with hepatic disease may bleed excessively, apply pressure to the venipuncture site until bleeding stops. If a hematoma develops at the site, apply warm soaks.

Interfering factors
None.

Incidence of thyroid autoantibodies in various disorders

The chart below indicates the percentage of people with thyroid disorders who have antithyroglobulin or antimicrosomal antibodies in the serum.

DISORDER	ANTITHYROGLOBULIN ANTIBODIES	ANTIMICROSOMAL ANTIBODIES
Hashimoto's disease	60% to 95%	70% to 90%
Idiopathic myxedema	75%	65%
Graves' disease	30% to 40%	50% to 85%
Adenomatous goiter	20% to 30%	20%
Thyroid carcinoma	40%	15%
Pernicious anemia	25%	10%

Antithyroid antibodies

In autoimmune disorders such as Hashimoto's thyroiditis and Graves' disease (hyperthyroidism), thyroglobulin, the major colloidal storage compound, is released into the blood. Because thyroxine usually separates from thyroglobulin before its release into the blood, thyroglobulin doesn't normally enter the circulation. When it does, antithyroglobulin antibodies are formed to attack this foreign substance; the ensuing autoimmune response damages the thyroid gland. The serum of a patient whose autoimmune system produces antithyroglobulin antibodies usually contains antimicrosomal antibodies, which react with the microsomes of the thyroid epithelial cells.

The tanned red cell hemagglutination test detects antithyroglobulin and antimicrosomal antibodies. In this assay, sheep red blood cells that have been pretreated with tannic acid and coated with thyroglobulin or microsomal fragments are mixed with a serum sample. The mixture agglutinates in the presence of these specific antibodies, and serial dilutions can quantify the antibody concentration. Another laboratory technique, indirect immunofluorescence, can detect antimicrosomal antibodies.

Purpose
■ To detect circulating antithyroglobulin antibodies when clinical evidence indicates Hashimoto's thyroiditis, Graves' disease, or another thyroid disorder.

Patient preparation
Explain to the patient that this test evaluates thyroid function. Advise him that he needn't restrict food or fluids. Tell him that this test requires a blood sample, who will perform the venipuncture and when, and that he may experience transient discomfort from the needle puncture and the pressure of the tourniquet.

Procedure
Perform a venipuncture, and collect the sample in a 7-ml *red-top* tube.

Precautions
None.

Reference values

The normal titer is less than 1:100 for both antithyroglobulin and antimicrosomal antibodies. (Low levels of these antibodies are normal in 10% of the general population and in 20% or more of people age 70 or older.)

Implications of results

The presence of antithyroglobulin or antimicrosomal antibodies in serum can indicate subclinical autoimmune thyroid disease, Graves' disease, or idiopathic myxedema. High titers (which may be in the millions) strongly suggest Hashimoto's thyroiditis. (See *Incidence of thyroid autoantibodies in various disorders.*) These antibodies may also occur in patients with other autoimmune disorders, such as system lupus erythematosus, rheumatoid arthritis, or autoimmune hemolytic anemia.

Post-test care

If a hematoma develops at the venipuncture site, apply warm soaks.

Interfering factors

None.

Serum thyroid-stimulating immunoglobulin

Thyroid-stimulating immunoglobulin (TSI), formerly called long-acting thyroid stimulator, appears in the blood of most patients with Graves' disease. This autoantibody reacts with the cell-surface receptors that usually combine with thyroid-stimulating hormone (TSH). TSI reacts with these receptors, activates intracellular enzymes, and promotes epithelial cell activity that functions outside the normal feedback regulation mechanism for TSH. It stimulates the thyroid gland to produce and excrete excessive amounts of thyroid hormones.

About 50% to 90% of people with thyrotoxicosis have elevated TSI levels. Positive test results strongly suggest Graves' disease but don't always correlate with overt signs of hyperthyroidism.

Purpose

- To aid evaluation of suspected thyroid disease
- To aid diagnosis of suspected thyrotoxicosis, especially in patients with exophthalmos
- To monitor treatment of thyrotoxicosis.

Patient preparation

Explain to the patient that this test evaluates thyroid function. Inform him that it requires a blood sample, who will perform the venipuncture and when, and that he may experience transient discomfort from the needle puncture and the pressure of the tourniquet.

Procedure

Perform a venipuncture, and collect the sample in a 5-ml *red-top* tube.

Precautions

- Handle the sample gently to prevent hemolysis.
- Send it to the laboratory promptly.
- Note on the laboratory request if the patient had a radioactive iodine scan within 48 hours of the test.

Normal findings

TSI doesn't normally appear in serum. However, it may be present in 5% of people without hyperthyroidism or exophthalmos.

Implications of results

Increased TSI levels are associated with exophthalmos, Grave's disease (thyrotoxicosis), and recurrence of hyperthyroidism.

Post-test care
If a hematoma develops at the venipuncture site, apply warm soaks to ease discomfort.

Interfering factors
■ Administration of radioactive iodine within 48 hours of the test may affect the accuracy of test results.
■ Hemolysis caused by excessive agitation of the sample may alter test results.

Lupus erythematosus cell preparation

Lupus erythematosus (LE) cell preparation is an in vitro procedure used in diagnosing systemic lupus erythematosus (SLE). (See *All about SLE.*) Although this test is less sensitive and reliable than either the antinuclear antibody (ANA) or the antideoxyribonucleic acid (DNA) antibody test, it's often used because it requires minimal equipment and reagents.

In this test, a blood sample is mixed with laboratory-treated nucleoprotein (the antigen). If the sample contains ANA, the ANA reacts with the nucleoprotein, causing swelling and rupture. Phagocytes from the serum then engulf the extruded nuclei, forming LE cells, which are then detected by microscopic examination of the sample.

Purpose
■ To aid diagnosis of SLE
■ To monitor treatment of SLE. (About 60% of successfully treated patients fail to show LE cells after 4 to 6 weeks of therapy.)

Patient preparation
Explain to the patient that this test helps detect antibodies to his own tissue. (See *Understanding autoantibodies in autoimmune disease,* pages 320 and 321.) If appropriate, inform him that the test will be repeated to monitor his response to therapy. Advise him that he needn't restrict food or fluids. Tell him the test requires a blood sample, who will perform the venipuncture and when, and that he may experience transient discomfort from the needle puncture and the pressure of the tourniquet.

Check the patient's medication history for drugs that may affect test results, such as isoniazid, hydralazine, and procainamide. If such drugs must be continued, be sure to note this on the laboratory request.

Procedure
Perform a venipuncture, and collect the sample in a 7-ml *red-top* tube.

Precautions
Handle the sample gently to prevent hemolysis.

Normal findings
No LE cells are normally present in serum.

Implications of results
The presence of at least two LE cells may indicate SLE. Although these cells occur primarily in SLE, they may also appear in chronic active hepatitis, rheumatoid arthritis, scleroderma, and certain drug reactions. Also, up to 25% of patients with SLE demonstrate no LE cells.

Apart from supportive clinical signs, a definitive diagnosis of SLE may require a confirming ANA or anti-DNA test. The ANA test detects autoantibodies in the serum of many SLE patients with negative LE cell tests. Anti-DNA antibodies appear in two-thirds of all SLE

All about SLE

Who gets it?	Systemic lupus erythematosus (SLE) is primarily a disease of young women, affecting five times as many women as men. In the United States, blacks and Hispanics have a higher incidence than whites.
What is it?	SLE is a chronic inflammatory disease of the connective tissue that produces biochemical and structural changes in the skin, joints, and muscles, usually with multiple organ involvement. It may eventually cause death from failure of vital organs, especially the kidneys. However, the disease is not always fatal; it may be controlled in some patients. Four or more of the following criteria help support the diagnosis: ■ facial erythema (butterfly rash) ■ alopecia ■ photosensitivity ■ Raynaud's phenomenon ■ pleuritis or pericarditis ■ hemolytic anemia, leukopenia, or thrombocytopenia ■ positive antinuclear antibody or LE cell test ■ chronic false-positive serologic test for syphilis ■ profuse proteinuria ■ cellular casts ■ discoid lupus erythematosus ■ nondeforming arthritis ■ oral or nasopharyngeal ulcerations ■ psychosis or seizures.
When does it first develop?	SLE typically first develops between ages 15 and 40, but it can occur at any age.
Why does it occur?	The cause is unknown. SLE is believed to stem from an autoimmune malfunction triggered by a viral, drug, environmental, or genetic stimulus.

patients but are rare in other conditions; thus, the presence of these antibodies is strong evidence of SLE.

Post-test care

■ Because many patients with SLE have compromised immune systems, keep a clean, dry bandage over the venipuncture site for at least 24 hours and check for infection.
■ If a hematoma develops at the venipuncture site, apply warm soaks.
■ If test results indicate SLE, tell the patient further tests may be required to monitor treatment.

Interfering factors

■ Hemolysis caused by rough handling of the sample may affect the accuracy of test results.
■ Certain drugs — most commonly isoniazid, hydralazine, and procainamide — can produce a syndrome resembling SLE. Other such drugs include para-aminosalicylic acid, chlorpromazine, clofibrate, phenytoin, griseofulvin, ethosuximide, gold salts, methyldopa, oral contraceptives, penicillin, propylthiouracil, phenylbutazone, methysergide, streptomycin, sulfonamides, tetracyclines, mephenytoin, quinidine, primidone, reserpine, and trimethadione.

Understanding autoantibodies in autoimmune disease

When the immune system produces autoantibodies against the antigenic determinants on and in cells, two types of autoimmune disease can result. *Organ-specific diseases,* such as pernicious anemia, occur when the targeted antigenic determinants are specific to an organ or tissue, or to certain cells or cell types. Lymphocytes invade the target organ, tissue, or cell and destroy targeted cells. *Non–organ-specific diseases,* such as myasthenia gravis, occur when the targeted antigenic determinants are shared with other cells (self-antigens). This causes deposition of immune complexes (Type III hypersensitivity) with subsequent lesions anywhere in the body.

Various diagnostic techniques are used to detect antibodies in autoimmune disease, including radioimmunoassay, hemagglutination, complement fixation, and immunofluorescence. The chart below lists common test methods and findings in various autoimmune diseases.

DISEASE	AFFECTED AREA	ANTIGEN	ANTIBODY	DIAGNOSTIC TECHNIQUE
Hashimoto's thyroiditis	Thyroid gland	Thyroglobulin, second colloid antigen, cytoplasmic microsomes, cell-surface antigens	Antibodies to thyroglobulin and to microsomal antigens	Radioimmunoassay, hemagglutination, complement fixation, immunofluorescence
Pernicious anemia	Hematopoietic system	Intrinsic factor	Antibodies to gastric parietal cells and vitamin B_{12} binding site of intrinsic factor	Immunofluorescence, radioimmunoassay
Pemphigus vulgaris	Skin	Desmosomes between prickle cells in the epidermis	Antibodies to intercellular substances of the skin and mucous membranes	Immunofluorescence
Myasthenia gravis	Neuromuscular system	Acetylcholine receptors of skeletal and heart muscle	Anti-acetylcholine antibodies	Immunoprecipitation radioimmunoassay
Autoimmune hemolytic anemia	Hematopoietic system	Red blood cells (RBCs)	Anti-RBC antibodies	Direct and indirect Coombs' test
Primary biliary cirrhosis	Small bile ducts in liver	Mitochondria	Antimitochondrial antibodies	Immunofluorescence of mitochondrial-rich cells (kidney biopsy)

	Understanding autoantibodies in autoimmune disease (continued)			
DISEASE	**AFFECTED AREA**	**ANTIGEN**	**ANTIBODY**	**DIAGNOSTIC TECHNIQUE**
Rheumatoid arthritis	Joints, blood vessels, skin, muscles, lymph nodes	Immuno-globulin G (IgG)	Antigamma-globulin anti-bodies	Sheep RBC agglutination, latex immuno-globulin agglu-tination, radio-immunoassay, immunofluo-rescence, immunodiffusion
Goodpas-ture's syndrome	Lungs and kidneys	Glomerular and lung basement membranes	Anti-basement membrane antibodies	Immunofluo-rescence of kidney biopsy sample, radio-immunoassay
Systemic lupus erythe-matosus	Skin, joints, muscles, lungs, heart, kidneys, brain, eyes	Deoxyribonu-cleic acid (DNA), nucleo-protein, blood cells, clotting factors, IgG, Wasserman antigen	Anti-nuclear antibodies, anti-DNA antibodies, anti-ds-DNA antibodies, anti-SS-DNA antibodies, anti-ribonu-cleoprotein antibodies, antigamma-globulin antibodies, anti-RBC antibodies, antilymphocyte antibodies, anti-platelet antibodies, antineuronal cell antibodies, anti-Sm antibodies	Counterelectro-phoresis, he-magglutination, radioimmuno-assay, immuno-fluorescence, Coombs' test

Cardiolipin antibodies

This test measures serum concentrations of IgG or IgM antibodies in relation to the phospholipid cardiolipin. These antibodies appear in some lupus erythematosus (LE) patients whose serum also contains a coagulation inhibitor (lupus anticoagulant). They also appear in some patients who do not fulfill all the diagnostic criteria for LE but who experience recurrent episodes of spontaneous thrombosis, fetal loss, or thrombocytopenia. Cardiolipin antibodies are measured by enzyme-linked immunosorbent assay.

Purpose

■ To aid diagnosis of cardiolipin antibody syndrome in patients with or without LE who experience recurrent episodes of spontaneous thrombosis, thrombocytopenia, or fetal loss.

Patient preparation

Explain the purpose of the test. Tell the patient that he needn't restrict food or fluids before the test. Inform him that the test requires a blood sample, who will perform the venipuncture and when, and that he may experience transient discomfort from the needle puncture and the pressure of the tourniquet.

Procedure

Perform a venipuncture, and collect the sample in a 5-ml *red-top* tube.

Precautions

Handle the sample gently to prevent hemolysis, and send it to the laboratory immediately.

Reference values

Cardiolipin antibody results are reported as dilution titers obtained by making 1:2 serial dilutions of serum. The highest dilution is reported. A 1:4 titer is a borderline result. A lower titer (1:2) is negative; a higher titer (1:8, 1:16), positive.

Implications of results

A positive result along with a history of recurrent spontaneous thrombosis, thrombocytopenia, or fetal loss suggests cardiolipin antibody syndrome. Treatment may involve anticoagulant or platelet-inhibitor therapy.

Post-test care

If a hematoma develops, apply warm soaks to ease discomfort.

Interfering factors

Hemolysis will affect results.

Rheumatoid factor

The rheumatoid factor (RF) test is the most useful immunologic test for confirming rheumatoid arthritis (RA). In this disease, "renegade" IgG antibodies, produced by lymphocytes in the synovial joints, react with other IgG or IgM molecules to produce immune complexes, complement activation, and tissue destruction. How IgG molecules become antigenic is still unknown, but they may be altered by aggregating with viruses or other antigens. These immune complexes can migrate from the synovial fluid to other areas of the body, causing vasculitis, subcutaneous nodules, or lymphadenopathy. The IgG or IgM molecules that react with altered IgG are called rheumatoid factors.

The sheep cell agglutination test and the latex fixation test can detect RF. In the sheep cell test, rabbit IgG absorbed onto sheep red blood cells (RBCs) is mixed with the patient's serum in serial dilutions; in the latex fixation test, human IgG absorbed onto latex particles is mixed with the patient's serum. Visible agglutination indicates the presence of RF. The last tube dilution to show visible agglutination is used as the titer. The sheep cell agglutination test is the better diagnostic method for confirming RA; the latex fixation test is the better screening method.

Purpose
- To confirm RA, especially when clinical diagnosis is doubtful.

Patient preparation
Explain to the patient that this test helps confirm RA. Advise him that he needn't restrict food or fluids before the test. Tell him that the test requires a blood sample, who will perform the venipuncture and when, and that he may experience transient discomfort from the needle puncture and the pressure of the tourniquet.

Procedure
Perform a venipuncture, and collect the sample in a 7-ml *red-top* tube.

Precautions
None.

Reference values
Normal RF titer is less than 1:20; normal rheumatoid screening test is nonreactive.

Implications of results
Positive RF titers are found in 80% of patients with RA. Titers above 1:80 strongly suggest a diagnosis of RA; titers between 1:20 and 1:80 are difficult to interpret because they occur in many other diseases, such as systemic lupus erythematosus, scleroderma, polymyositis, tuberculosis, infectious mononucleosis, leprosy, syphilis, sarcoidosis, chronic hepatic disease, subacute bacterial endocarditis, and chronic pulmonary interstitial fibrosis. In addition, 5% of the general population, including as many as 25% of the elderly, have positive RF titers.

Conversely, a negative RF titer doesn't rule out RA; 20% to 25% of patients with RA lack reactive RF titers, and RF itself isn't reactive until 6 months after the onset of active disease. Repeating the test is sometimes useful. However, a cor-

relation between RF and RA is inconclusive, and positive diagnosis always requires correlation with clinical status.

Post-test care
- Because a patient with RA may be immunocompromised from the disease or from corticosteroid therapy, keep the venipuncture site covered with a clean, dry bandage for 24 hours. Check regularly for signs of infection.
- If a hematoma develops at the venipuncture site, apply warm soaks.

Interfering factors
- Inadequately activated complement may cause false-positive results.
- Serum with high lipid or cryoglobulin levels may cause false-positive test results and requires repetition of the test after restriction of fat intake.
- Serum with high IgG levels may cause false-negative results through competition with IgG on the surface of latex particles or sheep RBCs used as substrate.

Cold agglutinins

Cold agglutinins are antibodies (usually of the IgM type) that cause red blood cells (RBCs) to aggregate at low temperatures. Transient elevations of these antibodies develop during certain infectious diseases, notably primary atypical pneumonia. (Small amounts may also occur in healthy people.) This test reliably detects such pneumonia within 1 to 2 weeks after onset.

Although cold agglutinins are inert at inner body temperatures, some become active in exposed areas of skin at 82.4° to 89.6° F (28° to 32° C), producing pallor and acrocyanosis (Raynaud's phenomenon), and numbness of hands and feet. Intense agglutination of a whole blood sample occurs on cooling to temperatures between 32° and 68° F (0° and 20° C), peaking at 39.2° F (4° C), and is reversible by rewarming to 98.6° F (37° C). However, after rewarming, complement remains on the cell and may produce hemolysis. Consequently, patients with high cold agglutinin titers, such as those with primary atypical pneumonia, may develop acute transient hemolytic anemia after repeated exposure to cold; patients with persistently high titers may develop chronic hemolytic anemia.

Purpose

■ To help confirm primary atypical pneumonia
■ To provide additional diagnostic evidence for cold agglutinin disease associated with many viral infections or lymphoreticular malignancy.

Patient preparation

Explain to the patient that this test detects antibodies in the blood that attack RBCs after exposure to low temperatures. If appropriate, inform him that the test will be repeated to monitor his response to therapy. Advise him that it isn't necessary to restrict food or fluids. Tell him that the test requires a blood sample, who will perform the venipuncture and when, and that he may experience transient discomfort from the needle puncture and the pressure of the tourniquet.

If the patient is receiving antimicrobial drugs, note this on the laboratory request because these drugs may interfere with the development of cold agglutinins.

Procedure

Perform a venipuncture, and collect the sample in a 7-ml *red-top* tube that has been *prewarmed* to 98.6° F (37° C).

Precautions

■ Handle the sample gently to prevent hemolysis, and send it to the laboratory immediately.

 ■ Don't refrigerate the sample; cold agglutinins will coat the RBCs, leaving none in the serum.

Reference values

Normal titers are less than 1:32, but they may be higher in elderly persons.

Implications of results

High titers may occur as primary phenomena or secondary to infections or lymphoreticular malignancy. Elevations may be present in infectious mononucleosis, cytomegalovirus infection, hemolytic anemia, multiple myeloma, scleroderma, malaria, cirrhosis, congenital syphilis, peripheral vascular disease, pulmonary embolism, trypanosomiasis, tonsillitis, staphylococcemia, scarlatina, influenza and, occasionally, in pregnancy. Chronically elevated titers are most commonly associated with pneumonia and lymphoreticular malignancy; an acute transient elevation commonly accompanies many viral infections.

In primary atypical pneumonia, cold agglutinins appear in serum in one-half to two-thirds of all patients during the first week of acute infection, even before antimycoplasmal antibodies can be detected by complement fixation or metabolic inhibition tests. Thus, titers usually become positive at 7 days, peak above 1:32 in 4 weeks, and disappear rapidly after 6 weeks. When sequential titers verify this pattern and clinical evidence of pneumonia exists, the diagnosis is confirmed.

Extremely high titers (1:1,000 to 1:1,000,000) can occur with idiopathic cold agglutinin disease that precedes development of lymphoma. Patients with titers this high are susceptible to intravascular agglutination, which causes significant clinical problems.

Post-test care

▪ If cold agglutinin disease is suspected, keep the patient warm. If the patient is exposed to low temperatures, agglutination may occur within peripheral vessels, possibly leading to frostbite, anemia, Raynaud's phenomenon or, rarely, focal gangrene.

▪ Watch for signs of vascular abnormalities, such as mottled skin, purpura, jaundice, or pallor; pain or swelling of extremities; and cramping of fingers and toes. Hemoglobinuria may result from severe intravascular hemolysis on exposure to severe cold.

▪ If a hematoma develops at the venipuncture site, ease discomfort by applying warm soaks.

Interfering factors

▪ Hemolysis caused by rough handling of the sample can falsely depress titers, as can refrigeration of the sample before serum is separated from RBCs.

▪ Antimicrobials can interfere with the development of cold agglutinins.

Cryoglobulins

Cryoglobulins are abnormal serum proteins that precipitate at low laboratory temperatures ($39.2° F [4° C]$) and redissolve after being warmed. Their presence in the blood (cryoglobulinemia) is usually associated with immune disorders, but cryoglobulins can also occur in the absence of known immunopathology. (See *Diseases associated with cryoglobulinemia,* page 326.)

Cryoglobulinemia occurs in three forms: Type I, which involves the reaction of a single monoclonal immuno-globulin; Type II, in which a monoclonal immunoglobulin shows antibody activity against a polyclonal immunoglobulin; and Type III, in which both components are polyclonal immunoglobulins. If patients with cryoglobulinemia are subjected to cold, they may experience Raynaud-like symptoms (pain, cyanosis, and coldness of fingers and toes), which generally result from precipitation of cryoglobulins in cooler parts of the body. In some patients, for example, cryoglobulins may precipitate at temperatures as high as $86° F (30° C)$; such temperatures are possible in some peripheral blood vessels.

The cryoglobulin test involves refrigerating a serum sample at $39.2° F (4° C)$ for at least 72 hours and observing for formation of a heat-reversible precipitate. Such a precipitate requires further study by immunoelectrophoresis or double diffusion to identify cryoglobulin components.

Purpose

▪ To detect cryoglobulinemia in patients with Raynaud-like vascular symptoms.

Patient preparation

Explain to the patient that this test detects antibodies in blood that may cause sensitivity to low temperatures. Instruct him to fast for 4 to 6 hours before the test. Tell him that the test requires a blood sample, who will perform the venipuncture and when, and that he may experience transient discomfort from the needle puncture and the pressure of the tourniquet.

Procedure

Perform a venipuncture, and collect the sample in a prewarmed 10-ml *red-top* tube.

Precautions

▪ Warm the syringe and collection tube to $98.6° F (37° C)$ before venipuncture,

Diseases associated with cryoglobulinemia

This chart indicates typical serum levels and diseases associated with the three types of cryoglobulins.

TYPE OF CRYOGLOBULIN	SERUM LEVEL	ASSOCIATED DISEASES
Type I Monoclonal cryoglobulin	> 5 mg/ml	▪ Myeloma ▪ Waldenström's macroglob-ulinemia ▪ Chronic lymphocytic leukemia
Type II Mixed cryoglobulin	> 1 mg/ml	▪ Rheumatoid arthritis ▪ Sjögren's syndrome ▪ Mixed essential cryoglobulinemia
Type III Mixed polyclonal cryoglobulin	< 1 mg/ml (50% below 80 µg/ml)	▪ Systemic lupus erythema-tosus ▪ Rheumatoid arthritis ▪ Sjögren's syndrome ▪ Infectious mononucleosis ▪ Cytomegalovirus infections ▪ Acute viral hepatitis ▪ Chronic active hepatitis ▪ Primary biliary cirrhosis ▪ Poststreptococcal glomeru-lonephritis ▪ Infective endocarditis ▪ Leprosy ▪ Kala-azar ▪ Tropical splenomegaly syndrome

and keep it at that temperature to prevent loss of cryoglobulins.
▪ Send the sample to the laboratory immediately.

Normal findings
Serum is negative for cryoglobulins.

Implications of results
Specific levels of cryoglobulins are characteristic of certain diseases. However, cryoglobulinemia doesn't always mean that clinical disease is present.

Post-test care
▪ Let the patient resume his usual diet.
▪ If the test is positive for cryoglobulins, tell the patient to avoid cold temperatures and contact with cold objects.
▪ If a hematoma develops at the venipuncture site, apply warm soaks.
▪ Observe for intravascular coagulation (decreased color and temperature in distal extremities, and increased pain).

Interfering factors
▪ Failure to adhere to dietary restrictions may affect the accuracy of test results.

■ Failure to keep the sample at 98.6° F (37° C) before centrifugation may cause loss of cryoglobulins.

■ Reading the sample before the end of the 72-hour precipitation period may cause test results to be reported incorrectly because some cryoglobulins take several days to precipitate.

Acetylcholine receptor antibodies

The acetylcholine receptor (AChR) antibodies test is the most useful test for confirming acquired (autoimmune) myasthenia gravis (MG), a disorder of neuromuscular transmission. In normal muscle contraction, acetylcholine (ACh) is released from the terminal end of the nerve and binds to AChR sites on the muscle motor end plate. In MG, however, antibodies block and destroy AChR sites, causing muscle weakness that can be either generalized or localized to the ocular muscles.

Two test methods — a binding assay and a blocking assay — are now available to determine the relative concentration of AChR antibodies in serum. In the binding assay, purified AChRs are complexed with ^{125}I-labeled α-bungarotoxin (a molecule that binds specifically to AChRs and blocks them). A serum sample is added to this complex; after incubation, antihuman immunoglobulin is added. Antibodies bind to AChR–^{125}I-labeled α-bungarotoxin complexes, which coprecipitate with the total human immunoglobulin. The amount of radioactivity is then measured to assay the available AChR sites. AChR-binding antibodies are found in about 90% of patients with generalized MG and in about 50% of those with localized MG.

When the AChR-binding assay is negative in a patient with MG symptoms, the AChR-blocking assay may be performed. In this test, the patient's serum is incubated with purified AChRs before ^{125}I-labeled α-bungarotoxin is added, to detect antibodies whose antigenic sites would otherwise be blocked. The blocking assay is relatively new, and its clinical significance is not yet fully known. However, it is specific for the autoimmune form of MG and is useful for research. Determination of AChR antibodies by either method also helps monitor immunosuppressive therapy for MG, although antibody levels do not usually parallel the severity of disease.

Purpose
■ To confirm a diagnosis of MG
■ To monitor the effectiveness of immunosuppressive therapy for MG.

Patient preparation
Explain to the patient that this test helps confirm MG or, when indicated, that it assesses the effectiveness of treatment for MG. Advise him that he needn't restrict food or fluids. Tell him that the test requires a blood sample, who will perform the venipuncture and when, and that he may experience transient discomfort from the needle puncture and the pressure of the tourniquet. Check the patient's medication history for immunosuppressive drugs that may affect test results, and note their use on the laboratory request.

Procedure
Perform a venipuncture, and collect the sample in a 7-ml *red-top* tube.

Precautions
Keep the sample at room temperature, and send it to the laboratory at once.

Reference values

Normal serum is negative or ≤0.03 nmol/L for AChR-binding antibodies and is negative for AChR-blocking antibodies.

Implications of results

Positive AChR antibodies in symptomatic adults confirm the diagnosis of MG. Patients with only ocular symptoms tend to have lower antibody titers than those with generalized symptoms.

Post-test care

▪ Because a patient with an autoimmune disease has a compromised immune system, check the venipuncture site for infection, and promptly report any change. Keep a clean, dry bandage over the site for at least 24 hours.
▪ If a hematoma develops at the venipuncture site, apply warm soaks.

Interfering factors

▪ Failure to maintain the sample at room temperature and to send it to the laboratory immediately may affect the accuracy of test results.
▪ Patients undergoing thymectomy, thoracic duct drainage, immunosuppressive therapy, or plasmapheresis may show reduced AChR-antibody levels.
▪ Patients with amyotrophic lateral sclerosis may show false-positive test results.

VIRAL TESTS

Rubella antibodies

Although rubella (German measles) is generally a mild viral infection in children and young adults, it can produce severe infection in a fetus, resulting in spontaneous abortion, stillbirth, or congenital rubella syndrome. Because rubella infection normally induces IgG and IgM antibody production, measuring rubella antibodies can determine present infection and immunity resulting from past infection.

Various methods of detecting rubella antibodies are available, including hemagglutination inhibition, passive hemagglutination, latex agglutination, enzyme immunoassay, fluorescence immunoassay, and radioimmunoassay. Suspected cases of congenital rubella may be confirmed if rubella-specific IgM antibodies are present in the infant's serum. Immune status in adults can be confirmed by an existing IgG-specific titer.

Exposure risk (when the immunity status is unknown) may be evaluated using two serum samples. The first sample should be drawn in the acute phase of clinical symptoms. If clinical symptoms are not apparent, the sample should be drawn as soon as possible after the suspected exposure. The second sample should be drawn 3 to 4 weeks later during the convalescent phase.

Purpose

▪ To diagnose rubella infection, especially congenital infection
▪ To determine susceptibility to rubella in women of childbearing age and in children.

Patient preparation

Explain that this test diagnoses or evaluates susceptibility to German measles. Inform the patient that she needn't restrict food or fluids before the test and that this test requires a blood sample (if a current infection is suspected, a second blood sample will be needed in 3 to 4 weeks to identify a rise in the titer). Explain who will perform the venipuncture and when and that she may experience transient discomfort from the needle puncture and the pressure of the tourniquet.

Procedure
Perform a venipuncture, and collect the sample in a 7-ml *red-top* tube.

Precautions
Handle the specimen gently to prevent hemolysis.

Reference values
Titer of 1:8 or less indicates little or no immunity against rubella; titer greater than 1:10 indicates adequate protection against rubella.

Implications of results
Demonstrable antibody levels normally appear 2 to 4 days after the onset of the rash, peak in 3 to 4 weeks, then slowly decline but remain detectable for life. In rubella infection, acute serum titers range from 1:8 to 1:16; convalescent serum titers, from 1:64 to 1:1,024+. A fourfold rise or greater from the acute to the convalescent titer indicates a recent rubella infection.

The presence of rubella-specific IgM antibodies indicates recent infection in an adult and congenital rubella in an infant.

Post-test care
■ If a hematoma develops at the venipuncture site, apply warm soaks.
■ When appropriate, instruct the patient to return for another blood test.
■ If a woman of childbearing age is found susceptible to rubella, explain that vaccination can prevent rubella and that she must wait at least 3 months after the vaccination before becoming pregnant or risk permanent damage or death to the fetus.
■ If a pregnant patient is found susceptible to rubella, instruct her to return for follow-up rubella antibody tests to detect possible subsequent infection.

■ If the test confirms rubella in a pregnant woman, be supportive and refer her for counseling, as needed.

Interfering factors
Hemolysis due to excessive agitation of the specimen may alter test results.

Hepatitis B surface antigen

Hepatitis B surface antigen (HBsAg) appears in the serum of patients with hepatitis B virus (formerly called serum hepatitis or long-incubation hepatitis). This antigen (also known as hepatitis-associated antigen and Australia antigen) can be detected by radioimmunoassay or, less commonly, by reverse passive hemagglutination during the extended incubation period and usually during the first 3 weeks of acute infection or if the patient is a carrier.

Because transmission of hepatitis is one of the gravest complications associated with blood transfusions, all donors must be screened for hepatitis B before their blood is stored. This test, required by the Food and Drug Administration, has helped reduce the incidence of hepatitis but it doesn't screen for hepatitis A (infectious hepatitis).

(For information on related tests, see *Viral hepatitis test panel*, pages 330 and 331, and *Serodiagnosis of acute viral hepatitis*, page 332.)

Purpose
■ To screen blood donors for hepatitis B
■ To screen persons at high risk for contracting hepatitis B (such as hemodialysis nurses)
■ To aid differential diagnosis of viral hepatitis.

Viral hepatitis test panel

The three types of viral hepatitis produce similar symptoms but differ in transmission mode, course of treatment, prognosis, and carrier status. When clinical history is insufficient for differentiation, serologic tests can aid diagnosis. Hepatitis A, B, and C antigens induce type-specific antibodies detectable by a variety of methods. The timing of the appearance and disappearance of these antibodies, in conjunction with clinical symptoms, helps to diagnose and stage acute and chronic forms of these distinct diseases.

Typical sequence of hepatitis A markers after exposure

Testing for hepatitis A: Present in blood and feces only briefly before symptoms appear, hepatitis A virus (HAV) may elude detection. However, anti-HAV, the antibody to hepatitis A virus, appears early in the acute phase of the disease, persists for many years after recovery, and ultimately gives the patient immunity. A single positive anti-HAV test may indicate previous exposure to the virus, but because this antibody persists so long in the bloodstream, only evidence of *rising* anti-HAV titers confirms hepatitis A as the cause of current or very recent infection. Determining recent infection relies on identifying the antibody as IgM (associated with recent infection). A negative anti-HAV test rules out hepatitis A.

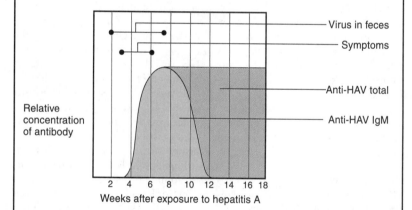

Weeks after exposure to hepatitis A

Relative concentration of antibody

Virus in feces
Symptoms
Anti-HAV total
Anti-HAV IgM

Typical sequence of hepatitis B and C markers after exposure

Testing for hepatitis B: Hepatitis B viral cells are composed of a core protein and a surface protein. The surface antigen (HBsAg) appears in serum during the long incubation period (up to 26 weeks) or during the early acute phase of infection (2 to 3 weeks) and normally peaks after symptoms begin. High levels of HBsAg continuing 3 or more months after onset of acute infection suggest chronic hepatitis or carrier status. Potential blood donors are screened for this antigen to prevent transmission of hepatitis B to recipients.

Another antibody that develops after exposure to hepatitis B is anti-HBc, induced by the core component of the B antigen. An early indicator of acute

Viral hepatitis test panel (continued)

infection, antibody (IgM) to core antigen (anti-HBc IgM) is rarely detected in chronic infection. Thus, it's also useful in distinguishing acute from chronic infection.

Anti-HBs, antibody to the surface component of the B virus, appears long after symptoms have subsided and after the HBsAg antigen itself has disappeared from blood. Detection of this antibody signals late convalescence or recovery from infection. Anti-HBs remains in the blood to provide immunity.

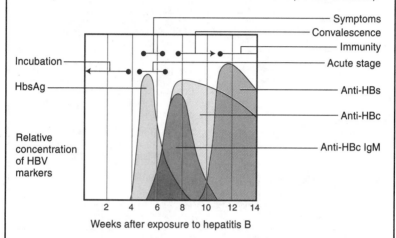

Testing for hepatitis C: The virus that causes hepatitis C (formerly called non-A, non-B hepatitis) was recently isolated. A serologic assay was developed to detect an antibody to a nonstructural protein of the virus. This antibody has been designated anti-HCV. Anti-HCV can occur relatively late in the infection, usually 16 to 24 weeks after the initial elevation of liver enzyme levels. The infection's progress can be monitored by periodic analysis of alanine aminotransferase and anti-HCV levels. The clinical symptoms and epidemiology are similar to that of hepatitis B, but the rate of chronic infection is much higher. The plasma of chronically infected HCV patients remains infectious.

Graphs reprinted with permission from Serodiagnostic Assessment of Acute Viral Hepatitis. *Abbott Park, Ill.: Abbott Laboratories, 1992.*

Patient preparation

Explain that the test helps identify a type of viral hepatitis. Inform the patient that he needn't restrict food or fluids before the test. Tell him that this test requires a blood sample, who will perform the venipuncture and when, and that he may experience transient discomfort from the needle puncture and the pressure of the tourniquet. Check the patient's history for hepatitis B vaccine. If the patient is giving blood, explain the donation procedure to him.

Serodiagnosis of acute viral hepatitis

The chart below helps evaluate positive test results in acute viral hepatitis.

TEST RESULTS			INTERPRETATION
HBsAg	Anti-HBc Igm	Anti-HAV Igm	
−	−	+	Recent acute hepatitis A infection
+	+	−	Acute hepatitis B infection
+	−	−	Early acute hepatitis B infection or chronic hepatitis B
−	+	−	Confirms acute or recent infection with hepatitis B virus
−	−	−	Possible hepatitis C (formerly non-A, non-B) infection, other viral infection, or liver toxin
+	+	+	Recent probable hepatitis A infection and superimposed acute hepatitis B infection; uncommon profile

KEY: + = positive   − = negative

Reprinted with permission of Abbott Laboratories, Abbott Park, Ill.

Procedure
Perform a venipuncture, and collect the sample in a 10-ml *red-top* tube.

Precautions
Wash your hands carefully after the procedure. Remember to wear gloves when drawing blood and to dispose of the needle properly.

Normal findings
Serum should be negative for HBsAg.

Implications of results
The presence of HBsAg in a patient with hepatitis confirms hepatitis B. In chronic carriers and persons with chronic active hepatitis, HBsAg may be present in serum several months after the onset of acute infection. It may also occur in more than 5% of patients with other diseases, such as hemophilia, Hodgkin's disease, and leukemia. If the antigen is found in donor blood, the blood must be discarded because of the high risk of transmitting hepatitis. Blood samples that test positive should be retested because inaccurate results do occur.

Post-test care
Notify the blood donor if test results are positive. Report confirmed viral hepatitis to public health authorities. This is a reportable disease in most states.

Interfering factors
Patients who have received the hepatitis B vaccine may test positive.

Epstein-Barr virus antibodies

Epstein-Barr virus (EBV), a member of the herpesvirus group, is the causative agent in heterophile-positive infectious mononucleosis, Burkitt's lymphoma, and nasopharyngeal carcinoma. Although the virus does not replicate in standard cell cultures, most EBV infections can be recognized by testing the patient's serum for heterophile antibodies (monospot test), which usually appear within the first 3 weeks of illness and then decline rapidly within a few weeks. (For more information about the monospot test, see *Monospot test for infectious mononucleosis,* page 334.)

In about 10% of adults and a larger percentage of children, the monospot test is negative despite primary infection with EBV. EBV has also been associated with lymphoproliferative processes in immunosuppressed people. These disorders occur with reactivated, rather than primary, EBV infections and, thus, are also monospot-negative.

Alternatively, EBV-specific antibodies, which develop to several antigens of the virus during active infection, can be measured with high sensitivity and specificity by indirect immunofluorescence tests. The test profile results of IgG, IgM, and IgA class antibodies directed to the EBV antigens, viral capsid antigen (VCA) and Epstein-Barr nuclear antigen (EBNA), can help determine whether the patient was infected recently or in the remote past.

Purpose

- To provide a laboratory diagnosis of heterophile- (or monospot-) negative cases of infectious mononucleosis
- To determine the antibody status to EBV of immunosuppressed patients with lymphoproliferative processes.

Patient preparation

Explain the purpose of the test. Inform the patient that this test requires a blood sample, who will perform the venipuncture and when, and that he may experience transient discomfort from the needle puncture and the pressure of the tourniquet.

Procedure

Perform a venipuncture, and collect 5 ml of sterile blood in a *red-top* tube. Allow the blood to clot for at least 1 hour at room temperature.

Precautions

- Handle the sample gently because excessive agitation will cause hemolysis of the sample.
- Transfer the serum to a sterile tube or vial, and send it to the laboratory promptly. If transfer must be delayed, store the serum at 39.2° F (4° C) for 1 or 2 days or at −4° F (−20° C) for longer periods to prevent bacterial contamination.

Normal findings

Serum from patients who have never been infected with EBV will have no detectable antibodies to the virus measured by either the monospot or indirect immunofluorescence test. The monospot test is positive only during the acute phase of EBV infection; the indirect immunofluorescence test will detect and discriminate between acute and past infection.

Implications of results

EBV infection can be ruled out if no antibodies to EBV antigens are detected in the indirect immunofluorescence test. A positive monospot test or an indirect immunofluorescence test that is either IgM-positive or EBNA-negative indicates acute EBV infection. However, a negative monospot result does not necessarily rule out acute or past infection with EBV. Conversely, IgG class

Monospot test for infectious mononucleosis

Several screening tests can detect the heterophil infectious mononucleosis (IM) antibody. One of these — the monospot test — converts the Paul-Bunnell and the Davidsohn's differential absorption tests into one rapid slide test without titration.

The monospot test relies on agglutination of horse red blood cells (RBCs) by heterophil antibodies. Because horse RBCs contain both Forssman and IM antigens, differential absorption of the patient's serum is necessary to distinguish between them. This is done by mixing the serum sample with guinea pig kidney antigen (containing only Forssman antigen) on one end of a slide and with beef RBC stroma (containing only IM antigen) on the other. Each absorbs only the heterophil antibody specific to it. After addition of horse RBCs to each spot, agglutination on the beef cell end of the slide indicates the presence of the IM heterophil antibody and confirms IM.

Monospot rivals the classic heterophil agglutination test for sensitivity. False-positive results may occur in lymphoma, hepatitis A and hepatitis B, leukemia, and pancreatic cancer.

antibody to VCA and EBNA antigens (IgM-negative) indicates remote (more than 2 months) infection with EBV. (Most cases of monospot-negative infectious mononucleosis are caused by cytomegalovirus infections.)

Post-test care
If a hematoma develops at the venipuncture site, apply warm soaks.

Interfering factors
Hemolysis will alter test results.

Serum respiratory syncytial virus antibodies

Respiratory syncytial virus (RSV), a member of the paramyxovirus group, is the major viral cause of severe lower respiratory tract disease in infants, but it may cause infections in persons of any age. RSV infections are most common and produce the most severe disease during the first 6 months of life. Initial infection involves viral replication in epithelial cells of the upper respiratory tract, but in younger children especially, the infection spreads to the bronchi, bronchioli, and even to the parenchyma of the lungs.

IgG and IgM class antibodies can be easily quantified using the indirect immunofluorescence test. Specific results for IgM are obtained only after separating this class of antibody from IgG. Prevalence of IgG antibodies to RSV is extremely high (greater than 95%), especially in adults.

Purpose
■ To diagnose infections caused by RSV.

Patient preparation
Explain the purpose of the test, and inform the patient that the test requires a blood sample, who will perform the venipuncture and when, and that he may experience transient discomfort

from the needle puncture and the pressure of the tourniquet.

Procedure

Perform a venipuncture to collect 5 ml of sterile blood in a *red-top* tube. Allow the blood to clot for at least 1 hour at room temperature.

Precautions

■ Handle the sample gently to prevent hemolysis.

■ Transfer the serum to a sterile tube or vial, and send it to the laboratory at once. If transfer must be delayed, store the serum at 39.2° F (4° C) for 1 to 2 days or at –4° F (–20° C) for longer periods to avoid bacterial contamination.

Normal findings

Serum from patients who have never been infected with RSV will have no detectable antibodies to the virus (less than 1:5). In infants, serologic diagnosis of RSV infections is difficult because of the presence of maternal IgG antibodies; thus, the presence of IgM antibodies is most significant.

Implications of results

RSV infection can be ruled out in patients whose serum samples have no detectable antibodies to the virus. The qualitative presence of IgM or a fourfold or greater increase in IgG antibodies indicates active RSV infection.

Post-test care

If a hematoma develops at the venipuncture site, apply warm soaks.

Interfering factors

Hemolysis of the sample may alter test results.

Serum herpes simplex antibodies

Herpes simplex virus (HSV), a member of the herpesvirus group, causes severe signs and symptoms, including genital lesions, keratitis or conjunctivitis, generalized dermal lesions, and pneumonia. Severe involvement is associated with intrauterine or neonatal infections and encephalitis; such infections are most severe in immunosuppressed patients.

Of the two closely related antigenic types, type 1 usually causes infections above the waistline; type 2 primarily involves the external genitalia. Primary contact with this virus occurs in early childhood as acute stomatitis or, more commonly, as an inapparent infection. More than 50% of adults have antibodies to HSV.

Sensitive assays, such as indirect immunofluorescence or enzyme immunoassay (but not complement fixation), are used to demonstrates IgM class antibodies to HSV or to detect a fourfold or greater increase in IgG class antibodies between acute- and convalescent-phase serum.

Purpose

■ To confirm infections caused by HSV.

Patient preparation

Explain the purpose of the test, and inform the patient that it will require a blood sample, who will perform the venipuncture and when, and that he may experience transient discomfort from the needle puncture and the pressure of the tourniquet.

Procedure

Perform a venipuncture, and collect 5 ml of sterile blood in a tube (color top to be designated by laboratory). Allow the blood to clot for at least 1 hour at room temperature.

Precautions
- Handle the sample gently to prevent hemolysis.
- Transfer the serum to a sterile tube or vial, and send it to the laboratory promptly. If transfer must be delayed for 1 or 2 days, store the serum at 39.2° F (4° C); if it must be delayed longer, store at –4° F (–20° C) to avoid bacterial contamination.

Normal findings
Serum from patients who have never been infected with HSV will have no detectable antibodies (less than 1:5). Patients with primary HSV infection will develop both IgM and IgG class antibodies. Reportedly, over 50% of adults have IgG class antibodies to HSV because of prior infection. Reactivated infections caused by HSV can be recognized serologically only by an increase in IgG class antibodies between acute- and convalescent-phase serum.

Implications of results
HSV infection can be ruled out in patients whose serum shows no detectable antibodies to the virus. The presence of IgM antibodies or a fourfold or greater increase in IgG antibodies indicates active HSV infection.

Post-test care
If a hematoma develops at the venipuncture site, apply warm soaks.

Interfering factors
Hemolysis will alter results.

Serum cytomegalovirus antibodies

After primary infection, cytomegalovirus (CMV) remains latent in white blood cells (WBCs). In an immunocompromised patient, CMV can be reactivated to cause active infection. The presence of CMV antibodies indicates past infection with this virus. CMV-seronegative organ transplant recipients and neonates (especially those born prematurely) are at high risk for active CMV infection if they're given blood or tissue from a seropositive donor.

Antibodies to CMV can be detected by several methods, including passive hemagglutination, latex agglutination, enzyme immunoassay, and indirect immunofluorescence. The complement fixation test is only 60% sensitive and thus should not be used to screen for CMV antibodies.

This screen for CMV antibodies is qualitative; it detects the presence of antibody at a single low dilution (for example, 1:5) to identify past infection with CMV. Quantitative methods can be used diagnostically by testing several dilutions of the serum specimen to indicate acute infection with CMV.

Purpose
- To detect past CMV infection in organ transplant donors and recipients
- To detect past CMV infection in immunocompromised patients and especially in premature neonates who receive transfused blood products.

Patient preparation
Explain the purpose of the test, and inform the patient (or the parents of the infant) that the test will require a blood sample. Tell the patient (or parents) who will perform the venipuncture and when and that he (or the infant) may

experience transient discomfort from the needle puncture and the pressure of the tourniquet.

Procedure

Perform a venipuncture to collect 5 ml of blood in a *red-top* tube. Allow the blood to clot for at least 1 hour at room temperature.

Precautions

- Handle the sample gently to prevent hemolysis.
- Transfer the serum to a sterile tube or vial, and send it to the laboratory at once. If transport must be delayed, store the serum at 39.2° F (4° C) for 1 or 2 days or at –4° F (–20° C) for longer periods to avoid bacterial contamination.

Normal findings

Serum from patients who have never been infected with CMV will show no detectable antibodies to the virus (less than 1:5). A positive specimen at this single dilution indicates that the patient has been infected with CMV and that his WBCs contain latent virus capable of being reactivated in an immunocompromised host.

Implications of results

Immunosuppressed patients who lack antibodies to CMV (a screening test less than 1:5) should receive blood products or organ transplants from donors who are also seronegative to avoid the morbidity and mortality associated with active infection with this virus. Patients with CMV antibodies (screening test greater than 1:5) are not given seronegative blood products.

Post-test care

None.

Interfering factors

Hemolysis may alter test results.

Human immunodeficiency virus antibodies

A number of test methods are used to detect antibodies to human immunodeficiency virus (HIV) in serum. Among the most common are enzyme immunoassay, fluorescence immunoassay, and enzyme-linked immunosorbent assay (ELISA). Each of these methods requires a blood sample. Patient preparation, normal findings, and post-test care are the same for all.

HIV transmission occurs by direct exposure of a person's blood to body fluids containing the virus. The virus may be transmitted when contaminated blood and blood products are exchanged from one person to another; during sexual intercourse with an infected partner; when I.V. drugs are shared; and during pregnancy or breast-feeding, from an infected mother to her child.

HIV causes acquired immunodeficiency syndrome (AIDS), which may be manifested in many forms. Female patients may present different symptoms than males.

Purpose

- To screen for HIV in high-risk groups
- To screen donated blood for HIV.

Patient preparation

Inform the patient that this test detects HIV infection. Provide adequate counselling about the reasons for performing the test (usually requested by the patient's doctor). If the patient has questions about his condition, provide full and accurate answers.

Tell the patient that this test requires a blood sample, who will perform the venipuncture and when, and that he may experience transient discomfort from the needle puncture and the pressure of the tourniquet.

Procedure
Perform a venipuncture, and collect the sample in a 10-ml *red-top* barrier tube. Barrier tubes help prevent contamination when pouring the serum.

Precautions
When drawing a blood sample, use standard precautions. Use gloves, dispose of needles properly, and use blood-fluid precaution labels on tubes, as necessary.

Normal findings
Test results should be nonreactive.

Implications of results
This test detects previous exposure to HIV. However, none of the test methods is 100% sensitive or specific, and all may produce false results. Therefore, a negative result does not necessarily mean that HIV antibodies are not present. For example, the tests don't identify individuals who have been exposed to the virus but who haven't yet developed antibodies. A positive test for the HIV antibody can't determine whether the person harbors actively replicating virus or when he will present signs and symptoms of AIDS.

A false-positive result may reflect a lack of specificity of the test method used. As a result, it is recommended that the Western blot test for HIV be performed on all persons with positive antibody tests. The Western Blot test for HIV is a confirmatory test because it detects the presence of specific viral proteins present in HIV.

Many apparently healthy people have been exposed to HIV and have circulating antibodies. *These are not false-positive results.* Furthermore, patients in the later stages of AIDS may exhibit no detectable antibodies in their serum because they can no longer mount an antibody response.

Post-test care
■ If a hematoma develops at the venipuncture site, apply warm soaks.
■ Keep test results confidential. When the results are received, give the patient another opportunity to ask questions.
■ Encourage the patient with a positive result to seek medical follow-up care, even if he's asymptomatic. Tell him to report early signs of AIDS, such as fever, weight loss, axillary or inguinal lymphadenopathy, rash, and persistent cough or diarrhea. Females should also report gynecologic symptoms.
■ Tell the patient to assume that he can transmit HIV to others. To prevent contagion, teach him safe sex precautions. Instruct him not to share razors, toothbrushes, or utensils (which may be contaminated with blood) and to clean such items with household bleach diluted 1:10 in water. Advise him not to donate blood, tissues, or organs. Urge the patient to inform his doctor and dentist about his condition so they can take proper precautions.

Interfering factors
None.

BACTERIAL AND FUNGAL TESTS

Antistreptolysin-O

Because streptococcal infections are often overlooked, serologic testing is valuable in patients with glomerulonephritis or acute rheumatic fever to confirm antecedent infection by showing a serologic response to streptococcal antigen. The antistreptolysin-O (ASO) test measures the relative serum concentrations of the antibody to streptolysin O, an oxygen-labile enzyme produced by group A beta-hemolytic streptococci.

In this test (also known as the streptococcal antibody test), a serum sample is diluted with commercially prepared streptolysin O and incubated. After the addition of rabbit or human red blood cells (RBCs), the tube is reincubated and examined visually. If hemolysis fails to develop, ASO has complexed with the antigen, inactivated it, and prevented RBC destruction, indicating recent beta-hemolytic streptococcal infection. The end point is read in Todd units, the reciprocal of the highest dilution (titer) that inhibits hemolysis.

Very high ASO titers occur in poststreptococcal diseases, such as rheumatic fever or glomerulonephritis. High titers may also occur in patients with uncomplicated streptococcal disease, but the incidence is lower and the titers are lower than in poststreptococcal diseases. Micro methods for detecting ASO, such as the Rapi/tex ASO latex agglutination test, currently screen for beta-hemolytic streptococcal infection.

Purpose
■ To confirm recent or ongoing infection with beta-hemolytic streptococci
■ To help diagnose rheumatic fever and poststreptococcal glomerulonephritis in the presence of clinical symptoms (see *Test for anti-DNase B,* page 340, for information about another method of diagnosing these two diseases)
■ To distinguish between rheumatic fever and rheumatoid arthritis when joint pains are present.

Patient preparation
Explain to the patient that this test detects an immune response to certain bacteria. Inform him that he needn't restrict food or fluids. Tell him that this test requires a blood sample, who will perform the venipuncture and when, and that he may experience transient discomfort from the needle puncture and the pressure of the tourniquet.

If the test is to be repeated at regular intervals to identify active and inactive states of rheumatic fever or to confirm acute glomerulonephritis, tell the patient that measuring changes in antibody levels helps determine the effectiveness of therapy.

Check the patient's medication history for drugs that may suppress the streptococcal antibody response. If such drugs must be continued, note this on the laboratory request.

Procedure
Perform a venipuncture, and collect the sample in a 7-ml *red-top* tube.

Precautions
Handle the sample gently to prevent hemolysis.

Reference values
Even healthy people have some detectable ASO titer from previous minor streptococcal infections. For adults, the normal ASO titer is less than 120 Todd units/ml; for school-age children, less than 170 Todd units/ml; and for preschoolers, less than 120 Todd units/ml.

Implications of results
High ASO titers usually occur only after prolonged or recurrent infections, but 15% to 20% of patients with poststreptococcal disease don't have high titers. Titers up to 250 Todd units may indicate inactive rheumatic fever. Titers of 500 to 5,000 Todd units suggest acute rheumatic fever or acute poststreptococcal glomerulonephritis. Serial titers, determined at 10- to 14-day intervals, provide more reliable information than a single titer. A rise in titer 2 to 5 weeks after the acute infection, which peaks 4

Test for anti-DNase B

The antideoxyribonuclease B (antiD-Nase B) test, a process similar to the antistreptolysin-O (ASO) test, detects antibodies to DNase B, a potent antigen produced by all group A streptococci.

For adults, normal anti-DNase B titer is less than 85 Todd units/ml; for school-age children, less than 170 Todd units/ml; and for preschoolers, less than 60 Todd units/ml.

Elevated anti-DNase B titers appear in 80% of patients with acute rheumatic fever, in 75% of those with poststreptococcal glomerulonephritis (following streptococcal pharyngitis), and in 60% of those with glomerulonephritis (following group A streptococcal pyoderma). This is a much higher percentage than those with ASO titer elevations (25%), making the test for anti-DNase B especially valuable in detecting a reaction to group A streptococcal pyoderma.

Other streptococcal antigens are of limited diagnostic value, or their use is controversial.

to 6 weeks after the initial rise, confirms poststreptococcal disease.

Post-test care

If a hematoma develops at the venipuncture site, apply warm soaks.

Interfering factors

■ False-negative results are likely in patients with streptococcal skin infections, who rarely have abnormal ASO titers even with poststreptococcal disease.
■ Antibiotic or corticosteroid therapy may suppress the streptococcal antibody response and thus alter test results.
■ Hemolysis due to rough handling of the sample may affect test results.

Febrile agglutination

Bacterial infections (such as tularemia, brucellosis, and the disorders caused by salmonella) and rickettsial infections (such as Rocky Mountain spotted fever and typhus) sometimes cause a fever of undetermined origin (FUO). In these infections and others in which micro-organisms are difficult to isolate from blood or excreta, febrile agglutination tests can provide important diagnostic information.

The Weil-Felix reaction for rickettsial disease, Widal's test for *Salmonella*, and tests for brucellosis and tularemia are essentially the same. In these tests, a serum sample is mixed with a few drops of prepared antigens in normal saline solution on a slide; the reaction is observed with the unaided eye. If agglutination occurs, antigen is added to serial dilutions of the patient's serum. Antibody titer is expressed as the reciprocal of the last dilution showing visible agglutination.

The *Weil-Felix reaction* establishes rickettsial antibody titers. Unlike other febrile agglutination tests, the Weil-Felix reaction doesn't use the causal agent as the antigen; instead it uses three forms of *Proteus* antigens (OX-19, OX-2, and OX-K) that cross-react with the various strains of rickettsiae.

In *Salmonella* infection — gastroenteritis and extraintestinal focal infections, both caused by *Salmonella enteritidis,* and enteric (typhoid) fever, caused by *Salmonella typhosa* — the

Salmonella organism presents flagellar (H) and somatic (O) antigens; *Widal's test* establishes their titers. Antibodies that agglutinate with H antigens form coarse, unstable aggregates that return to solution easily; those that agglutinate with O antigens form finer, more stable aggregates. The O antigens are considered more specific for *Salmonella* than H antigens. A third antigen — Vi, or envelope, antigen — may indicate typhoid carrier status, which often tests negative for H and O antigens. Widal's test isn't recommended for diagnosing *Salmonella* gastroenteritis because symptoms subside before the titer rises.

Slide-agglutination and *tube dilution tests,* using killed suspensions of the disease organism as antigens, establish titers for the gram-negative coccobacilli *Brucella* and *Francisella tularensis,* which cause brucellosis and tularemia, respectively.

Purpose
- To support clinical findings in diagnosing disorders caused by *Salmonella,* rickettsiae, *F. tularensis,* or *Brucella*
- To identify the cause of FUO.

Patient preparation
Explain to the patient that the test detects and measures microorganisms that may cause fever and other symptoms. Inform him that he needn't restrict food or fluids. Tell him that this test requires a blood sample, who will perform the venipuncture and when, and that he may experience transient discomfort from the needle puncture and the pressure of the tourniquet.

If appropriate, explain to the patient that this test requires a series of blood samples to detect a pattern of titers that is characteristic of the suspected disorder. Reassure him that a positive titer only suggests a disorder.

Note on the laboratory request when antimicrobial therapy (if any) began.

Procedure
Perform a venipuncture, and collect the sample in a 7-ml *red-top* tube.

Precautions
Use standard hospital isolation procedures when collecting and handling samples. Send samples to the laboratory immediately.

Reference values
Normal dilutions are as follows:
- *Salmonella* antibody: <1:80
- brucellosis antibody: <1:80
- tularemia antibody: <1:40
- rickettsial antibody: <1:40.

Implications of results
Observation of rising and falling titers is crucial for detecting active infection. If this is not possible, certain titer levels can suggest the disorder. For all febrile agglutinins, a fourfold increase in titers is strong evidence of infection.

The Weil-Felix reaction is positive for rickettsiae with antibodies to *Proteus* 6 to 12 days after infection; titers peak in 1 month and usually drop to negative in 5 or 6 months. However, this test cannot be used for diagnosing rickettsial pox or Q fever, because the antibodies of these diseases don't cross-react with *Proteus* antigens; the test shows positive titers in *Proteus* infections and, in such cases, is nonspecific for rickettsiae.

In *Salmonella* infection, H and O agglutinins usually appear in serum after 1 week, and titers rise for 3 to 6 weeks. O agglutinins usually fall to insignificant levels in 6 to 12 months; H agglutinins may remain elevated for years.

In brucellosis, titers usually rise after 2 or 3 weeks and reach their highest levels between 4 and 8 weeks. Absence of *Brucella* agglutinins doesn't rule out brucellosis. In tularemia, titers usually become positive in the second week of infection, exceed 1:320 by the third week, peak in 4 to 7 weeks, and usually decline gradually 1 year after recovery.

Post-test care
■ If a hematoma develops at the venipuncture site, apply warm soaks.
■ In FUO and suspected infection, contact the hospital infection control department. Isolation may be necessary.

Interfering factors
■ Failure to send the sample to the laboratory immediately may alter results.
■ Vaccination or continuous exposure to bacterial or rickettsial infection (resulting in immunity) causes high titers.
■ Many antibodies cross-react with bacteria that cause other infectious diseases. For example, tularemia antibodies cross-react with *Brucella* antigens.
■ Immunodeficient patients may show infectious symptoms but be unable to produce antibodies. In such cases, titers remain negative, even during infection.
■ Patients taking antibiotics show depressed titers early in the course of the disorder.
■ Patients with elevated immunoglobulin levels due to hepatic disease, or those who use drugs excessively, often have high *Salmonella* titers.
■ Patients who have had skin tests with *Brucella* antigen may show elevated *Brucella* titers.
■ Patients with *Proteus* infections may show positive Weil-Felix titers for rickettsial disease.

Fungal serology

Most fungal organisms enter the body as spores inhaled into the lungs or infiltrated through wounds in the skin or mucosa. If the body's defenses can't destroy the organisms initially, the fungi multiply to form lesions; blood and lymph vessels may then spread the mycoses throughout the body. Mycosis may be deep-seated or superficial. Deep-seated mycosis occurs primarily in the lungs; superficial mycosis, in the skin or the mucosal linings.

Most healthy people easily overcome initial mycotic infection, but the elderly and others with deficient immune systems are more susceptible to acute or chronic mycotic infection and to disorders secondary to such infection.

Although cultures are usually performed to diagnose mycosis by identifying the causative organism, serologic tests occasionally provide the sole evidence of mycosis. These tests are used to detect blastomycosis, coccidioidomycosis, histoplasmosis, aspergillosis, sporotrichosis, and cryptococcosis. Fungal serologic tests use immunodiffusion, complement fixation, precipitin, latex agglutination, or agglutination methods to demonstrate the presence of mycotic antibodies.

Purpose
■ To rapidly detect the presence of antifungal antibodies, aiding in the diagnosis of mycoses
■ To monitor the effectiveness of therapy for mycoses.

Patient preparation
Explain to the patient that this test aids diagnosis of certain fungal infections. If appropriate, explain that the test monitors his response to therapy and that it may be repeated during his illness. Instruct him to restrict food and fluids for 12 to 24 hours before the test. Tell him that this test requires a blood sample, who will perform the venipuncture and when, and that he may experience transient discomfort from the needle puncture and the pressure of the tourniquet.

Implications of abnormal fungal serologic tests

DISEASE AND NORMAL VALUES	CLINICAL SIGNIFICANCE OF ABNORMAL RESULTS
Blastomycosis Complement fixation: titers <1:8	Titers ranging from 1:8 to 1:16 suggest infection; titers >1:32 denote active disease. A rising titer in serial samples taken every 3 to 4 weeks indicates disease progression; a falling titer indicates regression. This test has limited diagnostic value because of the high percentage of false-negatives.
Immunodiffusion: negative	A more sensitive test for blastomycosis; detects 80% of infected people
Coccidioidomycosis Complement fixation: titers <1:2	Most sensitive test for this fungus. Titers ranging from 1:2 to 1:4 suggest active infection; titers >1:16 usually denote active disease. Test may remain negative in mild infections.
Immunodiffusion: negative	Most useful for screening, followed by complement fixation test for confirmation
Precipitin: titers <1:16	Good screening test; titers >1:16 usually indicate infection. About 80% of infected people show positive titers by 2 weeks; most revert to negative by 6 months. Early primary disease is shown by positive precipitin and negative complement fixation test. A positive complement fixation and negative precipitin test indicate chronic disease.
Histoplasmosis Complement fixation (histoplasmin): titers <1:8	Titers ranging from 1:8 to 1:16 suggest infection; titers >1:32 indicate active disease. Antibodies generally appear 10 to 21 days after initial infection. Test is positive in 10% to 15% of cases.
Complement fixation (yeast): titers <1:18	Titers ranging from 1:8 to 1:16 suggest infection; titers >1:32 indicate active disease. More sensitive than histoplasmin complement fixation test; gives positive results in 75% to 80% of cases. (Both histoplasmin and yeast antigens are positive in 10% of cases.) A rising titer in serial samples taken every 2 to 3 weeks indicates progressive infection; a decreasing titer indicates regression.
Immunodiffusion (histoplasmin): negative	Appearance of both H and M bands indicates active infection. If the M band appears first and lasts longer than the H band, the infection may be regressing. The M band alone may indicate early infection, chronic disease, or a recent skin test.
Aspergillosis Complement fixation: titers <1:8	Titers of >1:8 suggest infection; 70% to 90% of patients with known pulmonary aspergillosis or aspergillus allergy present antibodies, as does about 5% of the general population. This test cannot detect invasive aspergillosis because patients with this disease do not present antibodies; a biopsy is required.

(continued)

Implications of abnormal fungal serologic tests (continued)

DISEASE AND NORMAL VALUES	CLINICAL SIGNIFICANCE OF ABNORMAL RESULTS
Aspergillosis (continued) Immunodiffusion: negative	One or more precipitin bands suggests infection; precipitins appear in 95% of patients with pulmonary fungus balls and in 50% of those with allergic bronchopulmonary disorders. The number of bands is related to complement fixation titers; the more precipitin bands, the higher the titer.
Sporotrichosis Agglutination: titers <1:40	Titers >1:80 usually indicate active disease. The test usually is negative in cutaneous infections and positive in extracutaneous infections.
Cryptococcosis Latex agglutination for cryptococcal antigen: negative	About 90% of patients with cryptococcal meningoencephalitis present capsular antigen in cerebrospinal fluid (CSF) or serum. (Serum is positive less frequently than CSF.) Culturing is definitive because false-positive results do occur. (Presence of rheumatoid factor may cause a positive reaction.) Serum antigen tests are positive in 33% of patients with pulmonary cryptococcosis; a biopsy is usually required.

Procedure

Perform a venipuncture, and collect the sample in a 10-ml sterile *red-top* tube.

Precautions

Send the sample to the laboratory immediately. If transport must be delayed, store the sample at 39.2° F (4° C).

Normal findings

Depending on the test method, a negative finding or normal titer usually indicates the absence of mycosis.

Implications of results

The clinical significance of abnormal serologic test values varies, depending on which technique is used. (See *Implications of abnormal fungal serologic tests*, pages 343 and above.)

Post-test care

If a hematoma develops at the venipuncture site, apply warm soaks.

Interfering factors

■ Some antigens, such as the blastomycosis and histoplasmosis antigens, may cross-react to produce false-positive results or high titers.

■ Recent skin testing with fungal antigens may elevate titers.

■ Many mycoses depress the immune system, causing low titers or false-negative test results.

■ Failure to send a sterile sample to the laboratory immediately or to store the sample properly if transport is delayed may affect test results.

■ A nonfasting specimen may alter test results.

Serum *Candida* antibodies

Commonly present in the body, *Candida albicans* is a saprophytic yeast that can become pathogenic when the environment favors proliferation, or the host's defenses have been significantly weakened.

Candidiasis is usually limited to the skin and mucous membranes, but it may cause life-threatening systemic infection. Susceptibility to candidiasis is commonly associated with antibacterial, antimetabolic, or corticosteroid therapy and with immunologic defects, pregnancy, obesity, diabetes, and debilitating diseases. Oral candidiasis is common and benign in children; in adults, it may be the first sign of acquired immunodeficiency syndrome (AIDS).

Candidiasis is usually diagnosed by culture or histologic study. However, when such diagnosis cannot be made, identifying the *Candida* antibody may be helpful in diagnosing systemic candidiasis. Be aware that serologic testing for *Candida* antibodies is not reliable, and investigators continue to disagree about its usefulness.

Purpose
■ To aid diagnosis of candidiasis when culture or histologic study can't confirm diagnosis.

Patient preparation
Explain the purpose of the test to the patient, and tell him that he needn't restrict food or fluids. Inform him that the test requires a blood sample, who will perform the venipuncture and when, and that he may experience transient discomfort from the needle puncture and the pressure of the tourniquet.

Procedure
Perform a venipuncture and collect 5 ml of sterile blood in a *red-top* tube.

Precautions
■ Handle the sample gently to prevent hemolysis.
■ Send the sample to the laboratory promptly.
■ Note any recent antimicrobial therapy on the laboratory request.

Normal findings
A normal test result is negative for the *Candida* antigen. A positive test for the *C. albicans* antigen is common in patients with disseminated candidiasis but may also occur in 20% to 25% of normal people.

Implications of results
Because this test yields false-positive results in about 25% of people tested, interpretation of results is difficult.

Post-test care
If a hematoma develops at the venipuncture site, apply warm soaks.

Interfering factors
Hemolysis caused by excessive agitation of the sample will alter test results.

Bacterial meningitis antigen

This test, usually performed by latex agglutination, can detect specific antigens of *Streptococcus pneumoniae, Neisseria meningitidis,* and *Haemophilus influenzae* type B, the principal etiologic agents in meningitis. This test can be performed on samples of serum, cerebrospinal fluid (CSF), urine, pleural fluid, or joint fluid; however, the preferred specimen is either CSF or urine.

Purpose
- To identify the etiologic agent in meningitis
- To aid diagnosis of bacterial meningitis
- To aid diagnosis of meningitis when the Gram-stained smear and culture are negative.

Patient preparation
Explain the purpose of the test, and inform the patient that it requires a urine or CSF specimen. If a CSF specimen is required, describe how it will be obtained. Tell the patient who will perform the procedure and when and that he may experience transient discomfort from the needle puncture. Advise him that a headache is the most common adverse effect of lumbar puncture but that his cooperation during the test minimizes this effect. Make sure the patient or a family member has signed a consent form.

Procedure
As required, a 10-ml urine specimen or a 1-ml CSF specimen is collected in a sterile container.

Precautions
- Maintain specimen sterility during collection.
- Wear gloves when obtaining or handling all specimens.
- Make sure all caps are tightly fastened on specimen containers.
- Promptly send the specimen to the laboratory on a refrigerated coolant.

Normal findings
Results are negative for bacterial antigens.

Implications of results
Positive results identify the specific bacterial antigen: *S. pneumoniae, N. meningitidis, H. influenzae* type B, or group B streptococci in infants younger than 3 months.

Post-test care
None.

Interfering factors
- Results may be influenced by previous antimicrobial therapy.
- Failure to maintain sterility during collection of the specimen can interfere with accurate test results.

Lyme disease serology

Lyme disease is a multisystem disorder characterized by dermatologic, neurologic, cardiac, and rheumatic manifestations in various stages. Epidemiologic and serologic studies implicate a commonly tickborne spirochete, *Borrelia burgdorferi*, as the causative agent.

Serologic tests, both indirect immunofluorescent and enzyme-linked immunosorbent assays, measure antibody response to this spirochete and indicate current infection or past exposure. These assays can identify 50% of patient's with early-stage Lyme disease; nearly 100% of patients with later complications of carditis, neuritis, or arthritis; and 100% of patients in remission.

In an indirect immunofluorescent assay, *B. burgdorferi* is grown in culture, fixed to a microscope slide, and then incubated with a human serum sample. A fluorescein-labeled antiglobulin is then introduced into the antigen-antibody complex. Any human antibody that binds to the spirochete is detected by viewing (under an ultraviolet microscope) the fluorescent antiglobulin that attaches to it.

Purpose
■ To confirm diagnosis of Lyme disease.

Patient preparation
Explain to the patient that this test helps determine whether his symptoms are caused by Lyme disease. Instruct him to fast for 12 hours before the blood sample is drawn but to drink fluids as usual. Tell the patient that this test requires a blood sample, who will perform the venipuncture and when, and that he may experience transient discomfort from the needle puncture and the pressure of the tourniquet.

Procedure
Perform a venipuncture, and collect the sample in a 7-ml *red-top* tube.

Precautions
■ Handle the specimen carefully to prevent hemolysis.
■ Send the specimen to the laboratory immediately.

Reference values
Normal serum values are nonreactive.

Implications of results
A positive Lyme serologic test strongly suggests the diagnosis but is not definitive. Other treponemal diseases and high rheumatoid factor titers can cause false-positive results. Patients with other treponemal diseases demonstrate considerable cross-reactivity, and up to 20% of patients with high rheumatoid factor titers may have positive Lyme disease reactions.

In addition, a negative result does not rule out Lyme disease. More than 15% of patients with Lyme disease fail to develop antibodies.

Post-test care
If a hematoma develops at the venipuncture site, apply warm soaks.

Interfering factors
■ Analysis of serum with high lipid levels may cause inaccurate test results and requires repetition of the test after a period of restricted fat intake.
■ Blood samples contaminated with other bacteria can cause false-positive results.
■ Hemolysis caused by excessive agitation of the sample can affect the accuracy of test results.

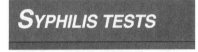

SYPHILIS TESTS

Venereal Disease Research Laboratory test

This flocculation test, commonly known as the VDRL test, is widely used to screen for primary and secondary syphilis. The test demonstrates the presence of reagin — an antibody relatively specific for *Treponema pallidum,* the spirochete that causes syphilis — in a serum sample after addition of an antigen consisting of cardiolipin and lecithin (two specific and reactive substances in beef heart muscle) and cholesterol. After the antigen complex is mixed with the serum on a slide, the sample is rotated and examined microscopically. If flocculation appears, the sample is diluted until no reaction occurs. The last dilution to reveal flocculation is taken as the titer.

Although the test has diagnostic significance during the first two stages of syphilis, transient or permanent biologic false-positive reactions can make accurate interpretation difficult. A biologic false-positive reaction can result from viral or bacterial infection, chronic systemic illness, or nonsyphilitic treponemal disease.

The VDRL test uses a serum sample but may also be performed on cerebrospinal fluid (CSF) to test for tertiary syphilis. However, the VDRL test of CSF is less sensitive than the fluorescent treponemal antibody absorption test. (See *Serodiagnostic tests for untreated syphilis.*) The rapid plasma reagin test can also be used to diagnose syphilis. (See *Rapid plasma reagin test,* page 350.)

Purpose

■ To screen for primary and secondary syphilis
■ To confirm primary or secondary syphilis in the presence of syphilitic lesions
■ To monitor response to treatment.

Patient preparation

Explain to the patient that this test detects syphilis. Tell him that he needn't restrict food, fluids, or medications but should abstain from alcohol for 24 hours before the test. Advise him that the test requires a blood sample, who will perform the venipuncture and when, and that he may experience transient discomfort from the needle puncture and the pressure of the tourniquet.

Procedure

Perform a venipuncture, and collect the sample in a 7-ml *red-top* tube.

Precautions

Handle the specimen carefully to prevent hemolysis.

Normal findings

Absence of flocculation is reported as a nonreactive test.

Implications of results

Definite flocculation is reported as a reactive test; slight flocculation is reported as a weakly reactive test. A reactive VDRL test occurs in about 50% of patients with primary syphilis and in nearly all patients with secondary syphilis. If syphilitic lesions exist, a reactive VDRL test is diagnostic. If no lesions are evident, a reactive VDRL test necessitates repeated testing. However, biologic false-positive reactions can be caused by conditions unrelated to syphilis, such as infectious mononucleosis, malaria, leprosy, hepatitis, systemic lupus erythematosus, rheumatoid arthritis, and nonsyphilitic treponemal diseases, such as pinta or yaws.

A nonreactive test doesn't rule out syphilis because *T. pallidum* causes no detectable immunologic changes in the serum for 14 to 21 days after infection. However, dark-field microscopic examination of exudate from suspicious lesions can provide early diagnosis by identifying the causative spirochetes.

A reactive VDRL test using a CSF specimen indicates neurosyphilis, which can follow the primary and secondary stages in untreated persons.

Post-test care

■ If a hematoma develops at the venipuncture site, apply warm soaks.
■ If the test is nonreactive or borderline but syphilis hasn't been ruled out, instruct the patient to return for follow-up testing. Explain that borderline test results don't necessarily mean he is free of the disease.
■ If the test is reactive, explain the importance of proper treatment. Teach the patient about venereal disease and how it is spread, and stress the need for antibiotic therapy. Also, prepare him for mandatory inquiries from public health authorities. If the test is reactive but the patient shows no clinical signs of syphilis, explain that many uninfected per-

Serodiagnostic tests for untreated syphilis

The fluorescent treponemal antibody absorption (FTA-ABS) test — which uses a strain of the *Treponema pallidum* antigen itself as a reagent — is more sensitive than the Venereal Disease Research Laboratory (VDRL) test or the rapid plasma reagin (RPR) test in detecting all stages of untreated syphilis (as shown in the graph below). However, the test's complexity and the incidence of false-positive results make it an impractical screening tool. The VDRL and RPR tests are preferred for wide-scale screening and also when primary- or secondary-stage disease is suspected. In advanced syphilis, when the VDRL test may be negative for more than one-third of infected people, the FTA-ABS test is preferred for sensitivity.

The VDRL test also can be used to monitor response to treatment. Untreated syphilis produces titers that are low in the primary stage (<1:32), elevated in the secondary stage (>1:32), and variable in the tertiary stage. Successful therapy markedly reduces titers, with two-thirds of patients reverting to a negative VDRL, especially during the first two stages of the disease. Third-stage therapy seldom produces a nonreactive VDRL, but maintenance of low-reactive values during the 6- to 12-month post-therapy period indicates success. A subsequent rise signals reinfection. By comparison, FTA-ABS test results usually remain positive following treatment.

A significant number of patients with infectious diseases show temporary false-positive VDRL test results. Chronic false-positive VDRL and FTA-ABS test readings are associated with the immune complex diseases.

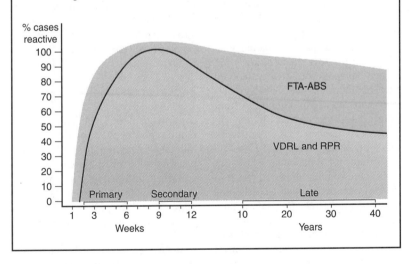

sons show false-positive reactions. However, stress the need for further specific tests to rule out syphilis.

Interfering factors
■ Ingestion of alcohol within 24 hours of the test can produce transient, nonreactive results.

■ A faulty immune system can cause nonreactive results.

■ Hemolysis of the sample can interfere with test results.

Rapid plasma reagin test

This rapid, macroscopic serologic test is an acceptable substitute for the VDRL test in diagnosing syphilis. The RPR test, available as a kit, uses a cardiolipin antigen to detect reagin, the antibody relatively specific for *Treponema pallidum,* the causative agent of syphilis.

In the RPR test, the patient's serum is mixed with cardiolipin on a plastic-coated card, rotated mechanically, and then examined with the unaided eye. If flocculation occurs, the test sample is diluted until no visible reaction occurs. The last dilution to show visible flocculation is the titer of the reagin antibody.

In the RPR test, like the VDRL test, normal serum shows no flocculation.

Fluorescent treponemal antibody absorption

The fluorescent treponemal antibody absorption (FTA-ABS or FTA) test uses indirect immunofluorescence to detect antibodies to the spirochete *Treponema pallidum* — the cause of syphilis — in serum. In this test, prepared *T. pallidum* is fixed on a slide, and the patient's serum is added after the addition of an absorbed preparation of Reiter treponema. This addition to the test serum prevents interference by antibodies from nonsyphilitic treponemas; Reiter treponema combines with most nonsyphilitic antibodies, making the FTA-ABS test specific for *T. pallidum.*

If syphilitic antibodies are present in the test serum, they will coat the treponemal organisms. The slide is then stained with fluorescein-labeled antiglobulin. This antiglobulin attaches to the coated spirochetes, which fluoresce when viewed under a microscope with ultraviolet light.

Although the FTA-ABS test is generally performed on a serum sample to detect primary or secondary syphilis, it requires a cerebrospinal fluid (CSF) specimen to detect tertiary syphilis. Because antibody levels remain constant for long periods, the FTA-ABS test is not recommended for monitoring response to therapy.

Two other tests can also detect *T. pallidum.* (See *Other tests for* Treponema pallidum.)

Purpose
▪ To confirm primary or secondary syphilis
▪ To screen for suspected false-positive results of the Venereal Disease Research Laboratory test.

Patient preparation
Explain to the patient that this test can confirm or rule out syphilis and doesn't require food or fluid restrictions. Tell him that the test requires a blood sample, who will perform the venipuncture and when, and that he may experience transient discomfort from the needle puncture and the pressure of the tourniquet.

Procedure
Perform a venipuncture, and collect the sample in a 7-ml *red-top* tube.

Precautions
Handle the sample gently to prevent hemolysis.

Other tests for Treponema pallidum

The microhemagglutination assay for *Treponema pallidum* antibody increases the specificity of syphilis testing by eliminating methodologic interference. In this assay, tanned sheep red blood cells are coated with *T. pallidum* antigen and are combined with absorbed test serum. Hemagglutination occurs in the presence of specific anti–*T. pallidum* antibodies in the serum.

In the enzyme-linked immunosorbent assay (ELISA), tubes coated with *T. pallidum* are washed and then treated with enzyme-labeled antihuman globulin. After the substrate for the enzymes is added to the tubes, the enzymatic activity is measured by quantitating the reaction product formed.

Normal findings
Reaction to the FTA-ABS test should be negative (no fluorescence).

Implications of results
The presence of treponemal antibodies in the serum — a reactive test result — does not indicate the stage or the severity of infection. (However, the presence of these antibodies in CSF is strong evidence of tertiary neurosyphilis.) Elevated antibody levels appear in 80% to 90% of patients with secondary syphilis. Higher antibody levels persist for several years, with or without treatment.

The absence of treponemal antibodies — a nonreactive test — doesn't necessarily rule out syphilis. *T. pallidum* causes no detectable immunologic changes in the blood for 14 to 21 days after initial infection. (A dark-field microscope may detect organisms earlier.) Low antibody levels or other nonspecific factors produce borderline findings. In such cases, repeated testing and a thorough review of the patient history may be productive.

Although the FTA-ABS test is specific, some patients with nonsyphilitic conditions — such as systemic lupus erythematosus, genital herpes, or increased or abnormal globulins — and pregnant women may show minimally reactive levels. In addition, the FTA-ABS test doesn't always distinguish between *T. pallidum* and certain other treponemas, such as those that cause pinta, yaws, and bejel.

Post-test care
■ If a hematoma develops at the venipuncture site, apply warm soaks.
■ If the test is reactive, explain the nature of syphilis, and stress the importance of proper treatment and the need to find and treat the patient's sexual partners. Also, prepare him for inquiries from the public health authorities.
■ If the test is nonreactive, or findings are borderline but syphilis has not been ruled out, instruct the patient to return for follow-up testing; explain that inconclusive results don't necessarily indicate he is free of the disease.

Interfering factors
Hemolysis caused by rough handling of the sample may affect test results.

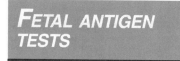

Fetal Antigen Tests

Carcinoembryonic antigen

Carcinoembryonic antigen (CEA), a glycoprotein secreted onto the glycocalyx surface of cells lining the GI tract, appears during the first or second trimester of fetal life. Production of CEA usually stops before birth but may begin again later if a neoplasm develops.

Because CEA levels are raised by biliary obstruction, alcoholic hepatitis, chronic heavy smoking, and other conditions as well as by benign or malignant neoplasms, this test can't be used as a general indicator of cancer. However, it is useful for staging colorectal cancer, assessing the adequacy of surgical resection, and monitoring the effectiveness of colorectal cancer therapy because serum CEA levels, measured by enzyme immunoassay, usually return to normal within 6 weeks if cancer treatment is successful. (See *Using CEA to monitor cancer treatment.*)

Purpose

■ To monitor the effectiveness of cancer therapy
■ To help stage colorectal cancer preoperatively and to test for its recurrence.

Patient preparation

Explain to the patient that the test detects and measures a special protein that's not normally present in adults. If appropriate, inform him that the test will be repeated to monitor the effectiveness of therapy.

Advise him that he needn't restrict food, fluids, or medications before the test. Tell him the test requires a blood sample, who will perform the venipuncture and when, and that he may experience transient discomfort from the needle puncture and the pressure of the tourniquet.

Procedure

Perform a venipuncture, and collect the sample in a 7-ml *red-top* tube.

Precautions

Handle the sample gently to prevent hemolysis, and send it to the laboratory immediately.

Reference values

Normal serum CEA values are less than 5 ng/ml in healthy nonsmokers. However, about 5% of the population has above-normal CEA concentrations.

Implications of results

If serum CEA levels are above-normal before surgical resection, chemotherapy, or radiation therapy, their return to normal within 6 weeks after therapy suggests successful treatment. Persistent elevation of CEA levels, however, suggests residual or recurrent tumor.

High CEA levels are characteristic in various malignant conditions, particularly endodermally derived neoplasms of the GI organs and the lungs, and in certain nonmalignant conditions, such as benign hepatic disease, hepatic cirrhosis, alcoholic pancreatitis, and inflammatory bowel disease. Elevated CEA concentrations may also result from nonendodermal cancers, such as breast cancer and ovarian cancer.

Post-test care

If a hematoma develops at the venipuncture site, apply warm soaks.

Interfering factors

■ Chronic cigarette smoking may elevate serum CEA levels, altering test results.
■ Hemolysis caused by rough handling may alter test results.

Using CEA to monitor cancer treatment

Because many patients in the early stages of colorectal cancer have normal or low levels of carcinoembryonic antigen (CEA), the CEA test does not screen successfully for early malignancy. It is a good tool, however, for monitoring response to cancer therapy.

Once a patient's serum CEA level has dropped following surgery, chemotherapy, or other treatment, any increase suggests recurrence of cancer or diminished effectiveness of treatment.

Both charts below illustrate CEA levels in patients during and after treatment for colorectal cancer. In the top chart, initial results show the usual dramatic drop in response to treatment; the subsequent rise in CEA indicates a diminishing response to chemotherapy. In the bottom chart, the progressive rise in CEA signals a recurrence of cancer 8 months before clinical symptoms or radiologic evidence.

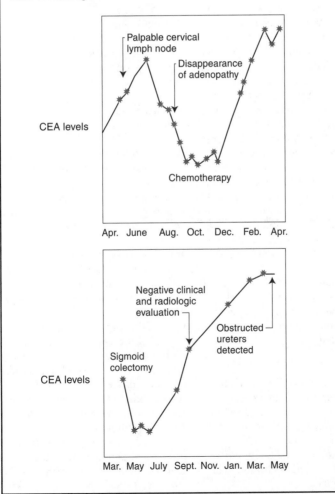

Alpha-fetoprotein

Alpha-fetoprotein (AFP) is a glycoprotein produced by fetal tissue and tumors that differentiate from midline embryonic structures. During fetal development, AFP levels in serum and amniotic fluid rise; because this protein crosses the placenta, it appears in maternal serum. In late stages of pregnancy, AFP concentrations in fetal and maternal serum and in amniotic fluid begin to diminish. During the first year of life, serum AFP levels continue to decline and usually remain low thereafter.

Fetal maternal serum AFP levels at 14 to 22 weeks' gestation may suggest fetal neural tube defects, such as spina bifida or anencephaly, but positive confirmation requires amniocentesis and ultrasonography. Other congenital anomalies may also be associated with high maternal serum AFP concentrations; evaluation for Down syndrome can be performed on serum samples from patients who are 15 to 20 weeks' pregnant. Elevated AFP levels in those persons who aren't pregnant may occur in malignancy, such as hepatocellular carcinoma, or in certain nonmalignant conditions, such as ataxia-telangiectasia; in these conditions, AFP assays are more useful for monitoring response to therapy than for diagnosis. AFP levels are best determined by enzyme-immunoassay on amniotic fluid or serum and should be used only as a tumor marker.

Purpose

■ To monitor the effectiveness of therapy in malignant diseases, such as hepatomas and germ cell tumors, and in certain nonmalignant disorders, such as ataxia-telangiectasia
■ To screen for the need for amniocentesis or high-resolution ultrasound in a pregnant female.

Patient preparation

Explain to the patient that this test monitors response to therapy or helps detect possible congenital defects in a fetus by measuring a specific blood protein. Advise the patient that she may need further testing. Tell her that she needn't restrict food, fluids, or medications before the test. Tell her that this test requires a blood sample, who will perform the venipuncture and when, and that she may experience transient discomfort from the needle puncture and the pressure of the tourniquet.

Procedure

Perform a venipuncture, and collect the sample in a 7-ml *red-top* tube. Record the patient's age, race, weight, and gestational period on the laboratory request.

Precautions

Handle the sample gently.

Reference values

When testing by immunoassay, AFP values are 0 to 6.4 IU/ml in males and nonpregnant females. For values in pregnant women, see *Alpha-fetoprotein values in pregnant women.*

Implications of results

Elevated maternal serum AFP levels may suggest a neural tube defect or other tube anomalies after 14 weeks' gestation. AFP levels rise sharply in approximately 90% of fetuses with anencephaly and in 50% of those with spina bifida. Definitive diagnosis requires ultrasonography and amniocentesis. High AFP levels may indicate intrauterine death or such anomalies as duodenal atresia, omphalocele, tetralogy of Fallot, or Turner's syndrome.

Elevated serum AFP levels in nonpregnant persons may indicate hepatocellular carcinoma (although low AFP levels don't rule it out) or germ cell tu-

Alpha-fetoprotein values in pregnant women

GESTATIONAL AGE (weeks)	MEDIAN VALUE IN WHITE WOMEN (IU/ml)	MEDIAN VALUE IN BLACK WOMEN (IU/ml)
14	19.9	23.2
15	23.2	26.9
16	27.0	31.1
17	31.5	35.9
18	36.7	41.6
19	42.7	48.0
20	49.8	55.6
21	58.1	64.2
22	67.8	74.2

mor of gonadal, retroperitoneal, or mediastinal origin. Serum AFP rises in ataxia-telangiectasia and, sometimes, in cancer of the pancreas, stomach, or biliary system. Transient modest elevations can occur in nonneoplastic hepatocellular disease, such as alcoholic cirrhosis and acute or chronic hepatitis.

In hepatocellular carcinoma, a gradual decrease in serum AFP levels indicates a favorable response to therapy. In germ cell tumors, serum AFP and human chorionic gonadotropin levels should be measured concurrently.

Post-test care
If a hematoma develops at the venipuncture site, apply warm soaks.

Interfering factors
- Hemolysis may alter test results.
- Multiple pregnancy may cause false-positive test results.

MISCELLANEOUS TEST

TORCH test

This test is performed to detect exposure to pathogens involved in congenital and neonatal infections. TORCH is an acronym for toxoplasmosis, rubella, cytomegalovirus, syphilis, and herpes simplex. These pathogens are commonly associated with congenital or neonatal infections that are not clinically apparent and may cause severe central nervous system impairment. This test confirms such infection serologically by detecting specific IgM-associated antibodies in infant blood.

Purpose
- To aid diagnosis of acute, congenital, and intrapartum infections.

Patient preparation
As appropriate, explain the purpose of the test and mention that the test re-

quires a blood sample. Tell the patient who will perform the venipuncture and when and that she may experience transient discomfort from the needle puncture and the pressure of the tourniquet.

Procedure
Obtain a 3-ml sample of venous or cord blood. Send it to the laboratory promptly for serologic testing.

Precautions
- Send the sample to the laboratory immediately.
- Don't freeze the sample.
- Handle the sample gently to prevent hemolysis.

Normal findings
Test results should be negative for TORCH agents.

Implications of results
Toxoplasmosis is diagnosed by sequential examination that shows rising antibody titers, changing titers, and serologic conversion from negative to positive; a titer of 1:256 suggests recent *Toxoplasma* infection. Approximately two-thirds of infected infants are asymptomatic at birth; one-third show signs of cerebral calcification and choroidoretinitis.

In infants less than 6 months old, rubella infection is associated with a marked and persistent rise in complement-fixing antibody titer over time. Persistence of rubella antibody in an infant after age 6 months strongly suggests congenital infection. Congenital rubella is associated with cardiac anomalies, neurosensory deafness, growth retardation and encephalitic symptoms. Detection of herpes antibodies in cerebrospinal fluid with signs of herpetic encephalitis, and persistent herpesvirus type 2 antibody levels confirm herpes simplex infection in a neonate without obvious herpetic lesions.

Post-test care
If a hematoma develops at the venipuncture site, apply warm soaks.

Interfering factors
Hemolysis caused by excessive agitation of the sample may affect the accuracy of test results.

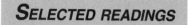

SELECTED READINGS

Diseases, 2nd ed. Springhouse, Pa.: Springhouse Corp., 1996.

Fischbach, F. *A Manual of Laboratory and Diagnostic Tests,* 5th ed. Philadelphia: Lippincott-Raven Pubs., 1996.

Guyton, A.C., and Hall, J.E. *Textbook of Medical Physiology,* 9th ed. Philadelphia: W.B. Saunders Co., 1996.

Henry, J.B., ed. *Clinical Diagnosis and Management by Laboratory Methods,* 19th ed. Philadelphia: W.B. Saunders Co., 1996.

Isselbacher, K.J., et al., eds. *Harrison's Principles of Internal Medicine,* 13th ed. New York: McGraw-Hill Book Co., 1994.

Leavelle, D., ed. *Mayo Medical Laboratories Interpretive Handbook.* Rochester, Minn.: Mayo Medical Laboratories, 1994.

Mayo Medical Laboratories 1996 Test Catalog. Rochester, Minn.: Mayo Medical Laboratories, 1996.

Nursing97 Drug Handbook. Springhouse, Pa.: Springhouse Corp., 1997.

Ravel, R.A. *Clinical Laboratory Medicine: Clinical Application of Laboratory Data,* 6th ed. St. Louis: Mosby–Year Book, Inc., 1995.

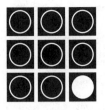

CHAPTER TWELVE

Urinalysis

Learning objectives

After completing this chapter, the reader will be able to:
- identify the components of the nephron unit and explain their functions
- describe the three mechanisms by which nephrons form urine
- list the common components of urine
- define the terms polyuria, oliguria, nocturia, and anuria
- state the causes, symptoms, and incidence of urinary calculi
- explain the importance of routine urinalysis
- state the purpose of each test discussed in the chapter
- prepare the patient physically and psychologically for each test
- describe the procedure for obtaining a specimen for each test
- specify appropriate precautions for accurately obtaining a specimen for each test
- implement appropriate post-test care
- state the reference values or findings for each test
- discuss the implications of abnormal test results
- list factors that may interfere with accurate test results.

INTRODUCTION

Routine urinalysis and special studies of renal function provide valuable information about the integrity of renal and urinary function and also serve as sensitive indicators of overall health. To understand the significance of such tests and their clinical applications, you need to know how urine is normally formed, what elements it contains, and the mechanisms that regulate urine volume.

Urine formation

The kidneys, through the activity of the nephrons, continuously remove metabolic wastes, drugs and other foreign substances, excess fluids, inorganic salts, and acid and base substances from the blood for eventual excretion in the urine. Each kidney has approximately 1 million *nephrons*; each nephron consists of a vascular ultrafilter called a *glomerulus* and a *renal tubule,* an epithelial-lined conduit for reabsorption of recy-

clable matter and secretion of foreign and waste substances. (See *Components of the nephron.*) The nephrons form urine through three mechanisms — *glomerular filtration, tubular reabsorption,* and *tubular secretion.*

Blood enters each kidney through the renal artery, passing through progressively smaller vascular channels and eventually entering the glomeruli through the afferent glomerular arterioles. These arterioles subdivide into clusters of capillary loops, each of which is partly enclosed in a membranous covering called Bowman's capsule. The walls of the capillaries are semipermeable, so dissolved substances can pass by simple filtration from the plasma through the glomerular capillaries and into the capsule space.

Blood leaves the glomeruli through the efferent glomerular arterioles and travels to a network of peritubular capillaries, which encircle the renal tubules. Glomerular filtrate leaves the Bowman's capsules and enters the proximal con-

Components of the nephron

Each kidney has about 1 million functional units called nephrons. In turn, each nephron contains a vascular ultrafilter called a glomerulus and a renal tubule, an epithelial-lined conduit made up of four sections (proximal convoluted tubule, loop of Henle, distal convoluted tubule, and collecting tubule). As the filtrate from the glomerulus travels through the renal tubules, reabsorption and secretion modify it to meet the body's needs. The end result is urine.

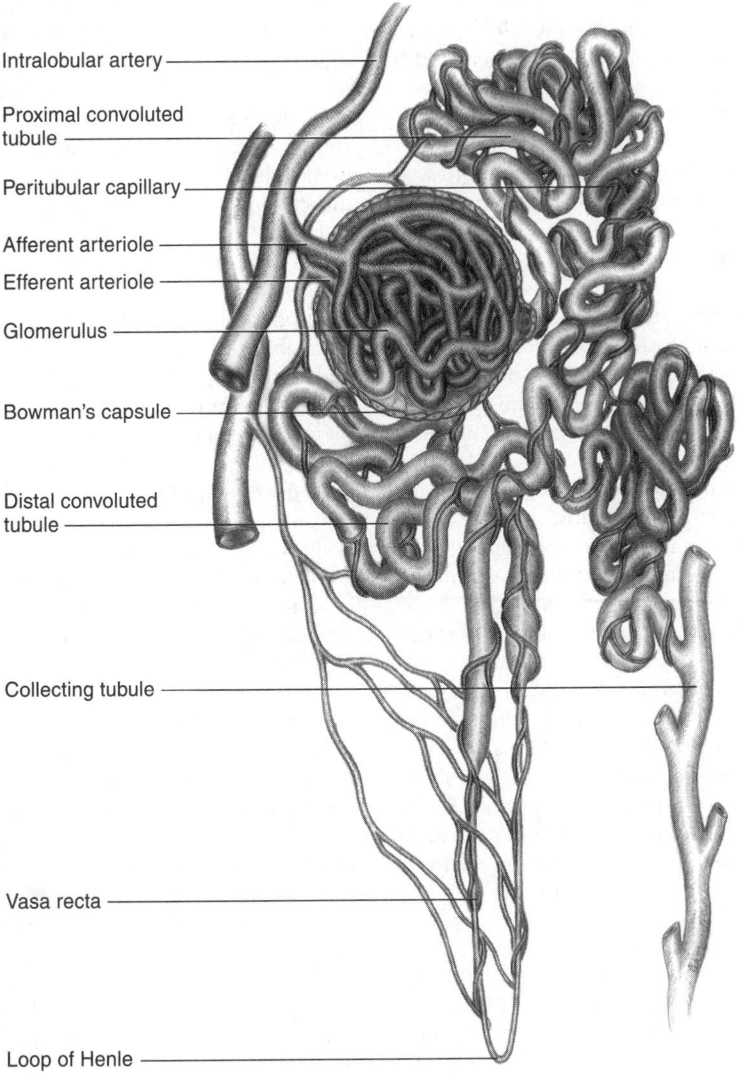

Intralobular artery

Proximal convoluted tubule

Peritubular capillary

Afferent arteriole

Efferent arteriole

Glomerulus

Bowman's capsule

Distal convoluted tubule

Collecting tubule

Vasa recta

Loop of Henle

voluted tubules, where approximately 65% is selectively reabsorbed by the peritubular capillaries. (Reabsorbed substances include water, glucose, some proteins, amino acids, acetoacetate ions, vitamins, and hormones.) The remaining 35% of the filtrate proceeds through the loops of Henle and the distal convoluted tubules, where sodium and water are reabsorbed as needed.

During secretion, fluid, solutes (such as potassium), uric acid, exogenous substances (such as drugs), and other waste materials move from the peritubular capillaries back into the glomerular filtrate. As the liquid filtrate evolves, it's continuously modified by filtration, reabsorption, and secretion. The end product is urine.

Urine composition

Although the actual composition of normal urine changes — depending on diet, physical activity, and emotional stress — it always includes water, urea, uric acid, and sodium chloride. Urine also usually contains other nonprotein nitrogen compounds, citric acid, other organic acids, catecholamines, sulfur-containing compounds, phosphate, potassium, calcium, magnesium, reducing substances, mucoproteins, vitamins, and hormones.

In the presence of disease, urine may contain protein, glucose, ketone bodies, hemoglobin, lipids, bacteria, pus, urobilinogen, bilirubin, or calculi. Microscopic examination of centrifuged urine sediment can detect cells, casts, crystals, bacteria, yeasts, parasites, spermatozoa, contaminants, and artifacts.

Urine volume

Urine volume, closely regulated by the kidneys, reflects overall fluid homeostasis. The volume depends on fluid intake, the concentration of solutes in the filtrate, cardiac output, hormonal influences, physical activity, and fluid loss through the lungs, large intestine, and skin. In adults, urine volume normally ranges from 800 to 2,000 ml/day and averages 1,200 to 1,500 ml/day. In children, volume ranges from 300 to 1,500 ml/day; however, a child's urine output is three to four times greater per kilogram of body weight than an adult's.

Polyuria, urine volume that exceeds 2,000 ml/day, is typical of many abnormal conditions. For example, it's a common effect of osmotic diuresis in diabetes mellitus, hyperparathyroidism, and infections. Polyuria can also result from insufficient secretion of antidiuretic hormone (ADH), as in pituitary diabetes insipidus, or from inability to respond to ADH, as in nephrogenic diabetes insipidus. Urine volume also increases from a lack of aldosterone, as in Addison's disease, which decreases renal reabsorption of sodium and water and decreases plasma volume. Polyuria follows the shift of interstitial fluid to plasma after burns or excessive intake or infusion of fluid. It also results from renal diseases in which the kidneys fail to concentrate urine and from the use of diuretics, alcohol, and caffeine.

Oliguria, the excretion of less than 500 ml of urine per day, can result from depressed sodium concentration in the filtrate because sodium normally promotes water excretion. It also follows any condition that decreases plasma volume — for example, when fluid shifts from plasma to the interstitial spaces, as in congestive heart failure; when fluid intake decreases; and when excess fluid escapes through extrarenal routes. Falling plasma volume and oliguria can follow dehydration due to prolonged vomiting, diarrhea, or profuse diaphoresis. Transfusion reactions, acute glomerulonephritis or pyelonephritis, and terminal chronic nephritis may cause oliguria and impair renal plasma flow and nephron function.

Anuria is the excretion of less than 100

ml of urine per day for 2 to 3 days despite high fluid intake. Anuria can follow oliguria in shock. It can also result from acute tubular necrosis caused by exposure to toxic agents, such as mercury bichloride, sulfonamides, and carbon tetrachloride, and from obstruction in bilateral hydronephrosis.

Nocturia, urine volume greater than 500 ml at night, with a specific gravity of less than 1.018, is characteristic of chronic glomerulonephritis and of heart or liver failure.

PHYSICAL AND CHEMICAL TESTS

Routine urinalysis

Routine urinalysis is important in screening for urinary and systemic disorders. These tests evaluate color, odor, and opacity (odor, though not usually documented on laboratory reports, may be noted under specimen comments); determine specific gravity and pH; detect and measure protein, glucose, and ketone bodies; and examine sediment for blood cells, casts, and crystals.

Diagnostic laboratory methods include visual examination, reagent strip screening, refractometry for specific gravity, and microscopic inspection of centrifuged sediment.

Purpose
▪ To screen urine for renal or urinary tract disease (See *Urine cytology*, page 362)
▪ To help detect metabolic or systemic disease unrelated to renal disorders.

Patient preparation
Explain that this test, which requires a urine specimen, aids diagnosis of renal or urinary tract disease and helps evaluate overall body function. Tell the patient he needn't restrict food or fluids but should avoid strenuous exercise before the test. Check the medication history for drugs that may affect test results.

Procedure
Collect a random urine specimen of at least 15 ml. If possible, obtain a first-voided morning specimen.

Precautions
▪ If the patient is being evaluated for renal colic, strain the specimen to catch stones or stone fragments. Place an unfolded 4" x 4" gauze pad or a fine-mesh sieve over the specimen container, and carefully pour the urine through it.
▪ Send the specimen to the laboratory immediately, or refrigerate it if analysis will be delayed longer than 1 hour.

Normal findings
See *Normal findings in routine urinalysis*, page 364.

Implications of results
Nonpathologic variations in normal values may result from diet, use of certain drugs, nonpathologic conditions, specimen collection time, and other factors. (See *Drugs that influence routine urinalysis results*, pages 365 and 366.) For example, specific gravity influences urine color and odor: as specific gravity increases, urine becomes darker and its odor becomes stronger.

Urine pH, which is greatly affected by diet and medications, influences the appearance of urine and the composition of crystals. An alkaline pH (above 7.0) — characteristic of a vegetarian diet — causes turbidity and formation of phosphate, carbonate, and amor-

Urine cytology

Epithelial cells line the urinary tract and exfoliate easily into the urine, so a simple cytologic examination of these cells can aid diagnosis of urinary tract disease. Although urine cytology is not performed routinely, it's useful for detecting cancer and inflammatory diseases of the renal pelvis, ureters, bladder, and urethra. It's especially useful for detecting bladder cancer in high-risk groups, such as smokers, people who work with aniline dyes (such as leather workers), and patients who have already received treatment for bladder cancer. Urine cytology can also determine whether bladder lesions that appear on X-rays are benign or malignant. This test can also detect cytomegalovirus infection and other viral disease.

To perform the test, the patient must collect a 100- to 300-ml clean-catch urine specimen 3 hours after his last voiding. (He should not use the first-voided specimen of the morning.) The urine specimen is sent to the cytology laboratory immediately so that it can be examined before the cells begin to degenerate.

Preparing the specimen

The specimen is prepared in one of the following ways and stained with Papanicolaou stain:

■ *Centrifuge:* After the urine is spun down, the sediment is smeared on a glass slide and stained for examination.

■ *Filter:* Urine is poured through a filter, which traps the cells so that they can be stained and examined directly.

■ *Cytocentrifuge:* After the urine is centrifuged, the sediment is resuspended and placed on slides, which are spun in a cytocentrifuge and stained for examination.

Implications of results

Normal urine is relatively free of cellular debris but should have some epithelial and squamous cells that appear normal under a microscope. Identification of malignant cells or any other signs of malignancy may indicate cancer of the kidney, renal pelvis, ureters, bladder, or urethra. It could also indicate a metastatic tumor.

An overgrowth of epithelial cells, an excess of red blood cells, or the presence of leukocytes or atypical cells may indicate a lower urinary tract inflammation, which can result from prostatic hyperplasia, urinary calculi, bladder diverticula, strictures, or malformation.

Large intranuclear inclusions may indicate a cytomegalovirus infection, which usually affects the renal tubular epithelium. This type of viral infection commonly occurs in cancer patients undergoing chemotherapy and transplant patients receiving immunosuppressant drugs. Cytoplasmic inclusion bodies may also indicate measles and may precede the characteristic Koplik's spots.

---

phous crystals. An acidic pH (below 7.0) — typical of a high-protein diet — causes turbidity and formation of oxalate, cystine, leucine, tyrosine, amorphous urate, and uric acid crystals.

Protein, normally absent from urine, may be present in a benign condition known as orthostatic (postural) proteinuria. Most common in patients age 10 to 20, this condition is intermittent — it appears after prolonged standing and disappears after recumbency.

Transient benign proteinuria can also occur with fever, exposure to cold, emotional stress, or strenuous exercise.

Sugars, usually absent from urine, may appear under normal conditions. The most common sugar in urine is glucose. Transient, nonpathologic glycosuria may result from emotional stress or pregnancy and may follow ingestion of a high-carbohydrate meal.

Centrifuged urine sediment contains cells, casts, crystals, bacteria, yeasts, and parasites. Red blood cells (RBCs) don't usually appear in urine without pathologic significance, but hard exercise can cause hematuria.

The following abnormal findings generally suggest pathologic conditions.

■ *Color:* Color change can result from diet, drugs, and many diseases.

■ *Odor:* In diabetes mellitus, starvation, and dehydration, a fruity odor accompanies formation of ketone bodies. In urinary tract infections, a common fetid odor is associated with *Escherichia coli.* Maple syrup urine disease and phenylketonuria also cause distinctive odors.

■ *Turbidity:* Turbid urine may contain RBCs or white blood cells (WBCs), bacteria, fat, or chyle and may reflect renal infection.

■ *Specific gravity:* Low specific gravity (<1.005) is characteristic of diabetes insipidus, acute tubular necrosis, and pyelonephritis. Fixed specific gravity, in which values remain 1.010 regardless of fluid intake, occurs in chronic glomerulonephritis with severe renal damage. High specific gravity (>1.035) occurs in nephrotic syndrome, dehydration, acute glomerulonephritis, congestive heart failure, liver failure, and shock.

■ *pH:* Alkaline urine pH may result from Fanconi's syndrome, urinary tract infection, and metabolic or respiratory alkalosis. Acidic urine pH is associated with renal tuberculosis, pyrexia, phenylketonuria, alkaptonuria, and acidosis.

■ *Protein:* Proteinuria may result from renal failure or disease (including nephrosis, glomerulosclerosis, glomerulonephritis, nephrolithiasis, and polycystic kidney disease) or possibly multiple myeloma.

■ *Sugars:* Glycosuria usually indicates diabetes mellitus but may result from pheochromocytoma, Cushing's syndrome, impaired tubular reabsorption, advanced renal disease, or increased intracranial pressure. Fructosuria, galactosuria, and pentosuria generally suggest rare hereditary metabolic disorders (except for lactosuria during pregnancy and lactation). However, an alimentary form of pentosuria and fructosuria may follow excessive ingestion of pentose or fructose. When the liver fails to metabolize these sugars, they spill into the urine because the renal tubules don't reabsorb them.

■ *Ketones:* Ketonuria occurs in diabetes mellitus when cellular energy needs exceed available cellular glucose. In the absence of glucose, cells metabolize fat for energy. Ketone bodies — the end products of incomplete fat metabolism — accumulate in plasma and are excreted in the urine. Ketonuria may also occur in starvation states and following diarrhea or vomiting.

■ *Bilirubin:* Bilirubin in urine may occur in liver disease resulting from obstructive jaundice or hepatotoxic drugs or toxins, or from fibrosis of the biliary canaliculi (as in cirrhosis).

■ *Urobilinogen:* Bilirubin is changed into urobilinogen in the duodenum by intestinal bacteria. The liver reprocesses the remainder into bile. Increased urobilinogen in the urine may indicate liver damage, hemolytic disease, or severe infection. Decreased levels may occur with biliary obstruction, inflammatory disease, antimicrobial therapy, severe diarrhea, or renal insufficiency.

■ *Cells:* Hematuria indicates bleeding within the genitourinary tract and may

Normal findings in routine urinalysis

ELEMENT	FINDINGS
Macroscopic	
Color	Straw to dark yellow
Odor	Slightly aromatic
Appearance	Clear
Specific gravity	1.005 to 1.035
pH	4.5 to 8.0
Protein	None
Glucose	None
Ketones	None
Bilirubin	None
Urobilinogen	Normal
Hemoglobin	None
Red blood cells	None
Nitrite (bacteria)	None
White blood cells	None
Microscopic	
Red blood cells	0 to 2/high-power field
White blood cells	0 to 5/high-power field
Epithelial cells	0 to 5/high-power field
Casts	None, except 1 to 2 hyaline casts/low-power field
Crystals	Present
Bacteria	None
Yeast cells	None
Parasites	None

result from infection, obstruction, inflammation, trauma, tumors, glomerulonephritis, renal hypertension, lupus nephritis, renal tuberculosis, renal vein thrombosis, renal calculi, hydronephrosis, pyelonephritis, scurvy, malaria, parasitic infection of the bladder, subacute bacterial endocarditis, polyarteritis nodosa, or hemorrhagic disorders. Strenuous exercise or exposure to toxic chemicals may also cause hematuria.

WBCs and white cell casts in urine suggest renal infection. An excess of WBCs in urine usually implies urinary tract inflammation, especially cystitis or pyelonephritis. Numerous epithelial

Drugs that influence routine urinalysis results

DRUGS THAT CHANGE URINE COLOR

Chlorzoxazone (orange to purple-red)
Deferoxamine mesylate (red)
Fluorescein sodium I.V. (yellow-orange)
Furazolidone (brown)
Iron salts (black)
Levodopa (dark)
Methylene blue (blue-green)
Metronidazole (dark)
Nitrofurantoin (brown)
Oral anticoagulants, indandione derivatives (orange)
Phenazopyridine (orange, red, or orange-brown)
Phenolphthalein (red to purple-red)
Phenolsulfonphthalein (pink or red)
Phenothiazines (dark)
Quinacrine (deep yellow)
Riboflavin (yellow)
Rifabutin (red-orange)
Rifampin (red-orange)
Sulfasalazine (orange-yellow)
Sulfobromophthalein (red)

DRUGS THAT CAUSE URINE ODOR

Antibiotics
Paraldehyde
Vitamins

DRUGS THAT INCREASE SPECIFIC GRAVITY

Albumin
Dextran
Glucose
Radiopaque contrast media

DRUGS THAT DECREASE pH

Ammonium chloride
Ascorbic acid
Diazoxide
Methenamine
Metolazone

DRUGS THAT INCREASE pH

Amphotericin B
Carbonic anhydrase inhibitors
Mafenide
Potassium citrate
Sodium bicarbonate

DRUGS THAT CAUSE FALSE-POSITIVE RESULTS FOR PROTEINURIA

Acetazolamide (Combistix)
Aminosalicylic acid (sulfosalicylic acid or Extons method)
Cephalothin in large doses (sulfosalicylic acid method)
Dichlorphenamide
Methazolamide
Nafcillin (sulfosalicylic acid method)
Sodium bicarbonate
Tolbutamide (sulfosalicylic acid method)
Tolmetin (sulfosalicylic acid method)

DRUGS THAT CAUSE TRUE PROTEINURIA

Aminoglycosides
Amphotericin B
Bacitracin
Cephalosporins
Cisplatin
Etretinate
Gold preparations
Isotretinoin

Proteinuria (continued)

Nonsteroidal anti-inflammatory drugs
Phenylbutazone
Polymyxin B
Sulfonamides
Trimethadione

DRUGS THAT CAN CAUSE EITHER TRUE PROTEINURIA OR FALSE-POSITIVE RESULTS

Penicillin in large doses (except with Ames reagent strips); however, some penicillins cause true proteinuria.
Sulfonamides (sulfosalicylic acid method)

DRUGS THAT CAUSE FALSE-POSITIVE RESULTS FOR GLYCOSURIA

Aminosalicylic acid (Benedict's test)
Ascorbic acid (Clinistix, Diastix, Tes-Tape)
Ascorbic acid in large doses (Clinitest tablets)
Cephalosporins (Clinitest tablets)
Chloral hydrate (Benedict's test)
Chloramphenicol (Clinitest tablets)
Isoniazid (Benedict's test)
Levodopa (Clinistix, Diastix, Tes-Tape)
Levodopa in large doses (Clinitest tablets)
Methyldopa (Tes-Tape)
Nalidixic acid (Benedict's test or Clinitest tablets)
Nitrofurantoin (Benedict's test)
Penicillin G in large doses (Benedict's test)
Phenazopyridine (Clinistix, Diastix, Tes-Tape)

(continued)

Drugs that influence routine urinalysis results (continued)

Glycosuria (continued)
Probenecid (Benedict's test, Clinitest tablets)
Salicylates in large doses (Clinitest tablets, Clinistix, Diastix, Tes-Tape)
Streptomycin (Benedict's test)
Tetracycline (Clinistix, Diastix, Tes-Tape)
Tetracyclines, due to ascorbic acid buffer (Benedict's test, Clinitest tablets)

DRUGS THAT CAUSE TRUE GLYCOSURIA

Ammonium chloride
Asparaginase
Carbamazepine
Corticosteroids
Dextrothyroxine
Lithium carbonate
Nicotinic acid (large doses)
Phenothiazines (long-term)
Thiazide diuretics

DRUGS THAT CAUSE FALSE-POSITIVE RESULTS FOR KETONURIA

Levodopa (Ketostix, Labstix)

Ketonuria (continued)
Phenazopyridine (Ketostix or Gerhardt's reagent strip shows atypical color)
Phenolsulfonphthalein (Rothera's test)
Phenothiazines (Gerhardt's reagent strip shows atypical color)
Salicylates (Gerhardt's reagent strip shows reddish color)
Sulfobromophthalein (Bili-Labstix)

DRUGS THAT CAUSE TRUE KETONURIA

Ether (anesthesia)
Insulin (excessive doses)
Isoniazid (intoxication)
Isopropyl alcohol (intoxication)

DRUGS THAT INCREASE WHITE BLOOD CELL COUNT

Allopurinol
Ampicillin
Aspirin (toxicity)
Kanamycin
Methicillin

DRUGS THAT CAUSE HEMATURIA

Amphotericin B
Coumarin derivatives
Methenamine in large doses
Methicillin
Para-aminosalicylic acid
Phenylbutazone
Sulfonamides

DRUGS THAT CAUSE CASTS

Amphotericin B
Aspirin (toxicity)
Bacitracin
Ethacrynic acid
Furosemide
Gentamicin
Griseofulvin
Isoniazid
Kanamycin
Neomycin
Penicillin
Radiographic agents
Streptomycin
Sulfonamides

DRUGS THAT CAUSE CRYSTALS (IF URINE IS ACIDIC)

Acetazolamide
Aminosalicylic acid
Ascorbic acid
Nitrofurantoin
Theophylline
Thiazide diuretics

cells suggest renal tubular degeneration.

■ *Casts:* These plugs of high-molecular-weight mucoprotein form in the renal tubules and collecting ducts by agglutination of protein cells or cellular debris and are flushed loose by urine flow. Excessive casts indicate renal disease.

Hyaline casts are associated with renal parenchymal disease, inflammation, and trauma to the glomerular capillary membrane; epithelial casts, with renal tubular damage, nephrosis, eclampsia, amyloidosis, and heavy metal poisoning; coarse and fine granular casts, with acute or chronic renal failure, pyelonephritis, and chronic lead intoxication; fatty and waxy casts, with nephrotic syndrome, chronic renal disease, and diabetes mellitus; RBC casts, with renal parenchymal disease (especially glomerulonephritis), renal infarction, sub-acute bacterial endocarditis, vascular disorders, sickle cell anemia, scurvy, blood dyscrasias, malignant hypertension, collagen disease, and acute inflammation; and WBC casts, with acute pyelonephritis and glomerulonephritis, nephrotic syndrome, pyogenic infection, and lupus nephritis.

■ *Crystals:* Some crystals normally appear in urine, but numerous calcium oxalate crystals suggest hypercalcemia. Cystine crystals (cystinuria) reflect an inborn error of metabolism.

■ *Other components:* Bacteria, yeast cells, and parasites in urinary sediment reflect genitourinary tract infection or contamination of external genitalia. Yeast cells, which may be mistaken for RBCs, are identifiable by their ovoid shape, lack of color, and variable size, and frequently by signs of budding. The most common parasite in urinary sediment is *Trichomonas vaginalis,* which causes vaginitis, urethritis, and prostatovesiculitis.

Post-test care
None.

Interfering factors
■ Failure to follow the proper collection procedure, to send the specimen to the laboratory immediately, or to refrigerate the specimen may affect the accuracy of test results.

■ Strenuous exercise before routine urinalysis may cause transient myoglobulinuria, resulting in inaccurate test results.

■ Many drugs influence the results of urinalysis.

Urinary calculi

Urinary calculi (commonly known as urinary stones) are insoluble substances that range in size from microscopic to several centimeters and may appear anywhere in the urinary tract. They're usually formed of the mineral salts calcium oxalate, calcium phosphate, magnesium ammonium phosphate, urate, or cystine. Calculi usually possess well-defined nuclei composed of bacteria, fibrin, blood clots, or epithelial cells that are enclosed in a protein matrix. Mineral salts accumulate around this matrix in layers, causing progressive enlargement.

Urinary calculi can result from reduced urinary volume, increased excretion of mineral salts, urinary stasis, pH changes, and decreased protective substances. They commonly form in the kidney, pass into the ureter, and are excreted in the urine. Because not all calculi pass spontaneously, they may require surgical extraction. Calculi don't always cause symptoms, but when they do, hematuria is most common. If calculi obstruct the ureter, they may cause severe flank pain, dysuria, urine retention, urinary frequency, and urinary urgency.

To test for urinary calculi, the patient must have all his urine carefully strained to remove any calculi. Qualitative chemical analysis then reveals the calculi's composition, which helps to identify their causes.

Purpose
■ To detect and identify calculi in the urine.

Patient preparation
Explain to the patient that the test detects urinary stones and that if such stones are found, laboratory analysis

Types and causes of calculi

A
Calcium oxalate calculi usually result from idiopathic hypercalciuria, a condition that reflects absorption of calcium from the bowel.

B
Calcium phosphate calculi usually result from primary hyperparathyroidism, which causes excessive resorption of calcium from bone.

C
Cystine calculi result from primary cystinuria, an inborn error of metabolism that prevents renal tubular reabsorption of cystine.

D
Urate calculi result from gout, dehydration (causing elevated uric acid levels), acidic urine, or hepatic dysfunction.

E
Magnesium ammonium phosphate calculi result from the presence of urea-splitting organisms, such as *Proteus*, which raises ammonia concentration and makes urine alkaline.

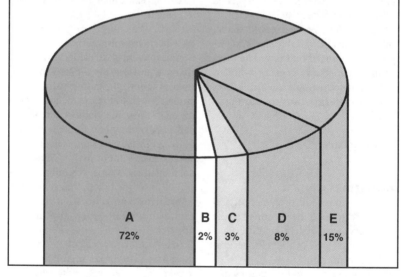

A	B	C	D	E
72%	2%	3%	8%	15%

will reveal their composition. Tell him the test requires that his urine be collected and strained. Advise him that he need not restrict food or fluids before the test. Reassure him that symptoms will subside immediately after any stones are excreted. Administer medication to control pain, as ordered.

Equipment
Strainer (unfolded 4" x 4" dressing or fine-mesh sieve) ✦ specimen container.

Procedure
After the patient voids into the strainer, inspect the strainer carefully because calculi may be minute. Calculi may look like gravel or sand. Document the appearance of the calculi and the number, if possible. Then place the calculi in a

properly labeled container, and send the container to the laboratory immediately for prompt analysis.

Precautions

If the patient has received analgesics, be sure to keep the strainer and urinal or bedpan within his reach because he may be drowsy and unable to get out of bed to void.

Normal findings

Calculi are not present in the urine.

Implications of results

More than half of all calculi in urine are of mixed composition, containing two or more mineral salts; calcium oxalate is the most common component. Determining the composition of calculi helps identify various metabolic disorders. (See *Types and causes of calculi.*)

Post-test care

▪ Observe for severe flank pain, dysuria, urine retention, urinary frequency, or urinary urgency. Hematuria should subside.
▪ Inform the patient of dietary restrictions intended to prevent formation of calculi.

Interfering factors

None.

TUBULAR FUNCTION TESTS

Urine osmolality

The kidneys normally concentrate or dilute urine according to fluid intake. When intake is excessive, the kidneys excrete more water in the urine; when intake is limited, they excrete less. To make such variation possible, the distal segment of the tubule varies its permeability to water in response to antidiuretic hormone, which, with renal blood flow, determines urine concentration or dilution.

This test measures the concentrating ability of the kidneys in acute and chronic renal failure. Osmolality is a more sensitive index of renal function than dilution techniques that measure specific gravity. It measures the number of osmotically active ions or particles present per kilogram of water. Osmolality is high in concentrated urine and low in dilute urine. It is determined by the effect of solute particles on the freezing point of the fluid.

Purpose

▪ To evaluate renal tubular function
▪ To detect renal impairment.

Patient preparation

Explain to the patient that this test evaluates kidney function. Tell him the test requires a urine specimen and collection of blood within 1 hour before or after the urine is collected. Withhold diuretics, as ordered.

Emphasize to the patient that his cooperation is necessary to obtain accurate results.

Procedure

Collect a random urine specimen, and draw a blood sample within 1 hour of urine collection. If a 24-hour urine collection is ordered, record the total urine volume on the laboratory request. (Preservatives are not required for a 24-hour container.)

Precautions

▪ Send each specimen to the laboratory immediately after collection.
▪ If the patient is unable to urinate into the specimen containers, provide him

with a clean bedpan, urinal, or toilet specimen pan. Rinse the collection device after each use.
■ If the patient is catheterized, empty the drainage bag before the test. Obtain the specimens from the catheter.

Reference values
For a random urine specimen, osmolality normally ranges from 50 to 1,400 mOsm/kg; for a 24-hour urine specimen, osmolality ranges from 300 to 900 mOsm/kg.

Implications of results
Decreased renal capacity to concentrate urine in response to fluid deprivation, or to dilute urine in response to fluid overload, may indicate tubular epithelial damage, decreased renal blood flow, loss of functional nephrons, or pituitary or cardiac dysfunction.

Post-test care
■ After collecting the final specimen, provide the patient with a balanced meal or a snack.
■ Make sure the patient voids within 8 to 10 hours after the catheter has been removed.

Interfering factors
■ Diuretics increase urine volume and dilution, thereby lowering specific gravity; nephrotoxic drugs cause tubular epithelial damage, thereby decreasing renal concentrating ability.
■ Patients who have been markedly overhydrated for several days before the test may have depressed concentration values; those who are dehydrated or have electrolyte imbalances may retain fluids, leading to inaccurate results.

Tubular reabsorption of phosphate

Because tubular reabsorption of phosphate is closely regulated by parathyroid hormone (PTH), measuring urine and plasma phosphate, with creatinine clearance, provides an indirect method of evaluating parathyroid function. PTH helps maintain optimum blood levels of ionized calcium and controls renal excretion of calcium and phosphate. Specifically, PTH stimulates reabsorption of calcium and inhibits reabsorption of phosphate from the glomerular filtrate. A regulatory feedback mechanism results in diminished PTH secretion as ionized calcium levels return to normal. In primary hyperparathyroidism, excessive secretion of PTH disrupts this calcium-phosphate balance.

This test is indicated to detect hyperparathyroidism in persons with clinical signs of this disorder and borderline or normal values for serum calcium, phosphate, and alkaline phosphatase.

Purpose
■ To evaluate parathyroid function
■ To aid diagnosis of primary hyperparathyroidism
■ To aid differential diagnosis of hypercalcemia.

Patient preparation
Explain to the patient that this test evaluates the function of the parathyroid glands and that it requires a blood sample and a 24-hour urine collection. Tell him who will perform the venipuncture and when and that he may experience transient discomfort from the needle puncture and the pressure of the tourniquet.

Instruct the patient to maintain a normal phosphate diet for 3 days before the test because low phosphate intake (less than 500 mg/day) may elevate tubular reabsorption values and a high-phosphate diet (3,000 mg/day or more) may lower them. Common dietary sources of phosphorus include legumes, nuts, milk, egg yolks, meat, poultry, fish, cereals, and cheese. These foods should be eaten in moderate amounts. Instruct the patient to fast from midnight the night before the test.

As ordered, withhold drugs that are known to influence test results, such as amphotericin B, thiazide diuretics, furosemide, and gentamicin. If these medications must be continued throughout the test period, note this on the laboratory request.

Procedure
First, perform a venipuncture, and collect the sample in a 10-ml *red-top* tube. Then instruct the patient to empty his bladder and discard the urine; record this as time zero. Collect a 24-hour urine specimen. (Occasionally, a 4-hour collection is ordered instead.)

After the venipuncture, allow the patient to eat, and encourage fluid intake to maintain adequate urine flow.

Precautions
- Handle the collection tube gently to prevent hemolysis, and send it to the laboratory immediately.
- Keep the urine specimen container refrigerated or on ice during the collection period. Tell the patient to avoid contaminating the specimen with toilet paper or stool.
- At the end of the collection period, label the specimen and send it to the laboratory immediately.

Normal findings
Renal tubules normally reabsorb 80% or more of phosphate.

Implications of results
Reabsorption of less than 74% of phosphate strongly suggests primary hyperparathyroidism, but additional studies are needed to confirm this diagnosis as the cause of hypercalcemia. Chest and bone X-rays and bone scans should be performed because bone metastasis is the most common cause of hypercalcemia. Depressed reabsorption occurs in a small number of patients with renal calculi but without parathyroid tumor. However, normal reabsorption occurs in roughly 20% of patients with parathyroid tumor. Increased reabsorption of phosphate may result from uremia, renal tubular disease, osteomalacia, sarcoidosis, or myeloma.

Post-test care
- If a hematoma develops at the venipuncture site, apply warm soaks.
- As ordered, resume the patient's regular diet and administration of any medications that were discontinued before the test.

Interfering factors
- Hemolysis caused by rough handling of the sample may alter test results.
- Failure to collect all urine during the test period may affect the accuracy of test results.
- The patient's failure to follow guidelines for diet restrictions and phosphate intake may alter test results.
- Amphotericin B and thiazide diuretics may diminish reabsorption; furosemide and gentamicin may enhance reabsorption.

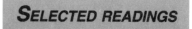

SELECTED READINGS

Black, J.M., and Matassarin-Jacobs, E., eds. *Luckmann and Sorensen's Medical-Surgical Nursing: A Psychophysiologic Approach,* 4th ed. Philadelphia: W.B. Saunders Co., 1993.

Fischbach, F. *A Manual of Laboratory and Diagnostic Tests,* 5th ed. Philadelphia: Lippincott-Raven Pubs., 1996.

Guyton, A.C., and Hall, J.E. *Textbook of Medical Physiology,* 9th ed. Philadelphia: W.B. Saunders Co., 1996.

Henry, J.B., ed. *Clinical Diagnosis and Management by Laboratory Methods,* 19th ed. Philadelphia: W.B. Saunders Co., 1996.

Karlowicz, K.A. *Urologic Nursing: Principles and Practice.* Philadelphia: W.B. Saunders Co., 1995.

Malarkey, L.M., and McMorrow, M.E. *Nurse's Manual of Laboratory Tests and Diagnostic Procedures.* Philadelphia: W.B. Saunders Co., 1996.

Phipps, W.J., et al. *Medical-Surgical Nursing: Concepts and Clinical Practice,* 5th ed. St. Louis: Mosby-Year Book, Inc., 1995.

Schumann, G.B. "The Growing Importance of Urinary Cytologic Testing," *Laboratory Medicine* 26(12): 801-09, December 1995.

Tilkian, S.M., et al. *Clinical and Nursing Implications of Laboratory Tests,* 5th ed. St. Louis: Mosby–Year Book, Inc., 1995.

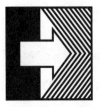

CHAPTER THIRTEEN

Urine enzymes

Learning objectives

After completing this chapter, the reader will be able to:
- explain the importance of measuring urine enzyme levels
- define the term enzyme
- discuss the role of cyclic adenosine monophosphate (cAMP) as an intracellular mediator
- state the purpose of each test discussed in the chapter
- prepare the patient physically and psychologically for each test
- describe the procedure for obtaining a specimen for each test
- list conditions that contraindicate the test for cAMP
- implement appropriate post-test care
- state the reference values for each test
- discuss the implications of abnormal test results
- list factors that may interfere with accurate test results.

INTRODUCTION

Enzymes are protein molecules that promote chemical reactions in the body without being destroyed or permanently changed themselves. They're present in all body tissues and fluids: tears, saliva, sweat, blood, urine, and digestive juices. Because enzyme actions are quite specific to tissue sites, abnormal enzyme levels often can identify and locate tissue damage or disease. Cellular damage or necrosis is likely to cause the release of a large aggregation of enzymes into the blood. When such enzymes saturate the serum, they exceed the renal threshold, and a significant quantity spill over into the urine. Because enzymes that circulate in the blood are normally reabsorbed by the renal tubules, with only small amounts excreted in the urine, increased enzyme levels in the urine may also signal renal dysfunction, especially impaired tubular reabsorption.

Because elevated urine levels may persist longer than serum levels (for example, of amylase), urine enzyme measurements can provide delayed or retrospective diagnosis. They also help monitor the progression of illness and the effec-tiveness of treatment in patients with confirmed disease.

Urine amylase, the most frequently performed urine enzyme test, can confirm acute pancreatitis and can aid diagnosis of chronic pancreatitis and salivary gland disorders. *Arylsulfatase A,* a rarely requested test, aids diagnosis of colorectal or bladder cancer, myeloid leukemia, and metachromatic leukodystrophy. *Lysozyme,* another rarely requested test, evaluates renal function, helps detect rejection or infarction of kidney transplants, and aids diagnosis of acute monocytic and granulocytic leukemia. *Cyclic adenosine monophosphate,* another enzyme detectable in urine, is measured after injection of parathyroid hormone to aid differential diagnosis of pseudohypoparathyroidism.

Because enzymes are especially affected by pH, specific gravity, and bacteria, reliable enzyme measurement requires certain precautions during urine collection. Such testing requires an uncontaminated timed urine specimen and an adequate patient intake of fluid. For a valid specimen, the collection container must contain the proper preservative, if one is designated by the laboratory, to maintain the required pH. Finally, the specimen must be refrigerated or packed in ice throughout the collection period to inhibit bacterial growth. Failure to meet any of these requirements may invalidate the test results.

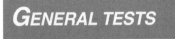

Urine amylase

Amylase is a starch-splitting enzyme produced primarily in the pancreas and salivary glands, usually secreted into the alimentary tract, and absorbed into the blood; small amounts of amylase are also absorbed into the blood directly from the pancreas and salivary glands. After glomerular filtration, amylase is excreted in the urine. If renal function is adequate, serum and urine levels usually rise in tandem. However, within 2 to 3 days after the onset of acute pancreatitis, serum amylase levels fall to normal, but urine amylase levels remain elevated for 7 to 10 days. One method of determining urine amylase levels is the dye-coupled starch method.

Purpose
■ To diagnose acute pancreatitis when serum amylase levels are normal or borderline
■ To aid diagnosis of chronic pancreatitis and salivary gland disorders.

Patient preparation
Explain to the patient that this test evaluates the function of the pancreas and the salivary glands. Inform him that he needn't restrict food or fluids. Tell him the test requires urine collection for 2, 6, 8, or 24 hours, and teach him how to collect a timed specimen. If a female

patient is menstruating, the test may have to be rescheduled.

As ordered, withhold morphine, meperidine, codeine, pentazocine, bethanechol, thiazide diuretics, indomethacin, and alcohol for 24 hours before the test. If these medications must be continued, note this on the laboratory request.

Procedure
Collect a 2-, 6-, 8-, or 24-hour specimen.

Precautions
■ Cover and refrigerate the specimen during the collection period. If the patient is catheterized, keep the collection bag on ice.
■ Instruct the patient not to contaminate the specimen with toilet tissue or stool.
■ Send the specimens to the laboratory as soon as the test is completed.

Reference values
Values differ from laboratory to laboratory, but urinary excretion of 10 to 80 amylase units/hour is generally considered normal.

Implications of results
Elevated amylase levels occur in acute pancreatitis; obstruction of the pancreatic duct, intestines, or salivary duct; carcinoma of the head of the pancreas; mumps; acute injury to the spleen; renal disease, with impaired absorption; perforated peptic or duodenal ulcers; and gallbladder disease.

Depressed levels occur in chronic pancreatitis, cachexia, alcoholism, cancer of the liver, cirrhosis, hepatitis, and hepatic abscess. (See *Serum and urine amylase values in acute pancreatitis,* page 376.)

Post-test care
None.

Serum and urine amylase values in acute pancreatitis

	SERUM	URINE
Normal	▪ 138 to 404 amylase units/L	▪ 10 to 80 amylase units/hour
Elevation	▪ Rises rapidly within 3 to 6 hours after onset of attack ▪ May rise to 40 times normal value ▪ Increase is not proportional to severity of attack	▪ Reflects rise in serum level, but lags 6 to 10 hours
Duration	▪ Peaks 20 to 30 hours after onset ▪ Returns to normal level within 2 or 3 days, although active inflammation of pancreas may persist ▪ Persistent elevation suggests pseudocyst, necrosis, or renal disease that inhibits amylase excretion	▪ Elevation persists for 7 to 10 days ▪ Allows retrospective diagnosis of acute or relapsing pancreatitis when serum level registers in normal range ▪ Persistent elevation in the absence of renal disease suggests pseudocyst formation

Interfering factors

▪ Heavy bacterial contamination of the specimen or blood in the urine may affect test results.

▪ Salivary amylase in the urine due to coughing or talking over the sample may raise urine amylase levels.

▪ Failure to collect all urine during the test period or to store the specimen properly may alter test results.

▪ Ingestion of morphine, meperidine, codeine, pentazocine, bethanechol, thiazide diuretics, indomethacin, or alcohol within 24 hours of the test may raise urine amylase levels. Fluoride may lower urine amylase levels.

Arylsulfatase A

Arylsulfatase A (ARS A), a lysosomal enzyme found in every cell except the mature erythrocyte, is principally active in the liver, the pancreas, and the kidneys, where exogenous substances are detoxified into ester sulfates. When ARS A is present in large amounts, it reverses this process by catalyzing the release of free phenylsulfates, such as benzidine and naphthaline, from the ester sulfates.

Although urine ARS A levels rise in transitional bladder cancer, colorectal cancer, and leukemia, research hasn't resolved whether elevated ARS A levels provoke malignant growths or are simply an enzymatic response to them. This test measures urine ARS A levels by colorimetric or kinetic techniques.

Purpose
▪ To aid diagnosis of bladder, colon, or rectal cancer; myeloid (granulocytic) leukemia; and metachromatic leukodystrophy (an inherited lipid storage disease).

Patient preparation
Explain to the patient that this test measures an enzyme that's present throughout the body. Advise him that he needn't restrict food or fluids before the test. Tell him the test requires 24-hour urine collection, and teach him how to collect a timed specimen. Test results are generally available in 2 or 3 days.

If a female patient is menstruating, the test may have to be rescheduled because increased numbers of epithelial cells in the urine raise ARS A levels.

Procedure
Collect a 24-hour urine specimen.

Precautions
▪ Tell the patient not to contaminate the urine specimen with toilet tissue or stool.
▪ Keep the collection container refrigerated or on ice during the collection period, and send the specimen to the laboratory as soon as the collection period is over. If the patient has an indwelling urinary catheter in place, keep the collection bag on ice for the duration of the test; the continuous urinary drainage apparatus should be changed before beginning the test.

Reference values
ARS A values normally range from 1.4 to 19.3 U/L in men, from 1.4 to 11 U/L in women, and over 1 U/L in children.

Implications of results
Elevated ARS A levels may result from bladder, colon, or rectal cancer or from myeloid leukemia. Decreased ARS A levels can result from metachromatic leukodystrophy. (In these patients, urine studies show metachromatic granules in the urinary sediment.)

Post-test care
None.

Interfering factors
▪ Failure to collect all urine during the test period may alter test results.
▪ Contamination of the urine specimen by stool or menses or by improper storage may alter test results.
▪ Surgery performed within 1 week before the test may raise ARS A levels.

Lysozyme

Lysozyme, a low-molecular-weight enzyme, is present in mucus, saliva, tears, skin secretions, and various internal body cells and fluids. This enzyme (also known as muramidase) splits, or lyses, the cell walls of gram-positive bacteria and, with complement and other blood factors, acts to destroy them. Lysozyme seems to be synthesized in granulocytes and monocytes, and it first appears in serum after destruction of such cells. When serum lysozyme levels exceed three times the normal rate, the enzyme appears in the urine. However, because renal tissue also contains lysozyme, renal injury alone can cause measurable excretion of this enzyme.

This test measures urine lysozyme levels turbidimetrically. Serum lysozyme values, using the same method, confirm the results of urine testing.

Purpose
- To aid diagnosis of acute monocytic or granulocytic leukemia and to monitor the progression of these diseases
- To evaluate proximal tubular function and to diagnose renal impairment
- To detect rejection or infarction of a kidney transplant.

Patient preparation
Explain to the patient that this test evaluates renal function and the immune system. Advise him that he needn't restrict food or fluids before the test. Tell him the test requires collection of a 24-hour urine specimen, and instruct him how to collect the specimen correctly. Test results should be available in 1 day.

If a female patient is menstruating, the test may have to be rescheduled.

Procedure
Collect a 24-hour urine specimen.

Precautions
- Tell the patient to avoid contaminating the urine specimen with toilet tissue or stool.
- Cover and refrigerate the specimen during the collection period. If the patient is catheterized, keep the collection bag on ice.
- Send the specimen to the laboratory as soon as the test is completed.

Reference values
Normally, urine lysozyme values are less than 3 mg/24 hours.

Implications of results
Elevated urine lysozyme levels are characteristic of impaired renal proximal tubular reabsorption, acute pyelonephritis, nephrotic syndrome, tuberculosis of the kidney, severe extrarenal infection, rejection or infarction of a kidney transplant, and polycythemia vera. Urine levels rise markedly after acute onset or relapse of monocytic or my-elomonocytic leukemia and rise moderately after acute onset or relapse of granulocytic (myeloid) leukemia.

Urine lysozyme levels remain normal or decrease in lymphocytic leukemia, and remain normal in myeloblastic and myelocytic leukemias.

Post-test care
None.

Interfering factors
- The presence of bacteria in the specimen decreases urine lysozyme levels; blood or saliva in the specimen raises lysozyme levels.
- Failure to collect all urine during the test period may alter test results.

STIMULATION TEST

Cyclic adenosine monophosphate

Formed from adenosine triphosphate by the action of the enzyme adenylate cyclase, the nucleotide cyclic adenosine monophosphate (cAMP) influences the protein synthesis rate within cells. (See *cAMP: The second messenger.*) Measuring urinary excretion of cAMP after I.V. infusion of a standard dose of parathyroid hormone (PTH) can show renal tubular resistance in a patient with hypoparathyroid symptoms and high levels of PTH. Such findings suggest Type I pseudohypoparathyroidism. This rare inherited disorder results from tissue resistance to PTH and produces hypocalcemia, hyperphosphatemia, and skeletal and constitutional abnormalities.

This test is contraindicated in patients with high calcium levels because PTH further raises calcium levels. It should

cAMP: The second messenger

Cyclic adenosine monophosphate (cAMP) is an intracellular mediator that relays hormone messages to target cells to effect programmed physiologic responses. It's the "second messenger" after the hormone itself.

Binding of a hormone with a specific receptor on the cell surface is believed to activate the enzyme adenylate cyclase in the cell membrane. This then leads adenosine triphosphate (ATP) to convert to cAMP within the cell. Then cAMP initiates functions specific to the cell, such as telling thyroid cells to produce hormone and kidney cells to increase tubule permeability. It also spurs cell enzymes to convert stored glucose into high-energy ATP needed for cell metabolism. Depletion of this ATP triggers formation of more cAMP.

As the messenger for parathyroid hormone, cAMP helps distinguish between pseudohypoparathyroidism and hypoparathyroidism. In a patient with hypoparathyroidism or in a healthy person, urine cAMP rises minutes after a dose of parathyroid hormone. But it fails to rise in pseudohypoparathyroidism.

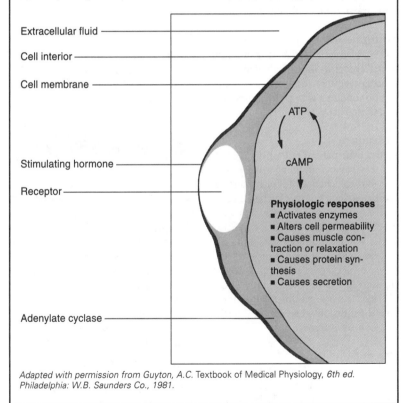

Extracellular fluid

Cell interior

Cell membrane

ATP

Stimulating hormone

cAMP

Receptor

Physiologic responses
- Activates enzymes
- Alters cell permeability
- Causes muscle contraction or relaxation
- Causes protein synthesis
- Causes secretion

Adenylate cyclase

Adapted with permission from Guyton, A.C. Textbook of Medical Physiology, *6th ed. Philadelphia: W.B. Saunders Co., 1981.*

be used cautiously in patients receiving digitalis glycosides and in those with sarcoidosis or renal or cardiac disease.

Purpose
- To aid differential diagnosis of pseudohypoparathyroidism.

Patient preparation

Explain to the patient that this test evaluates parathyroid function. Tell him it requires a 15-minute I.V. infusion of PTH and collection of a 3- to 4-hour urine specimen.

Perform a skin test to detect a possible allergy to PTH; keep epinephrine readily available in case of an adverse reaction. Just before the procedure is performed, instruct the patient not to touch the I.V. line or exert pressure on the arm receiving the infusion. Tell him he may experience transient discomfort from the needle puncture. Ask him to notify you if he feels severe burning or if the site becomes inflamed or swollen.

Equipment

PTH (300 units in refrigerated ampules) ✦ vial of sterile water (saline solution causes precipitate to form) ✦ urine collection container with hydrochloric acid as a preservative.

Procedure

Instruct the patient to empty his bladder. If he has an indwelling urinary catheter in place, change the collection bag. If ordered, send this specimen to the laboratory; otherwise, discard it. Prepare the PTH for infusion as directed, using sterile water for dilution. Start the I.V. infusion with dextrose 5% in water, and infuse the PTH over 15 minutes. Record the start of the infusion as time zero.

Collect a urine specimen 3 to 4 hours after the infusion. Then discontinue the infusion, as ordered.

Precautions

■ Tell the patient not to contaminate the specimen with toilet tissue or stool.
■ Send the specimen to the laboratory immediately or refrigerate it if transport is delayed. If the patient is catheterized, keep the collection bag on ice.

Reference values

A tenfold to twentyfold increase (3.6 to 4 μmol) in cAMP demonstrates a normal response or hypoparathyroidism.

Implications of results

Failure to respond to PTH, indicated by normal urinary excretion of cAMP, suggests type I pseudohypoparathyroidism.

Post-test care

■ Observe for symptoms of hypercalcemia: lethargy, anorexia, nausea, vomiting, vertigo, and abdominal cramps.
■ If a hematoma or irritation develops at the venipuncture site, apply warm soaks.

Interfering factors

Contamination or improper storage of the specimen or failure to acidify the urine with hydrochloric acid may alter test results.

SELECTED READINGS

Bennett, J.C., and Plum, F., eds. *Cecil Textbook of Medicine*, 20th ed. Philadelphia: W.B. Saunders Co., 1996.

Fischbach, F. *A Manual of Laboratory and Diagnostic Tests*, 5th ed. Philadelphia: Lippincott-Raven Pubs., 1996.

Guyton, A.C., and Hall, J.E. *Textbook of Medical Physiology*, 9th ed. Philadelphia: W.B. Saunders Co., 1996.

Henry, J.B., ed. *Clinical Diagnosis and Management by Laboratory Methods*, 19th ed. Philadelphia: W.B. Saunders Co., 1996.

Phipps, W.J., et al. *Medical-Surgical Nursing: Concepts and Clinical Practice*, 5th ed. St. Louis: Mosby–Year Book, Inc., 1995.

Tilkian, S.M., et al. *Clinical and Nursing Implications of Laboratory Tests*, 5th ed. St. Louis: Mosby–Year Book, Inc., 1995.

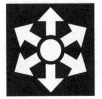

CHAPTER FOURTEEN

Urine hormones and metabolites

Learning objectives

After completing this chapter, the reader will be able to:
- identify the three chemical classes of hormones
- name the hormones and metabolites that are commonly measured in the urine and describe their principal functions
- list four common test methods used to measure urine hormone levels
- discuss the importance of a 24-hour urine specimen in determining urine hormone levels
- state the purpose of each test discussed in the chapter
- prepare the patient physically and psychologically for each test
- describe the procedure for obtaining a specimen for each test
- specify appropriate precautions for accurately obtaining a specimen for each test
- implement appropriate post-test care
- state the reference values for each test
- discuss the implications of abnormal test results
- list factors that may interfere with accurate test results.

INTRODUCTION

Hormones are potent, complex chemicals produced and secreted primarily by the endocrine glands to promote and regulate the activity of target organs and tissues. To directly determine circulating levels of hormones, laboratory methods commonly measure hormone concentrations in blood. But many hormones and their metabolites are also conveniently studied in urine.

Measuring urine hormone and metabolite levels provides a reliable estimate of the amount of circulating hormone. Moreover, timed, long-term urine measurements offer an advantage. Unlike a blood sample, which determines hormone levels only at the time of venipuncture, a 24-hour urine specimen reflects total daily secretion, offsets diurnal variations, and masks temporary fluctuations. (See *Key facts about urine hormones*.)

Chemical classes

Chemically, hormones can be classified into three groups: *steroids* (such as estrogens and androgens), *amines* (such as dopamine and epinephrine), and *proteins* (such as human chorionic gonadotropin). Each group has a marked structural specificity. This is especially true of steroid hormones — the ones most frequently tested in urine. A single structural change in the composition of a steroid hormone can dramatically alter the hormone's physiologic activity. For example, the introduction of a new hydroxyl group is responsible for the conversion of estradiol to estriol.

Hormone metabolites

Although hormones have specific and characteristic functions, they rarely act independently. Quite the contrary, hormones are linked in an intricate series of complex interactions, including positive and negative feedback mechanisms that enable them to function efficiently and maintain homeostasis. Perhaps the most important of these interactions is

Key facts about urine hormones

The chart below lists the secretion sites and methods of measuring the major hormones and their metabolites.

HORMONE OR METABOLITE	PRINCIPAL SECRETION SITE	METHOD OF PRINCIPAL QUANTITATION
Aldosterone	Adrenal cortex	Radioimmunoassay
Free cortisol	Adrenal cortex	Radioimmunoassay
Catecholamines	Adrenal medulla	Spectrophotofluorometry
Total estrogens	Gonads, placenta, adrenal glands	Spectrophotofluorometry
Estriol	Placenta, gonads, adrenal cortex	Radioimmunoassay
Human chorionic gonadotropin	Placenta	Hemagglutination inhibition (antigen-antibody reaction)
Pregnanetriol	Adrenal cortex	Spectrophotofluorometry
17-Hydroxycorticosteroids	Adrenal cortex	Chromatography, spectrophotofluorometry
17-Ketosteroids	Adrenal glands, testes	Spectrophotofluorometry
17-Ketogenic steroids	Adrenal cortex	Spectrophotofluorometry
Vanillylmandelic acid	Adrenal medulla	Spectrophotofluorometry
Homovanillic acid	Liver	Chromatography
5-Hydroxyindoleacetic acid	Intestinal wall, stomach	Colorimetry
Pregnanediol	Corpus luteum, adrenal cortex	Gas-liquid chromatography

the formation of hormone metabolites. These metabolites can be degradation products or essential precursors with individual hormonal effects.

Urine levels of hormone metabolites reflect the secretory rates of the hormones from which these metabolites are derived and serve as valuable diagnostic indicators when the hormones themselves aren't excreted in measurable quantities. Metabolite levels also provide important information about the integrity of degradation pathways. A case in point is the conversion of 17-OH progesterone to cortisol; when this met-

abolic process is blocked, as in adrenogenital syndrome (congenital adrenal hyperplasia), excessive amounts of pregnanetriol appear in the urine.

The hormones produced by the endocrine glands and their metabolites that are commonly measured in urine include the following:

■ *Adrenocortical hormones:* These hormones and metabolites are steroids that are synthesized and secreted primarily by the adrenal cortex. Formed from acetyl coenzyme A, cholesterol, and a variety of other precursors, adrenocortical hormones and metabolites fall into three major groups:

— *glucocorticoids* (17-hydroxycorticosteroids, particularly cortisol), which maintain carbohydrate, protein, and fat metabolism

— *mineralocorticoids,* principally aldosterone, which help regulate blood pressure and fluid and electrolyte balance

— *adrenal androgens* (sex hormones), the most potent of which is dehydroepiandrosterone, which aid development of male secondary sex characteristics.

Androgens are secreted in minute amounts and are usually measured as part of the 17-ketosteroids. The most inclusive test of adrenocortical hormones, however, measures urine levels of 17-ketogenic steroids.

■ *Adrenal medullary hormones:* The adrenal medullae synthesize and secrete the catecholamines *norepinephrine* and *epinephrine,* which help mediate stress. Although these hormones are less vital to life than the adrenocortical hormones, measuring them and their principal metabolite, *vanillylmandelic acid,* in urine can be extremely useful in detectincatecholamine-producing tumors.

■ *Dopamine and other amines:* A catecholamine secreted primarily by the basal ganglia of the brain, dopamine is the precursor of norepinephrine and epinephrine. When a pheochromocytoma, a catecholamine-secreting tumor, is suspected, measuring urine levels of dopamine and its major metabolite, *homovanillic acid,* can aid diagnosis. Urine levels of *serotonin,* an indole amine synthesized by the argentaffin cells of the intestinal mucosa, are reflected by the excretion of *5-hydroxyindoleacetic acid,* its primary metabolite, and aid diagnosis of certain carcinoid tumors.

■ *Gonadal and placental hormones:* Urine levels of gonadal and placental hormones, which are principally steroids, are clinically useful for detecting hormone-secreting tumors and pregnancy.

Early in pregnancy, the corpus luteum secretes greater amounts of progesterone and estrogen to maintain the pregnancy until the placenta can produce these hormones. Thus, urine levels of total estrogens, estriol, and pregnanediol help evaluate placental status and fetal well-being.

Human chorionic gonadotropin (hCG) may also be measured in the urine to detect pregnancy early. Soon after conception, the trophoblastic cells that develop into the chorionic villi of the placenta secrete hCG; thus, the presence of hCG in urine indicates pregnancy.

Four test methods useful

Quantitative assays of urine hormone levels are usually performed by using one or more of the following methods:

■ *Colorimetry* is based on the principle that some groups of hormones, when combined with certain chemical reagents, take on individual colors; the intensity of color indicates the degree of hormone concentration. A colorimeter or spectrophotometer measures the wavelength of maximum absorption.

■ *Fluorometry* reveals the characteristic fluorescence of hormones on placement in specific media. Under certain laboratory conditions, the wavelengths activated and emitted are specific for a given hormone and can be measured.

■ *Chromatography* determines the adsorption or fractionation of a hormone to a specific medium (solid or liquid). In *gas* chromatography, a urine specimen is mixed with an inert gas to create vapors that are passed over the medium. Adsorption of the hormone to the medium is measured. In *paper* chromatography, blotting or filter paper replaces the solid or liquid medium.

■ *Radioimmunoassay* involves combining a urine specimen with a radioactively tagged antigen (hormone) and its antibody. The unlabeled hormone being measured displaces the radioactively tagged hormone, which is then measured to determine the urine concentration of the hormone.

Special considerations

When measuring urine hormone levels, 24-hour urine specimens provide more accurate information than random urine specimens by compensating for diurnal variations in hormonal secretion. For the same reason, urine assays from a 24-hour specimen are often more accurate than serum hormone determinations. However, accurate results require strict adherence to collection procedures and precautions. Keep in mind the following points:

■ Before beginning a 24-hour urine collection, confer with the laboratory to determine if the test requires special collection procedures or precautions. In many cases, you'll need to enforce medication and diet restrictions to ensure accurate results. Many of these tests require dark collection containers and the addition of a preservative to the specimen. The specimen may have to be refrigerated or kept on ice during the collection period.

■ Make sure all urine voided during the 24-hour test period is collected. If a voiding is discarded accidentally, note this on the laboratory request, so the laboratory can take this lost specimen into consideration when determining the results of the test.

■ Because strenuous physical exercise and emotional stress can significantly alter the patient's hormone levels, encourage the patient to rest and relax before the test.

URINE HORMONE TESTS

Urine aldosterone

This test measures urine levels of aldosterone, the principal mineralocorticoid secreted by the zona glomerulosa of the adrenal cortex. Aldosterone promotes retention of sodium and excretion of potassium by the renal tubules, thereby helping to regulate blood pressure and fluid and electrolyte balance.

Aldosterone secretion is controlled by the renin-angiotensin system. Renin, an enzyme released in the kidneys in response to low plasma volume, stimulates production of angiotensin I, which is converted to angiotensin II, a powerful vasopressor that stimulates the adrenal cortex to secrete aldosterone. Potassium levels also affect aldosterone secretion: increased potassium stimulates the adrenal cortex, triggering substantial increase in aldosterone secretion to promote potassium excretion. This feedback mechanism is vital to maintaining fluid and electrolyte balance.

Urine aldosterone levels, measured through radioimmunoassay, are usually evaluated after measurement of serum electrolyte and renin levels.

Purpose

■ To aid diagnosis of primary and secondary aldosteronism.

Patient preparation

Explain to the patient that this test evaluates hormonal balance. Instruct him to maintain a normal sodium diet (3 g/day) before the test; to avoid sodium-rich foods, such as bacon, barbecue sauce, corned beef, bouillon cubes or powder, and olives; and to avoid strenuous physical exercise and stressful situations during the collection period. Tell him the test requires collection of a 24-hour urine specimen, and teach him the proper collection technique.

Check the patient's medication history for drugs that may affect aldosterone levels. Review your findings with the laboratory, then notify the doctor; he may want to restrict these medications before the test.

Procedure

Collect a 24-hour specimen in a bottle containing a preservative to keep the specimen at a pH of 4.0 to 4.5.

Precautions

Refrigerate the specimen or place it on ice during the collection period. Send the specimen to the laboratory as soon as the collection is completed.

Reference values

Normally, urine aldosterone levels range from 2 to 16 µg/24 hours.

Implications of results

Elevated urine aldosterone levels suggest primary or secondary aldosteronism. The primary form usually arises from an aldosterone-secreting adenoma of the adrenal cortex but may also result from adrenocortical hyperplasia.

Secondary aldosteronism, the more common form, results from external stimulation of the adrenal cortex, such as that produced when the renin-angiotensin system is activated by hypertensive and edematous disorders. The major systemic disorders that result in secondary aldosteronism are malignant hypertension, congestive heart failure, cirrhosis of the liver, nephrotic syndrome, and idiopathic cyclic edema.

Low urine aldosterone levels may result from Addison's disease, salt-losing syndrome, and toxemia of pregnancy. Aldosterone levels normally rise during pregnancy but rapidly decline following parturition.

Post-test care

■ Resume administration of any medications that were discontinued before the test, as ordered.
■ Tell the patient that he may resume normal physical activity restricted before the test.

Interfering factors

■ Antihypertensive drugs promote sodium and water retention and may suppress urine aldosterone levels. Diuretics and most steroids promote sodium excretion and may raise aldosterone levels. Some corticosteroids, such as fludrocortisone, mimic mineralocorticoid activity and consequently may lower aldosterone levels.
■ The patient's failure to maintain a normal dietary intake of sodium can influence test results. Failure to collect *all* urine during the 24-hour specimen collection period or to store the urine specimen properly can affect the accuracy of test results.
■ The patient's failure to avoid strenuous physical exercise and emotional stress before the test can stimulate adrenocortical secretions and thus increase aldosterone levels.
■ A radioactive scan performed within 1 week before the test may affect the accuracy of test results.

Urine free cortisol

Used as a screen for adrenocortical hyperfunction, this text measures urine levels of the portion of cortisol not bound to the corticosteroid-binding globulin transcortin. It is one of the best diagnostic tools for detecting Cushing's syndrome.

The major glucocorticoid secreted by the adrenal cortex in response to adrenocorticotropic hormone (ACTH) stimulation, cortisol helps regulate fat, carbohydrate, and protein metabolism; it also helps promote glyconeogenesis, anti-inflammatory response, and cellular permeability. Only about 10% of this hormone is unbound and physiologically active; this small portion is known as free cortisol. Urine cortisol concentrations increase significantly when the amount secreted exceeds the binding capacity of transcortin, which is normally almost saturated.

Radioimmunoassay determinations of free cortisol levels in a 24-hour urine specimen — unlike a single measurement of plasma cortisol — reflect overall secretion levels instead of diurnal variations. Concurrent measurements of plasma cortisol and ACTH, with urine 17-hydroxycorticosteroids and the dexamethasone suppression test, may be used to confirm the diagnosis.

Purpose
▪ To aid diagnosis of Cushing's syndrome.

Patient preparation
Explain to the patient that this test helps evaluate adrenal gland function. Advise him that he needn't restrict food or fluids before the test but should avoid stressful situations and excessive physical exercise during the collection period. Tell him the test requires collection of a 24-hour urine specimen, and teach him the proper collection technique.

Check the patient's recent drug history for medications that may interfere with test results, such as reserpine, phenothiazines, morphine, amphetamines, and prolonged steroid use. Review your findings with the laboratory and notify

the doctor; he may want to restrict such medications before the test.

Procedure
Collect a 24-hour specimen in a bottle containing a preservative to keep the specimen at a pH of 4.0 to 4.5.

Precautions
Refrigerate the specimen or place it on ice during the collection period.

Reference values
Normally, free cortisol values range from 24 to 108 µg/24 hours.

Implications of results
Elevated free cortisol levels may indicate Cushing's syndrome resulting from adrenal hyperplasia, adrenal or pituitary tumor, or ectopic ACTH production. Hepatic disease and obesity, which can raise plasma cortisol levels, generally don't appreciably raise urine levels of free cortisol.

This test is designed to screen for excessive secretion of free cortisol. Low levels have little diagnostic significance and don't necessarily indicate adrenocortical hypofunction.

Post-test care
▪ Tell the patient that he may resume normal activity restricted during the test.
▪ As ordered, resume administration of medications discontinued before the test.

Interfering factors
▪ Reserpine, phenothiazines, morphine, amphetamines, and prolonged steroid therapy may elevate free cortisol levels.
▪ Failure to collect all urine during the test period or to store the specimen properly may affect the accuracy of test results.

Urine catecholamines

This test uses spectrophotofluorometry to measure urine levels of the major catecholamines — dopamine, epinephrine, and norepinephrine. Dopamine is secreted by the central nervous system; epinephrine, by the adrenal medulla; and norepinephrine, by both. Catecholamines help regulate metabolism and prepare the body for the fight-or-flight response to stress. Certain tumors can also secrete catecholamines. One of the most common of these is a pheochromocytoma, which usually causes intermittent or persistent hypertension.

A 24-hour urine specimen is preferred for this test because catecholamine secretion fluctuates diurnally and in response to pain, heat, cold, emotional stress, physical exercise, hypoglycemia, injury, hemorrhage, asphyxia, and drugs. However, a random specimen may be useful for evaluating catecholamine levels after a hypertensive episode.

For a complete diagnostic workup of catecholamine secretion, urine levels of the catecholamine metabolites are measured concurrently. These metabolites — metanephrine, normetanephrine, homovanillic acid (HVA), and vanillylmandelic acid (VMA) — normally appear in the urine in greater quantities than the catecholamines. (See *Degradation pathway of the major catecholamines and metabolites.*)

Purpose

■ To aid diagnosis of pheochromocytoma in a patient with unexplained hypertension
■ To aid diagnosis of neuroblastoma, ganglioneuroma, and dysautonomia.

Patient preparation

Explain to the patient that this test evaluates adrenal function. Inform him that he needn't restrict food or fluids before the test but should avoid stressful situations and excessive physical activity during the collection period. Tell him that either a 24-hour or a random specimen is required, and explain the collection procedure.

Check the patient's drug history for medications that may affect catecholamine levels (such as those listed below). Review your findings with the laboratory; then notify the doctor. He may want to restrict such medications before the test.

Procedure

Collect a 24-hour urine specimen in a bottle containing a preservative to keep the specimen acidified to a pH of 3.0 or less. (If a random specimen is ordered, collect it immediately after a hypertensive episode.)

Precautions

Refrigerate a 24-hour specimen or place it on ice during the collection period. At the end of the collection period, send the specimen to the laboratory at once.

Reference values

Normally, urine epinephrine values range from undetectable to 20 µg/24 hours; norepinephrine, from undetectable to 80 µg/24 hours; and dopamine, from undetectable to 400 µg/24 hours.

Implications of results

In a patient with undiagnosed hypertension, elevated urine catecholamine levels following a hypertensive episode usually indicate a pheochromocytoma. With the exception of HVA — a metabolite of dopamine — catecholamine metabolites may also be elevated. Abnormally high HVA levels rule out a pheochromocytoma, because this tumor mainly secretes epinephrine, whose primary metabolite is VMA, not HVA. If tests indicate a pheochromocytoma,

Degradation pathway of the major catecholamines and metabolites

The brain synthesizes dopamine, the precursor of epinephrine and norepinephrine. Although some dopamine is excreted directly and some converts to norepinephrine, most of it converts in the liver to its metabolite, homovanillic acid (HVA), the form measured in urine.

Epinephrine is produced in the adrenal medulla; norepinephrine, in the storage vesicles of sympathetic nerve fibers. The liver metabolizes these two catecholamines into metanephrine and normetanephrine, respectively, and finally into vanillylmandelic acid (VMA). Some of the original hormones and their primary metabolites are excreted in urine, but VMA is by far the chief end product.

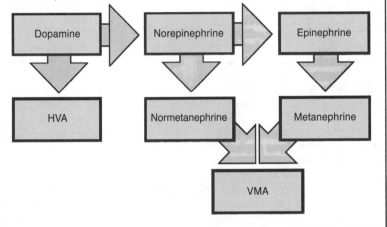

the patient may also be tested for multiple endocrine neoplasia.

Elevated catecholamine levels without marked hypertension may be due to a neuroblastoma or a ganglioneuroma, although HVA levels reflect these conditions more accurately. Neuroblastomas and ganglioneuromas primarily composed of immature cells secrete large quantities of dopamine and HVA. Myasthenia gravis and progressive muscular dystrophy commonly cause urine catecholamine levels to rise above normal, but this test is rarely performed to diagnose these disorders.

Consistently low-normal catecholamine levels may indicate dysautonomia, marked by orthostatic hypotension.

Post-test care
- Tell the patient that he may resume activity restricted during the test.
- As ordered, resume administration of medications withheld before the test.

Interfering factors
- Caffeine, insulin, nitroglycerin, aminophylline, ethanol, sympathomimetics, methyldopa, tricyclic antidepressants, chloral hydrate, quinidine, quinine, tetracycline, B-complex vitamins, isoproterenol, levodopa, and monoamine oxidase inhibitors may raise urine catecholamine levels.
- Clonidine, guanethidine, reserpine, and iodine-containing contrast media may lower urine catecholamine levels.

■ Phenothiazines, erythromycin, and methenamine compounds may raise or suppress catecholamine levels.

■ Failure to comply with drug restrictions, to collect all urine during the test period, or to store the specimen properly may affect test results.

■ Excessive physical exercise or emotional stress raises catecholamine levels.

Total urine estrogens

This test is a quantitative analysis of total urine levels of estradiol, estrone, and estriol — the major estrogens present in significant amounts in urine. In females who are past puberty, these estrogens are secreted by the theca interna cells of the ovarian follicle and by the corpus luteum; in pregnant women, by the placenta; and in postmenopausal women, primarily by the adrenal glands.

In males, two-thirds of estradiol and of estrone are derived from testosterone; the remaining third of estradiol and smaller quantities of estrone are secreted by the testes. In both sexes, the liver, which oxidizes or converts hormones to glucuronide and sulfate conjugates, is the major organ of estrogen metabolism.

Clinical indications for this test include tumors of ovarian, adrenocortical, or testicular origin. A common method of measuring total urine estrogen levels involves purification by gel filtration, followed by spectrophotofluorometry. Supplementary tests that may provide further information about ovarian function include cytologic examination of vaginal smears, measurement of urine levels of pregnanediol and follicle-stimulating hormone, and evaluation of response to an injection of progesterone.

Purpose

■ To evaluate ovarian activity and help determine the cause of amenorrhea and female hyperestrogenism

■ To aid diagnosis of testicular tumors

■ To assess fetoplacental status.

Patient preparation

Explain to the female patient that this test helps evaluate ovarian function; to the pregnant patient that this test helps evaluate fetal development and placental function; and to the male patient that this test helps evaluate testicular function. Inform all patients that the test requires collection of a 24-hour urine specimen and that no pretest restrictions of food or fluids are necessary. If the 24-hour specimen is to be collected at home, teach the patient the proper collection technique. Check the patient's medication history for use of drugs that may influence estrogen levels (such as those listed below).

Procedure

Collect a 24-hour specimen in a bottle containing a preservative to keep the specimen at a pH of 3.0 to 5.0. If the patient is pregnant, note the approximate week of gestation on the laboratory request. If the patient is a nonpregnant female, note the stage of her menstrual cycle.

Precautions

Refrigerate the specimen or keep it on ice during the collection period.

Reference values

In nonpregnant females, total urine estrogen levels rise and fall during the menstrual cycle, peaking shortly before midcycle, decreasing immediately following ovulation, increasing through the life of the corpus luteum, and decreasing greatly as the corpus luteum degenerates and menstruation begins.

Urine estrogen levels in a normal menstrual cycle

During a normal menstrual cycle, estrogen excretion levels have a primary peak at midpoint in the cycle (ovulatory phase) and another smaller increase just before the onset of menses (luteal or premenstrual phase), as shown below.

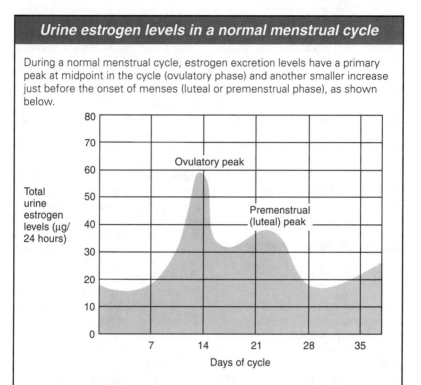

Adapted with permission from Mishell, D.R., et al. "Serum Gonadotropin and Steroid Patterns During the Normal Menstrual Cycle," American Journal of Obstetrics and Gynecology 111:60, Sept. 1, 1971.

(See *Urine estrogen levels in a normal menstrual cycle.*)

Normal values for nonpregnant females are as follows:
- *follicular phase:* 5 to 25 µg/24 hours
- *ovulatory phase:* 24 to 100 µg/24 hours
- *luteal phase:* 12 to 80 µg/24 hours.

In pregnant women, urine estrogen levels rise slowly in the first trimester, then rise rapidly and reach high levels as term nears. In postmenopausal females, values are less than 10 µg/24 hours; in males, 4 to 25 µg/24 hours.

Implications of results

Decreased total urine estrogen levels may reflect ovarian agenesis, primary ovarian insufficiency (due to Stein-Lev-enthal syndrome, for example), or secondary ovarian insufficiency (due to pituitary or adrenal hypofunction or metabolic disturbances).

Elevated total estrogen levels in nonpregnant females may indicate tumors of ovarian or adrenocortical origin, adrenocortical hyperplasia, or a metabolic or hepatic disorder. In males, elevated total estrogen levels are associated with testicular tumors.

Elevated total urine estrogen levels are normal during pregnancy; serial determinations should show a rising titer.

Post-test care

As ordered, resume administration of medications withheld before the test.

Interfering factors

■ Drugs that may influence total urine estrogen levels include steroids (such as estrogens, progesterone, and high-dose corticosteroids), methenamine mandelate, phenazopyridine, phenothiazines, tetracyclines, phenolphthalein, ampicillin, meprobamate, senna, cascara sagrada, and hydrochlorothiazide.

■ Failure to collect all urine during the 24-hour period, to refrigerate the specimen or keep it on ice, or to control pH properly may affect test results.

Urine placental estriol

This test monitors fetal viability by measuring urine levels of placental estriol, the predominant estrogen excreted in urine during pregnancy. Toward the end of the first trimester, placental constituents combine with estriol precursors from the fetal adrenal cortex and liver to steadily increase estriol production. This steady rise in estriol reflects a properly functioning placenta and, in most cases, a healthy, growing fetus. Normally, estriol is secreted in much smaller amounts by the ovaries in nonpregnant females, by the testes in males, and by the adrenal cortex in both sexes.

The usual clinical indication for this test is high-risk pregnancy, such as one complicated by maternal hypertension, diabetes mellitus, pregnancy-induced hypertension (preeclampsia), eclampsia, or a history of stillbirth. Serial testing is necessary to plot the expected rise in estriol levels or to show the absence of such a rise.

A 24-hour urine specimen is preferred for this test because estriol levels fluctuate diurnally. Radioimmunoassay is the usual test method. Generally, serum estriol levels are considered more reli-

able than urine levels. Serum levels aren't influenced by maternal glomerular filtration rate (GFR), nor are they as readily affected by drugs, some of which actually destroy urinary estriol.

Purpose

■ To assess fetoplacental status, especially in high-risk pregnancy.

Patient preparation

Explain to the patient that this test helps determine if the placenta is functioning properly, which is essential to the health of the fetus. Tell her she needn't restrict food or fluids. Advise her that a 24-hour urine specimen is required for this test, and teach her how to collect it. Emphasize that proper collection technique is necessary for test results to be valid. Check the patient's medication history for use of drugs that may affect urine estriol levels.

Procedure

Collect a 24-hour urine specimen in a bottle containing a preservative to keep the specimen at a pH of 3.0 to 5.0. Note the week of gestation on the laboratory request, and send the specimen to the laboratory.

Precautions

Refrigerate the specimen or keep it on ice during the collection period.

Reference values

Normal values vary considerably, but serial measurements of urine estriol levels, when plotted on a graph, should show a steadily rising curve. (See *Urine estriol levels in a typical pregnancy.*)

Implications of results

A 40% drop from baseline values occurring on 2 consecutive days strongly suggests placental insufficiency and impending fetal distress. A 20% drop over 2 weeks or failure of consecutive estriol

Urine estriol levels in a typical pregnancy

Because urine estriol levels rise as normal gestation proceeds (as shown below), any significant changes in serial urine determinations suggest abnormal conditions that may require prompt medical intervention.

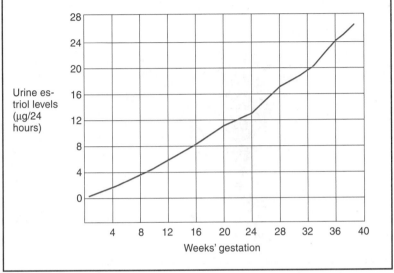

levels to rise in a normal curve similarly indicates inadequate placental function and undesirable fetal status. These developments may necessitate cesarean section, depending on the patient's condition and on other apparent signs of fetal distress.

A chronically low urine estriol curve may result from fetal adrenal insufficiency, congenital anomalies (such as anencephaly), Rh isoimmunization, or placental sulfatase deficiency. A high-risk pregnancy in which maternal GFR decreases, as in hypertension or diabetes mellitus, may cause a low-normal estriol curve. In such a case, the pregnancy may continue as long as no complications develop and estriol levels continue to rise. However, falling estriol levels or a sudden drop from baseline values indicates severe fetal distress.

High urine estriol levels are possible in multiple pregnancy.

Post-test care
As ordered, resume administration of medications discontinued before the test.

Interfering factors
■ Administration of the following drugs may influence urine estriol levels: steroid hormones (including estrogens, progesterone, and corticosteroids), methenamine mandelate, phenothiazines, ampicillin, phenazopyridine, tetracyclines, cascara sagrada, senna, phenolphthalein, hydrochlorothiazide, and meprobamate.
■ Maternal hemoglobinopathy, anemia, malnutrition, or hepatic or intestinal disease characteristically decreases estriol levels.

Site of hCG secretion

Human chorionic gonadotropin (hCG) is secreted by the trophoblastic cells of the chorionic villi at about 10 weeks' gestation. It then crosses the placenta into the maternal bloodstream.

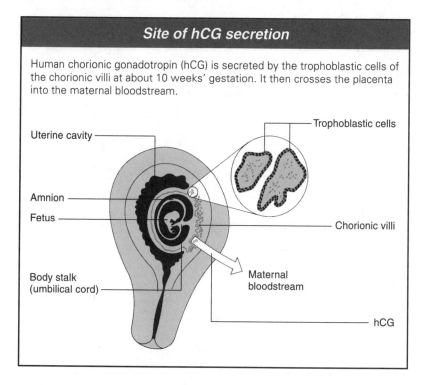

■ Failure to collect all urine during the 24-hour period may affect the accuracy of test results.
■ Failure to refrigerate the specimen or keep it on ice may alter test results.
■ Failure to maintain the prescribed pH level in the specimen may alter test results.

Urine human chorionic gonadotropin

As a qualitative analysis of urine levels of human chorionic gonadotropin (hCG), this test can detect pregnancy as early as 14 days after ovulation. Quantitative measurements can evaluate suspected hydatidiform mole or hCG-secreting tumors.

After conception, placental trophoblastic cells start to produce hCG, a glycoprotein that prevents degeneration of the corpus luteum at the end of the normal menstrual cycle. The corpus luteum then secretes large quantities of progesterone and estrogen, promoting early development of the endometrium, placenta, and fetus. Levels of hCG rise steadily and rapidly during the first trimester, peak around the 10th week of gestation, and subsequently taper off to less than 10% of peak levels. (See *Site of hCG secretion.*)

The most common method of evaluating hCG in urine is hemagglutination inhibition. This laboratory procedure, based on an antigen-antibody reaction, can provide both qualitative and quantitative information. The qualitative urine test is easier and less expensive than the serum hCG test (beta-subunit assay), so it's used more frequently to

OTC pregnancy tests

Many women today first learn they're pregnant through over-the-counter (OTC) home pregnancy tests. These tests confirm pregnancy by detecting the presence of human chorionic gonadotropin in the urine.

Several different kits are available. Some contain a second test to use if hormone levels aren't detectable at first. Each kit contains instruc-tions for performing the test and lists health conditions or drugs that might affect results.

False-positive or false-negative results can occur. Many kits include toll-free numbers to call for questions about the kit or the results. Follow-up care with a doctor is recommended for all positive results.

---

detect pregnancy. But the serum hCG test allows the earliest possible determination of pregnancy (as early as 7 days after conception).

Many women today use home pregnancy tests to initially determine whether they are pregnant. (See *OTC pregnancy tests*.)

Purpose
- To detect and confirm pregnancy
- To aid diagnosis of hydatidiform mole or hCG-secreting tumors.

Patient preparation
Explain to the patient that this test determines whether she is pregnant (if this isn't the test's purpose, offer an appropriate explanation). Tell her she needn't restrict food or fluids before the test. Inform her that the test requires a first-voided morning specimen or a 24-hour urine collection, depending on whether a qualitative or quantitative test will be performed. Check the patient's recent medication history for use of drugs that may affect hCG levels.

Procedure
To verify pregnancy (qualitative analysis), collect a first-voided morning specimen. If this is not possible, collect a random specimen.

For quantitative analysis of hCG, collect a 24-hour urine specimen.

Specify the date of the patient's last menstrual period on the laboratory request.

Precautions
Refrigerate the 24-hour specimen or keep it on ice during the collection period.

Reference values
In qualitative analysis, if agglutination fails to occur, test results are positive, indicating pregnancy.

In quantitative analysis, urine hCG levels in the first trimester of a normal pregnancy may be as high as 500,000 IU/ 24 hours; in the second trimester, they range from 10,000 to 25,000 IU/24 hours; and in the third trimester, from 5,000 to 15,000 IU/24 hours. Levels decline rapidly after delivery and are undetectable within a few days.

Measurable hCG shouldn't be found in the urine of males or nonpregnant females.

Implications of results
During pregnancy, elevated urine hCG levels may indicate multiple pregnancy or erythroblastosis fetalis; low levels may

indicate threatened abortion or ectopic pregnancy.

Measurable hCG levels in males and nonpregnant females may indicate choriocarcinoma, ovarian or testicular tumors, melanoma, multiple myeloma, or gastric, hepatic, pancreatic, or breast cancer.

Post-test care

As ordered, resume administration of medications discontinued before the test.

Interfering factors

- Gross proteinuria (more than 1 g/24 hours), hematuria, or an elevated erythrocyte sedimentation rate may produce false-positive results, depending on the laboratory method used.
- Early pregnancy, ectopic pregnancy, or threatened abortion may produce false-negative results.
- Phenothiazine use may result in false-negative or false-positive results.

URINE METABOLITE TESTS

Urine pregnanetriol

Using spectrophotometry, this test determines urine levels of pregnanetriol, the metabolite of the cortisol precursor 17-hydroxyprogesterone. Minute amounts of pregnanetriol are normally excreted in the urine. However, when cortisol biosynthesis is impaired at the point of 17-hydroxyprogesterone conversion, urinary excretion of pregnanetriol increases significantly. Such impairment results from the absence or deficiency of particular biosynthetic enzymes that convert 17-hydroxyproges-

terone to cortisol; in turn, low plasma cortisol levels interfere with the negative feedback mechanism that inhibits secretion of adrenocorticotropic hormone (ACTH). Consequently, excessive 17-hydroxyprogesterone accumulates in the plasma, leading to increased formation and excretion of pregnanetriol in urine.

Urine pregnanetriol levels may be measured concomitantly with urine 17-ketosteroids and urine 17-ketogenic steroids to assess androgen levels, which also rise with impaired cortisol biosynthesis. Elevated androgen levels, which occur in adrenogenital syndrome (congenital adrenal hyperplasia), result from conversion of excessive 17-hydroxyprogesterone to androgens and from hypersecretion of adrenal androgens in response to excessive ACTH stimulation.

Purpose

- To aid diagnosis of adrenogenital syndrome
- To monitor cortisol replacement.

Patient preparation

Explain to the patient (or to his parents if the patient is a child) that this test evaluates hormone secretion. Inform him that he needn't restrict food or fluids before the test. Tell him the test requires collection of a 24-hour urine specimen, and teach him the proper collection technique.

Procedure

Collect a 24-hour urine specimen in a bottle containing a preservative to keep the specimen at a pH of 4.0 to 4.5.

Precautions

Refrigerate the specimen or keep it on ice during the collection period. Send the specimen to the laboratory as soon as the collection is completed.

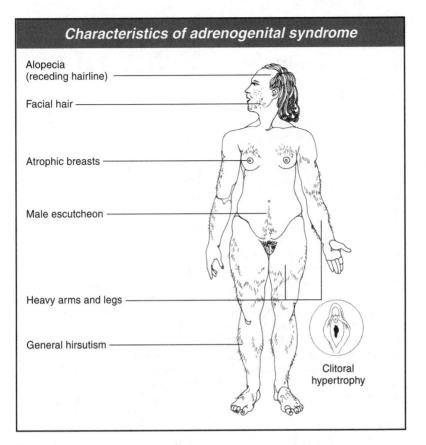

Characteristics of adrenogenital syndrome

Alopecia (receding hairline)

Facial hair

Atrophic breasts

Male escutcheon

Heavy arms and legs

General hirsutism

Clitoral hypertrophy

Reference values

The normal urine pregnanetriol values for males 16 years and over are 0.2 to 2 mg/24 hours; for females 16 years and over, 0 to 1.4 mg/24 hours.

Implications of results

Elevated urine pregnanetriol levels suggest adrenogenital syndrome, marked by excessive adrenal androgen secretion and resulting virilization. Females with this condition fail to develop normal secondary sex characteristics and show marked masculinization of external genitalia at birth. (See *Characteristics of adrenogenital syndrome.*) Males usually appear normal at birth but later develop signs of somatic and sexual precocity.

In monitoring treatment with cortisol replacement, elevated urine pregnanetriol levels indicate insufficient dosage of cortisol. When cortisol replacement adequately inhibits hypersecretion of ACTH and subsequent overproduction of 17-hydroxyprogesterone, pregnanetriol levels fall to normal.

Post-test care

None.

Interfering factors

Failure to collect all urine during the test period or to store the specimen properly may interfere with test results.

Urine 17-hydroxycorticosteroids

This test measures urine levels of 17-hydroxycorticosteroids (17-OHCS) — metabolites of the hormones that regulate glyconeogenesis. More than 80% of all urinary 17-OHCS are metabolites of cortisol, the primary adrenocortical steroid. Test findings thus reflect cortisol secretion and, indirectly, adrenocortical function.

Because cortisol secretion varies diurnally and in response to stress and many other factors, urine 17-OHCS levels are most accurately determined from a 24-hour specimen using column chromatography or spectrophotofluorometry with the Porter-Silber reagent. Levels of plasma cortisol, urine free cortisol, and urine 17-ketosteroids may be measured, and adrenocorticotropic hormone stimulation and suppression testing may be performed to confirm the results of this test.

Purpose
- To assess adrenocortical function.

Patient preparation
Explain to the patient that this test evaluates how his adrenal glands are functioning. Inform him that he needn't restrict food or fluids but should avoid excessive physical exercise and stressful situations during the testing period. Tell him the test requires collection of a 24-hour urine specimen, and teach him the proper collection technique.

Check the patient's medication history for drugs that may affect 17-OHCS levels. Review your findings with the laboratory and notify the doctor; he may restrict medications before the test.

Procedure
Collect a 24-hour urine specimen in a bottle containing a preservative to prevent deterioration of the specimen.

Precautions
Refrigerate the specimen or place it on ice during the collection period.

Reference values
- *Males:* 4.5 to 12 mg/24 hours
- *Females:* 2.5 to 10 mg/24 hours
- *Children age 8 to 12:* less than 4.5 mg/24 hours
- *Children under age 8:* less than 1.5 mg/24 hours.

Levels normally increase slightly during the first trimester of pregnancy. Patients who are obese or very muscular may excrete slightly higher amounts of 17-OHCS because of increased cortisol catabolism.

Implications of results
Elevated urine 17-OHCS levels may indicate Cushing's syndrome, adrenal carcinoma or adenoma, or pituitary tumor. Increased levels may also occur in patients with virilism, hyperthyroidism, or severe hypertension. Extreme stress induced by such conditions as acute pancreatitis and eclampsia also increases urine 17-OHCS levels.

Low urine 17-OHCS levels may indicate Addison's disease, hypopituitarism, or myxedema.

Post-test care
- Tell the patient that he may resume activities restricted during the test.
- Resume administration of any medications withheld before the test.

Interfering factors
- The following drugs may elevate urine 17-OHCS levels: meprobamate, phenothiazines, spironolactone, ascorbic acid, chloral hydrate, glutethimide, chlordiazepoxide, penicillin G, hydroxy-

zine, quinidine, quinine, iodides, and methenamine.

▪ The following drugs may suppress urine 17-OHCS levels: hydralazine, phenytoin, thiazide diuretics, ethinamate, nalidixic acid, and reserpine.

▪ Failure to follow drug restrictions, to collect all urine during the test period, or to store the specimen properly may interfere with test results.

Urine 17-ketosteroids

This test measure urine levels of 17-ketosteroids (17-KS) using spectrophotofluorometry. Steroids and steroid metabolites characterized by a ketone group on carbon 17 in the steroid nucleus, 17-KS originate primarily in the adrenal glands but also in the testes (which produce one-third of 17-KS in males) and the ovaries (which produce a minimal amount of 17-KS in females).

Although not all 17-KS are androgens, all cause androgenic effects. For example, excessive secretion of 17-KS may result in hirsutism and increased clitoral or phallic size; in utero, elevated 17-KS levels may cause a female fetus to develop a male urogenital tract.

Because 17-KS do not include all the androgens (such as testosterone, the most potent androgen), this test provides only a rough estimate of androgenic activity. To provide more information about androgen secretion, plasma testosterone and 17-KS fractionation tests may be performed. (See *17-KS fractionation values,* page 400.)

Purpose

▪ To aid diagnosis of adrenal and gonadal dysfunction

▪ To aid diagnosis of adrenogenital syndrome (congenital adrenal hyperplasia)

▪ To monitor cortisol therapy in the treatment of adrenogenital syndrome.

Patient preparation

Explain to the patient that this test evaluates hormonal balance. Inform him that he needn't restrict food or fluids before the test but should avoid excessive physical exercise and stressful situations during the collection period. Tell him the test requires 24-hour urine collection, and instruct him in the proper collection technique.

If the female patient is menstruating, urine collection may have to be postponed because blood in the specimen would interfere with test findings.

Check the patient's medication history for drugs that may affect test results. Review your findings with the laboratory and notify the doctor; he may want to restrict such drugs before the test.

Procedure

Collect a 24-hour urine specimen in a bottle containing a preservative to keep the specimen at a pH of 4.0 to 4.5.

Precautions

Refrigerate the specimen or place it on ice during the collection period. Send the specimen to the laboratory as soon as the collection is completed.

Reference values

▪ *Men:* 6 to 21 mg/24 hours

▪ *Women:* 4 to 17 mg/24 hours

▪ *Children age 11 to 14:* 2 to 7 mg/24 hours

▪ *Younger children and infants:* 0.1 to 3 mg/24 hours.

Implications of results

Elevated urine 17-KS levels may result from adrenal hyperplasia, carcinoma or adenoma, or adrenogenital syndrome. In women, elevated levels may also indicate ovarian dysfunction (such as polycystic ovarian disease [Stein-Lev-

17-KS fractionation values

Through gas-liquid chromatography, the 17-ketosteroid (17-KS) fractionation test shows which specific steroids in the 17-KS group are elevated or suppressed and thus aids differential diagnosis of conditions characterized by abnormal 17-KS levels. (All values in the chart below are expressed in number of milligrams per 24 hours.)

STEROID	ADULT MALES	ADULT FEMALES	MALES AGE 10 TO 15	FEMALES AGE 10 TO 15	BOTH SEXES AGE 0 TO 9
Androsterone	2.2 to 5.0	0.5 to 2.4	0.2 to 2.0	0.2 to 2.5	≤ 1
Dehydroepian-drosterone	0 to 2.3	0 to 1.2	< 0.4	< 0.4	< 0.2
Etiocholanolone	1.9 to 4.7	1.1 to 3.0	0.1 to 1.6	0.7 to 3.1	≤ 1
11-Hydroxyan-drosterone	0.5 to 1.3	0.2 to 0.6	0.1 to 1.1	0.2 to 1.0	≤ 1
11-Hydroxyetio-cholanolone	0.3 to 0.7	0.2 to 0.6	< 0.3	0.1 to 0.5	≤ 0.5
11-Ketoandro-sterone	0 to 0.1	0 to 0.2	< 0.1	< 0.1	< 0.1
11-Ketoetiocho-lanolone	0.2 to 0.7	0.2 to 0.6	0.2 to 0.6	0.1 to 0.6	≤ 0.7
Pregnanediol	0.6 to 1.6	0.2 to 2.4	0.1 to 0.7	0.1 to 1.2	< 0.5
Pregnanetriol	0.6 to 1.3	0.1 to 1.0	0.2 to 0.6	0.1 to 0.6	< 0.3
5-Pregnanetriol	0 to 0.3	0 to 0.3	< 0.3	< 0.3	< 0.2
11-Ketopreg-nanetriol	0 to 0.2	0 to 0.4	< 0.3	< 0.2	< 0.2

enthal syndrome] or lutein cell tumor of the ovary) or androgenic arrhenoblastoma. In men, elevated 17-KS levels may indicate interstitial cell tumor of the testis. Characteristically, 17-KS levels also rise during pregnancy, severe stress, chronic illness, or debilitating disease.

Depressed urine 17-KS levels may result from Addison's disease, panhypopituitarism, eunuchoidism, or castration and may occur in cretinism, myxedema, and nephrosis. When this test is used to monitor cortisol therapy for adrenogenital syndrome, 17-KS levels typically return to normal with adequate cortisol administration.

Post-test care
- Tell the patient that he may resume activities restricted during the test.
- As ordered, resume administration of medications withheld before the test.

Interfering factors
- Meprobamate, phenothiazines, spironolactone, and oleandomycin may elevate urine 17-KS levels. Estrogens, penicillin, ethacrynic acid, and phenytoin may suppress 17-KS levels. Nalidixic acid and quinine may elevate or suppress 17-KS levels.
- Failure to observe drug restrictions, to collect all urine, or to store the specimen properly may affect test results.

Urine 17-ketogenic steroids

Using spectrophotofluorometry, this test determines urine levels of 17-ketogenic steroids (17-KGS), which consist of the 17-hydroxycorticosteroids — such as cortisol and its metabolites — and other adrenocortical steroids, such as pregnanetriol, that can be oxidized in the laboratory to 17-ketosteroids.

Because 17-KGS represent such a large group of steroids, this test provides an excellent overall assessment of adrenocortical function. For accurate diagnosis of specific disease, 17-KGS must be compared with results of other tests, including plasma adrenocorticotropic hormone (ACTH), plasma cortisol, ACTH stimulation, single-dose metyrapone, and dexamethasone suppression.

Purpose
- To evaluate adrenocortical function
- To aid diagnosis of Cushing's syndrome and Addison's disease.

Patient preparation
Explain to the patient that this test evaluates adrenal function. Inform him that he needn't restrict food or fluids before the test but should avoid excessive physical exercise and stressful situations during the collection period. Tell him the test requires 24-hour urine collection, and teach him how to collect the specimen correctly.

Check the medication history for drugs that may affect 17-KGS levels. Review your findings with the laboratory, and notify the doctor; he may want to withhold medications before the test.

Procedure
Collect a 24-hour urine specimen in a bottle containing a preservative to keep the specimen at a pH of 4.0 to 4.5.

Precautions
Refrigerate the specimen or keep it on ice during the collection period. Send the specimen to the laboratory as soon as the collection is completed.

Reference values
- *Men:* 4 to 14 mg/24 hours
- *Women:* 2 to 12 mg/24 hours
- *Children age 11 to 14:* 2 to 9 mg/24 hours
- *Younger children and infants:* 0.1 to 4.0 mg/24 hours.

Implications of results
Elevated 17-KGS levels reflect hyperadrenalism, as in Cushing's syndrome; some cases of adrenogenital syndrome (congenital adrenal hyperplasia); and adrenal carcinoma or adenoma. Levels also rise with severe physical or emotional stress.

Low levels may reflect hypoadrenalism, as in Addison's disease, as well as panhypopituitarism, cretinism, and general wasting.

Post-test care
- Tell the patient that he may resume activities restricted before the test.
- As ordered, resume administration of drugs withheld before the test.

Interfering factors
- Urine 17-KGS levels may be elevated by ACTH therapy and by such drugs as meprobamate, phenothiazines, spironolactone, penicillin, oleandomycin, and hydralazine. Levels may be suppressed by estrogens, quinine, reserpine, thiazide diuretics, and long-term corticosteroid therapy. Nalidixic acid and dexamethasone may elevate or suppress urine 17-KGS levels.
- Failure to observe drug restrictions, to collect all urine, or to store the specimen properly may alter test results.

Urinary metabolite values in pheochromocytoma

Metabolite values in urine increase in patients with pheochromocytoma, as shown below.

METABOLITE	NORMAL EXCRETION RATE (mg/24 hours)	USUAL RANGE IN PHEOCHROMOCYTOMA (mg/24 hours)
Free catecholamines	< 0.1	0.2 to 4
Metanephrine and normetanephrine	< 1.3	2.5 to 40
Vanillylmandelic acid	< 6.8	10 to 250

Urine vanillylmandelic acid

Using spectrophotofluorometry, this test determines urine levels of vanillylmandelic acid (VMA), a phenolic acid. VMA, the most prevalent catecholamine metabolite in the urine, is the product of hepatic conversion of epinephrine and norepinephrine; urine VMA levels reflect endogenous production of these major catecholamines.

Like the test for urine total catecholamines, this test helps detect catecholamine-secreting tumors — especially pheochromocytoma — and helps evaluate the function of the adrenal medulla, the primary site of catecholamine production. A 24-hour urine specimen is preferred over a random specimen to overcome the effects of diurnal variations in catecholamine secretion. Other catecholamine metabolites — metanephrine, normetanephrine, and homovanillic acid (HVA) — may be measured at the same time. (See *Urinary metabolite values in pheochromocytoma.*)

Purpose
■ To help detect pheochromocytoma, neuroblastoma, and ganglioneuroma

■ To evaluate the function of the adrenal medulla.

Patient preparation
Explain to the patient that this test evaluates hormone secretion. Instruct him to restrict foods and beverages containing phenolic acid, such as coffee, tea, bananas, citrus fruits, chocolate, and vanilla, for 3 days before the test and to avoid stressful situations and strenuous physical activity during the urine collection period. Tell him the test requires collection of a 24-hour urine specimen, and teach him the proper collection technique.

Check the patient's medication history for drugs that may affect test results. Review your findings with the laboratory, and notify the doctor; he may want to restrict these drugs before the test.

Procedure
Collect a 24-hour urine specimen in a bottle containing a preservative to keep the specimen at a pH of 3.0.

Precautions
Refrigerate the specimen or keep it on ice during the collection period. Send the specimen to the laboratory as soon as the collection is completed.

Diagnosing catecholamine-secreting tumors

Although a pheochromocytoma is a catecholamine-producing tumor, causing hypersecretion of epinephrine and norepinephrine by the adrenal medulla, not every patient with this disorder has elevated urine catecholamine levels. Moreover, hypertension, a prime clue in this condition, is sometimes absent. Thus, an analysis of one or more catecholamine metabolites is helpful in confirming the diagnosis.

When catecholamine levels remain normal in the presence of hypertension, elevated vanillylmandelic acid (VMA) levels may signal a tumor. Or metanephrine may be high when VMA and catecholamines are essentially unchanged. VMA assay is also an alternative method when catecholamine analysis has been compromised by interfering food or drugs. Increased excretion of homovanillic acid (HVA) typically indicates malignant pheochromocytoma, although the incidence of malignancy is very low.

Measurement of urine VMA is also useful for diagnosing two neurogenic tumors — neuroblastoma, a common soft-tissue tumor that's a leading cause of death in infants and young children, and ganglioneuroma, a well-defined tumor of the sympathetic nervous system that occurs in older children and young adults. Both tumors primarily produce dopamine and thus show the expected high readings of dopamine's metabolite, HVA, especially in their malignant forms. But both tumors also show abnormal increases in urine VMA levels.

Reference values
Normally, urine VMA values range from 0.7 to 6.8 mg/24 hours.

Implications of results
Elevated urine VMA levels may result from a catecholamine-secreting tumor. Further testing, such as measurement of urine HVA levels to rule out pheochromocytoma, is necessary for a precise diagnosis. (See *Diagnosing catecholamine-secreting tumors.*) If a pheochromocytoma is confirmed, the patient may be tested for multiple endocrine neoplasia, an inherited condition commonly associated with pheochromocytoma. (Family members of a patient with confirmed pheochromocytoma should also be carefully evaluated for multiple endocrine neoplasia.)

Post-test care
■ As ordered, resume administration of medications withheld before the test.
■ Tell the patient that he may resume his normal diet and activities.

Interfering factors
■ Epinephrine, norepinephrine, lithium carbonate, and methocarbamol may raise urine VMA levels. Chlorpromazine, guanethidine, reserpine, monoamine oxidase inhibitors, and clonidine may lower VMA levels. Levodopa and salicylates may raise or lower them.
■ Failure to observe drug and dietary restrictions, to collect all urine during the test period, or to store the specimen properly may affect test results.
■ Excessive physical exercise or emotional stress may raise VMA levels.

Urine homovanillic acid

This test measures urine levels of homovanillic acid (HVA), a metabolite of dopamine, one of the three major catecholamines. Synthesized primarily in the brain, dopamine is a precursor of epinephrine and norepinephrine, the other principal catecholamines. The liver breaks down most dopamine into HVA for eventual excretion; a minimal amount of dopamine appears in the urine.

Using two-dimensional chromatography, urine HVA levels are usually measured simultaneously with the major catecholamines and other catecholamine metabolites — metanephrine, normetanephrine, and vanillylmandelic acid. The principal indication for this test is suspected neuroblastoma or ganglioneuroma, which usually affects children and adolescents.

Purpose
■ To aid diagnosis of neuroblastoma and ganglioneuroma
■ To rule out pheochromocytoma.

Patient preparation
Explain to the patient that this test assesses hormone secretion. Inform him that he needn't restrict food or fluids before the test but should avoid stressful situations and excessive physical exercise during the collection period. Tell him the test requires collection of a 24-hour urine specimen, and teach him the proper collection technique.

Check the patient's history for drugs that may affect test results. Review your findings with the laboratory, and notify the doctor; he may want to withhold these medications before the test.

Procedure
Collect a 24-hour urine specimen in a bottle containing a preservative to keep the specimen at a pH of 2.0 to 4.0.

Precautions
Refrigerate the specimen or keep it on ice during the collection period. Send the specimen to the laboratory as soon as the collection is completed.

Reference values
The normal urine HVA value for adults is less than 8 mg/24 hours. Normal values in children vary with age, as follows (values are expressed in micrograms per milligram of creatinine):
■ *age 15 to 17:* 0.5 to 2
■ *age 10 to 15:* 0.25 to 12
■ *age 5 to 10:* 0.5 to 9
■ *age 2 to 5:* 0.5 to 13.5
■ *age 1 to 2:* 4 to 23
■ *age 0 to 1:* 1.2 to 35.

Implications of results
Elevated urine HVA levels suggest neuroblastoma, a malignant soft-tissue tumor that develops in infants and young children, or ganglioneuroma, a tumor of the sympathetic nervous system that develops in older children and adolescents and rarely metastasizes. HVA levels don't usually rise in patients with pheochromocytoma, because this tumor secretes mainly epinephrine, which metabolizes primarily into vanillylmandelic acid. Thus, an abnormally high urine HVA level generally rules out pheochromocytoma.

Post-test care
■ As ordered, resume administration of medications withheld before the test.
■ Tell the patient that he may resume activities restricted during the test.

Interfering factors
■ Monoamine oxidase inhibitors decrease urine HVA levels by inhibiting

dopamine metabolism. Aspirin, methocarbamol, and levodopa may rise or lower HVA levels.

■ Failure to observe drug restrictions, to collect all urine during the test period, or to store the specimen properly may affect test results.

■ Excessive physical exercise or emotional stress during the collection period may raise HVA levels.

Urine 5-hydroxyindoleacetic acid

This test measures urine levels of 5-hydroxyindoleacetic acid (5-HIAA) and is used mainly to screen for carcinoid tumors (argentaffinomas). Urine 5-HIAA levels reflect plasma concentrations of serotonin (5-hydroxytryptamine). This powerful vasopressor is produced by argentaffin cells, primarily in the intestinal mucosa, and is metabolized through oxidative deamination into 5-HIAA. (See *Site of serotonin secretion,* page 406.)

Carcinoid tumors, found generally in the intestine or appendix, secrete an excessive amount of serotonin, which is reflected by high 5-HIAA levels. This test measures 5-HIAA levels by the colorimetric technique; a 24-hour urine specimen, which can detect small or intermittently secreting carcinoid tumors, is preferred.

Purpose
■ To aid diagnosis of carcinoid tumors.

Patient preparation
Explain to the patient what serotonin is and why this test is important. Instruct him not to eat foods containing serotonin, such as bananas, plums, pineapples, avocados, eggplants, tomatoes, and walnuts, for 4 days before the test. Tell him the test requires collection of a 24-hour urine specimen, and teach him the proper collection technique.

Check the patient's medication history for recent use of drugs that may affect test results. Review your findings with the laboratory, and notify the doctor; he may want to withhold these drugs before the test.

Procedure
Collect a 24-hour urine specimen in a bottle containing a preservative to keep the specimen at a pH of 2.0 to 4.0.

Precautions
Refrigerate the specimen or keep it on ice during the collection period. Send the specimen to the laboratory as soon as the collection is completed.

Reference values
Normally, urine 5-HIAA values are less than 6 mg/24 hours.

Implications of results
Markedly elevated urine 5-HIAA levels, possibly as high as 200 to 600 mg/24 hours, indicate a carcinoid tumor. However, since these tumors vary in their capacity to store and secrete serotonin, some patients with carcinoid syndrome (metastatic carcinoid tumors) may not have elevated levels. Repeated testing is often necessary.

Post-test care
■ As ordered, resume administration of medications withheld before the test.
■ Tell the patient that he may resume his normal diet.

Interfering factors
■ Melphalan, reserpine, and fluorouracil raise urine 5-HIAA levels. Ethanol, tricyclic antidepressants, monoamine ox-

Site of serotonin secretion

The argentaffin cells in the crypts of Lieberkühn (the indentations between the villi in the mucosa of the small intestine, as shown below) produce serotonin, which metabolizes into 5-hydroxyindoleacetic acid. High urine levels of this acid can signal the presence of serotonin-secreting argentaffinomas — carcinoid tumors that arise from the argentaffin cells.

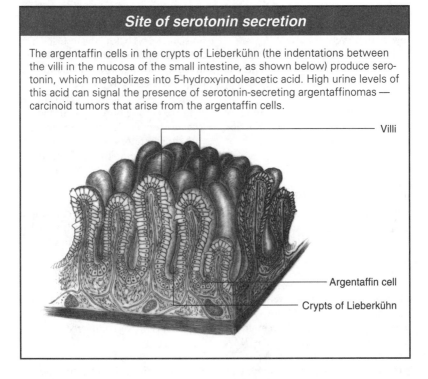

Villi

Argentaffin cell

Crypts of Lieberkühn

idase inhibitors, methyldopa, and isoniazid usually lower them.
■ Methenamine compounds, phenothiazines, salicylates, guaifenesin, mephenesin, methocarbamol, and acetaminophen may raise or lower 5-HIAA levels.
■ Failure to observe drug and dietary restrictions, to collect all urine during the test period, or to store the specimen properly may affect test results.
■ Severe GI disturbance or diarrhea may affect test results.

Urine pregnanediol

Using gas chromatography or radioimmunoassay, this test measures urine levels of pregnanediol, the chief metabolite of progesterone. Although biologically inert, pregnanediol has diagnostic significance because it reflects about 10% of the endogenous production of its parent hormone.

Progesterone is produced in nonpregnant females by the corpus luteum during the latter half of each menstrual cycle to prepare the uterus for implantation of a fertilized ovum. If implantation doesn't occur, progesterone secretion drops sharply; if implantation does occur, the corpus luteum secretes more progesterone to further prepare the uterus for pregnancy and to begin development of the placenta. Toward the end of the first trimester, the placenta becomes the primary source of progesterone secretion, producing the progressively larger amounts needed to maintain pregnancy.

Normally, urine levels of pregnanediol reflect variations in progesterone secretion during the menstrual cycle and during pregnancy. Direct measurement of plasma progesterone levels by radioimmunoassay may also be done. Pregnanediol is present in the urine as a metabolite of progesterone and is produced in small amounts by the adrenal cortex, the principal site of secretion in males, postmenopausal women, and menstruating females before ovulation.

Purpose
■ To evaluate placental function in pregnant females
■ To evaluate ovarian function in nonpregnant females.

Patient preparation
Explain to the patient that this test evaluates placental or ovarian function. Inform her that she needn't restrict food or fluids. Tell her the test requires a 24-hour urine specimen, and teach her the proper collection technique.

Check the patient's medication history for recent use of drugs that may affect pregnanediol levels.

Procedure
Collect a 24-hour urine specimen.

Precautions
■ Refrigerate the specimen or keep it on ice during the collection period.
■ If the patient is pregnant, note the approximate week of gestation on the laboratory request. For other premenopausal females, note the stage of the menstrual cycle.

Reference values
In nonpregnant females, urine pregnanediol values normally range from 0.5 to 1.5 mg/24 hours during the proliferative phase of the menstrual cycle. Pregnanediol levels begin to rise within 24 hours after ovulation and continue to rise for 3 to 10 days as the corpus lu-

teum develops. During this luteal phase, normal urine pregnanediol values range from 2 to 7 mg/24 hours. If fertilization does not occur, levels drop sharply as the corpus luteum degenerates, and menstruation begins.

During pregnancy, urine pregnanediol levels rise markedly, peaking around the 36th week of gestation and returning to prepregnancy levels by day 5 to day 10 postpartum. (See *Urine pregnanediol values in pregnancy,* page 408.)

Normal postmenopausal values range from 0.2 to 1 mg/24 hours. In males, levels rarely rise above 1.5 mg/24 hours.

Implications of results
During pregnancy, a marked decrease in urine pregnanediol levels based on a single 24-hour urine specimen, or a steady decrease in pregnanediol levels in serial measurements, may indicate placental insufficiency and requires immediate investigation. A precipitous drop in pregnanediol values may suggest fetal distress, as in threatened abortion or preeclampsia, or fetal death. However, pregnanediol levels are not reliable indicators of fetal viability, since they can remain normal even after fetal death as long as maternal circulation to the placenta remains adequate.

In nonpregnant females, abnormally low urine pregnanediol levels may occur with anovulation, amenorrhea, and other menstrual abnormalities. Low to normal pregnanediol levels may be associated with hydatidiform mole. Elevated levels may indicate luteinized granulosa or theca cell tumors, diffuse thecal luteinization, or metastatic ovarian cancer.

Adrenal hyperplasia or biliary tract obstruction may elevate urine pregnanediol values in males or females. Some forms of primary hepatic disease produce very low levels in both sexes.

Urine pregnanediol values in pregnancy

Serial determinations of average pregnanediol levels (middle line on chart) rise steadily until about 32 weeks' gestation, then level off. Excretion decreases 24 hours postpartum and drops to prepregnancy levels within 5 to 10 days. A wide range of normal values is possible — high-normal, low-normal, and average levels, as shown below.

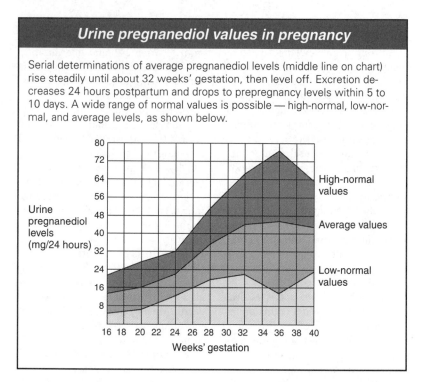

Post-test care
■ As ordered, resume administration of drugs withheld before the test.
■ Advise the pregnant patient that this test may be repeated several times to obtain serial measurements.

Interfering factors
■ Methenamine mandelate, methenamine hippurate, and drugs containing adrenocorticotropic hormone elevate urine pregnanediol levels. Progestogens and combination oral contraceptives characteristically lower them.
■ Failure to collect all urine during the collection period may alter test results.
■ Failure to refrigerate the specimen or to keep it on ice during the collection period may alter test results.

SELECTED READINGS

DeGroot, L.J., ed. *Endocrinology,* 3rd ed. Philadelphia: W.B. Saunders Co., 1995.

Guyton, A.C., and Hall, J.E. *Textbook of Medical Physiology,* 9th ed. Philadelphia: W.B. Saunders Co., 1996.

Henry, J.B., ed. *Clinical Diagnosis and Management by Laboratory Methods,* 19th ed. Philadelphia: W.B. Saunders Co., 1996.

Scott, J., et al. *Danforth's Obstetrics and Gynecology,* 7th ed. Philadelphia: Lippincott-Raven Pubs., 1994.

Vander, A.J. *Renal Physiology.* New York: McGraw-Hill Book Co., 1995.

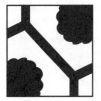

CHAPTER FIFTEEN

Urine proteins, protein metabolites, and pigments

INTRODUCTION

Laboratory analysis of urine specimens for abnormal levels of proteins, protein metabolites, and pigments is a significant factor in the detection and management of renal disorders and in the diagnosis of certain extrarenal or systemic diseases. Abnormalities that can be easily detected by analytical techniques include proteinuria and the presence of the pigments hemoglobin, bilirubin, urobilinogen, and the porphyrins. Examination of urine for protein metabolites is especially useful in evaluating renal function because healthy kidneys excrete these nonprotein nitrogenous (NPN) end products of protein metabolism.

Proteins

Normally, the protein content of urine is too small to be detected by routine screening procedures. Urine contains minute amounts of plasma proteins of low molecular weight or renal mucoproteins derived from the tubular cells. Benign proteinuria can result from changes in body position, as occurs in orthostatic proteinuria, or it can be associated with stress, exposure to cold, or fever.

Unusually high levels of proteins in urine, which are detectable by screening tests, nearly always indicate renal disease. Pathologic proteinuria can result from increased glomerular permeability due to a variety of causes, including glomerulonephritis, congestive heart failure, or renal tubular damage with defective reabsorption of protein. Infections of the lower urinary tract (cystitis, for example) can also cause proteinuria.

In most forms of renal disease marked by proteinuria, the predominant protein found in the urine is albumin because it's the smallest, the most easily filterable, and the most prevalent of all proteins. As kidney damage progresses, however, proteins of higher molecular weight — including the larger globulins — escape into the urine. The presence of certain abnormal proteins in the urine has special diagnostic significance; for example, Bence Jones protein in urine strongly suggests multiple myeloma.

Protein metabolites

Plasma contains more than 15 different NPN compounds, primarily urea, amino acids, creatine, creatinine, and uric acid. The kidneys normally excrete these nitrogenous waste products of protein metabolism, but diminished renal function causes these substances (including urea, uric acid, and creatinine) to accumulate in plasma. Consequently, renal dysfunction lowers the urine levels of these substances.

However, urine levels of urea and uric acid may change as a result of conditions other than renal disease — an important diagnostic consideration. Excessive purine catabolism, for example — which may be caused by a pathologic condition such as leukemia or simply by a high-purine diet — can raise both serum and urine uric acid levels because uric acid is a product of purine metabolism. Several factors, including dehydration, dietary ingestion of protein, and hepatic disease, can cause alteration in the levels of blood urea nitrogen and urine urea.

Because formation and urinary excretion of creatinine are more constant than urea and uric acid levels, serum and urine creatinine values provide a more reliable index of renal function. By comparing serum creatinine concentration with the total amount of creatinine excreted within a specified period, the creatinine clearance test shows how efficiently the kidneys are removing this substance from the blood. Values for this extremely important diagnostic test typically decrease when renal function is impaired.

Urinary excretion of amino acids is fairly constant in a healthy adult. However, metabolic disturbances can cause amino acids to accumulate in plasma and — when they exceed the renal threshold — to appear in the urine in excessive amounts. Urine amino acid screening can detect these overflow amino acids. Testing for the amino acid hydroxyproline helps detect disorders that affect bone metabolism. (For more information, see *Implications of abnormal protein and metabolite values,* page 412.)

Urine pigments

Pigments are involved in the biosynthesis of hemoglobin and its subsequent breakdown. A conjugated protein consisting of an iron-containing pigment (heme) and a protein (globin), *hemoglobin* normally appears in red blood cells, where its primary function is to carry oxygen from the lungs to body tissues. Hemoglobin is *not* a normal component of urine. However, when the amount of free hemoglobin in plasma exceeds the binding capacity of haptoglobin, as in severe intravascular hemolysis, hemoglobinuria results.

Myoglobin, which is closely related to hemoglobin in chemical composition, usually appears in cardiac and skeletal muscle; like hemoglobin, it doesn't usually appear in urine. Consequently, the presence of myoglobin in urine may indicate extensive muscle damage.

Porphyrins may be considered metabolic intermediates in heme synthesis, which takes place mainly in the marrow of the long bones and in the liver. Biosynthesis of heme begins with formation of delta-aminolevulinic acid and progresses through porphobilinogen to the precursors uroporphyrinogen, coproporphyrinogen, protoporphyrinogen and, finally, protoporphyrin, which chelates iron to form heme. Porphyrinogens are hematologically active. The inactive end products are normally excreted in small quantities: Protoporphyrin is excreted exclusively in feces; coproporphyrin and uroporphyrin, in feces or urine.

Metabolic defects in heme biosynthesis may cause inherited or acquired porphyrin disorders. Increased urinary ex-

Implications of abnormal protein and metabolite values

SUBSTANCE	NORMAL LEVELS IN URINE	IMPLICATIONS OF ABNORMAL LEVELS
Proteins		
Protein	< 150 mg/24 hours	*Increased:* urinary tract disorders; increased glomerular permeability; acute or chronic renal disease; other diseases, such as leukemia and toxemia
Bence Jones protein	Negative	*Increased:* multiple myeloma
Protein metabolites		
Amino acids	50 to 200 mg/24 hours	*Increased:* defective tubular reabsorption, resulting in increased renal excretion; congenital enzyme deficiencies, leading to metabolic disorders, such as phenylketonuria and cystinuria
Hydroxyproline	14 to 45 mg/24 hours for adults (higher for children and for women in the third trimester of pregnancy)	*Increased:* increased bone resorption caused by such disorders as Paget's disease, myeloma, or hyperthyroidism *Decreased:* drug treatment that decreases bone resorption
Creatinine	*Men:* 1 to 1.9 g/24 hours *Women:* 0.8 to 1.7 g/24 hours	*Decreased:* reduced renal blood flow, acute tubular necrosis, acute or chronic glomerulonephritis, advanced bilateral chronic pyelonephritis, advanced bilateral renal lesions, nephrosclerosis, severe dehydration, congestive heart failure (CHF)
Urea	Maximal clearance: 64 to 99 ml/minute	*Decreased:* reduced renal blood flow, acute or chronic glomerulonephritis, advanced bilateral chronic pyelonephritis, acute tubular necrosis, nephrosclerosis, advanced bilateral renal lesions, bilateral ureteral obstruction, CHF, dehydration
Uric acid	250 to 750 mg/24 hours (varies with purine intake)	*Increased:* chronic myeloid leukemia, polycythemia vera, multiple myeloma, pernicious anemia, lymphosarcoma and lymphatic leukemia during radiation therapy, defective tubular reabsorption, Wilson's disease *Decreased:* chronic glomerulonephritis, diabetic glomerulosclerosis, collagen disorders

cretion of specific porphyrins may aid diagnosis of a particular porphyrin disorder, perhaps in combination with results of fecal and erythrocyte porphyrin testing.

The breakdown of the heme fraction of hemoglobin results in the formation of *bilirubin*. In the liver, free bilirubin conjugates with glucuronic acid, which allows bilirubin to be filtered by the glomeruli (unconjugated bilirubin is not filterable). Bilirubin is normally excreted in bile as its principal pigment, but it is an abnormal element of urine. Conjugated bilirubin is present in urine when serum levels are elevated, as in biliary tract obstruction or hepatocellular damage, and is accompanied by jaundice.

Urobilinogen is formed in the intestine by bacterial action on conjugated bilirubin. Most urobilinogen is eventually excreted in feces, producing the stools' characteristic color. A small amount of urobilinogen is reabsorbed by the portal system and is excreted mainly in bile, although the kidneys do excrete some. Therefore, elevated urine urobilinogen levels may be an early indication of hepatic damage. Urine urobilinogen levels decrease in biliary obstruction because bilirubin doesn't reach the intestine.

Melanin, the main pigment of hair, skin, and the choroid of the eye, is formed from the metabolism of tyrosine. This pigment is not normally present in urine, but melanin-producing tumors (melanomas) may produce sufficient amounts of it to be detected in urine. In live metastasis, melanins and their precursors — melanogens — commonly appear in urine.

PROTEIN TESTS

Urine protein

This is a quantitative test for proteinuria. Normally, the glomerular membrane allows only proteins of low molecular weight to enter the filtrate. The renal tubules then reabsorb most of these proteins, normally excreting a small amount that's undetectable by a screening test. A damaged glomerular capillary membrane and impaired tubular reabsorption allow excretion of proteins in the urine.

A qualitative screening often precedes this test. (See *Random specimen screening for protein,* page 414.) A positive result requires quantitative analysis of a 24-hour urine specimen by acid precipitation tests. Electrophoresis can detect Bence Jones protein, hemoglobins, myoglobins, and albumin.

Purpose
■ To aid diagnosis of pathologic states characterized by proteinuria, primarily renal disease.

Patient preparation
Explain to the patient that this test detects proteins in the urine. Inform him that he needn't restrict food or fluids. Tell him that the test requires a 24-hour urine specimen, and teach him the correct collection technique.

Check the patient's medication history for drugs that may affect test results. Review your findings with the laboratory, and notify the doctor; he may want to restrict medications before the test.

Procedure
Collect a 24-hour urine specimen. A special specimen container can be obtained from the laboratory.

Random specimen screening for protein

Qualitative screening tests for proteinuria include reagent strips (dipsticks) and acids that precipitate proteins (sulfosalicylic acid or acetic acid with heat).

To perform such a test, collect a clean-catch urine specimen, preferably in the morning, when the urine is most concentrated and yields the most reliable information. A reagent strip (such as Chemstrips) is usually used. Dip the strip into the urine; remove excess urine by tapping the strip against a clean surface or the edge of the container. Hold the strip in a horizontal position to prevent mixing of chemicals from adjacent areas. Immediately place the strip close to the color block on the bottle and carefully compare colors. The results correspond to the number of milligrams per deciliter of protein (usually albumin, since strips are most sensitive to this protein). Results are as follows:

Negative = 0 to 5 mg/dl
Trace = 5 to 20 mg/dl
1+ = 30 mg/dl
2+ = 100 mg/dl
3+ = 300 mg/dl
4+ = 1,000 mg/dl

Normally, no detectable protein is present in a random specimen, although normal kidneys do excrete a minute amount. A positive result requires quantitative analysis of a 24-hour urine specimen.

Phenazopyridine can alter the color reaction of certain brands of reagent strips; so can high salt or alkaline content of the urine specimen. Acetazolamide and sodium bicarbonate can cause false-positive results with some reagent strips.

Precautions

- Tell the patient not to contaminate the urine with toilet tissue or stool.
- Refrigerate the specimen or place it on ice during the collection period.

Reference values

Normally, up to 150 mg of protein is excreted in 24 hours.

Implications of results

Proteinuria is characteristic of renal disease. When proteinuria is present in a single specimen, a 24-hour urine collection is required to identify specific renal abnormalities.

Proteinuria can result from glomerular leakage of plasma proteins (a major cause of protein excretion), from overflow of filtered proteins of low molecular weight (when they are present in excessive concentrations), from impaired tubular reabsorption of filtered proteins, and from the presence of renal proteins derived from the breakdown of kidney tissue.

Persistent proteinuria indicates renal disease resulting from increased glomerular permeability. Minimal proteinuria (less than 0.5 g/24 hours), however, is most often associated with renal disease in which glomerular involvement is not a major factor, such as chronic pyelonephritis.

Moderate proteinuria (0.5 to 4 g/24 hours) occurs in several types of renal disease — acute or chronic glomerulonephritis, amyloidosis, toxic nephropathies — and in diseases in which renal failure often develops as a late complication (such as diabetes and heart failure). Heavy proteinuria (more than 4 g/24 hours) is commonly associated with nephrotic syndrome.

Postural proteinuria

A benign form of proteinuria, postural (orthostatic) proteinuria occurs when a patient stands but not when he's recumbent. It can also happen when he assumes a lordotic position — from bending backward over a chair, for example. Generally, this condition is found in healthy children or young adults and has no pathologic significance, although it causes extensive proteinuria.

Postural proteinuria probably results from obstruction of renal venous outflow, which causes renal congestion and ischemia. To confirm this condition, diagnostic tests must rule out renal disease and clearly establish the absence of proteinuria during recumbency. In one test, the patient voids before retiring and remains recumbent for 12 hours. A urine specimen is collected as soon as he awakens and, for comparison, at specific times during the next 12 hours while he is ambulatory. In postural proteinuria, the specimen collected at the end of recumbency is free of proteins, but the ones collected during the ambulatory period contain proteins.

When accompanied by an elevated white blood cell (WBC) count, proteinuria indicates urinary tract infection; with hematuria, proteinuria indicates local or diffuse urinary tract disorders. Other pathologic states (such as infections and lesions of the central nervous system) can also result in detectable amounts of proteins in the urine.

Many drugs (such as amphotericin B, gold preparations, aminoglycosides, polymyxins, and trimethadione) inflict renal damage, causing true proteinuria. This makes the routine evaluation of urine proteins essential during treatment with these drugs.

In all forms of proteinuria, fractionation results obtained by electrophoresis provide more precise information than the screening test. For example, excessive hemoglobin in the urine indicates intravascular hemolysis; elevated myoglobin suggests muscle damage; albumin, increased glomerular permeability; and Bence Jones protein, multiple myeloma.

Not all forms of proteinuria have pathologic significance. Benign proteinuria can result from changes in body position. (See *Postural proteinuria.*) Functional proteinuria is associated with exercise, as well as emotional or physiologic stress, and is usually transient.

Post-test care
As ordered, resume administration of medications withheld before the test.

Interfering factors
■ Administration of tolbutamide, para-aminosalicylic acid, acetazolamide, sodium bicarbonate, penicillin, sulfonamides, iodine contrast media, or cephalosporins may cause false-positive results in acid precipitation tests.
■ Contamination of the urine specimen with heavy mucus, vaginal or prostatic secretions, or the presence of numerous WBCs can alter test results, regardless of laboratory method used.
■ Very dilute urine (which may result from forcing fluids) may depress protein values and cause false-negative results.

Urine Bence Jones protein

Bence Jones proteins are abnormal light-chain immunoglobulins of low molecular weight that are derived from the clone of a single plasma cell (monoclonal). This globulin appears in the urine of 50% to 80% of patients with multiple myeloma and in most patients with Waldenström's macroglobulinemia.

In most cases, these proteins — thought to be synthesized by malignant plasma cells in the bone marrow — are rapidly cleared from the plasma and don't usually appear in serum. When these proteins exceed renal tubular capacity to break down and reabsorb them, they overflow and are excreted in the urine (overflow proteinuria). Eventually, the renal tubular cells degenerate from the effort of reabsorbing excess amounts of protein. Consequently, protein precipitates and inclusions occur in the renal tubular cells. If renal failure results from such precipitation or from hypercalcemia, increased uric acid, or infiltration by abnormal plasma cells, more Bence Jones proteins and other proteins then appear in the urine because the dysfunctional nephrons no longer control protein excretion.

Urine screening tests, such as thermal coagulation and Bradshaw's test, can detect Bence Jones proteins, but urine immunoelectrophoresis is usually the method of choice for quantitative studies. Serum immunoelectrophoresis, which is sometimes used, is less sensitive than the urine tests. Nevertheless, both urine and serum studies are frequently used for patients suspected of having multiple myeloma.

Purpose
- To confirm the presence of multiple myeloma in patients with characteristic clinical signs, such as bone pain (especially in the back and thorax) and persistent anemia and fatigue.

Patient preparation
Explain to the patient that this test can detect an abnormal protein in the urine. Tell him the test requires an early-morning urine specimen, and teach him how to collect a clean-catch specimen.

Procedure
Collect an early-morning urine specimen of at least 50 ml.

Precautions
- Tell the patient not to contaminate the urine specimen with toilet tissue or stool.
- Send the specimen to the laboratory immediately. If transport is delayed, refrigerate the specimen.

Normal findings
Urine should contain no Bence Jones proteins.

Implications of results
The presence of Bence Jones proteins in urine suggests multiple myeloma or Waldenström's macroglobulinemia. Very low levels in the absence of other symptoms may result from benign monoclonal gammopathy. However, clinical evidence figures prominently in diagnosis of multiple myeloma.

Post-test care
None.

Interfering factors
- False-positive results may occur in connective tissue disease, renal insufficiency, and certain cancers.
- Contamination of the specimen with menstrual blood, prostatic secretions, or

semen may cause false-positive results.

■ Failure to send the specimen to the laboratory immediately or to keep the specimen refrigerated may produce a false-positive result because heat-coagulable protein denatures or decomposes at room temperature.

PROTEIN METABOLITE TESTS

Urine amino acid screening

This test screens for aminoaciduria — elevated urine amino acid levels — a condition that may result from inborn errors of metabolism due to the absence of specific enzymatic activities. (Normally, up to 200 mg of amino acids may be excreted in the urine in 24 hours.) Abnormal metabolism causes an excess of one or more amino acids to appear in plasma and, as the renal threshold is exceeded, in urine.

Aminoacidurias may be classified as primary (overflow) aminoacidopathies or secondary (renal) aminoacidopathies. The latter type is associated with conditions marked by defective tubular reabsorption from congenital disorders. A more specific defect, such as cystinuria, may cause one or more amino acids to appear in urine.

To screen neonates, children, and adults for congenital aminoacidurias, plasma or urine specimens may be used. The plasma test is the better indicator of overflow aminoaciduria; urine testing is used to confirm or monitor certain amino acid disorders and to screen for renal aminoacidurias.

Various laboratory techniques are available to screen for aminoacidurias, but chromatography is the preferred method. Positive findings on chromatography can be elaborated by fractionation, showing specific amino acid levels. Testing for specific amino acid levels is also necessary for infants or young children with acidosis, severe vomiting and diarrhea, and abnormal urine odor. Such testing is especially important in newborns, because early diagnosis of certain aminoacidurias may prevent mental retardation by allowing prompt treatment.

Purpose

■ To screen for renal aminoacidurias
■ To follow up plasma test findings when results of these tests suggest certain overflow aminoacidurias.

Patient preparation

Explain to the patient (or to his parents if the patient is an infant or a child) that this test helps detect amino acid disorders and that additional tests may be necessary. Inform him that he needn't restrict food or fluids before the test. Tell him the test requires a urine specimen.

Check the patient's medication history for drugs that may interfere with test results. If such drugs must be continued, note this on the laboratory request. (If the patient is a breast-fed infant, record any drugs that the mother is receiving.)

Procedure

If the patient is an infant, clean and dry the genital area, attach the collection device, and observe for voiding. Transfer urine — at least 20 ml — to a specimen container. If the patient is an adult or a child, collect a fresh random specimen.

Precautions

■ For an infant, apply adhesive flanges of the collection device securely to the skin to prevent leakage.

▪ Send the specimen to the laboratory immediately.

Normal findings
Patterns on thin-layer chromatography are reported as normal.

Implications of results
If thin-layer chromatography shows gross changes or abnormal patterns, blood and 24-hour urine quantitative column chromatography are performed to identify specific amino acid abnormalities and to differentiate overflow and renal aminoacidurias.

Post-test care
Remove the collection device carefully from an infant to prevent skin irritation.

Interfering factors
▪ Failure to send the urine specimen to the laboratory immediately may affect the accuracy of test results.
▪ Results are invalid in a neonate who has not ingested dietary protein in the 48 hours preceding the test.

Urine hydroxyproline

This test measures total urine levels of hydroxyproline, an amino acid found mainly in collagen (a component of skin and bone). Urine hydroxyproline levels are a good index of bone matrix turnover because levels increase when collagen breaks down during bone resorption.

Bone matrix turnover and hydroxyproline levels normally rise in children during periods of rapid skeletal growth. However, they also rise in disorders that increase bone resorption, such as Paget's disease, metastatic bone tumors, and certain endocrine disorders. This test helps diagnose these disorders, but it's more commonly used to monitor response to drug therapy in conditions marked by rapid bone resorption.

Hydroxyproline levels are most often determined colorimetrically on a timed urine sample; they may also be determined by ion-exchange or gas-liquid chromatography. A collagen-restricted diet is essential for this test because hydroxyproline levels reflect collagen intake. Free hydroxyproline, a small component of total hydroxyproline and a sensitive indicator of dietary collagen intake, may be measured to validate results.

Purpose
▪ To monitor the effectiveness of treatment for disorders characterized by bone resorption, primarily Paget's disease
▪ To aid diagnosis of disorders characterized by bone resorption.

Patient preparation
Explain to the patient that this test helps monitor treatment or detect an amino acid disorder related to bone formation. Advise him to avoid eating meat, fish, poultry, jelly, and any foods containing gelatin for 24 hours before the test and during the test period itself. Tell him the test requires a 2-hour or 24-hour urine specimen, as appropriate, and teach him the correct collection technique.

Note the patient's age and sex on the laboratory request. Check his medication history for drugs that may alter test results, and restrict such drugs as ordered.

Procedure
Collect a 2-hour or 24-hour urine specimen, as ordered, in a container that has a preservative to prevent degradation of hydroxyproline.

Precautions

Refrigerate the specimen or keep it on ice during the collection period, and send it to the laboratory immediately.

Reference values

■ *For 24-hour specimen:* 14 to 45 mg/ 24 hours (adults)
■ *For 2-hour specimen:* 0.4 to 5.0 mg/ 2-hour specimen (males); 0.4 to 2.9 mg/ 2-hour specimen (females).

Normal values for children are much higher and peak between ages 11 and 18. Values also rise during the third trimester of pregnancy, reflecting fetal skeletal growth.

Implications of results

Hydroxyproline levels should decrease slowly during therapy for bone resorption disorders. Elevated levels may indicate bone disease, metastatic bone tumors, or endocrine disorders that stimulate hormonal secretion.

Post-test care

As ordered, resume food and drugs withheld before the test.

Interfering factors

■ Ascorbic acid, vitamin D, aspirin, and glucocorticoids, as well as calcitonin and mithramycin (used to treat Paget's disease), can decrease levels.
■ Failure to observe restrictions, to collect all urine during the test period, or to store the specimen correctly may alter test results.
■ Psoriasis and burns can promote collagen turnover, elevating urine hydroxyproline levels.

Urine creatinine

This test measures urine levels of creatinine, the chief metabolite of creatine. Produced in amounts proportional to total body muscle mass, creatinine is removed from the plasma primarily by glomerular filtration and is excreted in the urine.

Because the body doesn't recycle it, creatinine has a relatively high, constant clearance rate, making it an efficient indicator of renal function. However, the creatinine clearance test, which measure both urine and plasma creatine clearance, is a more precise index than this test. A standard method of determining urine creatinine levels is based on Jaffé's reaction, in which creatinine treated with an alkaline picrate solution yields a bright orange-red complex.

Purpose

■ To help assess glomerular filtration
■ To check the accuracy of 24-hour urine collection based on the relatively constant levels of creatinine excretion.

Patient preparation

Explain to the patient that this test helps evaluate kidney function. Inform him that he needn't restrict fluids but should not eat an excessive amount of meat before the test and should avoid strenuous physical exercise during the collection period. Tell him the test usually requires a 24-hour urine specimen, and teach him the proper collection technique.

Check the patient's medication history for drugs that may affect creatinine levels. Review your findings with the laboratory, and then notify the doctor; he may restrict such drugs before the test.

Procedure

Collect a 24-hour urine specimen in a specimen bottle that contains a preservative to prevent degradation of creatinine.

Precautions

Refrigerate the specimen or keep it on ice during the collection period. When the collection is completed, send the specimen to the laboratory at once.

Reference values

Urine creatinine levels normally range from 0 to 40 mg/24 hours for men, and from 0 to 80 mg/24 hours for women.

Implications of results

Decreased urine creatinine levels may result from impaired renal perfusion (associated with shock, for example) or from renal disease due to urinary tract obstruction. Chronic bilateral pyelonephritis, acute or chronic glomerulonephritis, and polycystic kidney disease may also depress creatinine levels. Increased urine creatinine levels generally have little diagnostic significance.

Post-test care

▪ As ordered, resume medications withheld before the test.
▪ Tell the patient that he may resume his diet and normal activities.

Interfering factors

▪ Drugs that may affect urine creatinine levels include corticosteroids, gentamicin, tetracyclines, diuretics, and amphotericin B.
▪ Failure to observe pretest restrictions, to collect all urine during the test period, or to store the specimen properly may interfere with test results.

Creatinine clearance

Creatinine, an anhydride of creatine, is formed and excreted in constant amounts by an irreversible reaction and functions solely as the main end product of creatine. Creatinine production is proportional to total muscle mass and is relatively unaffected by normal physical activity, diet, or urine volume.

An excellent diagnostic indicator of renal function, the creatinine clearance test determines how efficiently the kidneys are clearing creatinine from the blood. The rate of clearance is expressed in terms of the volume of blood (in milliliters) that can be cleared of creatinine in 1 minute.

To arrive at this determination, the equation $C = (U \times V) \div P$ is used; C represents the clearance rate; U, the urine concentration of creatinine; V, the volume of urine collected during the test period (converted to ml/minute); and P, the plasma concentration of creatinine. Naturally, urine and plasma concentrations of creatinine must be expressed in the same units (usually mg/dl), so they cancel each other out in the equation.

A final adjustment must be made to allow for renal parenchymal mass, which differs in each patient. To do this, the clearance rate established in the above equation is multiplied by $(1.73 \div A)$, where 1.73 equals the body surface area (in square meters) of the average person, and A equals the patient's body surface area. Creatinine levels become abnormal when more than 50% of the total nephron units have been damaged.

Purpose

▪ To assess renal function (primarily glomerular filtration)
▪ To monitor progression of renal insufficiency.

Patient preparation

Explain to the patient that this test assesses kidney function. Inform him that he needn't restrict fluids but should not eat an excessive amount of meat before the test and should avoid strenuous physical exercise during the collection period. Tell him the test requires a timed urine specimen and at least one blood sample. Tell him how the urine specimen will be collected, who will perform the venipuncture and when, and that he may feel some discomfort from the needle puncture. Explain that more than one venipuncture may be necessary.

Check the patient's medication history for drugs that may affect creatinine clearance. Review your findings with the laboratory, and then notify the doctor; he may want to restrict these medications before the test.

Procedure

Collect a timed urine specimen at 2, 6, 12, or 24 hours in a bottle containing a preservative to prevent degradation of the creatinine.

Perform a venipuncture anytime during the collection period, and collect the sample in a 7-ml *red-top* tube.

Precautions

Refrigerate the specimen or keep it on ice during the collection period. When the collection is completed, send the specimen to the laboratory at once.

Reference values

At age 20, creatinine clearance normally ranges from 85 to 146 ml/minute/ 1.73 m² for men and from 81 to 134 ml/ minute/1.73 m² for women. Creatinine clearance normally decreases by 6 ml/ minute for each decade after age 20.

Implications of results

Low creatinine clearance may result from reduced renal blood flow (associated with shock or renal artery obstruc-

tion), acute tubular necrosis, acute or chronic glomerulonephritis, advanced bilateral chronic pyelonephritis, advanced bilateral renal lesions (as in polycystic kidney disease, cancer, or renal tuberculosis), or nephrosclerosis. Congestive heart failure and severe dehydration may also cause creatinine clearance to fall below normal.

High creatinine clearance rates generally have little diagnostic significance.

Post-test care

- If a hematoma develops at the venipuncture site, apply warm soaks to ease discomfort.
- As ordered, resume administration of medications withheld before the test.
- Tell the patient that he may resume his diet and normal activity.

Interfering factors

- Drugs that may affect creatinine clearance include amphotericin B, thiazide diuretics, furosemide, and aminoglycosides.
- A high-protein diet before the test and strenuous physical exercise during the collection period may increase creatinine excretion.
- Failure to observe pretest restrictions, to collect all urine during the test period, or to store the specimen properly may affect the accuracy of test results.

Urea clearance

The urea clearance test is a quantitative analysis of urine levels of urea, the main nitrogenous component in urine and the end product of protein metabolism. (See *How urea is formed*, page 422.) After filtration by the glomeruli, roughly 40% of the urea is reabsorbed by the renal tubules. Because of this reabsorp-

How urea is formed

Urea, the main nitrogenous component in urine, is the final product of protein metabolism. Amino acids absorbed by the intestinal villi pass from the portal vein into the liver. Because the liver stores only small amounts of amino acids — which are later returned to the blood for use in the synthesis of enzymes, hormones, or new protoplasm — the excess is converted into other substances, such as glucose, glycogen, and fat.

Before this conversion, the amino acids are deaminated — they lose their nitrogenous amino groups. These amino groups are then converted to ammonia. Because ammonia is very toxic, especially to the brain, it must be removed as quickly as it's formed. (Serious liver disease causes elevated blood ammonia levels and eventually leads to hepatic coma.)

In the liver, ammonia combines with carbon dioxide to form urea, which is released into the blood and ultimately secreted in urine.

---

tion, urea clearance was once considered a precise fraction (60%) of the glomerular filtration rate (GFR). However, because the reabsorption rate of urea varies with the amount of water reabsorbed, this test actually assesses overall renal function; the creatinine clearance test provides a more accurate evaluation of the GFR.

In urea clearance, blood urea content and the total amount of urea excreted in the urine are proportional only when the rate of urine flow is 2 ml/minute or higher (maximal clearance). At lower flow rates, the test's accuracy decreases. The equation for determining urea clearance is $C = (U \times V) \div P$; it's similar to the equation used for creatinine clearance.

Purpose

■ To assess overall renal function.

Patient preparation

Explain to the patient that this test evaluates kidney function. Instruct him to fast from midnight before the test and to abstain from exercise before and during the test. Tell him the test requires two timed urine specimens and one blood sample. Tell him how the urine specimens will be collected, who will perform the venipuncture and when, and that he may experience transient discomfort from the needle puncture.

Check the patient's medication history for drugs that may affect urea clearance. Review your findings with the laboratory, and then notify the doctor; he may want to restrict these medications before the test.

Procedure

Instruct the patient to empty his bladder and discard the urine. Then give him water to drink to ensure adequate urine output. Collect two specimens 1 hour apart, and mark the collection time on the laboratory request. Perform a venipuncture anytime during the collection period, and collect the sample in a 7-ml *red-top* tube.

Precautions

■ Because this is a clearance test, make sure the patient empties his bladder completely and that the total amount of urine is collected from each hour's specimen.

■ Send each specimen to the laboratory as soon as it is collected.

■ If the patient is catheterized, empty the drainage bag before beginning the specimen collection.

■ Handle the blood sample gently to prevent hemolysis, and send it to the laboratory immediately.

Reference values

Normally, urea clearance ranges from 64 to 99 ml/minute with maximal clearance. If the flow rate is less than 2 ml/minute, normal clearance is 41 to 68 ml/minute. (If the urine flow rate is less than 1 ml/minute, this test should not be performed.)

Implications of results

Low urea clearance values may indicate decreased renal blood flow (due to shock or renal artery obstruction), acute or chronic glomerulonephritis, advanced bilateral chronic pyelonephritis, acute tubular necrosis, or nephrosclerosis. Low clearance rates may also result from advanced bilateral renal lesions (as in polycystic kidney disease, renal tuberculosis, or cancer), bilateral ureteral obstruction, congestive heart failure, or dehydration.

High urea clearance rates are usually not diagnostically significant.

Post-test care

■ If a hematoma develops at the venipuncture site, apply warm soaks.

■ As ordered, resume administration of medications that were withheld before the test.

■ Tell the patient that he may resume his usual diet and activities.

Interfering factors

■ The patient's failure to empty his bladder completely — the most common error in this test — or to observe pretest restrictions will alter test results.

■ Caffeine, milk, or small doses of epinephrine increase urea clearance; antidiuretic hormone or large doses of epinephrine decrease urea clearance. Corticosteroids, amphotericin B, thiazide diuretics, and streptomycin may also affect test results.

■ Hemolysis caused by rough handling of the blood sample may affect test results.

Urine uric acid

A quantitative analysis of urine uric acid levels, this test supplements serum uric acid testing for identifying disorders that alter production or excretion of uric acid (such as leukemia, gout, and renal dysfunction). Derived from dietary purines in organ meats (liver, kidney, and sweetbread) and from endogenous nucleoproteins, uric acid (as urate) is found normally in the blood and in other tissues in amounts totaling about 1 g. Its primary site of formation is the liver, although the intestinal mucosa is also involved in urate production.

As the chief end product of purine catabolism, urate passes from the liver through the bloodstream to the kidneys, where roughly 50% is excreted daily in the urine. Renal urate metabolism is complex, involving glomerular filtration, tubular secretion, and a second reabsorption by the renal tubules.

The most specific laboratory method of detecting uric acid is spectrophotometric absorption after the specimen is treated with the enzyme uricase.

Purpose

■ To detect enzyme deficiencies and metabolic disturbances that affect uric acid production

▪ To help measure the efficiency of renal clearance.

Patient preparation

Explain to the patient that this test measures the body's production and excretion of a waste product known as uric acid. Inform him he needn't restrict food or fluids before the test. Tell him the test requires a 24-hour urine specimen, and teach him the proper collection technique.

Check the patient's medication history for recent use of drugs that may influence uric acid levels. If these medications must be continued, note this on the laboratory request.

Procedure

Collect a 24-hour urine specimen.

Precautions

Send the specimen to the laboratory as soon as the collection period is over.

Reference values

Normal urine uric acid values vary with diet but generally range from 250 to 750 mg/24 hours.

Implications of results

Elevated urine uric acid levels may result from chronic myeloid leukemia, polycythemia vera, multiple myeloma, early remission in pernicious anemia, as well as lymphosarcoma and lymphatic leukemia during radiation therapy. High levels also result from tubular reabsorption defects, such as Fanconi's syndrome and hepatolenticular degeneration (Wilson's disease).

Low urine uric acid levels occur in gout (when associated with normal uric acid production but inadequate excretion) and in severe renal damage, as occurs in chronic glomerulonephritis, diabetic glomerulosclerosis, and collagen disorders.

Post-test care

As ordered, resume administration of medications withheld before the test.

Interfering factors

▪ Drugs that decrease urine uric acid excretion include pyrazinamide and diuretics, such as benzthiazide, furosemide, and ethacrynic acid. Low doses of salicylates, phenylbutazone, and probenecid also lower uric acid levels; high doses of these drugs cause levels to rise above normal. Allopurinol, a drug used to treat gout, increases uric acid excretion.

▪ Urine uric acid concentrations rise with a high-purine diet and fall with a low-purine diet.

▪ Failure to observe drug restrictions or to collect all urine during the test period may alter test results.

PIGMENT TESTS

Urine hemoglobin

Free hemoglobin in the urine — an abnormal finding — may occur in hemolytic anemias, infection, or severe intravascular hemolysis from a transfusion reaction. It may also follow strenuous exercise. Contained in red blood cells (RBCs), hemoglobin consists of heme — an iron-protoporphyrin complex — and globin — a polypeptide. Hemoglobin combines with oxygen and carbon dioxide to allow RBCs to transport these gases between the lungs and the tissues.

Aging RBCs are constantly being destroyed by normal mechanisms within the reticuloendothelial system. However, when RBC destruction occurs within the circulation, as in intravascular

Bedside testing for urine blood pigments

To test a patient's urine for blood pigments at bedside, use one of the following methods.

Dipstick, Multistix, or Chemstrips

- Collect a urine specimen.
- Dip the stick into the specimen and withdraw it.
- After 30 seconds, compare the stick to the color chart. Blue indicates a positive reaction; the intensity of color indicates pigment concentration.

Occult tablet

- Collect a urine specimen.
- Put one drop of urine on the filter paper. Place the tablet on the urine, and then put two drops of water on the tablet.
- After 2 minutes, inspect the filter

paper around the tablet. Blue indicates a positive reaction; the intensity of color indicates pigment concentration.

Occult solution

- Collect a urine specimen.
- After placing one drop of urine on the filter paper, close the package and turn it over. Open the opposite side, and place two drops of solution on the filter paper.
- After 30 seconds, inspect the filter paper. Blue indicates a positive reaction; the intensity of color indicates pigment concentration.

Because these methods detect only blood pigments, immunochemical studies are necessary to differentiate hemoglobin from other blood pigments, such as myoglobin.

---

hemolysis, free hemoglobin enters the plasma and binds with haptoglobin, a plasma alpha$_2$ globulin. If the plasma level of hemoglobin exceeds that of haptoglobin, the excess of unbound hemoglobin is excreted in the urine (hemoglobinuria).

This test is based on the fact that heme proteins act like enzymes that catalyze oxidation of organic substances, such as guaiac or orthotolidine. This reaction produces a blue coloration; the intensity of color varies with the amount of hemoglobin present. Microscopic examination is required to identify intact RBCs in urine (hematuria), which can occur in the presence of unbound hemoglobin.

Testing for urine blood pigments can also be performed at the patient's bedside. (See *Bedside testing for urine blood pigments.*)

Purpose

- To aid diagnosis of hemolytic anemias, infection, or severe intravascular hemolysis from a transfusion reaction.

Patient preparation

Explain to the patient that this test detects excessive RBC destruction. Inform him that he needn't restrict food or fluids. Tell him the test requires a random urine specimen, and teach him the proper collection technique. If the female patient is menstruating, reschedule the test because contamination of the specimen with menstrual blood will alter test results.

Check the patient's medication history for drugs that may affect free hemoglobin levels. Review your findings with the laboratory, then notify the doctor; he may want to restrict these medications before the test.

Procedure

Collect a random urine specimen.

Precautions

Send the specimen to the laboratory immediately.

Normal findings

Hemoglobin should not be present in the urine.

Implications of results

Hemoglobinuria may result from severe intravascular hemolysis due to a blood transfusion reaction, burns, or a crushing injury; from acquired hemolytic anemias caused by chemical or drug intoxication or malaria; or from the hemolytic anemia known as paroxysmal nocturnal hemoglobinuria. Hemoglobinuria may also result from congenital hemolytic anemias, as in hemoglobinopathies or enzyme defects, and, less commonly, from cystitis, ureteral calculi, or urethritis.

Hemoglobinuria and hematuria occur in renal epithelial damage (as in acute glomerulonephritis or pyelonephritis), renal tumor, and tuberculosis.

Post-test care

As ordered, resume administration of medications discontinued before the test.

Interfering factors

■ Lysis of RBCs in stale or alkaline urine and contamination of the specimen with menstrual blood will alter test results.

■ Bacterial peroxidases in highly infected specimens can product false-positive test results.

■ Large doses of vitamin C or of drugs that contain vitamin C as a preservative (such as certain antibiotics) can inhibit reagent activity, producing false-negative results. Nephrotoxic drugs (such as amphotericin B) or anticoagulants (such as warfarin) may cause a positive result for hemoglobinuria or hematuria.

Urine myoglobin

This test detects the presence of myoglobin — a red pigment found in the cytoplasm of cardiac and skeletal muscle cells — in the urine. Myoglobin probably serves as a reservoir of oxygen, facilitating its movement within muscle. When muscle cells are extensively damaged, as by disease or severe crushing trauma, myoglobin is released into the blood, quickly cleared by renal glomerular filtration, and eliminated in the urine (myoglobinuria). For example, myoglobin appears in the urine within 24 hours after myocardial infarction. Because of the marked structural similarities of urine myoglobin and urine hemoglobin, they are not satisfactorily differentiated by qualitative assays.

The test method most commonly used to detect myoglobinuria is the differential precipitation test. Hemoglobin — bound to haptoglobin — precipitates when urine is mixed with ammonium sulfate, but myoglobin remains soluble and can be measured.

Purpose

■ To aid diagnosis of muscle disease
■ To detect extensive infarction of muscle tissue
■ To assess the extent of muscular damage from crushing trauma.

Patient preparation

Explain to the patient that this test detects a red pigment found in muscle cells and helps evaluate muscle injury or disease. Inform him that he needn't restrict food or fluids before the test. Tell him that this test requires a random urine specimen, and teach him the proper collection technique.

Procedure
Collect a random urine specimen.

Precautions
Send the specimen to the laboratory immediately.

Normal findings
Myoglobin should not appear in the urine.

Implications of results
Myoglobinuria occurs in acute or chronic muscular disease, alcoholic polymyopathy, familial myoglobinuria, and extensive myocardial infarction. It also results from severe trauma to the skeletal muscles (as in a crushing injury, extreme hyperthermia, or severe burns). Transient myoglobinuria ("march" myoglobinuria) may follow strenuous or prolonged exercise but disappears after rest.

Post-test care
None.

Interfering factors
▪ If this test is performed with Chemstrips or other reagent strips, recent ingestion of large amounts of vitamin C can inhibit the reaction, thereby interfering with test results.
▪ Extremely dilute urine can reduce test sensitivity.
▪ Contamination of urine with iodine during surgery may produce positive results.

Urine porphyrins

This test is a quantitative analysis of urine porphyrins (most notably, uroporphyrins and coproporphyrins) and their precursors (porphyrinogens, such as porphobilinogen [PBG]). Porphyrins are red-orange fluorescent compounds, consisting of four pyrrole rings, that are produced during heme biosynthesis. They are present in all protoplasm, figure in energy storage and utilization, and are normally excreted in urine in small amounts. Elevated urine levels of porphyrins or porphyrinogens, therefore, reflect impaired heme biosynthesis. Such impairment may result from inherited enzyme deficiencies (congenital porphyrias) or from defects caused by such disorders as hemolytic anemias and hepatic disease (acquired porphyrias).

Determining the specific porphyrins and porphyrinogens found in a urine specimen can help identify the impaired metabolic step in heme biosynthesis. Occasionally, a preliminary qualitative screening is performed on a random specimen; a positive finding on the screening test must be confirmed by the quantitative analysis of a 24-hour specimen. For correct diagnosis of a specific porphyria, urine porphyrin levels should be correlated with plasma and fecal porphyrin levels.

Purpose
▪ To aid diagnosis of congenital or acquired porphyrias.

Patient preparation
Explain to the patient that this test detects abnormal hemoglobin formation. Inform him that he needn't restrict food or fluids before the test. Tell him the test requires a 24-hour urine specimen, and

Urine porphyrin levels in porphyria

Defective heme biosynthesis increases levels of most urinary porphyrins and their corresponding precursors, as shown below.

PORPHYRIA	PORPHYRINS	
	Uroporphyrins	Coproporphyrins
Erythropoietic porphyria	Highly increased	Increased
Erythropoietic protoporphyria	Normal	Normal
Acute intermittent porphyria	Variable	Variable
Variegate porphyria	Normal or slightly increased; may be highly increased during acute attack	Normal or slightly increased; may be highly increased during acute attack
Coproporphyria	Not applicable	May be highly increased during acute attack
Porphyria cutanea tarda (assumed to be acquired in association with other hepatic diseases; genetic causes possible)	Highly increased	Increased

teach him the proper collection technique.

Check the patient's history for current pregnancy, menstruation, or drug use; such conditions may affect test results. Inform the laboratory and the doctor, who may reschedule the test or restrict drugs before the test.

Procedure

Collect a 24-hour urine specimen in a light-resistant specimen bottle containing a preservative to prevent degradation of the light-sensitive porphyrins and their precursors.

Precautions

▪ Refrigerate the specimen or keep it on ice during the collection period. Send it to the laboratory as soon as the collection is completed.
▪ If a light-resistant container isn't available, protect the specimen from light

exposure. If an indwelling urinary catheter is in place, put the collection bag in a dark plastic bag.

Reference values

Normal porphyrin and precursor values for urine fall in these ranges:
▪ *uroporphyrins:* in women, from 1 to 22 µg/24 hours; in men, from undetectable to 42 µg/24 hours
▪ *coproporphyrins:* in women, from 1 to 57 µg/24 hours; in men, from undetectable to 96 µg/24 hours
▪ *PBG:* in both sexes, up to 1.5 mg/24 hours.

Implications of results

Levels of most porphyrins and their precursors increase in patients with porphyria. Because heme synthesis occurs primarily in bone marrow and the liver, porphyrias are classified as erythropoi-

PORPHYRIN PRECURSORS	
Delta-aminolevulinic acid	**Porphobilinogen**
Normal	Normal
Normal	Normal
Highly increased	Highly increased
Highly increased during acute attack	Normal or slightly increased; highly increased during acute attack
Increased during acute attack	Increased during acute attack
Variable	Variable

etic or hepatic. (See *Urine porphyrin levels in porphyria.*)

Infectious hepatitis, Hodgkin's disease, central nervous system disorders, cirrhosis, and heavy metal, benzene, or carbon tetrachloride toxicity can also increase porphyrin levels.

Post-test care
As ordered, resume medications that were discontinued before the test.

Interfering factors
■ Elevated urine urobilinogen levels can interfere with test results by affecting the reagent used in the PBG screening test.
■ Oral contraceptives and griseofulvin can elevate urine porphyrin levels; rifampin turns urine red-orange, interfering with results.
■ Pregnancy and menstruation may increase porphyrin levels.

■ Barbiturates, chloral hydrate, chlorpropamide, sulfonamides, meprobamate, and chlordiazepoxide generally induce porphyria or porphyrinuria; they should be discontinued 10 to 12 days before the test, if possible.
■ If the urine specimen is left standing for a few hours, PBG levels decline.

Urine delta-aminolevulinic acid

Using the colorimetric technique, this quantitative analysis of urine delta-aminolevulinic acid (ALA) levels helps diagnose porphyrias, hepatic disease, and lead poisoning. (In an emergency, a simple qualitative screening test can be performed.) ALA, the basic precursor of the porphyrins, normally converts to porphobilinogen through the action of the enzyme ALA-dehydrase during heme synthesis. Impaired conversion, as in porphyrias and lead poisoning, causes urine ALA levels to rise before other chemical or hematologic changes occur.

Purpose
- To screen for lead poisoning
- To aid diagnosis of porphyrias and certain hepatic disorders, such as hepatitis and hepatic carcinoma.

Patient preparation
Explain to the patient that this test detects abnormal hemoglobin formation. If lead poisoning is suspected, tell the patient (or parents, since the patient is usually a child) that the test helps detect the presence of excessive lead in the body. Inform the patient (or parents) that he needn't restrict food or fluids. Tell him that the test requires a 24-hour urine specimen, and teach him (or his parents) the proper collection technique.

Check the patient's medication history for recent use of drugs that may alter ALA levels. Review your findings with the laboratory, and then notify the doctor; he may want to restrict these medications before the test.

Procedure
Collect a 24-hour urine specimen in a light-resistant bottle containing a preservative (usually glacial acetic acid) to prevent degradation of ALA.

Precautions
- Refrigerate the specimen or keep it on ice during the collection period. When the collection is completed, send the specimen to the laboratory at once.
- Protect the specimen from direct sunlight. If the patient has an indwelling

urinary catheter in place, insert the collection bag into a dark plastic bag.

Reference values
Normally, urine ALA values range from 1.5 to 7.5 mg/dl/24 hours.

Implications of results
Elevated urine ALA levels occur in lead poisoning, acute porphyria, hepatic carcinoma, and hepatitis.

Post-test care
Resume administration of medications withheld before the test, as ordered.

Interfering factors
- Barbiturates and griseofulvin cause porphyrins to accumulate in the liver and thus raise urine ALA levels. Vitamin E in pharmacologic doses may lower urine ALA levels.
- Failure to observe medication restrictions, to collect all urine during the test period, or to store the specimen properly may alter test results.

Urine bilirubin

This screening test, based on a color reaction with a specific reagent, detects abnormally high urine concentrations of direct (conjugated) bilirubin. The reticuloendothelial system produces the pigment bilirubin from hemoglobin breakdown. Bilirubin then combines with albumin, a plasma protein, and is transported to the liver as indirect (unconjugated) bilirubin.

In the liver, most indirect bilirubin joins with glucuronic acid to form bilirubin glucuronide and bilirubin diglucuronide — water-soluble compounds almost totally excreted into the bile. In the intestine, bacterial action converts direct bilirubin to urobilinogen. Normally, only a small amount of direct bilirubin — unbound or bound to albumin — returns to plasma. The kidneys filter the unbound portion, which may appear in trace amounts in the urine. Fat-soluble indirect bilirubin can't be filtered by the glomeruli and is never present in urine. Bilirubin in the urine may indicate liver disease caused by infections, biliary disease, or hepatotoxicity.

When combined with urobilinogen measurements, this test helps identify disorders that can cause jaundice. The analysis can be performed at bedside, using a bilirubin reagent strip, or in the laboratory. Highly sensitive spectrophotometric assays may be needed to detect trace amounts of urine bilirubin. This screening test doesn't detect such minute amounts.

Purpose
▪ To help identify the cause of jaundice.

Patient preparation
Explain to the patient that this test helps determine the cause of jaundice. Inform him that he needn't restrict food or fluids before the test. Tell him the test requires a random urine specimen, and let him know whether the specimen will be tested at bedside or in the laboratory. Bedside analysis can be performed immediately; laboratory analysis is completed in 1 day.

Procedure
Collect a random urine specimen in the container provided. For bedside analysis, use one of the following procedures:
▪ *Dipstrip:* Dip the reagent strip into the specimen and remove it immediately. After 20 seconds, compare the strip color with the color standards. Record the test results on the patient's chart.
▪ *Ictotest:* This test is easier to read and more sensitive than the dipstrip method. Place five drops of urine on the asbestos-cellulose test mat. If bilirubin is present, it will be absorbed into the mat. Next, put a reagent tablet on the wet area of the mat, and place two drops of water on the tablet. If bilirubin is present, a blue to purple coloration will develop on the mat. Pink or red indicates that no bilirubin is present — a negative test.

Precautions
▪ Use only a freshly voided specimen. Bilirubin disintegrates after 30 minutes' exposure to room temperature or light.
▪ If the specimen is to be analyzed in the laboratory, send it to the laboratory immediately. Record the time of collection on the patient's chart.
▪ If the specimen is tested at bedside, make sure 20 seconds elapse before you interpret the color change on the dipstrip. Also make sure lighting is adequate when you determine the color.

Normal findings
Normally, bilirubin is not found in urine in a routine screening test.

Implications of results
High concentrations of direct bilirubin in urine may be evident from the specimen's appearance (dark, with a yellow foam). To diagnose jaundice, however, the presence or absence of direct bilirubin in urine must be correlated with serum test results and with urine and fecal urobilinogen levels. (See *Comparing bilirubin and urobilinogen values,* pages 432 and 433.)

Post-test care
None.

Interfering factors
▪ Dipstrip testing, such as with Chemstrip or N-Multistix, is affected by large amounts of ascorbic acid and nitrite, which may lower bilirubin levels and cause false-negative test results.

Comparing bilirubin and urobilinogen values

Two types of hyperbilirubinemia — unconjugated (indirect) and conjugated (direct) — are associated with jaundice. Patients with unconjugated hyperbilirubinemia have an excess of unconjugated serum bilirubin, which normally makes up more than 80% of total serum bilirubin. Because unconjugated bilirubin is bound to albumin, it isn't water-soluble and is thus absent from urine. Conversely, patients with conjugated hyperbilirubinemia have an excess of conjugated serum bilirubin. Because conjugated bilirubin is protein-free, it can be filtered by the glomeruli and appears in urine.

To aid differential diagnosis of jaundice, urobilinogen assays are used to further distinguish the various hyperbilirubinemias. Normally, only trace amounts (1 to 4 mg daily) of this colorless compound — converted from conjugated bilirubin by intestinal bacteria — are reabsorbed into the bloodstream and excreted in urine. The rest (50 to 250 mg daily) is eliminated in feces. Because fecal urobilinogen measurements vary, an increase generally refers to levels above 250 mg daily; a decrease refers to levels below 5 mg daily.

This chart shows the changes in bilirubin and urobilinogen levels associated with both types of hyperbilirubinemia.

CAUSES OF JAUNDICE	SERUM		URINE		FECES
	Indirect bilirubin	Direct bilirubin	Bilirubin	Urobilinogen	Urobilinogen
Unconjugated hyperbilirubinemia					
Hemolytic disorders (hemolytic anemia, erythroblastosis fetalis)	Increased	Normal	Absent	May be increased	Increased
Gilbert's disease (constitutional hepatic dysfunction)	Moderately increased	Normal	Absent	Normal or decreased	Normal or decreased
Crigler-Najjar syndrome (congenital hyperbilirubinemia)	Markedly increased	Normal	Absent	Normal or decreased	Normal or decreased
Conjugated hyperbilirubinemia					
Extrahepatic obstruction (calculi, tumor, scar tissue in common bile duct or hepatic excretory duct)	Normal	Increased	Present	Decreased or absent	Decreased or absent
Hepatocellular disorders (viral, toxic, or alcoholic hepatitis; cirrhosis; parenchymal injury)	Increased	Increased	Present	Variable	Normal or decreased

Comparing bilirubin and urobilinogen values *(continued)*

CAUSES OF JAUNDICE	SERUM		URINE		FECES
	Indirect bilirubin	Direct bilirubin	Bilirubin	Urobi- linogen	Urobi- linogen
Conjugated hyperbilirubinemia *(continued)*					
Hepatocanalicular disorders or intrahepatic obstruction (drug-induced cholestasis; some familial defects, such as Dubin-Johnson and Rotor's syndromes; viral hepatitis; primary biliary cirrhosis)	Increased	Increased	Present	Variable	Normal or decreased

■ Phenazopyridine and phenothiazine derivatives, such as chlorpromazine and acetophenazine maleate, can cause false-positive results.

■ Exposure of the specimen to room temperature or light can lower bilirubin levels, due to bilirubin degradation.

Urine urobilinogen

This test detects impaired liver function by measuring urine levels of urobilinogen, the colorless, water-soluble product that results from the reduction of bilirubin by intestinal bacteria. Up to 50% of intestinal urobilinogen returns to the liver, where some of it is resecreted into bile and, eventually, into the intestine through enterohepatic circulation. Small amounts of the reabsorbed urobilinogen also enter general circulation for ultimate excretion in the urine (urobilinogenuria).

Eliminated in large amounts in the feces (50 to 250 mg/day) and in small amounts in the urine (1 to 4 mg/day), urobilinogen reflects bile pigment metabolism. Consequently, absent or altered urobilinogen levels can indicate hepatic damage or dysfunction. Urine urobilinogen can also indicate hemolysis of red blood cells, which increases bilirubin production and causes increased production and excretion of urobilinogen.

Quantitative analysis of urine urobilinogen involves addition of Ehrlich's reagent to a 2-hour urine specimen. The resulting color reaction is read promptly by spectrophotometry.

Purpose
■ To aid diagnosis of extrahepatic obstruction, such as blockage of the common bile duct
■ To aid differential diagnosis of hepatic and hematologic disorders.

Patient preparation
Explain to the patient that this test helps assess liver and biliary tract function.

Using a random specimen to test for urobilinogen

Quantitative tests for urinary urobilinogen excretion can be performed with reagent strips, such as Bili-Labstix or N-Multistix (dip-and-read test).

To perform such tests, collect a clean-catch urine specimen in a clean, dry container — preferably in the afternoon, when urine urobilinogen levels peak — and test the specimen immediately. A fresh urine specimen is essential for reliable results because urobilinogen is very unstable when exposed to room temperature and light.

Dip the strip into the urine, and as you remove it, start timing the reaction. Carefully remove excess urine by tapping the edge of the strip against the container or a clean, dry surface to prevent color changes along the edge of the test area. When using N-Multistix (or a similar product for multiple testing), hold the strip in a horizontal position to prevent mixing of chemicals from adjacent reagent areas. Place the strip near the color block on the bottle, and carefully compare the colors. Read the results at 45 seconds. The color results correspond to the

COLOR	VALUE
yellow-green to yellow (normal)	0.1 to 1 Ehrlich unit
yellow-orange (positive)	2 Ehrlich units
medium yellow-orange (positive)	4 Ehrlich units
light brown-orange (positive)	8 Ehrlich units
brown-orange (positive)	12 Ehrlich units

number of Ehrlich units per deciliter of urine, as shown above.

Normally, a random specimen contains small amounts of urobilinogen. This test cannot determine the absence of urobilinogen in the specimen being tested.

Para-aminosalicylic acid may cause unreliable results with this reagent strip test. Drugs containing azo dyes, such as Azo Gantrisin, mask test results by causing a golden color.

Inform him that he needn't restrict food or fluids, except for bananas, which he should avoid for 48 hours before the test. Tell him that the test may require a random specimen or a 2-hour urine specimen, and teach him how to collect the specimen.

Check the patient's history for drugs that may affect urine urobilinogen levels. Review your findings with the laboratory and the doctor, who may restrict such drugs before the test.

Procedure

Most laboratories request a random urine specimen; others prefer a 2-hour specimen, usually during the afternoon (ideally, between 1 p.m. and 3 p.m.), when urobilinogen levels peak. (See *Using a random specimen to test for urobilinogen.*)

Precautions

Send the specimen to the laboratory immediately. This test must be performed within 30 minutes of collection, since urobilinogen quickly oxidizes to an orange compound called urobilin.

Reference values

Normally, urine urobilinogen values in women range from 0.1 to 1.1 Ehrlich units/2 hours; in men, from 0.3 to 2.1 Ehrlich units/2 hours.

Implications of results

Absence of urine urobilinogen may result from complete obstructive jaundice or from treatment with broad-spectrum antibiotics, which destroy the intestinal bacterial flora. Low urine urobilinogen levels may result from congenital enzymatic jaundice (hyperbilirubinemia syndromes) or from treatment with drugs that acidify urine, such as ammonium chloride or ascorbic acid.

Elevated levels may indicate hemolytic jaundice, hepatitis, or cirrhosis.

Post-test care

▪ As ordered, resume administration of drugs restricted before the test.
▪ Tell the patient he may resume his usual diet.

Interfering factors

▪ The following drugs affect the test reagent and may affect the accuracy of test results: para-aminosalicylic acid, phenazopyridine, procaine, mandelate, phenothiazines, and sulfonamides.
▪ Highly alkaline urine, which may be caused by acetazolamide or sodium bicarbonate, may elevate urobilinogen levels.
▪ Bananas eaten up to 48 hours before the test may raise urobilinogen levels.

Urine melanin

This relatively rare test measures urine levels of melanin, the brown-black pigment that colors the skin, hair, and eyes. An end product of tyrosine metabolism, melanin is normally elaborated by specialized cells called melanocytes.

Cutaneous melanomas — malignant tumors that produce excessive amounts of melanin — develop most often around the head and neck but may also originate in mucous membranes (as in the rectum), the retinas, or the central nervous system, where melanocytes appear. Patients with these tumors may excrete melanin precursors — melanogens — in their urine. If the urine is left standing, exposure to air converts the melanogens to melanin in about 24 hours.

Thormählen's test uses sodium nitroprusside (nitroferricyanide) to detect melanogens or melanin in urine, based on characteristic color changes. More specific tests for melanin, such as chromatography, isolate and measure the pigment.

Purpose

▪ To aid in diagnosis of malignant melanomas.

Patient preparation

Explain to the patient what melanin is, and tell him this test detects its presence in urine. Inform him that he needn't restrict food or fluids before the test. Tell him the test requires a random urine specimen, and teach him the correct collection technique.

Procedure

Collect a random urine specimen.

Precautions

Send the specimen to the laboratory immediately.

Normal findings

Urine should not contain melanogens or melanin.

Implications of results

In the presence of a visible skin tumor, large quantities of melanin or melanogens in urine indicate advanced internal metastasis. Because malignant melanomas may also develop in internal organs, large quantities of melanin or melanogens in a urine specimen in the absence of a visible skin tumor indicate an internal melanoma.

Post-test care
None.

Interfering factors
Failure to send the urine specimen to the laboratory immediately may interfere with test results.

SELECTED READINGS

Guyton, A.C., and Hall, J.E. *Textbook of Medical Physiology,* 9th ed. Philadelphia: W.B. Saunders Co., 1996.

Henry, J.B., ed. *Clinical Diagnosis and Management by Laboratory Methods,* 19th ed. Philadelphia: W.B. Saunders Co., 1996.

Nursing97 Drug Handbook. Springhouse, Pa.: Springhouse Corp., 1997.

Ravel, R.A. *Clinical Laboratory Medicine: Clinical Application of Laboratory Data,* 6th ed. St. Louis: Mosby–Year Book, Inc., 1995.

Tietz, N.W. *Clinical Guide to Laboratory Tests,* 3rd ed. Philadelphia: W.B. Saunders Co., 1995.

Vander, A.J. *Renal Physiology.* New York: McGraw-Hill Book Co., 1995.

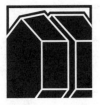

CHAPTER SIXTEEN

Urine sugars, ketones, and mucopolysaccharides

Learning objectives

After completing this chapter, the reader will be able to:

- describe the physiologic changes that cause excretion of glucose, ketone bodies, and mucopolysaccharides
- identify the laboratory methods used to screen for glycosuria, ketonuria, and mucopolysaccharidosis
- detect the pass-through phenomenon and understand its significance for determining glucose concentration
- state the purpose of each test discussed in the chapter

- prepare the patient physically and psychologically for each test
- describe the procedure for obtaining a specimen for each test
- specify appropriate precautions for accurately obtaining a specimen for each test
- implement appropriate post-test care
- state the reference values for each test
- discuss the implications of abnormal test results
- list factors that may interfere with accurate test results.

INTRODUCTION

This group of tests, used to detect excessive urinary excretion of glucose, ketones, and mucopolysaccharides, has great clinical significance because it encompasses some of the most common tests for diabetes. Several of these tests are sufficiently reliable and accessible to have become common screening procedures for detecting diabetes and for monitoring the response of diabetic patients to therapy.

Glycosuria significant

Because the renal tubules normally reabsorb glucose completely and return it to the blood, the presence of glucose in the urine (glycosuria) is abnormal and usually indicates a pathologic condition. Rarely, transient urinary traces of glucose and other reducing sugars (galactose, lactose, and pentoses) reflect a benign state, such as the third trimester of pregnancy or lactation, or occur as a metabolic complication of total parenteral nutrition.

Characteristically, however, glycosuria reflects decreased glucose reabsorption in the renal tubules or increased amounts of glucose entering the renal tubules per minute — almost invariably the result of blood glucose concentration above the threshold level (160 to 170 mg/dl of venous blood). Such glycosuria with hyperglycemia suggests diabetes mellitus, one of the most common metabolic disorders.

The severity and prevalence of diabetes mandate routine screening of urine specimens for glucose in neonates and in persons suspected of having diabetes as well as routine glucose testing to monitor the effectiveness of treatment with exogenous insulin in patients with controlled diabetes. In some patients, urine levels of glucose don't reflect blood levels. (See *Renal threshold and glucose testing.*)

Testing for glycosuria

Methods of detecting glucose in the urine include copper reduction tests (Benedict's test and Clinitest) and glucose oxidase tests (dip-and-read reagent

Renal threshold and glucose testing

Most patients with diabetes test their urine for sugars and ketones four times a day — before breakfast, lunch, dinner, and bedtime snack — using a second-voided specimen. A positive result usually indicates elevated blood glucose levels.

However, in some patients with diabetes (especially the elderly and young, well-controlled patients), urine levels don't reflect blood concentration. That's because glycosuria depends not only on the blood glucose level, but also on the renal threshold (blood glucose concentration above which the kidneys excrete glucose).

Thus, a patient with a low renal threshold may have a positive urine test even though his blood glucose level is low or normal. Consequently, to ensure the accuracy of urine test results, simultaneous blood glucose tests are sometimes necessary.

strips). In both methods, a color change indicates the presence of glucose or another reducing substance.

Benedict's test, the diagnostic test of choice in the past, a solution of cupric sulfate, sodium carbonate, and sodium citrate is added to a urine specimen and heated. After the solution cools, a color change indicates the presence of a reducing substance — probably glucose. Although this sensitive test can give a positive reaction to as little as 0.1% glucose concentration, it has important drawbacks: it's time-consuming, inconvenient (because of the need for a water bath and other laboratory apparatus), and nonspecific for glucose. Consequently, newer techniques using tablets and reagent strips have largely replaced Benedict's test.

In the *test tablet procedure* (Clinitest), a simplified version of Benedict's test, a commercially prepared tablet compounded of cupric sulfate, citric acid, sodium carbonate, and sodium hydroxide is added to a test tube containing water and urine. The reaction of the water and sodium hydroxide releases sufficient heat to activate the reduction of cupric ions in the presence of glucose. Comparing the resulting color change with reference color blocks provides the approximate level of the glucose in the specimen. This procedure is more convenient than Benedict's test, but it's less sensitive (0.2%) and is reactive to substances other than glucose.

Reagent test strips (Clinistix, Diastix, Chemstrip G strips, and Tes-Tape) are specific for glucose. In these tests, a commercially prepared plastic strip is impregnated with a mixture of enzymes and a chromogen and undergoes a chemical reaction that, in the presence of glucose, produces an oxidized form of the chromogen. A combination strip (such as Combistix) simultaneously tests for glucose, pH, and protein. Despite the possibility of false-negative and false-positive results, dip-and-read reagent strips are the most common screening method for routine qualitative checks for glycosuria.

Combining the Clinitest tablet test with one of the reagent strip tests offers a semiquantitative determination of glucose in urine. If a specimen tested with a Clinistix, Diastix, or Tes-Tape paper produces a positive reaction, testing another specimen with a Clinitest tablet can indicate the approximate glucose concentration by the intensity of the color change.

Ketone bodies

Substances designated ketone bodies (acetone bodies) include acetoacetic (diacetic) acid, acetone (formed by the spontaneous decarboxylation of acetoacetic acid), and beta-hydroxybutyric acid. Formed in the liver during fatty acid metabolism, ketone bodies circulate through the blood to the tissues for further oxidation. Normally, on the usual carbohydrate-protein-fat diet, less than 125 mg of such substances are excreted daily in the urine. Under conditions of absolute or relative carbohydrate deprivation, the metabolism of fat greatly accelerates. Such acceleration exceeds the liver's capacity to metabolize the fragments of acetyl coenzyme A derived from the fatty acid, causing formation and release of significant quantities of ketone bodies into the blood.

The extrahepatic tissues (such as the kidneys) have a great capacity for utilizing ketone bodies (ketolysis). However, when the rate of ketogenesis by the liver exceeds the rate of ketolysis in peripheral tissues, the blood concentration of ketone bodies rises (ketonemia), causing these bodies to appear in the urine (ketonuria). Ketonuria is characteristic in starvation and uncontrolled diabetes mellitus and offers clues to various causes of metabolic acidosis; it's usually unrelated to intrinsic urinary system disease.

Screening for ketonuria

Ketonuria is usually nonspecific, indicating urinary excretion of either acetoacetic acid, acetone, or beta-hydroxybutyric acid. Consequently, a test that identifies any one of these three ketones generally confirms ketonuria. Commercially prepared *dip-and-read reagent strips* (such as Ketostix) are available as screening tools. These reagent strips, which are impregnated with sodium nitroprusside, are specific for acetoacetic acid and sensitive to 10 mg/dl. When the strip is dipped into the specimen, the presence of acetoacetic acid produces a color change that can be compared to a standard color block to determine approximate concentrations.

The *tablet test* (Acetest) is another convenient screening procedure that is widely used because it works equally well with plasma or urine and reacts to concentrations as low as 5 mg/dl of acetone. (It's not specific for acetoacetic acid.) The Acetest tablet contains glycine, sodium nitroprusside, disodium phosphate, and lactose. Acetoacetic acid or acetone, in the presence of glycine, turns the tablet lavender-purple.

Two other tests, Rothera's test and Gerhardt's ferric chloride test, have been largely replaced by reagent strip and tablet tests. *Rothera's test* detects ketones through the reaction of a mixture of sodium nitroprusside and ammonium sulfate to a urine specimen. If the test is positive, a pink-purple ring develops at the interface of the reactants. This test is sensitive to acetoacetic acid levels of 1 to 5 mg/dl and to acetone levels of 10 to 25 mg/dl but is nonspecific for acetoacetic acid. It requires fresh preparations of the reagents daily and can't be readily performed outside the laboratory. In *Gerhardt's ferric chloride test*, a ferric chloride solution is added to a test tube of urine. If acetoacetic acid is present, the solution turns deep red. Although this test was popular for many years, it is neither specific (salicylates give a false-positive reaction) nor sensitive (25 to 50 mg/dl approaches the lower limit of sensitivity).

Hart's test is the only analytic method other than chromatography that's specific for beta-hydroxybutyric acid. After acidified urine is boiled to half its original volume, hydrogen peroxide is added. (Boiling also removes volatile fractions of acetoacetic acid and acetone.) If beta-hydroxybutyric acid is present, a red ring develops.

Mucopolysaccharides

These large-polymer compounds are present in various body tissues and fluids, including connective tissue, fetal and adult mucous membranes, and blood group substances. Mucopolysaccharides occur in the free state or are bound to small quantities of proteins. The most important mucopolysaccharides include dermatan sulfate (also known as chondroitin sulfate B), derived from fibroblasts; heparan sulfate (heparitin sulfate), derived from mast cells; keratosulfate (keratan sulfate), distributed in costal cartilage and the cornea; and hyaluronic acid, present in synovial fluid, the umbilical cord, and vitreous humor.

Normally, the mucopolysaccharides contribute viscosity and permeability to the tissues, controlling the intercellular migration of small molecules. Hyaluronic acid, for example, decreases fluid viscosity and enhances the lubricating property of synovial fluid. Ordinarily, only minute quantities (10 to 15 mg/day) of these compounds are excreted in the urine. However, in certain hereditary disorders known as mucopolysaccharidoses, excessive quantities of these glycoproteins can accumulate in the tissues, eventually resulting in abnormal levels excreted in the urine (100 to 500 mg/day). In such patients, the primary defect seems to be the genetically determined absence of the target enzymes that catabolize the mucopolysaccharides.

These genetic disorders are marked by severe clinical abnormalities that usually become apparent during the first decade of life, including mental retardation, aortic insufficiency, and pronounced skeletal deformities. The most common types of mucopolysaccharidosis are Hurler's, Hunter's, and Sanfilippo's syndromes.

Screening for mucopolysaccharidosis

Screening tests for mucopolysaccharidosis use an organic dye (toluidine blue) that changes color in the presence of large amounts of acid mucopolysaccharides. One convenient method uses litmus paper impregnated with the dye: A drop of urine is placed on the paper and treated with acidified methyl alcohol. If a blue dye spot persists, acid mucopolysaccharides are present. If the specimen is normal, no dye remains. However, up to 30% of spot tests produce false-negative results.

Another primarily qualitative test uses turbidimetry: Buffered urine is mixed with albumin at acid pH; if acid mucopolysaccharides are present, the solution grows uniformly turbid. (False-negative results occur in about 10% of these tests.) If spot or turbidity tests are positive, paper chromatography can identify the specific mucopolysaccharide. If the patient has Hurler's, Hunter's, or Sanfilippo's syndrome and his initial screening was negative, further tests are needed (paper or column chromatography, or electrophoresis).

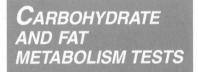

Copper reduction

The copper reduction test (also known as the Clinitest tablet test) measures the concentration of reducing substances in the urine through the reaction of these substances with a commercially prepared tablet — Clinitest. This test, which reacts to glucose and to other reducing substances (mostly sugars), has largely replaced Benedict's test. It is most valuable in providing the patient with overt or latent diabetes mellitus a simple method of monitoring his urine sugar levels at home. But it's sometimes used as a rapid laboratory screening tool.

Purpose
- To detect mellituria (sugars in the urine)
- To monitor urine glucose levels during insulin therapy (after determining that the sugar in the urine is glucose).

Patient preparation
Explain to the patient that this test determines his urine sugar level. If he has been recently diagnosed as diabetic, teach him how to perform the Clinitest tablet test. Have the patient void; then give him a drink of water. After 30 to 45 minutes, collect a second-voided urine specimen.

Check the patient's medication history for drugs that may interfere with test results.

Equipment
Specimen container ✦ 10-ml test tube ✦ medicine dropper ✦ Clinitest tablets ✦ Clinitest color chart.

Procedure
After collecting a second-voided specimen, perform the *five-drop Clinitest tablet test:* Hold the medicine dripper vertically, and instill five drops of urine from the specimen container into the test tube. Rinse the dropper with water, and add 10 drops of water to the test tube. Add one Clinitest tablet, and observe the color change, especially during effervescence — the pass-through phase. Wait 15 seconds after effervescence subsides, and gently agitate the test tube. If color develops at the 15-second interval, read the color against the Clinitest color chart, and record the results. Ignore any changes that develop after 15 seconds.

If rapid color changes occur in the pass-through phase of the five-drop test, record the results as over 2% without comparison to the color chart. Or perform a *two-drop Clinitest tablet test:* Hold the medicine dropper vertically, and instill two drops of urine into the test tube. Flush urine residue from the dropper with water; then add 10 drops of water to the test tube. Add one Clinitest tablet, and observe the color change during the pass-through phase. Wait 15 seconds after effervescence stops; then compare the color with the appropriate color reference chart, and record results.

Rapid color changes (bright orange to dark brown or green-brown) in the pass-through phase in a five-drop Clinitest reaction indicate glycosuria of 2% or more; in a two-drop Clinitest reaction, glycosuria up to 5% can be measured.

Precautions
- Instruct the patient not to contaminate the urine specimen with toilet tissue or stool.
- Tell the patient to make sure his hands are dry when handling Clinitest tablets and to avoid swallowing them or letting them come in contact with his eyes, mucous membranes, or clothing because sodium hydroxide and moisture produce caustic burns.
- Store tablets in a well-marked, child-proof bottle to prevent accidental ingestion.
- Don't use discolored (dark blue) tablets. The normal color of fresh tablets is light blue with darker blue flecks.
- During effervescence, the test tube becomes boiling hot. Hold it near the top to avoid burning your hand.

Normal findings
No sugars should be present in urine.

Implications of results

Glycosuria occurs in diabetes mellitus, adrenal and thyroid disorders, hepatic and central nervous system diseases, Fanconi's syndrome and other conditions involving low renal threshold, toxic renal tubular disease, heavy metal poisoning, glomerulonephritis, nephrosis, pregnancy, and total parenteral nutrition. It also occurs with administration of large amounts of glucose or niacin, long-term use of phenothiazines, and use of certain other drugs, such as asparaginase, corticosteroids, carbamazepine, ammonium chloride, thiazide diuretics, dextrothyroxine, and lithium carbonate.

Post-test care

■ Provide written guidelines and a flow sheet to help the patient record the Clinitest results and insulin taken at home.
■ Tell the patient when the next urine specimen is needed.

Interfering factors

■ Cephalosporins, nalidixic acid, and large doses of probenecid may produce false-positive results. Tetracycline and ascorbic acid may produce false-positive or false-negative results, depending on the test method.
■ Failure to use freshly voided urine or to flush urine residue from the medicine dropper may affect test results.
■ Failure to detect the pass-through phenomenon or to use the correct reference chart for color comparison of the specimen may influence test results.
■ Low renal threshold for glucose may alter test results.
■ Failure to use whole or fresh Clinitest tablets or to keep the tablet container tightly closed (to prevent absorption of light or moisture) may alter test results.
■ The presence of reducing substances other than glucose may influence test results. (See *Reducing substances that affect test results.*)

Reducing substances that affect test results

Aminosalicylic acid	Levodopa
Ascorbic acid	Maltose
Cephalosporins	Metolazone
Chloral hydrate	Nalidixic acid
Chloramphenicol	Nitrofurantoin
Creatinine	Penicillin G
Cysteine	Pentoses
Fructose	Probenecid
Galactose	Salicylates
Isoniazid	Streptomycin
Ketone bodies	Tetracycline
Lactose	Uric acid

Glucose oxidase

The glucose oxidase test — which involves the use of commercial, plastic-coated reagent strips (Clinistix, Diastix) or Tes-Tape — is a specific, qualitative test for glycosuria. Although indicated in routine urinalysis, this test is used primarily to monitor urine glucose levels in patients with diabetes. Because of its simplicity and convenience, the test can be performed by patients at home.

Purpose
■ To detect glycosuria
■ To monitor urine glucose levels during insulin therapy.

Patient preparation

Explain to the patient that this test determines urine glucose levels. If he's a newly diagnosed patient with diabetes, teach him how to perform the test himself. (See *Interpreting glucose oxidase test results,* page 445.) Have the patient void; then give him a drink of water. After 30 to 45 minutes, collect a second-voided urine specimen.

If the patient is receiving levodopa, ascorbic acid, phenazopyridine, salicylates, peroxides, or hypochlorites, use Clinitest tablets instead.

Equipment
Specimen container ✦ glucose test strips ✦ reference color blocks.

Procedure
Collect a second-voided specimen, and use one of the following procedures:
■ *Clinistix test:* Dip the test area of the reagent strip in the specimen for 2 seconds. Remove excess urine by tapping the strip against a clean surface or the side of the container, and begin timing. Hold the strip in the air, and "read" the color *exactly 10 seconds* after taking the strip out of the urine by comparing it with the reference color blocks on the container label. Record the results. Ignore color changes that develop after 10 seconds.
■ *Diastix test:* Dip the reagent strip in the specimen for 2 seconds. Remove excess urine by tapping the strip against the container, and begin timing. Hold the strip in the air, and compare the color to the color chart *exactly 30 seconds* after taking the strip out of the urine. Record the results. Ignore color changes that develop after 30 seconds.
■ *Tes-Tape:* Withdraw about 1½" (4 cm) of the reagent tape from the dispenser; dip ¼" (0.6 cm) in the specimen for 2 seconds. Remove excess urine by tapping the strip against the side of the container, and begin timing. Hold the tape in the air, and compare the color of the darkest part of the tape to the color chart *exactly 60 seconds* after taking the strip out of the urine. If the tape indicates 0.5% or higher, wait an additional 60 seconds to make the final color comparison. Record the results.

Precautions
■ Instruct the patient not to contaminate the urine specimen with toilet tissue or stool.
■ Keep the test strip container tightly closed to prevent deterioration of strips by exposure to light or moisture. Store it in a cool place (under 86° F [30° C]) to avoid heat degradation.
■ Don't use discolored or darkened Clinistix or Diastix strips, or dark yellow or yellow-brown Tes-Tape strips.

Normal findings
Glucose should not be present in urine.

Implications of results
Glycosuria occurs in diabetes mellitus, adrenal and thyroid disorders, hepatic and central nervous system diseases, Fanconi's syndrome and other conditions involving low renal threshold, toxic renal tubular disease, heavy metal poisoning, glomerulonephritis, nephrosis, pregnancy, and total parenteral nutrition. It also occurs with administration of large amounts of glucose or niacin, prolonged use of phenothiazines, and use of certain other drugs, such as asparaginase, corticosteroids, carbamazepine, ammonium chloride, thiazide diuretics, dextrothyroxine, and lithium carbonate.

Post-test care
■ Provide written guidelines and a flow sheet so the patient can record the test results and insulin taken at home.
■ Tell the patient when the next specimen is needed.

Interfering factors
■ Dilute, stale urine or bacterial contamination of the specimen may affect test results.
■ Reducing substances, such as levodopa, ascorbic acid, phenazopyridine, meth-

Interpreting glucose oxidase test results

Until recently, all glucose oxidase tests used the plus (+) symbol to indicate glycosuria. However, because the plus symbol did not reflect a standard glucose value, regulating insulin dosages was difficult. Therefore, some manufacturers have stopped using the plus symbol. As the chart below shows, Diastix doesn't use the plus symbol, but Tes-Tape does. These tests are semiquantitative.

Clinistix (not shown) has no quantitative value; it is strictly qualitative. Results for this test are reported as negative, light, medium, or dark.

TEST	0%	$\frac{1}{10}$%	$\frac{1}{4}$%	$\frac{1}{2}$%	1%	≥ 2%
Diastix	Negative	100 mg/dl	250 mg/dl	500 mg/dl	1,000 mg/dl	≥ 2,000 mg/dl
Tes-Tape	Negative	+	++	+++		++++

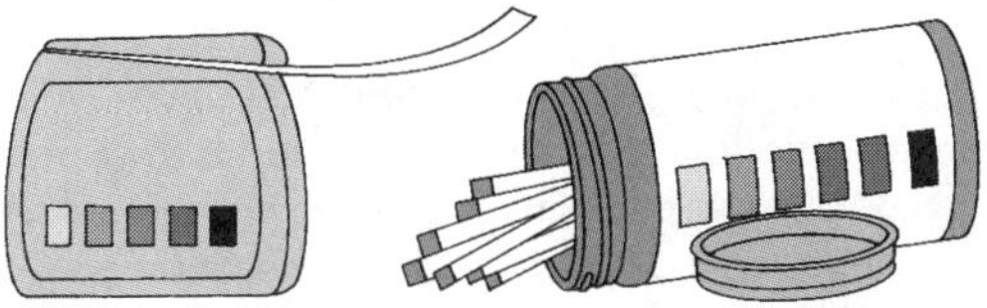

yldopa, and salicylates, may cause false-negative results.

■ Tetracyclines also produce false-negative results.

■ Use of reagent strips after the expiration date, failure to keep the reagent strip container tightly closed, or failure to record the reagent strip method used may alter test results.

Urine ketones

In this routine, semiquantitative screening test — which has largely replaced Rothera's and Gerhardt's tests — the action of urine on a commercially prepared product (Acetest tablet, Ketostix, or Keto-Diastix) measures the urine level of ketone bodies (also known as ketones). Each product measures a specific ketone body. For example, Acetest measures acetone, and Ketostix measures acetoacetic acid. Urine determinations reflect serum concentration.

Excessive accumulation of ketone bodies (acetoacetic acid, acetone, and beta-hydroxybutyric acid) — the byproducts of fat metabolism — follows carbohydrate deprivation, as occurs in starvation or diabetic ketoacidosis.

Purpose
■ To screen for ketonuria
■ To identify diabetic ketoacidosis and carbohydrate deprivation
■ To distinguish between a diabetic and a nondiabetic coma
■ To monitor control of diabetes mellitus, ketogenic weight reduction, and treatment of diabetic ketoacidosis.

Patient preparation

Explain to the patient that this test evaluates fat metabolism. If he's a newly diagnosed patient with diabetes, tell him how to perform the test. Instruct the patient to void; then give him a drink of water. About 30 minutes later, ask him for a second-voided urine specimen.

If the patient is taking levodopa or phenazopyridine or has recently received sulfobromophthalein, Acetest tablets must be used, since reagent strips will give inaccurate results.

Procedure

Collect a second-voided midstream specimen, and follow one of these procedures:

■ *Acetest:* Lay the tablet on a piece of white paper, and place one drop of urine on the tablet. After 30 seconds, compare the tablet color (white, lavender, or purple) with the color chart.

■ *Ketostix:* Dip the reagent stick into the specimen and remove it immediately. After 15 seconds, compare the stick color (buff or purple) with the color chart. Record the results as negative, small, moderate, or large amounts of ketones.

■ *Keto-Diastix:* Dip the reagent strip into the specimen, and remove it immediately. Tap the edge of the strip against the container or a clean, dry surface to remove excess urine. Hold the strip horizontally to prevent mixing the chemicals from the two areas. Interpret each area of the strip separately. After exactly 15 seconds, compare the color of the ketone section (buff or purple) with the appropriate color chart; after 30 seconds, compare the color of the glucose section. Ignore color changes that occur after the specified waiting periods. Record the results as negative or as positive for small, moderate, or large amounts of ketones.

Precautions

■ The specimen must be tested within 60 minutes after it is obtained or it must be refrigerated. Allow refrigerated specimens to return to room temperature before testing.

■ Don't use tablets or strips that have become discolored or darkened.

Normal findings

No ketones should be present in urine.

Implications of results

Ketonuria is present in uncontrolled diabetes mellitus and starvation; it also occurs as a metabolic complication of total parenteral nutrition.

Post-test care

■ If the test is to be performed at home, provide written guidelines and a flow sheet to help the patient record results.

■ Tell the patient when the next specimen is needed.

Interfering factors

■ Failure to keep the reagent container tightly closed to prevent absorption of light or moisture or bacterial contamination of the specimen causes false-negative results.

■ Levodopa, phenazopyridine, and sulfobromophthalein produce false-positive test results when Ketostix or Keto-Diastix is used.

Acid mucopolysaccharides

This quantitative test for mucopolysaccharidosis measures the urine level of acid mucopolysaccharides (AMPs), a group of polysaccharides or carbohydrates, in infants with a family history of the disease. When an inborn error metabolism causes enzymatic deficiencies, AMPs — especially dermatan sulfate and heparitin sulfate — accumulate in the tissues, producing a rare group of disorders called mucopolysaccharidoses. The severest form, Hurler's syndrome (gargoylism), results from deposition of these macromolecular complexes in several organs, particularly the heart and kidneys, and excretion of large amounts of mucopolysaccharides in the urine.

To measure AMPs, these compounds are precipitated out of the urine specimen with cetyltrimethylammonium bromide (CTAB). The CTAB is then extracted with ethanol. The glucuronic acid in the now-isolated AMPs is measured by the Dische carbazole reaction. The AMP value is then expressed as the number of milligrams of glucuronic acid. This number, divided by the amount of creatinine in the same specimen (which reflects the glomerular filtration rate), is a ratio that is used to overcome irregularities in the 24-hour urine collection.

Purpose
■ To diagnose mucopolysaccharidosis.

Patient preparation
Explain to the parents of the infant that this test helps determine the efficiency of carbohydrate metabolism. Inform them that they needn't restrict the child's food or fluids. Tell them that the test requires urine collection for 24 hours, and teach them the proper way to collect the specimen at home.

If the child is receiving therapy with heparin and must continue it, note this on the laboratory request.

Equipment
Pediatric urine collectors ✦ 24-hour collection container ✦ 20 ml of toluene (usually obtained from the laboratory).

Procedure
Obtain a 24-hour urine specimen. Add 20 ml of toluene as a preservative at the start of the collection period. Indicate the patient's age on the laboratory request, and send the specimen to the laboratory as soon as the 24-hour collection period is over.

Precautions
During the collection period, refrigerate the specimen or place it on ice.

Reference values
The normal AMP value for adults is <13.3 µg glucuronic acid/mg creatinine/ 24 hours. Children's values vary with age.

Implications of results
Elevated AMP levels reliably indicate mucopolysaccharidosis. Supplementary quantitative analysis and detailed blood studies can identify the specific enzyme that's defective.

Post-test care
Be sure to remove all adhesive from the urine collector from the infant's perineum. Wash the area gently with soap and water, and watch for irritation.

Interfering factors
■ Failure to collect all urine during the test period or to store the specimen properly may alter test results.
■ Heparin elevates urine AMP levels.

SELECTED READINGS

Guyton, A.C., and Hall, J.E. *Textbook of Medical Physiology*, 9th ed. Philadelphia: W.B. Saunders Co., 1996.

Henry, J.B., ed. *Clinical Diagnosis and Management by Laboratory Methods*, 19th ed. Philadelphia: W.B. Saunders Co., 1996.

Nursing97 Drug Handbook. Springhouse, Pa.: Springhouse Corp., 1997.

Tietz, N.W. *Clinical Guide to Laboratory Tests*, 3rd ed. Philadelphia: W.B. Saunders Co., 1995.

Vander, A.J. *Renal Physiology*. New York: McGraw-Hill Book Co., 1995.

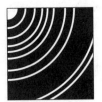

CHAPTER SEVENTEEN

Urine vitamins and minerals

Learning objectives

After completing this chapter, the reader will be able to:
- identify the class of vitamins that are most frequently measured in the urine
- describe the actions of five major minerals and three trace minerals that are usually measured in the urine
- identify dietary sources of major vitamins and minerals
- name the disorders that are associated with a deficiency of two or more of the major vitamins and minerals
- recognize the danger signs of severe potassium imbalance
- state the signs and symptoms of calcium, potassium, and magnesium imbalance
- state the purpose of each test discussed in the chapter
- prepare the patient physically and psychologically for each test
- describe the procedure for obtaining a specimen for each test
- specify appropriate precautions for accurately obtaining a specimen for each test
- implement appropriate post-test care
- state the reference values for each test
- discuss the implications of abnormal test results
- list factors that may interfere with accurate test results.

INTRODUCTION

A class of biochemical compounds essential for growth and metabolism, vitamins are classified into two groups according to their solubility. The *fat-soluble* vitamins include vitamins A, D, E, and K. The *water-soluble* group includes vitamins B_1 (thiamine) and B_2 (riboflavin), niacinamide (niacin or nicotinic acid), vitamin B_6 (pyroxidine), pantothenic acid, lipoic acid, folic acid, inositol, and vitamins B_{12} (cyanocobalamin) and C (ascorbic acid).

Fat-soluble vitamins

Fat-soluble vitamins require bile salts and lipids for intestinal absorption; much of the amount absorbed is stored — mainly in the liver; the rest is excreted in stool. Storage of these vitamins promotes excessive accumulation; for this reason, toxicity is more common than deficiency. Because fat-soluble vitamins aren't readily excreted in the urine, serum assay is the preferred method of measuring their concentrations within the body (see Chapter 9).

Water-soluble vitamins

Water-soluble vitamins are present in all living cells and act primarily as coenzymes or their precursors. Because water-soluble vitamins are easily absorbed, readily excreted, and stored only briefly (or not at all), they are characteristically vulnerable to deficiency.

Deficiency may result from inadequate diet, malabsorption, chronic alcoholism, or increased metabolic demands, as occurs in stress, pregnancy, lactation, or chronic illness. When correlated with the patient's clinical features, water-soluble vitamin levels in urine help evaluate metabolic disorders, malabsorption, and nutritional deficiency. For example, the urine test for vitamin B$_1$ helps detect neurologic disorders.

Minerals

Minerals are inorganic elements that are necessary for metabolism. Essential minerals — such as calcium, magnesium, and copper — participate in enzymatic catalysis directly and by binding with substrates to form metalloenzymes. Because minerals are stored in the body and tend to accumulate, toxicity is usually more common than deficiency. Minerals are classified according to their prevalence in the body: Major minerals are present in large amounts; trace elements are present in small amounts.

The following major minerals are commonly measured in the urine:

■ *Sodium* helps maintain osmotic pressure as well as water, electrolyte, and acid-base balance; with potassium, it also plays a part in transmission of nerve impulses and in muscle contractility. Sodium excretion is usually regulated by adrenocortical hormones, especially aldosterone.

■ *Chloride* helps control water, electrolyte, and acid-base balance and osmotic pressure; it's excreted mainly through the kidneys. Chloride levels usually parallel sodium levels.

■ *Potassium*, the major intracellular cation, helps maintain normal acid-base balance and neuromuscular function. Potassium excretion and concentration is regulated by the kidneys.

■ *Magnesium* activates several enzyme systems, aids cell metabolism, influences nucleic acid and protein metabolism, and enhances neuromuscular integration. Magnesium and calcium levels may be inversely related. Parathyroid hormone reduces magnesium excretion, but excessive secretion of aldosterone increases it.

■ *Calcium*, a vital component of bones and teeth, supports blood coagulation, muscle contractility, nerve impulse transmission, and cell wall permeability. It's excreted in urine as a result of excessive mobilization of bone calcium.

■ *Phosphorus* is necessary for mineralization of bones and teeth, energy metabolism, and fatty acid transport. Urine concentration of phosphorus is regulated by the renal tubules.

The following trace minerals may be measured in the urine:

■ *Iron* is needed for hemoglobin and myoglobin formation as well as cellular oxidation. It's stored in the body as hemosiderin and ferritin and is excreted in urine, stool, sweat, and menstrual flow.

■ *Copper* aids formation of hemoglobin and absorption of iron from the GI tract. It is a component of several enzymes for energy production and is excreted mainly in stool.

■ *Oxalate*, a salt of oxalic acid, combines with calcium in the digestive tract to form calcium oxalate, a component of urinary calculi.

These vitamins and minerals are found in many different foods. (See *Dietary sources of vitamins and minerals,* page 452.)

Tests that determine serum or urine concentrations of vitamins and minerals help assess nutritional status and detect metabolic disorders that cause deficiency or toxicity. Less common uses include assessing the effects of I.V. therapy or therapy with megavitamins or oral contraceptives, and monitoring the progression of debilitating diseases.

Serum analysis is generally preferred for determining mineral concentrations. However, urine levels are more significant in some cases — for instance, in detecting primary oxalosis.

Dietary sources of vitamins and minerals

NUTRIENT	FOOD SOURCES
Thiamine (vitamin B_1)	Pork, liver, dried yeast, whole-grain cereals, enriched cereals, nuts, legumes, potatoes
Pyridoxine (vitamin B_6)	Dried yeast, liver, whole-grain cereals, fish, legumes
Ascorbic acid (vitamin C)	Citrus fruits, tomatoes, potatoes, cabbage, green peppers
Sodium	Table salt, beef, pork, sardines, cheese, milk, eggs
Chloride	Table salt, seafood, milk, meat, eggs
Potassium	Potatoes, dried beans, squash, scallops, veal, dried figs, cantaloupes, bananas
Calcium	Milk, milk products, meat, fish, eggs, cereals, beans, fruit, vegetables
Phosphorus	Milk, cheese, meat, poultry, fish, whole-grain cereals, nuts, legumes
Magnesium	Seafood, soybeans, nuts, cocoa, whole-grain cereals, peas, dried beans, meat, milk
Copper	Liver, shellfish, nuts, dried legumes, poultry, whole-grain cereals
Iron	Liver, meat, egg yolks, beans, clams, peaches, whole or enriched grains, legumes
Oxalic acid	Strawberries, tomatoes, rhubarb, spinach

VITAMIN ASSAYS

Urine vitamin B_1

This test is used to detect a deficiency of vitamin B_1 (thiamine), a condition called beriberi. This water-soluble vitamin, which requires folic acid (folate) for effective uptake, is absorbed in the duodenum and excreted in the urine. Urine levels of vitamin B_1 reflect dietary intake and metabolic storage of thiamine. A coenzyme in decarboxylase reactions with citric acids, vitamin B_1 helps metabolize carbohydrates, fats, and proteins.

Rare in the United States, vitamin B_1 deficiency is most common in Asians because of their subsistence on polished rice. Vitamin B_1 deficiency may result from inadequate dietary intake (usually associated with alcoholism), impaired absorption (malabsorption syndrome), impaired utilization (hepatic disease), or conditions that increase the metabolic demand (pregnancy, lactation, fever, exercise, hyperthyroidism, surgery, and high carbohydrate intake). High dietary intake of fats and protein spares the vitamin B_1 necessary for tissue respiration.

The clinical effects of vitamin B_1 deficiency vary. Early deficiency produces nonspecific symptoms that may include fatigue, irritability, sleep disturbances, and abdominal and precordial discomfort. Severe deficiency states vary in several distinct patterns: Infantile beriberi produces abdominal pain, edema, irritability, vomiting, pallor and, possibly, seizures; wet, or edematous, beriberi (a complication of chronic alcoholism) produces severe neurologic symptoms — which may lead to Wernicke-Korsakoff syndrome and Korsakoff's psychosis — emaciation, and edema that rises from the legs. Beriberi also causes arrhythmias, cardiomegaly, and circulatory collapse.

Purpose
▪ To help confirm vitamin B_1 deficiency (beriberi) and to distinguish it from other causes of polyneuritis.

Patient preparation
Explain to the patient that this test evaluates the body's stores of vitamin B_1. Tell him the test requires a 24-hour urine specimen. Check his diet history to rule out a deficiency due to inadequate intake. If the patient is to collect the specimen, teach him the proper technique.

Procedure
Collect a 24-hour urine specimen.

Precautions
▪ Tell the patient not to contaminate the urine specimen with toilet tissue or stool.
▪ Refrigerate the specimen or place it on ice during the collection period.

Reference values
Normal urinary excretion ranges from 100 to 200 μg/24 hours.

Implications of results
Deficient urine levels of vitamin B_1 can result from inadequate dietary intake, hyperthyroidism, alcoholism, severe hepatic disease, chronic diarrhea, or prolonged diuretic therapy. Negative results indicate neuritis unrelated to deficiency.

Post-test care
Educate patients who are deficient in vitamin B_1 about good dietary sources of this vitamin: beef, pork, organ meats, fresh vegetables (especially peas and beans), and wheat and other whole grains.

Interfering factors
Failure to collect all urine during the test period or to store the specimen properly may alter test results.

Tryptophan challenge

Because direct assay of vitamin B_6 isn't currently available, measurement of urine xanthurenic acid after a challenge dose of tryptophan can confirm deficiency of vitamin B_6 long before symptoms appear. Although vitamin B_6 isn't directly involved in energy metabolism, it is essential for reactions that occur in protein metabolism and for amino acid synthesis.

Vitamin B_6 consists of three compounds — pyridoxine, pyridoxal, and pyridoxamine — that function as coenzymes in many biochemical reactions, including the conversion of tryptophan to niacin. Normally, this conversion prevents formation of xanthurenic acid; however, in a patient with vitamin B_6 deficiency, xanthurenic acid levels increase.

Vitamin B_6 deficiency can cause hypochromic microcytic anemia without iron deficiency and central nervous system disturbances. When normal magnesium levels accompany a vitamin B_6 deficiency, urinary citrate and oxalate solubility may decrease, causing formation of urinary calculi.

Purpose
- To detect vitamin B_6 deficiency.

Patient preparation
Explain to the patient that this test determines the body's stores of vitamin B_6. Tell him that after he receives an oral dose of medication, a 24-hour urine specimen will be collected. Check his medication history for current use of drugs that may cause vitamin B_6 deficiency.

Procedure
Administer L-tryptophan by mouth (usually, 50 mg/kg for children and up to 2 g/kg for adults). Have the patient void, discard the urine, and immediately begin collection of a 24-hour urine specimen.

Precautions
- Make sure the specimen bottle contains a crystal of thymol, a preservative.
- Tell the patient not to contaminate the urine specimen with toilet tissue or stool.
- Refrigerate the specimen or place it on ice during the collection period.

Reference values
Normal excretion of xanthurenic acid after a tryptophan challenge dose is less than 50 mg/24 hours.

Implications of results
Urine levels of xanthurenic acid exceeding 100 mg/24 hours indicate vitamin B_6 deficiency. This rare disorder may result from malnutrition, a malignant tumor, pregnancy, familial xanthurenic aciduria, or use of oral contraceptives, hydralazine, D-penicillamine, or isoniazid.

Post-test care
Inform the patient with vitamin B_6 deficiency that yeast, wheat, corn, liver, and kidneys are good sources of this vitamin.

Interfering factors
Failure to collect all urine during the test period or to store the specimen properly may alter test results.

Urine vitamin C

Through colorimetric measurement of urinary levels, this test determines body stores of vitamin C (also known as ascorbic acid). This water-soluble vitamin, which is easily absorbed by the intestine, acts as a reversible reducing agent in metabolic processes, aids collagen formation, and helps maintain connective and osteoid tissues.

Analysis of urinary vitamin C levels is particularly useful in diagnosing scurvy, an extreme deficiency of vitamin C characterized by the degeneration of connective and osteoid tissues, dentin, and endothelial membranes. Scurvy is considered uncommon in the United States today. (See *History of scurvy.*) However, it may appear in alcoholics, in people who are on low-residue or low-citrus diets, and in infants who have been weaned to cow's milk that does not contain a vitamin C supplement.

Purpose
- To aid diagnosis of scurvy, scurvylike conditions, and metabolic disorders that

History of scurvy

Scurvy was probably the first disease to be recognized as a dietary deficiency. Rare now, scurvy was common in the past in places where fresh fruits and vegetables — major sources of vitamin C — weren't accessible in the winter. Known as the "plague of the seas," scurvy was most prevalent in sailors because perishable foods couldn't be stored aboard ship. This deficiency also occurred as a result of famine and war-induced food scarcity.

When Vasco da Gama took his first trip around the Cape of Good Hope in 1497, more than half his crew died of scurvy. Several centuries later, in 1747, Scottish naval surgeon James Lind found that he could cure sailors with scurvy by giving them lemons and oranges.

In an effort to duplicate Dr. Lind's success, in 1797, lime juice was distributed to the crews of British navy ships during long sea voyages — thus, the nickname "limeys" for British sailors.

interfere with oxidative processes, such as malnutrition.

Patient preparation
Explain to the patient that this test detects vitamin C deficiency. Inform him that he needn't restrict food or fluids before the test and that the test requires a 24-hour urine collection. If the specimen is to be collected at home, teach the patient the proper urine collection technique.

Procedure
Collect a 24-hour urine specimen.

Precautions
- Tell the patient not to contaminate the specimen with toilet tissue or stool.
- Refrigerate the specimen or place it on ice during the collection period.

Reference values
Normal urine vitamin C excretion is 30 mg/24 hours.

Implications of results
Decreased urine vitamin C levels are common in patients with infection, cancer, burns, or other stress-producing conditions. Diminished levels may also indicate malnutrition, malabsorption, renal deficiency, or prolonged I.V. therapy without vitamin C replacement. Severe vitamin C deficiency causes scurvy.

Post-test care
Advise the patient with vitamin C deficiency that citrus fruits, tomatoes, potatoes, cabbage, and strawberries are good dietary sources of vitamin C.

Interfering factors
Improper specimen collection may affect test results.

MINERAL ASSAYS

Urine sodium and chloride

This test determines urine levels of sodium, the major extracellular cation, and of chloride, the major extracellular anion. Less significant than serum levels (and, consequently, performed less frequently), urine sodium and chloride measurement is used to evaluate renal conservation of these two electrolytes and to confirm serum sodium and chloride values.

Sodium and chloride help maintain osmotic pressure and water and acid-base balance. After these ions are absorbed by the intestinal tract, they're regulated by the kidneys and rise and fall in tandem. The kidneys conserve constant serum levels of sodium and chloride — even at the risk of dehydration or edema — or excrete excessive amounts.

Purpose

- To help evaluate fluid and electrolyte imbalance
- To monitor the effects of a low-salt diet
- To help evaluate renal and adrenal disorders.

Patient preparation

Explain to the patient that this test helps determine the balance of salt and water in his body. Advise him that no special restrictions are necessary and that the test requires a 24-hour urine specimen. If the specimen is to be collected at home, teach the patient the proper collection technique. Check the patient's medication history for drugs that may influence test results.

Procedure

Collect a 24-hour urine specimen.

Precautions

Tell the patient not to contaminate the specimen with toilet tissue or stool.

Reference values

Although levels of sodium and chloride in the urine vary greatly with dietary salt intake and perspiration, the normal range for urine sodium excretion is 30 to 280 mEq/24 hours; for urine chloride excretion, 110 to 250 mEq/24 hours; and for urine sodium-chloride excretion, 5 to 20 g/24 hours.

Implications of results

Usually, urine sodium and chloride levels are parallel, rising and falling in tandem. Abnormal sodium and chloride levels may indicate the need for more specific tests. Elevated urine sodium levels may reflect increased salt intake, adrenal failure, salicylate toxicity, diabetic acidosis, salt-losing nephritis, or water-deficient dehydration. Decreased urine sodium levels suggest decreased salt intake, primary aldosteronism, acute renal failure, or congestive heart failure.

Elevated urine chloride levels may result from water-deficient dehydration, salicylate toxicity, diabetic acidosis, adrenocortical insufficiency (Addison's disease), or salt-losing renal disease. Decreased levels may result from excessive diaphoresis, congestive heart failure, or hypochloremic metabolic alkalosis due to prolonged vomiting or gastric suctioning.

To evaluate fluid-electrolyte imbalance, results must be correlated with serum electrolyte findings.

Post-test care

None.

Interfering factors

- Failure to collect all urine during the test period may alter test results.
- Ammonium chloride and potassium chloride elevate urine chloride levels.
- Sodium bicarbonate and thiazide diuretics raise urine sodium levels; steroids suppress them.

Urine potassium

This quantitative test measures urine levels of potassium, a major intracellular cation that helps regulate acid-base balance and neuromuscular function. Potassium imbalance may cause such signs and symptoms as muscle weakness, nausea, diarrhea, confusion, hypotension, and electrocardiogram (ECG) changes; a severe imbalance may lead to cardiac arrest.

A serum potassium test is usually performed to detect hyperkalemia (abnormally high levels) or hypokalemia (abnormally low levels). A urine potassium test may be performed to evaluate hypokalemia when a history and physical examination fail to uncover the cause. Because kidneys regulate potassium balance through potassium excretion in the urine, measuring urine potassium levels can determine whether hypokalemia results from a renal disorder, such as renal tubular acidosis, or an extrarenal disorder, such as malabsorption syndrome. If results suggest a renal disorder, additional renal function tests may be ordered.

Purpose
■ To determine whether hypokalemia is caused by renal or extrarenal disorders.

Patient preparation
Explain to the patient that this test evaluates his kidney function. Advise him that no special dietary restrictions are necessary and that the test requires a 24-hour urine specimen. If the specimen is to be collected at home, teach him the correct collection technique. Check his medication history for drugs that may alter test results. If they must be continued, note this on the laboratory request.

Procedure
Collect a 24-hour urine specimen.

Precautions
■ Tell the patient not to contaminate the specimen with toilet tissue or stool.
■ Refrigerate the specimen or place it on ice during the collection period.
■ After collection, send the specimen to the laboratory immediately or refrigerate it.

Reference values
Normal potassium excretion is 25 to 125 mEq/24 hours, with an average potassium concentration of 25 to 100 mEq/L. In a patient with hypokalemia and normal kidney function, potassium concentration will be less than 10 mEq/L, indicating that potassium loss is most likely the result of a GI disorder such as malabsorption syndrome.

Implications of results
In a patient with hypokalemia lasting more than 3 days, urine potassium levels above 10 mEq/L indicate renal losses that may result from such disorders as aldosteronism, renal tubular acidosis, or chronic renal failure. However, extrarenal disorders, such as dehydration, starvation, Cushing's disease, or salicylate intoxication, may also elevate urine potassium levels.

Post-test care
 ■ Monitor the hypokalemic patient for diminished reflexes; rapid, weak, irregular pulse; confusion; hypotension; anorexia; muscle weakness; and paresthesias. Watch for ECG alterations, especially a flattened T wave, ST-segment depression, and U-wave elevation. Severe potassium imbalance may lead to ventricular fibrillation, respiratory paralysis, and cardiac arrest.

■ Administer potassium supplements and monitor serum levels, as ordered.

- Provide dietary supplements and nutritional counseling, as ordered.
- Replace volume loss with I.V. or oral fluids, as ordered.
- Resume medications withheld before the test, as ordered.

Interfering factors
- Excess dietary potassium raises urine potassium levels.
- Excessive vomiting or stomach suctioning produces test results that don't reflect actual potassium depletion.
- Potassium-wasting medications, such as ammonium chloride, thiazide diuretics, and acetazolamide, raise potassium levels.
- Failure to collect all urine during the test period or to store the specimen properly may alter test results.

Urine calcium and phosphates

This test measures the urine levels of calcium and phosphates, elements essential for the formation and resorption of bone. Urine calcium and phosphate levels generally parallel serum levels.

Normally absorbed in the upper intestine and excreted in feces and urine, calcium and phosphates help maintain tissue and fluid pH, electrolyte balance in cells and extracellular fluids, and permeability of cell membranes. Calcium promotes enzymatic processes, aids blood coagulation, and lowers neuromuscular irritability; phosphates aid carbohydrate metabolism. Factors that affect the calcium level and, indirectly, the phosphate level include parathyroid hormone level, calcitonin, and plasma proteins.

Purpose
- To evaluate calcium and phosphate metabolism and excretion
- To monitor treatment of calcium or phosphate deficiency.

Patient preparation
Explain to the patient that this test measures the amount of calcium and phosphates in the urine. Encourage him to be as active as possible before the test. Tell him the test requires 24-hour urine specimen collection. If the specimen is to be collected at home, teach him the correct collection technique.

As ordered, provide the Albright-Reifenstein diet (which contains about 130 mg of calcium/24 hours) for 3 days before the test, or provide a copy of the diet for the patient to follow at home. Note recent use of thiazide diuretics, sodium phosphate, or glucocorticoids on the laboratory request.

Procedure
Collect a 24-hour urine specimen.

Precautions
Tell the patient not to contaminate the specimen with toilet tissue or stool.

Reference values
Normal values depend on dietary intake. Males excrete less than 275 mg of calcium/24 hours; females, less than 250 mg/24 hours. Normal excretion of phosphates is less than 1,000 mg/24 hours.

Implications of results
Many disorders can affect urine calcium and phosphate levels. (See *Disorders that affect urine calcium and phosphate levels.*)

Post-test care
Observe a patient with low urine calcium levels for tetany.

Disorders that affect urine calcium and phosphate levels

The following disorders can cause changes in urine calcium or phosphate levels.

DISORDER	URINE CALCIUM LEVEL	URINE PHOSPHATE LEVEL
Hyperparathyroidism	Elevated	Elevated
Vitamin D intoxication	Elevated	Suppressed
Metastatic carcinoma	Elevated	Normal
Sarcoidosis	Elevated	Suppressed
Renal tubular acidosis	Elevated	Elevated
Multiple myeloma	Elevated or normal	Elevated or normal
Paget's disease	Normal	Normal
Milk-alkali syndrome	Suppressed or normal	Suppressed or normal
Hypoparathyroidism	Suppressed	Suppressed
Acute nephrosis	Suppressed	Suppressed or normal
Chronic nephrosis	Suppressed	Suppressed
Acute nephritis	Suppressed	Suppressed
Renal insufficiency	Suppressed	Suppressed
Osteomalacia	Suppressed	Suppressed
Steatorrhea	Suppressed	Suppressed

Interfering factors

■ Failure to collect all urine during the test period may affect the accuracy of test results.

■ Thiazide diuretics decrease excretion of calcium. Prolonged inactivity and ingestion of corticosteroids, sodium phosphate, or calcitonin increase excretion. Vitamin D increases phosphate absorption and excretion.

■ Parathyroid hormone increases urinary excretion of phosphates and decreases urinary excretion of calcium.

Urine magnesium

This test measures the urine level of magnesium, an important cation absorbed in the intestinal tract and excreted in the urine. Measurement of urine magnesium was rarely used in the past, but it's becoming more widely used because magnesium deficiency is detectable earlier in urine than in serum. The test is used to rule out magnesium deficiency as the cause of neurologic symptoms and to help evaluate glomerular function in suspected renal disease.

Magnesium is found primarily in the bones and in intracellular fluid; a small amount is present in extracellular fluid. This element activates many enzyme

Signs and symptoms of magnesium imbalance

A deficiency or excess of magnesium can affect various body systems and cause numerous signs and symptoms, as shown below.

BODY SYSTEM	HYPOMAGNESEMIA	HYPERMAGNESEMIA
Neuromuscular system	■ Hyperirritability, tetany, leg and foot cramps, Chvostek's sign (facial muscle spasms induced by tapping the area over the branches of the facial nerve)	■ Diminished reflexes, muscle weakness, flaccid paralysis, respiratory muscle paralysis that may cause respiratory distress
Central nervous system	■ Confusion, delusions, hallucinations, seizures	■ Drowsiness, flushing, lethargy, confusion, diminished sensorium
Cardiovascular system	■ Arrhythmias, vasomotor changes (vasodilation and hypotension) and, occasionally, hypertension	■ Bradycardia, weak pulse, hypotension, heart block, cardiac arrest (common with serum levels of 25 mEq/L)

systems, helps transport sodium and potassium across cell membranes, affects nucleic acid and protein metabolism, and influences intracellular calcium levels through its effect on secretion of parathyroid hormone. Magnesium deficiency usually results from poor absorption, often due to increased absorption of calcium; magnesium absorption increases as dietary intake of calcium increases.

Purpose

■ To rule out magnesium deficiency in patients with symptoms of central nervous system irritation
■ To detect excessive urinary excretion of magnesium
■ To help evaluate glomerular function in renal disease.

Patient preparation

Explain to the patient that this test determines urine magnesium levels. Advise him that no special restrictions are necessary and that the test requires a 24-hour urine specimen.

Inquire whether the patient is receiving magnesium-containing antacids, ethacrynic acid, thiazide diuretics (for example, spironolactone), or aldosterone. If he is, be sure to note this on the laboratory request.

Procedure

Collect a 24-hour urine specimen.

Precautions

Tell the patient not to contaminate the urine specimen with toilet tissue or stool.

Reference values

Normal urinary excretion of magnesium is less than 150 mg/24 hours (atomic absorption).

Implications of results

Low urine magnesium levels may result from malabsorption, acute or chronic diarrhea, diabetic acidosis, dehydration, pancreatitis, advanced renal failure, primary aldosteronism, or decreased dietary intake of magnesium.

Elevated urine magnesium levels may result from early chronic renal disease, adrenocortical insufficiency (Addison's disease), chronic alcoholism, or chronic ingestion of magnesium-containing antacids.

Magnesium imbalances cause a variety of clinical effects. (See *Signs and symptoms of magnesium imbalance.*)

Post-test care
None.

Interfering factors
- Failure to collect all urine during the test period may affect the accuracy of test results.
- Ethacrynic acid, thiazide diuretics, aldosterone, or excessive amounts of magnesium-containing antacids elevate urine magnesium levels.
- Spironolactone lowers urine magnesium levels.
- Increased calcium intake reduces urinary excretion of magnesium.

Urine copper

This test measures the urine level of copper, an essential trace element and a component of several metalloenzymes and proteins necessary for hemoglobin synthesis and oxidation reduction. Urine normally contains only a small amount of free copper; plasma, only trace amounts. Most copper in plasma is bound to and transported by an alpha$_2$ globulin (plasma protein) called ceruloplasmin. When copper is unbound, the ions can inhibit many enzyme reactions, resulting in copper toxicity.

Urine copper levels are frequently measured to detect Wilson's disease, a rare, inborn error of metabolism that's most common among persons of eastern European Jewish, southern Italian, or Sicilian ancestry. Wilson's disease is marked by decreased ceruloplasmin, increased urinary excretion of copper, and accumulation of copper in the interstitial tissues of the liver and brain. The cause of this disorder is unclear. Early detection and treatment (with a low-copper diet and D-penicillamine) are vital to prevent irreversible changes, such as nerve tissue degeneration and cirrhosis of the liver. (See *Assessing Wilson's disease,* page 462.)

Purpose
- To help detect Wilson's disease
- To screen infants with a family history of Wilson's disease.

Patient preparation
Explain to the patient that this test determines the amount of copper in urine. Inform him that no special restrictions are necessary and that the test requires a 24-hour urine specimen. If it's to be collected at home, explain the proper collection technique.

Procedure
Collect a 24-hour urine specimen.

Precautions
Tell the patient not to contaminate the urine specimen with toilet tissue or stool.

Reference values
Normal urinary excretion of copper ranges from 15 to 60 µg/24 hours.

Implications of results
Elevated urine copper levels usually indicate Wilson's disease (a liver biopsy helps establish this diagnosis). High copper levels may also occur in neph-

Assessing Wilson's disease

The primary purpose of the copper test is to assess Wilson's disease. Usually, the first symptoms of this rare, inherited disorder are neurologic — rigidity, tremors, incoordination, and ataxia. Later, liver insufficiency may develop with jaundice, ascites, and cirrhosis.

Kayser-Fleischer ring, a green or rust-colored ring around the cornea (shown below) caused by copper deposits, confirms Wilson's disease.

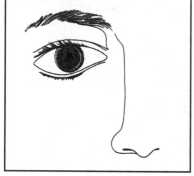

rotic syndrome, chronic active hepatitis, biliary cirrhosis, and rheumatoid arthritis.

Post-test care
None.

Interfering factors
- Failure to collect all urine during the test period may affect the accuracy of test results.
- Administration of D-penicillamine causes elevated urine levels of copper.

Urine hemosiderin

This test measures the urine level of hemosiderin — a colloidal iron oxide and one of the two forms of storage iron deposited in body tissue. When iron storage mechanisms fail to manage iron overload, excess iron may escape to cells unaccustomed to high iron concentrations, leading to toxic effects. Particularly vulnerable to such toxicity are the liver, myocardium, bone marrow, pancreas, kidneys, and skin, which tend to develop tissue damage known as hemochromatosis. This disorder may occur in a rare hereditary form known as primary hemochromatosis and in exogenous forms. Elevated tissue storage of iron without associated tissue damage is called hemosiderosis and is often confused with hemochromatosis.

Purpose
- To aid diagnosis of hemochromatosis.

Patient preparation
Explain to the patient that this test helps determine if the body is accumulating excessive amounts of iron. Inform him that no special restrictions are necessary and that the test requires a urine specimen.

Procedure
Collect a random urine specimen of approximately 30 ml.

Precautions
Seal the container securely, and send the specimen to the laboratory at once.

Normal findings
Hemosiderin is not found in urine.

Implications of results
The presence of hemosiderin, appearing as yellow-brown granules in urinary

sediment, indicates hemochromatosis; liver or bone marrow biopsy is necessary to confirm primary hemochromatosis. Hemosiderin may also suggest pernicious anemia, chronic hemolytic anemia, multiple blood transfusions, and paroxysmal nocturnal hemoglobinuria due to excessive iron injections or dietary intake of iron.

Post-test care
None.

Interfering factors
Failure to send the specimen to the laboratory immediately may alter test results.

Urine oxalate

This test measures urine levels of oxalate, a salt of oxalic acid. Oxalate is an end product of metabolism and is excreted almost exclusively in the urine. Most important, the test detects hyperoxaluria, a disorder in which oxalate accumulates in the soft and connective tissue, especially in the kidneys and bladder, causing chronic inflammation and fibrosis. Calcium oxalate deposits are the most common cause of renal calculi, which may produce kidney damage.

Purpose
▪ To detect primary hyperoxaluria in infants
▪ To rule out hyperoxaluria in renal insufficiency.

Patient preparation
Explain to the patient (or to the parents if the patient is a child) that this test determines if the urine contains excess oxalate. Instruct him to restrict intake of tomatoes, strawberries, rhubarb, and spinach for about 1 week before the test. Tell him the test requires a 24-hour urine specimen and that the laboratory requires at least 2 days to complete the analysis.

Procedure
Collect a 24-hour urine specimen in a light-resistant container with hydrochloric acid.

Precautions
Tell the patient not to urinate directly into the 24-hour specimen container and not to contaminate the urine specimen with toilet tissue or stool.

Reference values
Urine oxalate levels up to 40 mg/24 hours are considered normal.

Implications of results
Elevated urine oxalate levels (hyperoxaluria) result from excessive metabolic production of oxalate or increase oxalate intake. Levels as high as 100 to 400 mg/24 hours can occur.

Primary hyperoxaluria, a rare inborn metabolic disorder, causes excessive production and urinary excretion of oxalate. In this type of hyperoxaluria, elevated urine oxalate levels typically precede elevated serum levels.

Secondary hyperoxaluria can result from pancreatic insufficiency, diabetes mellitus, cirrhosis, pyridoxine deficiency, Crohn's disease, ileal resection, ingestion of antifreeze (ethylene glycol) or stain-remover, or a reaction to a methoxyflurane anesthetic.

Post-test care
None.

Interfering factors
▪ Failure to collect all urine during the test period or to store the specimen properly may alter test results.

■ Ingestion of strawberries, tomatoes, rhubarb, or spinach increases urine oxalate levels.

SELECTED READINGS

Diseases, 2nd ed. Springhouse, Pa.: Springhouse Corp., 1996.

Fischbach, F. *A Manual of Laboratory and Diagnostic Tests,* 5th ed. Philadelphia: Lippincott-Raven Pubs., 1996.

Henry, J.B., ed. *Clinical Diagnosis and Management by Laboratory Methods,* 19th ed. Philadelphia: W.B. Saunders Co., 1996.

Illustrated Manual of Nursing Practice, 2nd ed. Springhouse, Pa.: Springhouse Corp., 1994.

Long, B.C., et al. *Medical-Surgical Nursing: A Nursing Process Approach,* 3rd ed. St. Louis: Mosby–Year Book, Inc., 1993.

Nursing97 Drug Handbook. Springhouse, Pa.: Springhouse Corp., 1997.

Phipps, W.J., et al. *Medical-Surgical Nursing: Concepts and Clinical Practice,* 5th ed. St. Louis: Mosby–Year Book, Inc., 1995.

Tietz, N.W. *Clinical Guide to Diagnostic Tests,* 3rd ed. Philadelphia: W.B. Saunders Co., 1995.

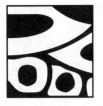

CHAPTER EIGHTEEN

Histology

Learning objectives

After completing this chapter, the reader will be able to:
- state three requirements of accurate histologic diagnosis
- describe five types of tissue biopsies
- explain how specimens are prepared for histologic examination
- describe frozen section tissue analysis
- identify the common sites of bone marrow aspiration and biopsy
- state the purpose of each test discussed in the chapter
- prepare the patient physically and psychologically for each test
- specify appropriate precautions for obtaining a specimen for each test
- recognize signs of an adverse reaction and respond appropriately
- implement appropriate post-test care
- identify the normal findings of each test
- discuss the implications of abnormal test results
- list factors that may interfere with accurate test results.

INTRODUCTION

Histology, the study of the microscopic structure of tissues and cells, is vital to confirm malignant disease and has made biopsy — extraction of a living tissue specimen — a common procedure. New tissue preparation techniques and needle designs have made biopsy more accessible — even allowing rapid specimen removal from deep tissues without surgery.

Accurate histologic diagnosis requires a representative or complete tissue specimen, procured with good technique to prevent damage; proper specimen handling and storage, usually in a fixative; and knowledge of the tissue's origin, the suspected diagnosis, previous biopsies at the site, and any current treatments.

Types of biopsy

In *incisional biopsy,* a scalpel, a cutting or aspiration needle, or a punch is used to remove a portion of tissue from large, multiple, hidden lesions. Fine-needle aspiration differs slightly from tradi-tional needle biopsy. It provides a smaller specimen, requires cytologic (not histologic) studies, and is usually performed on outpatients for breast biopsies. Incision of a hidden lesion is called a closed, or blind, biopsy. In *excisional biopsy,* a scalpel is used to remove abnormal tissue from the skin or subcutaneous tissue.

When such tissue can be easily and completely removed, excisional biopsy is preferred because it combines diagnosis and treatment. (For more information, see *Common types of tissue biopsy,* pages 468 and 469.)

A biopsy is commonly performed in a doctor's office or an outpatient surgical clinic; when the patient is already hospitalized, it's performed at the bedside or in a treatment room. It can also be done in the operating room, using open technique. An open biopsy is usually performed if results of a closed biopsy or other tests suggest the need for complete excision of a tissue mass. During open biopsy, a tissue specimen is obtained (usually under general anesthesia) and sent immediately to the histology laboratory for rapid analysis. Test results are relayed to the operating room, and a decision is made about subsequent surgery.

Tissue preparation critical

Because a decomposed tissue specimen is diagnostically useless, fixation — a process that arrests cellular structures and prevents decomposition — is very important in slide preparation. Inadequately fixed tissue breaks down immediately after removal from the body, losing one or more components. To prevent this, biopsy specimens are placed immediately in fixing fluid to kill and harden the tissue, and make it resistant to damage by reagents used to process it for microscopic study. The most common fixative solution is 10% neutral buffered formaldehyde; however, some laboratories require different fixatives and procedures for specimen fixation.

Temperature also influences specimen preservation: Cold slows decomposition and heat speeds it. If a fixative isn't immediately available, refrigeration of the specimen temporarily prevents deterioration. However, even a refrigerated specimen deteriorates significantly after 24 hours.

When a tissue specimen arrives in the histology department, a histologist numbers and labels it and a pathologist examines it, recording its weight, length, width, color, contents, unusual markings, and hollowness. After sectioning, the pathologist selects representative cuts of tissue and places them in numbered capsules for processing. To prevent tissue loss in processing, small pieces of tissue, such as those obtained from needle biopsies or curettage, are placed in embedding bags, wrapped in lens paper, or placed between wet sponges before being inserted in the capsules. A histologist then places the capsules in an automatic processor that moves them through a fixing fluid, through ascending strengths of dehydrating fluids, through a clearing fluid, and finally, into melted paraffin, which infiltrates the tissue. This procedure generally takes place overnight.

After processing, the tissue, now embedded in paraffin, is ready for cutting and staining. Special stains color various cellular components and permit identification. One stain that's used routinely — hematoxylin-eosin stain — is an example of this: Hematoxylin stains the nucleus, while eosin stains the cytoplasm. After staining, the histologist seals the tissues under labeled coverslips and delivers them to the pathologist for diagnosis. Because of these preparations, a stat tissue report generally takes 24 hours.

Rapid analysis: Frozen sections

Frozen sections, an alternative method of preparing tissue for study, permit rapid, accurate analysis of potentially malignant tissue during surgery. In this method, an individual tissue specimen is sent directly from the operating room to the histology department, where a pathologist grossly examines the tissue, sections it, and selects a representative section for quick freezing. Freezing fixes the tissue, hardening it to allow cutting into microscopic sections. After rapid staining, the pathologist analyzes the tissue for malignant cells and tissue margins, which indicate adequate excision, and reports findings to the surgeon, who then closes the wound or further excises malignant tissue.

Generally, this technique allows pathologic diagnosis within 10 to 15 minutes after excision. Results from frozen section analysis are usually reliable, but standard analysis on tissue from the same specimen must verify the diagnosis. Frozen sections can eliminate the need for two separate surgical and anesthetic procedures (one for biopsy, the second for treatment) and spare the pa-

Common types of tissue biopsy

BIOPSY TYPE AND TARGET TISSUE	EQUIPMENT
Excision Surgical removal of entire lesion from any tissue; may be excised under local anesthetic	Scalpel
Shaving Tissue shaved from raised surface lesion on the skin	Scalpel
Needle Removal of a core of tissue from bone, bone marrow, breast, lung, pleura, lymph node, liver, kidney, prostate, synovial membrane, or thyroid	Cutting needle (such as Cope's needle or Vim-Silverman needle)
Aspiration Aspiration of tissue sample from bone marrow or breast	Flexible or fine aspiration needle, needle guide, and aspiration syringe
Punch incision Removal of tissue specimen from core of lesion in skin or cervix	Punch (such as Tischler forceps)

ADVANTAGES AND DISADVANTAGES

- *Advantage:* combines diagnosis and treatment of lesion
- *Disadvantage:* may require major surgery under general anesthesia

---

- *Advantages:* generally safe; combines diagnosis and treatment of benign lesion; yields good cosmetic results
- *Disadvantages:* may require excision or other treatment if lesion is malignant; may cause seeding of malignant cells

---

- *Advantages:* avoids need for surgery; usually furnishes a representative specimen; preserves cell architecture
- *Disadvantages:* may require excision or other treatment based on histologic results; may be traumatic to surrounding tissues; may not furnish a representative specimen; may cause seeding of malignant cells

---

- *Advantages:* avoids need for surgery; aspiration of fluid from a breast cyst combines diagnosis and treatment; fine-needle aspiration causes less pain and can be done on outpatients
- *Disadvantages:* disturbs cell architecture; permits study of individual cells but not of intercellular structure; may not furnish a representative specimen; may cause seeding of malignant cells (less likely with fine-needle aspiration

---

- *Advantages:* avoids need for surgery; furnishes a representative specimen
- *Disadvantages:* may cause seeding of malignant cells when part of mass is removed; may require excision or other treatment based on histologic results

tient the anxiety of waiting for the biopsy report.

GLAND BIOPSIES

Breast biopsy

Although mammography, thermography, and ultrasonography aid diagnosis of breast masses, only histologic examination of breast tissue obtained by biopsy can confirm or rule out cancer. Needle biopsy or fine-needle biopsy can provide a core of tissue or a fluid aspirate, but needle biopsy should be restricted to fluid-filled cysts and advanced malignant lesions. Both methods have limited diagnostic value because of the small and perhaps unrepresentative specimens they provide. Open biopsy provides a complete tissue specimen, which can be sectioned to allow more accurate evaluation. All three techniques require only a local anesthetic and can often be performed on outpatients; however, open biopsy may require a general anesthetic if the patient is fearful or uncooperative.

A new advance in stereotactic biopsy has recently become available in some medical centers. (See *Latest advance in breast biopsy,* page 470.)

Breast biopsy is indicated for patients with palpable masses, suspicious areas in mammography, bloody discharge from the nipples, or persistently encrusted, inflamed, or eczematoid breast lesions. During mammography and before biopsy, a probe may be placed to help identify the precise site of the biopsy.

Breast tissue analysis often includes an estrogen and progesterone receptor assay to help select therapy if the mass

---

Latest advance in breast biopsy

A new diagnostic procedure that improves the accuracy of breast biopsies has recently become available in a few medical centers in the United States. The Advanced Breast Biopsy Instrument procedure, which involves computers linked to X-rays, offers patients less pain and chance of deformity than conventional biopsies, requires only local anesthesia, and can be completed in about an hour.

In the new procedure, doctors use the computer to pinpoint the exact location of the area to be biopsied. Using computer coordinates, a probing tube is then inserted into the breast to remove a tissue specimen. Test results usually take less than 2 days.

Until now, doctors have had to rely on two-dimensional X-rays to locate the calcium deposits they wanted to biopsy and could not be absolutely sure if they were cutting into the correct area.

The new method provides 100% accuracy, surgeons who have used it say, allowing them to determine the exact three-dimensional location of the calcium deposits while the patient lies face down on a raised operating table. A rotating camera under the table provides X-rays of the breast from every angle. Doctors can then match up the coordinates to make sure they extract a specimen from the correct area.

---

proves malignant. This assay measures quick-frozen tumor tissue to determine binding capacity of its estrogen and progesterone receptors.

Purpose

■ To differentiate between benign and malignant breast tumors.

Patient preparation

Obtain a complete medical history, including when the patient first noticed the lesion, the presence or absence of pain or nipple discharge, a change in the lesion's size, association with the patient's menstrual cycle, and nipple or skin changes, such as the characteristic "orange-peel" skin that may indicate an underlying inflammatory carcinoma.

Describe the procedure to the patient, and explain that this test permits microscopic examination of a breast tissue specimen. Offer her emotional support, and assure her that breast masses don't always indicate cancer.

If the patient is to receive a local anesthetic, tell her that she needn't restrict food, fluids, or medication prior to the biopsy. If she's to receive a general anesthetic, advise her to fast from midnight the night before the test until after the biopsy. Tell her who will perform the biopsy and where and that it will take 15 to 30 minutes. Also explain to her that pretest studies, such as blood tests, urine tests, and chest X-rays, may be required.

Make sure the patient has signed a consent form. Check the patient history for hypersensitivity to anesthetics.

Procedure

For needle biopsy: Instruct the patient to undress to the waist. After guiding her to a sitting or recumbent position, with her hands at her sides, tell her to remain still. The biopsy site is prepared, a local anesthetic is administered, and the syringe (luer-lock syringe for aspiration, Vim-Silverman needle for tissue specimen) is introduced into the lesion. Fluid aspirated from the breast is expelled into a properly labeled, heparinized tube; the tissue specimen is placed in a labeled specimen bottle containing normal saline solution or formaldehyde. (With fine- needle aspiration, a slide is made for cytology and viewed immediately under a microscope.) Pressure is exerted on the biopsy site, and after bleeding stops, an adhesive bandage is applied. (Since breast fluid aspiration is not considered diagnostically accurate, some doctors aspirate fluid only from cysts. If such fluid is clear yellow and the mass disappears, the aspiration procedure is both diagnostic and therapeutic, and the aspirate is discarded. If aspiration yields no fluid, or if the lesion recurs two or three times, an open biopsy is then considered appropriate.)

For open biopsy: After the patient receives a general or local anesthetic, an incision is made in the breast to expose the mass. The examiner may then *incise* a portion of tissue or *excise* the entire mass. If the mass is smaller than $\frac{3}{4}$" (2 cm) in diameter and appears benign, it's usually excised; if it is larger or appears malignant, a specimen is usually incised before the mass is excised. (Incisional biopsy generally provides an adequate specimen for histologic analysis.) The specimen is placed in a properly labeled specimen bottle containing 10% formaldehyde solution. Tissue that appears malignant is sent for frozen section and receptor assays. (Receptor assay specimens must not be placed in formaldehyde.) The wound is sutured, and an adhesive bandage is applied.

Precautions
▪ Open breast biopsy is contraindicated in patients with conditions that preclude surgery.

▪ Send the specimen to the laboratory immediately.

Normal findings
Breast tissue normally consists of cellular and noncellular connective tissue, fat lobules, and various lactiferous ducts. It's pink, more fatty than fibrous, and shows no abnormal development of cells or tissue elements.

Implications of results
Abnormal breast tissue may exhibit a wide range of malignant or benign pathology. Breast tumors are common in women and account for 32% of female cancers; they are rare in men (0.2% of male cancers). Benign conditions include fibrocystic disease, adenofibroma, intraductal papilloma, mammary fat necrosis, and plasma cell mastitis (mammary duct ectasia). Malignant tumors include adenocarcinoma, cystosarcoma, intraductal carcinoma, infiltrating carcinoma, inflammatory carcinoma, medullary or circumscribed carcinoma, colloid carcinoma, lobular carcinoma, sarcoma, and Paget's disease.

The receptor assays evaluate tumors for estrogen and progesterone protein and assign a positive or negative value to the estrogen and progesterone receptors. This positive or negative value assists in the prognosis and treatment of breast cancer.

Post-test care
▪ If the patient has received a local anesthetic during needle or open biopsy, check vital signs and provide medication for pain, as ordered. Watch for and report bleeding, tenderness, or redness at the biopsy site.

▪ If the patient has received a general anesthetic, check vital signs every 30 minutes for the first 4 hours, every hour for the next 4 hours, and then every 4 hours. Administer an analgesic as or-

dered. Watch for and report bleeding, tenderness, or redness at the biopsy site.
■ An ice bag to the biopsy site may provide comfort. Instruct the patient to wear a support bra at all times until healing is complete.
■ Provide emotional support to the patient who is awaiting diagnosis. If the biopsy confirms cancer, the patient will require follow-up tests, including radiographic tests, blood studies, bone scans, and urinalysis, to determine appropriate treatment.

Interfering factors

Failure to obtain an adequate tissue specimen or to place the specimen in the proper solution container may interfere with test results.

Prostate gland biopsy

Prostate gland biopsy is the needle excision of a prostate tissue specimen for histologic examination. A perineal, transrectal, or transurethral approach may be used; the transrectal approach is usually used for high prostatic lesions. Indications include potentially malignant prostatic hypertrophy and prostatic nodules.

Purpose

■ To confirm prostate cancer
■ To determine the cause of prostatic hypertrophy.

Patient preparation

Describe the procedure to the patient, answer his questions, and tell him the test provides a tissue specimen for microscopic study. Tell him who will perform the biopsy and where, that he'll receive a local anesthetic, and that the procedure takes less than 30 minutes.

Make sure the patient has signed a consent form. Check the patient history for hypersensitivity to the anesthetic or to other drugs. For a transrectal approach, prepare the bowel by administering enemas until the return is clear. And, as ordered, administer an antibacterial to minimize the risk of infection. Just before the biopsy, check vital signs and administer a sedative, as ordered. Instruct the patient to remain still during the procedure and to follow instructions.

Procedure

For perineal approach: Place the patient in the proper position (left lateral, knee-chest, or lithotomy), and clean the perineal skin. After the local anesthetic is administered, a 2-mm incision may be made into the perineum. The examiner immobilizes the prostate by inserting a finger into the rectum, and introduces the biopsy needle into a prostate lobe. The needle is rotated gently, pulled out about 5 mm, and reinserted at another angle. The procedure is repeated at several areas. Specimens are placed immediately in a labeled specimen bottle containing 10% formaldehyde solution. Pressure is exerted on the puncture site, which is then bandaged.

For transrectal approach: This approach may be performed on outpatients without an anesthetic. Place the patient in a left lateral position. A curved needle guide is attached to the finger palpating the rectum. The biopsy needle is pushed along the guide, into the prostate. As the needle enters the prostate, the patient may experience pain. The needle is rotated to cut off the tissue and then is withdrawn.

An alternate method of transrectal detection is the automated cone biopsy, in which the doctor uses a spring-powered device with an inner trocar needle to cut through prostatic tissue. This relatively new technique is quick and reportedly painless. With both transrectal methods, the specimen is placed immediately in a labeled specimen bottle containing 10% formaldehyde solution.

For transurethral approach: An endoscopic instrument is passed through the urethra, permitting direct viewing of the prostate and passage of a cutting loop. The loop is rotated to chip away pieces of tissue and is then withdrawn. The specimen is placed immediately in a labeled specimen bottle containing 10% formaldehyde solution.

Precautions

Complications may include transient, painless hematuria and bleeding into the prostatic urethra and bladder.

Normal findings

The prostate gland normally consists of a thin, fibrous capsule surrounding the stroma, which is made up of elastic and connective tissues and smooth-muscle fibers. The epithelial glands, found in these tissues and muscle fibers, drain into the chief excreting ducts.

Implications of results

Histologic examination can confirm cancer. Bone scans, bone marrow biopsy, and measurement of prostate-specific antigen and serum acid phosphatase values determine its extent. Acid phosphatase levels usually rise in metastatic prostate cancer and tend to be low in cancer that is confined to the prostatic capsule.

Histologic examination can also detect benign prostatic hyperplasia, prostatitis, tuberculosis, lymphomas, and rectal or bladder cancers.

Post-test care

■ Check vital signs immediately after the procedure, every 2 hours for 4 hours, and then every 4 hours.
■ Observe the biopsy site for a hematoma and for signs of infection, such as

redness, swelling, and pain. Watch for urine retention or urinary frequency and for hematuria.

Interfering factors

Failure to obtain an adequate tissue specimen or to place the specimen in formaldehyde solution may affect the accuracy of test results.

Thyroid biopsy

Thyroid biopsy is the excision of a thyroid tissue specimen for histologic examination. This procedure is indicated for patients with thyroid enlargement or nodules (even if serum triiodothyronine [T_3] and serum thyroxine [T_4] levels are normal), breathing and swallowing difficulties, vocal cord paralysis, weight loss, hemoptysis, or a sensation of fullness in the neck. It's commonly performed when noninvasive tests, such as thyroid ultrasonography and scans, are abnormal or inconclusive.

A thyroid tissue specimen may be obtained with a hollow needle under local anesthesia or during open (surgical) biopsy under general anesthesia. Fine-needle aspiration with a cytologic smear examination can aid in diagnosis and replace an open biopsy. Open biopsy, performed in the operating room, is more complex and provides more direct information than needle biopsy. In open biopsy, the surgeon obtains a tissue specimen from the exposed thyroid and sends it to the histology laboratory for rapid analysis. This method also permits immediate excision of suspicious thyroid tissue.

Coagulation studies should always precede thyroid biopsy.

Purpose

- To differentiate between benign and malignant thyroid disease
- To help diagnose Hashimoto's disease, hyperthyroidism, and nontoxic nodular goiter.

Patient preparation

Describe the procedure to the patient, and answer any questions he may have. Explain that this test permits microscopic examination of a thyroid tissue specimen. Inform the patient that he needn't restrict food or fluids (unless he'll receive a general anesthetic). Tell him who will perform the biopsy and where, that it takes 15 to 30 minutes, and that results should be available in 1 day. Make sure the patient has signed a consent form. Check for hypersensitivity to anesthetics or analgesics.

Tell the patient he'll receive a local anesthetic to minimize pain during the procedure but may experience some pressure when the tissue specimen is procured. Advise him that he may have a sore throat the day after the test. Administer a sedative to the patient 15 minutes before the biopsy, as ordered.

Procedure

For needle biopsy, place the patient in the supine position, with a pillow under his shoulder blades. (This position pushes the trachea and thyroid forward and allows the neck veins to fall backward.) Prepare the skin over the biopsy site. As the examiner prepares to inject the local anesthetic, warn the patient not to swallow. After the anesthetic is injected, the carotid artery is palpated, and the biopsy needle is inserted parallel to and about 1" (2.5 cm) from the thyroid cartilage to prevent damage to the deep structures and the larynx. When the specimen is obtained, the needle is removed, and the specimen is immediately placed in formaldehyde.

Apply pressure to the biopsy site to stop bleeding. If bleeding continues for more than a few minutes, press on the site for up to 15 minutes more. Apply an adhesive bandage. Bleeding may persist in a patient with abnormal prothrombin time (PT) or abnormal activated partial thromboplastin time (APTT) or in a patient with a large vascular thyroid and distended veins.

Precautions

- Thyroid biopsy should be used cautiously in patients with coagulation defects, as indicated by abnormal PT or APTT.
- Because cell breakdown in the tissue specimen begins immediately after excision, the specimen must be placed in formaldehyde solution immediately.

Normal findings

Histologic examination of normal tissue shows fibrous networks dividing the gland into pseudolobules that consist of follicles and capillaries. Cuboidal epithelium lines the follicle walls and contains the protein thyroglobulin, which stores T_4 and T_3.

Implications of results

Malignant tumors appear as well-encapsulated, solitary nodules of uniform but abnormal structure. Papillary carcinoma is the most common type of thyroid cancer. Follicular carcinoma, a less common form, strongly resembles normal cells.

Benign conditions such as nontoxic nodular goiter demonstrate hypertrophy, hyperplasia, and hypervascularity. Distinct histologic patterns characterize subacute granulomatous thyroiditis, Hashimoto's disease, and hyperthyroidism.

Because many malignant thyroid tumors are multicentric and small, a negative histologic report doesn't necessarily rule out cancer.

Post-test care

■ To make the patient more comfortable, place him in semi-Fowler's position. Tell him he may avoid undue strain on the biopsy site by putting both hands behind his neck when he sits up.

■ Watch for signs of bleeding, tenderness, or redness at the biopsy site. Observe for difficulty breathing due to edema or hematoma, with resultant tracheal collapse. Also check the back of the neck and the patient's pillow for bleeding every hour for 8 hours. Report bleeding immediately.

■ Keep the biopsy site clean and dry.

Interfering factors

Failure to obtain a representative tissue specimen or to place the specimen in formaldehyde solution immediately may affect the accuracy of test results.

Lymph node biopsy

Lymph node biopsy is the surgical excision of an active lymph node or the needle aspiration of a nodal specimen for histologic examination. Both techniques usually use local anesthesia and sample the superficial nodes in the cervical, supraclavicular, axillary, or inguinal region. Excision is the preferred technique because it provides a larger specimen.

Usually flat and bean-shaped, lymph nodes swell during infection but return to normal size as infection clears. When nodal enlargement is prolonged and accompanied by backache, leg edema, breathing and swallowing difficulties and, later, weight loss, weakness, severe itching, fever, night sweats, cough, hemoptysis, or hoarseness, a biopsy is indicated. Generalized or localized lymph node enlargement is typical of such diseases as chronic lymphocytic leukemia,

Hodgkin's disease, non-Hodgkin's lymphoma, infectious mononucleosis, and rheumatoid arthritis.

A complete blood count, liver function studies, liver and spleen scans, and X-rays should precede this test.

Purpose

■ To determine the cause of lymph node enlargement

■ To distinguish between benign and malignant lymph node tumors

■ To stage metastatic cancer.

Patient preparation

Describe the procedure to the patient, and ask if he has any questions. Explain that this test allows microscopic study of lymph node tissue. For excisional biopsy, instruct the patient to restrict food from midnight and to drink only clear liquids. (If a general anesthetic is needed for deeper nodes, he must also restrict fluids.) For a needle biopsy, inform him that he needn't restrict food or fluids. Tell him who will perform the biopsy and where, that the procedure takes 15 to 30 minutes, and that the analysis takes 1 day to complete.

Make sure the patient has signed a consent form. Check the patient history for hypersensitivity to the anesthetic. If the patient will receive a local anesthetic, explain that he may experience discomfort during the injection. Just before the biopsy, record baseline vital signs.

Procedure

For excisional biopsy: Prepare the skin over the biopsy site, and drape the area for privacy. The anesthetic is then administered. The examiner makes an incision, removes an entire node, and places it in a properly labeled bottle containing normal saline solution. Then the wound is sutured, and a sterile dressing is applied.

For needle biopsy: After preparing the biopsy site and administering a local anesthetic, the examiner grasps the node between his thumb and forefinger, inserts the needle directly into the node, and obtains a small core specimen. Then he removes the needle and places the specimen in a properly labeled bottle containing normal saline solution. Pressure is exerted on the biopsy site to control bleeding, and an adhesive bandage is applied.

Precautions

Storing the tissue specimen in normal saline solution instead of in 10% formaldehyde solution allows part of the specimen to be used for cytologic impression smears, which are studied along with the biopsy specimen.

Normal findings

The normal lymph node is encapsulated by collagenous connective tissue and is divided into smaller lobes by tissue strands called *trabeculae.* It has an outer *cortex,* composed of lymphoid cells and nodules or follicles containing lymphocytes, and an inner *medulla,* composed of reticular phagocytic cells that collect and drain fluid.

Implications of results

Histologic examination of the tissue specimen distinguishes between malignant and nonmalignant causes of lymph node enlargement. Lymphatic malignancy accounts for up to 5% of all cancers and is now thought to be bimodal. Hodgkin's disease, a lymphoma affecting the entire lymph system, is the leading cancer affecting adolescents and young adults. Lymph node malignancy may also result from metastatic cancer.

When histologic results aren't clear or nodular material isn't involved, mediastinoscopy or laparotomy can provide another nodal specimen. Occasionally,

lymphangiography can furnish additional diagnostic information.

Post-test care

- Check vital signs and watch for bleeding, tenderness, and redness at the biopsy site.
- Tell the patient that he may resume his usual diet.

Interfering factors

- Improper specimen storage or failure to obtain a representative tissue specimen may alter test results.
- Inability to differentiate nodal pathology may affect the accuracy of test results.

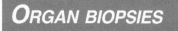

ORGAN BIOPSIES

Skin biopsy

Skin biopsy is the removal of a small piece of tissue, under local anesthesia, from a lesion suspected of being malignant. A specimen for histologic examination may be secured by one of three techniques — shave, punch, or excision. A *shave biopsy* cuts the lesion above the skin line and leaves the lower layers of dermis intact, permitting further biopsy at the site. A *punch biopsy* removes an oval core from the center of a lesion. An *excision biopsy,* the procedure of choice, removes the entire lesion; it's indicated for rapidly expanding lesions; for sclerotic, bullous, or atrophic lesions; and for examination of a lesion's border and surrounding normal skin.

Lesions suspected of being malignant usually have changed color, size, or appearance or have failed to heal properly after injury. Fully developed lesions should be selected for biopsy whenever

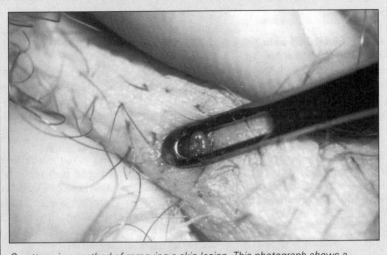

Curettage is a method of removing a skin lesion. This photograph shows a curette cupping a suspected molluscum lesion for biopsy. After the tissue is removed and properly prepared, it's examined microscopically for characteristic molluscum cells, which confirm the diagnosis of skin cancer.

possible because they provide more diagnostic information than those that are resolving or in early developing stages. For example, if the skin shows blisters, the biopsy should include the most mature ones.

Purpose
■ To provide differential diagnosis of basal cell carcinoma, squamous cell carcinoma, malignant melanoma, and benign growths
■ To diagnose chronic bacterial or fungal skin infections.

Patient preparation
Describe the procedure to the patient, and answer any questions he may have. Explain that the biopsy provides a sample of skin for microscopic study. Inform him that he needn't restrict food or fluids. Tell him who will perform the procedure and where, that he'll receive a local anesthetic to minimize pain dur-

ing the procedure, and that the biopsy takes approximately 15 minutes.

Make sure the patient has signed a consent form. Check the patient history for hypersensitivity to the local anesthetic.

Procedure
Position the patient comfortably, and clean the biopsy site. Then the local anesthetic is administered.

For shave biopsy: The protruding growth is cut off at the skin line with a #15 scalpel, and the tissue is placed immediately in a properly labeled specimen bottle containing 10% formaldehyde solution. Pressure is applied to the area to stop the bleeding.

For punch biopsy: The skin surrounding the lesion is pulled taut, and the punch is firmly introduced into the lesion and rotated to obtain a tissue specimen. The plug is lifted with forceps or a needle and is severed as deeply into the fat layer as possible. The specimen is placed in a properly labeled specimen bottle containing 10% formaldehyde solution or, if indicated, in a sterile container. The method used to close the wound depends on the size of the punch. A 3-mm punch biopsy requires only an adhesive bandage; a 4-mm punch biopsy requires one suture; and a 6-mm punch biopsy requires two sutures.

For excision biopsy: A #15 scalpel is used to excise the lesion completely; the incision is made as wide and as deep as necessary. The examiner removes the tissue specimen and places it immediately in a properly labeled specimen bottle containing 10% formaldehyde solution. Pressure is applied to the site to stop the bleeding. The wound is closed using 4-0 sutures. If the incision is large, skin graft may be required.

Precautions
Send the specimen to the laboratory immediately.

Normal findings
Normal skin consists of squamous epithelium (epidermis) and fibrous connective tissue (dermis).

Implications of results
Histologic examination of the tissue specimen may reveal a benign or malignant lesion. Benign growths include cysts, seborrheic keratoses, warts, pigmented nevi (moles), keloids, dermatofibromas, and multiple neurofibromas. Malignant skin cancers include basal cell carcinoma, squamous cell carcinoma, and malignant melanoma. Basal cell carcinoma occurs on hair-bearing skin, the most common location being the face — including the nose and its folds. Squamous cell carcinoma most often appears on the lips, mouth, and genitalia. Malignant melanoma, the most deadly skin cancer, can spread

throughout the body by way of the lymphatic system and the blood vessels.

Cultures can detect chronic bacterial and fungal infections in which flora are relatively sparse.

Post-test care
■ Check the biopsy site for bleeding.
■ If the patient experiences pain at the biopsy site, administer medication, as ordered.
■ Advise the patient with sutures to keep the area clean and as dry as possible. Tell him the facial sutures will be removed in 3 to 5 days; trunk sutures, in 7 to 14 days. Instruct the patient with adhesive strips to leave them in place for 14 to 21 days or until they fall off.

Interfering factors
■ Improper selection of the biopsy site may affect test results.
■ Failure to use the appropriate fixative or to use a sterile container when it's indicated may alter test results.

Small-bowel biopsy

Small-bowel biopsy helps evaluate diseases of the intestinal mucosa, which may cause malabsorption or diarrhea. Using a capsule, it produces larger specimens than does endoscopic biopsy and allows removal of tissue from areas beyond an endoscope's reach. (See *Endoscopic biopsy of the GI tract.*)

Several types of capsules are available, all similar in design and use. The Carey capsule, for example, has a spring-loaded, two-piece capsule that's 8 mm in diameter and 2.6 cm long. A mercury-weighted bag is attached to one end of the capsule; a thin polyethylene tube about 150 cm long is attached to the other end. Once the bag, capsule, and

Endoscopic biopsy of the GI tract

Endoscopy allows direct visualization of the GI tract and any site that requires biopsy of tissue samples for histologic analysis. This relatively painless procedure can detect cancer, lymphoma, amyloidosis, candidiasis, and gastric ulcers; can support a diagnosis of Crohn's disease, chronic ulcerative colitis, gastritis, esophagitis, and melanosis coli in laxative abuse; and can monitor progression of Barrett's esophagus, multiple gastric polyps, colon cancer and polyps, and chronic ulcerative colitis. Its complications, notably hemorrhage, perforation, and aspiration, are rare.

Preparation

Careful patient preparation is vital for this procedure. Describe the procedure to the patient, and reassure him that he'll be able to breathe with the endoscope in place. Instruct him to fast for at least 8 hours before the procedure. (For lower GI biopsy, clean the bowel, as ordered.) Make sure the patient has signed a consent form.

Just before the procedure, sedate the patient, as ordered. He should be relaxed but not asleep, because his cooperation promotes smooth passage of the endoscope. Spray the back of his throat with a local anesthetic to suppress his gag reflex. Have suction equipment and bipolar cauterizing electrodes available to prevent aspiration and excessive bleeding.

Procedure

After the doctor passes the endoscope into the upper or lower GI tract and visualizes a lesion, node, or other abnormal area, he pushes a biopsy forceps through a channel in the endoscope until this, too, can be seen. Then he opens the forceps, positions it at the biopsy site, and closes it on the tissue. The closed forceps and tissue specimen are removed from the endoscope, and the tissue is taken from the forceps.

The specimen is placed mucosal side up on fine-mesh gauze or filter paper and then inserted in a labeled specimen bottle containing fixative. When all specimens have been collected, the endoscope is removed. Specimens are sent to the laboratory immediately.

---

tube are in place in the small bowel, suction applied to the tube causes the mucosa to enter the capsule. Continued suction closes the capsule, cutting off the piece of tissue within.

This test verifies the diagnosis of some diseases, such as Whipple's disease, and may help confirm others, such as tropical sprue. Capsule biopsy is an invasive procedure, but it causes little pain and complications are rare.

Purpose

■ To help diagnose diseases of the intestinal mucosa.

Patient preparation

Describe the procedure to the patient, and ask if he has any questions. Explain that this test helps identify intestinal disorders. Instruct him to restrict food and fluids for at least 8 hours before the test. Tell him who will perform the biopsy and where and that the procedure takes 45 to 60 minutes but causes little discomfort.

Make sure the patient has signed a consent form. Ensure that coagulation tests have been performed and that the results are recorded on the patient's chart. Withhold aspirin and anticoagulants, as ordered. If these must be continued, note this on the laboratory request.

Procedure

Check the tubing and the mercury bag for leaks. Lightly lubricate the tube and the capsule with a water-soluble lubricant, and moisten the mercury bag with water. Spray the back of the patient's throat with a local anesthetic, as ordered, to decrease gagging during passage of the tube. Ask the patient to sit upright. The capsule is placed in his pharynx, and he is asked to flex his neck and swallow as the doctor advances the tube about 50 cm. (If a local anesthetic is used to control the gag reflex, the patient must not receive any fluids to help him swallow the capsule.) Place the patient on his right side; the doctor then advances the tube another 50 cm. The tube's position must be checked by fluoroscopy or by instilling air through the tube and listening with a stethoscope for air to enter the stomach.

Next, the tube is advanced 5 to 10 cm at a time to pass the capsule through the pylorus. Talk to the patient about food to stimulate the pylorus and help the capsule pass. When fluoroscopy confirms that the capsule has passed the pylorus, keep the patient on his right side to allow the capsule to move into the second and third portions of the small bowel. Tell the patient that he may hold the tube loosely to one side of his mouth if it makes him more comfortable. Capsule position is checked again by fluoroscopy.

When the capsule is at or beyond the ligament of Trietz, the biopsy sample can be taken. (The doctor will determine the biopsy site.) Place the patient in the supine position so the capsule's position can be verified fluoroscopically. A 100-ml glass syringe is placed on the end of the tube, and steady suction is applied to close the capsule and cut

off a tissue specimen. Suction is maintained on the syringe as the tube and capsule are removed; then the suction is released. This opens the capsule and exposes the specimen, mucosal side down. The specimen is gently removed with forceps, placed mucosal side up on a piece of mesh, and placed in a biopsy bottle with required fixative. Send the specimen to the laboratory at once.

Precautions

- Keep suction equipment nearby to prevent aspiration if the patient vomits.
- Do not allow the patient to bite the tubing.
- Handle the tissue specimen carefully and place it correctly on the slide, as ordered.
- Biopsy is contraindicated in uncooperative patients, those taking aspirin or anticoagulants, and those with uncontrolled coagulation disorders.

Normal findings

A normal small-bowel biopsy specimen consists of fingerlike villi, crypts, columnar epithelial cells, and round cells.

Implications of results

Small-bowel tissue that reveals histologic changes in cell structure may indicate Whipple's disease, abetalipoproteinemia, lymphoma, lymphangiectasia, eosinophilic enteritis, and such parasitic infections as giardiasis and coccidiosis. Histologic abnormalities may also suggest celiac disease, tropical sprue, infectious gastroenteritis, intraluminal bacterial overgrowth, folate and B_{12} deficiency, radiation enteritis, and malnutrition, but such disorders require further studies.

Post-test care

- As ordered, resume diet after confirming return of the gag reflex.
- Complications are rare. However, watch for signs of hemorrhage, bacte-

remia with transient fever and pain, and bowel perforation. Tell the patient to report abdominal pain or bleeding.

Interfering factors
■ Mechanical failure of the biopsy capsule or any hole in the tubing can prevent removal of a tissue specimen.
■ Incorrect handling or positioning of the specimen may alter test results.
■ Failure to fast before the biopsy may yield a poor specimen or cause vomiting and aspiration.
■ Failure to place the specimen in a fixative or a delay in transport to the laboratory may alter test results.

Percutaneous liver biopsy

Percutaneous biopsy of the liver is the needle aspiration of a core of tissue for histologic analysis. This procedure is performed under local or general anesthesia using a special needle. (See *Using a Menghini needle.*) Such analysis can identify hepatic disorders after ultrasonography, computed tomography scans, and radionuclide studies have failed to detect them. Because many patients with hepatic disorders have coagulation defects, testing for hemostasis should precede liver biopsy.

Purpose
■ To diagnose hepatic parenchymal disease, malignant tumors, and granulomatous infections.

Patient preparation
Describe the procedure to the patient, and ask if he has any questions. Explain that this test helps diagnose liver disorders. Instruct the patient to restrict food and fluids for 4 to 8 hours before the

Using a Menghini needle

In percutaneous liver biopsy, a Menghini needle attached to a 5-ml syringe containing normal saline solution is introduced through the chest wall and intercostal space (1). Negative pressure is created in the syringe. Then the needle is pushed rapidly into the liver (2) and pulled out of the body entirely (3) to obtain a tissue specimen.

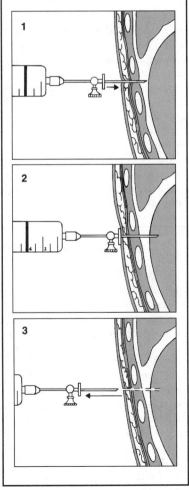

test, as ordered. Tell him who will perform the biopsy and where, that the biopsy needle remains in the liver about 1 second, and that the entire procedure takes about 10 to 15 minutes.

Make sure the patient has signed a consent form. Check the patient history for hypersensitivity to the local anesthetic. Make sure prothrombin time, partial thromboplastin time, and platelet count tests have been performed and that the results are recorded on the patient's chart. A blood sample is usually drawn for baseline assessment of hematocrit.

Just before the biopsy, tell the patient to void. After he does, record vital signs. Inform him that he will receive a local anesthetic but may experience pain similar to that of a punch in his right shoulder as the biopsy needle passes the phrenic nerve.

Procedure

For aspiration biopsy using a Menghini needle, place the patient in the supine position, with his right hand under his head. Instruct him to maintain this position and remain as still as possible during the procedure. The liver is palpated, the biopsy site is selected and marked, and the anesthetic is then injected.

The needle flange is set to control the depth of penetration, and 2 ml of sterile normal saline solution are drawn into the syringe. The syringe is attached to the biopsy needle, and the needle is introduced into the subcutaneous tissue, through the right eighth or ninth intercostal space, between the anterior and posterior axillary lines. One ml of normal saline solution is injected to clear the needle and the plunger; then the plunger is drawn back to the 4-ml mark to create negative pressure.

At this point in the procedure, ask the patient to take a deep breath, exhale, and hold his breath at the end of expiration

to prevent any movement of the chest wall. As the patient holds his breath, the biopsy needle is quickly inserted into the liver and withdrawn in 1 second. After the needle is withdrawn, tell the patient to resume normal respirations.

The tissue specimen is then placed in a properly labeled specimen cup containing 10% formaldehyde solution. This is done by releasing negative pressure while the point of the needle is in the formaldehyde solution. Again, 1 ml of normal saline solution is injected to clear the needle of the tissue specimen. Apply pressure to the biopsy site to halt bleeding.

Precautions

■ Percutaneous liver biopsy is contraindicated in a patient with a platelet count below 100,000/µl; prothrombin time longer than 15 seconds; empyema of the lungs, pleurae, peritoneum, biliary tract, or liver; vascular tumor; hepatic angioma; hydatid cyst; or tense ascites. If extrahepatic obstruction is suspected, ultrasonography or subcutaneous transhepatic cholangiography should rule out this condition before the biopsy is considered.

■ Pain in the abdomen or dyspnea following the biopsy may indicate perforation of an abdominal organ or pneumothorax, respectively. In such cases, complete a thorough assessment and notify the doctor at once.

■ Instruct the patient to hold his breath while the needle is in place.

■ Send the specimen to the laboratory immediately.

Normal findings

The normal liver consists of sheets of hepatocytes supported by a reticulin framework.

Implications of results

Examination of the hepatic tissue may reveal diffuse hepatic disease, such as cirrhosis or hepatitis, or granulomatous infections, such as tuberculosis. Primary malignant tumors include hepatocellular carcinoma, cholangiocellular carcinoma, and angiosarcoma, but hepatic metastases are more common.

Nonmalignant findings with a known focal lesion require further studies, such as laparotomy or laparoscopy with biopsy.

Post-test care
■ Position the patient on his right side for 2 hours, with a small pillow or sandbag under the costal margin to provide extra pressure. Advise bed rest for 24 hours.
■ Check the patient's vital signs every 15 minutes for 1 hour, then every 30 minutes for 4 hours, and every 4 hours thereafter for 24 hours. Throughout, observe carefully for signs of shock.
■ Watch for bleeding or signs of bile peritonitis-tenderness and rigidity around the biopsy site. Be alert for symptoms of pneumothorax: rising respiration rate, depressed breath sounds, dyspnea, persistent shoulder pain, and pleuritic chest pain. Report such complications promptly.
■ If the patient experiences pain, which may persist for several hours after the test, administer an analgesic as ordered.
■ Tell the patient he may resume his normal diet.

Interfering factors
Failure to obtain a representative specimen, to place the specimen in the proper preservative, or to transport the specimen to the laboratory immediately may affect the accuracy of test results.

Percutaneous renal biopsy

Percutaneous renal biopsy is the needle excision of a core of kidney tissue to obtain a specimen for histologic examination, using light, electron, and immunofluorescent microscopy. Such examination provides valuable information about glomerular and tubular function. Acute and chronic glomerulonephritis, pyelonephritis, renal vein thrombosis, amyloid infiltration, and systemic lupus erythematosus produce characteristic histologic changes in the kidneys.

Complications of percutaneous renal biopsy may include bleeding, hematoma, arteriovenous fistula, and infection. Despite the risk of these complications, this procedure is considered safer than open biopsy, which is usually the preferred method for removing a tissue specimen from a solid lesion. However, more recent noninvasive procedures, especially renal ultrasonography and computed tomography scans, have replaced percutaneous renal biopsy in many hospitals.

In some cases, a renal tissue specimen is obtained by a brush biopsy of the urinary tract. (See *Brush biopsy of the urinary tract,* page 484.)

Purpose
■ To aid diagnosis of renal parenchymal disease
■ To monitor progression of renal disease and to assess the effectiveness of treatment.

Patient preparation
Describe the procedure to the patient, and ask him if he has any questions. Explain that this test helps diagnose kidney disorders. Instruct the patient to restrict food and fluids for 8 hours be-

Brush biopsy of the urinary tract

Retrograde brush biopsy of the urinary tract may be used to obtain a renal tissue specimen when X-rays show a lesion in the renal pelvis or calyx. It can also be used to obtain specimens from other areas of the urinary tract. However, this procedure is contraindicated in patients with acute urinary tract infection or an obstruction at or below the biopsy site.

Preparation

To prepare the patient for brush biopsy, describe the procedure and tell him he may feel some discomfort. Inform him who will perform the biopsy and when, and reassure him that it will take only 30 to 60 minutes. Make sure the patient has signed an appropriate consent form.

Because this procedure requires use of a contrast agent and a general, local, or spinal anesthetic, check the patient's history for hypersensitivity to anesthetics, contrast media, or iodine-containing foods (such as shellfish). Just before the biopsy, administer a sedative, as ordered.

Procedure

After the patient has received a sedative and an anesthetic, place him in the lithotomy position. Using a cystoscope, the doctor passes a guide wire up the ureter and passes a urethral catheter over the guide wire. A contrast medium is instilled through the catheter, which is positioned next to the lesion under fluoroscopic guidance. The contrast medium is washed out with normal saline solution to prevent cell distortions from the dye. A nylon or steel brush is passed up the catheter and the lesion is brushed. This procedure is repeated at least six times, using a new brush each time.

As each brush is removed from the catheter, a smear is made for Papanicolaou staining and the brush tip is cut off and placed in formaldehyde for 1 hour. The biopsy material is then removed from the brush tip for histologic examination. When the last brush is withdrawn, the catheter is irrigated with normal saline solution to remove additional cells. These cells are also sent for histologic examination.

Results differentiate between malignant and benign lesions, which may appear the same on X-rays.

Because brush biopsy may cause such complications as perforation, hemorrhage, sepsis, or contrast medium extravasation, carefully monitor the patient's vital signs. Be sure to record the time, color, and amount of voiding, being alert for hematuria and abdominal or flank pain. Report any abnormal findings to the doctor immediately, and administer analgesics and antibiotics, as ordered.

fore the test. Tell him who will perform the biopsy and where, that the procedure takes only 15 minutes, and that the needle is in the kidney for only a few seconds.

Tell the patient that blood and urine specimens are collected and tested before the biopsy and that other tests, such as excretory urography, ultrasonography, or an erect film of the abdomen, may be ordered to help determine the biopsy site.

Make sure the patient has signed a consent form. Check the patient history for hemorrhagic tendencies and hypersensitivity to the local anesthetic. As ordered, 30 minutes to 1 hour before the biopsy, administer a mild sedative to help the patient relax. Inform him that he'll receive a local anesthetic but may experience a pinching pain when the needle is inserted through the back into the kidney. Check vital signs, and tell the patient to void just before the test.

Procedure

Place the patient in a prone position on a firm surface, with a sandbag beneath his abdomen. Tell him to take a deep breath while his kidney is being palpated. A 7" 20G needle is used to inject the local anesthetic into the skin at the biopsy site. Instruct the patient to hold his breath and remain immobile as the needle is inserted just below the angle formed by the intersection of the lowest palpable rib and the lateral border of the sacrospinal muscle. The needle is directed through the back muscles, the deep lumbar fascia, the perinephric fat, and the kidney capsule.

After the needle is inserted, tell the patient to take several deep breaths. If the needle swings smoothly during deep breathing, it has penetrated the kidney capsule. After the penetration depth is marked on the needle shaft, instruct the patient to hold his breath and remain as still as possible while the needle is withdrawn, injecting the local anesthetic into the back tissues.

After a small incision is made in the anesthetized skin, instruct the patient to hold his breath and remain immobile while the Vim-Silverman needle with stylet is inserted through the incision, down the tract of the infiltrating needle, to the measured depth. Then tell the patient to breathe deeply. If the characteristic needle swing occurs, instruct him to hold his breath and remain still while the tissue specimen is obtained. The specimen is examined immediately under a hand lens to ensure that it contains tissue from both the cortex and the medulla; then the tissue is placed on a saline-soaked gauze pad and inserted in a properly labeled container.

If an adequate tissue specimen has not been obtained, the procedure is repeated immediately. After an adequate specimen is secured, apply pressure to the biopsy site for 3 to 5 minutes to stop superficial bleeding. Then apply a pressure dressing.

Precautions

■ Percutaneous renal biopsy is contraindicated in a patient with a renal tumor, a severe bleeding disorder, markedly reduced plasma or blood volume, severe hypertension, hydronephrosis, perinephric abscess, advanced renal failure with uremia, or only one kidney.

 ■ Instruct the patient to hold his breath and remain still whenever the needle or prongs are advanced into or retracted from the kidney.

■ Send the tissue specimen to the laboratory immediately.

Normal findings

A section of normal kidney tissue shows Bowman's capsule (the area between two layers of flat epithelial cells), the glomerular tuft, and the capillary lumen. The tubule sections differ, depending on the area of tubule involved. The proximal tubule is one layer of epithelial cells with microvilli that form a brush border. The descending loop of Henle has flat, squamous epithelial cells, unlike the ascending, distal convoluted, and collecting tubules, which are lined with squamous epithelial cells.

Implications of results

Histologic examination of renal tissue can reveal malignancy or renal disease. Malignant tumors include Wilms' tumor, usually present in early childhood, and renal cell carcinoma, most prevalent in persons over age 40. Characteristic histologic changes can indicate disseminated lupus erythematosus, amyloid infiltration, acute and chronic glomerulonephritis, renal vein thrombosis, and pyelonephritis.

Post-test care

■ Instruct the patient to lie flat on his back without moving for at least 12 hours to prevent bleeding. Check vital signs every 15 minutes for 4 hours, then every 30 minutes for 4 hours, then every hour for 4 hours, and finally every 4 hours. Report any changes.

■ Examine all urine for blood; small amounts may be present after biopsy but should disappear within 8 hours. Occasionally, hematocrit may be monitored after the procedure to screen for internal bleeding.

■ Encourage the patient to drink fluids to initiate mild diuresis, which minimizes colic and obstruction from blood clotting within the renal pelvis.

■ Tell the patient he may resume his normal diet.

■ Discourage the patient from engaging in strenuous activities for several days after the procedure to prevent possible bleeding.

Interfering factors

Failure to obtain an adequate tissue specimen, to store the specimen properly, or to send the specimen to the laboratory immediately may affect test results.

Lung biopsy

In a lung biopsy, a specimen of pulmonary tissue is excised by closed or open technique for histologic examination. Closed technique, performed under local anesthesia, includes both needle and transbronchial biopsies; open technique, performed under general anesthesia in the operating room, includes both limited and standard thoracotomies.

Needle biopsy is appropriate when the lesion is readily accessible or when it originates in the lung parenchyma, is confined to it, or is affixed to the chest wall; this procedure provides a much smaller specimen than the open technique. Transbronchial biopsy, the removal of multiple tissue specimens through a fiber-optic bronchoscope, is appropriate for diffuse infiltrative pulmonary disease, tumors, or when severe debilitation contraindicates open biopsy. Open biopsy is appropriate for the study of a well- circumscribed lesion that may require resection.

Generally, a lung biopsy is recommended after chest X- rays, a computed tomography (CT) scan, and bronchoscopy have failed to identify the cause of diffuse parenchymal pulmonary disease or a pulmonary lesion. Possible complications of lung biopsy include bleeding, infection, and pneumothorax.

Purpose

■ To confirm a diagnosis of diffuse parenchymal pulmonary disease and pulmonary lesions.

Patient preparation

Describe the procedure to the patient, and answer any questions he may have. Explain that this test assesses the condition of the lungs. Instruct the patient to fast after midnight before the procedure. (Sometimes clear liquids are permitted the morning of the test.) Tell him who will perform the biopsy and where and that it takes 30 to 60 minutes. Also tell him that a chest X-ray and blood studies (prothrombin time, activated partial thromboplastin time, and platelet count) will be performed before the biopsy.

Make sure the patient has signed a consent form. Check the patient history for hypersensitivity to the local anesthetic. Administer a mild sedative, as ordered, 30 minutes before the biopsy to help the patient relax. Tell him he'll receive a local anesthetic but may experience a sharp, transient pain when the biopsy needle touches the lung.

Procedure

After the biopsy site is selected, lead markers are placed on the patient's skin, and X-rays are ordered to verify their correct placement. Place the patient in a sitting position, with arms folded on a table in front of him; instruct him to maintain this position, remaining as still as possible, and to refrain from coughing. The skin over the biopsy site is prepared, and the area is draped. To prevent damage to the intercostal nerves and vessels, a local anesthetic is injected with a 25G needle just above the lower rib. Using a 22G needle, the examiner anesthetizes the intercostal muscles and parietal pleura, makes a small incision (2 to 3 mm) with a scalpel, and introduces the biopsy needle through the incision, chest wall, and pleura, into the tumor or pulmonary tissue.

If the intercostal space at the incision site is wide, the needle is inserted at a 90-degree angle; if the ribs overlap and the intercostal space is narrow, at a 45-degree angle. When the needle is in the tumor or pulmonary tissue, the specimen is obtained and the needle is withdrawn. The specimen is divided immediately: The tissue for histologic examination is placed in a properly labeled bottle containing 10% neutral buffered formaldehyde solution; the tissue for microbiologic culture is placed in a sterile container.

Pressure is exerted on the biopsy site to stop the bleeding, and then a small bandage is applied.

Precautions

- Needle biopsy is contraindicated in patients with a lesion that has separated from the chest wall or that is accompanied by emphysematous bullae, cysts, or gross emphysema and in patients with coagulopathy, hypoxia, pulmonary hypertension, or cardiac disease with cor pulmonale.
- During biopsy, observe for signs of respiratory distress — shortness of breath, elevated pulse rate, and cyanosis (late sign); if such signs develop, report them immediately.
- Because coughing or movement during the biopsy can cause tearing of the lung by the biopsy needle, keep the patient calm and still.

Normal findings

Pulmonary tissue should exhibit uniform texture of the alveolar ducts, alveolar walls, bronchioles, and small vessels.

Implications of results

Histologic examination of a pulmonary tissue specimen can reveal squamous cell or oat cell carcinoma and adenocarcinoma. Such examination supplements the results of microbiologic cultures, deep-cough sputum specimens, chest X-rays, bronchoscopy, and the patient's physical examination in confirming cancer or parenchymal pulmonary disease.

Post-test care

- Check vital signs for 15 minutes for 1 hour, every hour for 4 hours, then every 4 hours. Watch for bleeding, shortness of breath, elevated pulse rate, diminished breath sounds on the biopsy side and, eventually, cyanosis. Make sure the chest X-ray is repeated immediately after the biopsy is completed.
- Tell the patient he may resume his normal diet.

Interfering factors

Failure to obtain a representative tissue specimen or to store the specimen in the appropriate containers may affect test results.

Pleural biopsy

Pleural biopsy is the removal of pleural tissue, by needle biopsy or open biopsy, for histologic examination. Needle pleural biopsy is performed under local anesthesia. It generally follows thoracentesis — aspiration of pleural fluid — which is performed when the cause of the effusion is unknown, but it can be performed separately.

Open pleural biopsy, performed in the absence of pleural effusion, permits direct visualization of the pleura and the underlying lung. It's performed in the operating room.

Purpose

- To differentiate between nonmalignant and malignant disease
- To diagnose viral, fungal, or parasitic disease and collagen vascular disease of the pleura.

Patient preparation

Describe the procedure to the patient and answer his questions. Explain that this test permits microscopic examination of pleural tissue. Tell him who will perform the biopsy and where, that it takes 30 to 45 minutes to perform, and that the needle remains in the pleura less than 1 minute. Also tell him that blood studies will precede the biopsy and that chest X-rays will be taken before and after the biopsy.

Make sure the patient has signed a consent form. Check the patient history for hypersensitivity to the local anesthetic. Tell him that he'll receive an anesthetic and should experience little pain. Just before the procedure, record vital signs.

Procedure

Seat the patient on the side of the bed, with his feet resting on a stool and his arms supported by the overbed table or upper body. Tell him to hold this position and to remain still during the procedure. If he is unable to sit up, position him in a side-lying position with the side to be biopsied up. Prepare the skin and drape the area. The local anesthetic is then administered.

For Vim-Silverman needle biopsy: The needle is inserted through the appropriate intercostal space into the biopsy site, with the outer tip distal to the pleura and the central portion pushed in deeper and held in place. The outer case is inserted about $3/8$" (1 cm), the entire assembly rotated 360 degrees, and the needle and tissue specimen are withdrawn.

For Cope's needle biopsy: The trocar is introduced through the appropriate intercostal space into the biopsy site. The sharp obturator is then removed and a hooked stylet is inserted through the trocar. The opened notch is directed against the pleura, along the intercostal space, and is slowly withdrawn. While the outer tube is held stationary, the inner tube is twisted to cut off the tissue specimen, and the assembly is withdrawn. (See *Using Cope's needle.*)

The specimen is immediately put in 10% neutral buffered formaldehyde solution in a labeled specimen bottle. Then the skin around the biopsy site is cleaned and an adhesive bandage is applied.

Precautions

- Pleural biopsy is contraindicated in patients with severe bleeding disorders.
- Send the specimen to the laboratory immediately.

Using Cope's needle

Cope's needle, which is used to obtain a pleural biopsy specimen, consists of three parts: a sharp obturator (A) and a cannula (B), which when fitted together are called a trocar, and a blunt-ended, hooked stylet (C). The trocar is used to gain access to the pleural cavity. Then the obturator is removed, leaving the cannula in place. The stylet is passed through the cannula to excise a tissue specimen, as shown below.

Normal findings

The normal pleura consists primarily of mesothelial cells, flattened in a uniform layer. Layers of areolar connective tissue — containing blood vessels, nerves, and lymphatics — lie below.

Implications of results

Histologic examination of the tissue specimen can reveal malignant disease; tuberculosis; or viral, fungal, parasitic, or collagen vascular disease. Primary neoplasms of the pleura are generally fibrous and epithelial.

Post-test care

▪ Check the patient's vital signs every 15 minutes for 1 hour, then every hour for 4 hours or until stable. Make sure the chest X-ray is repeated immediately after the biopsy.

▪ Instruct the patient to lie on his unaffected side to promote healing of the biopsy site.

▪ Watch for signs of respiratory distress (shortness of breath), shoulder pain, and other complications, such as pneumothorax (immediate) and pneumonia (delayed).

Interfering factors

Failure to use the proper fixative or to obtain an adequate specimen may alter results.

Cervical punch biopsy

Cervical punch biopsy is the excision by sharp forceps of a tissue specimen from

Endometrial and ovarian biopsies

METHOD	PURPOSE	SPECIAL CONSIDERATIONS
Endometrial biopsy		
▪ Dilatation and curettage (D&C) ▪ Endometrial washing (by jet irrigation, aspiration, or brushing)	▪ To evaluate uterine bleeding ▪ To diagnose suspected endometrial cancer ▪ To diagnose a missed abortion	▪ Time of menstrual cycle affects accuracy of biopsy results. ▪ Type of specimen obtained depends on patient's age and disorder. ▪ Endometrial washing requires no anesthesia and can be done in a doctor's office. ▪ D&C by endometrial washing may follow a negative biopsy. ▪ Specimens obtained by D&C may be processed as frozen sections.
Ovarian biopsy		
▪ Transrectal or transvaginal fine-needle biopsy ▪ Aspiration biopsy during laparoscopy	▪ To detect an ovarian tumor ▪ To determine the spread of cancer	▪ Fine-needle biopsy may follow palpation, laparoscopy, or computed tomography that detects an abnormal ovary. ▪ Aspiration during laparoscopy is particularly useful for young women who are infertile or who have lesions that appear benign.

the cervix for histologic examination. Generally, multiple biopsies are done to obtain specimens from all areas with abnormal tissue or from the squamocolumnar junction and other sites around the cervical circumference.

This procedure is indicated for women with suspicious cervical lesions and should be performed when the cervix is least vascular (usually 1 week after menses). Biopsy sites are selected by direct visualization of the cervix with a colposcope — the most accurate method — or by Schiller's test, which stains normal squamous epithelium a dark mahogany but fails to color abnormal tissue. (For information on other biopsies done to detect gynecologic disorders, see *Endometrial and ovarian biopsies*.)

Purpose
▪ To evaluate suspicious cervical lesions
▪ To diagnose cervical cancer.

Patient preparation
Describe the procedure to the patient, and explain that it provides a cervical tissue specimen for microscopic study. Tell her who will perform the biopsy and where and that it takes about 15 minutes. Tell the patient that she may experience mild discomfort during and after the biopsy. Advise the outpatient to have someone accompany her home after the biopsy.

Make sure the patient has signed a consent form. Just before the biopsy, ask her to void.

Procedure

Place the patient in the lithotomy position. Tell her to relax as the unlubricated speculum is inserted.

For direct visualization: The colposcope is inserted through the speculum, the biopsy site is located, and the cervix is cleaned with a swab soaked in 3% acetic acid solution. The biopsy forceps are then inserted through the speculum or the colposcope, and tissue is removed from any lesion or from selected sites, starting from the posterior lip to avoid obscuring other sites with blood. Each specimen is immediately put in 10% formaldehyde solution in a labeled bottle. To control bleeding after biopsy, the cervix is swabbed with 5% silver nitrate solution (cautery or sutures may be used instead). If bleeding persists, the examiner may insert a tampon.

For Schiller's test: An applicator stick saturated with iodine solution is inserted through the speculum. This stains the cervix to identify lesions for biopsy.

Record the patient's and clinician's names and the biopsy sites on the laboratory request.

Precautions

Send the specimens to the laboratory immediately.

Normal findings

Cervical tissue should be composed of columnar and squamous epithelial cells, loose connective tissue, and smooth-muscle fibers, with no dysplasia or abnormal cell growth.

Implications of results

Histologic examination of a cervical tissue specimen identifies abnormal cells and differentiates the tissue as intraepithelial neoplasia or invasive cancer. If the cause of an abnormal Papanicolaou (Pap) test isn't demonstrated by cervical biopsy, or if the specimen shows advanced dysplasia or carcinoma in situ, a cone biopsy is performed in the operating room under general anesthesia. A cone biopsy garners a larger tissue specimen and allows a more accurate evaluation of dysplasia.

Post-test care

- Instruct the patient to avoid strenuous exercise for 8 to 24 hours after the biopsy. Encourage the outpatient to rest briefly before leaving the office.
- If a tampon was inserted after the biopsy, tell the patient to leave it in place for 8 to 24 hours, as ordered. Inform her that some bleeding may occur, but tell her to report heavy bleeding (heavier than menstrual) to the doctor. Warn the patient to avoid using tampons, which can irritate the cervix and provoke bleeding, according to her doctor's directions.
- Tell the patient to avoid douching and to refrain from intercourse for up to 2 weeks, or as directed, if she has undergone such treatments as cryotherapy or laser treatment during the procedure.
- Inform the patient that a foul-smelling, gray-green vaginal discharge is normal for several days after the biopsy and may persist for 3 weeks.

Interfering factors

Failure to obtain representative specimens or to place them in the preservative immediately may alter results.

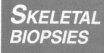

Bone biopsy

Bone biopsy is the removal of a piece or a core of bone for histologic examination. It's performed either by using a special drill needle under local anesthesia or by surgical excision under general anesthesia. Bone biopsy is indicated in patients with bone pain and tenderness after a bone scan, a computed tomography scan, X-rays, or arteriography reveals a mass or deformity. Excision provides a larger specimen than drill biopsy and permits immediate surgical treatment if rapid histologic analysis of the specimen reveals a malignant tumor. In the presence of tumors, bone bows slightly, thickens, and sometimes fractures — the result of increased osteoblastic or osteoclastic activity, or both.

Possible complications of bone biopsy include bone fracture, damage to surrounding tissue, and infection (osteomyelitis).

Purpose

▪ To distinguish between benign and malignant bone tumors.

Patient preparation

Describe the procedure to the patient, and answer any questions. Explain that this test permits microscopic examination of a bone specimen. If the patient is to have a drill biopsy, inform him that he needn't restrict food or fluids. If the patient is to have an open biopsy, instruct him to fast overnight before the test. Tell him who will perform the biopsy and where and that it should take no longer than 30 minutes.

Tell the patient that he will receive a local anesthetic but will still experience discomfort and pressure when the biopsy needle enters the bone. Explain that a special drill forces the needle into the bone; if possible, show him a photograph of the bone drill to make the biopsy seem less ominous. Stress the importance of his cooperation during the biopsy.

Make sure the patient has signed a consent form; if the patient is a minor, ask a responsible parent or guardian to do so. Check the patient history for hypersensitivity to the local anesthetic.

Procedure

For drill biopsy: Position the patient properly, and shave and prepare the biopsy site. After the local anesthetic is injected, the doctor makes a small incision (usually about 3 mm) and pushes the biopsy needle with pointed trocar into the bone, using firm, even pressure. Once the needle is engaged in the bone, it is rotated about 180 degrees while steady pressure is maintained. When the bone core is obtained, the trocar is withdrawn by reversing the drilling motion, and the specimen is placed in a properly labeled bottle containing 10% formaldehyde solution.

Apply pressure to the site with a sterile gauze pad. When bleeding stops, remove the gauze and apply a topical antiseptic (povidone-iodine ointment) and an adhesive bandage or other sterile covering to close the wound and prevent infection.

For open biopsy: After the patient is anesthetized, shave the biopsy site, clean it with surgical soap, and then disinfect it with an iodine wash and alcohol. The doctor makes an incision, removes a piece of bone, and sends it to the histology laboratory immediately for analysis. Further surgery can then be performed, depending on bone specimen findings.

Precautions

■ Bone biopsy should be performed cautiously in patients with coagulopathy.
■ Send the specimen to the laboratory immediately.

Normal findings

Bone tissue consists of fibers of collagen, osteocytes, and osteoblasts. It can be classified as one of two histologic types: compact or cancellous. Compact bone has dense, concentric layers of mineral deposits, or lamellae. Cancellous bone has widely spaced lamellae, with osteocytes and red and yellow marrow lying between them.

Implications of results

Histologic examination of a bone specimen can reveal benign or malignant tumors. Benign tumors, generally well circumscribed and nonmetastasizing, include osteoid osteoma, osteoblastoma, osteochondroma, unicameral bone cyst, benign giant cell tumor, and fibroma.

Malignant tumors spread irregularly and rapidly. The most common types are multiple myeloma and osteosarcoma; the most lethal is Ewing's sarcoma. Most malignant tumors metastasize to bone through the blood and lymph systems from the breast, lungs, prostate, thyroid, or kidneys.

Post-test care

■ Check vital signs and the dressing at the biopsy site, as ordered. Ask the doctor how much drainage is expected, and notify him if drainage is excessive.
■ If the patient experiences pain at the biopsy site, administer an analgesic, as ordered.

 ■ For several days after the biopsy, watch for indications of bone infection: fever, headache, pain on movement, and tissue redness or abscess at or near the biopsy site. Notify the doctor if these symptoms develop.

■ Advise the patient that he may resume his usual diet.

Interfering factors

Failure to obtain a representative bone specimen, to use the proper fixative, or to send the specimen to the laboratory immediately may alter test results.

Bone marrow aspiration and biopsy

Bone marrow, the soft tissue contained in the medullary canals of long bone and in the interstices of cancellous bone, may be removed by aspiration or needle biopsy under local anesthesia. In aspiration biopsy, a fluid specimen in which pustulae of marrow are suspended is removed from the bone marrow. In needle biopsy, a core of marrow — cells, not fluid — is removed. These methods are often used concurrently to obtain the best possible marrow specimens.

Because bone marrow is the major site of hematopoiesis, the histologic and hematologic examination of its contents provides reliable diagnostic information about blood disorders. Marrow removed from the bone may be red or yellow. Red marrow, which constitutes about 50% of an adult's marrow, actively produces red blood cells; yellow marrow contains fat cells and connective tissue, and is inactive. Because yellow marrow can become active in response to the body's needs, an adult has a large hematopoietic capacity. An infant's marrow is mainly red and, consequently, reflects a small hematopoietic capacity.

Bleeding and infection may result from bone marrow biopsy at any site, but the most serious complications occur at the sternum. Such complications

Common sites of bone marrow aspiration and biopsy

The *posterior superior iliac spine* (1) is usually the preferred site because no vital organs or vessels are located nearby. With the patient in a lateral position with one leg flexed, the clinician inserts the needle several centimeters lateral to the iliosacral junction, entering the bone plane crest with the needle directed downward and toward the anterior inferior spine, or entering a few centimeters below the crest at a right angle to the surface of the bone.

The *sternum* (2) involves the greatest risks but is commonly used for marrow aspiration because it's near the surface, the cortical bone is thin, and the marrow cavity contains numerous cells and relatively little fat or supporting bone. For this procedure, the patient is supine on a firm bed or examining table with a small pillow beneath the shoulders to elevate the chest and lower the head. The clinician secures the needle guard 3 to 4 mm from the tip of the needle to avoid accidental puncture of the heart or a major vessel. Then he inserts the needle at the midline of the sternum at the second intercostal space.

The *spinous process* (3) is the preferred site if multiple punctures are necessary, marrow is absent at other sites, or the patient objects to sternal puncture. For this procedure, the patient sits on the edge of the bed, leaning over the bedside stand; or, if he's uncooperative, he may be placed in the prone position with restraints. The clinician selects the spinous process of the third or fourth lumbar vertebra and inserts the needle at the crest or slightly to one side, advancing the needle in the direction of the bone plane.

The *tibia* (4) is the site of choice for infants under age 1. The infant is placed in a prone position on a bed or examining table with a sandbag beneath the leg. The foot is taped to the surface of the table, or an assistant holds the leg stationary by placing a hand under it. The clinician inserts the needle about ⅜" (1 cm) below the tibial tuberosity and slightly toward the medial side, being careful to angle the needle point toward the foot to avoid epiphyseal injury.

are rare but include puncture of the heart and major vessels — causing severe hemorrhage — and puncture of the mediastinum — causing mediastinitis or pneumomediastinum.

Purpose
- To diagnose thrombocytopenia, leukemias, granulomas, and aplastic, hypoplastic, and pernicious anemias
- To diagnose primary and metastatic tumors
- To determine the cause of infection
- To aid staging of disease, such as Hodgkin's disease
- To evaluate the effectiveness of chemotherapy and help monitor myelosuppression.

Patient preparation
Describe the procedure to the patient, and answer any questions. Explain that the test permits microscopic examination of a bone marrow specimen. Inform the patient that he needn't restrict food or fluids before the test. Tell him who will perform the biopsy and where and that it usually takes only 5 to 10 minutes. Inform him that more than one bone marrow specimen may be required and that a blood sample will be

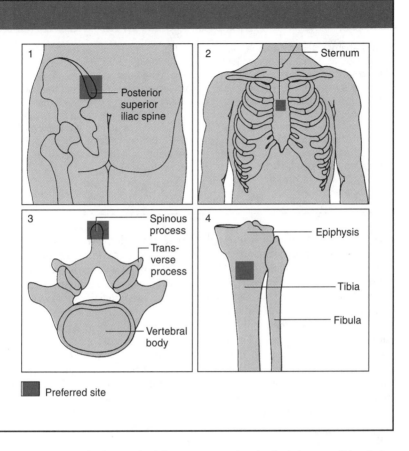

1 — Posterior superior iliac spine

2 — Sternum

3 — Spinous process — Transverse process — Vertebral body

4 — Epiphysis — Tibia — Fibula

Preferred site

collected before the biopsy for laboratory testing.

Make sure the patient has signed a consent form; if the patient is a minor, ask a responsible parent or guardian to do so. Check the patient history for hypersensitivity to the local anesthetic. After checking with the doctor, tell the patient which bone — sternum, anterior or posterior iliac crest, vertebral spinous process, rib, or tibia — will be the biopsy site. (See *Common sites of bone marrow aspiration and biopsy.*) Inform him that he will receive a local anesthetic but will feel pressure on insertion of the biopsy needle and a brief, pulling pain on removal of the marrow.

As ordered, administer a mild sedative 1 hour before the test.

Preparation of children requires additional steps. (See *Preparing children for bone marrow biopsy,* page 496.)

Procedure

After positioning the patient, instruct him to remain as still as possible. Offer emotional support during the biopsy by talking to him quietly, describing what is being done, and answering any questions.

For aspiration biopsy: After the skin over the biopsy site is prepared and the area is draped, the local anesthetic is injected. With a twisting motion, the

---

Preparing children for bone marrow biopsy

To prepare a child for a bone marrow biopsy, give him his own biopsy kit: a syringe without a needle, cotton balls, and adhesive bandages. Act out the procedure by using a doll or a stuffed animal as a model. This will help you gain the child's confidence and answer any questions he may have. Be sure to prepare him by describing the kinds of pressure and discomfort he will feel during the procedure.

Before the biopsy, explain the equipment on the tray to the child. Encourage the parents to get involved by helping you hold the child still and reassuring him. Tell the child that he'll feel some pain when the clinician aspirates the bone marrow and that it's OK to cry or yell if he wants to, but the pain will go away quickly.

---

marrow aspiration needle is inserted through the skin, the subcutaneous tissue, and the cortex of the bone. The stylet is removed from the needle, and a 10- to 20-ml syringe is attached. The examiner aspirates 0.2 to 0.5 ml of marrow, then withdraws the needle. Pressure is applied to the site for 5 minutes while the marrow slides are being prepared. (If the patient has thrombocytopenia, pressure is applied for 10 to 15 minutes.) The biopsy site is cleaned again, and a sterile adhesive bandage is applied.

If an adequate marrow specimen has not been obtained on the first attempt, the needle may be repositioned within the marrow cavity, or may be removed and reinserted in another site within the anesthetized area. If the second attempt fails, a needle biopsy may be necessary.

For needle biopsy: After preparing the biopsy site and draping the area, the examiner marks the skin at the site with an indelible pencil or marking pen. A local anesthetic is then injected intradermally, subcutaneously, and at the surface of the bone. Then the biopsy needle is inserted into the periosteum, and the needle guard is set, as indicated.

The needle is advanced with a steady boring motion, until the outer needle

passes through the cortex of the bone. The inner needle with trephine tip is inserted into the outer needle, and the stylet is removed. By alternately rotating the inner needle clockwise and counterclockwise, the examiner directs the needle into the marrow cavity and then removes a tissue plug. The needle assembly is withdrawn, and the marrow is expelled into a labeled bottle containing Zenker's solution. After the biopsy site is cleaned, a sterile adhesive bandage or a pressure dressing is applied.

Precautions

■ Bone marrow biopsy is contraindicated in patients with severe bleeding disorders.

■ Send the tissue specimen or slides to the laboratory immediately.

Normal findings

Yellow marrow contains fat cells and connective tissue; red marrow contains hematopoietic cells, fat cells, and connective tissue. In addition, special stains that detect hematologic disorders produce these normal findings: the iron stain, which measures hemosiderin (storage iron), has a +2 level; the Sudan black B (SBB) stain, which shows granulocytes, is negative; and the periodic acid–Schiff (PAS) stain, which detects glycogen reactions, is negative.

Implications of results

Histologic examination of a bone marrow specimen can help detect myelofibrosis, granulomas, lymphomas, or cancer. Hematologic analysis, including the differential count and the myeloid-erythroid ratio, can implicate a wide range of disorders. (See *Bone marrow: Normal values and implications of abnormal findings,* pages 498 and 499.)

In an iron stain, decreased hemosiderin levels may indicate a true iron deficiency. Increased levels may accompany other types of anemias or blood disorders. A positive SBB stain can differentiate acute myelogenous leukemia from acute lymphoblastic leukemia (negative SBB), or it may indicate granulation in myeloblasts. A positive PAS stain may indicate acute or chronic lymphocytic leukemia, amyloidosis, thalassemia, lymphoma, infectious mononucleosis, iron-deficiency anemia, or sideroblastic anemia.

Post-test care

■ Check the biopsy site for bleeding and inflammation.
■ Observe the patient for signs of hemorrhage and infection: rapid pulse rate, low blood pressure, and fever.

Interfering factors

Failure to obtain a representative specimen, to use a fixative (for histologic analysis), or to send the specimen to the laboratory immediately may alter test results.

Synovial membrane biopsy

Biopsy of the synovial membrane is the needle excision of a tissue specimen for histologic examination of the thin epithelial layer lining the diarthrodial joint capsules. In a large joint, such as the knee, preliminary arthroscopy can aid selection of the biopsy site. Synovial membrane biopsy is performed when analysis of synovial fluid — a viscous, lubricating fluid contained within the synovial membrane — proves nondiagnostic or when the fluid itself is absent.

Purpose

■ To diagnose gout, pseudogout, bacterial infections and lesions, and granulomatous infections
■ To aid diagnosis of rheumatoid arthritis, systemic lupus erythematosus (SLE), or Reiter's syndrome
■ To monitor joint pathology.

Patient preparation

Describe the procedure to the patient, and ask if he has any questions. Explain that this test helps to diagnose certain joint disorders. Inform him that he needn't restrict food or fluids. Tell him who will perform the procedure and where, that the procedure takes about 30 minutes, and that test results are usually available in 1 or 2 days. Advise him that he'll receive a local anesthetic to minimize discomfort but will experience transient pain when the needle enters the joint. Tell him that complications are rare but may include infection and bleeding into the joint.

Make sure the patient has signed a consent form. Check the patient history for hypersensitivity to the local anesthetic.

Inform the patient which site — knee (most common), elbow, wrist, ankle, or

Bone marrow: Normal values and implications of abnormal findings		

CELL TYPES	NORMAL MEAN VALUES		
	Adults	Children	Infants
Normoblasts, total	25.6%	23.1%	8.0%
Pronormoblasts	0.2% to 1.3%	0.5%	0.1%
Basophilic	0.5% to 2.4%	1.7%	0.34%
Polychromatic	17.9% to 29.2%	18.2%	6.9%
Orthochromatic	0.4% to 4.6%	2.7%	0.54%
Neutrophils, total	56.5%	57.1%	32.4%
Myeloblasts	0.2% to 1.5%	1.2%	0.62%
Promyelocytes	2.1% to 4.1%	1.4%	0.76%
Myelocytes	8.2% to 15.7%	18.3%	2.5%
Metamyelocytes	9.6% to 24.6%	23.3%	11.3%
Bands	9.5% to 15.3%	0	14.1%
Segmented	6.0% to 12.0%	12.9%	3.6%
Eosinophils	3.1%	3.6%	2.6%
Basophils	0.01%	0.06%	0.07%
Lymphocytes	16.2%	16.0%	49.0%
Plasma cells	1.3%	0.4%	0.02%
Megakaryocytes	0.1%	0.1%	0.05%
Myeloid-erythroid ratio	2.3%	2.9%	4.4%

shoulder — has been chosen for the biopsy (usually, the most symptomatic joint is selected). Administer a sedative, if ordered, to help him relax.

Procedure

Place the patient in the proper position, clean the biopsy site, and drape the area. After the local anesthetic is injected into the joint space, the trocar is forcefully thrust into the joint space, away from the site of anesthetic infiltration, to minimize the possibility of artifacts. The biopsy needle is inserted through the trocar. The hooked notch side of the biopsy needle is positioned against the synovium, and suction is applied with a 50-ml luer-lock syringe.

While the trocar is held stationary, the biopsy needle is twisted to cut off a tis-

IMPLICATIONS OF ABNORMAL FINDINGS	
Elevated values	**Depressed values**
Polycythemia vera	Vitamin B_{12} or folic acid deficiency; hypoplastic or aplastic anemia
Acute myeloblastic or chronic myeloid leukemia	Lymphoblastic or acute monocytic leukemia; aplastic anemia
Bone marrow carcinoma, lymphadenoma, myeloid leukemia, eosinophilic leukemia, pernicious anemia (in relapse)	
No relationship between basophil count and symptoms	No relationship between basophil count and symptoms
B- and T-cell chronic lymphocytic leukemia, other lymphatic leukemias, lymphoma, mononucleosis, aplastic anemia, macroglobulinemia	
Myeloma, collagen disease, infection, antigen sensitivity, malignancy	
Old age, chronic myeloid leukemia, polycythemia vera, megakaryocytic myelosis, infection, idiopathic thrombocytopenic purpura, thrombocytopenia	Pernicious anemia
Myeloid leukemia, infection, leukemoid reactions, depressed hematopoiesis	Agranulocytosis, hematopoiesis after hemorrhage or hemolysis, iron deficiency anemia, polycythemia vera

sue segment. Then the needle is withdrawn, and the specimen is placed in a properly labeled sterile container or a specimen bottle containing heparin or absolute ethyl alcohol. By changing the angle of the biopsy needle, several specimens can be obtained without reinserting the trocar. The trocar is then removed, the biopsy site cleaned, and a pressure bandage is applied.

Precautions
Send the container with absolute ethyl alcohol to the histology laboratory immediately. Send the sterile container to the microbiology laboratory.

Normal findings
The synovial membrane contains cells that are identical to those found in other connective tissue. The membrane

surface is relatively smooth, except for villi, folds, and fat pads that project into the joint cavity. The membrane tissue produces synovial fluid and contains a capillary network, lymphatic vessels, and a few nerve fibers. Pathology of the synovial membrane also affects the cellular composition of the synovial fluid.

Implications of results

Histologic examination of synovial tissue can diagnose coccidioidomycosis, gout, pseudogout, hemochromatosis, tuberculosis, sarcoidosis, amyloidosis, pigmented villonodular synovitis or synovial tumors. Such examination can also aid diagnosis of rheumatoid arthritis, SLE, and Reiter's syndrome.

Post-test care

■ Watch for signs of bleeding into the joint (swelling and tenderness) every hour for 4 hours, then every 4 hours for 12 hours.

■ Administer medication, as ordered, if the patient experiences pain at the biopsy site.

■ Instruct the patient to rest the joint from which the tissue specimen was removed for 1 day before resuming normal activities.

Interfering factors

Failure to obtain several biopsy specimens, to obtain the specimens away from the infiltration site of the anesthetic, to store the specimens in the appropriate solution, or to send them to the laboratory immediately may alter test results.

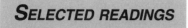

Selected Readings

Corbett, J.V. *Laboratory Tests and Diagnostic Procedures with Nursing Diagnoses*, 4th ed. Stamford, Conn.: Appleton & Lange, 1995.

Diseases, 2nd ed. Springhouse, Pa.: Springhouse Corp., 1996.

Groenwald, S.L. *Cancer Nursing*, 3rd ed. Boston: Jones and Bartlett, 1993.

Guyton, A.C., and Hall, J.E. *Textbook of Medical Physiology*, 9th ed. Philadelphia: W.B. Saunders Co., 1996.

Kee, J.L. *Laboratory and Diagnostic Tests*, 4th ed. Stamford, Conn.: Appleton & Lange, 1995.

Pagana, K., and Pagana, T.J. *Diagnostic Testing and Nursing Implications: A Case Study Approach,* 4th ed. St. Louis: Mosby–Year Book, Inc., 1994.

Porth, C. *Pathophysiology: Concepts of Altered Health States*, 4th ed. Philadelphia: Lippincott-Raven Pubs., 1994.

Ravel, R.A. *Clinical Laboratory Medicine: Clinical Application of Laboratory Data*, 6th ed. St. Louis: Mosby–Year Book, Inc., 1995.

Wallach, J.B. *Interpretation of Diagnostic Tests: A Synopsis of Laboratory Medicine*, 6th ed. Boston: Little, Brown & Co., 1996.

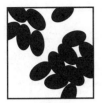

CHAPTER NINETEEN

Microbes and parasites

Learning objectives

After completing this chapter, the reader will be able to:
- discuss the importance of staining procedures
- describe culture and sensitivity testing
- define four classes of protozoa
- explain how protozoa are transmitted
- state the characteristics of helminths
- explain the anatomy and physiology of the lymphatic system
- explain the purpose of each test discussed in the chapter

- prepare the patient physically and psychologically for each test
- describe the procedure for obtaining a specimen for each test
- specify appropriate precautions for safe administration of each test
- recognize signs of an adverse reaction and respond appropriately
- implement appropriate post-test care
- identify the normal findings of each test
- discuss the implications of abnormal test results
- list factors that may interfere with accurate test results.

INTRODUCTION

Microbiology is the study of microorganisms — bacteria, fungi, viruses, and protozoa — that are so small they require special techniques, such as staining or electron microscopy, to reveal their sizes, shapes, and cellular structures.

Gram stain

The Gram staining method, the most common and useful staining procedure, separates bacteria into two classifications, according to the composition of their cell walls: gram-positive organisms, which retain crystal violet stain after decolorization, and gram-negative organisms, which lose the purple stain but counterstain red with safranin.

Microscopic examination of a Gram-stained smear frequently allows tentative identification of the suspected organism. Examining a direct Gram smear of the specimen for inflammatory cells, such as neutrophils and macrophages, can also provide clues about the type of infection present and consequent mobilization of the immune system. For example, a large number of segmented neutrophils in a smear of cerebrospinal fluid suggests bacterial meningitis; a large number of mononuclear cells suggests viral, fungal, or tubercular meningitis.

Acid-fast stain

Another staining procedure, the acid-fast method, helps identify organisms of the genus *Mycobacterium*. Since mycobacteria (including pathogens of tuberculosis and leprosy) are acid-fast, they retain carbolfuchsin stain after treatment with an acid-alcohol solution. This technique is particularly useful for identifying mycobacteria in sputum specimens, which may contain many different organisms.

Confirmation by culture

Although stained smears provide rapid, valuable diagnostic leads, they only tentatively identify a pathogen. For example, detection of acid-fast organisms in sputum doesn't conclusively diagnose tuberculosis; nor does a negative acid-fast smear preclude the possibility of tuberculosis. Generally, visualization of an acid-fast microorganism requires the presence of 10,000 to 100,000 microbes per gram of sputum or per milliliter of body fluid.

Confirmation requires culturing and identifying the microbes. Since this process depends on a particular organism's growth rate and nutritional requirements, growing microbes in culture takes longer than microscopic examination of a stained smear. For instance, slow-growing mycobacteria may need weeks of incubation before growth appears. Nevertheless, sufficient growth must take place before further microscopic and biochemical studies can identify the organism.

Sensitivity testing

After a microbe is isolated, its susceptibility to specific antimicrobials and the extent of infection must be determined before choosing antimicrobial therapy. Some pathogens, such as *Streptococcus pneumoniae* (pneumococci), *Streptococcus pyogenes,* and *Neisseria meningitidis,* usually have predictable sensitivity patterns; other pathogens, such as most gram-negative bacilli *(Escherichia coli, Enterobacter, Salmonella, Shigella, Klebsiella, Proteus,* and *Pseudomonas),* enterococci (such as *Streptococcus faecalis),* and *Staphylococcus* species, require testing to determine antimicrobial susceptibility.

These tests also help determine the dosage needed to inhibit or kill an organism in vivo. However, in vitro tests can't account for pharmacologic properties of the selected antimicrobial, such as toxicity, protein binding, absorption, and excretion; nor can they establish the immune status of the host or the nature of the underlying pathologic process.

Thus, in vitro antimicrobial susceptibility studies provide only an approximate guide; the patient's clinical response determines the precise dosage.

In the Kirby-Bauer disk-diffusion method, the most widely used qualitative test, disks of filter paper are impregnated with exact amounts of different antimicrobial agents and are added to an agar plate that has been seeded with the test organism. After overnight incubation, zones of inhibition around the disks demonstrate the sensitivity patterns of the organism. A *resistant* strain isn't inhibited by a therapeutic amount of an antimicrobial; a *moderately susceptible* strain may be inhibited by high dosages of the antimicrobial; a *sensitive* strain is inhibited or killed by the recommended dosage of an antimicrobial; and an *intermediate* or *indeterminate* strain is equivocally susceptible.

Quantitative sensitivity testing may be necessary for patients with bacterial endocarditis, bacteremia, or impaired renal function; for those who fail to respond to antimicrobial therapy; or for those who have a relapse during therapy. Quantitative sensitivity testing requires the dilution technique, in which serial dilutions of the antimicrobial are inoculated with the organism and incubated to determine the minimal inhibitory concentration and the minimum lethal concentration for the tested isolate.

The antibacterial serum level determination test can help evaluate the effectiveness of antimicrobial therapy. This test consists of titrating serum drawn at peak levels (when the antibacterial level is highest) or at trough levels (when the antibacterial level is lowest, before the next antimicrobial dose) against dilutions of the infecting organism.

Parasitology

Transmission of parasites — organisms that live in or on other biological species to take nourishment from them — is affected by such factors as sanitation, diet, and climate. In countries with good sanitation and effective infection control, the incidence of parasitic disease is relatively low. The clinically important groups of parasites are protozoa (single-cell organisms), helminths (worms), and arthropods (insects and arachnids, such as spiders, mites, and ticks).

Protozoa

Protozoa are classified according to their means of locomotion:

■ *Sarcodina* (amoebae) move on temporary cytoplasmic protrusions called pseudopodia. Most species of amoebae appear in humans in the motile, feeding stage (trophozoite form) and the infective stage (cyst form). Of these species, only *Entamoeba histolytica* causes significant disease.

■ *Mastigophora* (flagellates) propel themselves by long filamentous appendages called flagella. The most common pathogenic species of flagellates in the United States are *Giardia lamblia*, which infests the intestinal tract, and *Trichomonas vaginalis*, which infests the genital tract. Hemoflagellates, an important subgroup, include the genera *Trypanosoma* and *Leishmania*.

■ *Ciliophora* (ciliates and suctorians) move on hundreds of hairlike projections that cover their bodies. The only pathogenic ciliate is *Balantidium coli*, the largest protozoan parasite affecting humans and the cause of balantidial dysentery.

■ *Sporozoa*, which are immobile in the adult stages, include tissue and blood parasites, such as *Toxoplasma gondii*, *Pneumocystis carinii*, *Cryptosporidium*, and *Plasmodium* (the cause of malaria). (See *Four pathogenic protozoa*.)

Transmission of protozoa usually results from ingestion of parasitic cysts contained in fecally contaminated food, water, or soil; other modes of transmission include sexual intercourse (*Trichomonas vaginalis*), mechanical vectoring by flies and other insects (*E. histolytica*, *G. lamblia*), or the bites of blood-sucking insects (*Trypanosoma, Plasmodium*, and *Leishmania*).

Helminths

Both types of helminths — Platyhelminthes (flatworms) and Nemathelminthes (roundworms) — are usually visible to the naked eye, but confirmation of infestation requires microscopic examination of ova because the worms themselves are rarely passed. Flatworms include tapeworms, which inhabit the intestinal tract, and leaf-shaped flukes, which appear in the intestinal tract, bile ducts, and blood. Although some species of tapeworms, such as *Taenia saginata* and *Diphyllobothrium latum* are common in the United States, all fluke infections are rare.

Pathogenic species of the slender roundworms include blood and tissue parasites, such as *Wuchereria bancrofti* and *Onchocerca volvulus* (which rarely cause infection in the United States), and intestinal parasites, such as *Ascaris lumbricoides, Necator americanus, Enterobius vermicularis, Trichuris trichiura*, and *Strongyloides stercoralis* (which are indigenous to the United States).

Arthropods

Arthropods include flies, spiders, mites, ticks, crayfish, crabs, lice, fleas, beetles, gnats, and mosquitoes. Although some arthropods, such as lice and the itch mite *Sarcoptes scabiei*, are true parasites, most are vectors (carriers) of parasitic disease. Two kinds of vectors transmit such infections: A mechanical vector, such as an insect, simply carries parasites from one person or object to another; a biological vector, such as a mosquito, acts as a host, allowing parasites to develop and multiply before passing them to another host.

Four pathogenic protozoa

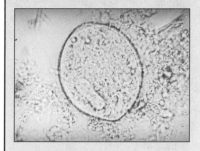

Balantidium coli: *This is the largest intestinal protozoan found in humans and the only pathogenic ciliate. In this photograph of an unstained B. coli tro-phozoite taken from a stool specimen, food vacuoles and an anterior cyto-stome are visible.*

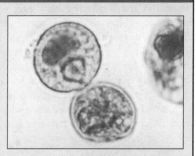

Entamoeba histolytica: *This is the most common human pathogen of the six species of* Entamoeba *protozoa. Notice the large chromatoid bodies, diffused glycogen, and delicate chro-matin beads on the inner surface of the nuclear membrane that distinguish these infective cysts from nonpatho-genic amoebae.*

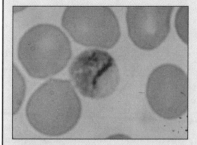

Plasmodium malariae: *This organism attacks mature erythrocytes. The tro-phozoite shown in the photograph dis-plays the granular band of dark brown or black pigment acquired during growth of this sporozoan.*

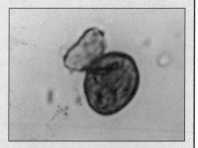

Giardia lamblia: *These flagellates commonly infest the intestinal tract. The photograph shows an ellipsoid cyst with a smooth, well-defined wall and multiple nuclei. Notice the tropho-zoites — forms in the feeding stage — within the cyst.*

Testing procedures

All protozoan parasites, helminth eggs and larvae, and some arthropods re-quire microscopic identification. Wet films of unstained material can detect various stages of intestinal parasites; the addition of iodine stains protozoan cysts. Permanent stains, such as Giemsa stain, help identify species of blood and tissue parasites and reveal the cytologic detail necessary to identify protozoan parasites. Preservation with formalin (formaldehyde), followed by concentra-tion procedures, can detect small num-bers of ova, as in helminth infections.

Serologic tests are available for detect-ing at least 24 protozoan and helminth infections, especially those that cause high antibody levels (such as amebiasis, trichinosis, echinococcosis, and toxoplasmosis) and clinically occult infections (such as filariasis or cysticercosis). The degree of sensitivity and specificity of such testing varies with the disease and the serologic method.

Culturing is available for only a few protozoan parasites and larvae and is performed mainly for research purposes. A culture may be performed if infection with *E. histolytica, Trichomonas vaginalis, Trypanosoma cruzi, Naegleria, Acanthamoeba,* or *Leishmania* is suspected and conventional methods fail to confirm it.

CULTURES FOR BACTERIA AND VIRUSES

Urine culture

Laboratory examination and culture of urine are necessary for evaluation of urinary tract infections (UTIs) — most commonly bladder infections. Although urine in the kidneys and bladder is normally sterile, a small number of bacteria are usually present in the urethra and, consequently, may pass into the urine. Nevertheless, bacteriuria generally results from prevalence of a single type of bacteria. Indeed, the presence of more than two distinct bacterial species in a urine specimen strongly suggests contamination during collection. However, a single negative culture doesn't always rule out infection, as in chronic, low-grade pyelonephritis. Urine cultures also identify pathogenic fungi, such as *Coccidioides immitis.* (See *Culture sites for common pathogenic fungi.*)

Significant results of urine culture are possible only after quantitative examination. To distinguish between true bacteriuria and contamination, it's necessary to know the number of organisms in a milliliter of urine, estimated by a culture technique known as a "colony count." In addition, a quick centrifugation test can determine where a UTI originates. (See *Quick centrifugation test,* page 508.)

Clean-voided midstream collection, rather than suprapubic aspiration or catheterization, is now the method of choice for obtaining a urine specimen.

Purpose
- To diagnose UTI
- To monitor microorganism colonization after urinary catheter insertion.

Patient preparation
Explain to the patient that this test helps detect UTI. Advise him that it requires a urine specimen and that he needn't restrict food or fluids. Teach him how to collect a clean-voided midstream specimen, and emphasize the importance of cleaning the external genitalia thoroughly. Or, if appropriate, explain catheterization or suprapubic aspiration to the patient, and inform him that he may experience some discomfort during specimen collection.

Tell the patient with suspected urogenital tuberculosis that specimen collection may be required on three consecutive mornings. Check the patient history for current use of antimicrobial drugs.

Equipment
Gloves ✦ sterile specimen cup ✦ premoistened, antiseptic towelettes. Commercial clean-catch urine kits are available; many include instructions in several languages.

Culture sites for common pathogenic fungi

ORGANISM	CULTURE SITES
Aspergillus species*	Skin, respiratory secretions, nasal sinuses, ear, gastric washings
*Blastomyces dermatitidis**	Respiratory secretions, skin, oropharyngeal ulcer, bone, prostate
Candida species*	Mucous membranes, skin, gastric washings, blood, stool, sputum, body fluids, bone
Cladosporium species*	Respiratory exudates, skin, nails, nose, cornea
*Coccidioides immitis**	Sputum, skin, cerebrospinal fluid (CSF), joint fluid, urine
*Cryptococcus neoformans**	Respiratory tract, CSF, blood, urine, cornea, ocular orbit, vitreous humor
Epidermophyton floccosum	Skin, nails
*Histoplasma capsulatum**	Sputum, blood, CSF, pleural fluid, vaginal secretions, larynx
Microsporum species	Skin, hair
Mucor species	Wound specimens, sputum, ear, cornea, vitreous humor, stool
Paracoccidioides brasiliensis	Mucous membrane lesions, including those of the nose, gingiva, and, less commonly, conjunctiva
Penicillium species	Bronchial washings, skin, ear, cornea, urine
Pseudallescheria boydii	Sputum, skin, cornea, gastric washings
*Sporothrix schenckii**	Sputum, skin, joint fluid, CSF, ear, conjunctiva, maxillary sinuses
Trichophyton species	Skin, hair, nails
Zygomycetes species (not *Mucor*)	Nasal mucosa, palate, sinuses, lung fluid, GI tract

* Serum tests are available for these fungi.

Adapted with permission from Baron, E.J., and Finegold, S.M. Bailey and Scott's Diagnostic Microbiology, 8th ed. St. Louis: Mosby–Year Book, Inc., 1990, and from Koneman, E.W., and Roberts, G.D. "Mycotic Disease" in Clinical Diagnosis and Management, 18th ed. Edited by Henry, J.B. Philadelphia: W.B. Saunders Co., 1991.

Procedure

Collect a urine specimen as ordered. Record the suspected diagnosis, the collection time and method, current antimicrobial therapy, and fluid- or drug-induced diuresis on the laboratory request.

Precautions

- Use gloves when performing the procedure and handling specimens.
- Collect at least 3 ml of urine, but don't fill the specimen cup more than halfway.
- Seal the cup with a sterile lid, and send

it to the laboratory at once. If transport is delayed for more than 30 minutes, store the specimen at 39.2° F (4° C) or place it on ice, unless a urine transport tube containing preservative is used.

Normal findings

Culture results of sterile urine are normally reported as "no growth," which usually indicates the absence of UTI.

Implications of results

Bacterial counts of 100,000 or more organisms of a single microbe species per milliliter indicate probable UTI. Counts under 100,000/ml may be significant, depending on the patient's age, sex, history, and other individual factors. However, counts under 10,000/ml usually suggest that the organisms are contaminants, except in symptomatic patients, those with urologic disorders, or those whose urine specimens were collected by suprapubic aspiration. A special test for acid-fast bacteria can isolate *Mycobacterium tuberculosis*, thus indicating tuberculosis of the urinary tract.

Isolation of more than two species of organisms, or of vaginal or skin organisms, usually suggests contamination and requires a repeat culture. Prolonged

catheterization or urinary diversion may cause polymicrobial infection.

Post-test care
None.

Interfering factors
- Improper collection technique may contaminate the specimen.
- Fluid- or drug-induced diuresis and antimicrobial therapy may lower bacterial counts.
- Improper preservation or delays in sending the specimen to the laboratory may lead to inaccurate counts.

Stool culture

Bacteriologic examination of the feces is valuable for identifying pathogens that cause overt GI disease — such as typhus and dysentery — and carrier states. Normally, feces contains many species of bacterial flora and several potentially pathogenic organisms. The most common pathogenic organisms of the GI tract are *Shigella, Salmonella,* and *Campylobacter jejuni.* Less common pathogenic organisms include *Vibrio cholerae, Clostridium botulinum, C. difficile, Clostridium perfringens, Staphylococcus aureus,* enterotoxigenic *Escherichia coli, Bacillus cereus, Yersinia enterocolitica, Aeromonas hydrophila,* and *Vibrio parahaemolyticus.* (See *Pathogens of the GI tract.*) Identifying these organisms is vital to treat the patient, to prevent possibly fatal complications (especially in a debilitated patient), and to confine these severe infectious diseases. A sensitivity test may follow isolation of the pathogen.

Some viruses, such as rotavirus and parvovirus, may also cause GI symp-

Pathogens of the GI tract

The presence of the following pathogens in a stool culture may indicate certain disorders:

Aeromonas hydrophila: gastroenteritis, which causes diarrhea, especially in children

Bacillus cereus: food poisoning, acute gastroenteritis (rare)

Campylobacter jejuni: gastroenteritis

Clostridium botulinum: food poisoning and infant botulism (a possible cause of sudden infant death syndrome)

Toxin-producing *Clostridium difficile:* pseudomembranous enterocolitis

Clostridium perfringens: food poisoning

Enterotoxigenic *Escherichia coli:* gastroenteritis (resembles cholera or shigellosis)

Salmonella: gastroenteritis, typhoid fever, nontyphoidal salmonellosis, paratyphoid fever

Shigella: shigellosis, bacillary dysentery

Staphylococcus aureus: food poisoning, suppression of normal bowel flora from antimicrobial therapy

Vibrio cholerae: cholera

Vibrio parahaemolyticus: food poisoning, especially seafood

Yersinia enterocolitica: gastroenteritis, enterocolitis (resembles appendicitis), mesenteric lymphadenitis, ileitis.

---

toms. However, these viruses can be detected only by immunoassay or electron microscopy. Stool culture may detect other viruses, such as enterovirus, which can cause aseptic meningitis.

Purpose
- To identify pathogenic organisms causing GI disease
- To identify carrier states.

Patient preparation
Explain to the patient that this test helps determine the cause of GI distress and may establish whether he is a carrier of infectious organisms. Inform him that he needn't restrict food or fluids. Tell him the test may require the collection of a stool specimen on 3 consecutive days.

Check the patient history for dietary patterns, recent antimicrobial therapy, and recent travel that might suggest an endemic infection or infestation.

Equipment
Gloves ✦ half-pint, waterproof container with tight-fitting lid, or sterile swab and commercial sterile collection and transport system ✦ tongue blade ✦ bedpan (if needed).

Procedure
Collect a stool specimen directly in the container. If the patient isn't ambulatory, collect it in a clean, dry bedpan; then, using a tongue blade, transfer the specimen to the container. If you must collect the specimen by rectal swab, insert the swab past the anal sphincter, rotate it gently, and withdraw it. Then place the swab in the appropriate container.

Check with the laboratory for the proper collection procedure before obtaining a specimen for a virus test.

Remember to label the specimen with the patient's name, doctor's name, hospital number, and date and time of collection.

Precautions

- If the patient uses a bedpan or a diaper, avoid contaminating the stool specimen with urine.
- Send the specimen to the laboratory immediately; be sure to include mucoid and bloody portions. The specimen must always represent the first, middle, and last portion of the feces passed.
- Use gloves when performing the procedure and handling the specimen. Be sure to put the specimen container in a leakproof bag before sending it to the laboratory.
- Indicate the suspected cause of the patient's GI disorder and current antimicrobial therapy on the laboratory request.

Normal findings

More than 95% of normal fecal flora consist of anaerobes, including non-spore-forming bacilli, clostridia, and anaerobic streptococci. The remainder consist of aerobes, including gram-negative bacilli (predominantly *E. coli* and other Enterobacteriaceae, plus small amounts of *Pseudomonas*), gram-positive cocci (mostly enterococci), and a few yeasts.

Implications of results

Isolation of some pathogens (such as *Salmonella, Shigella, Campylobacter, Yersinia,* and *Vibrio*) indicates bacterial infection in patients with acute diarrhea and may require antimicrobial sensitivity tests. Since normal fecal flora may include *C. difficile, E. coli,* and other organisms, isolation of these may require further tests to demonstrate invasiveness or toxin production.

Isolation of such pathogens as *C. botulinum* indicates food poisoning; however, the pathogens must also be isolated from the contaminated food. In a patient undergoing long-term antimicrobial therapy, isolation of large numbers of *S. aureus* or such yeasts as *Candida* may indicate infection. (Asymptomatic carrier states are also indicated by these enteric pathogens.) Isolation of enteroviruses may indicate aseptic meningitis.

If a stool culture shows no unusual growth, detection of viruses by immunoassay or electron microscopy may diagnose nonbacterial gastroenteritis. A highly increased polymorphonuclear leukocyte count in fecal material may indicate an invasive pathogen.

Post-test care
None.

Interfering factors

- Improper collection technique or contamination of the specimen by urine may injure or destroy some enteric pathogens.
- Antimicrobial therapy may decrease bacterial growth in the specimen.
- Failure to transport the specimen promptly or, if delivery is delayed, to use a transport medium that stabilizes pH (such as a buffered glycerol medium) may result in loss of some enteric pathogens or overgrowth of nonpathogenic organisms.

Throat culture

A throat culture is used primarily to isolate and identify group A beta-hemolytic streptococci *(Streptococcus pyogenes),* thus allowing early treatment of pharyngitis and prevention of sequelae, such as rheumatic heart disease and glomerulonephritis. It's also used to screen for carriers of *Neisseria meningitidis.* In rare instances, a throat culture may be used to identify *Corynebacterium diphtheriae* or *Bordetella pertussis.* Although a throat culture may also be used to identify *Candida albicans,* direct potassium hydroxide preparation usually provides the same information faster.

A throat culture requires swabbing the throat, streaking a culture plate, and allowing the organisms to grow for isolation and identification of pathogens. A Gram-stained smear may provide preliminary identification, which may guide clinical management and determine the need for further tests. Culture results must be interpreted in light of clinical status, recent antimicrobial therapy, and amount of normal flora.

Purpose
■ To isolate and identify pathogens, particularly group A beta-hemolytic streptococci
■ To screen asymptomatic carriers of pathogens, especially *N. meningitidis.*

Patient preparation
Explain to the patient that this test helps identify the microorganisms that could be causing his symptoms or a carrier state. Inform him that he needn't restrict food or fluids before the test. Tell him who will perform the procedure and when. Reassure him that the test takes less than 30 seconds and that test results should be available in 2 or 3 days.

Describe the procedure, and warn him that he may gag during the swabbing. Check the patient history for recent antimicrobial therapy. Determine immunization history if it's pertinent to the preliminary diagnosis. Procure the throat specimen before beginning any antimicrobial therapy.

Equipment
Gloves ✦ sterile swab and culture tube with transport medium, or commercial collection and transport system.

Procedure
Tell the patient to tilt his head back and close his eyes. With the throat well illu-minated, check for inflamed areas, using a tongue blade. Swab the tonsillar areas from side to side; include any inflamed or purulent sites. *Don't* touch the tongue, cheeks, or teeth with the swab. Immediately place the swab in the culture tube. If a commercial sterile collection and transport system is used, crush the ampule and force the swab into the medium to keep it moist.

Note recent antimicrobial therapy on the laboratory request. Label the specimen with the patient's name, doctor's name, date and time of collection, and origin of the specimen. Also indicate the suspected organism, especially *C. diphtheriae* (requires two swabs and a special growth medium), and *N. meningitidis* (requires enriched selective media).

Rapid nonculture antigen testing methods can detect group A streptococcal antigen in as little as 10 minutes. Cultures should be performed on all negative specimens.

Precautions
■ Use gloves when performing the procedure and handling specimens.
■ Send the specimen to the laboratory immediately. Unless a commercial sterile collection and transport system is used, keep the container upright during transport.

Normal findings
Throat flora normally include non-hemolytic and alpha-hemolytic streptococci, *Neisseria* species, staphylococci, diphtheroids, some *Haemophilus* species, pneumococci, yeasts, and enteric gram-negative organisms.

Implications of results
Possible pathogens cultured include group A beta-hemolytic streptococci (*S. pyogenes*), which can cause scarlet fever or pharyngitis; *C. albicans,* which can cause thrush; *C. diphtheriae,* which can cause diphtheria; and *B. pertussis,* which

can cause whooping cough. The laboratory report should indicate the prevalent organisms and the quantity of pathogens cultured.

Post-test care
None.

Interfering factors
- Failure to report recent or current antimicrobial therapy on the laboratory request may cause false-negative results.
- Failure to use the proper transport media may affect the accuracy of results.
- A delay of more than 15 minutes in sending the specimen to the laboratory may yield inaccurate results.

Nasopharyngeal culture

This test evaluates nasopharyngeal secretions for the presence of pathogenic organisms. Direct microscopic inspection of a Gram-stained smear of the specimen provides preliminary identification of organisms, which may guide clinical management and determine the need for additional testing. Streaking a culture plate with the swab and allowing any organisms present to grow permits isolation and identification of pathogens. Cultured pathogens may then require susceptibility testing to determine appropriate antimicrobial therapy.

Nasopharyngeal cultures are often useful for identifying *Bordetella pertussis* and *Neisseria meningitidis,* especially in very young, elderly, or debilitated patients. They can also be used to isolate viruses, especially carriers of influenza virus A and B. However, because the laboratory procedure required for such testing is complex, time-consum-

ing, and costly, this culture is performed infrequently.

Purpose
- To identify pathogens causing upper respiratory tract symptoms
- To identify proliferation of normal nasopharyngeal flora, which may prove pathogenic in debilitated and other immunocompromised persons
- To detect asymptomatic carriers of infectious organisms, such as *N. meningitidis* and *B. pertussis.*

Patient preparation
Describe the procedure to the patient, and explain that this test isolates the cause of nasopharyngeal infection and allows identification of the organism and testing for antimicrobial susceptibility. Tell him that secretions will be obtained from the back of the nose and the throat, using a cotton-tipped swab, and who will perform this procedure. Warn him that he may experience slight discomfort and may gag, but reassure him that obtaining the specimen takes less than 15 seconds. Inform him that initial test results are available in 48 to 72 hours but that viral test results take longer.

Equipment
Gloves ✦ penlight ✦ sterile, flexible wire swab ✦ small, sterile, open-ended glass Pyrex tube or sterile nasal speculum ✦ tongue blade ✦ culture tube ✦ transport medium (broth).

Procedure
Put on gloves. Ask the patient to cough before you begin collecting the specimen. Then position the patient with his head tilted back.

Using a penlight and a tongue blade, inspect the nasopharyngeal area. Next, gently pass the swab through the nostril and into the nasopharynx, keeping the swab near the septum and floor of the nose. (See *Obtaining a nasopharyngeal specimen*.) Or place the Pyrex tube in the patient's nostril, and carefully pass the swab through the tube into the nasopharynx. Rotate the swab for 5 seconds; then place it in the culture tube with transport medium. Remove the Pyrex tube. Label the specimen appropriately, including the date and time of collection, the origin of the material, and the suspected organism.

Ideally, a fresh culture medium should be inoculated with specimens for *B. pertussis* at the patient's bedside because of this organism's susceptibility to environmental changes. If the specimen is for isolation of a virus, verify the laboratory's recommended collection techniques.

Precautions
▪ Use gloves when performing the procedure and handling the specimen.
▪ Don't let the swab touch the sides of the patient's nostril or his tongue to prevent specimen contamination.
▪ Note recent antimicrobial therapy or chemotherapy on the laboratory request.
▪ Keep the container upright.
▪ Tell the laboratory if *Corynebacterium diphtheriae* or *B. pertussis* is suspected; these organisms need special growth media.
▪ Refrigerate a viral specimen according to your laboratory's procedure.

Normal findings
Flora that are commonly found in the nasopharynx include nonhemolytic streptococci, alpha-hemolytic streptococci, *Neisseria* species (except *N. meningitidis* and *N. gonorrhoeae*), coagulase-negative staphylococci such as *Staphylococcus epidermidis*, and occasionally, the coagulase-positive *Staphylococcus aureus*.

> ## Obtaining a nasopharyngeal specimen
>
> When the swab passes into the nasopharynx, gently but quickly rotate it to collect a specimen. Then remove the swab, taking care not to injure the nasal mucous membrane.
>
>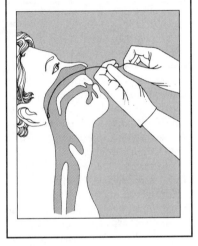

Implications of results
Pathogens may include group A beta-hemolytic streptococci; occasionally groups B, C, and G beta-hemolytic streptococci; *B. pertussis; C. diphtheriae; S. aureus;* and large numbers of pneumococci, *Haemophilus influenzae,* or *Candida albicans.*

Post-test care
None.

Interfering factors
▪ Recent antimicrobial therapy decreases bacterial growth.
▪ Improper collection technique may contaminate the specimen.
▪ Failure to place the specimen in transport medium allows the specimen to dry out and the bacteria to deteriorate.

- Failure to send the specimen to the laboratory immediately after collection permits proliferation of organisms.
- Failure to keep a viral specimen cold allows the viruses to deteriorate.

Sputum culture

Bacteriologic examination of sputum — material raised from the lungs and bronchi during deep coughing — is an important aid in managing lung disease. During passage through the throat and oropharynx, sputum specimens are commonly contaminated with indigenous bacterial flora, such as alpha-hemolytic streptococci, *Neisseria* species, diphtheroids, some *Haemophilus* species, pneumococci, staphylococci, and yeasts such as *Candida*.

Pathogenic organisms most often found in sputum include *Streptococcus pneumoniae, Mycobacterium tuberculosis, Klebsiella pneumoniae* (and other Enterobacteriaceae), *Haemophilus influenzae, Staphylococcus aureus,* and *Pseudomonas aeruginosa.* Other pathogens, such as *Pneumocystis carinii, Legionella* species, *Mycoplasma pneumoniae,* and respiratory viruses, may exist in the sputum and can cause lung disease, but they usually require serologic or histologic diagnosis rather than diagnosis by sputum culture.

The usual method of specimen collection is expectoration (which may require ultrasonic nebulization, hydration, physiotherapy, or postural drainage); other methods include tracheal suctioning and bronchoscopy. (See *Using an in-line trap.*)

A Gram stain of expectorated sputum must be examined to ensure that it's a representative specimen of secretions from the lower respiratory tract (many white blood cells [WBCs], few epithelial cells) rather than one contaminated by oral flora (few WBCs, many epithelial cells). Careful examination of an acid-fast smear of sputum may provide presumptive evidence of a mycobacterial infection, such as tuberculosis.

Purpose

- To isolate and identify the cause of a pulmonary infection, thus aiding diagnosis of respiratory diseases (most frequently bronchitis, tuberculosis, lung abscess, and pneumonia).

Patient preparation

Explain to the patient that this test helps to identify the organism causing respiratory tract infection. Tell him the test requires a sputum specimen and who will perform the procedure. If the suspected organism is *M. tuberculosis,* tell him that specimens may need to be collected on at least 3 consecutive mornings.

Test results are usually available in 48 to 72 hours. However, since cultures for tuberculosis take up to 2 months, diagnosis of this disorder is usually based on clinical symptoms, a smear for acid-fast bacilli, a chest X-ray, and response to a purified protein derivative skin test.

If the specimen is to be collected by expectoration, encourage fluid intake the night before collection to help sputum production. Teach the patient how to expectorate by taking three deep breaths and forcing a deep cough. Emphasize that sputum isn't the same as saliva, which will be rejected for culturing. Tell him not to brush his teeth or use mouthwash before the specimen collection, although he may rinse his mouth with water.

If the specimen is to be collected by tracheal suctioning, tell the patient he'll experience discomfort as the catheter passes into the trachea.

If the specimen is to be collected by bronchoscopy, instruct the patient to fast for 6 hours before the procedure. Make sure he or a responsible member of the family has signed a consent form. Tell him he'll receive a local anesthetic just before the test to minimize discomfort during passage of the tube.

Equipment

For expectoration: sterile, disposable, impermeable container with a tight-fitting cap ✦ 10% sodium chloride, acetylcysteine, propylene glycol, or sterile or distilled water aerosols, to induce cough, as ordered ✦ leakproof bag.

For tracheal suctioning: size 16 or 18 French suction catheter ✦ water-soluble lubricant ✦ sterile gloves ✦ sterile specimen container or in-line specimen trap ✦ normal saline solution.

For bronchoscopy: bronchoscope ✦ local anesthetic ✦ sterile needle and syringe ✦ sterile specimen container ✦ normal saline solution ✦ bronchial brush ✦ sterile gloves.

Procedure

For expectoration: Put on gloves. Instruct the patient to cough deeply and expectorate into the container. If the cough is nonproductive, use chest physiotherapy or nebulization to induce sputum, as ordered. Using aseptic technique, close the container securely. Dispose of equipment properly; seal the container in a leakproof bag before sending it to the laboratory.

For tracheal suctioning: Administer oxygen to the patient before and after the procedure, as necessary. Attach the sputum trap to the suction catheter. Using sterile gloves, lubricate the catheter with normal saline solution, and pass the catheter through the patient's nostril, without suction. (The patient will cough when the catheter passes through the larynx.) Advance the catheter into the trachea. Apply suction for

Using an in-line trap

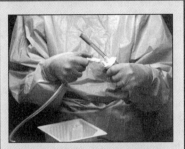

Push the suction tubing onto the male adapter of the in-line trap.

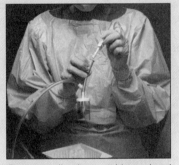

Put on sterile gloves; with one hand, insert the suction catheter into the rubber tubing of the trap. Then suction the patient.

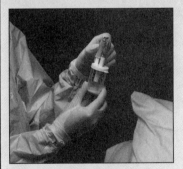

After suctioning, disconnect the in-line trap from the suction tubing and catheter. To seal the container, connect the rubber tubing to the female adapter of the trap.

no longer than 15 seconds to obtain the specimen. Stop suction, and gently remove the catheter. Discard the catheter and gloves in the proper receptacle. Then detach the in- line sputum trap from the suction apparatus and cap the opening.

For bronchoscopy: After a local anesthetic is sprayed into the patient's throat or the patient gargles with a local anesthetic, the bronchoscope is inserted through the pharynx and trachea into the bronchus. Secretions are then collected with a bronchial brush or aspirated through the inner channel of the scope, using an irrigating solution (such as normal saline solution) if necessary. After the specimen is obtained, the bronchoscope is removed.

Label the container with the patient's name. Include on the laboratory request the nature and origin of the specimen, the date and time of collection, the initial diagnosis, and any current antimicrobial therapy.

Precautions
▪ Tracheal suctioning is contraindicated in patients with esophageal varices or cardiac disease.

 ▪ In a patient with asthma or chronic bronchitis, watch for aggravated bronchospasms with use of more than 10% concentration of sodium chloride or acetylcysteine in an aerosol.

▪ During tracheal suctioning, suction for only 5 to 10 seconds at a time. *Never* suction longer than 15 seconds. If the patient becomes hypoxic or cyanotic, remove the catheter immediately, and administer oxygen.
▪ Use gloves when performing the procedure and handling specimens.
▪ Since the patient may cough violently during suctioning, wear gloves and a mask to avoid exposure to pathogens.
▪ *Don't* use more than 20% propylene

glycol with water as an inducer for a specimen scheduled for tuberculosis culturing, since higher concentrations inhibit the growth of *M. tuberculosis.* (If propylene glycol isn't available, use 10% to 20% acetylcysteine with water or sodium chloride.)
▪ Send the specimen to the laboratory immediately after collection.

Normal findings
Flora commonly found in the respiratory tract include alpha-hemolytic streptococci, *Neisseria* species, and diphtheroids. However, the presence of normal flora doesn't rule out infection.

Implications of results
Because sputum is invariably contaminated with normal oropharyngeal flora, a culture isolate must be interpreted in light of the patient's overall clinical condition. Isolation of *M. tuberculosis* is always a significant finding.

Post-test care
▪ Provide good mouth care.
▪ After tracheal suctioning, offer the patient a drink of water.
▪ After bronchoscopy, observe the patient carefully for signs of hypoxemia (cyanosis), laryngospasm (laryngeal stridor), bronchospasm (paroxysms of coughing or wheezing), pneumothorax (dyspnea, cyanosis, pleural pain, tachycardia), perforation of the trachea or bronchus (subcutaneous crepitus), or trauma to respiratory structures (bleeding). Also, check for difficulty breathing or swallowing. *Don't* give liquids until the gag reflex returns.

Interfering factors
▪ Improper collection or handling of the specimen may alter test results.
▪ Failure to report current or recent antimicrobial therapy may cause falsenegative results.
▪ Sputum collected over an extended

period may cause pathogens to deteriorate or become overgrown by commensals and will not be accepted as a valid specimen by most laboratories.

Blood culture

A blood culture is performed by inoculating a culture medium with a blood sample and incubating it for isolation and identification of the causative pathogens in bacteremia (bacterial invasion of the bloodstream) and septicemia (systemic spread of such infection). Blood culture can identify about 67% of pathogens within 24 hours and up to 90% within 72 hours.

Bacteria from local tissue infection usually invade the bloodstream through the lymphatic system by way of the thoracic duct. (See *The lymphatic system,* page 518.) Occasionally, they enter the bloodstream directly through infusion lines, thrombophlebitis, or bacterial endocarditis from prosthetic heart valve replacements. Bacteremia may be transient, intermittent, or continuous. The timing of specimen collection for blood cultures varies; it usually depends on the type of bacteremia (intermittent or continuous) suspected and on whether drug therapy needs to be started regardless of test results.

Purpose
■ To confirm bacteremia
■ To identify the causative organism in bacteremia and septicemia.

Patient preparation
Explain to the patient that this procedure may identify the organism causing his symptoms. Inform him that he needn't restrict food or fluids before the test. Tell him how many samples the test will require; who will perform the venipunctures and when; and that he may experience transient discomfort from the needle punctures and the pressure of the tourniquet.

Equipment
Gloves ✦ tourniquet ✦ small adhesive bandages ✦ alcohol swabs ✦ povidone-iodine swabs ✦ 10- to 20-ml syringe for an adult; 6-ml syringe for a child ✦ three or four sterile needles ✦ two blood culture bottles, one vented (aerobic) and one unvented (anaerobic), with nutritionally enriched broths and sodium polyethanol sulfonate [SPS] added; or bottles with resin; or a lysis-centrifugation tube.

Procedure
Put on gloves. After cleaning the venipuncture site with an alcohol swab, clean it again with a povidone-iodine swab, starting at the site and working outward, in a circular motion. Wait at least 1 minute for the skin to dry, and remove the residual iodine with an alcohol swab. (Or you can remove the iodine after venipuncture.) Apply the tourniquet.

Perform a venipuncture; draw 10 to 20 ml of blood for an adult or 2 to 6 ml for a child. Clean the diaphragm tops of the culture bottles with alcohol or iodine, and change the needle on the syringe. If you're using broth, add blood to each bottle until you obtain a 1:5 or 1:10 dilution. For example, add 10 ml of blood to a 100-ml bottle. (Size of the bottle may vary depending on hospital protocol.) If you're using a special resin, such as Bactec resin medium or Antimicrobial Removal Device, add blood to the resin in the bottles and invert them gently to mix. Draw the blood directly into a special collection-processing tube, if you're using the lysis-centrifugation technique (Isolator). Next, indicate the tentative diagnosis on the

The lymphatic system

The lymphatic system — a network of capillary and venous channels — returns excess interstitial fluids and proteins to the blood. Materials flowing through these channels pass into the thoracic and right lymph ducts. The thoracic duct, the larger of the two, drains the lymphatic vessels from all but the upper right quadrant. This lymphatic drainage (commonly called lymph, the tissue fluid absorbed in the lymphatic vessels) then flows into the junction of the left internal jugular and left subclavian veins. The right lymph duct drains interstitial fluid from the upper right quadrant into the right subclavian vein.

Bacteria from local tissue infection usually enter the bloodstream through this system. When functioning properly, however, the lymphatic system provides a strong defense against bacteria and viruses. Before lymph reenters the bloodstream, afferent lymphatic vessels transport it to lymph nodes or glands — clusters of lymphatic tissues throughout the body — where numerous lymphocytes destroy microorganisms and foreign particles.

If the lymphatic system fails to destroy harmful particles before they enter the bloodstream, white blood cells (WBCs) in the spleen, liver, and bone marrow act as another defense mechanism. As blood circulates through the body, it flows into the spleen, where it's filtered. There, residing lymphocytes ingest abnormal or foreign cells while normal cells pass through. Bacteria that accompany digested food particles into the portal vein — which supplies the liver — are ingested by reticulum cells. Likewise, WBCs formed in the bone marrow protect the body from invading bacteria.

Macrophages constitute still another defense system. These WBCs in the tissues, lymph nodes, and red bone marrow are usually immobile, but they migrate to inflamed areas, where they ingest and destroy infective particles.

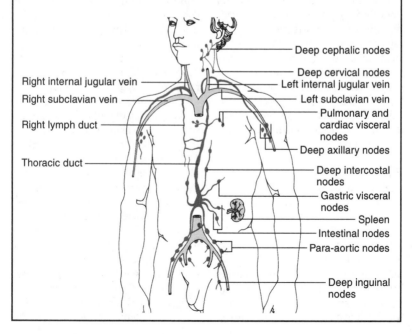

laboratory request, and note any current or recent antimicrobial therapy.

Precautions
- Use gloves when performing the procedure and handling the specimens.
- Send each sample to the laboratory immediately after collection.

Normal findings
Blood cultures are normally sterile.

Implications of results
Positive blood cultures don't necessarily confirm pathologic septicemia. Mild, transient bacteremia may occur during the course of many infectious diseases or may complicate other disorders. Persistent, continuous, or recurrent bacteremia reliably confirms the presence of serious infection. To detect most causative agents, blood cultures are ideally performed on 2 consecutive days.

Isolation of most organisms takes about 72 hours; however, negative cultures are held for 1 week or more before being reported negative. For example, negative reports for suspected *Brucella* infection are held for about 4 weeks.

Common blood pathogens include *Neisseria meningitidis*, *Streptococcus pneumoniae* and other *Streptococcus* species, *Haemophilus influenzae*, *Staphylococcus aureus*, *Pseudomonas aeruginosa*, *Brucella*, Bacteroidaceae, and Enterobacteriaceae. Although 2% to 3% of cultured blood samples are contaminated by skin bacteria, such as *Staphylococcus epidermidis*, diphtheroids, and *Propionibacterium*, these organisms may be clinically significant when isolated from multiple cultures or from immunocompromised patients.

Post-test care
If a hematoma develops at the venipuncture site, apply warm soaks.

Interfering factors
- Improper collection technique may contaminate the sample.
- Previous or current antimicrobial therapy may give false-negative results.
- Removal of culture bottle caps at bedside may prevent anaerobic growth; use of incorrect bottle and media may prevent aerobic growth.

Wound culture

A wound culture consists of microscopic analysis of a specimen from a lesion to confirm infection. Wound cultures may be aerobic (for detection of organisms that usually require oxygen to grow and typically appear in a superficial wound) or anaerobic (for organisms that need little or no oxygen and appear in areas of poor tissue perfusion, such as postoperative wounds, ulcers, or compound fractures). Indications for wound culture include fever as well as inflammation and drainage in damaged tissue.

Purpose
- To identify an infectious microbe in a wound.

Patient preparation
Explain to the patient that this test identifies infectious microbes. Advise him that a drainage specimen from the wound will be withdrawn by a syringe or removed on cotton swabs. Tell him who will perform the procedure and when.

Equipment
Sterile cotton swabs and sterile culture tube, or commercial sterile collection and transport system (for aerobic culture) ♦ sterile cotton swabs or sterile 10-

Anaerobic specimen collector

Some anaerobes die when they're exposed to the slightest bit of oxygen. To facilitate anaerobic collection and culturing, tubes filled with carbon dioxide (CO_2) or nitrogen are used for oxygen-free transport.

The anaerobic specimen collector shown here consists of a rubber-stoppered tube filled with CO_2, a small inner tube, and a swab attached to a plastic plunger. The drawing on the left shows the tube before specimen collection. The small inner tube containing the swab is held in place by the rubber stopper.

After specimen collection (right), the swab is quickly replaced in the inner tube and the plunger depressed. This separates the inner tube from the stopper, forcing it into the larger tube, and thus exposes the specimen to the CO_2-rich environment. Keep the tube upright.

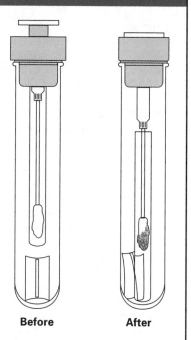

Before   **After**

---

ml syringe with 21G needle, and special culture tube containing carbon dioxide or nitrogen (for anaerobic culture) ✦ sterile gloves ✦ alcohol wipes ✦ sterile gauze and povidone-iodine solution.

Procedure

Using gloves, prepare a sterile field and clean the area around the wound with antiseptic solution.

For aerobic culture: Express the wound and swab as much exudate as possible, or insert the swab deep into the wound and gently rotate. Immediately place the swab in the aerobic culture tube.

For anaerobic culture: Insert the swab deep into the wound, gently rotate it, and immediately place it in the anaerobic culture tube; or insert the needle into the wound, aspirate 1 to 5 ml of exudate into the syringe, and immediately inject the exudate into the anaerobic culture tube. (See *Anaerobic specimen collector.*) If the needle is covered with a rubber stopper, the aspirate may be sent to the laboratory in the syringe.

Record on the laboratory request recent antimicrobial therapy, the source of the specimen, and the suspected organism. Also, label the specimen container appropriately with the patient's name, the doctor's name, the hospital number, and the wound site and time of specimen collection.

Precautions

▪ Clean the area around the wound thoroughly to limit contamination of the culture by normal skin flora, such as diphtheroids, *Staphylococcus epidermidis,* and alpha-hemolytic streptococci. However, *don't* clean the area around a perineal wound.

- Make sure no antiseptic enters the wound.
- Obtain exudate from the entire wound, using more than one swab.
- Because some anaerobes die in the presence of even a small amount of oxygen, place the specimen in the culture tube quickly, take care that no air enters the tube, and check that double stoppers are secure.
- Keep the specimen container upright, and send it to the laboratory within 15 minutes to prevent growth or deterioration of microbes.
- Use gloves during the procedure and when handling the specimen, and take necessary isolation precautions when sending the specimen to the laboratory.

Normal findings

No pathogenic organisms should be present in a clean wound.

Implications of results

The most common aerobic pathogens in wounds are *Staphylococcus aureus*, group A beta-hemolytic streptococci, *Proteus*, *Escherichia coli* and other Enterobacteriaceae, and some *Pseudomonas* species; the most common anaerobic pathogens are some *Clostridium* and *Bacteroides* species.

Post-test care

Dress the wound as ordered.

Interfering factors

- Failure to report recent or current antimicrobial therapy may cause false-negative results.
- Poor collection technique (for example, exposing some specimens to oxygen) may contaminate or invalidate the specimen.
- Failure to use the proper transport media may cause the specimen to dry up and the bacteria to die, affecting the accuracy of test results.

Gastric culture

This test requires aspiration of gastric contents and cultivation of any microbes present to identify mycobacterial infection. Performed in conjunction with a chest X-ray and a purified protein derivative skin test, gastric culture is especially useful when a sputum sample can't be obtained by expectoration or nebulization. Gastric aspiration also provides a specimen for rapid presumptive identification of bacteria (by Gram stain) in neonatal septicemia.

Purpose

- To aid diagnosis of mycobacterial infections
- To identify the infecting bacteria in neonatal septicemia.

Patient preparation

Explain to the patient (or to the parents if the patient is a child) that gastric culture helps diagnose tuberculosis. Instruct him to fast for 8 hours before the test. Tell him who will perform the procedure and that it may have to be performed on 3 consecutive mornings. Instruct the patient to remain in bed each morning until the specimen has been collected to prevent premature emptying of stomach contents.

Describe the procedure to the patient. Tell him the nasogastric (NG) tube may make him gag but passes more easily if he relaxes and follows instructions about breathing and swallowing. Just before the procedure, obtain baseline heart rate and rhythm, and place the patient in high-Fowler's position.

Inform the patient (or his parents) that test results may take 2 months because acid-fast bacteria generally grow slowly. Check his history for recent antimicrobial therapy.

Equipment

Water-soluble lubricating jelly ✦ sterile water ✦ size 16 or 18 French disposable, plastic NG tube ✦ 50-ml sterile syringe ✦ sterile specimen container ✦ sterile gloves ✦ emesis basin ✦ stethoscope ✦ clamp (if necessary).

Procedure

As soon as the patient awakens in the morning, put on gloves, perform nasogastric intubation and obtain gastric washings. Clamp the tube before quickly removing it. Note recent antimicrobial therapy on the laboratory request, along with the site and time of collection. Label the specimens with the patient's name, the doctor's name, and the hospital number.

Precautions

■ Gastric intubation is contraindicated in pregnancy, esophageal disorders (varices, stenosis, diverticula, or malignant neoplasms), recent severe gastric hemorrhage, aortic aneurysm, heart failure, and myocardial infarction.

■ If possible, obtain the specimen before the start of antimicrobial therapy.

■ Watch for signs that the tube has entered the trachea — coughing, cyanosis, or gasping.

■ *Never* inject fluid into an NG tube unless you're sure the tube is correctly placed in the patient's stomach. During lavage, use sterile, distilled water to decrease risk of contamination with saprophytic mycobacteria.

■ Because some patients develop arrhythmias during this procedure, check the pulse rate for irregularities.

■ Use gloves when performing the procedure and handling specimens.

■ Make sure the specimen container is tightly capped. Wipe the outside of the container with disinfectant, and send it to the laboratory (upright in a plastic bag) immediately.

■ Handle the NG tube with gloved hands, and dispose of all equipment carefully to prevent staff contamination.

Normal findings

The culture specimen should be free of pathogenic mycobacteria.

Implications of results

Isolation and identification of the organism *Mycobacterium tuberculosis* indicates the presence of active tuberculosis; other species of *Mycobacterium,* such as *M. bovis, M. kansasii,* and *M. avium-intracellulare* complex, may cause pulmonary disease that is clinically indistinguishable from tuberculosis. Treatment of these mycobacterial diseases may be difficult and commonly requires susceptibility studies to determine effective antimicrobial therapy. Pathogenic bacteria that cause neonatal septicemia may also be identified through culture.

Post-test care

■ As ordered, resume administration of medications discontinued before the test.

■ Instruct the patient not to blow his nose for at least 4 hours to prevent bleeding.

■ Tell the patient that he may resume his normal diet.

Interfering factors

■ Failure to observe an 8-hour fast before the test may decrease the amount of bacteria by diluting stomach contents or removing contents through digestion.

■ Certain drugs, such as tetracycline and aminoglycosides, can weaken bacilli, causing false-negative culture results.

■ The presence of saprophytic mycobacteria in gastric contents may cause false-positive acid-fast smears because these bacteria can't be microscopically distinguished from pathogenic mycobacteria.

Duodenal contents culture

This test requires duodenal intubation, aspiration of duodenal contents, and cultivation of any microbes present to isolate and identify a duodenal or biliary pathogen. Occasionally, a specimen may be obtained during surgery (such as a cholecystectomy) or duodenoscopy. Duodenal contents (pancreatic and duodenal enzymes and bile) are normally almost sterile, but they're subject to infection by many pathogens, such as *Escherichia coli, Staphylococcus aureus,* and *Salmonella.* Such microbial infection of the biliary tract and duodenum can result in duodenitis, cholecystitis, or cholangitis.

Purpose

■ To detect bacterial infection of the biliary tract and duodenum; to differentiate between such infection and gallstones
■ To rule out bacterial infection as the cause of persistent GI symptoms (epigastric pain, nausea, vomiting, and diarrhea).

Patient preparation

Explain to the patient that this tests helps to determine the cause of his symptoms. Instruct him to restrict food and fluids for 12 hours before the test. Tell him who will perform the procedure and where it will be done.

Describe the intubation procedure to the patient. Assure him that although this procedure is uncomfortable, it isn't dangerous. Explain that passage of the tube may make him gag, but following the examiner's instructions about proper positioning, breathing, swallowing, and relaxing will minimize discomfort. Suggest to the patient that he empty his bladder before the procedure to increase his comfort.

Equipment

Gloves ✦ double-lumen tube with olive tip ✦ water-soluble lubricating jelly ✦ 30-ml sterile syringe ✦ emesis basin ✦ sterile specimen container ✦ adhesive tape.

Procedure

After the nasoenteric tube is inserted, place the patient in the left lateral decubitus position, with his feet elevated, to allow peristalsis to move the tube into the duodenum. The pH of a small amount of aspirated fluid determines tube position: If the tube is in the stomach, pH is lower than 7.0; if the tube is in the duodenum, pH is higher than 7.0. Correct tube position can also be confirmed by fluoroscopy. After confirmation, duodenal contents are aspirated.

Transfer the specimen to a sterile container, and label it with the patient's name, doctor's name, and date and time of collection.

Precautions

■ Use gloves when performing procedures and handling specimens.
■ Duodenal intubation is contraindicated in pregnancy, acute pancreatitis or cholecystitis, esophageal disorders (varices, stenosis, diverticula, or malignant neoplasms), recent severe gastric hemorrhage, aortic aneurysm, congestive heart failure, or myocardial infarction.
■ Collect the specimen for culture before antimicrobial therapy begins.
■ Withdraw the tube slowly (6" to 8" [15 to 20 cm] every 10 minutes) until it reaches the esophagus; then clamp the tube and remove it quickly. Notify the doctor if the tube can't be withdrawn easily; *never* force the tube.
■ Send the specimen to the laboratory immediately.

Normal findings

A duodenal contents culture normally contains small amounts of polymorphonuclear leukocytes and epithelial cells with no pathogens. The bacterial count is usually less than 100,000/ml.

Implications of results

Generally, bacterial counts of 100,000/ml or more, or the presence of any number of pathogens, such as *Salmonella*, indicates infection. Susceptibility testing may be required. Numerous polymorphonuclear leukocytes, copious mucous debris, and bile- stained epithelial cells in the bile fluid suggest inflammation of the biliary tract; many segmented neutrophils and exfoliated epithelial cells suggest inflammation of the pancreas, the duodenum, or bile ducts. The presence of bile sand indicates cholelithiasis or calculi in the biliary tract.

Differential diagnosis requires further testing, including oral or I.V. cholecystography; white blood cell count; cholangiography; measurement of serum bilirubin, alkaline phosphatase, serum amylase, and urine urobilinogen; and culture of surgical material.

Post-test care

■ After duodenal intubation or duodenoscopy, observe the patient carefully for signs of perforation from tube passage, such as dysphagia, epigastric or shoulder pain, dyspnea, or fever.
■ After duodenoscopy, monitor vital signs until the patient is stable; keep the bed rails up, and enforce bed rest until the patient is fully alert.
■ As ordered, resume diet discontinued before the test.

Interfering factors

■ Failure to observe a 12-hour fast can dilute the specimen, which decreases the bacterial count.

■ Improper collection technique can contaminate the specimen.

Culture for gonorrhea

Although a stained smear of genital exudate can confirm gonorrhea in 90% of males with characteristic symptoms, a culture is often necessary, especially in asymptomatic females. Possible culture sites include the urethra (usual site in males), endocervix (usual site in females), anal canal, and oropharynx.

Gonorrhea, the most prevalent venereal disease, almost always results from sexual transmission of *Neisseria gonorrhoeae*. Its most common effect in females is a greenish yellow cervical discharge, but in many females, it causes no signs or symptoms at all — a factor that contributes to the epidemic prevalence of this infection. In males, gonorrhea generally causes painful urination and a mucopurulent urethral discharge, symptoms of acute anterior urethritis.

Purpose

■ To confirm gonorrhea.

Patient preparation

Describe the procedure to the patient, and explain that this test confirms gonorrhea. Inform the patient who will perform the test and when and that results are usually available within 24 to 72 hours.

Instruct the female patient not to douche for 24 hours before the test. Tell the male patient not to void for an hour before the test. Warn him that males sometimes experience nausea, sweating, weakness, and fainting from fear or discomfort when the cotton swab or wire loop is introduced into the urethra.

Equipment

Sterile gloves ✦ sterile cotton swabs or sterile gauze ✦ wire bacteriologic loop or thin urogenital alginate swabs (for male patient) ✦ vaginal speculum ✦ modified Thayer-Martin medium in plates (or Transgrow medium in specimen bottles if laboratory isn't readily available) ✦ ring forceps ✦ cotton balls.

Procedure

For endocervical culture: Place the patient in the lithotomy position, drape her, and instruct her to take deep breaths. Using gloved hands, insert a vaginal speculum that has been lubricated only with warm water. Clean mucus from the cervix, using cotton balls in ring forceps. Then insert a dry, sterile cotton swab into the endocervical canal, and rotate it from side to side. Leave the swab in place for several seconds for optimum absorption of organisms.

For urethral culture: Place the patient in the supine position, and drape him appropriately. Clean the urinary meatus with sterile gauze or a cotton swab; then insert a thin urogenital alginate swab or a wire bacteriologic loop $\frac{3}{8}$" to $\frac{3}{4}$" (1 to 2 cm) into the urethra, and rotate it from side to side. Leave it in place for several seconds for optimum absorption of organisms. If permitted, the patient may milk the urethra, bringing urethral secretions to the meatus for collection on a cotton swab.

For rectal culture: After obtaining an endocervical or urethral specimen (while the patient is still on the examining table), insert a sterile cotton swab about 1" (2.5 cm) into the anal canal, move it from side to side, and leave it in place for several seconds for optimum absorption. If the swab is contaminated with feces, discard it and repeat the procedure with a clean swab.

For throat culture: Position the patient with his head tilted back and his eyes closed. Check his throat for inflamed areas, using a tongue blade. Rub a sterile swab from side to side over the tonsillar areas, including any inflamed or purulent sites. Be careful not to touch the teeth, cheeks, or tongue with the swab.

After collecting any of these specimens, roll the swab in a Z pattern in a plate containing modified Thayer-Martin medium. Then cross- streak the medium with a sterile wire loop or the tip of the swab, and cover the plate. Label the specimen with the patient's name and room number (if applicable), the doctor's name, and the date and time of collection.

If laboratory facilities aren't readily available, uncap the Transgrow medium specimen bottle just before inserting the swab of test material into the bottle. Keep the bottle upright to minimize loss of carbon dioxide. With the swab, absorb the excess moisture in the bottle; then roll the swab across the Transgrow medium. Discard the swab, and place the lid on the bottle. Label the bottle appropriately.

Precautions

■ Use gloves when performing procedures and handling specimens.

■ Place the male patient in the supine position to prevent falling if vasovagal syncope occurs during introduction of the cotton swab or wire loop into the urethra. Observe him for profound hypotension, bradycardia, pallor, and sweating.

■ Collect a urethral specimen at least 1 hour after the patient has voided to prevent loss of urethral secretions.

■ After collecting the specimens, carefully dispose of gloves, swabs, and speculum to prevent staff exposure to any organisms.

■ Immediately send the specimen to the laboratory or arrange for transport of the Transgrow bottle because the specimen must be subcultured within 24 to 48 hours.

Normal findings

No *N. gonorrhoeae* organisms should appear in the culture.

Implications of results

A positive culture confirms a diagnosis of gonorrhea.

Post-test care

■ Advise the patient to avoid intercourse and all sexual contact until test results are available. Explain that treatment usually begins after confirmation of a positive culture, except in a patient with symptoms of gonorrhea or in a person who has had intercourse with someone known to have gonorrhea.

■ Advise the patient that a repeat culture is required 1 week after treatment is completed to evaluate the effectiveness of therapy.

■ Inform the patient that positive culture findings must be reported to the local health department.

Interfering factors

■ Improper collection technique may provide a nonrepresentative or contaminated specimen.

■ Fecal material may contaminate a rectal culture.

■ In males, voiding within 1 hour of specimen collection washes secretions out of the urethra, making fewer organisms available for culture.

■ In females, douching within 24 hours of specimen collection washes out cervical secretions, making fewer organisms available for culture.

Culture for *Chlamydia trachomatis*

The most common cause of sexually transmitted disease in the United States is *Chlamydia trachomatis*, an obligate intracellular parasite that must be cultivated in the laboratory by infection of susceptible cells.

In this procedure, the elementary bodies of *C. trachomatis* attach to specific receptor sites on McCoy cells and are engulfed by the cytoplasm of the cells where the organisms divide within inclusion bodies. After 48 hours of incubation, chlamydia-infected cells can be detected by fluorescein isothiocyanate-conjugated monoclonal antibodies (FITC-MoAb) or by iodine stain. Optimal conditions for recovery of *C. trachomatis* include infection of McCoy cells in shell vials, centrifugation at 700 x G, incubation for 48 hours, and staining with FITC-MoAb rather than iodine.

Recovery of *C. trachomatis* is considered the laboratory method of choice, although rapid nonculture (antigen detection) procedures are available for processing specimens from most clinical sites. Strains of *C. psittaci* and *C. pneumoniae* are not detected in these cell cultures without specific technical manipulations and reagents for detecting these species.

Purpose

■ To confirm infections caused by *C. trachomatis*.

Patient preparation

Explain the purpose of the test and the procedure for collecting the specimen to the patient. If the specimen will be collected from the genital tract, instruct the patient not to urinate for 3 to 4 hours before the specimen is taken. Instruct a female patient not to douche for 24 hours before the test.

Equipment

Gloves ✦ sterile cotton swabs ✦ wire bacteriologic loop or thin urogenital alginate swabs (for male patient) ✦ vaginal speculum ✦ sucrose phosphate (2SP) transport medium ✦ microbiologic transport swab or cytobrush.

Procedure

Obtain a specimen of the epithelial cells from the infected site. In adults, these sites may include the eye, urethra, endocervix, or rectum. Epithelial cells are collected from the urethra rather than from the purulent exudate that may be present.

You can obtain a urethral specimen by inserting a cotton-tipped applicator ¾" to 2" (2 to 5 cm) into the urethra. To collect a specimen from the endocervix, use a microbiologic transport swab or cytobrush. Then extract the specimen into sucrose phosphate (2SP) transport medium. Specimens collected from the throat, eye, and nasopharynx, and aspirates from infants should be extracted into 2SP transport medium. Send the specimens to the laboratory at 39.2° F (4° C).

If the anticipated time between specimen collection and inoculation into cell culture is more than 24 hours, freeze the 2SP transport medium and send it to the laboratory with dry ice.

Note: If you suspect that your patient has been sexually abused, test all specimens for *C. trachomatis* by culture rather than antigen detection methods.

Precautions

■ Place the male patient in the supine position to prevent him from falling if he develops vasovagal syncope when the cotton swab or wire loop is introduced into the urethra. Observe him for pro-

found hypotension, bradycardia, pallor, and sweating.

■ Use gloves when performing procedures and handling specimens.

■ Collect a urethral specimen at least 1 hour after the patient has voided to prevent loss of urethral secretions.

■ After collecting the specimens, carefully dispose of gloves, swabs, and speculum to prevent staff exposure to the organism.

Normal findings

No *C. trachomatis* should appear in the culture.

Implications of results

A positive culture confirms *C. trachomatis.*

Post-test care

■ If the culture confirms infection, provide counseling for the patient regarding treatment of sexual partners.

■ Advise the patient to avoid all sexual contact until test results are available.

Interfering factors

■ Use of an antimicrobial within a few days before collection of the specimen may prevent recovery of *C. trachomatis.*

■ Improper collection technique may provide a nonrepresentative or contaminated specimen.

■ Fecal material may contaminate a rectal culture.

■ In males, voiding within 1 hour of specimen collection washes secretions out of the urethra, making fewer organisms available for culture.

■ In females, douching within 24 hours of specimen collection can interfere with results by washing out cervical secretions, making fewer organisms available for culture.

Culture for herpes simplex virus

Herpes simplex virus (HSV), a herpesvirus, produces a wide spectrum of disorders, including keratitis, gingivostomatitis, encephalitis and, commonly, disseminated disease in immunocompromised individuals.

Of the six members of the herpesvirus group (Epstein-Barr virus, cytomegalovirus [CMV], varicella-zoster virus [VZV], human herpesvirus-6, and the two closely related serotypes of HSV — type 1 and type 2), only CMV, VZV, and HSV replicate in the standard cell cultures used in diagnostic laboratories. Of these herpesviruses, HSV replicates most rapidly in cell cultures. Approximately 50% of HSV strains can be detected by characteristic cytopathic effects (CPE) within 24 hours after the laboratory receives the specimen; the rest require 5 to 7 days to be detected because they're present in low titers in specimens.

Alternatively, early antigens of HSV can be detected by monoclonal antibodies in shell vial cell cultures within 16 hours after receipt of the specimen with the same sensitivity and specificity as standard tube cell cultures.

Purpose
■ To confirm diagnosis of HSV infection by culturing the virus from specimens.

Patient preparation
Explain that the test will be performed to detect infection by HSV. Specimens should be collected from suspected lesions during the prodromal and acute stages of clinical infection to ensure the best chance of recovering a virus in cell cultures.

Procedure
Collect a specimen for culture in the appropriate collection device.

For throat, skin, eye, or genital area: Use a microbiologic transport swab.

For body fluids or other respiratory specimens (washings, lavage): Use a sterile screw-capped jar.

Specimens should be transported to the laboratory as soon as possible after collection. If the anticipated time between collection and inoculation of cell cultures is more than 3 hours, the specimen should be stored and transported at 39.2° F (4° C).

Precautions
■ Wear gloves when obtaining and handling all specimens.
■ Do not freeze the specimen or allow it to dry up.

Normal findings
HSV is rarely recovered from immunocompetent patients who show no overt signs of disease. However, like other herpesviruses, HSV can be shed intermittently from immunocompromised patients without apparent disease. For epidemiologic purposes, HSV detected by CPE in standard tube cell cultures must be confirmed and identified by transfer of infected cells to slides with subsequent immunologic serotyping as type 1 or type 2. In the shell vial assay, this step occurs as part of the initial detection of the virus.

Implications of results
HSV detected in specimens taken from dermal lesions, the eye, cerebrospinal fluid, or tissue are highly significant. Specimens from the upper respiratory tract may be associated with intermittent shedding of the virus, particularly in an immunocompromised patient.

Post-test care
None.

Interfering factors

Administration of antiviral drugs before specimen collection may interfere with detection of the virus.

Rapid monoclonal test for cytomegalovirus

Cytomegalovirus (CMV), a member of the herpesvirus group, can cause systemic infection in congenitally infected infants and in immunocompromised patients, such as transplant recipients, patients receiving chemotherapy for neoplastic disease, and those with acquired immunodeficiency syndrome (AIDS).

In the past, CMV infections were detected in the laboratory by recognizing the distinctive cytopathic effects (CPE) that the virus produced in conventional tube cell cultures. In this slow method of detecting CMV, CPE cultures grow in about 9 days. The faster shell vial assay (rapid monoclonal test) is based on the availability of a monoclonal antibody specific for the 72 kd protein of CMV synthesized during the immediate early stage of viral replication.

Through indirect immunofluorescence, CMV- infected fibroblasts are recognized by their dense, homogeneous staining confined to the nucleus. Because of the smooth, regular shape of the nucleus and the surrounding nuclear membrane, infected cells are readily differentiated from nonspecific background fluorescence that may be present in some specimens.

Purpose

■ To obtain rapid laboratory diagnosis of CMV infection, especially in immunocompromised patients who currently have, or are at risk for developing, systemic infections caused by this virus.

Patient preparation

Explain the purpose of the test, and describe the procedure for collecting the specimen, which will depend on the laboratory used.

Procedure

Specimens should be collected during the prodromal and acute stages of clinical infection to maximize the chances of detecting CMV. Each type of specimen requires a specific collection device, as listed below:

■ *for throat:* microbiologic transport swab

■ *for urine or cerebrospinal fluid:* sterile screw-capped tube or vial

■ *for bronchoalveolar lavage tissue:* sterile screw-capped jar

■ *for blood:* sterile tube with anticoagulant (heparin).

Precautions

■ Transport the specimen to the laboratory as soon as possible after the collection. If the anticipated time between collection and inoculation into shell vial cell cultures is longer than 3 hours, store the specimen at 39.2° F (4° C). Don't freeze the specimen or allow it to become dry.

■ Use gloves when obtaining and handling all specimens.

Normal findings

CMV should not appear in a culture specimen.

Implications of results

CMV can be detected in urine and throat specimens from patients who are asymptomatic. However, detection from these sites indicates active, asymptomatic infection, which may herald symptomatic involvement, especially in immunocompromised patients. Detection of CMV in specimens of blood, tissue, and bronchoalveolar lavage generally indicates systemic infection and disease.

Post-test care
None.

Interfering factors
Administration of antiviral drugs before collection of the specimen may interfere with detection of CMV.

Stool examination for rotavirus antigen

Rotavirus (previously referred to as orbivirus, reovirus-like agent, duovirus, and gastroenteritis virus) is the most frequent cause of infectious diarrhea in infants and young children, associated with approximately 50% of pediatric hospitalizations for gastroenteritis.

Clinical features of rotavirus infection include diarrhea, vomiting, fever, and abdominal pain. This infection is most prevalent in children ages 3 months to 2 years during the winter months. In contrast to the severe clinical illness it causes in hospitalized infants, rotavirus may cause only mild symptoms in adults.

Human rotaviruses do not replicate efficiently in the usual laboratory cell cultures. Therefore, detection of the typical virus particles in stool specimens by electron microscopy has been replaced by sensitive, specific enzyme immunoassays that can provide results within minutes or a few hours (depending on the assay) after the specimen is received in the laboratory.

Purpose
■ To obtain a laboratory diagnosis of rotavirus gastroenteritis.

Patient preparation
Explain the purpose of the test to the patient or to the parents if the patient is a child. Inform him that the test requires a stool specimen. The specimens should be collected during the prodromal and acute stages of clinical infection to ensure detection of the viral antigens by enzyme immunoassay.

Procedure
A stool specimen (1 g in a screw-capped tube or vial) is preferred for detecting rotaviruses. If a microbiologic transport swab is used, it must be heavily stained with feces to be diagnostically productive for rotavirus.

Precautions
■ Avoid using collection containers with preservatives, metal ions, detergents, or serum, which may interfere with the assay.
■ Store stool specimens for up to 24 hours at 35.6° F to 46.4° F (2° C to 8° C). If a longer period of storage or shipment is necessary, freeze the specimens at −4° F (−20° C) or colder. Repeated freezing and thawing will cause the specimen to deteriorate and yield misleading results.
■ Don't store the specimen in a self-defrosting freezer.
■ Use gloves when obtaining or handling all specimens.

Normal findings
The detection of rotavirus by enzyme immunoassay is evidence of current infection with the organism.

Implications of results
Rotavirus can infect all age-groups, but the disease is generally more severe in young children than in adults.

Rotavirus infections are easily transmitted in group settings, such as day-care centers and nursing homes. Transmission is presumed to occur from person to person by the fecal-oral route. Nosocomial spread of this viral infection can have significant medical and economic effects in a hospital setting.

Post-test care
Monitor the patient's intake and output to avoid dehydration caused by vomiting and diarrhea.

Interfering factors
Collecting the specimen in containers with preservatives, metal ions, detergents, or serum may interfere with detection of the virus.

TESTS FOR OVA AND PARASITES

Stool examination

Examination of a stool specimen can detect several types of intestinal parasites. Some of these parasites live in nonpathogenic symbiosis; others cause intestinal disease. In the United States, the most common parasites include the roundworms *Ascaris lumbricoides* and *Necator americanus* (commonly called hookworm); the tapeworms *Diphyllobothrium latum, Taenia saginata* and, rarely, *Taenia solium*; the amoeba *Entamoeba histolytica*; and the flagellate *Giardia lamblia. Cyclospora* can also be detected in stool examination for ova and parasites.

Detection of pinworm requires a different collection method. (See *Collection procedure for pinworm*.)

Purpose
■ To confirm or rule out intestinal parasitic infection and disease.

> ## Collection procedure for pinworm
>
> The ova of the pinworm *Enterobius vermicularis* seldom appear in feces because the female migrates to the anus and deposits her ova there. To collect them, place a piece of cellophane tape, sticky side out, on the end of a tongue blade, and press it firmly on the anal area. Then transfer the tape, sticky side down, to a slide (kits with tape and a slide or a sticky paddle are available). Because the female usually deposits her ova at night, collect the specimen early in the morning, before the patient bathes or defecates.

Patient preparation
Explain to the patient that this test detects intestinal parasitic infection. Instruct him to avoid treatments with castor or mineral oil, bismuth, magnesium or antidiarrheal compounds, barium enemas, and antibiotics for 7 to 10 days before the test. Tell him the test requires three stool specimens — one every other day or every third day. Up to six specimens may be required to confirm the presence of *E. histolytica*.

If the patient has diarrhea, record recent dietary and travel history. Check the patient history for use of antiparasitic drugs, such as tetracycline, paromomycin, metronidazole, and iodoquinol, within 2 weeks of the test.

Equipment
Gloves ✦ waterproof container with tight-fitting lid ✦ bedpan (if necessary) ✦ tongue blade.

Procedure
Put on gloves and collect a stool specimen directly in the container. If the pa-

tient is bedridden, collect the specimen in a clean, dry bedpan; then, using a tongue blade, transfer it into a properly labeled container. Note on the laboratory request the date and time of collection and the specimen consistency. Also record recent or current antimicrobial therapy and any pertinent travel or dietary history.

Precautions

▪ Do not contaminate the stool specimen with urine, which can destroy trophozoites.

▪ Don't collect stool from a toilet bowl because water is toxic to trophozoites and may contain organisms that interfere with test results.

▪ Send the specimen to the laboratory immediately. If a liquid or soft stool specimen can't be examined within 30 minutes of passage, place some of it in a preservative; if a formed stool specimen can't be examined immediately, refrigerate it or place it in preservative.

▪ If the entire stool can't be sent to the laboratory, include macroscopic worms or worm segments as well as bloody and mucoid portions of the specimen.

▪ Use gloves when performing the procedure and handling the specimen, disposing of equipment, sealing the container, and transporting the specimen. Dispose of gloves after specimen collection and transport.

Normal findings

No parasites or ova should appear in stool.

Implications of results

The presence of *E. histolytica* confirms amebiasis; *G. lamblia*, giardiasis. However, the extent of infection depends on the degree of tissue invasion. If amebiasis is suspected but stool examinations are negative, specimen collection after saline catharsis using buffered sodium biphosphate or during sigmoidoscopy may be necessary. If giardiasis is suspected but stool examinations are negative, examination of duodenal contents may be necessary.

Because injury to the host is difficult to detect — even when helminth ova or larvae appear — the number of worms is usually correlated with the patient's clinical symptoms to distinguish between helminth infestation and helminth diseases. Eosinophilia may also indicate parasitic infection. Helminths may migrate from the intestinal tract, producing pathologic changes in other parts of the body. For example, the roundworm *Ascaris* may perforate the bowel wall, causing peritonitis, or may migrate to the lungs, causing pneumonitis. Hookworms can cause hypochromic microcytic anemia secondary to bloodsucking and hemorrhage, especially in patients with iron-deficient diets. The tapeworm *D. latum* may cause megaloblastic anemia by removing vitamin B_{12}.

Post-test care

As ordered, resume administration of medications discontinued before the test.

Interfering factors

▪ Improper collection technique or the presence of urine may cause false-negative results.

▪ Collection of too few specimens may cause false-negative results.

▪ Failure to transport the specimen promptly or to refrigerate or preserve it if transport is delayed may influence test results.

▪ Excessive heat or excessive cold can destroy parasites.

▪ Failure to observe pretest drug restrictions may interfere with microscopic analysis or reduce the number of parasites.

Examination of urogenital secretions

Microscopic examination of urine or vaginal, urethral, or prostatic secretions can detect urogenital infection by *Trichomonas vaginalis* — a parasitic, flagellate protozoan that's usually transmitted sexually. This test is performed more often on females than on males because more females exhibit symptoms. Males with trichomoniasis may have symptoms of urethritis or prostatis.

Purpose
■ To confirm trichomoniasis.

Patient preparation
Explain that this test can identify the cause of urogenital infection. Tell the female patient that it requires a specimen of vaginal secretion or urethral discharge and that she should not douche before the test. Tell the male patient that a specimen of urethral or prostatic secretion is required. Inform the patient who will perform the procedure and when.

Equipment
Gloves ✦ cotton swab ✦ test tube containing a small amount of normal saline solution (0.85% sodium chloride) ✦ vaginal speculum ✦ specimen cup (for urine specimen).

Procedure
For vaginal secretion: With the patient in the lithotomy position, insert an unlubricated vaginal speculum, and collect the discharge with a cotton swab. Then place the swab in the tube containing normal saline solution, and remove the speculum. Another method is to smear the specimen on a glass slide, allow it to air dry, and then transport it to the laboratory.

For prostatic material: After prostatic massage, collect secretions with a cotton swab, and place the swab in normal saline solution.

For urethral discharge: Collect the discharge with a cotton swab, and place the swab in normal saline solution.

For urine: Include the first portion of a voided random specimen (not midstream).

Label the specimen appropriately, including the date and time of collection.

Precautions
■ Remember to use gloves when performing procedures and handling specimens.
■ If possible, obtain the urogenital specimen before treatment with a trichomonacide begins.
■ Send the specimen to the laboratory immediately because trichomonads can be identified only while still motile.

Normal findings
Trichomonads are normally absent from the urogenital tract. In approximately 25% of females and most infected males, trichomonads may be present without associated pathology.

Implications of results
The presence of trichomonads confirms trichomoniasis.

Post-test care
Provide perineal care.

Interfering factors
■ Failure to send the specimen to the laboratory immediately causes trichomonads to lose their motility.
■ Improper collection technique may interfere with detection.
■ Collection of the specimen after trichomonacide therapy begins decreases the number of parasites in the specimen.

Examination of duodenal contents

This test evaluates duodenal contents for the presence of parasites in a specimen obtained by duodenal intubation and aspiration or by the string (Entero) test. Such parasites include trophozoites of *Giardia lamblia*; the ova and larvae of *Strongyloides stercoralis*; and the ova of *Necator americanus* or *Ancylostoma duodenale* in various stages of cleavage. This test can also detect ova of the liver flukes *Clonorchis sinensis* and *Fasciola hepatica* in the biliary tract. (Liver fluke infestations are rare in the United States.)

Examination of duodenal contents for ova and parasites is performed only in a symptomatic patient with negative stool examinations.

Purpose

■ To detect parasitic infection when stool examinations are negative.

Patient preparation

Explain to the patient that this test detects parasitic infection of the GI tract. Instruct him to restrict food and fluids for 12 hours before the test. Tell him who will perform the test and when. If the test will be done with a nasoenteric tube, warn him that he may gag during the tube's passage, but reassure him that following the examiner's instructions about positioning, breathing, and swallowing will minimize discomfort. Just before the procedure, instruct the patient to empty his bladder.

Equipment

Gloves ✦ double-lumen tube with olive tip (or weighted gelatin capsule with string attached, for string test) ✦ water-soluble jelly ✦ 30-ml sterile syringe ✦ emesis basin ✦ sterile specimen container ✦ ½" adhesive tape.

Procedure

For a nasoenteric tube: After inserting the tube, place the patient in a left lateral decubitus position, with his feet elevated, to allow peristalsis to move the tube into the duodenum. The pH of a small amount of aspirated fluid determines tube position: If the tube is in the stomach, pH is lower than 7.0; if it's in the duodenum, pH is higher than 7.0. Fluoroscopy can also determine correct positioning. When tube position is confirmed, residual duodenal contents are aspirated. Transfer the entire specimen to a sterile container; label it appropriately.

For an Entero test capsule with string: Tape the free end of the string to the patient's cheek. Then tell him to swallow the capsule (on the other end of the string) with water. Leave the string in place for 4 hours; then pull it out gently and place it in a sterile container. Label the container appropriately.

Precautions

■ Use gloves when performing the procedure and handling specimens.
■ Duodenal intubation is contraindicated during pregnancy and in patients with acute cholecystitis, acute pancreatitis, esophageal disorders (varices, stenosis, diverticula, or malignant neoplasms), recent severe gastric hemorrhage, aortic aneurysm, or congestive heart failure.
■ When possible, obtain the specimen before the start of drug therapy.
■ Send the specimen to the laboratory immediately.
■ Withdraw the tube slowly (6" to 8" [15 to 20 cm] every 10 minutes) to the esophagus; then clamp the tube and remove it quickly. *Never* force the tube.

Normal findings

No ova or parasites should be present.

Implications of results

Finding *G. lamblia* indicates giardiasis, which may cause malabsorption syndrome; *S. stercoralis* suggests strongyloidiasis; *A. duodenale* and *N. americanus* imply hookworm disease; and *C. sinensis* and *F. hepatica* signify histopathologic changes in the bile ducts.

Post-test care

- Dispose of equipment properly.
- Provide mouth care and offer water.
- Observe carefully for signs of perforation, such as dysphagia or fever.
- As ordered, have the patient resume his normal diet.

Interfering factors

- Failure of the patient to observe the 12-hour fast can dilute the specimen.
- Previous drug therapy or delay in sending the specimen may alter results.

Sputum examination

This test evaluates a sputum specimen for parasites. Such infestation is rare in the United States but may result from exposure to *Entamoeba histolytica, Ascaris lumbricoides, Echinococcus granulosus, Strongyloides stercoralis, Paragonimus westermani,* or *Necator americanus.* The specimen is obtained by expectoration or tracheal suctioning.

Purpose

- To identify pulmonary parasites.

Patient preparation

Explain to the patient that this test helps identify parasitic pulmonary infection. Tell him the test requires a sputum specimen or, if necessary, tracheal suctioning. Inform him that early morning collection is preferred because secretions accumulate overnight.

For expectoration, encourage fluid intake the night before collection to increase sputum production. Teach the patient how to expectorate by taking three deep breaths and forcing a deep cough. For tracheal suctioning, tell him he'll experience discomfort from the catheter.

Equipment

For expectoration: sterile, disposable, impermeable container with screw cap or tight-fitting cap ✦ nebulizer, intermittent positive-pressure breathing ventilator, and 10% sodium chloride, acetylcysteine, or sterile or distilled water aerosols to induce cough, as ordered.

For tracheal suctioning: size 16 or 18 French suction catheter ✦ sterile gloves ✦ sterile specimen container or sputum trap ✦ sterile normal saline solution.

Procedure

For expectoration: Instruct the patient to breathe deeply a few times and then to cough deeply and expectorate into the container. If the cough is nonproductive, use chest physiotherapy or heated aerosol spray (nebulization), as ordered. Close the container securely and clean the outside of it. Dispose of equipment properly, and take proper precautions in sending the specimen to the laboratory.

For tracheal suctioning: Administer oxygen before and after the procedure, if necessary. Attach a sputum trap to the suction catheter. While wearing a sterile glove, lubricate the tip of the catheter, and pass it through the patient's nostril, without suction. (The patient will cough when the catheter passes into the larynx.) Advance the catheter into the trachea. Apply suction for no longer than 15 seconds to obtain the specimen. Stop suction, and gently remove the catheter. Discard the catheter and glove in a proper receptacle. Then detach the sputum trap from the suction apparatus and cap the opening. Label all specimens carefully.

Precautions

■ Use gloves when performing procedures and handling specimens.
■ Tracheal suctioning is contraindicated in patients with esophageal varices or cardiac disease.

 ■ In a patient with asthma or chronic bronchitis, watch for aggravated bronchospasms with use of more than 10% concentration of sodium chloride or acetylcysteine in an aerosol.
■ During tracheal suctioning, suction for only 5 to 10 seconds at a time. *Never* suction for more than 15 seconds. If the patient becomes hypoxic or cyanotic, remove the catheter immediately, and administer oxygen.
■ Send the specimen to the laboratory immediately, or place it in preservative.

Normal findings

No parasites or ova should be present.

Implications of results

The parasite identified indicates the type of pulmonary infection and the presence of adult-stage intestinal infection:
■ *E. histolytica* trophozoites: pulmonary amebiasis
■ *A. lumbricoides* larvae and adults: pneumonitis
■ *E. granulosus* cysts of larval stage: hydatid disease
■ *S. stercoralis* larvae: strongyloidiasis
■ *P. westermani* ova: paragonimiasis
■ *N. americanus* larvae: hookworm disease.

Post-test care

■ Provide good mouth care.

■ After suctioning, offer the patient water and monitor vital signs every hour until stable.

Interfering factors

■ Recent therapy with anthelmintics or amebicides may alter test results.
■ Improper collection may produce a nonrepresentative specimen, thereby affecting test results.
■ Delay in sending the specimen to the laboratory may alter test results.

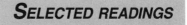
SELECTED READINGS

Baron, E.J., et al. *Bailey and Scott's Diagnostic Microbiology,* 9th ed. St. Louis: Mosby–Year Book, Inc., 1994.

Diseases, 2nd ed. Springhouse, Pa.: Springhouse Corp., 1996.

Fischbach, F. *A Manual of Laboratory and Diagnostic Tests,* 5th ed. Philadelphia: Lippincott-Raven Pubs., 1996.

Guyton, A.C., and Hall, J.E. *Textbook of Medical Physiology,* 9th ed. Philadelphia: W.B. Saunders Co., 1996.

Henry, J.B., ed. *Clinical Diagnosis and Management by Laboratory Methods,* 19th ed. Philadelphia: W.B. Saunders Co., 1996.

Mayo Medical Laboratories 1996 Test Catalog. Rochester, Minn.: Mayo Medical Laboratories, 1996.

Nursing97 Drug Handbook. Springhouse, Pa.: Springhouse Corp., 1997.

Ravel, R.A. *Clinical Laboratory Medicine: Clinical Application of Laboratory Data,* 6th ed. St. Louis: Mosby–Year Book, Inc., 1995.

Ryan, K.J., ed. *Sherris Medical Microbiology: An Introduction to Infectious Diseases,* 3rd ed. Stamford, Conn.: Appleton & Lange, 1994.

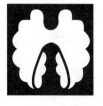

CHAPTER TWENTY

Thyroid

Learning objectives

After completing this chapter, the reader will be able to:
- describe the five categories of thyroid function tests
- explain the anatomy and physiology of the thyroid
- state the usual sequence of thyroid testing procedures
- list common disorders caused by thyroid dysfunction
- state the purpose of each test discussed in the chapter
- prepare the patient physically and psychologically for each test
- describe the procedure for performing each test
- specify appropriate precautions for safe administration of each test
- recognize signs of an adverse reaction and respond appropriately
- implement appropriate post-test care
- identify the normal findings of each test
- discuss the implications of abnormal test results
- list factors that may interfere with accurate test results.

INTRODUCTION

A number of sensitive and specific laboratory tests are available to evaluate thyroid function and hormone use. These tests make diagnosis of thyroid dysfunction possible even in patients with marginal or obscure thyroid abnormalities. However, since no one test diagnoses all thyroid disorders and interpretation of test results may be complicated by many factors, a combination of laboratory tests is usually required to ensure accurate diagnosis.

Laboratory tests of thyroid function can be classified into the following categories:
- *direct tests of thyroid function* that measure thyroid hormone synthesis and excretion, such as the radioactive iodine uptake test
- *tests that measure concentration and binding of the thyroid hormones* and other iodinated materials in the blood, such as serum free thyroxine and T_3 resin uptake (see Chapter 5), and protein-binding iodine

- *tests that assess the metabolic effects of thyroid hormones on the tissues,* such as serum cholesterol, basal metabolic rate (BMR), and Achilles reflex time (however, BMR and Achilles reflex time have largely been replaced by other tests)
- *tests that evaluate hormonal regulating mechanisms,* such as the thyroid-stimulating hormone test (see Chapter 5) and the thyroid suppression and stimulation tests
- *tests that evaluate anatomic detail of the thyroid gland* and aid in evaluation of thyroid masses, such as radionuclide thyroid imaging and thyroid ultrasonography.

Thyroid disorders

Thyroid dysfunction can cause several disorders, most commonly hyperthyroidism, hypothyroidism, thyroiditis, and goiter.

Hyperthyroidism, which affects females four times more often than males, results from excessive secretion of thyroid hormone. Conversely, *hypothyroidism* results from inadequate production of thyroid hormone. *Thyroiditis* may occur as an acute inflammation, as a subacute viral inflammation that generally subsides spontaneously, or as a chronic disorder (Hashimoto's disease). *Simple goiter* results from inadequate intake of iodine and tends to occur in certain geographic areas.

Benign adenomas and malignant tumors cause one-third of all thyroid enlargements. Well-encapsulated and noninvasive, a benign adenoma usually causes no symptoms until it grows large enough to cause respiratory distress by compressing the trachea. Malignant thyroid tumors are rare, accounting for fewer than 1% of all cancer deaths. However, large doses of radiation to the head and neck may predispose a person to develop thyroid nodules and cancer later in life, and prolonged thyroid-stimulating hormone production may lead to malignant transformation of benign adenomas.

Testing procedures

Measurement of serum hormone levels — primarily triiodothyronine (T_3) and thyroxine (T_4) — is usually the first step in thyroid evaluations. Abnormal hormone levels indicate the need for visualization of the thyroid gland to assess function and detect anatomic abnormalities. (See *Thyroid anatomy and physiology*, page 540.)

Thyroid tests can determine the thyroid gland's size, identify tumors or cysts, and measure the thyroid's ability to retain iodine (essential for thyroid hormone synthesis). Such tests, which often include the radioactive iodine uptake test, T_3 resin uptake study, radionuclide thyroid imaging, and thyroid ultrasonography, are commonly performed as part of a series to provide a complete analysis.

Radioactive iodine tests

Measuring thyroid uptake of radioactive iodine reflects the gland's ability to handle stable dietary iodine and allows direct evaluation of thyroid function. This measurement is especially significant in assessment of thyroid hyperfunction, thyrotoxicosis factitia, and subacute thyroiditis. In the radioactive iodine uptake test, the patient's thyroid is scanned at specific intervals after oral administration of a radioisotope of iodine (usually ^{131}I) to help determine the degree of iodine retention.

Three radioisotopes of iodine — ^{123}I, ^{125}I, and ^{131}I — are useful because they differ in terms of half-life and amount of radiation emitted. All are synthetic isotopes and are indistinguishable from the naturally occurring stable isotope, ^{127}I. All emit gamma radiation, which allows their external measurement in sites of concentration, such as the thyroid gland or aberrant thyroid tissue.

Radionuclide thyroid imaging

Thyroid imaging, which uses radionuclides to locate sites of radioactive iodine accumulation, is valuable in diagnosis and management of thyroid disease. In this test, the patient is given a radiopharmaceutical; then a gamma camera is placed near the anterior portion of his neck, where it assesses and processes the radioactivity of the radionuclide, producing a precise image of the thyroid gland.

Radionuclide thyroid imaging provides information on overall thyroid size and shape. More important, it can define areas of hyperfunction (hot spots) or hypofunction (cold spots) and is especially valuable in detecting cancer. Palpable nodules shown to be nonfunctioning may be malignant. Conversely, functioning nodules, particularly if they are more active than surrounding tissue, are unlikely to be malignant. Radionuclide thyroid imaging may also reveal substernal goiters; the location of ectopic thyroid tissue in the tongue, chest, or ovary; and functioning metastases of

Thyroid anatomy and physiology

The thyroid gland is located in the neck, just below the cricoid cartilage. Its two lateral lobes straddle the trachea, usually connected by an isthmus that crosses in front of the trachea. The right lobe is a bit larger and higher in the neck than the left. About 50% of people have a third, pyramidal lobe rising from the isthmus. Occasionally, this lobe is the site of a malignant tumor.

Visualization of the thyroid can determine abnormalities in gland size and ability to absorb iodine as well as the presence and quality of tumors and cysts. The parathyroid glands, two upper and two lower, sit behind the thyroid and are so closely involved in its tissue that they're often inadvertently removed during thyroid surgery, causing hypoparathyroidism.

Thyroid tissue is composed of follicles filled with colloid, a substance consisting primarily of an iodine-containing protein known as *thyroglobulin*. Normally, the thyroid weighs about 20 g, but certain disorders, such as goiter, can grossly enlarge it to more than several hundred grams.

The thyroid controls the body's metabolism primarily through the secretion of two hormones, *thyroxine* (T_4) and triiodothyronine (T_3). T_4 regulates body metabolism and helps control physical and mental development, resistance to infection, and vitamin requirements. Its production is regulated by release of thyroid-stimulating hormone, a pituitary hormone, and the ingestion of iodine and protein. T_4 may also be converted to T_3, a more potent hormone, by deiodination. T_3 is essential for maintaining metabolic rates in all cells. A third thyroid hormone, *thyrocalcitonin*, is a polypeptide whose function is limited to lowering plasma phosphate and calcium levels.

Anterior thyroid

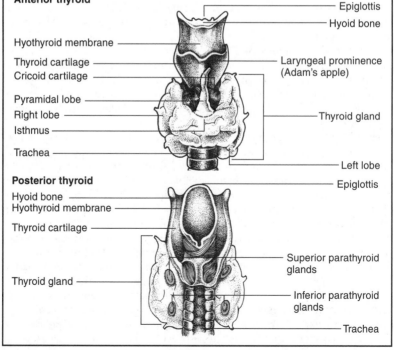

Epiglottis
Hyoid bone
Hyothyroid membrane
Thyroid cartilage
Cricoid cartilage
Laryngeal prominence (Adam's apple)
Pyramidal lobe
Right lobe
Isthmus
Thyroid gland
Trachea
Left lobe

Posterior thyroid
Epiglottis
Hyoid bone
Hyothyroid membrane
Thyroid cartilage
Superior parathyroid glands
Inferior parathyroid glands
Thyroid gland
Trachea

thyroid cancer. Accurate interpretation of thyroid imaging results requires careful correlation with findings on palpation.

Ultrasonography

Thyroid ultrasonography allows visualization of the thyroid gland through high-frequency sound waves that are converted to images on an oscilloscope screen. This test is especially useful for distinguishing cystic from solid thyroid nodules. When used during pregnancy, thyroid ultrasonography doesn't expose the fetus to radioactive materials.

Magnetic resonance imaging

A noninvasive procedure, magnetic resonance imaging (MRI) uses magnetic energy to obtain images of the posterior and substernal thyroid. This test helps to detect tumors or tissue abnormalities in these areas. Because the MRI scanner records magnetic signals and translates them into detailed pictures, this test involves no exposure to radiation.

SCANNING

Radioactive iodine uptake

The radioactive iodine uptake (RAIU) test evaluates thyroid function by measuring the amount of orally ingested ^{123}I or ^{131}I that accumulates in the thyroid gland after 6 and 24 hours. An external single counting probe measures the radioactivity in the thyroid as a percentage of the original dose, thus indicating the ability of the gland to trap and retain iodine.

This test accurately diagnoses hyperthyroidism (about 90%) but is less accurate for hypothyroidism. When performed concurrently with radionuclide thyroid imaging and the T_3 resin uptake test, the RAIU test helps differentiate Graves' disease from hyperfunctioning toxic adenoma. Indications for this test include abnormal results of chemical tests used to evaluate thyroid function (see Chapter 5).

Patients with suspected Hashimoto's disease may undergo the perchlorate suppression test in addition to the RAIU. (See *Perchlorate suppression test*, page 542.)

Purpose

- To evaluate thyroid function
- To aid diagnosis of hyperthyroidism or hypothyroidism
- To help distinguish between primary and secondary thyroid disorders (in combination with other tests).

Patient preparation

Explain to the patient that this test assesses thyroid function. Instruct him to fast from midnight before the test. Tell him that after he receives the radioactive iodine capsule or liquid, he'll be scanned 6 and 24 hours later to determine the amount of radioactive substance present in the thyroid gland — an indicator of thyroid function. Assure him that the test is painless and that the small amount of radiation used for the procedure is harmless.

Check the patient history for past or present iodine exposure, which may interfere with test results. If the patient previously had radiologic tests using contrast media or nuclear medicine procedures, or if he's currently receiving iodine preparations or thyroid medications, note this on the X-ray request.

Since the amount of iodine used in this test is similar to the amount obtained through dietary intake, a history

Perchlorate suppression test

This test is used to evaluate patients with suspected Hashimoto's disease or to demonstrate an enzyme deficiency within the thyroid gland. Because potassium perchlorate competes with and displaces the iodide ions that are not organified, this study can identify defects in the iodide organification process within the thyroid.

In this procedure, a small dose of radioactive iodine is administered orally. A radioactive iodine uptake test is performed 1 and 2 hours afterward. After the 2-hour uptake test, the patient receives 400 mg to 1 g of potassium perchlorate orally. Uptake tests are performed every 15 minutes for the first hour after the dose and then every 30 minutes for the next 2 to 3 hours.

The results of the uptake tests performed after administration of potassium perchlorate are compared with those of the 2-hour uptake test before perchlorate was administered. In a normal person, the uptake of radioactive iodine will not change significantly after administration of perchlorate. Patients with either Hashimoto's disease or an enzyme deficiency will experience a decrease in uptake. Those with an enzyme deficiency will experience a drop in their uptake of more than 15% after administration of perchlorate.

---

of iodine hypersensitivity is not considered a contraindication to the test.

Equipment
Oral dose of ^{123}I or ^{131}I (radiologist determines the exact dosage) + external single counting probe.

Procedure
At 6 and 24 hours after an oral dose of radioactive iodine is administered, the patient's thyroid is scanned by placing the anterior portion of his neck in front of an external single counting probe. The amount of radioactivity that the probe detects is compared to the amount in the original dose to determine the percentage of radioactive iodine retained by the thyroid.

Precautions
This test is contraindicated during pregnancy and lactation because of possible teratogenic effects.

Reference values
After 6 hours, 3% to 16% of the radioactive iodine should have accumulated in the thyroid; after 24 hours, 8% to 29%. The remaining radioactive iodine is excreted in the urine.

Local variations in the normal range of iodine uptake may stem from regional differences in dietary iodine intake or procedural differences among individual laboratories.

Implications of results
Below-normal percentages of iodine uptake may indicate hypothyroidism, subacute thyroiditis, or iodine overload. Above-normal percentages may indicate hyperthyroidism, early Hashimoto's disease, hypoalbuminemia, ingestion of lithium, or iodine-deficient goiter.

However, in hyperthyroidism, the rate of turnover may be so rapid that the 24-hour measurement appears falsely normal.

Post-test care

■ As ordered, instruct the patient to resume a light diet 2 hours after taking the oral dose of ^{123}I or ^{131}I.

■ After the study is complete, tell the patient to resume his normal diet.

Interfering factors

■ Renal failure, diuresis, severe diarrhea, X-ray contrast media studies, ingesting iodine preparations (including iodized salt, cough syrups, and some multivitamins), or using other drugs (thyroid hormones, thyroid hormone antagonists, salicylates, penicillins, antihistamines, anticoagulants, corticosteroids, and phenylbutazone) can decrease iodine uptake, thereby affecting the accuracy of test results.

■ An iodine-deficient diet or ingestion of phenothiazines can increase iodine uptake, affecting the accuracy of test results.

Radionuclide thyroid imaging

This test allows visualization of the thyroid gland by a gamma camera after administration of a radioisotope — usually ^{123}I, ^{131}I, or technetium Tc 99m (^{99m}Tc) pertechnetate. The first two radioisotopes are used most often because of their short half-lives (which limit exposure to radiation) and because of their ability to measure thyroid function.

Thyroid imaging is usually recommended after discovery of a palpable mass, enlarged gland, or asymmetrical goiter. This test is usually performed concurrently with measurement of serum triiodothyronine (T_3) and serum thyroxine (T_4) levels, and thyroid uptake

tests. Later, thyroid ultrasonography may be done.

Purpose

■ To assess the size, structure, and position of the thyroid gland

■ To evaluate thyroid function in conjunction with other thyroid tests.

Patient preparation

Explain to the patient that this test helps determine the cause of thyroid dysfunction. If he's scheduled to receive an oral dose of ^{123}I or ^{131}I, instruct him to fast from midnight the night before the test; he needn't fast if he's to receive an I.V. injection of ^{99m}Tc pertechnetate. Tell the patient that after he receives the radioisotope, his thyroid will be viewed with a gamma camera. Assure him that neither the radioisotope nor the equipment will expose him to dangerous radiation levels and that the actual imaging takes only 30 minutes.

Ask the patient if he has undergone tests that used radiographic contrast media within the past 60 days. Note such tests or the use of drugs that may interfere with iodine uptake on the X-ray request.

As ordered, 2 to 3 weeks before the test, discontinue administration of thyroid hormones, thyroid hormone antagonists, and iodine preparations (Lugol's solution, some multivitamins, and cough syrups). One week before the test, discontinue phenothiazines, corticosteroids, salicylates, anticoagulants, and antihistamines, as ordered. Also, instruct the patient to avoid ingesting iodized salt, iodinated salt substitutes, and seafood during this period, as ordered.

As ordered, give ^{123}I or ^{131}I orally. Alternatively, you or a laboratory technician may be asked to give ^{99m}Tc pertechnetate intravenously, depending on your training and the hospital's protocol. Record the date and the time of administration. The patient receiving an oral

T_3 thyroid suppression test

The T_3 (Cytomel) thyroid suppression test helps determine whether areas of excessive iodine uptake in the thyroid (hot spots) are autonomous (as in some cases of Graves' disease) or reflect pituitary overcompensation (as in iodine-deficient goiter). Autonomous hot spots function independently of pituitary control. However, hot spots caused by iodine deficiency stem from reduced T_4 production, which decreases T_3 production and increases thyroid-stimulating hormone (TSH) production. Increased TSH production, in turn, overstimulates the thyroid and causes excessive iodine uptake.

After a baseline reading of thyroid function is obtained by a radioactive iodine uptake (RAIU) test, 100 mcg of synthetic T_3 (Cytomel) is administered for 7 days. (Normally, T_3 acts through a negative feedback mechanism to suppress pituitary release of TSH; TSH suppression then suppresses thyroid function and iodine uptake.) During the last 2 days of Cytomel administration, RAIU tests are repeated to assess thyroid response.

Suppression of RAIU to at least 50% of baseline indicates that the hot spot is under pituitary control and suggests iodine deficiency as the cause of increased iodine uptake. Failure to suppress RAIU by 50% suggests autonomous thyroid hyperfunction, resulting perhaps from Graves' disease or a toxic thyroid nodule.

radioisotope should fast for another 2 hours after it's administered.

Equipment
Radionuclide solution (^{123}I or ^{131}I for oral administration or ^{99m}Tc pertechnetate for I.V. administration) ✦ scanning equipment ✦ gamma camera.

Procedure
The test is performed 24 hours after oral administration of ^{123}I or ^{131}I or 20 to 30 minutes after I.V. injection of ^{99m}Tc pertechnetate. Just before the test, tell the patient to remove his dentures and any jewelry that could interfere with visualization of the thyroid.

The patient's thyroid gland is palpated. Then, with the patient in a supine position and his neck extended, the gamma camera is placed over the anterior portion of his neck. The radioactive substance within the thyroid gland projects an image of the gland on an oscilloscope screen and X-ray film.

Three views of the thyroid are obtained: one straight-on anterior view and two bilateral oblique views.

Precautions
Radionuclide thyroid imaging is contraindicated during pregnancy and lactation.

Normal findings
Radionuclide thyroid imaging should reveal a thyroid gland that is about 2" (5 cm) long and 1" (2.5 cm) wide, with a uniform uptake of the radioisotope and without tumors. The gland should be butterfly-shaped, with the isthmus located at the midline. Occasionally, a third lobe called the pyramidal lobe may be present; this is a normal variant.

Implications of results
During radionuclide thyroid imaging, hyperfunctioning nodules (areas of excessive iodine uptake) appear as black regions called *hot spots*. The presence of

Thyroid imaging results in thyroid disorders

The chart below shows the characteristic findings in radionuclide imaging tests that are associated with various thyroid disorders as well as the possible causes of those disorders.

CONDITION	FINDINGS	CAUSES
Hypothyroidism	■ Glandular damage or absent gland	■ Surgical removal of gland ■ Inflammation ■ Radiation ■ Neoplasm (rare)
Hypothyroid goiter	■ Enlarged gland ■ Decreased uptake (of radioactive iodine) if glandular destruction is present ■ Increased uptake possible from congenital error in thyroxine synthesis	■ Insufficient iodine intake ■ Hypersecretion of thyroid stimulating hormone (TSH) caused by thyroid hormone deficiency
Myxedema (cretinism in children)	■ Normal or slightly reduced gland size ■ Uniform pattern ■ Decreased uptake	■ Defective embryonic development, resulting in congenital absence or underdevelopment of thyroid gland ■ Maternal iodine deficiency
Hyperthyroidism (Graves' disease)	■ Enlarged gland ■ Uniform pattern ■ Increased uptake	■ Unknown, but may be hereditary ■ Production of thyroid-stimulating immunoglobulins
Toxic nodular goiter	■ Multiple hot spots	■ Long-standing simple goiter
Hyperfunctioning adenomas	■ Solitary hot spot	■ Adenomatous production of triiodothyronine and thyroxine, suppressing TSH secretion and producing atrophy of other thyroid tissue
Hypofunctioning adenomas	■ Solitary cold spot	■ Cyst or nonfunctioning nodule
Benign multinodular goiter	■ Multiple nodules with variable or no function	■ Local inflammation ■ Degeneration
Thyroid carcinoma	■ Usually a solitary cold spot with occasional or no function	■ Neoplasm

hot spots requires a follow-up T_3 (Cytomel) thyroid suppression test to determine if the hyperfunctioning areas are autonomous. (See *T_3 thyroid suppression test* and *Thyroid imaging results in thyroid disorders*.)

Hypofunctioning nodules (areas of little or no iodine uptake) appear as

---

Parathyroid ultrasonography

On ultrasonography, the parathyroid glands appear as solid masses, 5 mm or smaller in size, with an echo pattern of less amplitude than thyroid tissue. Glandular enlargement is usually characteristic of tumor growth or of hyperplasia. Normally, on a scan, the parathyroid glands are indistinguishable from the nearby neurovascular bundle.

---

white or light gray regions called *cold spots*. If a cold spot appears, thyroid ultrasonography may be performed later to rule out cysts; in addition, fine-needle aspiration and biopsy of such nodules may be performed to rule out a malignant tumor.

Post-test care

▪ As ordered, resume administration of any medications that were discontinued before the test.
▪ Instruct the patient to resume his normal diet.

Interfering factors

▪ An iodine-deficient diet and use of phenothiazines increase uptake of radioactive iodine.
▪ Renal disease; ingestion of iodinized salt, iodine preparations, iodinated salt substitutes, or seafood; and use of thyroid hormones, thyroid hormone antagonists, aminosalicylic acid, corticosteroids, multivitamins, or cough syrups containing inorganic iodides decrease uptake of radioactive iodine. Severe diarrhea and vomiting can also decrease uptake by impairing GI absorption of radioiodine.

ULTRASONOGRAPHY

Thyroid ultrasonography

In this safe, noninvasive procedure, ultrasonic pulses are emitted from a piezoelectric crystal in a transducer, directed at the thyroid gland, and reflected back to the transducer. These pulses are then converted electronically to produce structural visualization on an oscilloscope screen.

When a mass is located by palpation or by thyroid imaging, thyroid ultrasonography can differentiate between a cyst and a tumor larger than $3/8''$ (1 cm) with about 85% accuracy. This test is particularly useful in the evaluation of thyroid nodules during pregnancy because it doesn't expose the fetus to the radioactive iodine used in other diagnostic procedures.

Ultrasonography can also be performed on the parathyroid glands. (See *Parathyroid ultrasonography.*)

Purpose

▪ To evaluate thyroid structure
▪ To differentiate between a cyst and a solid tumor
▪ To monitor the size of the thyroid gland during suppressive therapy.

Patient preparation

Describe the procedure to the patient, and explain that it defines the size and shape of the thyroid gland. Inform him that he needn't restrict food or fluids before the test. Tell him who will perform the procedure and where and that it takes approximately 30 minutes. Re-

How ultrasonography works

During ultrasonography, the technician guides a transducer over the pertinent area of the patient's body. The transducer sends an ultrasound beam, composed of sound waves, through the tissue. These sound waves travel at varying speeds, depending on the density of the tissue they're passing through. For example, sound waves travel through bone at 13,200' (4,000 m)/second; through muscle, at 5,230' (1,585 m)/second.

After passing through the tissue, the sound waves reflect back to the transducer, where they're converted into electrical impulses. Then these impulses are amplified and displayed on a screen. Because the densities of the cyst and tumor differ, sound waves pass through them at different speeds. The image on the display screen reflects this difference.

assure him that the procedure is painless and safe.

Equipment
Ultrasound equipment ✦ camera and film, or videotape ✦ water-soluble contact solution.

Procedure
The patient is placed in a supine position, with a pillow under his shoulder blades to hyperextend his neck. Next, his neck is coated with water-soluble gel. The transducer then scans the thyroid, projecting its echographic image on the oscilloscope screen. (See *How ultrasonography works.*) The image on the screen is photographed for subsequent examination. Accurate visualization of the anterior portion of the thyroid requires use of a short-focused transducer.

Precautions
None.

Normal findings
Thyroid ultrasonography should exhibit a uniform echo pattern throughout the gland.

Implications of results
Cysts appear as smooth-bordered, echo-free areas with enhanced sound transmission; adenomas and carcinomas appear either solid and well demarcated, with identical echo patterns, or — less frequently — solid, with cystic areas. Carcinoma infiltrating the gland may not be well demarcated.

Identification of a tumor is generally followed up by fine-needle aspiration or an excisional biopsy to determine malignancy.

Post-test care
Thoroughly clean the patient's neck to remove the contact solution.

Interfering factors
None.

SELECTED READINGS

Folio, L.R., et al. "Split-screen Contiguous Ultrasound Imaging," *Radiologic Technology* 66(4):255, March-April 1995.

Guyton, A.C., and Hall, J.E. *Textbook of Medical Physiology*, 9th ed. Philadelphia: W.B. Saunders Co., 1996.

Henry, J.B., ed. *Clinical Diagnosis and Management by Laboratory Methods*, 19th ed. Philadelphia: W.B. Saunders Co., 1996.

Isselbacher, K.J., et al., eds. *Harrison's Principles of Internal Medicine*, 13th ed. New York: McGraw-Hill Book Co., 1994.

"Lab Test Tips: Evaluating Thyroxine Levels," *Nursing95* 25(9):74, September 1995.

Ravel, R.A. *Clinical Laboratory Medicine: Clinical Application of Laboratory Data*, 6th ed. St. Louis: Mosby–Year Book, Inc., 1995.

Statland, B.E. "Thyroid Testing in the Sick Patient," *Medical Laboratory Observer* 26(12):9, December 1994.

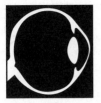

CHAPTER TWENTY-ONE

Eye

Learning objectives

After completing this chapter, the reader will be able to:
- explain the anatomy and physiology of the eye
- identify pertinent interview questions for a patient history
- describe a systematic approach to physical assessment of the eye
- define four common eye conditions related to age
- identify common ophthalmic abbreviations
- state the purpose of each test discussed in the chapter
- prepare the patient physically and psychologically for each test

- describe the procedure for performing each test
- specify appropriate precautions for safe administration of each test
- recognize signs of an adverse reaction and respond appropriately
- implement appropriate post-test care
- identify the normal findings of each test
- discuss the implications of abnormal test results
- list factors that may interfere with accurate test results.

INTRODUCTION

Tests to diagnose eye disorders fall into three categories. *Subjective tests,* such as visual acuity tests and the tangent screen examination, require oral responses from the patient that must be interpreted by the examiner. These tests need to be correlated with *objective tests,* such as tonometry and ophthalmoscopy, in which the examiner obtains measurements or directly visualizes the interior of the eye. When severe abnormalities result from ocular disease or trauma, the ophthalmologist can resort to *special procedures,* such as computed tomography. Understanding the diagnostic application and significance of these tests begins with review of the anatomic structure and physiology of the eye.

Outer layer

The cornea and sclera constitute the outermost portion of the eye's three layers. The *cornea,* a transparent structure composed of avascular tissue, lies in the anterior portion of the eye. It bends light rays that enter the eye and helps to focus the images on the retina. Adjoining the cornea is the *sclera,* an opaque, white, fibrous coat covering the posterior five-sixths of the eye through which nerves and blood vessels pass in order to penetrate the eye's interior.

Middle layer

The middle vascular layer, known as the *uveal tract,* consists of the iris, the ciliary body, and the choroid. The *iris,* the colored part of the eye, is composed of muscle fibers that regulate the amount of light admitted to the eye's interior through the pupil, the circular opening in its center. Behind the iris lies the *lens,* a biconvex, transparent structure that can change its shape to focus light rays precisely on the retina. The *ciliary body* produces aqueous humor and permits flexibility of the lens for clearer vision. The highly vascular and pigmented *choroid* supplies blood to the retina and conducts blood and nerve impulses to the eye's anterior structures.

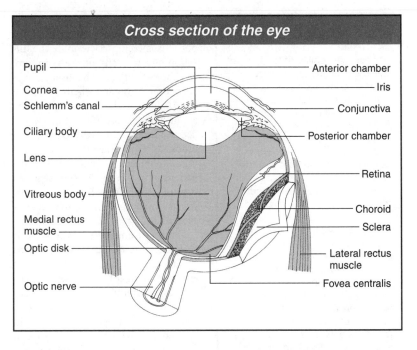

Cross section of the eye

Pupil — Anterior chamber
Cornea — Iris
Schlemm's canal — Conjunctiva
Ciliary body — Posterior chamber
Lens — Retina
Vitreous body — Choroid
Medial rectus muscle — Sclera
Optic disk — Lateral rectus muscle
Optic nerve — Fovea centralis

Inner layer

The third layer of the eye, the *retina,* consists of a complicated network of rods, cones, and other nerve cells lined with pigment epithelium. In the posterior portion of the retina lies the *fovea;* composed entirely of cones, the fovea is the area of most acute vision.

Chambers and their fluids

The iris forms a curtain that divides the space between the cornea and the lens into the anterior and posterior chambers of the eye. *Aqueous humor* secreted by the ciliary processes in the posterior chamber flows through the pupil into the anterior chamber. This fluid nourishes the internal eye structures and maintains constant pressure within the eyeball. Defective drainage of aqueous humor can increase intraocular pressure and eventually cause glaucoma.

The *vitreous body* is surrounded by the retina and the optic nerve and constitutes four-fifths of the back of the eye.

It is filled with *vitreous humor* — a clear, avascular, gelatinous substance. Vitreous humor helps maintain the transparency and shape of the eye. (See *Cross section of the eye.*)

How the eye moves

The eye rests on a cushion of fat within its bony orbit, which also contains the eye's appendages — eyelids, lacrimal system, and conjunctiva. Six extraocular muscles attached to the sclera control the movements of the eyeball. Although each has at least one specific action, these muscles never act independently. Complex muscular interactions allow the eyes to move in different directions and make possible coordinated use of both eyes.

Progressive change

The eye is a dynamic organ that changes progressively throughout life. Because the elasticity of the lens greatly affects its ability to change its shape, changes

Presbyopia

Normally, the ability of the lens to change its shape and to accommodate to focus on objects closer than 20' (6 m) gradually decreases with age. This process, known as presbyopia, is so inexorable that determination of the convex lens strength needed for correction can usually be estimated on the basis of age. Even a patient with normal vision eventually needs the aid of lenses for close work.

Presbyopia usually begins between ages 42 and 47 and progresses steadily, so a 75-year-old patient requires a stronger correction than a 45-year-old patient.

Because presbyopia is a normal part of aging, failure to wear corrective lenses doesn't affect its progression. However, after correction, a patient should be reexamined every 1 to 2 years because he'll probably need new lenses at such intervals.

in visual acuity from adolescence to adulthood are quite common, as the lens becomes increasingly less elastic.

Presbyopia, impaired near vision caused by loss of the natural elasticity of the lens, occurs commonly in middle age. This disorder often requires the use of reading glasses. (See *Presbyopia*.) In older persons, eye tissue may degenerate and seriously affect vision, especially in those with chronic diseases such as diabetes. *Cataracts* — degenerative clouding of the lens — commonly afflict elderly patients.

Examination

A thorough eye examination begins with a patient history, including documentation of medical conditions and eye surgery. Identify the patient's chief complaint, such as discharge, pain, itch-

ing, blurred vision, blind spots, vertigo, difficulty in distinguishing color, or poor visual acuity. Determine the duration and intensity of the symptom. Ask the patient about his occupation's effect on his eyes and whether he's had facial pain or headaches. In addition, ask about systemic diseases that may cause ocular changes, such as diabetes, thyroid problems, hypertension, and acquired immunodeficiency syndrome. Note the patient's current medication regimen because many drugs have ophthalmic effects. Tailor questions to the patient's age and ability.

The next step in the examination is visual acuity testing, using standardized vision charts such as the Snellen chart and the Jaeger card. After assessing acuity, look for clinical features, such as redness, excessive tearing or blinking, displacement of the eye within the orbit, and asymmetry of ocular and facial structures. External examination assesses pupillary light reflexes, inspects anterior segments, and evaluates extraocular muscle function and ocular alignment. The interior structures of the eye are inspected with an ophthalmoscope and a slit-lamp biomicroscope. Tonometry, which measures intraocular pressure, is done to diagnose glaucoma. (See *Common ophthalmic abbreviations.*)

Observe the patient's appearance and posture. Odd clothing combinations may indicate a color vision defect. Be alert to nonverbal behavior, such as squinting or abnormal eye movements. Head tilting may signal that the patient is compensating for a defect (for example, to focus double images into one image). Extend your hand as the patient approaches you to check depth perception.

Abnormalities detected by routine procedures may require more refined tests. Suspected abnormalities can often be located more precisely with orbital radiography, computed tomography, or

Common ophthalmic abbreviations

When recording the patient's responses during eye examinations, use the following ophthalmic abbreviations.

AC	anterior chamber	**OS**	left eye *(oculus sinister)*
c̅c̅	with spectacles	**OU**	both eyes *(oculi uter-*
CF	count fingers (visual		*que)*
	acuity)	**PERRLA**	pupils equal, round,
EOM	extraocular muscles		reactive to light, and
HM	hand motion (visual		accommodation
	acuity)	**PH**	pinhole
IOP	intraocular pressure	**s̅c̅**	without spectacles
LP	light perception	**VF**	visual field
NLP	no light perception	Δ	prism diopters
NPC	near point of conver-	**D**	lens diopters
	gence	**(+)**	convex lens
OD	right eye *(oculus dexter)*	**(–)**	concave lens

ocular ultrasonography (or a combination of these tests).

Nursing considerations

In several routine tests, the doctor may request ophthalmic drugs. *Cycloplegics* cause paralysis of accommodation and are often required before refraction. *Mydriatics* cause pupillary dilation and are commonly used to inspect intraocular structures. Generally, two instillations are required to induce maximum mydriasis. To help prevent contamination, avoid touching the eye dropper to the eye or lids during instillation.

 Never instill dilating drops in a patient who has, or is suspected of having, angle-closure glaucoma. In such a patient, pupillary dilation could trigger an acute attack of angle closure.

To ensure the patient's cooperation during an eye examination, provide a thorough explanation of each test and reassure him that the procedures are painless. These measures are essential with tests that require subjective responses from the patient.

The first section of this chapter deals with subjective tests; the second section focuses on objective tests. The final section covers definitive diagnostic procedures that are usually performed in a hospital or radiology department.

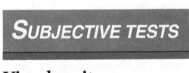

SUBJECTIVE TESTS

Visual acuity

Part of a routine eye examination, a visual acuity test evaluates the patient's ability to distinguish the form and detail of an object. In this test, the patient is asked to read letters on a standardized visual chart, known as the Snellen chart, from a distance of 20' (6 m). Charts showing the letter E in various positions and sizes are used for young children and other people who can't read. The smaller the symbol the patient can identify, the sharper his visual acuity. A patient's near, or reading, vision may be tested as well, using a standardized chart such as the Jaeger card.

The Snellen test should be performed on all patients with eye complaints. It's also performed by doctors and by school or occupational health nurses on people who have no complaints. Near-vision testing is routine for those complaining of eyestrain or reading difficulty and for everyone over age 40. Results serve as a baseline for treatments, follow-up examinations, and referrals.

Purpose
- To test distance and near visual acuity
- To identify refractive errors in vision.

Patient preparation
Explain to the patient that these tests evaluate distant and near vision and take only a few minutes. If he wears glasses, tell him to bring them with him.

Equipment
Standardized eye charts (Snellen chart or E chart to test distance visual acuity; Jaeger card to test near visual acuity) ✦ occlusion supplies (handheld occluder, disposable tissues for insertion between patient's eyes and glasses [particularly useful for geriatric or pediatric patients who can't or won't use a handheld occluder], or disposable eyepatches) ✦ standard 20' (6 m) room or equipment to simulate correct distance (such as mirrors or chart with proportionately reduced letters) ✦ illumination (10 to 30 footcandles).

Procedure
For distance visual acuity: Have the patient sit 20' (6 m) away from the eye chart. If he's wearing glasses, tell him to remove them so his uncorrected vision can be tested first. Begin with the right eye, unless vision in the left eye is known to be more acute. Have the patient occlude the left eye and then read the smallest line of letters he can see on the chart. Encourage him to try to read lines he can't see clearly, because intelligent guesses usually indicate the patient can recognize some of the symbols' details.

Visual acuity is reported as a fraction: The numerator is the distance from the chart, and the denominator is the distance at which a normal eye can read this line. Record the number of the smallest line the patient can read as the denominator. If he makes an error on a line, record the results with a minus number. For example, if the patient reads the 20/40 line but makes one error, record his vision as 20/40–1. If he reads the 20/40 line and one symbol on the following line, record his vision as 20/40+1.

Have the patient occlude the right eye, and repeat the test with the left eye. However, to minimize recall, use a different set of symbols or have the patient read the lines backward.

If the patient wears glasses, test his corrected vision using the same procedure. If he normally wears glasses but doesn't have them with him, note this on the test results. In recording the patient's responses, indicate which eye was tested and whether it was tested with or without correction.

If the patient can't read the largest letter on the chart, further testing is necessary to determine what he can see. (See *Special procedures for testing vision.*)

For near visual acuity: Have the patient remove his glasses and occlude the left eye. Ask him to read the Jaeger card (a card with print in graded sizes) at his customary reading distance. Test both eyes with and without corrective lenses. In reporting near visual acuity, specify both the size of the smallest print legible to the patient and the nearest distance at which reading is possible.

Precautions
None.

Special procedures for testing vision

The following additional tests may be performed if the patient can't identify the largest letter on the Snellen chart:

■ *Pinhole test:* If the patient's visual acuity is less than 20/20, perform the pinhole test to determine whether reduced visual acuity is due to refractive error or organic disease. In this test, the patient is asked to look through a pinhole in the center of a disk at the visual acuity chart; the same effect can be achieved by punching a pinhole in a card. Looking through the tiny opening eliminates peripheral light rays and improves the patient's vision if impairment is due to refractive error. If impairment results from organic disease, vision fails to improve.

■ *Changing the distance:* If the patient can't identify the largest letter or symbol on the chart (line 20/200), tell him to walk toward the chart until he can correctly identify it. Record the distance at which the patient can identify the symbol as the numerator. For example, 2/200 means the patient can identify at 2' (60 cm) a symbol that a person with normal vision can identify at 200' (60 m).

■ *Counting fingers:* If the patient can't identify the largest symbol at any distance, hold up your fingers at various distances in front of his eyes. When the patient correctly identifies the number of fingers in front of him, note the distance — for example, 4'/CF.

■ *Hand motion:* If the patient can't identify the number of fingers at any distance, wave your hand in front of his eyes at various distances. If he can detect hand movement, note the distance — for example, 2'/HM.

■ *Light projection:* If the patient can't identify hand motion at any distance, darken the room, and tell him to look straight ahead. Shine a penlight in each quadrant — nasal, temporal, superior, and inferior — of each eye. Note in which quadrants the patient can perceive light — for example, light projection/superior and nasal quadrants.

■ *Light perception:* If the patient can't perceive light projection at all, ask if he can tell whether the light is on or off. If the patient has no light perception, note "NLP"; otherwise, note that light perception exists.

Normal findings

Most charts for distance visual acuity are read at 20' (6 m). If the patient's vision is normal, results are expressed as 20/20, which means that the smallest symbol he can identify at 20' is the same symbol the normal eye can identify from the same distance.

The normal value for near visual acuity is 14/14, where the first 14 represents the distance in inches and the second 14 represents the correct identification of symbols that a person with normal vision can identify at 14" (35 cm).

Implications of results

People who can read the 20/20 line on the Snellen chart are considered to have normal distance visual acuity. If the denominator is more than 20, the patient's visual acuity is less than normal. For example, 20/40 vision means the patient reads at 20' (6 m) what a person with normal vision can read at 40' (12 m). A patient with 20/200 visual acuity or less in the best corrected eye is considered legally blind.

If the denominator is less than 20, the patient's distance visual acuity is better than normal. For example, 20/15 vision means the patient reads at 20' what a person with normal visual acuity can see at 15' (4.5 m).

Normal near visual acuity is usually recorded as 14/14 because standard testing charts, like the Jaeger card, are typically held 14" (35 cm) from the patient's eyes. Decreased near visual acuity is indicated by a larger denominator. For example, 14/20 near vision means the patient reads at 14" what a person with normal vision reads at 20" (50 cm). Most charts aren't designed to measure better-than-normal near vision.

Patients with less-than-normal visual acuity require further testing, including refraction and a complete ophthalmologic examination to determine whether visual loss is due to injury, disease, or a need for corrective lenses.

Normal or better-than-normal visual acuity doesn't necessarily indicate normal vision, however. For example, a visual field defect may be present if the patient consistently misses the letters on one side of all the lines. A field defect is certainly present if the patient states that one or more of the letters disappears or becomes illegible when he is looking at a nearby letter. Such findings indicate the need for further visual field testing, such as the Amsler grid test and the tangent screen examination.

Post-test care
None.

Interfering factors
■ The patient's failure to cooperate or to bring his glasses to the examination will interfere with test results.
■ If the patient's glasses were improperly prescribed or are outdated in their degree of correction, he may have better visual acuity without them.

Amsler grid

Composed of a central black dot and horizontal and vertical lines that form 5-mm squares, the Amsler grid helps detect central scotomas — blind or partially blind spots in the macular area of the retina. The macula is responsible for the central visual field and has the greatest visual acuity of any retinal segment. The Amsler grid test can also detect microscopic areas of macular or perimacular edema that cause visual distortions. However, because this test is only a screening procedure, it must be supplemented with other tests, such as ophthalmoscopy, visual field testing, and fluorescein angiography, to determine the cause of abnormal vision.

Purpose
■ To detect central scotomas
■ To evaluate the stability or progression of macular disease.

Patient preparation
Explain to the patient that this test evaluates his central field of vision and takes 5 to 10 minutes to perform. If he normally wears corrective lenses, instruct him to keep them on during the test.

Equipment
Amsler grid ◆ occlusion supplies (handheld occluder, disposable tissues for insertion between the patient's eyes and glasses, or disposable eyepatches).

Procedure
Occlude one of the patient's eyes. Hold the Amsler grid at his customary reading distance, approximately 11" to 12" (28 to 30 cm) in front of the unoccluded eye. Tell the patient to stare at the central dot on the Amsler grid; then ask these questions:

Amsler grid: Normal and abnormal views

On the left is a normal view of an Amsler grid. On the right is an Amsler grid as it might look to a patient with a central scotoma due to a macular hole. The center dot is entirely absent, as are the lines around it. The lines of the periphery of the scotoma appear bowed in an asymmetrical pattern.

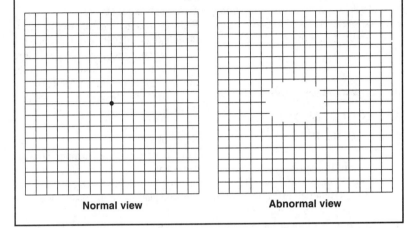

Normal view   **Abnormal view**

- Can you see the black dot in the center?
- When you look directly at the dot, can you see all four sides of the grid? All the little squares?
- Do all the lines appear ruler-straight?
- Is there any blurring, distortion, or movement?

If the patient answers yes to any of these questions, ask him to elaborate. Give him a pencil and paper, and encourage him to outline and describe the specific areas that appear distorted.

After recording the patient's observations, occlude the other eye and repeat the procedure.

Precautions
- Remind the patient to keep his unoccluded eye fixed on the central black dot on the grid.
- Perform this test with the patient's pupils undilated, before examining the fundus or conducting the refraction test.

Normal findings
The patient should be able to see the central black dot and, while staring at the dot, all four sides of the grid and all the little squares. All the lines should appear ruler-straight. He should not see any blurring, distortion, or missing squares. (See *Amsler grid: Normal and abnormal views.*)

Implications of results
Inability to see the black dot in the center of the grid suggests a central scotoma. If any of the lines do not appear ruler-straight to the patient, metamorphopsia (distorted perception of objects) may be indicated. Blurring, distortion, or movement may signal an imminent scotoma. Abnormal findings indicate the need for further evaluation by ophthalmoscopy, visual field testing, and fluorescein angiography.

Post-test care
None.

Interfering factors

- The patient's inability to see the Amsler grid because of poor eyesight or failure to cooperate or to keep his unoccluded eye fixed on the central dot will interfere with test results.
- Bleaching of the retina with the bright light of a retinoscope or an ophthalmoscope before the test will impair the patient's ability to see the Amsler grid.

Tangent screen examination

The area within which objects can be seen as the eye fixates on a central point is called the visual field. It consists of a central field — a 25-degree area surrounding the fixation point — and a peripheral field — the remainder of the area within which objects can be visualized. The tangent screen examination evaluates a patient's central visual field through systematic movement of a test object across a tangent screen, usually a piece of black felt with concentric circles and lines radiating from a central fixation point, much like a spider web.

Monocular visual field examinations are important in detecting and following the progression of ocular diseases, such as glaucoma and optic neuritis. They are also used to detect and evaluate neurologic disorders, such as brain tumors and cerebrovascular accidents. Localization of a specific visual field defect often points to the underlying pathology. However, the tangent screen examination provides only a general evaluation of the patient's visual field, however. Abnormal findings warrant further examination with a perimeter to evaluate areas of the peripheral visual field. (Perimeters are used almost exclusively by ophthalmologists.) Another test that can assess visual field is the confrontation test. (See *Confrontation test.*)

Purpose

- To detect central visual field loss and evaluate its progression or regression.

Patient preparation

Explain to the patient that this test evaluates his central field of vision and takes about 30 minutes to perform. Reassure him that it causes no pain but requires his full cooperation. If he normally wears corrective lenses, tell him to wear them during the test.

Equipment

Tangent screen ✦ black-tipped straight pins ✦ handheld occluder, disposable tissues for insertion between the patient's eyes and glasses, or disposable eyepatches ✦ test objects (usually 1- to 10-mm objects that can be inserted into a black wand) ✦ visual field recording charts ✦ stick or other object (to assist the patient in signaling).

Procedure

Have the patient sit comfortably about 3' (1 m) from the tangent screen so that the eye being tested is directly in line with the central fixation target on the screen. Occlude the patient's left eye, and tell him that while he fixates on the central target, you'll move a test object into his visual field. The test object is white on one side and black on the other; its diameter varies in size from 1 to 10 mm, depending on the patient's visual acuity (for example, if he has 20/20 vision, the test object should have a diameter of 1 mm).

Tell him not to look for the test object, but to wait for it to appear and then to signal when he sees it. Stand to the side of the eye being tested. Move the test object inward from the periphery of the screen at 30-degree intervals, as represented by the radiating lines on the

Confrontation test

If a tangent screen or perimeter isn't available, or if the patient can't cooperate for other tests, use this simple method to evaluate the visual field. Sit about 2' (60 cm) from the patient, directly in front of him, and test his right eye first. Have him occlude his left eye, and tell him to look at your right eye and maintain fixation during the test. Explain that you'll hold up fingers or a fist in various positions. When he sees your hand, he should tell you what he can see — a fist or the number of fingers. Instruct him not to look for your hand, but to stare at your eye and signal when your hand appears.

Occlude your right eye. In each quadrant, hold up your hand midway between yourself and the patient. Move it from nonseeing to seeing areas. Alternate between presenting fingers and a fist. You and the patient should see your hand at the same time, and the patient should correctly identify what you're presenting.

If the patient responds correctly in all quadrants, present fingers on both sides of fixation to test horizon-tal, vertical, and oblique meridians. If the patient responds correctly, wiggle the index finger of each hand in the horizontal, vertical, and oblique meridians, and ask the patient if one finger is clearer than the other. If the patient reports that both fingers appear equally clear, occlude and fixate the opposite eyes, and repeat the procedure to test the left visual field.

However, if the patient reports that one finger is clearer than the other, you'll need to pinpoint the questionable area. To do this, simultaneously hold fingers above and below the area, and ask the patient which finger he sees better. Then proceed to test the other eye. If any areas of the visual field remain questionable, the patient should be tested with a tangent screen or a perimeter.

Although the confrontation test is a simple means of screening a patient's visual field for gross abnormalities, it can't replace quantitative methods of evaluation. Also, the examiner's own visual field must be normal to produce valid test results.

---

screen. Using black-tipped straight pins, plot the points on the screen at which the patient can see the object. When connected, these points define areas of equal visual acuity. The boundaries of a visual field for a specific target size and distance is called an isopter. To guarantee the adequacy of fixation, the blind spot (projection of optic nerve into the visual field) should be clearly identified.

After the boundaries of the patient's central visual field have been plotted, test how well he can see within his visual field. To do this, turn the test object to the black side. Then turn it over within each 30-degree interval, and ask the

patient to signal when he sees the test object. Plot suspicious areas — those in which the patient has failed to identify the test object — for size, shape, and density. Record the patient's visual field on the recording chart, marked in degrees, and note any abnormal areas within the field.

Because isopters vary with the patient's age, visual acuity, and pupil size; the size and color of the test object; and the distance between the patient and the screen, careful recording of all measurements is essential.

Occlude the patient's right eye, and repeat the test.

Complete bitemporal hemianopia

These illustrations show the results of an examination of the peripheral visual field with a perimeter. The heavy black line encloses the normal visual field. The white area within it represents the limited visual field in a person with complete bitemporal hemianopia, a serious eye disorder that's usually caused by lesions of the optic chiasm.

Left eye   **Right eye**

Precautions

Remind the patient that he must maintain fixation on the central target on the tangent screen; watch his eyes carefully to make sure he is following your instructions.

Normal findings

The central visual field normally forms a circle, extending 25 degrees superiorly, nasally, inferiorly, and temporally. The physiologic blind spot lies 12 to 15 degrees temporal to the central fixation point, approximately 1.5 degrees below the horizontal meridian. It extends approximately 7.5 degrees in height and 5.5 degrees in width. The test object should be visible throughout the patient's entire central visual field, except within the physiologic blind spot.

Implications of results

Visual field defects appear in a variety of forms and may arise from many causes. For example, inability to see the test object within the temporal half of the central visual field may indicate bitemporal hemianopia. Lesions of the optic chiasm (commonly caused by pituitary tumor), craniopharyngiomas in the young, and meningiomas or aneurysm of the circle of Willis in adults can cause bitemporal hemianopia. (See *Complete bitemporal hemianopia.*) Hemianopia may also occur after a cerebrovascular accident (CVA). Although bilateral homonymous hemianopia is uncommon, it may follow multiple thrombosis in the posterior cerebral circulation. Plotting visual fields after a CVA helps to locate cerebrovascular lesions.

When a disease, such as glaucoma, involves the optic nerve, an enlarged blind spot, a central scotoma, or a centrocecal scotoma may result. A ring scotoma (a scotoma 10 or more degrees away from the fixation point) is characteristic of retinitis pigmentosa, a slowly progressive disease that leads to night blindness. The peripheral area beyond this ring is usually spared. Retinal detachments can be outlined as well.

Repeat tangent screen examinations can help evaluate progression or regression of a diagnosed disorder.

Post-test care
None.

Interfering factors
If the patient is uncooperative or has severe loss of vision that causes him to have difficulty seeing even the largest test object, the test results will be invalid.

Color vision

The human eye perceives color through the cones of the retina, which are also responsible for central visual acuity. The most widely accepted theories of color vision propose that these retinal cones contain three different photosensitive pigments, each of which absorbs light of different wavelengths. Specifically, these pigments are sensitive to red, green, and blue — the primary colors of light. Mixtures of these three pigments allow perception of other colors.

Color vision tests assess the ability to recognize differences in color. They're commonly used to evaluate patients with suspected retinal disease or with a family history of color vision deficiency. A color vision deficiency may be inherited — a sex-linked recessive trait affecting approximately 8% to 10% of males and less than 1% of females —

or acquired as a result of disease. These tests are also used to screen applicants for jobs in which accurate color perception is vital, as in the military and electronics fields.

The most common color vision tests use pseudoisochromatic plates made up of dot patterns of the primary colors superimposed on backgrounds of randomly mixed colors. A patient with normal color vision can identify the dot pattern; a patient with a color vision deficiency can't distinguish between the pattern and the background. Basic color vision tests merely indicate the presence of a deficiency; more sophisticated tests can determine the degree of deficiency.

Purpose
■ To detect color vision deficiency.

Patient preparation
Explain to the patient that this test evaluates color perception, takes only a few minutes, and causes no pain. If he normally wears glasses or contact lenses, tell him to wear them during the test.

Equipment
Color vision test kit (Hardy-Rand-Rittler [H-R-R] or Ishihara pseudoisochromatic plates) ◆ occlusion supplies (handheld occluder, disposable tissues for insertion between the patient's eyes and glasses, or disposable eyepatches) ◆ pointer (an artist's paintbrush is recommended because secretions from the patient's fingertip may discolor the plates).

Procedure
After seating the patient comfortably, occlude one of his eyes. Hold the test book approximately 14" (35 cm) in front of his unoccluded eye, and give him the pointer.

Explain to the patient what patterns or symbols he may see. Show him the sample plates — which can be deciphered by most patients — and tell him you'll ask him to identify the symbols and then to trace them with the pointer. Inform him that some symbols are more difficult to see than others.

Conduct the test, eliciting immediate responses from the patient. Record the responses according to the instructions included with the test kit. When testing the other eye (or repeating the test, if necessary), rotate the plates 90 to 180 degrees to minimize recall.

Precautions
To prevent discoloration of the plates, keep the test book closed when it isn't being used and turn the pages by their edges.

Normal findings
A person with normal color vision — a trichromat — can identify all the patterns or symbols.

Implications of results
A patient with deficient color vision — an anomalous trichromat — can't identify all the patterns or symbols. This deficiency may be diagnosed more precisely by noting the combinations of colors that elicit incorrect responses. For example, *protanopia* is a deficiency of the retinal cone pigment that is sensitive to red. A patient with protanopia has difficulty discriminating between red/green and blue/green. A patient with *deuteranopia*, a deficiency of the retinal pigment sensitive to green, can't distinguish between green/purple and red/purple. *Tritanopia*, a deficiency of the pigment sensitive to blue, causes the patient to have difficulty discriminating between blue/green and yellow/green.

Achromatopsia — true color blindness — is a rare disease inherited as a Mendelian autosomal dominant or autosomal recessive trait. Patients with achromatopsia, called monochromats,

see all colors as shades of gray. These patients may also have impaired visual acuity, nystagmus, and photophobia due to reduced or absent cone function.

Inherited color deficiency affects both eyes; acquired deficiency may affect only one eye. Patients with acquired deficiencies may complain of inability to recognize colors that were formerly recognizable.

Abnormalities of the ocular media, retina, or optic nerve can cause deficient color vision. For this reason, a patient with an acquired color vision deficiency or an inherited deficiency accompanied by a loss of visual acuity should be referred for a complete ophthalmologic examination to determine the source of the deficiency.

Post-test care
None.

Interfering factors
- Failure to cooperate, inability to see the plates because of reduced visual acuity or failure to wear glasses, or improper lighting will affect test results.
- Errors in the testing procedure, such as inaccurately recording the patient's responses or allowing too much time for a response, will alter test results.

Refraction

Refraction — the bending of light rays by the cornea, aqueous humor, lens, and vitreous humor in the eye — enables images to focus on the retina and directly affects visual acuity. This test, done routinely during a complete eye examination or whenever a patient complains of a change in vision, defines the refractive error and determines the degree of correction required to improve visual

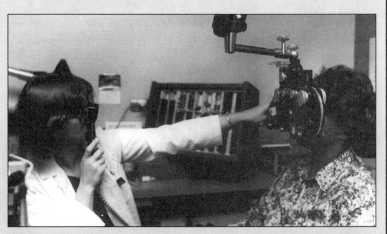

The ophthalmologist uses the retinoscope to project a beam of light into the eye of a patient wearing trial lens glasses. By manipulating the retinoscope beam, the ophthalmologist can illuminate retinal movement and test optic refraction.

acuity with corrective lenses. The ophthalmologist generally performs a refraction both objectively, by using a retinoscope, and subjectively, by asking the patient about his visual acuity while placing trial lenses before his eyes.

Purpose

■ To diagnose refractive error and prescribe corrective lenses, if necessary.

Patient preparation

Explain to the patient that this test helps determine whether he needs corrective lenses. Tell him eyedrops may be instilled to dilate the pupils and that the test takes 10 to 20 minutes. Reassure him that the test is painless and safe.

Check the patient's history for angle-closure glaucoma. Also check for previous use of and hypersensitivity to dilating eyedrops.

Equipment

Retinoscope ✦ trial lens set ✦ cycloplegic eyedrops ✦ Snellen chart ✦ occlusion supplies (handheld occluder, disposable

tissues for insertion between the patient's eyes and glasses, or disposable eyepatches).

Procedure

After cycloplegic eyedrops are administered (if ordered), the examiner directs the light of the retinoscope at the pupillary opening. Through the aperture at the top of the instrument, he looks for an orange glow — the retinoscopic, or red, reflex, which represents the reflection of light from the retinoscope — and notes its brightness, clarity, and uniformity. Moving the retinoscope's light across the pupil, he observes the reflex for any movement. The examiner then places trial lenses before the patient's eyes and adjusts the lens power to make the reflex clear, bright, and uniform and to neutralize its motion. The lens power necessary to make this adjustment is recorded.

Objective findings can be refined by altering the trial lenses and having the patient read lines on a standardized visual chart. This helps determine which

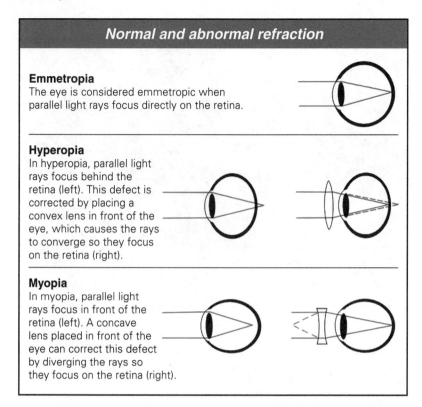

Normal and abnormal refraction

Emmetropia
The eye is considered emmetropic when parallel light rays focus directly on the retina.

Hyperopia
In hyperopia, parallel light rays focus behind the retina (left). This defect is corrected by placing a convex lens in front of the eye, which causes the rays to converge so they focus on the retina (right).

Myopia
In myopia, parallel light rays focus in front of the retina (left). A concave lens placed in front of the eye can correct this defect by diverging the rays so they focus on the retina (right).

---

lens or combination of lenses provides the best correction of his visual acuity.

Precautions

 Don't administer dilating eyedrops to a patient who has angle-closure glaucoma or to any patient who has had a hypersensitivity reaction to such drops.

Normal findings

Refractive power, measured in diopters, is greatest at the cornea (approximately 44 diopters) because of its curvature. The aqueous humor has the same refractive power as the cornea and is considered to be the same medium. The lens, normally a convex structure, has a refractive power of approximately 10 to 14 diopters but can alter this power by changing its shape. This phenomenon is known as accommodation and occurs when the eye views objects closer than 20' (6 m).

The vitreous humor, a gelatinous medium, has little refractive power and mainly transmits light. In the absence of accommodation, the average refractive power of the human eye is 58 diopters.

Ideally, the eyes have no refractive error (emmetropia). Parallel light rays emanating from a point source can be focused directly on the retina to produce a clear image.

Implications of results

Most patients show some degree of refractive error (ametropia). *Hyperopia,* or farsightedness, occurs when the eyeball is too short and parallel light rays focus behind the retina. Examination with the retinoscope shows a red reflex moving in the same direction as the retinoscope's light. A patient with hyperopia sees clearly at a distance but experiences blurring of near objects.

Myopia, or nearsightedness, occurs when the eyeball is too long and parallel light rays focus in front of the retina. Retinoscopic examination reveals reflex motion opposite to movement of the retinoscope's light. A patient with myopia sees near objects clearly but experiences blurring of distant images. (See *Normal and abnormal refraction.*)

When light rays entering the eye are not refracted uniformly and a clear focal point on the retina is not attained, the patient has *astigmatism.* This disorder is usually caused by unequal curvature of the cornea and is typically associated with some degree of hyperopia or myopia.

Post-test care
If corrective lenses are prescribed, advise the patient that images may appear blurred the first time he wears the lenses but eventually his eyes will adjust to the prescription. If the patient has worn glasses or contact lenses previously, tell him to wear only his new prescription lenses, since changing back and forth from the old prescription to the new one will prevent his eyes from making the required adjustment to the new lenses.

Interfering factors
Inadequate paralysis of accommodation or pupil dilation or the patient's failure to cooperate with the test will interfere with test results.

OBJECTIVE TESTS

Exophthalmometry

This test determines the relative forward protrusion of the eye from its orbit by using an exophthalmometer to measure the distance from the apex of the cornea to the lateral orbital margin. The exophthalmometer is a horizontal calibrated bar with movable carriers on both sides. These carriers hold mirrors inclined at a 45-degree angle that reflect both the scale readings and the corneal apex in profile.

Exophthalmometry provides information that's useful in detecting and evaluating thyroid disease, tumors of the eye, and any condition that displaces the eye in the orbit.

Purpose
■ To measure the amount of forward protrusion of the eye
■ To evaluate the progression or regression of exophthalmos.

Patient preparation
Explain to the patient that this test determines the degree of eye protrusion.

Equipment
Exophthalmometer.

Procedure
Ask the patient to sit upright facing you, with his eyes on the same level as yours. Hold the horizontal bar of the exophthalmometer in front of the patient's eyes, parallel to the floor. Move the device's two small concave carriers against the lateral orbital margins, and carefully record the calibrated bar reading. This baseline reading should be used during follow-up examinations. If the patient has already been measured with an ex-

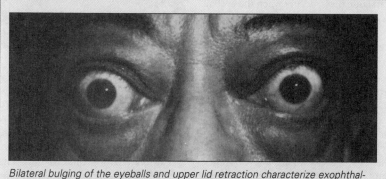

Bilateral bulging of the eyeballs and upper lid retraction characterize exophthalmos, which usually results from a thyroid disorder. Exophthalmometry evaluates the severity of exophthalmos.

ophthalmometer, set the calibrated bar at the baseline reading. Tighten the locking screws on the mirrors to keep them properly positioned.

Measure each eye separately. First, instruct the patient to fixate his right eye on your left eye. Using the inclined mirrors, superimpose the apex of the right cornea on the millimeter scale, and record the reading, which represents the eye's relative forward displacement from its orbit. Then tell the patient to fixate his left eye on your right eye, and repeat the procedure.

Precautions
For follow-up examinations, set the calibrated bar at the baseline reading.

Reference values
Normally, readings range from 12 to 20 mm. Measurements for each eye are similar, usually differing by 1.5 mm or less and rarely by more than 3 mm.

Implications of results
A difference between the eyes of more than 3 mm may indicate exophthalmos or enophthalmos. A single reading that exceeds 20 mm may indicate exophthalmos; readings under 12 mm may indicate enophthalmos.

A patient with exophthalmos should receive a thorough ophthalmologic examination, since the underlying cause may be local in origin. Any mass in the orbital cavity, edematous or hemorrhagic conditions, inflammatory diseases (such as periostitis or cellulitis), hyperostosis of the orbit, or other conditions causing a reduction in orbit size will result in exophthalmos. However, it may also result from a systemic disorder, such as thyroid disease, as well as xanthomatosis or a blood dyscrasia, in which case a complete medical examination is indicated. In such cases, exophthalmos is usually bilateral.

Enophthalmos may result from traumatic injury, such as a fractured orbital floor. Less commonly, it may be congenital or associated with inflammation.

Post-test care
Refer the patient to an appropriate specialist as needed.

Interfering factors
Failure to set the calibrated bar of the exophthalmometer at the baseline distance will interfere with test results.

Slit-lamp examination

The slit lamp, an instrument equipped with a special lighting system and a binocular microscope, allows an ophthalmologist to visualize in detail the anterior segment of the eye, which includes the eyelids, eyelashes, conjunctiva, sclera, cornea, tear film, anterior chamber, iris, crystalline lens, and vitreous face. To evaluate normally transparent or near-transparent ocular fluids and tissues, the size, shape, intensity, and depth of the light source as well as the magnification of the microscope may be altered. If any abnormalities are noted, special devices may be attached to the slit lamp to allow more detailed investigation. (See *Other slit-lamp procedures,* page 568.)

Purpose
▪ To detect and evaluate abnormalities of the anterior segment tissues and structures.

Patient preparation
Explain to the patient that this examination evaluates the front portion of the eyes. Tell him that the test takes 5 to 10 minutes and requires that he remain still. Reassure him that the examination is painless.

Contact lenses are removed before the test, unless the test is being performed to evaluate the fit of the contact lens. If dilating eyedrops have been ordered, check the patient's history for adverse reactions to mydriatics or for the presence of angle-closure glaucoma before administering. For a routine eye examination, dilating drops aren't used because the slit lamp's bright light would hurt the dilated eyes. However, some diseases require pupillary dilation before a slit-lamp examination. Iritis, for example, a painful condition aggravat-ed by pupillary constriction, requires pupillary dilation to alleviate pain and allow the ophthalmologist to examine the eyes with adequate illumination.

Equipment
Slit lamp ✦ mydriatics, as ordered.

Procedure
After seating the patient in the examining chair, with both his feet on the floor, ask him to place his chin on the rest and his forehead against the bar. Dim the lights in the room. The ophthalmologist examines the patient's eyes — starting with the lids and lashes and progressing to the vitreous face — altering light and magnification as necessary. In some cases, a special camera can be attached to the slit lamp to photograph portions of the eye.

Precautions
 Don't instill mydriatic drops into the eyes of a patient who has angle-closure glaucoma or has had a hypersensitivity reaction to the drops.

Normal findings
Slit-lamp examination should reveal no abnormalities of anterior segment tissues and structures.

Implications of results
Slit-lamp examination may detect pathologic conditions — such as corneal abrasions and ulcers, lens opacities, iritis, and conjunctivitis — and irregular corneal shapes — as in keratoconus. A parchmentlike consistency of the lid skin, with redness, minor swelling, and moderate itching, may indicate a hypersensitivity reaction. If a corneal abrasion or ulcer is detected, a fluorescein stain may be applied to allow better viewing of the area. If a tearing deficiency is suspected, the ophthalmologist may exam-

Other slit-lamp procedures

If a slit-lamp examination reveals any abnormalities, the following tests may be performed to elicit more information.

Fluorescein staining

When a patient complains of a scratching sensation or when corneal or conjunctival abnormalities are suspected, fluorescein staining provides a better view of the anterior portion of the eye than the basic slit-lamp examination. Because the corneal layers and conjunctiva are transparent, the slit lamp can't detect minute scratches or breaks in tissue. By staining the eye's surface with a sodium fluorescein dye and observing the resulting fluorescence through a cobalt blue filter (a special attachment to the slit lamp), the ophthalmologist can visualize corneal and conjunctival injuries — such as abrasions, foreign bodies, damage from ultraviolet light, and drying due to exposure — as well as their area, depth, and pattern. (Such injuries have specific staining patterns that aid diagnosis.)

To stain the eye's surface, the tip of a sterile fluorescein strip is moistened with sterile normal saline solution, and the strip is touched to the patient's lower conjunctival sac. The patient is asked to close his eyes gently, and a film of fluorescein dye spreads over the corneal and conjunctival surfaces. Surface defects absorb more dye than normal areas. When the corneal epithelium is broken or scratched, for example, the underlying Bowman's membrane stains bright green. Injuries or chemical insults to the conjunctiva or cornea also fluoresce green.

Hruby lens

A –55 diopter lens placed in front of — not on — the eye permits binocular, magnified examination of the posterior vitreous and retina, when used with the slit lamp. The pupils must be widely dilated for the examination. Following mydriasis and placement of the lens, a pencil of light from the slit lamp is directed through the center of the lens toward the posterior portion of the eye. Pathologies can be further studied by direct or indirect ophthalmoscopy.

Gonioscopy

The angle of the anterior chamber may be evaluated by using focal illumination, a microscope, and a special contact lens. This special lens (goniolens) eliminates the corneal curvature, allowing light to be reflected from the angle of the anterior chamber so that its structures can be seen in detail.

Before the lens is placed on the eye, the cornea is anesthetized and a thin layer of fluid (usually 2% methylcellulose solution) is applied to the contact surface of the lens to separate the lens from the cornea. The goniolens deflects the beam of light from the slit lamp into the opposite angle of the anterior chamber, revealing the image of the angle structure.

Gonioscopy is essential in evaluating glaucoma, especially when caused by angle closure, because prompt action is needed to prevent further rise in pressure.

ine the eye after applying a fluorescein or rose bengal stain; he may also perform the Schirmer tearing test. Some abnormal findings may indicate impending disorders. For example, early-stage lens opacities may signal the development of cataracts.

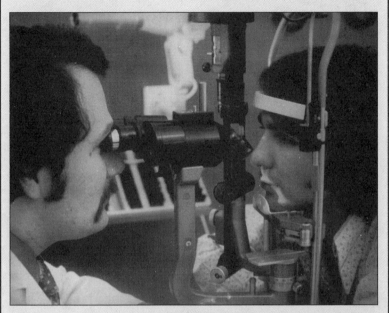

The patient shown at right is undergoing a slit-lamp biomicroscopic examination. The slit lamp directs an intense, narrow beam of light on optic tissue, allowing the ophthalmologist to see the patient's cornea and lens as layers of different optical densities, not transparent structures. This method permits accurate detection of pathologic conditions in the eye's anterior segment.

Post-test care

If dilating drops were instilled, tell the patient that his near vision will be blurred for 40 minutes to 2 hours.

Interfering factors

Poor patient cooperation will affect test results.

Schirmer tearing test

The Schirmer test assesses the function of the major lacrimal glands, which are responsible for reflex tearing in response to stressful situations, such as the presence of a foreign body. Reflex tearing is stimulated by the insertion of a strip of filter paper into the lower conjunctival sac, followed by measurement of the amount of moisture absorbed by the paper. (See *Proper filter placement in Schirmer test,* page 570.) Both eyes are tested simultaneously.

A variation of this test evaluates the function of the accessory lacrimal glands of Krause and Wolfring by instillation of a topical anesthetic before insertion of the filter papers. The anesthetic inhibits reflex tearing by the major lacrimal glands, ensuring measurement of only the basic tear film that is normally produced by the accessory glands. This tear film usually maintains adequate corneal moisture under normal circumstances.

This illustration shows the proper placement of the filter paper for the Schirmer test. The filter paper should be inserted into the inferior conjunctival sac of each eye.

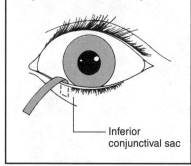

Inferior
conjunctival sac

Purpose

■ To measure tear secretion in persons with a suspected tearing deficiency.

Patient preparation

Explain to the patient that this test measures secretion of tears. Tell him the test requires that a strip of filter paper be placed in the lower part of each eye for 5 minutes. Reassure him that the procedure is painless.

If the patient wears contact lenses, ask him to remove them before the test. If an anesthetic is instilled, he won't be able to reinsert the lenses for 2 hours after the test.

Equipment

Schirmer test kit (standardized sterile strips of individually wrapped filter paper in millimeter-ruled envelopes) ✦ topical anesthetic (such as proparacaine) for evaluation of accessory lacrimal glands.

Procedure

Seat the patient in the examining chair, with his head against the headrest. To remove the test strip from the wrapper, bend the rounded wick end at the indentation, and cut open the envelope at the other end. Tell the patient to look up; then gently lower the inferior eyelid. Hook the bent end of the strip over the inferior eyelid at the junction of the medial and nasal segments. Insert one strip in each eye, and note the time of insertion. Tell the patient not to squeeze or rub his eyes, but to blink normally or to keep his eyes closed lightly.

After 5 minutes, remove the strips from the patient's eyes, and measure the length of the moistened area from the indentation, using the millimeter scale on the envelope. Report the results as a fraction: the numerator is the length of the moistened area; the denominator is the time the strips were left in place. Also note which eye was tested. Thus, if a strip inserted in the right conjunctival sac for 5 minutes shows 8 mm of moisture, the correct notation is OD (*oculus dexter,* or right eye), 8 mm/5 minutes.

To measure the function of the accessory lacrimal glands of Krause and Wolfring, instill one drop of topical anesthetic into each conjunctival sac before inserting the Schirmer strips.

Precautions

To prevent patient discomfort, be careful not to touch the cornea while inserting the test strip.

Normal findings

A Schirmer test strip should show at least 15 mm of moisture after 5 minutes. However, because tear production decreases with age, normal test results in patients over age 40 may range from 10 to 15 mm. Both eyes usually secrete the same amount of tears.

Implications of results

Although the Schirmer tearing test is a simple and efficient method of measuring the rate of tear secretion, up to 15%

of the patients tested have false-positive or false-negative results. Since the test is rapid and simple, it may be repeated and findings compared. Additional testing, such as a slit-lamp examination with fluorescein or rose bengal stain, is necessary to corroborate results.

A positive result confirmed by additional testing indicates a definite tearing deficiency, which may result from aging or, more seriously, from Sjögren's syndrome, a systemic disease of unknown origin that is most common among postmenopausal women. Tearing deficiency may also arise secondarily to systemic diseases, such as lymphoma, leukemia, and rheumatoid arthritis. Regardless of the cause, tearing deficiency is a matter of clinical concern because it can lead to corneal erosions, scarring, and secondary infection.

Post-test care

If a topical anesthetic was instilled, advise the patient not to rub his eyes for at least 30 minutes after instillation because this can cause a corneal abrasion. Patients who wear contact lenses should not reinsert them for at least 2 hours.

Interfering factors

■ If the patient closes his eyes too tightly during the test, tearing will increase.
■ Reflex tearing due to contact of the test strip with the cornea affects test results.

Tonometry

Tonometry allows indirect measurement of intraocular pressure and serves as an effective screen for early detection of glaucoma, a common cause of blindness. Intraocular pressure rises when the production of aqueous humor — the clear fluid secreted continuously by the ciliary process in the eye's posterior chamber — exceeds the rate of drainage. This rise in pressure causes the eyeball to harden and become more resistant to extraocular pressure.

Indentation tonometry tests this resistance by measuring how deeply a known weight depresses the cornea; *applanation tonometry* provides the same information by measuring the amount of force required to flatten a known area of the cornea. (See *Applanation tonometry,* page 572.) Both procedures necessitate corneal anesthetization and careful examination technique. Tonometry should never be performed on a patient with a corneal ulcer or infection except by a skilled examiner, and then only in an emergency, such as suspected acute angle-closure glaucoma.

The diagnostic significance of tonometry is readily apparent because glaucoma — which can be treated if detected early enough — is the second leading cause of permanent blindness in the United States and the leading cause of blindness in blacks. This test should be performed routinely on people over age 40, since glaucoma strikes 2% of people past this critical age.

Patients with intraocular pressure problems can now monitor their pressure at home with a portable tonometer. Nurses may perform tonometry in emergency or occupational health settings. Findings must be confirmed by visual field testing and ophthalmoscopy.

Purpose

■ To measure intraocular pressure
■ To aid diagnosis and follow-up evaluation of glaucoma.

Patient preparation

Explain to the patient that this test measures the pressure within his eyes. Tell him the test takes only a few minutes and requires that his eyes be anesthetized. Reassure him that the procedure

Applanation tonometry

The most precise test of intraocular pressure, applanation tonometry measures the force required to flatten a certain area of the cornea. The applanation tonometer (usually the Goldmann tonometer) is mounted on a slit-lamp biomicroscope.

This test is performed with minimal corneal trauma and may be done after a routine slit-lamp examination. However, since the slit-lamp biomicroscope is used only by an ophthalmologist, applanation tonometry is less available than indentation tonometry for large-scale screening of the general population.

To perform this test, a topical anesthetic is instilled, and the tear film is stained with fluorescein drops or a moistened fluorescein paper strip is inserted into the lower conjunctival sac. The patient is seated as for a slit-lamp examination and is instructed to look straight ahead. The examiner moves the slit lamp forward until the tonometer comes in contact with the cornea. Through the eyepiece of the slit lamp, the examiner sees two fluorescein semicircles. He adjusts the tension dial on the tonometer until the inner, straight-edged margins of the semicircles touch.

The reading on the tension dial provides a direct indication of the patient's intraocular pressure.

---

is painless. If the patient wears contact lenses, instruct him to remove them before the procedure and leave them out for 2 hours after the test or until the anesthetic wears off completely.

Ask the patient to assume a supine position. Make sure he's relaxed because anxiety can raise intraocular pressure. Have him loosen or remove restrictive clothing around his neck, which can also raise intraocular pressure. Instruct him not to cough or squeeze his eyelids together. Explain that his cooperation will ensure accurate test results.

Equipment

Indentation tonometer (the Schiøtz tonometer is the most popular), sterilized or used with disposable sterile tonofilms ✦ topical anesthetic.

Procedure

Ask the patient to look down. Raise his superior eyelid with your thumb, and place one drop of the topical anesthetic at the top of the sclera. The solution spreads over the entire sclera when the patient blinks.

Check the tonometer for a zero reading on the steel test block that comes with the instrument. Make sure the plunger moves freely. The first measurement on each eye is obtained with the 5.5-g weight.

Have the patient look up and stare at a spot on the ceiling. Then ask him to open his mouth, take a deep breath, and exhale slowly. This distracts him, preventing forceful closure of the lids. After this initial breath, tell the patient to breathe normally during the test.

With the thumb and forefinger of one hand, hold the lids of his right eye open against the orbital rim. Hold the tonometer vertically with the thumb and forefinger of the other hand, and rest the footplate on the apex of the cornea. Be especially careful to avoid resting your fingers on the cornea or pressing on the cornea, since this increases intraocular pressure. With the footplate in place, check the indicator needle for a rhythmic transmission caused by the ocular pulse. Then record the calibrated scale reading that converts to a measurement of intraocular pressure. If the reading doesn't exceed 4, add an additional weight (7.5, 10, or 15 g) to obtain a reliable result.

Repeat the procedure on the left eye, and record the time when the test was performed.

Precautions

 To avoid corneal abrasion, hold the tonometer still. Don't touch the lashes; this could trigger a blink response or Bell's phenomenon (upward movement of the eyes with forced closure of the lids), which can cause the footplate to move and scratch the cornea.

Reference values

Intraocular pressure normally ranges from 12 to 20 mm Hg, with diurnal variations. The highest point is reached at the time of waking; the lowest point, in the evening.

Implications of results

Elevated intraocular pressure requires further testing for glaucoma. Since intraocular pressure varies diurnally, findings must be supplemented with serial measurements obtained at different times on different days.

Indentation tonometry alone can't diagnose glaucoma; applanation tonometry, visual field testing, and ophthalmoscopy must confirm the diagnosis.

Post-test care

■ Because an anesthetic was instilled, tell the patient not to rub his eyes for at least 20 minutes after the test to prevent corneal abrasion. If the patient wears contact lenses, tell him not to reinsert them for at least 2 hours.

■ If the tonometer moved across the cornea during the test, tell the patient he may feel a slight scratching sensation in the eye when the anesthetic wears off.

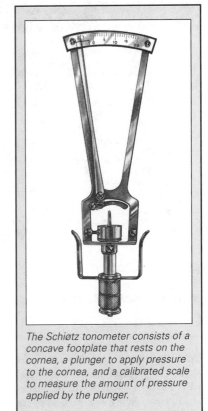

The Schiøtz tonometer consists of a concave footplate that rests on the cornea, a plunger to apply pressure to the cornea, and a calibrated scale to measure the amount of pressure applied by the plunger.

This sensation should disappear within 24 hours, since most corneal abrasions resulting from tonometry affect only the corneal epithelium, which regenerates within 24 hours without scarring.

Interfering factors

■ Deformed corneal curvature prevents proper placement of the footplate.

■ Corneoscleral rigidity or flaccidity, as determined by an ophthalmologist, may cause falsely elevated or depressed readings, since the Schiøtz tonometer measures the pressure required for corneal indentation.

■ Poor patient cooperation or careless examination technique interferes with test results.

Comparing direct and indirect ophthalmoscopes

FEATURES	DIRECT OPHTHALMOSCOPE	INDIRECT OPHTHALMOSCOPE
Image	True	Rotated 180 degrees
Intensity of illumination	Medium to high	Dazzling
Magnification	15x	2x to 4x
Field of vision (disk diameters)	2	8
Affected by major refractive errors	Yes	No
Good view despite opacities in the media	No	Yes
Stereopsis	No (monocular)	Yes (binocular)
Easy to use	Yes	No

Ophthalmoscopy

Ophthalmoscopy — an important part of routine physical examinations and eye evaluations — allows magnified examination of living vascular and nerve tissue of the fundus, including the optic disk, retinal vessels, macula, and retina. The instrument used in this test — either the direct or the indirect ophthalmoscope — is considered one of the most important diagnostic tools in ophthalmology.

Most examiners use the direct ophthalmoscope — a small, handheld instrument consisting of a light source, a viewing device, a reflecting device to channel light into the patient's eyes, and spherical lenses to correct refractive error of the patient or examiner. The direct model is easier to use than the indirect model. (See *Comparing direct and indirect ophthalmoscopes.*) If a slit lamp is not available, the examiner may also use the ophthalmoscope to examine the cornea, iris, and lens.

Purpose

- To detect and evaluate eye disorders as well as ocular manifestations of systemic disease.

Patient preparation

Explain to the patient that this test permits examination of the back of the eye. Tell him who will perform the test and where and that it takes less than 5 minutes. Advise him that eyedrops may be instilled to dilate the pupils for a clearer examination, but reassure him that he'll feel no discomfort during the test.

Check the patient's history for previous use of dilating eyedrops, possible hypersensitivity to the eyedrops, and angle-closure glaucoma.

Equipment

Direct ophthalmoscope ✦ mydriatic eyedrops ✦ disposable tissues.

Procedure

Routine examination of the ocular media and fundus is usually possible without dilating the pupil if there is sufficient light in the ophthalmoscope and

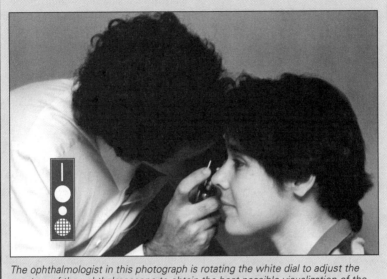

The ophthalmologist in this photograph is rotating the white dial to adjust the aperture of the ophthalmoscope to obtain the best possible visualization of the patient's eye. The aperture controls the amount of light directed onto the retina. The large aperture usually allows the best visualization of the fundus, but only when the pupils are dilated. The small aperture allows visualization to be dilated beyond 3 to 4 mm. The grid permits an estimate of the size of fundal lesions. The slit helps determine the size of such lesions as tumors and swollen disks.

room lighting is subdued. However, if indicated, mydriatic eyedrops may be used; usually two instillations are needed to achieve maximum mydriasis.

Have the patient sit upright in the examination chair. Darken the room to keep irregular reflections from interfering with the examination. Sit about 2' (60 cm) away from the patient, at his eye level. Examine the patient's right eye first, holding the ophthalmoscope in your right hand and in front of your right eye. Position your right index finger on the lens selection dial to facilitate rapid lens changes, and sit slightly to the patient's right. Set the illuminated dial to zero, and tell the patient to look straight ahead at a specific object 20' (6 m) away — for example, a large symbol on a standardized vision chart. Tell him to keep his eyes fixed on the object throughout the examination.

Remaining on the patient's right side, move forward slightly, until you're about 6" (15 cm) away from him.

Direct the light beam into the pupil; select the proper lens aperture on the ophthalmoscope, and look through it for the red reflex. (You can see this without magnification; it represents a red reflection from the fundus.) Keeping this reflection in view and reminding the patient to maintain fixation, move slowly toward the patient until you're 1½" to 2½" (4 to 5 cm) from him. Rotate the lenses on the scope to focus on the optic disk, and note its size, shape, and color.

Next, look for a white, central depression in the disk — the physiologic cup. Observe the retinal vessels that emerge from the optic disk. They normally bifurcate and extend toward all quadrants

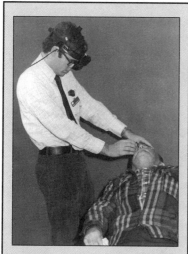

A more expensive and more sophisticated instrument than the direct ophthalmoscope, the indirect ophthalmoscope is used with a convex lens, which the ophthalmologist holds a few inches from the patient's eye, and a headlamp, which provides a strong source of illumination. The lens focuses light reflected from the retina, producing an image that is rotated 180 degrees but is unaffected by refractive errors or opacities in the media.

Because the indirect ophthalmoscope provides a wide-angle, stereoscopic view of the peripheral retina, many surgeons depend on it for preoperative diagnosis and during retinal detachment surgery.

of the retina. Follow each vessel as far as possible to the periphery.

Examine the macula — a yellowish depression lying approximately two disk diameters away from and slightly below the center of the optic disk — and its center, the fovea. To examine the extreme periphery, tell the patient to look up, down, and to each side. Examine the superior, inferior, temporal, and nasal portions of the retina, respectively.

Repeat the procedure to examine the patient's left eye, moving slightly to the patient's left side and holding the ophthalmoscope in your left hand and in front of your left eye. Adjust the lens selection dial to account for a different refractive state, if necessary.

Precautions

NURSING ALERT ■ Don't administer dilating eyedrops to a patient who has angle-closure glaucoma or a history of hypersensitivity reactions to the drops.
■ Make sure the patient maintains fixation throughout the procedure.

Normal findings

With the beam of light from the ophthalmoscope directed into the patient's pupil, the red reflex should be visible through the aperture. The slightly oval optic disk, measuring approximately 1.5 mm vertically, lies to the nasal side of the fundus center. Although its color varies, it's usually pink, with darker edges at its nasal border. The physiologic cup, a pale depression in the center of the disk, varies in size; it tends to be larger in patients with myopia and smaller in those with hyperopia.

The semitransparent retina surrounds the optic disk. Branching out from the disk are the retinal vessels, including venules and the slightly smaller arterioles. Vessel diameter progressively decreases with distance from the optic disk. Retinal arterioles generally have a medium red color; venules appear dark red or blue.

The macula, a small avascular area that appears darker than the surrounding retina, is located approximately 2½" disk diameters temporal from the optic disk and slightly beneath the horizontal meridian. In its center lies a small, even darker spot — the fovea. A tiny light reflex can be seen at the center of the fovea, caused by reflection of the ophthalmoscopic light from the concave inner surface of the area.

Implications of results

An absent or diminished red reflex may be due to gross corneal lesions, dense opacities of the aqueous or vitreous humor (such as from blood following hemorrhage), cataracts, or a detached retina. Cloudy vitreous humor that obscures the fundus may be due to inflammatory disease of the optic disk, retina, or uvea. Fundal lesions should be sketched or photographed for further study.

Optic neuritis causes the optic disk to become elevated and more vascular; small hemorrhages may also occur. Optic nerve atrophy causes the disk to appear white. Papilledema, which may result from increased intracranial pressure, causes abnormal elevation of the disk, blurring of disk margins, engorged vessels, and hemorrhages. In glaucoma, the physiologic cup may appear enlarged and gray, with white edges. A milky-white retina characterizes the acute phase of central retinal artery occlusion; the fovea, in contrast to the ischemic macula, appears as a bright red spot. Central retinal vein occlusion is marked by widespread retinal hemorrhaging, patches of white exudate, and disk elevation. Retinal detachments appear as gray, elevated areas, possibly with areas of red vascular choroid exposed by retinal tears. A choroidal tumor appears as a dark lesion.

The integrity of retinal vessels is commonly evaluated to aid diagnosis of systemic disease. Hypertension, for example, causes vasospasm, sclerosis, and eventual occlusion of retinal arterioles, leading to retinal edema and hemorrhage, and papilledema. Diabetes mellitus may be complicated by retinal fibroses, patches of white exudate, and microaneurysms. Other systemic disorders present similar findings.

Interpretation of ophthalmoscopic findings depends largely on the examiner's knowledge and experience, since an abnormality can arise from several sources. After an ophthalmologic evaluation, referral for complete medical evaluation may be necessary.

Post-test care

None.

Interfering factors

■ Poor patient cooperation or conditions that prohibit a good view of the fundus, such as insufficient dilation, dense cataracts, cloudy media, or gross nystagmus, may affect test results.
■ Proper examination conditions (darkened room, adequate light source on ophthalmoscope) are essential to accurate diagnosis.

Fluorescein angiography

In this test, rapid-sequence photographs of the fundus are taken with a special camera after I.V. injection of sodium fluorescein, a contrast medium. The fluorescein dye and the use of sophisticated photographic equipment enhance the visibility of microvascular structures of the retina and choroid, allowing evaluation of the entire retinal vascular bed, including retinal circulation. (See *Phases of retinal circulation*, page 579.)

Purpose

■ To document retinal circulation as an aid in evaluating intraocular abnormalities, such as retinopathy, tumors, and circulatory or inflammatory disorders.

Patient preparation

Tell the patient that this test evaluates the small blood vessels in the eyes and takes about 30 minutes.

Make sure the patient or a responsible family member has signed a consent form, if required. Check the patient's history for glaucoma and hypersensitivity reactions, especially to contrast media and dilating eyedrops. If ordered, tell a patient with glaucoma not to use miotic eyedrops on the day of the test.

Explain to the patient that eyedrops will be instilled to dilate his pupils and that a dye will be injected into his arm. Tell him that his eyes will be photographed with a special camera before and after the injection. Stress that these are photographs, *not* X-rays. Warn him that his skin and urine may appear yellow, but these effects disappear within 24 to 48 hours.

Equipment
Fundus camera and film ✦ mydriatic eyedrops ✦ alcohol swabs ✦ tourniquet ✦ 21G scalp-vein needle ✦ 5- to 10-ml syringe ✦ 2 ml of 25% or 5 ml of 10% sodium fluorescein ✦ small sterile dressing ✦ emesis basin ✦ emergency resuscitation kit.

Procedure
Administer mydriatic eyedrops, as ordered. Usually, two instillations are necessary to achieve maximum mydriasis in 15 to 40 minutes. After mydriasis, seat the patient comfortably in the examining chair, facing the camera. Have him loosen or remove any restrictive clothing around his neck. Then ask him to place his chin on the chin rest and his forehead against the bar. Instruct him to keep his teeth together, to open his eyes as widely as possible, to stare straight ahead, and to breathe and blink normally.

The antecubital vein is prepared and punctured, but the dye isn't injected yet. A few preinjection photographs may be taken at this time. Tell the patient to keep his arm extended; if necessary, use an arm board.

When ordered, the dye is injected rapidly into the vein. Remind the patient to maintain his position and fixation. The patient may briefly experience nausea and a feeling of warmth. Reassure him as needed, and observe for hypersensitivity reactions, such as vomiting, dry mouth, metallic taste, sudden increased salivation, sneezing, light-headedness, fainting, and hives. Rarely, anaphylactic shock may result.

As the dye is injected, 25 to 30 photographs are taken in rapid sequence (1 second apart). The needle and syringe are removed carefully; pressure and a dressing are applied to the injection site. If late-phase photographs are needed, tell the patient to sit and relax for 20 minutes; then reposition him for 5 to 10 photographs. If ordered, photographs may be taken up to 1 hour after the injection.

Precautions
▪ Don't leave the patient unattended. Mild side effects, such as nausea, vomiting, sneezing, paresthesia of the tongue, and dizziness, may occur. Serious side effects (laryngeal edema, bronchospasm, and respiratory arrest) are possible. Have emergency resuscitation equipment at hand. If a reaction occurs, have the patient note it for his allergy history.
▪ Make sure the needle is in the vein correctly, since extravasation of the dye around the injection site is painful.

Normal findings
After rapid injection into the antecubital vein, sodium fluorescein reaches the retina in 12 to 15 seconds (*filling phase*). As the choroidal vessels and choriocapillaries fill, the background of the retina fluoresces, taking on an evenly mottled appearance known as the *choroidal flush*. Then the dye fills the arteries (*arterial phase*). The *arteriovenous phase* lasts from the complete filling of the

Phases of retinal circulation

These six angiograms chronicle the phases of retinal circulation in the right eye: filling phase (A), early arterial phase (B), laminar venous filling phase (C), full venous phase (D), late venous phase (E), and recirculation phase (F).

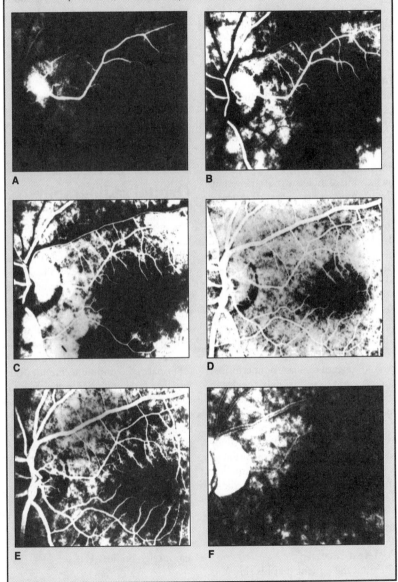

arteries and capillaries to the earliest evidence of dye in the veins. The *venous phase* lasts from the time the arteries begin to empty to the time the veins fill and empty. Finally, the *recirculation phase* occurs 30 to 60 minutes after the injection, when the fluorescein — if at all present — is barely detectable in the retinal vessels. Normally, there is no leakage from the retinal vessels.

Implications of results

The varying and complex findings after fluorescein angiography require interpretation by a highly skilled ophthalmologist with extensive experience in the diagnosis of retinal disorders. Abnormalities in the early filling phase may include microaneurysms, arteriovenous shunts, and neovascularization. Angiography may identify arterial occlusion by showing delayed or absent flow of the dye through the arteries, stenosis, and prolonged venous drainage. Venous occlusion may be associated with dilation of the vessels and fluorescein leakage.

Chronic obstruction may produce recanalization and collateral circulation. In hypertensive retinopathy, abnormalities may include areas of increased vascular tortuosity, microaneurysms around zones of capillary nonperfusion, and generalized suffusion of the dye in the retina. Aneurysms and capillary hemangiomas may leak fluorescence and are often surrounded by hard, yellow exudate. Tumors exhibit variable fluorescein patterns, depending on histologic type. Retinal edema, or inflammation and fibrous tissue may show variable degrees of fluorescence. Papilledema produces vascular leakage in the disk area.

Post-test care

- Remind the patient that his skin and urine will be slightly discolored for 24 to 48 hours after the test.
- Tell the patient that his near vision will

be blurred for up to 12 hours and that he should avoid direct sunlight and driving during this time.

Interfering factors

Inadequate view of the fundus, resulting from insufficient pupillary dilation, a cataract, media opacity, or inability of the patient to keep his eyes open and to maintain fixation will affect test results.

SPECIAL PROCEDURES

Orbital radiography

The orbit is a deep-set cavity that contains the eye, lacrimal gland, blood vessels, nerves, muscles, and fat. It is enclosed anteriorly by the eyeball and the eyelids. Since portions of the orbit are composed of thin bone that is easily fractured, X-rays of these structures are commonly taken following facial trauma. X-rays are also useful in diagnosing ocular and orbital pathology.

Special radiographic techniques can visualize foreign bodies in the orbit or the eye that can't be seen with an ophthalmoscope. To further define abnormalities, tomograms may be taken concurrently with standard X-rays. Computed tomography and ultrasonography can provide further information.

Purpose

- To aid in diagnosis of orbital fractures and pathology
- To help locate intraorbital or intraocular foreign bodies.

Patient preparation

Explain to the patient that this test assesses the condition of the bones around the eye. Tell him that several X-rays will be taken of his eye, who will perform the test and where, and that the procedure takes about 15 minutes. Reassure him that this test is usually painless unless he has suffered facial trauma, in which case positioning may cause some discomfort.

Tell the patient he'll be asked to turn his head from side to side and to flex or extend his neck to achieve correct positioning. Instruct him to remove all metal objects and jewelry in the X-ray field.

Procedure

The patient is placed in a supine position on the radiographic table or is seated in a chair, and is instructed to remain still while the X-rays are taken. A standard series of orbital X-rays usually includes a lateral view, a posteroanterior view, a submentovertex (base) view, stereo Waters' views (views from both sides), Towne's (half-axial) projection, and optic canal projections. If enlargement of the superior orbital fissure is suspected, apical views are also obtained. Before the patient leaves the radiography department, the films are developed and checked for quality.

Precautions

None.

Normal findings

Each orbit is composed of a roof, a floor, and medial and lateral walls. The bones that form the roof and floor are very thin; the floor may be only 1 mm thick or less. The medial wall is slightly thicker than the roof and floor, except for the portion formed by the ethmoid bone. The medial walls of both orbits parallel each other. The lateral wall — the thickest part of the orbit — is strongest at the orbital rim. The lateral walls of both orbits project toward each other; if they were straight and extended farther into the head, they would meet at a 90-degree angle.

The superior orbital fissure lies in the back of the orbit, between the lateral wall and the roof, and is actually a gap between the greater and the lesser wings of the sphenoid bone. The optic canal, found at the apex of the orbit, is an opening in the lesser wing of the sphenoid bone, through which the optic nerve and ophthalmic artery pass. (See *Radiographic view of orbital structures,* page 582.)

Implications of results

Orbital fractures resulting from facial trauma usually occur in the floor and in the ethmoid bone, since these structures are extremely thin.

To detect abnormalities, the size and shape of the orbital structures on the affected side are compared with those on the other side. Enlargement of an orbit, for example, generally indicates the presence of a lesion that has caused exophthalmos from increased intraorbital pressure. Any growing tumor can produce these changes. Specifically, superior orbital fissure enlargement can result from orbital meningioma, intracranial conditions (such as pituitary tumors) or, more characteristically, vascular anomalies. Optic canal enlargement may result from extraocular extension of a retinoblastoma or, in children, from optic nerve glioma.

In adults, only prolonged pathology can increase orbital size. In children, however, even a rapidly growing lesion can cause orbital enlargement because of the incomplete development of the orbital bones. A decrease in the size of the orbit may follow childhood enucleation of the eye or such conditions as congenital microphthalmia.

Destruction of the orbital walls may indicate a malignant neoplasm or infection. A benign tumor or cyst produces a clear-cut local indentation of the or-

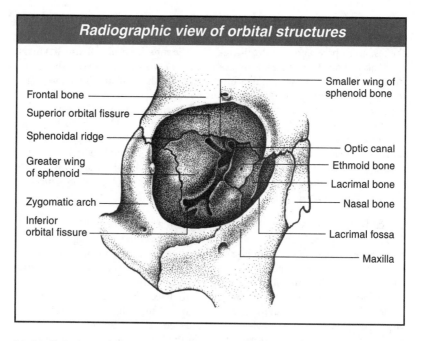

Radiographic view of orbital structures

Frontal bone

Superior orbital fissure

Sphenoidal ridge

Greater wing of sphenoid

Zygomatic arch

Inferior orbital fissure

Smaller wing of sphenoid bone

Optic canal

Ethmoid bone

Lacrimal bone

Nasal bone

Lacrimal fossa

Maxilla

bital wall. Lesions of adjacent structures may produce radiographic changes due to orbital enlargement and erosion.

Increased bone density may be seen in such conditions as osteoblastic metastasis, sphenoid ridge meningioma, or Paget's disease. To confirm orbital pathology, however, radiographic findings must be supplemented with results from other appropriate tests and procedures.

Post-test care
None.

Interfering factors
None.

Orbital computed tomography

Orbital computed tomography (CT) allows visualization of abnormalities not readily seen on standard X-rays, delineating their size, position, and relationship to adjoining structures. The orbital CT scan — a series of tomograms reconstructed by a computer and displayed as anatomic slices on an oscilloscope screen — identifies space-occupying lesions earlier and more accurately than other radiographic techniques. In addition, it provides three-dimensional images of orbital structures, especially the ocular muscles and the optic nerve.

Contrast enhancement may be used in CT scans to define ocular tissues and evaluate a patient with a suspected circulatory disorder, hemangioma, or subdural hematoma. CT scans also permit precise diagnosis of many intracranial lesions that affect vision.

Purpose
- To evaluate pathologies of the orbit and eye — especially expanding lesions and bone destruction

■ To evaluate fractures of the orbit and adjoining structures
■ To determine the cause of unilateral exophthalmos.

Patient preparation

Tell the patient that this test visualizes the anatomy of the eye and its surrounding structures. Unless contrast enhancement is scheduled, inform him that he needn't restrict food or fluids. If contrast enhancement is scheduled, withhold food and fluids from the patient for 4 hours before the test.

Tell the patient that a series of X-rays will be taken of his eye, and inform him who will perform the test and where. Reassure him that the test will cause him no discomfort and will take 15 to 30 minutes to perform.

Tell the patient he'll be positioned on an X-ray table and that the head of the table will be moved into the scanner, which will rotate around his head and make loud, clacking sounds. If a contrast agent will be used for the procedure, tell the patient he may feel flushed and warm and may experience a transient headache, a salty taste, and nausea or vomiting after the dye is injected. Reassure him that these reactions to the contrast medium are typical.

Make sure the patient or a responsible member of the family has signed a consent form. Check the patient history for hypersensitivity reactions to iodine, shellfish, or radiographic dyes. Instruct the patient to remove jewelry, hairpins, or other metal objects in the X-ray field to allow for precise imaging of the orbital structures.

Procedure

The patient is placed in a supine position on the radiographic table, with his head immobilized by straps, and is asked to lie still. The head of the table is then moved into the scanner, which rotates around the patient's head, taking X-rays.

The information obtained is stored on magnetic tapes, and the images are displayed on an oscilloscope screen, which may be photographed if a permanent record is desired.

After this series of X-rays has been taken, contrast enhancement is performed, if ordered. The contrast agent is injected and a second series of scans is recorded.

Precautions

Use of contrast enhancement, if ordered, is contraindicated in patients with known hypersensitivity reactions to iodine, shellfish, or radiographic dyes used in other tests.

Normal findings

Orbital structures are evaluated for size, shape, and position. Dense orbital bone provides a marked contrast to less dense periocular fat. The optic nerve and the medial and lateral rectus muscles are clearly defined. The rectus muscles appear as thin dense bands on each side, behind the eye. The optic canals should be equal in size.

Implications of results

Orbital CT scans can identify intra- and extraorbital space-occupying lesions that obscure the normal structures or cause orbital enlargement, indentation of the orbital walls, or bone destruction. They can also help determine the type of lesion. For example, infiltrative lesions, such as lymphomas and metastatic carcinomas, appear as irregular areas of density. However, encapsulated tumors, such as benign hemangiomas and meningiomas, appear as clearly defined masses of consistent density. CT scans can also visualize intracranial tumors that invade the orbit, thickening of the optic nerve that may occur with gliomas, meningiomas, and secondary tumors that may cause enlargement of the optic canal.

In evaluating fractures, CT scans allow a complete three-dimensional view of the affected structures. In determining the cause of unilateral exophthalmos, they can show early erosion or expansion of the medial orbital wall that may arise from lesions in the ethmoidal cells. They can also detect space-occupying lesions in the orbit or paranasal sinuses that cause exophthalmos as well as thickening of the medial and lateral rectus muscles in exophthalmos due to Graves' disease.

Enhancement with a contrast agent can yield important information when the dye circulates through abnormal ocular tissues.

Post-test care

None, if test was performed without contrast enhancement. If a contrast agent was used, watch for residual adverse reactions, including headache, nausea, and vomiting. Tell the patient he may resume his usual diet if he's not experiencing such reactions.

Interfering factors

Movement of the head during scanning or failure to remove radiopaque objects from the X-ray field may cause unclear images, interfering with test results.

Ocular ultrasonography

Ocular ultrasonography involves the transmission of high-frequency sound waves through the eye and the measurement of their reflection from ocular structures. An A-scan converts the resulting echoes into waveforms whose crests represent the positions of different structures, providing a linear dimensional picture. The B-scan converts the echoes into patterns of dots that form a two-dimensional, cross-sectional image of the ocular structure.

Because the B-scan is easier to interpret than the A-scan, it is used more often to evaluate the structures of the eye and to diagnose abnormalities. However, the A-scan is more valuable in measuring the axial length of the eye and characterizing the tissue texture of abnormal lesions. Thus, a combination of A- and B-scans produces the most useful test results.

Illustrating the eyes' structures through ultrasound is especially helpful in evaluating a fundus clouded by an opaque medium, such as a cataract. In such a patient, this test can identify pathologies that are normally undetectable through ophthalmoscopy.

Ophthalmologists may also perform this test before surgery — for example, cataract removal — to ensure the integrity of the retina. If an intraocular lens is to be implanted, ultrasound may be used preoperatively to measure the length of the eye and the curvature of the cornea as a guide for the surgeon. Unlike computed tomography, ocular ultrasonography is readily available and provides information immediately.

In addition to its diagnostic capabilities, ocular ultrasonography can also identify intraocular foreign bodies and determine their position in relation to ocular structures as well as assess the severity of resulting ocular damage.

Purpose

- To aid in evaluating the fundus in an eye with an opaque medium, such as a cataract
- To aid diagnosis of vitreous disorders and retinal detachment
- To diagnose and differentiate between intraocular and orbital lesions and to follow their progression through serial examinations
- To locate intraocular foreign bodies.

Patient preparation

Describe the procedure to the patient, and explain that this test evaluates the eye's structures. Inform him that he needn't restrict food or fluids before the test. Tell the patient who will perform the test and where. Reassure him that it is safe and painless and takes about 5 minutes to perform.

Tell the patient that a small transducer will be placed on his closed eyelid and that the transducer transmits high-frequency sound waves that are reflected by the structures in the eye. Inform him that he may be asked to move his eyes or change his gaze during the procedure and that his cooperation is required to ensure accurate test results.

Equipment

Ultrasound transducer ✦ water-soluble gel ✦ eye cup (for A-scan) ✦ oscilloscope and photographic equipment.

Procedure

Place the patient in the supine position on an X-ray table. For the B-scan, the patient is asked to close his eyes, and a water-soluble gel (such as Goniosol) is applied to his eyelid. The transducer is then placed on the eyelid. For the A-scan, the patient's eye is numbed with anesthetizing drops, and a clear plastic eye cup is placed directly on the eyeball. A water-soluble gel is then applied to the eye cup, and the transducer is positioned on this medium. The transducer then transmits high-frequency sound waves into the patient's eye, and the resulting echoes are transformed into images or waveforms on the oscilloscope screen, which may be photographed.

Precautions

None.

Normal findings

The optic nerve and the posterior lens capsule produce echoes that take on characteristic forms on A- and B-scan images. The posterior wall of the eye appears as a smooth, concave curve; retrobulbar fat can also be identified. The lens and vitreous humor, which don't produce echoes, can also be identified. Normal orbital echo patterns depend on the position of the transducer and the position of the patient's gaze during the procedure. (See *Normal B-scan*, page 586.)

Implications of results

In eyes clouded by a vitreous hemorrhage, the organization of the hemorrhage can be identified by the degree of density that appears on the image. In some instances, the cause of the hemorrhage, the prognosis, and associated abnormalities can also be determined.

Other vitreous abnormalities, such as massive vitreous organization and vitreous bands, may also be detected by ultrasonography. Retinal detachment, commonly found in a patient with an opaque medium, characteristically produces a dense, sheetlike echo on a B-scan. The extent of retinal or choroidal detachment can be defined by transmitting ultrasound waves through the quadrants of the patient's eye.

Ocular ultrasonography can be used to diagnose and differentiate intraocular tumors according to size, shape, location, and texture. The most common tumors identified are melanomas, metastatic tumors, and hemangiomas. This test can also identify retinoblastomas and measure the dimensions of other tumors detectable by ophthalmoscopy.

Hemangiomas and cystic lesions produce characteristic ultrasound patterns. Other orbital lesions detectable by ultrasound include meningiomas, neurofibromas, gliomas, neurilemomas, and the inflammatory changes associated with Graves' disease.

Normal B-scan

This is a normal B-scan using the lid contact method. The posterior lens capsule is visible, but the cornea and iris are not because of obscuring echoes from the eyelid.

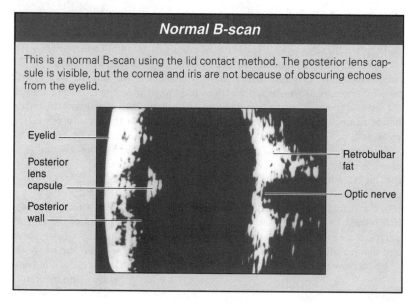

Eyelid

Posterior lens capsule

Posterior wall

Retrobulbar fat

Optic nerve

Post-test care
Make sure the water-soluble gel is removed from the patient's eyelid.

Interfering factors
None.

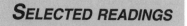

SELECTED READINGS

Carlson, N.B., et al. *Clinical Procedures for Ocular Examination,* 2nd ed. Stamford, Conn.: Appleton & Lange, 1996.

Diseases, 2nd ed. Springhouse, Pa.: Springhouse Corp., 1996.

Ignatavicius, D.D., et al., eds. *Medical-Surgical Nursing: A Nursing Process Approach,* 2nd ed. Philadelphia: W.B. Saunders Co., 1995.

Lewis, S.M., et al. *Medical-Surgical Nursing: Assessment and Management of Clinical Problems,* 4th ed. St. Louis: Mosby–Year Book, Inc., 1996.

Roy, F.H. *Ocular Differential Diagnosis,* 6th ed. Baltimore: Williams & Wilkins Co., 1996.

Smeltzer, S.C., and Bare, B.G. *Brunner and Suddarth's Textbook of Medical-Surgical Nursing,* 8th ed. Philadelphia: Lippincott–Raven Pubs., 1996.

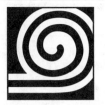

CHAPTER TWENTY-TWO

Ear

Learning objectives

After completing this chapter, the reader will be able to:
- explain the anatomy and physiology of the ear
- distinguish sensorineural from conductive hearing loss
- identify screening programs used to detect hearing impairment in children
- list categories of job-related hearing loss
- explain how to use an audiometer
- state guidelines for communicating effectively with the hearing impaired
- describe common abnormalities of the tympanic membrane
- evaluate eustachian tube function
- state the purpose of each test discussed in the chapter
- prepare the patient physically and psychologically for each test
- describe the procedure for performing each test
- specify appropriate precautions for safe administration of each test
- recognize signs of an adverse reaction and respond appropriately
- implement appropriate post-test care
- identify the normal findings of each test
- discuss the implications of abnormal test results
- list factors that may interfere with accurate test results.

INTRODUCTION

Auditory tests can detect hearing impairment and reveal the presence of lesions or disorders requiring treatment. For equilibrium disorders, vestibular tests, which primarily investigate the function of the labyrinthine structures of the inner ear, can locate a vestibular lesion. However, only a complete otologic and neurologic workup can provide full diagnostic information.

Anatomy and physiology

The ear has three parts — the external ear, the middle ear, and the inner ear — and is innervated by several sensory nerves. The external ear consists of the auricle, or pinna (the visible flap), and the external ear canal. These structures direct and transmit sound waves toward the tympanic membrane (eardrum). The external ear canal also serves as a resonating tube, amplifying sound frequencies between 2,000 and 6,000 Hz.

These frequencies are critical for perceiving consonants. Cerumen (earwax) combines the secretions of the canal's sebaceous and ceruminous glands. The tympanic membrane separates the external and the middle ear; disease can significantly alter the concavity of the drumhead (umbo) and its position relative to the ear canal.

The middle ear, which lies directly behind the tympanic membrane, is a small air space in the tympanic region of the temporal bone. Three small bones — the malleus (hammer), incus (anvil), and stapes (stirrup) — make up the auditory ossicles. The vibrations of these bones transmit sound waves from the tympanic membrane to the inner ear through a membrane called the oval window. The eustachian tube's connection to the nasopharynx makes it a direct route for middle ear infection.

The inner ear contains the sensory end organs for hearing and balance. The temporal bone surrounds and protects these interconnected, fluid-filled membranous structures. The auditory end organ, or cochlea, is a coiled tube that is divided into three compartments; vibration of the ossicles sets the fluid in these compartments into motion. The middle compartment, or cochlear duct, contains the organ of Corti. Here, sensitive hair cells convert fluid disturbance into neural impulses, which travel along the eighth cranial nerve to the brain.

The vestibular organs include the utricle, the saccule, and the semicircular canals. Changes in body orientation disturb the fluid in the canals (the equilibrium) and stimulate vestibular hair cells, called cristae or maculae. These hair cells dispatch messages to the brain, enabling muscles to respond to position changes.

Types of hearing loss

Hearing loss can result from injury to or disease of any part of the auditory system. For example, foreign objects, impacted cerumen, or growths can obstruct the external ear canal; perforation may damage the tympanic membrane; and various diseases may affect the delicate parts of the middle and inner ear.

Conductive hearing loss results from impairment of sound transmission through the external ear canal, tympanic membrane, and oval window of the middle ear because these parts conduct mechanical vibrations to the inner ear or sensorineural system. Such loss may result from impacted cerumen, a perforated tympanic membrane, accumulation of pus or serous fluid in the middle ear (as in otitis media), or impaired ossicular mobility (as in otosclerosis). In audiometric testing, a conductive loss is associated with better conduction thresholds in bone than in air because bone-conducted sound, or skull vibration, doesn't pass through the external or middle ear, whereas air conducted sound does; a lesion in the conductive system thus depresses only air conduction thresholds.

Sensorineural hearing loss indicates a lesion in the inner ear (cochlear lesion) or in the eighth cranial nerve or higher neural pathways (retrocochlear lesion). It's important to distinguish between cochlear and retrocochlear lesions because the latter may prove life-threatening. Cochlear hearing loss may result from Ménière's disease, ototoxic agents, or viral labyrinthitis; retrocochlear loss, from tumors or multiple sclerosis.

Mixed hearing loss results from a combined sensorineural–conductive dysfunction. *Central hearing loss* results from damage to the brain's auditory receptors.

Audiologic tests

A thorough otoscopic examination of the external ear, ear canal, and tympanic membrane should precede auditory and vestibular tests. After otoscopy, a basic audiologic examination includes pure tone audiometry to measure thresholds for air- and bone-conducted sound; the spondee threshold; word discrimination tests; and acoustic immittance measurements, such as tympanometry, acoustic reflexes, and eustachian tube function. Tuning fork tests may be omitted.

An audiologic examination reveals the degree and type of hearing loss. When the examination or the patient's history suggests that a lesion is present, site-of-lesion, vestibular, and radiographic tests may be ordered. Site-of-lesion tests distinguish between cochlear and retrocochlear lesions; vestibular tests, such as electronystagmography and falling and past-pointing tests, help detect and locate vestibular lesions; numerous radiographic techniques, such as standard X-rays, computed tomography (CT) scans, magnetic resonance imaging, and pneumoencephalography, may detect or confirm a lesion and identify its type.

Evaluating ear structures

Because the ear is so complex, a thorough examination of all its structures requires a battery of diagnostic tests. For example, otoscopy provides direct visualization of the external ear canal and tympanic membrane; acoustic immittance tests evaluate middle ear and eustachian tube function; and electronystagmography and falling and past-pointing tests evaluate the vestibular system. Pure tone audiometry and tuning fork tests evaluate conductive and sensorineural function and help determine the cause and extent of hearing loss.

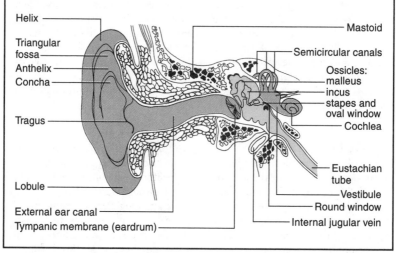

Standard X-rays can reveal congenital malformations of the middle or inner ear, mastoid inflammation, cholesteatoma, and acoustic tumors. CT scans also help detect neural degeneration, hydrocephalus, brain abscesses, and central tumors that disrupt auditory and vestibular function. (See *Evaluating ear structures*.)

Screening infants and toddlers

A significant percentage of hearing-impaired children (20% to 30%) acquire their hearing loss during infancy or early childhood. Because the first 3 years of life are the most important period for language and speech development, early identification of high-risk infants and surveillance throughout infancy and early childhood are important. The Joint Committee on Infant Hearing recommends that hearing-impaired infants be identified and start treatment within the first 6 months of life. Three years is the average age for identification; about 70% of infants and children with deficits are identified by their parents.

All infants in the neonatal intensive care unit as well as high-risk infants should be screened. High-risk infants include those who are born prematurely; those with a family history of hearing impairment, congenital anomalies of the face and skull, low birth weight, or hyperbilirubinemia; and those whose mothers had an intrauterine infection. Screening may include the auditory brain stem response (ABR), evoked otoacoustic emissions (EOAE), and behavioral testing. The ABR objectively measures the integrity of the auditory system through the brain stem with low- and high-frequency stimuli. This test is expensive and must be conducted by trained personnel. The EOAE is less expensive because it doesn't require scalp electrodes and can be performed by less skilled personnel; however, it produces significantly more false-positive results than does the ABR. Behavioral testing can be done on infants as young as 6 months old.

Let the parents know that they should report any hearing concerns and that speech and language development will be evaluated during their routine well-baby checkups. Children who don't reach appropriate language milestones during their first 18 months should be promptly referred for further hearing evaluation.

Screening schoolchildren

Screening programs in nursery and elementary schools aim to identify children with hearing losses that interfere with language development and general learning. These tests, performed by a nurse or an audiologist and graded pass-fail, simply demonstrate the need for more precise testing. School screening programs can be successful only if they provide audiologic or medical referrals, involve consultation with parents, and dispense information to teachers.

The American Speech-Language-Hearing Association (ASHA) recommends annual hearing impairment screening for all children in preschool through grade 3 because this age-group has a high incidence of hearing loss. ASHA also recommends testing children with:
- speech or language problems
- learning difficulties or special needs
- classroom behavior problems, such as inattention to auditory signals, unusual visual alertness, and confusion

- a history of allergies, repeated colds or earaches, mumps, or meningitis
- recent placement in a new school.

Screening should take place early in the school year to allow enough time for follow-up testing and referral. If comprehensive screening isn't possible, the testing of high-risk groups should take priority.

If you're performing hearing screening tests, present pure tones at levels established by state public health regulations to each child individually. If a child does not respond to any single tone, he has failed the test. This child should be retested later that day or within 1 week. Remember that many children who fail the initial screening test pass the second test after reinstruction. If a child fails twice, refer him to an audiologist for a complete workup.

When notifying parents of test results, explain that screening doesn't confirm hearing loss but suggests the need for further evaluation. Provide referrals for audiologic and medical services. If a doctor or an audiologist confirms hearing loss, help the parents, teachers, and child understand the implications.

Although pure tone screening is a valuable tool, many children with active middle ear pathology pass the test. To identify such pathology, ASHA recommends an otologic examination, pure-tone bone conduction screening, or acoustic immittance tests.

Screening adults

Aging can lead to gradual bilateral hearing loss. More than 50% of people over age 50 experience presbycusis, which results from degeneration of the middle ear. Often accompanied by tinnitus, this hearing loss is primarily sensorineural, bilateral, and irreversible.

Adults can also suffer noise-induced hearing loss in the workplace and from loud music, hunting, power tools, and fire alarms. Occupational and lifestyle

Hearing loss or malingering?

Some patients with an apparent hearing loss may be malingering to gain some financial or psychological advantage. You can often identify such patients by watching for behavioral cues.

Watch the patient in the waiting room; he may converse normally with the receptionist but not with you or the examiner. Abnormal behavior on speech tests often suggests malingering. The patient may refuse to guess, take long pauses before responding, or provide only half-word responses to spondee (easily understood, bisyllabic, equally stressed) words. The pure tone average and spondee threshold should agree; if they differ by 12 dB or more, malingering is possible.

If test results are questionable, instruct the patient again. Emphasize that he should respond to the softest tone he can detect. Give the equipment a quick listening check. If the problem persists, reschedule the test. Don't confront the patient with your suspicions of malingering, but give him a chance to yield gracefully. If these maneuvers fail, refer him to an audiologist.

---

hazards necessitate thorough history taking. Adults are often reluctant to seek diagnosis or treatment, so encourage hearing screening and, if necessary, treatment.

Preventing environmental hearing impairment

High noise levels can cause changes in heart rate and blood pressure as well as annoyance, decreased productivity, distress, and hearing impairment. Workers' compensation claims for hearing-related disability and passage of the Occupational Safety and Health Act and other legislation have stimulated the development of industrial programs for hearing conservation.

Job-related hearing loss has been divided into two general categories of severity: permanent threshold shift (PTS) and temporary threshold shift (TTS). In PTS, hearing loss is permanent and typically results from years of exposure to noise. It may also result from acoustic trauma, in which one or more intense sounds damage the tympanic membrane, ossicles, or organ of Corti. TTS, which causes temporary deafness, may result from any sound that is intense enough to cause ringing in the ears, a sensation of fullness in the ears, or difficulty in one-on-one conversation. The temporary deafness caused by TTS may last for hours to weeks, but repeated, intermittent exposure to such noise can cause permanent hearing loss. Be sure to consider TTS when evaluating an employee for permanent hearing loss because TTS and PTS produce a similar audiometric pattern. Accurate audiograms can be obtained only after at least 16 hours have elapsed since exposure to intense noise.

Noise hazard includes not just loudness but also frequency and duration of noise. Impact noises, such as riveting and jackhammering, produce sensorineural impairment more readily than does constant noise. Because noise levels may fluctuate considerably during the workday and some people are more susceptible to noise than others, official guidelines for hazardous noise in the workplace necessarily represent a compromise between complete protection and agreed-on thresholds of hearing loss.

Measures of sound

Frequency and intensity are the two measures of sound. *Frequency,* measured in hertz (Hz), is the number of sound vibrations per second. Although the ear can detect frequencies of 20 to 20,000 Hz, those between 500 and 2,000 Hz are the most important for speech recognition in a quiet environment.

Intensity is measured in decibels (dB). One decibel is roughly the smallest difference in intensity that the human ear can detect. Audiometric testing is measured in dB HL (hearing level). A whisper registers 10 to 15 dB HL, average conversation registers 50 to 60 dB HL, and a shout registers 70 to 80 dB HL.

Some industries require their employees to wear protective devices, such as earplugs or earmuffs. As part of the hearing conservation program, nurses should encourage the use of such protective devices and promote routine screening for hearing loss to monitor their effectiveness. The tendency of teenagers and young adults to use headphones and loud sound systems in confined spaces such as a car and to listen to rock and rap music for long periods can also lead to hearing deficits.

Some patients whose test results suggest hearing loss may be malingering or unable to understand the test procedures. (See *Hearing loss or malingering?*)

Audiometry
Pure tone audiometry is the standard test of hearing level. The audiometer, an instrument that evaluates hearing, should meet the specifications established by the American National Standards Institute and should deliver precisely calibrated tones at octave frequencies between 250 and 8,000 Hz. Such tones can be delivered by air or bone conduction. A normal tracing for this test is between −10 dB and +10 dB at all frequencies. Three conditions are necessary for valid audiometry: an accurately functioning and calibrated audiometer, a suitable test environment, and

a well-trained examiner. This test is conducted by an audiologist. (See *Measures of sound.*)

Otoscopy

Otoscopy is the direct visualization of the external auditory canal and the tympanic membrane through an otoscope. This test is the basic element of a physical examination of the ear and should be performed before other auditory or vestibular tests. Otoscopy indirectly provides information about the eustachian tube and the middle ear cavity.

Purpose
- To detect foreign bodies, cerumen, or stenosis in the external canal
- To detect external or middle ear pathology, such as infection of tympanic membrane perforation.

Patient preparation
Describe the procedure to the patient, and explain that this test permits visualization of the ear canal and tympanic

Pneumatic otoscopy

This test demonstrates the tympanic membrane's capacity to adjust to changes in air pressure in the middle ear. A separate device may be used to perform the test (left), or the otoscope may be fitted with a pneumatic bulb (right). Once a tight seal is achieved on insertion of the speculum, air pressure from the bulb forces the tympanic membrane to flex inward or outward.

Suction reveals pinhole perforations in the tympanic membrane when middle ear secretions issue from them. A perforated tympanic membrane is unable to move because suction can't be maintained; adhesions or fluid in the middle ear may also prevent normal movement. A tympanic membrane previously perforated but now healed may appear abnormally flaccid.

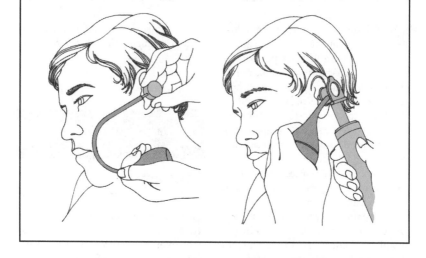

membrane. Reassure him that the examination is usually painless and takes less than 5 minutes to perform. Inform him that his ear will be pulled upward and backward to straighten the canal and to facilitate insertion of the otoscope. If the patient will undergo pneumatic otoscopy, tell him that he may experience dizziness with nystagmus (a positive fistula sign). (See *Pneumatic otoscopy.*)

Procedure

When assembling the otoscope, test the lamp and attach the largest speculum that fits comfortably into the patient's ear; the speculum straightens and dilates the ear canal. With the patient seated, tilt his head slightly away from you so that the ear to be examined is pointed upward. (If the patient is restless or unable to sit up during the procedure, he may lie down, as long as the ear is positioned upward. However, in conditions such as serous otitis media, recumbency may displace the accumulated fluid in the middle ear, making the condition harder to detect.)

Pull the auricle up and back (pull downward if the patient is under age 3); then insert the otoscope gently into the ear canal with a downward and forward motion. If insertion is difficult, replace the speculum with a smaller one. If you still feel resistance, withdraw the otoscope and tell the doctor. When the oto-

Otoscopic view of tympanic membrane

The normal tympanic membrane is shiny and pearl gray or pale pink. It reflects the light of the otoscope as a cone of light (shown below).

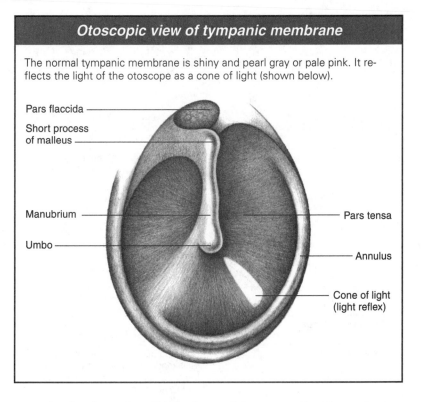

scope is placed comfortably, look through the lens and gently advance the speculum ⅜" to ½" (1 to 1.5 cm) until you see the tympanic membrane. Obtain as full a view as possible, and note redness, swelling, lesions, discharge, foreign bodes, or scaling in the canal. Check the tympanic membrane for color, contours, perforation, and a cone of light that appears at the 5-o'clock position in the right ear and at the 7-o'clock position in the left; this is a reflection of the otoscope lamp. (See *Otoscopic view of tympanic membrane.*)

Locate the *malleus,* which should be partially visible through the translucent tympanic membrane. Consisting of the short process, manubrium mallei, and umbo, the malleus extends downward to the center of the tympanic membrane. Examine the membrane itself

and the surrounding fibrous rim (annulus).

Precautions

■ The otoscope should be advanced slowly and gently through the medial portion of the ear canal to avoid irritation of the canal lining, especially if an infection is suspected.
■ Continuing to insert an otoscope against resistance may cause a perforation or damage.

Normal findings

The normal tympanic membrane is thin, translucent, shiny, and slightly concave. It appears as a pearl gray or pale pink disk that reflects light in its inferior portion. The short process, manubrium mallei, and umbo should be visible but not prominent.

Common abnormalities of the tympanic membrane

Visual examination of the tympanic membrane may reveal abnormal findings. This chart lists some of the more common findings as well as their typical causes.

ABNORMAL FINDINGS	USUAL CAUSE
Bright red	Inflammation (otitis media)
Yellowish	Pus or serum behind the tympanic membrane (acute or chronic otitis media)
Bubble behind tympanic membrane	Serous fluid in middle ear (serous otitis media)
Absent light reflection	Bulging tympanic membrane (acute otitis media)
Absent or diminishing landmarks	Thickened tympanic membrane (chronic otitis media, otitis externa, or tympanosclerosis)
Oval dark areas	Perforated or scarred tympanic membrane (otitis media or trauma)
Prominent malleus	Retracted tympanic membrane (nonfunctional eustachian tube)
Reduced mobility	Stiffened middle ear system (serous otitis media or, more rarely, middle ear adhesions); negative pressure; middle ear fluid

Implications of results

Scarring, discoloration, or retraction or bulging of the tympanic membrane indicates pathology. Movement of the tympanic membrane in tandem with respiration suggests abnormal patency of the eustachian tube. (See *Common abnormalities of the tympanic membrane.*)

Post-test care

None.

Interfering factors

■ Obstruction of the ear canal by cerumen or foreign matter obscures the tympanic membrane.
■ A recumbent position during otoscopy can mask serous otitis media.

Tuning fork tests

Despite their limitations, the Weber, Rinne, and Schwabach tuning fork tests are quick, valuable screening tools for detecting hearing loss and providing preliminary information about its type. The *Weber test* determines whether a patient lateralizes the tone of the tuning fork to one ear. The *Rinne test* compares air and bone conduction in both ears. The *Schwabach test* compares the patient's bone conduction response with that of the examiner, who is assumed to have normal hearing.

Although the results of these tests are most reliable when a low-frequency tuning fork is used, they're not definitive because they depend on subjective factors, such as the examiner's ability to strike the fork with equal force each time and the patient's ability to report audible tones correctly. Also, the Weber test results may be misleading, and the Rinne test frequently doesn't detect a mild conductive loss (10 to 35 dB). Thus, abnormal test results require confirmation by pure tone audiometry.

Purpose

- To screen for or confirm hearing loss
- To help distinguish between conductive and sensorineural hearing loss.

Patient preparation

Describe the procedure to the patient, and explain that these tests help detect hearing loss and give information on the type of loss. Tell him who will perform the tests, and reassure him that the tests are painless and take only a few minutes.

Advise the patient that his concentration and prompt responses are essential to ensure accurate results. Have him use hand signals to indicate whether a tone is louder in his right ear or in his left ear and when he stops hearing the tone. Inform him that tuning fork tests are not definitive and that further testing may be necessary to confirm abnormal results.

Procedure

Using a low-frequency tuning fork (256 or 512 Hz), practice achieving a consistent tone. You can vibrate the tuning fork by gently striking one prong against your elbow or the heel of your hand, by stroking the prongs upward, or by pinching them together. (See *How to use the tuning fork,* pages 598 and 599.)

For the Weber test: Vibrate the fork and place its base on the midline of the skull at the forehead. Ask the patient if he hears the tone in his left ear, right ear, or equally in both. Record the results as

"Weber left," "Weber right," or "Weber midline," respectively.

For the Rinne test: To test bone conduction, hold the tuning fork between your thumb and index finger, and place the base of the vibrating fork against the patient's mastoid process. Then, to test air conduction, move the still-vibrating prongs next to — but not touching — the external ear. Ask the patient which location has the louder or longer sound. Repeat the procedure for the other ear. Record the results as "Rinne positive" if the patient hears air-conducted sound louder or longer and "Rinne negative" if he hears bone-conducted sound louder or longer.

For the Schwabach test: Hold the tuning fork between your thumb and index finger, place the base of the vibrating tuning fork against the left mastoid process, and ask the patient if he hears the tone. If he does, immediately place the tuning fork on *your* left mastoid process and listen for the tone. Alternate the tuning fork between the patient's left mastoid process and your own until one of you stops hearing the sound; record the length of time that the other continues to hear it. Then repeat the procedure on the right mastoid process.

Record the name of the test, the result, and the vibrating frequency of the tuning fork.

Precautions

Strike the tuning fork with equal force each time. Hold the fork at its base to allow the prongs to vibrate freely.

Normal findings

In the Weber test, a patient with normal hearing hears the same tone equally loud in both ears — a Weber-midline result. In the Rinne test, a patient hears the air-conducted tone louder or longer than the bone-conducted tone — a Rinne-positive result. In the Schwabach

How to use the tuning fork

You'll use a tuning fork to perform the Weber, Rinne, and Schwabach tests. These photos will help you place the tuning fork properly.

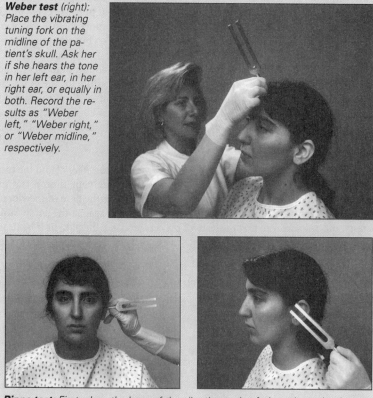

Weber test *(right): Place the vibrating tuning fork on the midline of the patient's skull. Ask her if she hears the tone in her left ear, in her right ear, or equally in both. Record the results as "Weber left," "Weber right," or "Weber midline," respectively.*

Rinne test: *First, place the base of the vibrating tuning fork on the patient's mastoid process to test bone conduction (left); then hold the prongs ½" (1 cm) from the ear canal to test air conduction (right).*

test, both the patient and the examiner hear the tone equally long.

Implications of results

In the Weber test, lateralization of the tone to one ear suggests a conductive loss on that side or a sensorineural loss on the other side. Physiologically, lateralization results from the tone being louder in one ear (Stenger effect) or from the tone reaching one ear sooner than the other (phase effect). If one ear has a sensorineural loss, the Stenger effect causes lateralization to the unaffected ear; if one ear has a conductive loss, either the Stenger or the phase effect produces lateralization to that ear. If a patient's hearing loss is unilateral, the Weber test may suggest the type of loss. When a patient's hearing loss is bilater-

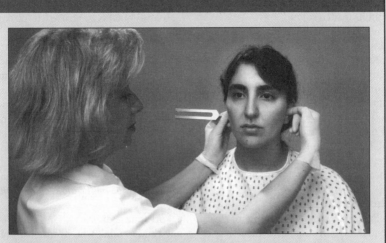

Schwabach test: *First place the vibrating tuning fork on the patient's right mastoid process (top) and then on your own (bottom). Continue alternating the fork until one of you stops hearing the sound, and record how long the sound is heard. Repeat the procedure on the left mastoid process.*

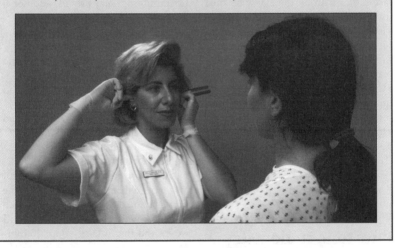

al, this test may help to identify the ear with the better bone conduction.

In the Rinne test, hearing the bone-conducted tone louder or for a longer duration than the air-conducted tone indicates a conductive loss. With a unilateral hearing loss, the tone may be heard louder when conducted by bone, but in the opposite ear. This is a false-negative Rinne. A sensorineural loss is indicated when the sound is heard louder by air conduction.

In the Schwabach test, prolonged duration of the tone, compared with that of the examiner, suggests a conductive loss; conversely, shortened duration indicates a sensorineural loss. A conductive loss attenuates (decreases the energy of) air-conducted sound in a room with ambient noise, enabling patients with this type of loss to hear bone-conducted sound longer than the examiner can hear such sound.

A patient with abnormal results on any or all tuning fork tests should be retested. Similar results on retesting require formal pure tone audiometry to confirm the hearing loss and determine its type and severity.

Post-test care

Refer the patient for further audiologic testing if tuning fork tests suggest a hearing loss.

Interfering factors

■ Failure to strike the tuning fork with equal force or to hold it correctly during the procedure interferes with accuracy.

■ Striking the tuning fork on a hard surface rather than on the elbow or knee invalidates results.

■ Failure to use either the 256-Hz (more sensitive) or the 512-Hz frequency tuning forks will affect the accuracy of test results.

■ Undetected hearing loss in the examiner invalidates results of the Schwabach test.

■ Inaccurate patient response because of poor understanding of his task interferes with accurate testing.

Pure tone audiometry

This test, performed with an audiometer, provides a record of the thresholds — the lowest intensity levels — at which a patient can hear a set of test tones introduced through earphones or a bone conduction (sound) vibrator. These tones, called pure tones, have their energy concentrated at discrete frequencies. Octave frequencies between 125

and 8,000 Hz are used to obtain air conduction thresholds; frequencies between 250 and 4,000 Hz are used to obtain bone conduction thresholds.

Comparison of air and bone conduction thresholds can suggest a conductive, sensorineural, or mixed hearing loss but not the cause of the loss; further audiologic and vestibular tests and X-rays may provide the cause. Pure tone audiometry results may also suggest the need for referral to an audiologist for evaluation of communication difficulties and planning of appropriate rehabilitation. (See *Implications of pure tone average.*)

Pure tone audiometry is indicated for any child or adult who needs quantitative hearing assessment. Although this test has no contraindications, results depend on patient cooperation. Acoustic immittance may provide additional information.

Purpose

■ To determine the presence, type, and degree of hearing loss

■ To assess communication abilities and rehabilitation needs

■ To accurately determine pure tone and speech reception threshold.

Patient preparation

Describe the procedure to the patient, and explain that this test determines the presence and degree of hearing loss. Tell him who will perform the test and where and that it takes about 20 minutes.

Inform him that each ear will be tested separately, starting with the ear in which he has better hearing. Advise him that he'll hear tones at various intensities and that he'll be instructed to give a signal (or press the response button) each time he hears the tone. Emphasize that he should respond even if the tone is faint. Just before the test, ask the patient to remove all obstructions to prop-

Implications of pure tone average

The patient's pure tone average helps determine his degree of hearing loss as well as the audibility of speech in a quiet environment.

PURE TONE AVERAGE	DEGREE OF HEARING LOSS	SPEECH AUDIBILITY
0 to 25 dB	Normal limits	No significant difficulty
26 to 40 dB	Mild	Difficulty with faint or distant speech
41 to 55 dB	Moderate	Difficulty with conversational speech
56 to 70 dB	Moderately severe	Speech must be loud; difficulty with group conversation
71 to 90 dB	Severe	Difficulty with loud speech; understands only shouted or amplified speech
91+ dB	Profound	May not understand amplified speech

er earphone placement. If he has been exposed to loud noises (loud enough to cause tinnitus or make face-to-face communication difficult) within the past 16 hours, postpone the test.

Equipment

Otoscope ✦ calibrated audiometer with earphones and bone conduction vibrator ✦ quiet test environment (sound-treated room).

Procedure

The patient's ear canal is checked with the otoscope for impacted cerumen. Next, the examiner presses a finger first on the auricle and then on the tragus to rule out possible closure of the canal under pressure from the earphones. If the canal tends to close, a stiff-walled plastic tube is carefully inserted into the canal, and this modification is recorded on the audiogram; children and elderly patients are most likely to require this modification.

The earphones are positioned so that they line up opposite the ear canals, and the headband is tightened. The examiner familiarizes the patient with the test tone by presenting it to his better ear for less than 1 second at a level 15 to 25 dB above the expected threshold. If he responds to the tone, air conduction testing is begun at 1,000 Hz, and intensity is decreased in 10-dB steps until the patient fails to respond. Then intensity is increased in 5-dB steps until he hears the tone again. After he responds to the ascending run, intensity is decreased in 10-dB steps. Sequences of 10-dB decrements and 5-dB increments are repeated until the patient responds to at least two of three presentations at a single level. The threshold level is the lowest decibel level at which the response rate is at least 50%.

Using this procedure, tones are presented to the better ear in this order: 1,000 Hz, 2,000 Hz, 4,000 Hz, 8,000 Hz, 1,000 Hz, 500 Hz, and 250 Hz. After testing the better ear, the poorer ear is tested. In each ear, test or retest differences may be ±5 dB. If the difference between the first and second threshold at 1,000 Hz is greater than 10 dB, test results are unreliable; equipment should be checked for malfunction, and the

Evaluating results of pure tone audiometry

Pure tone audiometry can determine sensorineural, conductive or mixed hearing loss. This chart shows the level of bone and air conduction thresholds for each type of hearing loss.

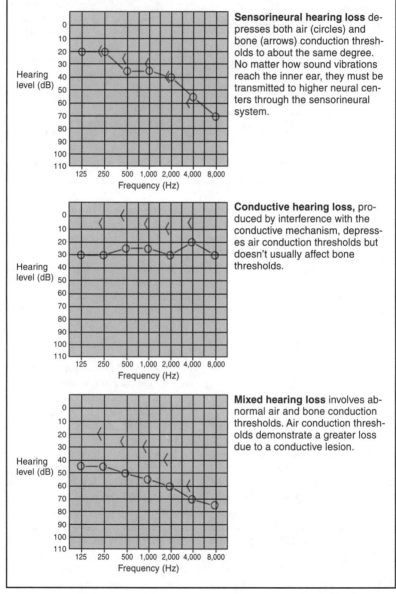

Sensorineural hearing loss depresses both air (circles) and bone (arrows) conduction thresholds to about the same degree. No matter how sound vibrations reach the inner ear, they must be transmitted to higher neural centers through the sensorineural system.

Conductive hearing loss, produced by interference with the conductive mechanism, depresses air conduction thresholds but doesn't usually affect bone thresholds.

Mixed hearing loss involves abnormal air and bone conduction thresholds. Air conduction thresholds demonstrate a greater loss due to a conductive lesion.

Preventing crossover

A sufficiently intense test tone presented to one ear causes the skull to vibrate. The tone then passes by bone conduction to the opposite ear (crossover). For air conduction testing, this crossover generally occurs when the test tone exceeds 40 dB HL (125 to 750 Hz) or 50 dB HL (1,000 to 8,000 Hz). During bone conduction, crossover occurs at all levels.

Crossover can be prevented by masking the ear not being tested with narrow-band noise from the audiometer. If crossover isn't prevented, test results will underestimate the degree of hearing loss.

Because of the difficulty involved, masking is generally performed by an audiologist.

patient should be reinstructed and re-tested.

For *bone conduction* testing, the earphones are removed and the vibrator is placed on the mastoid process of the better ear (the auricle shouldn't touch the vibrator). Ascending and descending tones are used as in air conduction testing, using 250 Hz, 500 Hz, 1,000 Hz, 2,000 Hz, and 4,000 Hz.

Precautions
Record on the audiogram any modifications to the standard testing procedure, such as insertion of a plastic tube into the ear canal to avoid ear canal collapse.

Normal findings
The normal range of hearing sensitivity is 0 to 25 dB for adults and 0 to 15 dB for children. However, normal test results do not rule out pathology; a mild middle ear infection or other pathology may exist but not interfere with auditory function.

Implications of results
The pure tone average — the average of pure tone air conduction thresholds obtained at 500 Hz, 1,000 Hz, and 2,000 Hz — quantifies the degree of hearing loss. When these three thresholds vary widely, the mean of the best

two — the Fletcher average — indicates the degree of hearing loss.

The relationship between threshold responses for air and bone conduction tones determines the type of hearing loss. In sensorineural loss, both thresholds are depressed; in conductive loss, air thresholds are depressed but bone thresholds are unchanged; in mixed hearing loss, both thresholds are abnormal, with air conduction more depressed than bone conduction. (See *Evaluating results of pure tone audiometry*.)

Post-test care
If test results aren't reliable or if they're hindered by possible crossover, refer the patient for further testing. (See *Preventing crossover*.)

Interfering factors
- Impacted cerumen or a closed ear canal can cause a 35- to 40-dB artifactual conductive hearing loss.
- A patient who confuses vibrotactile with auditory sensation or tinnitus with the signal will give invalid responses.
- Cracked or poorly fitting earphones result in low-frequency leakage and falsely elevated thresholds.
- An uncalibrated audiometer or background noise can invalidate test results.

■ Presentation of extraneous cues to the patient, such as a rhythmic pattern of test tones or hand movement near the attenuator dial, can invalidate results.

■ An uncooperative or inattentive patient may give invalid responses.

Acoustic immittance

Immittance tests evaluate middle ear function by measuring the flow of sound energy into the ear (admittance) and the opposition to that flow (impedance). Not all sound energy that impinges on the tympanic membrane reaches the inner ear; some reflects into the external ear canal. The relationship between incident and reflected sound energy determines the admittance, which depends on the resistance, stiffness, and mass of the auditory system. Normally, stiffness is the predominant factor in the middle ear.

Admittance is commonly measured by two tests: tympanometry and acoustic reflexes. Each of these tests uses an electronic tone generator, an air pressure manometer, and a tone probe that delivers both sound and air pressure stimuli to the ear canal and tympanic membrane through an airtight seal. *Tympanometry* measures middle ear admittance in response to changes in air pressure in the ear canal; the *acoustic reflexes test* measures the change in admittance produced by contraction of the stapedius muscle as it responds to an intense sound. Stapedial contraction stiffens the tympanic membrane and ossicular chain, causing a measurable change in middle ear admittance. Reflex decay, part of the acoustic reflexes test, is a function of eighth nerve adaptation or fatigue in response to a reflex-eliciting stimulus.

Admittance tests help diagnose middle ear pathology, lesions in the seventh (facial) or eighth cranial nerve, and eustachian tube dysfunction. They can also help verify the presence of a labyrinthine fistula and identify pseudohypoacusis (nonorganic hearing loss). Because admittance tests require little patient cooperation, they can reliably test young children and mentally or physically handicapped patients.

Purpose

Tympanometry:

■ To assess the continuity and admittance of the middle ear

■ To evaluate the status of the tympanic membrane.

Acoustic reflexes and reflex decay:

■ To distinguish between cochlear and retrocochlear lesions

■ To differentiate eighth nerve or peripheral brain stem lesions from intra-axial brain stem lesions

■ To locate seventh nerve lesions relative to stapedius muscle innervation

■ To confirm conductive hearing loss

■ To help confirm pseudohypoacusis.

Patient preparation

Describe the procedure to the patient, and explain that these tests evaluate the condition of the middle ear. Inform him who will perform the tests and where and that each test takes 2 to 3 minutes.

Instruct the patient not to move, speak, or swallow while admittance is being recorded, and caution him not to startle during the loud tone reflex–eliciting measurement. Advise him that changes in ear canal pressure rarely cause transient vertigo, and tell him to report any discomfort or dizziness. Reassure him that although the probe may cause discomfort, it won't harm his ear.

Equipment

Admittance meter ✦ calibrated probe cavity to calibrate the meter (supplied

Performing acoustic immittance tests

With the probe tip sealed in the external meatus, the examiner can deliver both sound and air pressure stimuli to the ear canal and tympanic membrane.

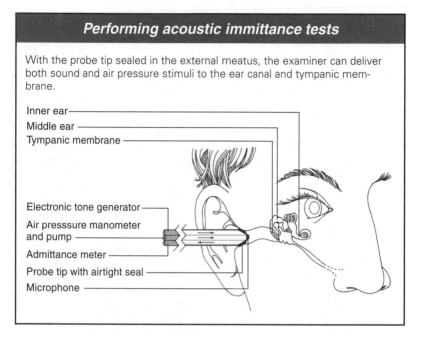

Inner ear

Middle ear

Tympanic membrane

Electronic tone generator

Air presssure manometer and pump

Admittance meter

Probe tip with airtight seal

Microphone

---

by manufacturer) ✦ strip chart recorder (optional) ✦ probe tips and cuffs (to seal probe in ear canal) ✦ silicone putty (for difficult seal) ✦ otoscope with speculum ✦ wire (to clean bores of probe) ✦ pure tone audiometer (to provide stimulus for acoustic reflex [optional]).

Procedure

A quick otoscopic examination is performed to verify that no impacted cerumen or other obstruction is present in the ear canal. The size and shape of the canal are checked to select the appropriate-size probe cuff, which is then attached to the probe. The probe tip is inserted into the ear canal while pulling upward and backward on the auricle; a proper seal can maintain a negative pressure of −200 daPa. If necessary, silicone putty is applied to ensure a snug, leakproof seal; care must be taken to avoid clogging the probe tip with putty. (See *Performing acoustic immittance tests.*)

For tympanometry: After a seal is obtained, the admittance meter sensitivity and probe tone level are set (if they're not automatic). The patient is informed when the test is about to begin. Air pressure is then changed, and the admittance is recorded. If recording is manual, at least six measurements between −200 and +200 daPa are taken. Additional measurements are taken if admittance changes are large. Although the direction of air pressure change (positive to negative or vice versa) is arbitrary, the direction is kept consistent throughout the test.

If a flat tympanogram is obtained (no change in admittance), the possibility that the probe tip may have rested against the canal wall or that it was clogged with cerumen must be ruled out with ear canal volume measurements. The probe is moved slightly and the tympanogram is observed for a large admittance change. The probe tip is removed, cleaned, and reinserted, and the test is repeated.

For acoustic reflexes test: A broad-band noise or a pure tone (500 to 4,000 Hz) is presented monaurally; a monaural stimulus causes bilateral reflex activation. Depending on the equipment available, the change in admittance in the stimulated ear (ipsilateral measurement) or in the opposite ear (contralateral or trans–brain stem measurement) is monitored. The results for the stimulated ear are recorded, regardless of whether monitoring is ipsilateral or contralateral.

The patient is told that stimuli will be presented. Reflex threshold is determined by presenting stimuli in ascending steps of 10 dB; when the first reflex occurs, decrease the level by 10 dB and start an ascending run in 5-dB steps. The lowest-level stimulus that elicits a reflex is recorded. Then reflex decay is measured contralaterally at 500 and 1,000 Hz by presenting the stimulus at 10 dB above the reflex threshold for 10 seconds; the magnitude of the reflex during the first second of stimulation is the baseline. Reflex magnitude at 5 or 10 seconds is compared with baseline at 1 second; significant reflex decay occurs when reflex magnitude declines to less than one-half of baseline.

Precautions

■ Obtain medical clearance before performing admittance tests on patients with head trauma or a possible labyrinthine fistula and on those who've recently had middle ear surgery.

■ Check equipment carefully. If the probe tip is clogged with cerumen or debris, the measured admittance won't change, even when the probe isn't coupled to the ear. To clean the probe, carefully insert a wire through each bore, wipe the wire, and then withdraw it.

■ If you can't obtain a seal even though the probe seems well seated, look for leakage elsewhere in the air system. Check the system by putting your finger over the probe tip and cuff and determining whether nonzero pressure can be maintained. If it can't, seal the air outlet behind the meter with your finger and check admittance. Then check each subsequent link in the system for possible leakage.

■ Although the capability for monitoring acoustic reflexes both ipsilateral and contralateral to the stimulated ear is diagnostically useful, ipsilateral measurement is subject to equipment artifact. To check for this, put the probe tip in a calibrated cavity supplied by the manufacturer. Presentation of the reflex stimulus in this cavity should not change the measured admittance.

Normal findings

In tympanometry, the normal middle ear air pressure range is ±100 daPa. The overall shape of the tympanogram is smooth and symmetrical. (See *Interpreting tympanograms.*)

In acoustic reflexes, the normal trans–brain stem reflex threshold levels for pure tones range from 70 to 100 dB HL; ipsilateral thresholds are 3 to 12 dB lower. Reflex decay is normally slight — no more than one-half of baseline over 10 seconds.

Implications of results

A flat tympanogram, indicating no change in admittance with changing air pressure, can result from fluid in the middle ear, a perforated tympanic membrane, or impacted cerumen. Large changes in admittance can reflect tympanic membrane scarring or disarticulated ossicular chain. If the eustachian tube is patent, admittance may change with the patient's respiration, resulting in periodic fluctuations on the tympanogram. (See *Evaluating eustachian tube function,* page 608.) Fluctuations synchronous with the patient's pulse sug-

Interpreting tympanograms

Tympanograms can be classified according to shape, amplitude, and pressure, as depicted in the chart below.

TYMPANOGRAM	SHAPE	AMPLITUDE	PRESSURE
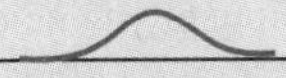	Normal	Normal	Normal
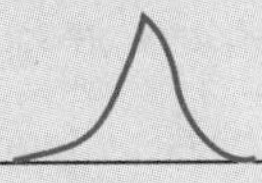	Peaked	Flaccid	Normal
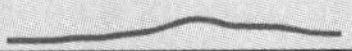	Normal	Stiff	Normal
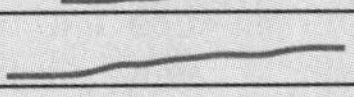	Flat	Stiff	Absent-negative
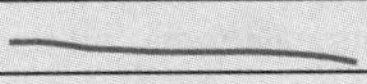	Flat	Stiff	Absent-negative
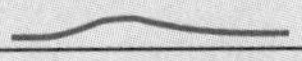	Normal	Stiff	–125 daPa
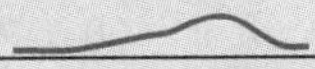	Normal	Normal	+90 daPa
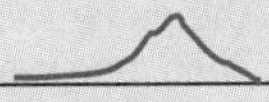	Notched	Flaccid	Normal
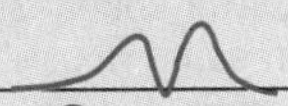	Deep, broad notching	Flaccid	Normal
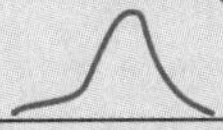	Normal	Flaccid	–200 daPa
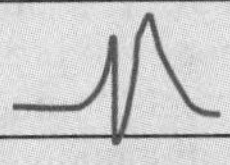	Deep, broad notching	Flaccid	–200 daPa
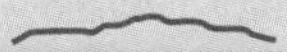	Vascular perturbation	Stiff	Normal

–300   0   +300
Pressure in daPa
(0.983 daPa = 1 mm H_2O)

gest a glomangioma in the middle ear space.

The absence of acoustic reflexes may indicate poor residual sensitivity in the stimulated ear (hearing loss greater than 70 dB); a conductive loss of sufficient magnitude (greater than 25 dB) to prevent adequate stimulus levels from reaching the inner ear; damage to the eighth nerve in the stimulated ear or lower brain stem; absence of the stapedius muscle in the probe ear; a conductive loss greater than 5 dB in the probe ear; or damage to the seventh nerve of the probe ear central to the innervation of the stapedius muscle.

Reflexes can't be monitored if middle ear reconstructive surgery has removed the stapedius muscle or if the muscle is congenitally absent. A suprastapedial lesion of the seventh nerve paralyzes the stapedius. Thus, the presence of the reflex in a patient with seventh nerve pathology suggests that the lesion is inferior or peripheral to stapedial innervation.

Evaluating eustachian tube function

An oxygen-absorbing mucosal lining covers the middle ear cavity and mastoid air cells. The eustachian tube periodically opens to ensure the middle ear's oxygen supply. If this tube is blocked, negative air pressure in the middle ear results, causing edema and a buildup of effusions.

Three-step procedure

Testing eustachian tube function in an ear with an intact tympanic membrane generally involves three steps: inducing negative (preferable) or positive pressure in the middle ear cavity (verified tympanometrically); having the patient swallow or yawn to open the tube; and recording another tympanogram to determine if this maneuver altered middle ear pressure. Because it's difficult to artificially induce sufficient negative pressure, this test doesn't duplicate the most critical conditions for eustachian tube function. The test also can't be performed if the tympanogram is abnormally shaped and middle ear pressure isn't known.

Implications of results

If the patient's tympanogram shows a well-defined peak, peak admittance pressure is a useful indicator of eustachian tube function. Normal pressure (±100 daPa) usually means that the middle ear is properly ventilated and that the eustachian tube is functioning adequately; if pressure is abnormal, the examiner asks the patient to swallow or yawn several times and repeats the tympanogram to verify that negative pressure isn't transient.

If the patient has a perforated tympanic membrane or a ventilatory tube in place, the ear canal and middle ear form a single cavity; pressure within this cavity can be varied directly with the admittance meter air system. The examiner creates a negative pressure of –100 daPa in the cavity, asks the patient to swallow four to six times, and watches the manometer for changes in air pressure. If pressure doesn't return to within ±50 daPa, the procedure is repeated with +100 daPa and again with +200 daPa. Positive pressure isn't as accurate as negative pressure, but it does suggest the degree of eustachian tube dysfunction.

Tympanometry can also verify abnormal patency or opening of the eustachian tube. If the eustachian tube is open, air pressure in the middle ear cavity fluctuates with respiration, and this can be recorded with the admittance meter.

Ipsilateral stimulation and monitoring don't require transmission of stimulus information across the brain stem. Comparison of ipsilateral and trans–brain stem findings may help distinguish eighth nerve and peripheral brain stem lesions from intra-axial brain stem lesions.

A change in reflex magnitude in response to a sustained stimulus suggests an eighth nerve or a brain stem lesion.

Using the first second of stimulation as the baseline magnitude, reflex decay to less than one-half of baseline in 5 to 10 seconds is a significant sign of a retrocochlear lesion. (See *Correlating tympanogram findings with selected disorders.*)

If cochlear sensitivity is poor, reflexes are absent; therefore, if reflex thresholds are better than voluntary thresholds, suspect malingering. In such a case, re-emphasize the importance of this test

Correlating tympanogram findings with selected disorders

FEATURE	FINDING	ASSOCIATED DISORDERS
Shape	Altered smoothness	▪ Tympanic membrane abnormality ▪ Ossicular discontinuity ▪ Vascular tumor
	Flat	▪ Serous otitis media ▪ Perforated tympanic membrane ▪ Canal wall or cerumen artifact ▪ Middle ear tumor
	Peaked	▪ Tympanic membrane abnormality ▪ Ossicular discontinuity
Amplitude	Increased	▪ Tympanic membrane abnormality ▪ Ossicular discontinuity
	Normal	▪ Blocked eustachian tube ▪ Early acute otitis media
	Reduced	▪ Ossicular fixation ▪ Serous otitis media ▪ Cholesteatoma, polyps, granuloma ▪ Glomangioma
Pressure	Positive	▪ Early acute otitis media
	Normal	▪ Ossicular fixation or adhesive fixation ▪ Ossicular discontinuity ▪ Middle ear tumor ▪ Tympanic membrane abnormality
	Negative	▪ Blocked eustachian tube ▪ Early serous otitis media

to the patient, inform him that the admittance meter reveals his actual ability to hear, and ask for his complete cooperation.

Post-test care
None.

Interfering factors
▪ Clogged tone probe, poor air seal, or movement of the probe tip during measurement interferes with accurate testing.
▪ The patient's talking, swallowing, or startling during measurement interferes with accurate testing.

Spondee threshold

This simple, reliable, and widely used test (also known as the speech reception threshold and the spondaic word threshold) determines the faintest level at which a patient correctly repeats 50% of a live or recorded set of spondee words presented to him through earphones in a quiet environment. Spondees are two-syllable words that are accented equally on each syllable, such as baseball, airplane, and birthday. The spondees selected for the test are familiar words that are uniformly audible and dissimilar in phonetic construction. The spondee threshold test is commonly performed after pure tone audiometry to check the validity of audiometric hearing thresholds; the pure tone (Fletcher) average should agree with the spondee threshold within 10 dB.

Purpose

- To measure the degree of hearing loss for speech recognition
- To distinguish true hearing loss from nonorganic hearing loss (pseudohypoacusis)
- To confirm the results of pure tone audiometry for frequencies most important for speech recognition.

Patient preparation

Describe the procedure to the patient, and explain that this test evaluates his ability to hear conversational speech. Tell him that the test is performed by an audiologist and takes about 5 minutes. Inform him that a series of two-syllable words will be transmitted to him through earphones while he's in a soundproof booth. Tell him to repeat each word after he hears it and to guess if he isn't sure of a word. Inform him that the volume of each word spoken becomes progressively softer as the test continues and that each ear will be tested separately.

If the patient has difficulty understanding English, provide him with a printed list of words before the test and, if necessary, help him learn them. Advise him that he won't be able to refer to the list during the test.

Equipment

Calibrated speech audiometer ✦ earphones ✦ recorded spondee list ✦ soundproof booth.

Procedure

The patient is instructed to enter the soundproof booth, and the audiologist places the earphones securely over the patient's ears. The ear with better hearing acuity is tested first, with the sound level set about 20 dB above the patient's pure tone threshold. After familiarizing the patient with the spondees, the spondee threshold is determined in a manner similar to that for determining the pure tone threshold. The intensity is decreased and then increased until it reaches the faintest level at which the patient has a 50% correct response rate.

After determining the spondee threshold of the better ear, the procedure is repeated for the other ear.

Precautions

Although the spondee threshold provides a direct and reliable measure of hearing loss for speech in most adults, it cannot measure it reliably in young children and in people with language difficulties.

Normal findings

The spondee threshold should fall within ±10 dB of the pure tone threshold. However, this relationship may vary in patients with precipitous sloping hearing losses and in those whose tests demonstrate irregular audiometric configuration.

Implications of results

If the spondee threshold differs by more than 10 dB from the pure tone threshold, the patient may be unable to respond to the lowest audible levels or may be malingering. In such cases, the instructions are repeated to the patient and the test is performed again. A patient with abnormal test results should be referred to an audiologist for tests of malingering or nonorganic hearing loss.

Post-test care
None.

Interfering factors
Young children and people who are unfamiliar with the English language or the terminology used in the test may give inaccurate responses.

Word recognition

Word recognition tests measure a person's ability to recognize and repeat a series of monosyllabic words presented by a live or recorded voice at suprathreshold levels (about 40 dB above the spondee threshold) in a quiet environment. The phonetically balanced test words represent the relative frequency with which sounds occur in English. Commonly used word recognition tests include the PAL PB-50 (Psychoacoustics Laboratories, Harvard University, Cambridge, Mass.), the CID W-22 (Central Institute for the Deaf, St. Louis), and the NU auditory test #4 or #6 (Northwestern University, Evanston, Ill.).

Most speech energy is contained in vowel sounds and concentrated in low frequencies; less energy is contained in consonant sounds and high frequencies. Because consonants distinguish most words (such as pin, thin, and bin), a patient with high-frequency hearing loss misses consonant cues and commonly complains that he hears speech but doesn't understand it.

Word recognition is tested because patients with similar audiogram results may have markedly different word recognition abilities. Poor word recognition is the result of the distortion imposed by hearing loss. In real-life situations, nonauditory factors, such as the ability to read lips and use contextual information, are important for understanding speech.

Purpose
- To evaluate the clarity of speech reception at suprathreshold levels
- To determine the need for and potential benefits of a hearing aid or speech reading instruction
- To help locate auditory tract and central nervous system lesions.

Patient preparation
Describe the procedure to the patient, and explain that these tests assess his ability to hear and understand speech presented at above-normal tones and help determine if he would benefit from a hearing aid. Tell him that the test will be performed by an audiologist and that each ear will be tested separately. Advise the patient that a series of short words will be transmitted to him through earphones while he's in a soundproof booth. Tell him to repeat each word after he hears it and to guess when unsure.

If he's wearing a hearing aid, ask him to remove it.

Equipment
Calibrated speech audiometer and earphones ✦ standardized word list.

Procedure
After the patient is seated in a soundproof booth, earphones are placed on his ears. The live voice or recorded word list is presented at a sensation level about 40 dB greater than the patient's spondee threshold or at a level the patient considers comfortable. The number of correct responses is recorded and converted to a percentage score.

Precautions
None.

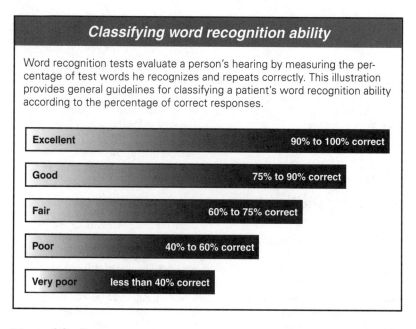

Classifying word recognition ability

Word recognition tests evaluate a person's hearing by measuring the percentage of test words he recognizes and repeats correctly. This illustration provides general guidelines for classifying a patient's word recognition ability according to the percentage of correct responses.

Excellent	90% to 100% correct
Good	75% to 90% correct
Fair	60% to 75% correct
Poor	40% to 60% correct
Very poor	less than 40% correct

Normal findings

A person with normal hearing can correctly repeat at least 90% of the test words. (See *Classifying word recognition ability*.)

Implications of results

Test scores may vary by as much as 12% as a result of sampling error or normal test-retest differences. If the score for one ear differs from that for the other ear by more than 12% or if the scores are significantly poorer than expected (compared with the pure tone audiogram), a retrocochlear lesion may be present.

Patients with conductive hearing loss can have excellent word recognition if speech is loud enough. Sensorineural loss may distort neural representation of sound and cause poor recognition. Amplification allows hearing-impaired people to hear speech at conversational levels. A hearing aid may improve understanding by amplifying frequencies that are important for distinguishing speech sounds. Some people may also benefit from increased awareness of environmental sounds.

If test scores suggest (or the patient reports) difficulty hearing or understanding speech, refer the patient for aural rehabilitation; if scores suggest a retrocochlear lesion, refer the patient for neuro-otologic examination.

Post-test care

None.

Interfering factors

■ The characteristics of the test equipment (particularly the earphones) or changes in the presentation level of the word list may affect test scores.

■ Scores obtained using earphones at a particular presentation level may not agree with those obtained using a hearing aid at the same level.

Site-of-lesion tests

When the patient history or pure tone audiometry suggests the presence of a lesion, site-of-lesion tests can be performed to locate it. Indications from the patient history include difficulty understanding speech that's disproportionate to the degree of pure tone loss; dizziness, tinnitus, or sudden or fluctuating hearing loss; or other neural symptoms. The primary indication from pure tone audiometry is a difference between ears in the sensorineural components. However, not all lesions impair pure tone sensitivity. Because the auditory system contains many neural pathways in the brain stem and cortex, a pure tone signal can bypass a lesion and be carried by relatively few neural fibers. More difficult stimuli, presented in the site-of-lesion tests, are required to test auditory system function and to reveal the effects of lesions.

Site-of-lesion tests help distinguish cochlear from retrocochlear lesions and can often localize lesions in the retrocochlear system at the eighth nerve, in the extra-axial (peripheral) or intra-axial brain stem, and in the cortex. Some commonly used site-of-lesion tests include alternate binaural loudness balance (ABLB), simultaneous binaural midplane localization (SBMPL), tone decay, Békésy audiometry, masking level differences (MLD), difficult speech discrimination tasks, auditory brain stem electrical response measures (ABR), and competing message (CM) tasks.

When performing site-of-lesion tests, the intensity of the test signal is distinguished from the sensation level. Intensity is the hearing level (HL) shown on the audiometer dial, and sensation level (SL) is the number of decibels above the patient's threshold for that signal. For example, a patient with a threshold of 0 dB HL hears a 60-dB HL tone at 60 dB SL; a patient with a 40-dB HL threshold (or a 40-dB hearing loss) hears the same tone at 20 dB SL. The distinction between HL and SL is diagnostically important because a person with a cochlear hearing loss often performs as well as a person with normal hearing if intensity levels are held constant; sensation levels, however, may be quite different.

By itself, the site-of-lesion test battery cannot diagnose a disorder, but it can suggest the location and extent of damage to the auditory system. Air and bone conduction thresholds and aural immittance tests must rule out or measure the extent of conductive hearing loss before site-of-lesion tests can be performed.

Purpose
- To distinguish cochlear from retrocochlear hearing loss
- To localize lesions in the retrocochlear component of the auditory system.

Patient preparation
Explain to the patient that these tests help locate the probable cause of hearing impairment. Inform him that they're performed by an audiologist, who will thoroughly explain each procedure before it is done, and that they take about 90 minutes.

Procedure
Earphones are used for each test.

For ABLB: A tone is alternately presented to one ear and then the other. The tone in one ear is held at a constant intensity of 90 dB HL; the other tone is varied. The patient indicates when the tones sound equally loud to both ears.

For SBMPL: A 90–dB HL tone is presented to one ear and tones of varying intensity are simultaneously presented to the other ear. The patient indicates when he perceives a single tone in the center of his head.

For tone decay: A tone is presented at or near threshold and the patient indicates how long he can hear it. If the tone becomes inaudible or changes to a buzzing or hissing sound, the tone is raised 5 dB, which produces a tone that the patient should again be able to hear. The process is repeated until the patient hears the tone continuously for 60 seconds.

For Békésy audiometry: In this test, the patient controls the tone intensity by depressing a response button whenever he hears a tone. When the tone softens and disappears, he releases the button; the tone then becomes louder. The patient repeats this procedure for several minutes, and the resulting audiometric tracing shows excursions above and below the actual threshold. The audiometer is set to sweep across frequencies or to record at one frequency. When the test is being used for site-of-lesion studies, first the threshold for a pulsing tone is determined and then the threshold for a continuous tone is determined. Test results conform to one of five types of curves.

For MLD: A 500-Hz tone and a narrow-band masking noise are presented to both ears at once. The noise is held at a constant intensity, and the patient's threshold for the tonal stimulus in that noise is determined. Then the phase of the tone to one ear is changed by 180 degrees. This minimal change, which can't be heard by either ear individually, makes the tone subjectively louder for the binaural system. A new threshold is then obtained at this level. Although MLD is quite sensitive to small neural lesions, it must be used cautiously because peripheral losses can affect the results. The test can also use spondaic words in noise instead of a tone in noise.

For difficult speech discrimination tasks: An example of this type of test is speech discrimination in white noise. A speech stimulus is presented to one ear and the result is scored; then white noise and speech stimulus are simultaneously presented to the same ear and the result is scored. The two scores are compared; then the task is repeated for the other ear and its scores compared. Finally, each ear's score is compared with the other's and with normal range.

For ABR: Electrodes are placed at the vertex of the patient's scalp (active), the mastoid process or earlobe of the stimulated ear (reference), and the mastoid process or earlobe of the opposite ear (ground). Stimuli in the form of clicks or rapid rise time (1 millisecond) tone pips are presented at 10/second until 2,000 time-locked responses are collected and averaged.

The origins of the peaks are complex, but primary contributors may be the eighth nerve (Wave I), cochlear nucleus (Wave II), superior olive (Wave III), and lateral lemniscus and inferior colliculus (Waves IV and V). To estimate thresholds, responses to stimuli are collected at decreasing intensities until Wave V disappears from the trace. Cochlear and retrocochlear lesions are differentiated by presenting click stimuli at high intensities and comparing the absolute latencies of waves I, III, and V, and the interwave latency differences between ears and to normal data.

For CM tasks: In these tests, a different message is presented to each ear, and the patient is asked to discriminate between the messages. In a gross measure test, such as the Northwestern University test #20, speech discrimination words are presented to one ear and the patient is asked to repeat them. Then speech discrimination words are presented to the same ear and short sentences are simultaneously presented to the other ear, and the patient is asked to repeat the words and ignore the sentences. The patient's scores on each task are then compared.

Auditory brain stem electrical response

In this test, auditory neural activity is recorded as it passes from the peripheral or cochlear end organ through the brain stem to the cortex. (The test reflects presentation of auditory stimuli in the form of 4,000-Hz tone pips at 75 dB HL.) Wave I is associated with the acoustic nerve response, and wave V is associated with an upper brain stem response. Waves I and V are considered the most clinically useful.

Because this test is repeated for accuracy, each graph below shows two sets of waveforms. Both waveforms follow the same pattern, confirming test results.

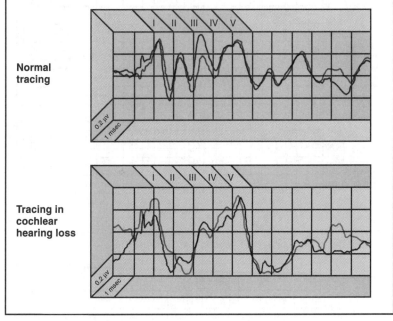

Normal tracing

Tracing in cochlear hearing loss

In a precise message test, such as the dichotic nonsense syllables test, carefully aligned nonsense syllables are presented to both ears at once, and the patient is asked to repeat or write both syllables. The number of syllables correctly identified in one ear is compared with the number of syllables correctly identified in the other ear as well as with a normal range.

Precautions
Patient cooperation is essential for accurate test results.

Normal findings
For normal findings, see *Auditory brain stem electrical response,* above, and *Békésy audiometry,* pages 616 and 617.

Implications of results
Site-of-lesion tests can rule out cochlear and retrocochlear lesions. If a lesion is present, these tests help distinguish its type. (See *Interpreting site-of-lesion test results,* pages 618 and 619.)

Post-test care
None.

(Text continues on page 619.)

Békésy audiometry

In this test, pure tone frequencies are presented in a sweep of 100 to 10,000 Hz, changing at one octave per minute. They're presented first as pulsed tones (broken tracings), then as continuous tones (solid tracings). The patient controls tone intensity by pushing a response button whenever he hears a tone. Except in cases of functional hearing loss, the pulsed tone always has a better pure tone threshold than the continuous tone. Test results fall into one of five categories, four of which are shown here.

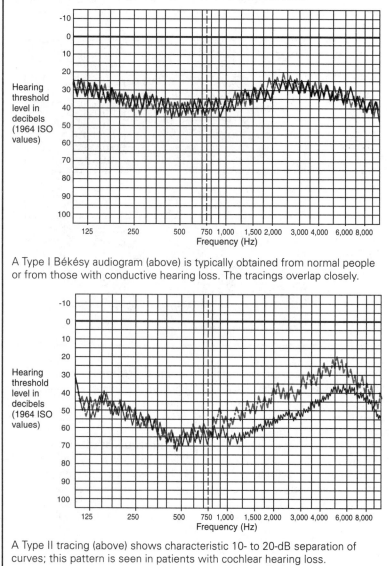

A Type I Békésy audiogram (above) is typically obtained from normal people or from those with conductive hearing loss. The tracings overlap closely.

A Type II tracing (above) shows characteristic 10- to 20-dB separation of curves; this pattern is seen in patients with cochlear hearing loss.

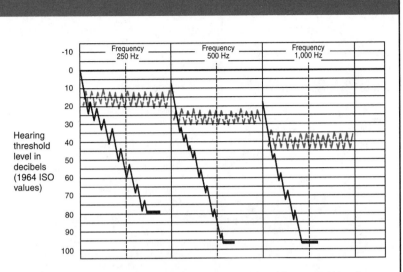

Type III tracings similar to the one above may appear with retrocochlear lesions. This tracing, conducted at three discrete frequencies, shows a rapid decline in threshold only for the continuous tone.

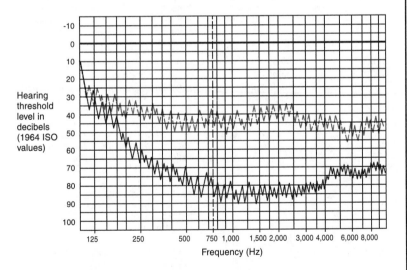

A Type IV tracing (above) indicates marked curve separation with the continuous tone tracing reaching a plateau more than 20 dB below that for the pulsed tone. This pattern may be seen in patients with neural or severe cochlear lesions.

Interpreting site-of-lesion test results

The site-of-lesion test battery can suggest the location and extent of damage to the auditory system. This chart shows the specific findings for each test and the implications of these findings.

TEST	FINDINGS	IMPLICATIONS
Alternate binaural loudness balance	Patient interprets two sounds of equal intensity as being equally loud.	■ *Cochlear lesion:* tones sound equally loud at 90 dB HL; recruitment, a sudden growth in loudness in the recruiting ear, occurs ■ *Retrocochlear lesion:* no recruitment; difference between ears at 90 dB HL equals or exceeds the difference between ears at threshold levels
Simultaneous binaural midplane localization	Single tone heard in center of head when both tone intensities are equal.	■ *Cochlear lesion:* response same as normal ■ *Retrocochlear lesion:* tones never sound centered; or both ears may require significantly different intensities for midline perception; may indicate nerve or intra-axial brain stem lesion
Tone decay	Patient may require 0 to 10 dB above threshold to perceive tone for 60 seconds.	■ *Cochlear lesion:* may require a tone up to 30 dB above threshold ■ *Retrocochlear lesion:* may require a tone more than 30 dB above threshold
Békésy audiometry	Type I audiogram tracings generally overlap in both pulsed and continuous mode.	■ *Type I:* same as normal with conductive hearing loss ■ *Type II:* continuous tracing falls 10 to 20 dB below pulsed tracing; may indicate cochlear loss ■ *Type III:* pulsed tracing continues at threshold level; continuous tracing drops to equipment limits; may indicate auditory fatigue or possible neural lesion, such as acoustic neuroma ■ *Type IV:* pulsed tracing continues at threshold level; continuous tracing drops more than 20 dB and plateaus; may occur with neural or severe cochlear lesions ■ *Type V:* pulsed tracing drops below continuous tracing; suggests uncooperative patient (no physiologic explanation)

Interpreting site-of-lesion test results (continued)

TEST	FINDINGS	IMPLICATIONS
Masking level difference	Tone heard subjectively louder in antiphasic mode; threshold difference between homophasic and antiphasic conditions is about 12 dB.	■ Little or no difference between conditions may suggest eighth nerve or intra-axial brain stem lesion.
Difficult speech discrimination tasks (in white noise)	Scores in quiet and in noise differ by 40% or less.	■ Difference of more than 40% between scores may indicate a lesion anywhere in the auditory system.
Auditory brain stem electrical response	Series of five potentials: wave I appears 2 msec after stimulus; other waves follow at 1-msec intervals. Waves diminish as stimulus level is lowered; wave V, occurring within 10 dB of behavioral threshold, disappears last.	■ *Cochlear lesion:* normal response at high intensities; depending on the degree and configuration of cochlear loss, wave V may occur slightly later than normal, and earlier waves may be distorted. ■ *Retrocochlear lesion:* possibly absent or late waves at high intensities; possibly increased interval between waves I and V; possibly decreased amplitude of wave V to less than one-half that of wave I
Gross competing message tasks (Northwestern University test #20)	Same score with and without competing message	■ *Cortical damage:* poor scores from ear opposite the damage
Precise competing message tasks (dichotic nonsense syllables test)	About 80% in right ear; about 65% in left ear	■ *Cortical damage:* poor scores from ear opposite the damage; better-than-normal scores from other ear ■ *Lesions of left hemisphere:* possibly low scores from both ears ■ *Lesions of the corpus callosum:* possibly lower scores from left ear

Interfering factors

■ Severe hearing loss can interfere with accurate testing.

■ Poor electrode placement or equipment failure can interfere with the ABR test.

■ If the patient is tense or uncooperative, the test results may be unreliable.

■ Cochlear or brain stem lesions interfere with competing message tests.

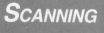
Computed tomography of the ear

Computed tomography (CT) combines the use of a computer and X-rays passed through the body at different angles to produce clear cross-sectional images of body tissues. High-resolution computed tomography (HRCT) is the most commonly used diagnostic procedure for assessing cochlear abnormalities and determining which patients are potential candidates for cochlear implants. It is also the procedure of choice for differentiating between cholesteatoma and chronic otitis media.

Purpose
- To investigate the cause of bilateral hearing loss
- To confirm cochlear abnormalities
- To differentiate between chronic inflammation and cholesteatoma
- To evaluate ossification of cochlea coils before cochlear implantation
- To evaluate sensorineural damage
- To diagnose paragangliomas of the temporal bone
- To detect bone abnormalities and tumors.

Patient preparation
Describe the procedure to the patient. Explain that he'll be secured to the scan table because even the slightest movement during imaging can lead to a blurred picture. Inform him that his head will be moved into the scanner, an air-conditioned chamber that looks like a giant metal doughnut. Tell him that the technician will be able to see him at all times and that they'll be able to communicate with each other during the procedure. Tell him that the study takes 15 to 20 minutes and that he may hear a humming sound as the machine takes the images. Tell him he'll need to remove all metal objects before the test.

If a contrast agent will be used, tell the patient he'll receive it through an I.V. line. Make sure he doesn't have a history of allergy to iodine products.

Procedure
The protocol for each HRCT depends on the purpose of the test. Most HRCT studies are done in the transverse and coronal planes. A contrast medium is not required for evaluating ossification of the cochlea coils or studying the petrous portion of the temporal bone.

The patient is taken to the radiology department and placed on the scan table with his head toward the machine. The mobile scan table allows easy transfer and accurate positioning in the machine. A trained technician conducts the study under the supervision of a radiologist. The technician explains the details of the procedure to the patient to reassure him and gain his cooperation.

Numerous low-dosage X-ray beams pass through the patient's body at different angles for a fraction of a second as the scanner rotates around him. Detectors in the scanner record the number of X-rays absorbed by different tissues, and a computer transforms this data into an image, which is interpreted by the radiologist. The temporal bones are imaged separately in the transverse and coronal planes. Because contrast already exists between bone, air, and soft tissue in the middle and inner ears, the use of a contrast medium is unnecessary in many cases.

Precautions
If a contrast medium will be used, ask the patient if he has a history of iodine sensitivity.

Normal findings

A CT scan of the ear should reveal normal ear structures that are free from cochlear or soft-tissue abnormalities, tumors, and bone deformities.

Implications of results

A CT scan can reveal cholesteatomas, cochlear abnormalities, paragangliomas in the temporal bone. It can also detect abnormal appearance, size, shape, position, and symmetry of internal ear structures and also help determine the appropriateness of a cochlear implant.

Post-test care

None.

Interfering factors

▪ The patient's inability to lie still during the scan may interfere with the test's accuracy.
▪ Failure to remove all metal objects may affect the test's accuracy.

Magnetic resonance imaging of the ear

Magnetic resonance imaging (MRI) is a noninvasive test used to assess cranial nerves and bone. This diagnostic technique provides high-quality, cross-sectional images of the body without X-rays or other radiation. In some instances, it can replace the auditory brain stem electrical response.

Because of improvements in equipment and more highly trained personnel, this test is quicker and more economical to perform than it was in the past. Advances have also led to the use of fast-spin echo (FSE) MRIs for otologic assessment, especially when a retrocochlear lesion is suspected.

For studies of the inner ear and its connections, MRI complements high-resolution computed tomography by providing more accurate assessment of intracranial and infracranial extension as well as the patency of the jugular bulb.

Purpose

▪ To assess the cause of sudden unilateral sensorineural hearing loss
▪ To show early nonossified soft-tissue scarring in the membranous labyrinth
▪ To investigate lesions of the petrous apex
▪ To diagnose vestibular schwannomas as small as 2 mm
▪ To visualize cranial nerves VII and VIII, especially when anticipating excision of an auditory neuroma.

Patient preparation

Explain to the patient that MRI is valuable in studying the head and the internal structures of the ear. Tell him that the MRI machine emits a loud, banging noise when it's operating. Advise him that the test may require the use of an I.V. contrast medium, which seldom causes adverse reactions. Tell him that the procedure takes about 15 minutes when a contrast medium is not used. (FSE MRI takes even less time.) Have the patient remove all jewelry (including his watch) and metal objects, such as hairpins and barrettes. Tell him to inform the doctor if he is fitted with a pacemaker, hearing aid, or other electrical device because these items can interfere with the scanner.

Procedure

The protocol for each MRI depends on the purpose of the test. After the patient is prepared and placed on the MRI table, the technician, under the direction of the doctor, sets the parameters that will provide optimum spatial resolution in a reasonable scan time. The patient's head is moved into a large, hollow, cylindrical magnet. The machine surrounds the patient with short bursts of powerful magnetic fields and radio waves. These bursts stimulate hydrogen atoms in the patient's system to emit signals, which are detected and analyzed by the computer to create images that resemble "slices" of the patient's body.

Normal findings

The cranial nerves and bone should appear normal.

Implications of results

MRI can detect viral labyrinthitis, increased intracranial pressure, paragangliomas, and other disorders. If a large lesion is identified in a vascular or cranial nerve area, angiography may be necessary to prevent difficulties during surgery to remove the paraganglioma.

Post-test care

None.

Interfering factors

Failure to remove all metal objects may affect test accuracy.

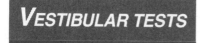

VESTIBULAR TESTS

Falling and past-pointing tests

Falling and past-pointing tests, performed as part of a neuro-otologic examination, screen for vestibular or cerebellar dysfunction in a patient who complains of dizziness, disequilibrium, or nystagmus. These tests evaluate balance and coordination as the patient performs various maneuvers with eyes open and closed. Abnormal results suggest the need for further evaluation.

Purpose

■ *Falling test:* To help identify vestibular or cerebellar disorders that affect the entire body.
■ *Past-pointing test:* To help identify vestibular or cerebellar disorders that affect the arms.

Patient preparation

Describe the tests to the patient, and explain that they help evaluate his sense of balance and identify neurologic dysfunction. Reassure him that someone will stand next to him to ensure that he doesn't fall.

Assess the patient's general physical condition, which influences his ability to perform the maneuvers. Check his history for use of drugs that affect the central nervous system (CNS) and for recent alcohol consumption.

Procedure

For the falling test: Instruct the patient to perform as many of the following maneuvers as possible, and observe for marked swaying or falling. First, ask him to stand with feet together, arms at his sides, and eyes open for 20 seconds; then tell him to maintain this position for another 20 seconds with eyes closed (Romberg test). Next, have the patient stand on one foot for 5 seconds, then on the other foot for 5 seconds; instruct him to repeat the procedure with eyes closed. Then tell him to stand heel to toe for 20 seconds with eyes open, then to maintain the same position with eyes closed for another 20 seconds. Finally, instruct him to walk forward and backward in a straight line, heel to toe, first with eyes open and then with eyes closed.

For the past-pointing test: With the patient seated and facing you, hold out your index finger at his shoulder level. Instruct him to touch your finger with his right index finger. Then tell him to lower his arm, close his eyes, and touch your finger again. Have the patient repeat the entire maneuver using his left index finger. Observe the degree and direction of past-pointing.

Precautions

■ The falling and past-pointing tests, or parts of them, are contraindicated in patients who are physically unable to perform all or some of the required maneuvers.

■ During the falling test, the examiner should stand close to the patient to catch him if he falls. If the patient is tall or heavy, someone should assist the examiner.

Normal findings

In the falling test, a healthy person maintains his balance with eyes both open and closed. In the past-pointing test, a healthy person touches the examiner's finger with eyes both open and closed.

Implications of results

A peripheral vestibular lesion can cause swaying or falling in the direction opposite to the nystagmus when the patient's eyes are closed; a cerebellar lesion causes swaying or falling when eyes are open or closed. A labyrinthine disorder can lead to past-pointing in the opposite direction to the nystagmus when the patient's eyes are closed; a cerebellar lesion can lead to past-pointing when the patient's eyes are open or closed; and a lateralized lesion can lead to past-pointing only with the arm on the affected side.

Post-test care

None.

Interfering factors

Use of alcohol or drugs that affect the CNS — such as stimulants, antianxiety agents, sedatives, and medications to relieve vertigo — affects the accuracy of test results.

Electronystagmography

In electronystagmography, eye movements in response to specific stimuli are recorded on graph paper and used to evaluate the interactions of the vestibular system and the muscles controlling eye movement in what is known as the *vestibulo-ocular reflex.* Nystagmus, the involuntary back-and-forth eye movement caused by this reflex, results from the vestibular system's attempts to maintain visual fixation during head movement. When the head turns in one direction, the eyes deviate slowly in the opposite direction; on reaching their deviation limit, they quickly return to the center. If the head continues to turn, the pattern of eye movement continues. (See *Glossary of eye movement terms,* page 624.)

The nystagmus cycle has two parts: Slow deviation against the direction of the turn (the slow phase) is controlled by the vestibular system; rapid return to center (the fast phase) is controlled by the central nervous system (CNS). Nystagmus is described as "beating" in the direction of the fast phase. Thus, a head turn to the right yields a right-beating nystagmus, with its slow phase to the left and its fast phase to the right.

Nystagmus accompanying a head turn is normal; prolonged nystagmus after a head turn is abnormal. Because of the interaction of the vestibular and ocular systems, abnormal nystagmus can result from lesions of either system; such lesions can be peripheral (end organ or vestibular nerve involvement) or central (cerebellar or brain stem involvement). Abnormal nystagmus is the

Glossary of eye movement terms

Conjugate deviation: drawing of the eyes to one side in unison.

Directional preponderance: difference in beat intensity in one direction versus the other direction.

Nystagmus: involuntary, rhythmic, back-and-forth movement of the eyes, usually composed of a slow deviation in one direction and a rapid return in the other; *fast phase of nystagmus:* the quick, jerky component of nystagmus controlled by the central nervous system; *horizontal nystagmus:* nystagmus in the horizontal plane, either left- or right-beating; *inverted nystagmus:* nystagmus that beats in the direction opposite to that anticipated; *positional nystagmus:* a persistent nystagmus that appears on assumption of a particular head position; *posi-*

tioning nystagmus: a transient nystagmus occurring immediately after a change in head position; *rotary nystagmus:* a nystagmus that rotates about the axis of the eye; *slow phase of nystagmus:* the vestibular phase of nystagmus or the slow deviation of the eyes from the midline; *spontaneous nystagmus:* a nystagmus occurring in the absence of stimuli; *vertical nystagmus:* nystagmus occurring in the vertical plane, either up- or down-beating.

Saccades: rapid, involuntary, jerky movements that occur simultaneously in both eyes when they change their fixation to a new point.

Unilateral weakness: decreased intensity of nystagmus after one auditory stimulus as compared with the other.

main sign of vestibular disturbances, such as dizziness and vertigo.

Electronystagmography is the technique for monitoring nystagmus; the battery of tests used to elicit nystagmus includes calibration, gaze, pendulum tracking, optokinetics, positional methods, and caloric tests. Electronystagmography relies on the corneoretinal potential — the difference of 1 mV between the positive charge of the cornea and the negative charge of the retina — to record nystagmus through electrodes placed near the eyes. As the eyes move horizontally or vertically, the electrodes pick up the corneoretinal potential and feed it to a recorder, which amplifies the signal and charts it. This method permits the recording of nystagmus in dimly lit surroundings, with the patient's eyes open or closed.

Purpose
- To help identify the cause of dizziness, vertigo, or tinnitus
- To help diagnose unilateral hearing loss of unknown origin
- To confirm the presence and location (central, peripheral, or both) of a lesion
- To assess neurologic disorders.

Patient preparation
Describe the tests to the patient, and explain that they evaluate visual and balance control mechanisms. Instruct him to observe the following pretest restrictions, if ordered: to abstain from stimulants, antianxiety agents, sedatives, antivertigo drugs, and alcohol for 24 to 48 hours before the test; to abstain from tobacco and beverages containing caffeine the day of the test; and to avoid eating a heavy meal immediately before

the test because caloric testing may cause transient nausea.

Tell the patient who will perform the tests, that he'll receive appropriate instructions before each test, and that the tests take 60 to 90 minutes to perform. Reassure him that someone will be nearby during all the tests to prevent him from falling.

If the patient wears glasses, tell him to bring them with him. Emphasize the importance of fully documenting his experience to ensure an accurate diagnosis. Provide emotional support because the test can be uncomfortable at times. Remind the patient that he must cooperate fully to achieve accurate test results.

Obtain a complete patient history, including psychological and physical condition, recent medication history, and a description of symptoms, including the nature of the sensation, its first occurrence, and its frequency, severity, and duration. Also include data on related problems, such as hearing loss, tinnitus, fullness in the ears, ear infection or surgery, and headaches; visual disorders or head trauma; weakness, numbness, slurred speech, difficulty swallowing, or confusion; and neck or back conditions that limit the patient's ability to assume the positions required for the positional test portion of electronystagmography.

Just before the test, perform an otoscopic examination. If the patient's ear canals are filled with cerumen, clean them.

Equipment
Two-channel differential amplifier with high- and low-frequency filters ✦ strip-chart record ✦ electrodes (one for ground, and two for horizontal and two for vertical recordings) ✦ electrode paste ✦ adhesive tape ✦ cotton and 70% alcohol ✦ examination table with headrest and adjustable back.

For water caloric tests: two water pans ✦ water pump and hose, with foot switch control ✦ two thermostatically controlled heaters: one set at 86° F (30° C), the other set at 111.2° F (44° C) ✦ timer ✦ emesis basin ✦ fingercot (to protect middle ear if patient has a perforated tympanic membrane).

For air caloric tests: air pump and hose, with foot switch control ✦ timer ✦ air heater with thermostat.

For ice water caloric tests: 20 ml of ice water ✦ irrigating syringe.

Procedure
The electronystagmography test sequence discussed here is representative. Although the sequence may vary, caloric tests are usually performed last. When performing the tests, indicate the name of the test, and note whether the recording stylus has been recentered or whether any unusual event occurs during the test. Tell the patient to follow all instructions. For the ocular tests, allow an adequate opportunity for him to learn the tasks. For the positional tests, do *not* permit him to practice the positions before the recording because this movement may fatigue him and yield inaccurate results.

Because the corneoretinal potential is labile, calibrate the equipment at the start of the test battery and before each caloric test. Avoid touching the gain knob on the amplifier except for calibration; however, you may adjust the balance knob, as needed, without affecting calibration. If the stylus becomes pinned to one side of the graph and cannot be centered, you may need to reposition the electrodes. (See *Electrode placement for electronystagmography,* page 626.)

For the calibration test: Have the patient sit upright on the examination table with his head against the headrest and his eyes directed toward a light bar that's located 6' to 10' (2 to 3 m) away.

Electrode placement for electronystagmography

To ensure accurate electronystagmography results, electrodes must be positioned properly. However, before placing the electrodes, the patient's skin must be prepared as follows. First, the contact points of each electrode are scrubbed with an alcohol-saturated cotton pad and air-dried. A small amount of electrode paste is then rubbed into the patient's skin at each contact point. Just before placement, an adhesive collar is placed on the electrode and the electrode cup is filled with paste. Next, the backing is peeled from the adhesive collar and the electrode is pressed firmly against the patient's skin.

The ground electrode, which minimizes line noise interference, is positioned in the neutral position in the center of the patient's forehead, midway between the eyes. If horizontal nystagmus is being recorded, two lateral electrodes are placed as close to the outer canthus of each eye as possible without interfering with eye closure. If vertical nystagmus is being recorded, two additional electrodes are positioned directly above and below the center of one eye. (Generally, only one eye is monitored for vertical nystagmus.) It is important that the eye is not artificial or paralyzed and that there is not disconjugate movement between the eyes.

After the electrodes are positioned, the impedance in each pair is determined; if impedance exceeds 10,000 ohms, the electrode is reapplied. The electrode paste must be allowed to stabilize for 5 minutes before starting the test.

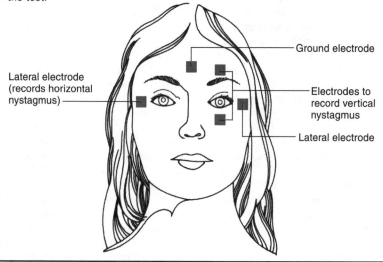

Lateral electrode (records horizontal nystagmus)

Ground electrode

Electrodes to record vertical nystagmus

Lateral electrode

Tell him to hold his head still and to follow the light only with his eyes. Center the stylus, set the paper speed to 5 mm/second, and start the recorder. Move the light so that the patient's eyes deviate 10 degrees to the right of center. By adjusting gain and balance, fix the stylus sensitivity so that the 10-degree deviation of the eyes corresponds to a 10-mm deflection of the stylus on the chart. Move the light back to the center, then to the left, and readjust the stylus position until its deflection again matches eye deviation.

To detect ocular dysmetria, move the light in this sequence: center, 10 degrees right, center, and 10 degrees left, stopping in each position for about 2 seconds. Repeat this sequence until you get two cycle tracings that represent the patient's best tracking ability.

For the gaze nystagmus test: Remove the visual target from the previous test. Place the patient in a comfortable seated or supine position, and have him close his eyes. To keep his mind off the eye motion itself, give him a mental arithmetic task to perform while you record spontaneous eye motion for 30 seconds.

To record center-gaze nystagmus, have the patient look straight ahead with his eyes fixed on the center light. Record for 30 seconds. Then tell him to close his eyes without changing their position; record for another 30 seconds. On the chart, mark the transition point from open to closed eyes.

To record right-gaze nystagmus, tell the patient to look at the center light, and start the stylus near the right margin of the chart. Instruct him to move his eyes to the right on cue and to fix them on a light 25 degrees to the right of center; record for 30 seconds. Then tell the patient to close his eyes but to maintain eye position; record for 30 seconds. Mark the transition from open to closed eyes. To record left-gaze nystagmus, proceed as above but have the patient look at a light set at 20 degrees and then at 30 degrees to the left of center. Start the stylus near the left margin of the chart.

For the pendulum tracking test: Have the patient look straight ahead. Activate the pendulum movement or a light that mimics this movement, and ask the patient to follow the target with his eyes. Record until you obtain 20 seconds of tracings that reflect the patient's best tracking ability. Then tell the patient to close his eyes while looking straight ahead, and record his eye movements for 30 seconds.

For the optokinetics test: Tell the patient to look straight ahead. If there is a velocity channel, set it to read *left*-beating nystagmus. Adjust the stimulus to travel across the patient's visual field, from left to right, at about 20 degrees/second. Instruct the patient to follow the target across his visual field until it disappears, then to snap his eyes back to meet the next target and follow it across, and so on. Continue recording until you've obtained 20 seconds of the patient's best responses. Then instruct him to look straight ahead with his eyes closed, and record for another 30 seconds.

Repeat the procedure, setting the velocity channel to read *right*-beating nystagmus and adjusting the stimulus to move from right to left. Mark the transition from right to left on the chart.

For positional tests: Obtain a baseline recording for about 5 seconds before having the patient assume each of the nine test positions, and identify each transition on the chart.

■ Erect to head right: Instruct the patient to sit erect with his eyes forward and closed. On cue, have him turn his head quickly to the right as far as he can. Instruct him to maintain this posture; record for 30 seconds or until nystagmus subsides. (If it doesn't subside, stop recording after 90 seconds.) Then have the patient slowly turn his head back to center. If nystagmus occurs, repeat the maneuver. If dizziness occurs, note this on the chart.

■ Erect to head left: Repeat the preceding maneuver with the patient's head turned to the left.

■ Erect to supine: Lower the back of the examination table to the horizontal position. Instruct the patient to sit erect at one end with his eyes closed and centered. On cue, have him quickly lie flat on his back; record for 30 seconds or until nystagmus subsides, or stop recording after 90 seconds if nystagmus continues. If nystagmus occurs, repeat the maneuver.

- Supine to erect: Repeat as above but have the patient quickly sit erect from a supine position.
- Supine to lateral right: Have the patient lie supine with eyes closed and head supported by a pillow. Instruct him to turn his body and head quickly to the right; record for 30 seconds or until nystagmus subsides, or stop recording after 90 seconds if nystagmus continues. Instruct the patient to return slowly to the supine position; repeat the maneuver if nystagmus occurred.
- Supine to lateral left: Repeat the procedure described above with the patient quickly turning his body and head to the left.
- Erect to head hanging: Remove the headrest from the examination table. Instruct the patient to sit erect with eyes forward and closed. Position him so that his head will clear the other end of the table when he lies down. On cue, instruct him to lie back quickly, letting his head hang over the edge; record for 30 seconds or until nystagmus subsides, or stop recording after 90 seconds if nystagmus continues. Repeat the maneuver if nystagmus occurred. Record on the chart any sensation reported by the patient.
- Head hanging to erect: Repeat as above but have the patient move from the head-hanging position to an erect position.
- Erect to head hanging right/left: Repeat as above but as the patient moves from the erect to the head-hanging position, tell him to turn his head to the right. Then ask him to repeat the movement but to turn his head to the left.

For the water caloric test: Have the patient lie supine with his head elevated 30 degrees so that his lateral semicircular canals are perpendicular to the floor. Place a towel and emesis basin under his ear to collect the water as it drains from the ear. Except as noted below, instruct the patient to close his eyes during and after stimulation. Inform him when stimulation is about to begin, so he isn't startled by the sudden rush of water in his ear.

Introduce water into the ear canal so that it hits the tympanic membrane directly, and continue the stimulation for 30 seconds. Then begin the recording immediately; give the patient some mental tasks to keep him alert. After about 60 seconds, tell him to open his eyes and fix them on a target, such as his raised thumb. After 10 seconds, tell him to close his eyes; continue recording until the nystagmus subsides or for a total of 3 minutes. Record on the chart any sensation that the patient reports as well as the transition from open to closed eyes. Wait 5 minutes before starting the next caloric stimulation. Repeat the test if the stimulation seems inadequate; recalibrate before starting the next test.

Repeat the preceding procedure with each of these stimuli: 86° F (30° C) to the right ear (set velocity channel for left-beating nystagmus), 86° F to the left ear (set velocity channel for right-beating nystagmus), 111.2° F (44° C) to the right ear (set velocity channel for right-beating nystagmus), and 111.2° F to the left ear (set velocity channel for left-beating nystagmus). Be sure to recalibrate each time.

If the patient has a punctured tympanic membrane, insert a fingercot into the canal to protect the middle ear, and change temperatures to 87° F (30.5° C) for the cool stimulus and 120.2° F (49° C) for the warm stimulus. Alternatively, use air calorics to obtain the same information. Deliver 8 L of air at 85.2° F

(29.5° C) and 122° F (50° C) to each ear separately over 60 seconds.

If the patient fails to respond to standard caloric stimulation, use ice water calorics. Use a blunt syringe to irrigate the ear with 20 ml of ice water. Then record the results as you would with standard calorics. After completing caloric testing, carefully lift the electrodes from the patient's face. To avoid spreading the electrode paste, advise the patient not to rub his eyes. Wipe the paste from his skin.

Precautions

 ■ Electronystagmography is contraindicated in patients with pacemakers because the equipment may interfere with pacemaker function.

■ If the patient has a back or neck condition that could be aggravated by rapid changes in position, check with the doctor to determine if any of the positional tests should be omitted.

 ■ Don't use the usual water caloric tests if the patient has a perforated tympanic membrane. If there is any question about the condition of the membrane, make sure a doctor has examined the patient and authorized the test. Modified air or water caloric tests with fingercots in place may also be substituted. When fingercots are used in such tests, be certain that their placement in each ear is equidistant from the tympanic membrane so that both labyrinths are stimulated equally.

Normal findings

For normal responses to the battery of electronystagmography tests, see *Results of electronystagmography,* pages 630 to 633.

Implications of results

Electronystagmography results are reported as normal, borderline, or abnormal. Abnormal results are further described as indicating a peripheral, central, or undetermined (nonlocalized) lesion.

A peripheral lesion may involve the end organ or the vestibular branch of the eighth cranial nerve and may result from conditions such as ototoxity and eighth nerve tumors. A central lesion may involve the brain stem, cerebellum, cerebrum, or any of the connecting structures and may result from demyelinating diseases, tumors, or circulatory disorders.

Post-test care

Observe for signs of weakness, dizziness, and nausea. If the patient experiences such symptoms, help him to an area where he can sit comfortably or lie down until he recovers.

Interfering factors

■ Use of CNS stimulants, depressants, or medications to relieve vertigo may suppress nystagmus, produce gaze or positional nystagmus, or reduce the patient's ability to concentrate on the test tasks.

■ Poor eyesight may reduce the patient's ability to perform ocular tests and to suppress nystagmus visually.

■ Drowsiness may suppress any nystagmus that might otherwise occur and may produce wide, pendular eye movements that could affect the accuracy of test results.

■ Blinking the eyes may mimic nystagmus, and thus affecting the accuracy of test results.

■ Loose or poorly applied electrodes invalidate test findings.

■ Poor patient cooperation influences test results.

(Text continues on page 634.)

Results of electronystagmography

TEST AND NORMAL FINDINGS	ABNORMAL FINDINGS	USUAL IMPLICATIONS
Calibration Square wave pattern indicates accurate, repeatable eye movement (1)	*Ocular dysmetria:* results from inability of the ocular system to exert fine control over eye movements; results in "overshoots" or "undershoots" in pattern (2)	Lesion in cerebellum or cerebellar–brain stem pathways
Spontaneous nystagmus (No external stimulus) Eyes open: no nystagmus; eyes closed: some weak horizontal < 7 degrees/second) or vertical < 10 degrees/second) nystagmus (4)	*Ocular nystagmus:* diminishes at a particular angle of gaze and with convergence of eyes; with upward gaze, it's horizontal	Most prevalent as a congenital, nonlesional disorder; some forms caused by poor vision
	Vestibular nystagmus: horizontal direction; suppressed with visual fixation; unidirectional beats; fast and slow components (3)	Peripheral or central (brain stem or cerebellar) lesion
	Central nystagmus: unclassified as above	Central lesion
Positional (head in position) **Positioning** (head in movement to the position usually taken together)	*Type I — persistent, direction-changing nystagmus:* duration, > 1 minute; beats in different directions, depending on head position	Nonlocalized lesion
	Type II — persistent, direction-fixed nystagmus: duration, > 1 minute; beats in same direction, regardless of head position; intensity may vary	Nonlocalized lesion
Eyes open: no nystagmus; eyes closed: weak nystagmus < 7 degrees/second) in one or more positions (5)	*Type III — transitory, fixed, or changeable direction nystagmus:* duration, < 1 minute; benign paroxysmal nystagmus is most common form, marked by a latent period, transient burst of nystagmus, severe vertigo, and fatigue on repeating the position (6A, 6B)	Peripheral lesion; occurs in elderly, after head trauma, with middle ear pathology. Nystagmus that changes direction during a position may indicate cerebellar or brain stem damage. (Drug effects must be ruled out.)
Pendulum tracking	Sinusoidal tracking with superimposed saccades or nystagmus	End organ or brain stem pathology
Sinusoidal waveform for stimuli with excursions of 40 degrees and eye speeds of 40 to 50 degrees/second (7)	Disrupted (ataxic) sinusoidal tracking (8)	Brain stem pathology (If spontaneous nystagmus wasn't present before the test, there should be none after it when eyes are closed. Its presence is a nonlocalizing sign.)

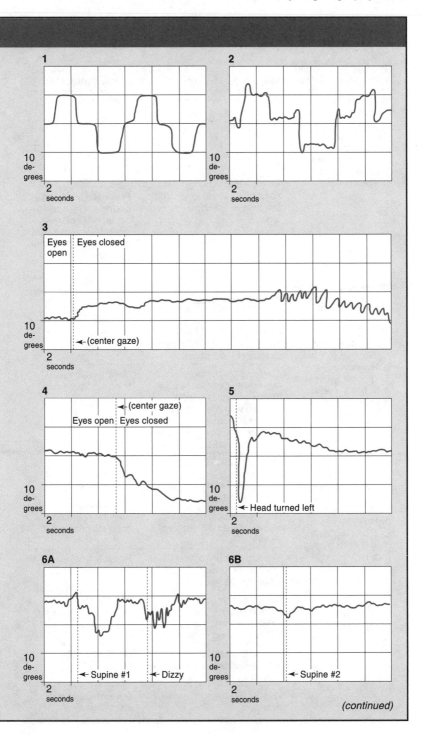

(continued)

Results of electronystagmography *(continued)*		
TEST AND NORMAL FINDINGS	**ABNORMAL FINDINGS**	**USUAL IMPLICATIONS**
Optokinetics Stimulus followed up to 30 degrees/second; clear triangular wave pattern; similar pattern for stimuli traveling in both directions (9)	Difference in slow-phase velocities resulting from stimuli to left and right > 20 degrees/ second	Nonlocalized lesion
	Disconjugate eye movements or reduced velocity in both directions (10)	Cerebellar or brain stem pathology
	Asymmetry in velocities in the direction of spontaneous nystagmus	Peripheral lesion producing strong spontaneous vestibular nystagmus; drug use; inattention; old age. (When eyes are closed, nystagmus should cease; persistence is a sign of nonlocalized pathology.)
Gaze nystagmus (eyes deviated from center) Eyes closed: weak nystagmus (< 7 degrees/second). End point nystagmus may occur when eyes are deviated to their limit (11)	*Peripheral gaze nystagmus:* horizontal or horizontal-rotary; inhibited by visual fixation; beats strongest with gaze in direction of fast phase	Peripheral lesion
	Central gaze nystagmus: bilateral nystagmus that beats in different directions; suppressed with eyes closed; may change direction even if gaze stays constant or may move in horizontal, vertical, oblique, and rotary direction (12)	Central lesion (Drug effects must be ruled out.)
Water calorics Eyes closed: nystagmus occurs in all conditions; suppressed by visual fixation (13). With cold stimuli, nystagmus beats to opposite ear; with warm stimuli, it beats to same ear. (Acronym COWS — cold opposite, warm same — helps to recall this phenomenon.)	*Unilateral weakness:* > 20% difference in maximum slow-phase velocities	Peripheral lesion of weaker side
	Bilateral weakness: slow-phase velocity < 7 degrees/ second	Bilateral peripheral or brain stem lesion
	Hyperexcitability of vestibular system: slow-phase velocity > 50 degrees/second	Possibly CNS lesion or anxious patient
	Directional preponderance: more than 30% difference in slow-phase velocities for right- and left-beating nystagmus	Peripheral or cerebellar–brain stem lesions
	Failure to suppress fixation: visual fixation fails to reduce nystagmus by at least 20% (14)	Cerebellar or brain stem pathology
	Inverted or distorted nystagmus	Cerebellar or brain stem pathology

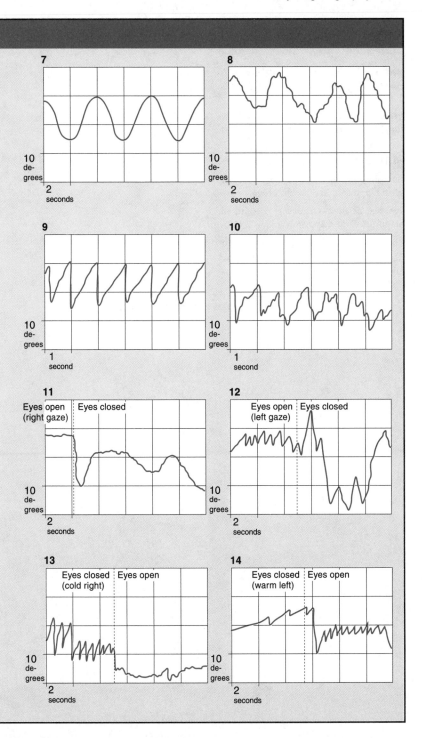

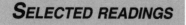
SELECTED READINGS

Becker, W., et al. *Ear, Nose and Throat Diseases: A Pocket Reference,* 2nd ed. New York: Thieme Med. Pubs., 1994.

Browning, G.G. *Updated ENT,* 3rd ed. Newton, Mass.: Butterworth-Heinemann, 1994.

Bull, T.R. *Color Atlas of ENT Diagnosis,* 3rd ed. St. Louis: Mosby–Year Book, Inc., 1995.

English, G.M., ed. *Otolaryngology.* Philadelphia: Lippincott-Raven Pubs., 1996.

Lee, K.J. *Essential Otolaryngology,* 6th ed. Stamford, Conn.: Appleton & Lange, 1995.

Phelps, P.D. "Fast Spin Echo MRI in Otology," *Journal of Laryngology and Otology,* 108(5):383-94, May 1994.

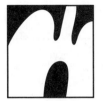

CHAPTER TWENTY-THREE

Respiratory system

Learning objectives

After completing this chapter, the reader will be able to:
- explain the physiology of respiration and list its control mechanisms
- describe the procedures for evaluating pulmonary dysfunction
- state the characteristics of pulmonary transudate and exudate
- explain the staging system for lung cancer
- describe six common radiographic views of the chest and list anatomic landmarks
- state the purpose of each test discussed in the chapter
- prepare the patient physically and psychologically for each test
- describe the procedure for performing each test
- specify appropriate precautions for safe administration of each test
- recognize signs of an adverse reaction and respond appropriately
- implement appropriate post-test care
- identify the normal findings of each test
- discuss the implications of abnormal test results
- list factors that may interfere with accurate test results.

INTRODUCTION

The pulmonary and circulatory systems are designed to provide the body with a continuous supply of oxygen and a quick, efficient removal of carbon dioxide. The pulmonary system controls the exchange of gases between the atmosphere and blood, and the circulatory system transports these gases between the lungs and cells. A dysfunction in either system disrupts homeostasis and causes anoxia and even cell death. The tests described in this chapter are designed to identify and assess such dysfunction.

Pulmonary physiology

The organs involved in the exchange of gases between the atmosphere and blood are the nose, pharynx, larynx, trachea, bronchi, and lungs. The trachea branches into primary bronchi, secondary bronchi, bronchioles, terminal bronchioles, and finally, alveolar sacs. The walls of the alveolar sacs are lined with small outpouchings called alveoli and are covered by a capillary network of arterioles and venules. The alveoli are the functional units of the lungs that are responsible for the exchange of gases between the air and blood. (See *Pulmonary gas exchange*.)

Three concurrent processes permit gas exchange during respiration.
- *Ventilation* is the movement of air between the atmosphere and the alveoli. This process is the result of the contraction and relaxation of the respiratory muscles (primarily the diaphragm), which alternately compress and distend the lungs, causing the decrease and increase of pressure within the alveoli. Inspiration occurs when the pressure in the alveoli is less than atmospheric pressure, and expiration occurs when the pressure in the alveoli is greater than atmospheric pressure.

Pulmonary gas exchange

Grapelike clusters of alveoli are the sites of gas exchange in the lungs. Each alveolus is served by two systems: the capillary network, which transports mixed venous blood to the alveolar membrane, and the tracheobronchial tree (trachea, bronchi, and bronchioles), which delivers air to the alveolar space. When the venous blood passes through the alveolar membrane, it releases carbon dioxide and takes in oxygen. Then the oxygenated blood travels to the heart. From there, it circulates throughout the body, releasing oxygen and taking in carbon dioxide and cellular waste before returning to the lungs.

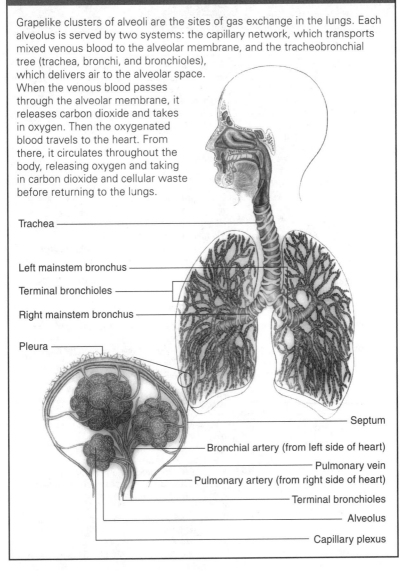

Trachea

Left mainstem bronchus

Terminal bronchioles

Right mainstem bronchus

Pleura

Septum

Bronchial artery (from left side of heart)

Pulmonary vein

Pulmonary artery (from right side of heart)

Terminal bronchioles

Alveolus

Capillary plexus

■ *Diffusion* is the process by which oxygen and carbon dioxide cross the alveolocapillary membrane. Oxygen (at a higher concentration in alveolar air than in blood) and carbon dioxide (at a higher concentration in blood than in alveolar air) move from their respective region of higher concentration to one of lower concentration.

Evaluating pulmonary function and structure

TEST	PURPOSE
Volumetric tests	**Assess function**

Lung capacity
  Vital capacity
  Inspiratory capacity
  Functional residual capacity
  Total lung capacity
  Forced vital capacity
  Flow-volume curve
  Forced expiratory volume
  Peak expiratory flow
  Forced expiratory flow
  Maximal voluntary ventilation
	■ Evaluates ventilatory function of lungs and chest wall; screens for pulmonary disorders
	■ Helps classify pulmonary disorders as restrictive or obstructive
	■ Evaluates severity of pulmonary disorders
	■ Evaluates response to therapy

Lung volume
  Total volume
  Minute volume
  CO_2 response
  Inspiratory reserve volume
  Expiratory reserve volume
  Residual volume
  Thoracic gas volume
	■ Evaluates ventilatory function of lungs and chest wall; screens for pulmonary disorders
	■ Helps classify pulmonary disorders as restrictive or obstructive
	■ Evaluates severity of pulmonary disorders
	■ Evaluates response to therapy

Endoscopic tests	**Assess structure**
Bronchoscopy	■ Directly examines larger airways of tracheobronchial tree
Mediastinoscopy	■ Directly examines mediastinum for biopsy (usually supplements bronchoscopy)
Thoracoscopy	■ Directly examines pleural cavity
Radiographic and scanning tests	**Assess structure, function, and vascular status**
Chest radiography	■ Visualizes appearance and status of respiratory system
Paranasal sinus radiography	■ Visualizes appearance and status of paranasal sinus
Fluoroscopy	■ Visualizes thoracic organs in motion
Tomography	■ Supplements radiographs; visualizes target areas in a series of planes to reveal occult pathology
Bronchography	■ Visualizes size and appearance of tracheobronchial tree
Pulmonary angiography	■ Visualizes pulmonary vascular system
Lung perfusion scan	■ Visualizes distribution of blood flow patterns in lungs
Ventilation scan	■ Evaluates ventilatory function
Thoracic computed tomography	■ Locates suspected neoplasms, mediastinal nodes, and pleural involvement

- *Perfusion* is the movement of blood through vessels that supply blood to an organ or tissue.

Primary controls

The following mechanisms are the primary controls of respiration.

- The *nervous system* adjusts the rate of respiration to satisfy physiologic demands. The respiratory center in the brain, located in the medulla oblongata and the pons, directs the contraction and relaxation of respiratory muscles.
- The *Hering-Breuer reflex* controls the depth and rhythm of respiration and prevents overinflation of the lungs. This reflex occurs in response to nerve impulses transmitted from stretch receptors in the bronchi and bronchioles to the respiratory center in the brain.
- *Carbon dioxide, oxygen, and hydrogen ion concentrations* determine the rate of respiration by acting directly on the respiratory center in the brain or on chemoreceptors located in the carotid arteries and the aorta.

Together, these control mechanisms keep blood oxygen and carbon dioxide levels remarkably stable.

Pulmonary assessment

Clinical evaluation of a patient with suspected pulmonary dysfunction begins with a physical examination and a thorough patient history. A *chest X-ray* usually is performed after initial assessment and, depending on its results, may be followed by collection of a *sputum specimen* to determine whether the dysfunction results from cancer, bacteria, or parasites. *Arterial blood gas analysis* can evaluate the patient's ability to exchange a sufficient amount of carbon dioxide for oxygen.

Pulmonary function tests may then identify obstructive or restrictive ventilatory defects. Such tests measure lung capacity and volume and are useful in screening patients preoperatively to evaluate surgical risk. (See *Evaluating pulmonary function and structure.*)

Endoscopic examinations permit direct observation of structures in the thorax. Such examinations may serve both diagnostic and therapeutic purposes. For example, they allow the removal of foreign bodies (with a rigid bronchoscope), secretions, and blood.

Finally, *radiographic and scanning tests* serve a variety of purposes, from screening for asymptomatic cancer to determining perfusion and ventilation abnormalities. These tests visualize the entire pulmonary system or can provide a three-dimensional view of a specific area.

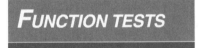

FUNCTION TESTS

Pulmonary function

Pulmonary function tests (including volume, capacity, and flow rate tests) are a series of measurements that evaluate ventilatory function through spirometric measurements; they are performed on patients with suspected pulmonary dysfunction. Of the seven tests that are performed to determine volume, tidal volume (VT) and expiratory reserve volume (ERV) are direct spirographic measurements (see *Reading a spirogram,* page 640); minute volume (MV), carbon dioxide (CO_2) response, inspiratory reserve volume (IRV), and residual volume (RV) are calculated from the results of other pulmonary function tests; and thoracic gas volume (TGV) is calculated from body plethysmography.

Reading a spirogram

To plot a spirogram, or lung signature, you need to know the patient's tidal volume (V_T) and his maximum inspiration (A) and expiration (B) capabilities, which constitute forced vital capacity (FVC). After you've plotted these, you can use the spirogram to calculate inspiratory reserve volume (IRV), expiratory reserve volume (ERV), residual volume (RV), inspiratory capacity (IC), functional residual capacity (FRC), and total lung capacity (TLC).

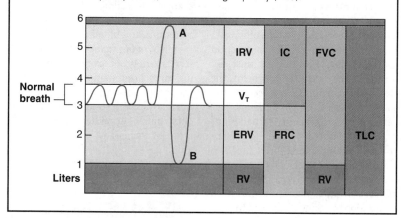

Of the pulmonary capacity tests, vital capacity (VC), inspiratory capacity (IC), functional residual capacity (FRC), total lung capacity (TLC), and forced expiratory flow (FEF) may be measured directly or calculated from the results of other tests. Forced vital capacity (FVC), flow-volume curve, forced expiratory volume (FEV), peak expiratory flow rate (PEFR), and maximal voluntary ventilation (MVV) are direct spirographic measurements. The diffusing capacity for carbon monoxide (DL_{CO}) is calculated from the amount of carbon monoxide exhaled.

Purpose

- To determine the cause of dyspnea
- To assess the effectiveness of specific therapeutic regimen
- To determine whether a functional abnormality is obstructive or restrictive
- To measure pulmonary dysfunction
- To evaluate the patient before surgery.

Patient preparation

Explain to the patient that these tests evaluate pulmonary function. Instruct him not to eat a heavy meal before the tests and not to smoke for 4 to 6 hours before the tests. Tell him who will perform these tests and where, and explain the operation of a spirometer. Inform him that the accuracy of the tests depends on his cooperation. Assure him that the procedure is painless and that he will be able to rest between tests.

Inform the laboratory if the patient is taking an analgesic that depresses respiration. As ordered, withhold bronchodilators and intermittent positive-pressure breathing therapy.

Just before the test, tell the patient to urinate and to loosen tight clothing. If he wears dentures, tell him to wear them during the test to help form a seal around the mouthpiece. Advise him to put on the noseclip so that he can adjust to it before the test.

Equipment

For direct spirography: spirometer ✦ recording paper ✦ noseclip ✦ mouthpiece.

For body plethysmography: body plethysmograph ✦ mouthpiece ✦ transducer.

Procedure

Tidal volume: The patient is told to breathe normally into the mouthpiece 10 times.

Expiratory reserve volume: The patient is told to breathe normally for several breaths and then to exhale as completely as possible.

Vital capacity: The patient is told to inhale as deeply as possible and to exhale into the mouthpiece as completely as possible. This procedure is repeated three times, and the test result showing the largest volume is used.

Inspiratory capacity: The patient is instructed to breathe normally for several breaths and then to inhale as deeply as possible.

Functional residual capacity: The patient is told to breathe normally into a spirometer that contains a known concentration of an insoluble gas (usually helium or nitrogen) in a known volume of air. After a few breaths, the concentrations of gas in the spirometer and the lungs reach equilibrium. The FRC is calculated by subtracting the spirometer volume from the original volume.

Thoracic gas volume: The patient is put in an airtight box or body plethysmograph and told to breathe through a tube connected to a transducer. At end-expiration, the tube is occluded, the patient is told to pant, and changes in intrathoracic and plethysmographic pressure are measured. The results are used to calculate total TGV and FRC.

Forced vital capacity and *forced expiratory volume:* The patient is instructed to inhale as slowly and deeply as possible and then asked to exhale into the mouthpiece as quickly and completely as possible. This procedure is repeated three times, and the largest volume is recorded. The volume of air expired at 1 second (FEV_1), at 2 seconds (FEV_2), and at 3 seconds (FEV_3) during all three repetitions is also recorded. (See *Restrictive vs. obstructive lung disease*, page 642.)

Maximal voluntary ventilation: The patient is instructed to breathe into the mouthpiece as quickly and deeply as possible for 15 seconds.

Diffusing capacity for carbon monoxide: The patient is told to inhale a gas mixture with a low concentration of carbon monoxide and then to hold his breath for 10 seconds before exhaling.

Precautions

 Pulmonary function tests are contraindicated in patients with acute coronary insufficiency, angina, or recent myocardial infarction. During such tests, watch for respiratory distress, changes in pulse rate and blood pressure, coughing, and bronchospasm.

Reference values

Normal values are predicted for each patient based on age, height, weight, and sex and are expressed as a percentage:

- *VT:* 5 to 7 mg/kg of body weight
- *ERV:* 25% of VC
- *IC:* 75% of VC
- *FEV_1:* 83% of VC (after 1 second)
- *FEV_2:* 94% of VC (after 2 seconds)
- *FEV_3:* 97% of VC (after 3 seconds).

Restrictive vs. obstructive lung disease

A spirogram helps determine whether a patient's lung disorder is restrictive or obstructive. As these graphs of forced vital capacity (FVC) maneuvers show, FVC, forced expiratory volume (FEV), and forced expiratory flow (FEF) are reduced in restrictive disease. But FEV is reduced less in restrictive disease, which doesn't change airway resistance. In obstructive disease, all of these parameters are reduced because the patient takes a longer time per unit to exhale.

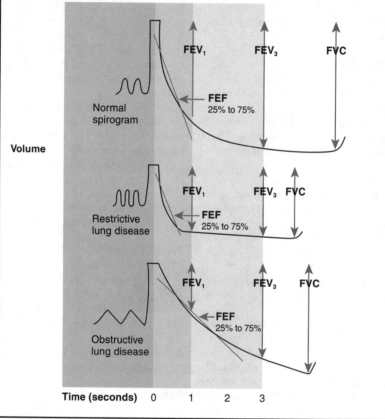

Values such as these can be calculated at bedside with a portable spirometer. Results are usually considered abnormal if they're less than 80% of these values.

Implications of results

See *Interpreting pulmonary function tests.*

Post-test care

As ordered, resume medications, diet, and activities discontinued before the tests.

Interfering factors

■ Lack of patient cooperation, hypoxia, and metabolic disturbances can make testing difficult or impossible.

Interpreting pulmonary function tests

TEST	METHOD OF CALCULATION	IMPLICATIONS
Tidal volume (V_T): amount of air inhaled or exhaled during normal breathing	Determine the spirographic measurement for 10 breaths and divide by 10.	Decreased V_T may indicate restrictive disease and requires further testing, such as full pulmonary function studies or chest radiography.
Minute volume (MV): total amount of air expired per minute	Multiply V_T by the respiration rate.	Normal MV can occur in emphysema; decreased MV may indicate other diseases such as pulmonary edema. Increased MV can occur with acidosis, increased carbon dioxide (CO_2), decreased partial pressure of oxygen (Po_2), exercise, and low compliance states.
CO_2 response: increase or decrease in MV after breathing various CO_2 concentrations	Plot changes in MV against increasing inspired CO_2 concentrations.	Reduced CO_2 response may occur in emphysema, myxedema, obesity, hypoventilation syndrome, and sleep apnea.
Inspiratory reserve volume (IRV): amount of air inspired after normal inspiration	Subtract V_T from inspiratory capacity (IC).	Abnormal IRV alone doesn't indicate respiratory dysfunction; IRV decreases during normal exercise.
Expiratory reserve volume (ERV): amount of air exhaled after normal expiration	Direct spirographic measurement	ERV varies, even in healthy people, but it usually decreases in obese people.
Residual volume (RV): amount of air remaining in the lungs after forced expiration	Subtract ERV from functional residual capacity (FRC).	RV greater than 35% of total lung capacity (TLC) after maximal expiratory effort may indicate obstructive disease.
Vital capacity (VC): total volume of air that can be exhaled after maximum inspiration	Direct spirographic measurement or add V_T, IRV, and ERV	Normal or increased VC with decreased flow rates may indicate any condition that reduces functional pulmonary tissue, such as pulmonary edema. Decreased VC with normal or increased flow rates may indicate decreased respiratory effort resulting from neuromuscular disease, drug overdose, or head injury; decreased thoracic expansion; or limited movement of diaphragm.

(continued)

Interpreting pulmonary function tests (continued)

TEST	METHOD OF CALCULATION	IMPLICATIONS
Inspiratory capacity (IC): amount of air that can be inhaled after normal expiration	Direct spirographic measurement or add IRV and V_T.	Decreased IC indicates restrictive disease
Thoracic gas volume (TGV): total volume of gas in lungs from both ventilated and non-ventilated airways	Body plethysmography	Increased TGV indicates air trapping, which may result from obstructive disease.
Functional residual capacity (FRC): amount of air remaining in lungs after normal expiration	Nitrogen washout, helium dilution technique, or add ERV and RV	Increased FRC indicates overdistention of lungs, which may result from obstructive pulmonary disease.
Total lung capacity: total volume of lungs when maximally inflated	Add V_T, IRV, ERV, and RV; or FRC and IC; or VC and RV.	Low TLC indicates restrictive disease; high TLC indicates overdistended lungs caused by obstructive disease.
Forced vital capacity (FVC): measurement of the amount of air exhaled forcefully and quickly after maximum inspiration	Direct spirographic measurement; expressed as a percentage of the total volume of gas exhaled	Decreased FVC indicates flow resistance in respiratory system from obstructive disease such as chronic bronchitis or from restrictive disease such as pulmonary fibrosis.
Flow-volume curve (also called flow-volume loop): greatest rate of flow (Vmax) during FVC maneuvers versus lung volume change	Direct spirographic measurement at 1-second intervals; calculated from flow rates (expressed in liters/second) and lung volume changes (expressed in liters) during maximal inspiratory and expiratory maneuvers	Decreased flow rates at all volumes during expiration indicate obstructive disease of the small airways, such as emphysema. A plateau of expiratory flow near TLC, a plateau of inspiratory flow at mid-VC, and a square wave pattern through most of VC indicate obstructive disease of large airways. Normal or increased peak expiratory flow, decreased flow with decreasing lung volumes, and markedly decreased VC indicate restrictive disease.
Forced expiratory volume (FEV): volume of air expired in the 1st, 2nd, or 3rd second of FVC maneuver	Direct spirographic measurement; expressed as percentage of FVC	Decreased FEV_1 and increased FEV_2 and FEV_3 may indicate obstructive disease; decreased or normal FEV_1 may indicate restrictive disease.

Interpreting pulmonary function tests (continued)

TEST	METHOD OF CALCULATION	IMPLICATIONS
Forced expiratory flow (FEF): average rate of flow during middle half of FVC	Calculated from the flow rate and the time needed for expiration of middle 50% of FVC	Low FEF (25% to 75%) indicates obstructive disease of the small and medium-sized airways.
Peak expiratory flow rate (PEFR): Vmax during forced expiration	Calculated from flow-volume curve or by direct spirographic measurement using a pneumotachometer or electronic tachometer with a transducer to convert flow to electrical output display	Decreased PEFR may indicate a mechanical problem, such as upper airway obstruction, or obstructive disease. PEFR is usually normal in restrictive disease but decreases in severe cases. Because PEFR is effort-dependent, it's also low in a person who has poor expiratory effort or doesn't understand the procedure.
Maximal voluntary ventilation (MVV) (also called maximum breathing capacity [MBC]): greatest volume of air breathed per unit of time	Direct spirographic measurement	Decreased MVV may indicate obstructive disease; normal or decreased MVV may indicate restrictive disease such as myasthenia gravis.
Diffusing capacity for carbon monoxide (DL_{CO}): milliliters of carbon monoxide diffused per minute across the alveolo-capillary membrane	Calculated from analysis of amount of carbon monoxide exhaled compared with amount inhaled	Decreased DL_{CO} because of thickened alveolocapillary membrane occurs in interstitial pulmonary diseases, such as pulmonary fibrosis, asbestosis, and sarcoidosis; it's reduced in emphysema because of the loss of alveolocapillary membrane.

■ Pregnancy or gastric distention may displace lung volume.

■ A narcotic analgesic or sedative can decrease inspiratory and expiratory forces.

■ Bronchodilators may temporarily improve pulmonary function.

FLUID ANALYSIS

Pleural fluid

The pleura, a two-layer membrane covering the lungs and lining the thoracic cavity, maintains a small amount of lubricating fluid between its layers to minimize friction during respiration. Increased fluid in this space — the result of diseases such as cancer and tuberculosis or of blood or lymphatic disorders — can cause respiratory difficulty.

In pleural fluid aspiration (also known as thoracentesis), the thoracic wall is punctured to obtain a specimen of pleural fluid for analysis or to relieve pulmonary compression and resultant respiratory distress. The specimen is examined for color, consistency, glucose and protein content, cellular composition, and the enzymes lactate dehydrogenase (LD) and amylase; it's also examined cytologically for malignant cells and cultured for pathogens. Locating the fluid before thoracentesis — by physical examination and chest X-ray or ultrasonography — reduces the risk of puncturing the lung, liver, or spleen.

Purpose
■ To provide a fluid specimen to determine the cause and nature of pleural effusion
■ To permit better radiographic visualization of a lung with large effusions.

Patient preparation
Explain to the patient that this test assesses the space around the lungs for fluid. Inform him who will perform the test and where and that he needn't restrict food or fluids.

Inform the patient that a chest X-ray or ultrasound study may precede the test to help locate the fluid. Check the patient's history for hypersensitivity to local anesthetics. Warn him that he may feel a stinging sensation on injection of the anesthetic and some pressure during withdrawal of the fluid. Advise him not to cough, breathe deeply, or move during the test to minimize the risk of injury to the lung.

Equipment
Sterile collection bottles ✦ sterile gloves ✦ adhesive tape ✦ sterile thoracentesis tray (a prepackaged, disposable tray with the following: 70% alcohol or povidone-iodine solution ✦ drapes ✦ local anesthetic [usually 1% lidocaine] ✦ sterile 5-ml syringe for local anesthetic ✦ 25G needle ✦ 50-ml syringe for removing fluid ✦ 17G aspiration needle ✦ sterile specimen bottle or tube ✦ three-way stopcock or sterile tubing to prevent air from entering the pleural cavity ✦ small sterile dressing).

Procedure
Record baseline vital signs. Shave the area around the needle insertion site, if necessary. Position the patient properly to widen the intercostal spaces and allow easier access to the pleural cavity; make sure he's well supported and comfortable. If possible, seat him at the edge of the bed with a chair or stool supporting his feet and his head and arms resting on a padded overbed table. If he can't sit up, position him on his unaffected side with the arm on the affected side elevated above his head. (See *Positioning the patient for thoracentesis.*) Remind him not to cough, breathe deeply, or move suddenly during the procedure.

After the patient is properly positioned, the doctor disinfects the skin, drapes the area, injects a local anesthetic into the subcutaneous tissue, and inserts the thoracentesis needle above the rib to avoid lacerating intercostal vessels. When the needle reaches the pocket of fluid, he attaches the 50-ml syringe and the stopcock and opens the clamps on the tubing to aspirate fluid into the container. During aspiration, check the patient for signs of respiratory distress, such as weakness, dyspnea, pallor, cyanosis, changes in heart rate, tachypnea, diaphoresis, blood-tinged frothy mucus, and hypotension.

Positioning the patient for thoracentesis

To prepare the patient for thoracentesis, place him in one of the three positions shown below: sitting on the edge of the bed with arms on an overbed table; sitting up in bed with arms on an overbed table; or lying partially on the side, partially on the back with arms over the head. These positions serve to widen the intercostal spaces and permit easy access to the pleural cavity. Using pillows as shown will make the patient more comfortable.

Sitting up in bed

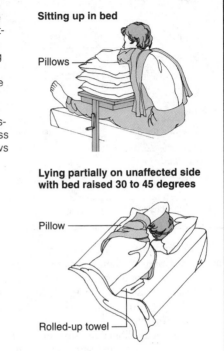

Pillows

Lying partially on unaffected side with bed raised 30 to 45 degrees

Pillow

Rolled-up towel

Sitting on edge of bed

Pillow

After the needle is withdrawn, apply slight pressure and a small adhesive bandage to the puncture site. Label the specimen, and record the date and time of the test and the amount, color, and character of the fluid (clear, frothy, purulent, bloody) on the laboratory request. Note any signs of distress the patient exhibited during the procedure. Document the exact location from which fluid was removed because this information may aid diagnosis.

Precautions

NURSING ALERT

■ Thoracentesis is contraindicated in patients with a history of bleeding disorders.
■ Use strict aseptic technique.
■ Note the patient's temperature and use

of antimicrobial therapy, if applicable, on the laboratory request.
■ Send the specimen to the laboratory immediately.

Normal findings

The pleural cavity should maintain negative pressure and contain less than 20 ml of serous fluid.

Implications of results

Pleural effusion results from the abnormal formation or reabsorption of pleural fluid. Certain characteristics classify pleural fluid as either a transudate (a low-protein fluid that has leaked from normal blood vessels) or an exudate (a protein-rich fluid that has leaked from blood vessels with increased permeability).

Characteristics of pulmonary transudate and exudate

The following characteristics help classify pleural fluid as either a transudate or an exudate.

CHARACTERISTIC	TRANSUDATE	EXUDATE
Appearance	Clear	Cloudy, turbid
Specific gravity	<1.016	>1.016
Clot (fibrinogen)	Absent	Present
Protein	<3 g/dl	>3 g/dl
White blood cells	Few lymphocytes	Many lymphocytes; may be purulent
Red blood cells	Few	Variable
Glucose	Equal to serum level	May be less than serum level
Lactate dehydrogenase	Low	High

Pleural fluid may contain blood (hemothorax), chyle (chylothorax), or pus and necrotic tissue. Blood-tinged fluid may indicate a traumatic tap; if so, the fluid should clear as aspiration progresses.

Transudative effusion usually results from diminished colloidal pressure, increased negative pressure within the pleural cavity, ascites, systemic and pulmonary venous hypertension, congestive heart failure, hepatic cirrhosis, and nephritis.

Exudative effusion results from disorders that increase pleural capillary permeability (possibly with changes in hydrostatic or colloid osmotic pressures), lymphatic drainage interference, infections, pulmonary infarctions, and neoplasms. Exudative effusion in association with depressed glucose levels, elevated LD levels, rheumatoid arthritis cells, and negative smears, cultures, and cytologic examination may indicate pleurisy associated with rheumatoid arthritis. (See *Characteristics of pulmonary transudate and exudate.*)

The most common pathogens that appear in culture studies of pleural fluid include *Mycobacterium tuberculosis,* *Staphylococcus aureus, Streptococcus pneumoniae* and other streptococci, *Haemophilus influenzae* and, in the case of a ruptured pulmonary abscess, anaerobes such as bacteroides. Cultures are usually positive during the early stages of infection; however, antibiotic therapy may produce a negative culture despite a positive Gram stain and grossly purulent fluid. Empyema may result from complications of pneumonia, pulmonary abscess, perforation of the esophagus, and penetration from mediastinitis. A high percentage of neutrophils suggests septic inflammation; predominating lymphocytes suggest tuberculosis or fungal or viral effusions.

Serosanguineous fluid may indicate pleural extension of a malignant tumor. Elevated LD levels in a nonpurulent, nonhemolyzed, nonbloody effusion may also suggest a malignant tumor. Pleural fluid glucose levels that are 30 to 40 mg/dl lower than blood glucose levels may indicate cancer, bacterial infection, nonseptic inflammation, or metastasis. Increased amylase levels occur with pleural effusions associated with pancreatitis.

Recognizing complications of thoracentesis

You can identify the following potential complications of thoracentesis by watching for their characteristic signs and symptoms:

- *pneumothorax:* apprehension, increased restlessness, cyanosis, sudden breathlessness, tachycardia, chest pain
- *tension pneumothorax:* dyspnea, chest pain, tachycardia, hypoten-sion, absent or diminished breath sounds on affected side
- *subcutaneous emphysema:* local tissue swelling, crackling on palpation of site
- *infection:* fever, rapid pulse rate, pain
- *mediastinal shift:* labored breathing, cardiac arrhythmias, cardiac distress, pulmonary edema (pink, frothy sputum; paradoxical pulse).

Post-test care

- Reposition the patient comfortably on the affected side or as ordered by the doctor. Tell him to remain on this side for at least 1 hour to seal the puncture site. Elevate the head of the bed to facilitate breathing.
- Monitor vital signs every 30 minutes for 2 hours, then every 4 hours until they are stable.
- Tell the patient to call a nurse immediately if he experiences difficulty breathing.
- Watch for signs of pneumothorax, tension pneumothorax, fluid reaccumulation and, if a large amount of fluid was withdrawn, pulmonary edema or cardiac distress due to mediastinal shift. Usually, a post-test X-ray is ordered to detect these complications before clinical symptoms appear. (See *Recognizing complications of thoracentesis.*)
- Check the puncture site for fluid leakage. A large amount of leakage is abnormal. Also check the site and surrounding area for subcutaneous emphysema.

Interfering factors

- Failure to use aseptic technique may contaminate the specimen.
- Antimicrobial therapy before aspiration of fluid for culture may decrease the number of bacteria, making isolation of the infecting organism difficult.
- Failure to send the specimen to the laboratory immediately may affect the accuracy of test results.

Sweat

The sweat test quantitatively measures electrolyte concentrations (primarily sodium and chloride) in sweat, usually through pilocarpine iontophoresis (pilocarpine is a sweat inducer). This test is used almost exclusively in children to confirm cystic fibrosis, a congenital condition that raises the sodium and chloride electrolyte levels in sweat.

Purpose

- To confirm cystic fibrosis
- To exclude the diagnosis in siblings of those with cystic fibrosis.

Patient preparation

Because the patient is generally a child, explain the test to him as simply as possible (if he's old enough to understand). Inform the patient and his parents that there are no restrictions of diet, medications, or activity before the test. Tell the patient who will perform the test and where and that it takes 20 to 45 minutes (depending on the equipment used).

Tell the child he may feel a slight tickling sensation during the procedure but won't feel any pain. If he becomes nervous or frightened during the test, try to distract him with a book, television, or another appropriate diversion.

Encourage the parents to assist with preparations and to stay with their child during the test. Their presence will minimize the child's anxiety.

Equipment

Analyzer ✦ two skin chloride electrodes (positive and negative) ✦ distilled water ✦ two standardizing solutions (chloride concentrations) ✦ sterile 2" x 2" gauze pads (kept in airtight container) ✦ pilocarpine pads ✦ forceps (for handling pads) ✦ straps (for securing electrodes) ✦ gram scale ✦ normal saline solution.

Procedure

With distilled water, wash the area to be tested, and dry it. (The flexor surface of the right forearm is commonly used or, when the patient's arm is too small to secure electrodes, as with an infant, the right thigh.) Place a gauze pad saturated with premeasured pilocarpine solution on the positive electrode; place a gauze pad saturated with normal saline solution on the negative electrode. Apply both electrodes to the area to be tested, and secure them with straps.

Lead wires to the analyzer — which are attached in a manner similar to that used for ECG electrodes — are given a current of 4 mA in 15 to 20 seconds. This process (iontophoresis) is continued at 15- to 20-second intervals for 5 minutes. After iontophoresis, remove both electrodes. Discard the pads, clean the patient's skin with distilled water, and then dry it.

Using forceps, place a dry gauze pad or filter paper (previously weighed on a gram scale) on the area where the pilo-

carpine was used. Cover the pad or filter paper with a slightly larger piece of plastic, and seal the edges of the plastic with waterproof adhesive tape. Leave the gauze pad or filter paper in place for about 45 minutes. (The appearance of droplets on the plastic usually indicates induction of an adequate amount of sweat.)

Remove the pad or filter paper with the forceps, place it immediately in the weighing bottle, and insert the stopper in the bottle. The difference between the first and second weights indicates the weight of the sweat specimen collected.

Precautions

■ Always perform iontophoresis on the right arm (or right thigh) rather than on the left. *Never* perform iontophoresis on the chest, especially in a child, because the current can induce cardiac arrest.

■ To prevent electric shock, use battery-powered equipment, if possible.

■ Make sure that at least 100 mg of sweat is collected in 45 minutes.

■ Stop the test immediately if the patient complains of a burning sensation, which usually indicates that the positive electrode is exposed or positioned improperly. Adjust the electrode, and continue the test.

■ Carefully seal the gauze pad or filter paper in the weighing bottle, and send the bottle to the laboratory at once.

Reference values

Normal sodium values in sweat range from 10 to 30 mEq/L. Normal chloride values range from 10 to 35 mEq/L.

Implications of results

Abnormal sodium values range from 50 to 130 mEq/L. Abnormal chloride values range from 50 to 110 mEq/L. Sodium and chloride concentrations of 50 to 60 mEq/L strongly suggest cystic fibrosis. Concentrations greater than 60 mEq/L with typical clinical features confirm the diagnosis. Only a few conditions other than cystic fibrosis cause elevated sweat electrolyte levels — most notably, untreated adrenal insufficiency as well as type I glycogen storage disease, vasopressin-resistant diabetes insipidus, meconium ileus, and renal failure. However, cystic fibrosis is the only condition that raises sweat electrolyte levels above 80 mEq/L.

In females, sweat electrolyte levels fluctuate cyclically: Chloride concentrations usually peak 5 to 10 days before onset of menses, and most women retain fluid before menses. Males also show fluctuations (up to 70 mEq/L).

Post-test care

▪ Wash the tested area with soap and water, and dry it thoroughly.
▪ If the area looks red, reassure the patient that this is normal and that the redness will disappear within a few hours.
▪ Tell the patient that he may resume his usual activities.

Interfering factors

▪ Dehydration and edema, especially in the area of collection, may interfere with test results.
▪ Failure to obtain an adequate amount of sweat (common in neonates) prevents proper testing.
▪ Presence of pure salt depletion (common during hot weather) may cause false-normal test results.
▪ Failure to clean the skin thoroughly or to use sterile gauze pads may cause false elevations.
▪ Failure to seal the gauze pad or filter paper carefully may falsely elevate electrolyte levels because of evaporation.
▪ Unstable clinical conditions allow erroneous interpretation of test results.

ENDOSCOPY

Direct laryngoscopy

Direct laryngoscopy, the visualization of the larynx by the use of a fiber-optic endoscope or laryngoscope passed through the mouth and pharynx to the larynx, usually follows indirect laryngoscopy, the more common procedure. (See *Indirect laryngoscopy*, page 652.) Direct laryngoscopy permits visualization of areas that are inaccessible through indirect laryngoscopy. It's indicated for children; for patients with strong gag reflexes due to anatomic abnormalities; for those with symptoms of pharyngeal or laryngeal disease, such as stridor and hemoptysis; and for those who have had no response to short-term symptomatic therapy. The procedure may include the collection of secretions or tissue for further study and the removal of foreign bodies.

This test is usually contraindicated in patients with epiglottitis because trauma can quickly cause edema and airway obstruction; when the test is necessary in such patients, it may be performed in the operating room with resuscitative equipment available.

Purpose

▪ To detect lesions, strictures, or foreign bodies in the larynx
▪ To aid diagnosis of laryngeal cancer
▪ To remove benign lesions or foreign bodies from the larynx
▪ To examine the larynx when the view provided by indirect laryngoscopy is inadequate.

Patient preparation

Explain to the patient that this test determines laryngeal abnormalities. Instruct him to fast for 6 to 8 hours be-

Indirect laryngoscopy

Indirect laryngoscopy, normally an office procedure, allows visualization of the larynx using a warm laryngeal mirror positioned at the back of the throat, a head mirror held in front of the mouth, and a light source.

The patient sits erect in a chair and sticks out his tongue as far as possible. The tongue is grasped with a piece of gauze and held in place with a tongue blade. If the patient's gag reflex is sensitive, a local anesthetic may be sprayed on the pharyngeal wall. Then the larynx is observed at rest and during phona-tion. A simple excision of polyps may also be performed during this procedure.

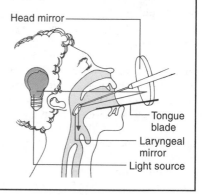

Head mirror

Tongue blade

Laryngeal mirror

Light source

---

fore the test. Tell him who will perform the laryngoscopy and that it will be done in a dark operating room.

Inform the patient that he'll receive a sedative to help him relax, medication to reduce secretions and, during the procedure, a general or local anesthetic. Also, reassure him that this procedure won't obstruct the airway.

Make sure the patient or a responsible member of his family has signed a consent form. Check the patient's history for hypersensitivity to the anesthetic. Obtain baseline vital signs. Administer the sedative and other medication to the patient, as ordered (usually 30 minutes to 1 hour before the test). Just before the test, instruct the patient to remove dentures, contact lenses, and jewelry, and tell him to urinate.

Equipment

Laryngoscope ✦ sedative ✦ atropine ✦ local anesthetic (spray or jelly, as ordered) or general anesthetic ✦ sterile container for microbiology specimen ✦ sterile gloves ✦ Coplin jar with 95% ethyl alcohol for cytology smears ✦ container with 10% formaldehyde solution for histol-ogy specimen ✦ forceps for biopsy ✦ emesis basin ✦ resuscitative equipment.

Procedure

Place the patient in the supine position. Encourage him to relax with his arms at his sides and to breathe through his nose. A general anesthetic is administered or the patient's mouth and throat are sprayed with local anesthetic. The patient's head is positioned and held while the doctor introduces the laryngoscope through the patient's mouth. The larynx is examined for abnormalities, and a specimen or secretions may be removed for further study. Minor surgery, such as removal of polyps, may be performed at this time. Place specimens for histology, cytology, and microbiology in their respective containers.

Precautions

Send the specimens to the laboratory immediately.

Normal findings

A normal larynx shows no evidence of inflammation, lesions, strictures, or foreign bodies.

Implications of results

The combined results of direct laryngoscopy, biopsy, and radiography may indicate laryngeal cancer. Direct laryngoscopy may show benign lesions, strictures, or foreign bodies and, with a biopsy, may distinguish laryngeal edema from a radiation reaction or a tumor.

Post-test care

■ As ordered, place the conscious patient in semi-Fowler's position; place the unconscious patient on his side with his head slightly elevated to prevent aspiration.

■ Monitor vital signs according to your facility's protocol. Immediately report any adverse reaction to the anesthetic or sedative (tachycardia, palpitations, hypertension, euphoria, excitation, and rapid, deep respirations).

■ Apply an ice collar to prevent or minimize laryngeal edema.

■ Provide an emesis basin, and instruct the patient to spit out saliva rather than swallow it. Observe sputum for blood, and notify the doctor immediately if excessive bleeding occurs.

■ If the patient has a biopsy, instruct him to refrain from clearing his throat and coughing, which could dislodge the clot at the biopsy site and cause hemorrhaging. Also, advise him to avoid smoking until vital signs are stable and there is no evidence of complications.

■ Immediately report subcutaneous crepitus around the patient's face and neck — a possible indication of tracheal perforation.

 ■ Observe the patient with epiglottitis for signs of airway obstruction. Immediately report signs of respiratory difficulty due to laryngeal edema or laryngospasm, such as laryngeal stridor and dyspnea. Keep emergency resuscitation equipment and a tracheotomy tray nearby for 24 hours.

■ Restrict food and fluids until the gag reflex returns (usually 2 hours). Then tell the patient he may resume his usual diet, beginning with sips of water.

■ Reassure the patient that voice loss, hoarseness, and sore throat are temporary. Provide throat lozenges or a soothing liquid gargle when his gag reflex returns.

Interfering factors

Failure to place the specimens in the appropriate containers or to send them to the laboratory at once may interfere with accurate test results and diagnosis.

Bronchoscopy

Bronchoscopy is the direct visualization of the larynx, trachea, and bronchi through a standard metal or fiber-optic bronchoscope, a slender flexible tube with mirrors and a light at its distal end. A brush, biopsy forceps, or a catheter may be passed through the bronchoscope to obtain specimens for cytologic examination.

A flexible fiber-optic bronchoscope is used most often because it's smaller, allows a better view of the segmental and subsegmental bronchi, and carries less risk of trauma than a rigid bronchoscope. However, a large, rigid bronchoscope must be used to remove foreign objects, excise endobronchial lesions, and control massive hemoptysis.

Possible complications of bronchoscopy include hypoxemia, cardiac arrhythmias, bleeding, infection, bronchospasm, and pneumothorax.

Purpose

■ To visually examine a tumor, obstruction, secretion, or foreign body in the tracheobronchial tree, as demonstrated on chest X-ray

■ To help diagnose bronchogenic carcinoma, tuberculosis, interstitial pulmonary disease, or fungal or parasitic pulmonary infection by obtaining a specimen for bacteriologic and cytologic examination

■ To locate a bleeding site in the tracheobronchial tree

■ To remove foreign bodies, malignant or benign tumors, mucous plugs, or excessive secretions from the tracheobronchial tree.

Patient preparation

Describe the procedure to the patient, and explain that this test allows the doctor to examine the lower airways. Instruct the patient to fast for 6 to 12 hours before the test. Tell him who will perform the test and where, that the room will be darkened, and that the procedure takes 45 to 60 minutes. Advise him that test results are usually available in 1 day — except for a tuberculosis report, which may take up to 6 weeks.

Tell the patient that chest X-rays and certain blood studies (prothrombin time, activated partial thromboplastin time, platelet count and, possibly, arterial blood gas analysis) will be performed before the bronchoscopy. Advise him that he may receive a sedative I.V. to help him relax. If the procedure is not being performed under a general anesthetic, inform the patient that a local anesthetic will be sprayed into his nose and mouth to suppress the gag reflex. Warn him that the spray has an unpleasant taste and that he may experience some discomfort during the procedure. Reassure him that his airway won't be blocked during the procedure and that oxygen will be administered through the bronchoscope.

Make sure the patient or a responsible family member has signed the consent form. Check the patient history for hypersensitivity to the anesthetic, and obtain baseline vital signs. Administer the preoperative sedative, as ordered. If the patient is wearing dentures, instruct him to remove them just before the test.

Equipment

Flexible fiber-optic bronchoscope ✦ sedative ✦ local anesthetic (spray, jelly, or liquid, as ordered) ✦ sterile gloves ✦ sterile container for microbiology specimen ✦ container with 10% formaldehyde solution for histology specimen ✦ Coplin jar with 95% ethyl alcohol for cytology smears ✦ six glass slides (all frosted, if possible, or with frosted tips) ✦ emesis basin ✦ hand-held resuscitation bag with face mask ✦ oral and endotracheal airways ✦ laryngoscope ✦ oxygen setup ✦ ventilating bronchoscope (for a patient who requires controlled mechanical ventilation).

Procedure

Place the patient in the supine position on a table or bed, or have him sit upright in a chair. Tell him to remain relaxed, with his arms at his sides, and to breathe through his nose. Provide supplemental oxygen by nasal cannula, if ordered.

After the local anesthetic is sprayed into the patient's throat and takes effect (usually in 1 to 2 minutes), the doctor introduces the bronchoscope (possibly tipped with lidocaine jelly) through the patient's mouth or nose. When the bronchoscope is just above the vocal cords, about 3 to 4 ml of 2% to 4% lidocaine is flushed through the inner channel of the scope to the vocal cords to anesthetize deeper areas.

The doctor inspects the anatomic structure of the trachea and bronchi, observes the color of the mucosal lining, and notes masses or inflamed areas. Then he may use biopsy forceps to remove a tissue specimen from a suspect area, a bronchial brush to obtain cells from the surface of a lesion, or suction apparatus to remove foreign bod-

Features of the bronchoscope

The bronchoscope, inserted through the nostril into the bronchi, has four channels (see inset): two light channels (A) that provide a light source; one visualizing channel (B) to see through; and one open channel (C) that accommodates biopsy forceps, cytology brush, suction apparatus, lavage device, anestl

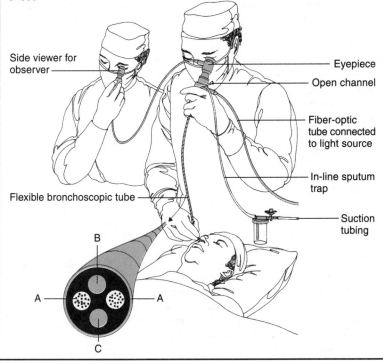

Side viewer for observer

Eyepiece

Open channel

Fiber-optic tube connected to light source

In-line sputum trap

Flexible bronchoscopic tube

Suction tubing

B

A — A

C

ies or mucous plugs. Bronchoalveolar lavage may be performed to diagnose the infectious causes of infiltrates in immunocompromised patients or to remove thickened secretions, as occur in cystic fibrosis. After the tissue, mucus, or secretion is collected, place the specimens for microbiology, histology, and cytology in their respective containers, and label them properly.

Bronchoscopy requires fluoroscopic guidance for distal evaluation of lesions or for a transbronchial biopsy in alveolar areas. (See *Features of the bronchoscope*.)

Precautions

NURSING ALERT ▪ A patient with severe respiratory failure who can't breathe adequately by himself should be placed on a ventilator before bronchoscopy.

▪ Send the specimens to the laboratory immediately.

Normal findings

The trachea, a $4\frac{1}{2}"$ (11-cm) tube lined with ciliated mucosa extending from the larynx to the bronchi, normally consists of smooth muscle containing C-shaped rings of cartilage at regular intervals.

The bronchi appear structurally similar to the trachea; the right bronchus is slightly larger and more vertical than the left. Smaller segmental bronchi branch off from the main bronchi.

Implications of results

Abnormalities of the bronchial wall include inflammation, swelling, protruding cartilage, ulceration, tumors, and enlargement of the mucous gland orifices or submucosal lymph nodes.

Abnormalities of endotracheal origin include stenosis, compression, ectasia (dilation of tubular vessel), irregular bronchial branching, and abnormal bifurcation due to diverticulum.

Abnormal substances in the trachea or bronchi include blood, secretions, calculi, and foreign bodies.

Results of tissue and cell studies may indicate interstitial pulmonary disease, bronchogenic carcinoma, tuberculosis, or other pulmonary infections. Bronchogenic carcinomas include epidermoid or squamous cell carcinoma, small-cell (oat cell) carcinoma, adenocarcinoma, and large-cell (undifferentiated) carcinoma. Bronchoscopy findings must be correlated with radiographic and cytologic findings as well as with clinical signs and symptoms.

Post-test care

■ Monitor vital signs. Notify the doctor immediately if the patient has an adverse reaction to the anesthetic or sedative.

■ As ordered, place the conscious patient in semi-Fowler's position; place the unconscious patient on his side with the head of the bed slightly elevated to prevent aspiration.

■ Provide an emesis basin, and instruct the patient to spit out saliva rather than swallow it. Observe sputum for blood, and notify the doctor immediately if excessive bleeding occurs.

■ Tell the patient who had a biopsy to refrain from clearing his throat and coughing, which could dislodge the clot at the biopsy site and cause hemorrhaging.

■ Immediately report subcutaneous crepitus around the patient's face and neck — a possible indication of tracheal or bronchial perforation.

NURSING ALERT ■ Watch for and immediately report symptoms of respiratory difficulty due to laryngeal edema or laryngospasm, such as laryngeal stridor and dyspnea. Observe for signs of hypoxemia (cyanosis), pneumothorax (dyspnea, cyanosis, diminished breath sounds on affected side), bronchospasm (dyspnea, wheezing), and bleeding (hemoptysis).

■ Restrict food and fluids until the gag reflex returns (usually in 2 hours). Then let the patient resume his usual diet, beginning with sips of clear liquid or ice chips.

■ Reassure the patient that hoarseness, loss of voice, and sore throat after this procedure are only temporary. Provide lozenges or a soothing liquid gargle to ease discomfort when his gag reflex returns.

Interfering factors

Failure to place the specimens in the appropriate containers or to send them to the laboratory immediately may interfere with accurate test results and diagnosis.

Mediastinoscopy

Mediastinoscopy is an operative procedure that allows doctors to see mediastinal structures directly — through a mediastinoscope with a built-in light source — and permits palpation and biopsy of paratracheal and carinal lymph nodes. The mediastinum is the cavity behind the sternum that separates the lungs. Its major components include the heart and its vessels as well as the trachea, esophagus, thymus, and lymph nodes. Mediastinoscopic examination of the nodes, which receive lymphatic drainage from the lungs, can detect lymphoma (including Hodgkin's disease) and sarcoidosis and can help in staging lung cancer. (See *Staging lung cancer,* pages 658 and 659.) Mediastinoscopy is also indicated when such tests as sputum cytology, lung scans, radiography, and bronchoscopic biopsy fail to confirm a diagnosis.

The right side of the mediastinum is easily explored, and because mediastinoscopy can diagnose bronchogenic carcinoma at an early stage, this procedure is now replacing the scalene fat pad biopsy. Exploring the left side is more hazardous because of the aorta's proximity. Although rare, complications of this test include pneumothorax, perforated esophagus, infection, hemorrhage, and left recurrent laryngeal nerve damage. Scarring from a previous mediastinoscopy contraindicates this test.

Purpose
■ To detect bronchogenic carcinoma, lymphoma, and sarcoidosis
■ To determine staging of lung cancer.

Patient preparation
Describe the procedure to the patient and answer his questions. Explain that this test evaluates the lymph nodes and other structures in the chest. Instruct the patient to fast after midnight before the test. Tell him who will perform the procedure and where, that he'll be given a general anesthetic, and that the procedure takes about 1 hour. Tell him he may have temporary chest pain, tenderness at the incision site, or a sore throat (from

intubation). Reassure him that complications are rare with this procedure.

Make sure the patient or a responsible family member has signed a consent form. Check the patient history for hypersensitivity to the anesthetic. As ordered, give a sedative the night before the test and again before the procedure.

Equipment
Mediastinoscope ✦ light carriers ✦ suction tubes ✦ long aspiration needle ✦ cup biopsy forceps ✦ laryngeal scissors ✦ spreader.

Procedure
After the endotracheal tube is in place, a small transverse suprasternal incision is made. Using finger dissection, the surgeon forms a channel and palpates the lymph nodes. The mediastinoscope is inserted, and tissue specimens are collected and sent to the laboratory for frozen section examination. If analysis confirms malignancy of a resectable tumor, thoracotomy and pneumonectomy may follow immediately.

Precautions
None.

Normal findings
Lymph nodes should appear as small, smooth, flat oval bodies of lymphoid tissue.

Implications of results
Malignant lymph nodes usually indicate inoperable — but not always untreatable — lung or esophageal cancer or lymphomas (such as Hodgkin's disease). Staging of lung cancer helps determine the therapeutic regimen. (For example, multiple nodular involvement can contraindicate surgery.)

Post-test care
■ Monitor vital signs, and check the dressing for bleeding or fluid drainage.

Staging lung cancer

CLASSIFICATION	DEFINITION
Primary tumor (T)	
TO	No evidence of primary tumor.
TX	Tumor proven by malignant cells in bronchopulmonary secretions but not visualized by X-ray or bronchoscopy.
TIS	Carcinoma in situ.
T1	Tumor 3 cm or less in diameter, surrounded by normal lung or visceral pleura.
T2	Tumor more than 3 cm in diameter, or tumor of any size that invades the visceral pleura or extends to the hilar region. Tumor lies within a lobar bronchus or at least 2 cm from the carina. Any associated atelectasis or obstructive pneumonitis involves less than an entire lung.
T3	Tumor of any size that extends into neighboring structures, such as the chest wall, diaphragm, or mediastinum; that involves a main bronchus less than 2 cm from the carina; or that occurs with atelectasis or obstructive pneumonitis of an entire lung or with pleural effusion.
Regional lymph nodes (N)	
NO	No demonstrable metastasis to regional lymph nodes.
N1	Metastasis to peribronchial or ipsilateral hilar lymph nodes.
N2	Metastasis to mediastinal lymph nodes.
Distant metastasis (M)	
MO	No distant metastasis
MI	Distant metastasis, such as to scalene, cervical, or contralateral hilar lymph nodes as well as to brain, bones, lung, or liver.

STAGE GROUPING

T, N, and M factors may be combined into the following groups or stages:

Occult carcinoma

TX NO MO	Bronchopulmonary secretions contain malignant cells; no other evidence of the primary tumor or of metastasis.

Stage I

TIS NO MO	Carcinoma in situ.
T1 NO MO	Tumor classified as T1 without metastasis to the regional lymph nodes.
T1 N1 MO	Tumor classified as T1 with metastasis to the ipsilateral hilar lymph nodes only.
T2 NO MO	Tumor classified as T2 without metastasis to nodes or distant metastasis.

(*Note:* TX N1 MO and TO N1 MO also fall under stage I but are difficult, if not impossible, to diagnose.)

Staging lung cancer *(continued)*	
STAGE GROUPING *(continued)*	
Stage II	
T2 N1 MO	Tumor classified as T2 with metastasis to ipsilateral hilar lymph nodes only.
Stage III	
T3 (with any N or M)	Any tumor more extensive than T2.
N3 (with any T or M)	Any tumor with metastasis to mediastinal lymph nodes.
M1 (with any T or N)	Any tumor with distant metastasis.

■ Observe for signs of complications: fever (mediastinitis); crepitus (subcutaneous emphysema); dyspnea, cyanosis, and diminished breath sounds (pneumothorax); tachycardia and hypotension (hemorrhage).

■ Administer the prescribed analgesic, as needed.

Interfering factors
None.

Thoracoscopy

Thoracoscopy is an operative procedure that allows doctors to see the pleural space by inserting an endoscope directly into the chest wall. Used for both diagnostic and therapeutic purposes, it can sometimes replace traditional thoracotomy. This procedure reduces morbidity (by avoiding open chest surgery) and postoperative pain, decreases surgical and anesthesia time, and allows faster recovery. Complications, although rare, include hemorrhage, nerve injury, perforation of the diaphragm, air emboli, and tension pneumothorax.

Purpose
■ To diagnose pleural disease
■ To obtain a biopsy specimen from the mediastinum
■ To treat pleural conditions, such as cysts, blebs, and effusions
■ To perform wedge resections.

Patient preparation
Explain the procedure to the patient. Tell him that an open thoracotomy may be needed for diagnosis or treatment and that general anesthesia may be necessary. Advise him not to eat or drink for 10 to 12 hours before the procedure.

Make sure appropriate preoperative tests (such as pulmonary function and coagulation tests, electrocardiogram, and chest X-ray) have been performed. Obtain a signed consent form.

Tell the patient that he'll have a chest tube and drainage system in place after surgery. Reassure him that analgesics will be available and that complications are rare.

Equipment
Monitors ✦ VCR ✦ camera ✦ light source ✦ insufflator ✦ cautery ✦ suction and irrigation equipment ✦ trocars ✦ endostaplers ✦ endosutures.

Procedure

The doctor anesthetizes the patient and inserts a double-lumen endobronchial tube. The lung on the operative side is collapsed, and a small intercostal incision is made through which a trocar is inserted. A lens is then inserted to view the area and assess thoracoscopy access. Two or three more small incisions are made, and trocars are placed for insertion of suctioning and dissection instruments. The camera lens and instruments are moved from site to site as needed.

After thoracoscopy, the lung is reexpanded and a chest tube is placed through one incision site. The other incisions are closed with adhesive strips and dressed. A water-sealed drainage system is attached to the chest tube.

Precautions

▪ Thoracoscopy is contraindicated in patients who have coagulopathies or lesions near major blood vessels, who have had previous thoracic surgery, or who can't be adequately oxygenated with one lung.
▪ Send specimens to the laboratory immediately.

Normal findings

The pleural cavity, a potential space, should contain a small amount of lubricating fluid that facilitates movement of the lung and chest wall. The parietal and visceral layers should be lesion-free and able to separate from each other.

Implications of results

Lesions adjacent to or involving the pleura or mediastinum can be seen and biopsied for diagnosis and determination of treatment. After accumulated fluid is removed, sterile talc can be blown into the pleural space to promote sclerosing and prevent future accumu-lations. Blebs can be removed by wedge resection to reduce the risk of repeated spontaneous pneumothorax.

Post-test care

▪ Monitor vital signs every 15 minutes for 1 hour and then every 4 hours.
▪ Assess respiratory status and the patency of the chest drainage system.
▪ Give analgesics, as needed, for pain.

Interfering factors

▪ Excessive bleeding during the procedure may necessitate open thoracotomy.
▪ Extensive or inaccessible pathology may prevent thoracoscopy.

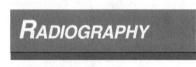

RADIOGRAPHY

Chest radiography

In chest radiography (commonly known as chest X-ray), X-ray beams penetrate the chest and react on specially sensitized film. Because normal pulmonary tissue is radiolucent, abnormalities such as infiltrates, foreign bodies, fluids, and tumors appear as densities on the film. A chest X-ray is most useful when compared with the patient's previous films because it allows the radiologist to detect changes.

Although chest radiography was once routinely performed as a cancer screening test, the associated expense and exposure to radiation have caused many authorities to question its usefulness for this purpose. The American Cancer Society recommends sputum culture rather than chest radiography — even for patients at high risk.

Purpose

- To detect pulmonary disorders, such as pneumonia, atelectasis, pneumothorax, pulmonary bullae, and tumors
- To detect mediastinal abnormalities, such as tumors, and cardiac disease
- To determine correct placement of pulmonary artery catheters, endotracheal tubes, and chest tubes
- To determine the location of foreign bodies (such as coins or broken central lines) swallowed or aspirated
- To determine the location and size of a lesion
- To help assess pulmonary status
- To evaluate response to interventions.

Patient preparation

Describe the procedure to the patient, and explain that this test assesses his respiratory status. Inform him that he needn't restrict food or fluids. Tell him who will perform the test and where and when it will be done.

Provide a gown without snaps, and instruct the patient to remove all jewelry in the X-ray field. Tell him that he'll be asked to take a deep breath and hold it momentarily while the film is being taken to provide a clearer view of pulmonary structures.

Equipment

X-ray machine (stationary or portable).

Procedure

For a stationary X-ray machine: The patient stands or sits in front of the machine, so that films can be taken of the posteroanterior and left lateral views.

For a portable X-ray machine (used at patient's bedside): Help to position the patient. Because an upright chest X-ray is preferable, move the patient to the top of the bed if he can tolerate it. Elevate the head of the bed for maximum upright positioning. (See *Common radiographic views,* pages 662 and 663.) Move cardiac monitoring cables, oxygen tubing, I.V. tubing from subclavian lines, pulmonary artery catheter lines, and safety pins as far as possible out of the X-ray field.

Precautions

- Chest radiography is usually contraindicated during the first trimester of pregnancy, but if it's necessary, place a lead apron over the patient's abdomen to shield the fetus.
- If the patient is intubated, check that no tubes have been dislodged during positioning.
- To avoid exposure to radiation, leave the room or the immediate area while the films are being taken. If you must stay in the area, wear a lead-lined apron.

Normal findings

See *Clinical implications of chest X-ray findings,* pages 664 and 665.

Implications of results

For accurate diagnosis, radiography findings must be correlated with additional radiologic and pulmonary tests as well as with physical assessment findings. Pulmonary hyperinflation with low diaphragm and generalized increased radiolucency may suggest emphysema but may also appear in a healthy person's X-rays.

Post-test care

None.

Interfering factors

- Portable chest X-rays taken in the anteroposterior position may show larger cardiac shadowing than other X-rays because the distance from the anterior structures to the beam is shorter. Portable chest X-rays — primarily those taken to detect atelectasis, pneumonia, pneumothorax, and mediastinal shift or to evaluate treatment — may be less reliable than stationary X-rays.

(Text continues on page 665.)

Common radiographic views

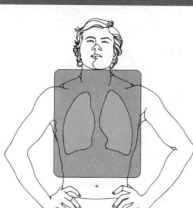

Frontal

Performed with the X-ray beam positioned posteriorly and anteriorly and with the patient in an upright position. Posteroanterior (PA) view is the most common frontal view; it's preferred over the anteroposterior (AP) view because the heart is anteriorly situated in the thorax and magnified less in a PA view than in an AP view. The frontal views show greater lung area than the other views because of the lower diaphragm position.

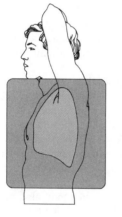

Lateral

Performed with the X-ray beam directed toward the patient's side. The left lateral (LL) view is the most common lateral view; it's preferred over the right lateral (RL) view because the heart is left of midline and magnified less in an LL view than in an RL view. Lateral views visualize lesions not apparent on a PA view.

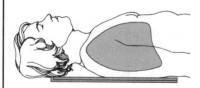

Recumbent

Performed with the X-ray beam overhead and with the patient supine. This view helps distinguish free fluid from encapsulated fluid and from an elevated diaphragm.

Oblique

Performed with the X-ray beam angled between the frontal and lateral views. This view helps evaluate intrathoracic disorders, pleural disease, esophageal abnormalities, hilar masses, and mediastinal masses. (Occasionally it's also used to localize lesions within the chest.)

Lordotic

Performed with the X-ray beam directed through the axis of the middle thoracic lobe and with the patient leaning back against the film plate. This view evaluates the apices of the lungs (usually obscured by bony structures) and helps localize sites of tuberculosis.

Decubitus

Performed with the X-ray beam parallel to the floor and with the patient in one of several horizontal positions (supine, prone, or side). This view demonstrates the extent of pulmonary abscess or cavity, the presence of free pleural fluid or pneumothorax, and the mobility of mediastinal mass when the patient changes positions.

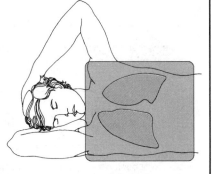

Clinical implications of chest X-ray findings

ANATOMIC STRUCTURE AND NORMAL APPEARANCE	ABNORMALITY	IMPLICATIONS
Trachea Visible midline in the anterior mediastinal cavity; translucent tube-like appearance	▪ Deviation from midline ▪ Narrowing, with hourglass appearance and deviation to one side	▪ Tension pneumothorax, atelectasis, pleural effusion, consolidation, mediastinal nodes; in children, enlarged thymus ▪ Substernal thyroid
Heart Visible in the anterior left mediastinal cavity; solid appearance due to blood contents; edges may be clear in contrast with surrounding air density of the lung	▪ Shift ▪ Hypertrophy of right heart ▪ Cardiac borders obscured by stringy densities ("shaggy heart")	▪ Atelectasis, pneumothorax ▪ Cor pulmonale, congestive heart failure ▪ Cystic fibrosis
Aortic knob Visible as water density; formed by the aortic arch	▪ Solid densities, possibly indicating calcifications ▪ Tortuous shape	▪ Atherosclerosis ▪ Atherosclerosis
Mediastinum (mediastinal shadow) Visible as the space between the lungs; shadowy appearance that widens at the hilum of the lungs	▪ Deviation to nondiseased side; deviation to diseased side by traction ▪ Gross widening	▪ Pleural effusion or tumor, fibrosis or collapsed lung ▪ Neoplasms of esophagus, bronchi, lungs, thyroid, thymus, peripheral nerves, lymphoid tissue; aortic aneurysm; mediastinitis; cor pulmonale
Ribs Visible as thoracic cavity encasement	▪ Break or misalignment ▪ Widening of intercostal spaces	▪ Fractured sternum or ribs ▪ Emphysema
Spine Visible midline in the posterior chest; straight bony structure	▪ Spinal curvature ▪ Break or misalignment	▪ Scoliosis, kyphosis ▪ Fractures
Clavicles Visible in upper thorax; intact and equidistant in properly centered X-ray films	▪ Break or misalignment	▪ Fractures

Clinical implications of chest X-ray findings (continued)

ANATOMIC STRUCTURE AND NORMAL APPEARANCE	ABNORMALITY	IMPLICATIONS
Hila (lung roots) Visible above the heart, where pulmonary vessels, bronchi, and lymph nodes join the lungs; appear as small, white, bilateral densities	▪ Shift to one side ▪ Accentuated shadows	▪ Atelectasis ▪ Pneumothorax, emphysema, pulmonary abscess, tumor, enlarged lymph nodes
Mainstem bronchus Visible; part of the hila with translucent, tube-like appearance	▪ Spherical or oval density	▪ Bronchogenic cyst
Bronchi Usually not visible	▪ Visible	▪ Bronchial pneumonia
Lung fields Usually not visible throughout, except for the blood vessels	▪ Visible ▪ Irregular, patchy densities	▪ Atelectasis ▪ Resolving pneumonia, infiltrates, silicosis, fibrosis, metastatic neoplasm
Hemidiaphragm Rounded, visible; right side $\frac{3}{8}$" to $\frac{3}{4}$" (1 to 2 cm) higher than left	▪ Elevation of diaphragm (difference in elevation can be measured on inspiration and expiration to detect movement) ▪ Flattening of diaphragm ▪ Unilateral elevation of either side ▪ Unilateral elevation of left side only	▪ Active tuberculosis, pneumonia, pleurisy, acute bronchitis, active disease of abdominal viscera, bilateral phrenic nerve involvement, atelectasis ▪ Asthma, emphysema ▪ Possibly unilateral phrenic nerve paresis ▪ Perforated ulcer (rare), gas distention of stomach, splenic flexure of colon, free air in abdomen

▪ Films taken with the patient in a supine position will not show fluid levels. (However, decubitus views can demonstrate fluid levels.)

▪ Because chest X-ray findings vary with the patient's age and sex, these factors should be considered when the films are evaluated.

▪ The patient's inability to take a full inspiration may interfere with interpretation of X-rays.

▪ Underexposure or overexposure of the films may result in poor-quality X-rays.

Paranasal sinus radiography

The paranasal sinuses — air-filled cavities lined with mucous membrane — lie within the maxillary, ethmoid, sphenoid, and frontal bones. Sinus abnormalities resulting from inflammation, trauma, cysts, mucoceles, granulomatosis, and other conditions include distorted bony sinus walls, altered mucous membranes, and fluid or masses within the cavities.

In paranasal sinus radiography, X-rays or electromagnetic waves penetrate the paranasal sinuses, forming a film image that differentiates sinus structures. The air that normally fills the paranasal sinuses appears black on film, but fluid in a sinus appears as a clouded-to-opaque density and may reveal an air-fluid level. A bone fracture is visible as a linear, radiolucent defect; cysts, polyps, and tumors are visible as soft-tissue masses projecting into the sinus.

If surrounding facial structures superimposed on the paranasal sinuses interfere with visualization of relevant areas, computed tomography scans may be indicated for further evaluation and diagnosis.

Purpose
■ To detect unilateral or bilateral abnormalities, possibly indicating trauma or disease
■ To confirm diagnosis of neoplastic or inflammatory paranasal sinus disease
■ To determine the location and size of a malignant tumor.

Patient preparation
Describe the procedure to the patient, and explain that this test helps evaluate abnormalities of the paranasal sinuses. Tell him who will perform the test, where and when it will be performed, and that it usually takes 10 to 15 minutes to complete.

Tell the patient that his head may be immobilized in a foam vise during the test to help him maintain the correct position but that the vise doesn't hurt. Explain that he'll be asked to sit upright and to avoid moving while the X-rays are being taken to prevent blurring of the image and to allow visualization of air-fluid levels, if present. Emphasize the importance of his cooperation. Instruct him to remove dentures, jewelry, and any metal objects in the X-ray field.

Equipment
Franklin radiographic head unit ✦ X-ray machine.

Procedure
The patient sits upright (possibly with his head in a foam vise) between the X-ray tube and a film cassette. During the test, the X-ray tube is positioned at specific angles and the patient's head is placed in various standard positions while his paranasal sinuses are filmed from different angles. If necessary, assist with positioning the patient.

Precautions
■ Paranasal sinus radiography is usually contraindicated during pregnancy; when it's necessary, a lead-lined apron placed over the patient's abdomen can shield the fetus.
■ To avoid exposure to radiation, leave the room or the immediate area during the test; if you must stay in the area, wear a lead-lined apron.

Normal findings
The paranasal sinuses should be radiolucent and filled with air, which appears black on paranasal sinus films.

Implications of results
See *Sinus X-ray findings.*

Sinus X-ray findings

This chart lists the abnormal radiographic findings associated with various sinus disorders.

DISORDER	ABNORMAL FINDINGS
Paranasal sinus trauma or fracture	■ Edema or hemorrhage in mucous membrane lining or sinus cavity ■ Clouded sinus air cells ■ Air-fluid level ■ Radiolucent, linear bone defects ■ Irregular, overriding bone edges ■ Depression or displacement of bone fragments ■ Foreign bodies
Acute sinusitis	■ Swollen, inflamed mucous membrane ■ Inflammatory exudate ■ Hazy to opaque sinus air cells ■ Air-fluid level
Chronic sinusitis	■ Thickened mucous membrane ■ Hazy to opaque sinus air cells ■ Air-fluid level ■ Thickening or sclerosis of bony wall of affected sinus
Wegener's granulomatosis	■ Clouded to opaque sinus air cells ■ Destruction of bony sinus wall
Malignant neoplasm	■ Rounded or lobulated soft-tissue mass projecting into sinus ■ Destruction of bony sinus wall
Benign bone tumor	■ Distortion of bony sinus wall in specific patterns
Cyst, polyp, or benign tumor	■ Rounded or lobulated soft-tissue mass projecting into sinus
Mucocele	■ Clouded sinus air cells ■ Destruction of bony sinus wall resulting in various degrees of radiolucency

Post-test care
None.

Interfering factors
■ Failure to remove dentures, jewelry, and metal objects within the X-ray field or the presence of numerous metallic foreign bodies in or around the paranasal sinuses may affect the accuracy of test results.

■ If the patient moves during filming, the X-rays may have to be repeated.

■ The patient's inability to sit upright during filming may necessitate performing the test on an X-ray table. This impairs visualization and diminishes the diagnostic value of the test.

■ Superimposition of surrounding facial structures on the film may impair visualization of the paranasal sinuses.

Fluoroscopy

In fluoroscopy, a continuous stream of X-rays passes through the patient, casting shadows of the heart, lungs, and diaphragm on a fluorescent screen. Because fluoroscopy exposes the patient to high levels of radiation and reveals less detail than does standard chest radiography, it's indicated only when diagnosis requires visualization of physiologic or pathologic motion of thoracic contents — for example, to rule out paralysis in patients with diaphragmatic elevation.

Purpose

- To assess lung expansion and contraction during quiet breathing, deep breathing, and coughing
- To assess movement and paralysis of the diaphragm
- To detect bronchiolar obstructions and pulmonary disease.

Patient preparation

Describe the procedure to the patient, and explain that this test assesses respiratory structures and their motion. Tell him who will perform the test and where and that it usually takes 5 minutes.

Tell the patient that he'll be asked to follow specific instructions, such as to breathe deeply and to cough, while X-ray images depict his breathing. Instruct him to remove all metallic objects (including jewelry) in the X-ray field.

Equipment

X-ray machine (X-ray transformer/ X-ray tube). A portable fluoroscopy unit may be used on intubated patients in the intensive care unit so that they don't have to be transported to the radiology department.

Procedure

If necessary, assist with positioning the patient. Move cardiac monitoring cables, I.V. tubing from subclavian lines, pulmonary artery catheter lines, and safety pins as far as possible from the X-ray field. During the test, the patient's cardiopulmonary motion is observed on a screen. Special equipment may be used to intensify the images, or a videotape recording of the fluoroscopy may be made for later study.

Precautions

- Fluoroscopy is contraindicated during pregnancy.
- If the patient is intubated, check that no tubes have been dislodged during positioning.
- To avoid exposure to radiation, leave the room or the immediate area during the test; if you must stay in the area, wear a lead-lined apron.

Normal findings

Normal diaphragmatic movement is synchronous and symmetrical. Normal diaphragmatic excursion ranges from $\frac{3}{4}$" to $1\frac{5}{8}$" (2 to 4 cm).

Implications of results

Diminished diaphragmatic movement may indicate pulmonary disease. Increased lung translucency may indicate loss of elasticity or bronchiolar obstruction. In elderly people, the lowest part of the trachea may be displaced to the right by an elongated aorta. Diminished or paradoxical diaphragmatic movement may indicate diaphragmatic paralysis, which sometimes occurs after open-heart surgery; however, fluoroscopy may not detect such paralysis in patients who compensate for diminished diaphragm function by forcefully contracting their abdominal muscles to aid expiration.

Post-test care
None.

Interfering factors
Failure to remove all metal objects within the X-ray field may interfere with accurate test results.

Chest tomography

Tomography (also known as laminagraphy, planigraphy, stratigraphy, and body-section roentgenography) provides clearly focused radiographic images of selected body sections otherwise obscured by the shadow of overlying or underlying structures. In this procedure, the X-ray tube and film move around the patient (the linear tube sweep) in opposite directions, producing exposures in which a selected body plane appears sharply defined and the areas above and below it are blurred.

Because tomography emits high radiation levels, it's used only for further evaluation of chest lesions and has been replaced by computed tomography scanning.

Purpose
■ To demonstrate pulmonary densities (for cavitation, calcification, and presence of fat), tumors (especially those obstructing the bronchial lumen), and lesions (especially those located deep within the mediastinum, such as lymph nodes at the hilum).

Patient preparation
Describe the procedure to the patient, and explain that this test helps evaluate structures within the chest. Inform him that he needn't restrict food or fluids before the test. Tell him who will perform the test and where and that it takes 30 to 60 minutes.

Warn the patient that the equipment is noisy because of rapidly moving metal-on-metal parts and that the X-ray tube swings overhead. Advise him to breathe normally during the test but to remain immobile; tell him that foam wedges will be used to help him maintain a comfortable, motionless position. Suggest that he close his eyes to prevent involuntary movement. Instruct him to remove all metal objects, including jewelry, within the X-ray field.

Equipment
Tomograph.

Procedure
The patient is placed in the supine position or in different degrees of lateral rotation on the X-ray table. The X-ray tube then swings over the patient, taking numerous films from different angles.

For lung tomography, the X-ray tube is usually moved in a linear direction but may be moved in a hypocycloid, circular, elliptic, trispiral, or figure-eight pattern. Pluridirectional films aid diagnosis of mediastinal lesions and tumors.

Precautions
■ Tomography is contraindicated during pregnancy.
■ To avoid exposure to radiation, leave the room or the immediate area during the test; if you must stay in the area, wear a lead-lined apron.

Normal findings
In a normal chest tomogram, structures should appear as they would in a normal chest X-ray film.

Implications of results
Central calcification in a nodule suggests a benign lesion; an irregularly bordered tumor suggests cancer; a sharply

defined tumor suggests a granuloma or a benign lesion. Evaluation of the hilum can help differentiate blood vessels from nodes; identify bronchial dilation, stenosis, and endobronchial lesions; and detect tumor extension into the hilar lung area. Tomography can also identify extension of a mediastinal lesion to the ribs or spine.

Post-test care
None.

Interfering factors
■ Failure to remove all metal objects within the X-ray field may interfere with accurate test results.
■ The patient's inability to lie still may interfere with test results and require additional X-ray films, resulting in greater exposure to radiation.

Bronchography

Bronchography is X-ray examination of the tracheobronchial tree after instillation of a radiopaque iodine contrast agent through a catheter or bronchoscope into the tracheal and bronchial lumens. The contrast agent coats the bronchial tree, permitting visualization of anatomic deviations. Infrequently used since the development of computed tomography scanning, bronchography of a localized lung area may be accomplished by instilling contrast dye through a fiber-optic bronchoscope placed in the area to be filmed.

Purpose
■ To help detect bronchiectasis and map its location for surgical resection
■ To provide permanent films of pathologic findings.

Patient preparation
Explain to the patient that this test helps evaluate abnormalities of the bronchial structures. Instruct him to fast for 12 hours before the test and to perform good oral hygiene the night before and the morning of the test. Tell him who will perform the test and where and when it will be performed.

Make sure the patient or a responsible member of the family has signed the consent form. Check the patient's history for hypersensitivity to anesthetics, iodine, and contrast dyes. If the patient has a productive cough, administer an expectorant and perform postural drainage 1 to 3 days before the test, as ordered.

If the procedure is to be performed under a local anesthetic, tell the patient he'll receive a sedative to help him relax and to suppress the gag reflex. Prepare him for the unpleasant taste of the anesthetic spray. Warn him that he may experience some difficulty breathing during the procedure, but reassure him that his airway won't be blocked and that he'll receive enough oxygen. Tell him that the catheter or bronchoscope will pass more easily if he relaxes. Just before the test, instruct the patient to remove his dentures and to urinate.

If bronchography is to be performed under general anesthesia, inform the patient that he'll receive a sedative before the test to help him relax.

Equipment
X-ray machine ♦ tilting table ♦ sedative ♦ anesthetic ♦ catheter or bronchoscope ♦ radiopaque or water-soluble contrast agent ♦ emergency resuscitation equipment.

Procedure
After a local anesthetic is sprayed into the patient's mouth and throat, a bronchoscope or catheter is passed into the trachea, and the anesthetic and contrast

agent are instilled. The patient is placed in various positions during the test to promote movement of the contrast agent into different areas of the bronchial tree. After radiographs are taken, the dye is removed through postural drainage and having the patient cough it up.

Precautions

■ Bronchography is contraindicated during pregnancy, in people with hypersensitivity to iodine or contrast agents and, usually, in people with respiratory insufficiency.

 ■ Observe the patient with asthma for laryngeal spasm secondary to the instillation of the contrast agent.

■ Observe the patient with chronic obstructive pulmonary disease for airway occlusion secondary to the instillation of the contrast agent.

Normal findings

The right mainstem bronchus is shorter, wider, and more vertical than the left bronchus. Successive branches of the bronchi become smaller in diameter and are free of obstruction or lesions.

Implications of results

Bronchography may demonstrate bronchiectasis or bronchial obstruction due to tumors, cysts, cavities, or foreign objects. Findings must be correlated with the physical examination, the patient history, and perhaps other pulmonary studies.

Post-test care

■ Watch for signs of laryngeal spasms (dyspnea) or edema (hoarseness, dyspnea, laryngeal stridor) secondary to traumatic intubation.

■ Immediately report signs of an allergic reaction to the contrast agent or anesthetic, such as itching, dyspnea, tachy-

cardia, palpitations, excitation, hypotension or hypertension, and euphoria.

■ Withhold food, fluid, and oral medications until the gag reflex returns (usually within 2 hours). Fluid intake before the gag reflex returns may cause aspiration.

■ Encourage gentle coughing and postural drainage to facilitate clearing of the contrast agent. A postdrainage film is usually taken in 24 to 48 hours.

■ Watch for signs of chemical or secondary bacterial pneumonia — such as fever, dyspnea, crackles, or rhonchi — the result of incomplete expectoration of the contrast agent.

■ If the patient has a sore throat, reassure him that it's only temporary, and provide throat lozenges or a liquid gargle when his gag reflex returns.

■ Advise the outpatient to postpone resuming his usual activities until the next day.

Interfering factors

■ The presence of secretions or failure to position the patient properly may inhibit the contrast agent from adequately filling the bronchial tree.

■ Inability to suppress coughing will interfere with bronchiolar filling and retention of the contrast medium.

Pulmonary angiography

Pulmonary angiography (also known as pulmonary arteriography) is the radiographic examination of the pulmonary circulation after injection of a radiopaque contrast agent into the pulmonary artery or one of its branches. This procedure is usually used to confirm symptomatic pulmonary emboli when scans prove nondiagnostic (especially before anticoagulant therapy) or are contraindicated. It also provides accurate preoperative evaluation of patients with congenital heart disease.

Possible complications include arterial occlusion, myocardial perforation or rupture, ventricular arrhythmias from myocardial irritation, and acute renal failure from hypersensitivity to the contrast agent; bleeding, hematoma formation, or infection may occur at the catheter site.

Purpose

- To detect pulmonary embolism in a patient who is symptomatic but whose lung scan is equivocal
- To evaluate pulmonary circulation abnormalities
- To evaluate pulmonary circulation preoperatively in a patient with congenital heart disease
- To locate a large embolus before surgical removal.

Patient preparation

Describe the procedure to the patient, and explain that this test permits evaluation of the blood vessels to help identify the cause of his symptoms. Instruct him to fast for 8 hours before the test, or as ordered. Tell him who will perform the test and where and that it takes about $1\frac{1}{2}$ hours.

Tell the patient that a small puncture will be made in the blood vessel of his right arm, where blood samples are usually drawn, or in his right groin at the femoral vein and that a local anesthetic will be used to numb the area. Inform him that a small catheter will then be inserted into the blood vessel and passed into the right side of the heart to the pulmonary artery. Tell him that the contrast agent will then be injected into this artery to allow visualization of blood flow to the lungs. Warn him that he may have an urge to cough, feel flushed, or experience a salty taste for 3 to 5 min-

utes after the injection. Inform him that his heart rate will be monitored continuously during the procedure and that he should tell the doctor or nurse if he is having any concerns.

Make sure the patient, a responsible family member, or a person with medical power of attorney has signed the consent form. Check the patient history for hypersensitivity to anesthetics, iodine, seafood, radiographic contrast agents, or anticoagulants. Obtain or check laboratory tests (including prothrombin time, partial thromboplastin time, platelet count, and blood urea nitrogen [BUN] and serum creatinine levels), and notify the radiologist of any abnormal results. I.V. hydration may need to be considered, depending on the patient's renal and cardiac status. The radiologist may want to discontinue a heparin drip 3 to 4 hours before the test.

Equipment

Angiography tray ✦ 50 ml of contrast medium ✦ imaging equipment ✦ angiography catheters and guide wires ✦ monitoring equipment (electrocardiogram, arterial oxygen saturation, blood pressure, pulmonary artery pressure) ✦ emergency resuscitation equipment.

Procedure

After the patient is placed in a supine position, the local anesthetic is injected and the cardiac monitor is attached to the patient. A puncture is made at the procedure site, and a catheter is introduced into the antecubital or femoral vein. As the catheter passes through the right atrium, the right ventricle, and the pulmonary artery, pressures are measured and blood samples are drawn from various regions of the pulmonary circulation. The contrast agent is then injected and circulates through the pulmonary artery and lung capillaries while X-rays are taken.

Precautions

- Pulmonary angiography is contraindicated during pregnancy.
- Monitor for ventricular arrhythmias due to myocardial irritation from passage of the catheter through the heart chambers.
- Observe for signs and symptoms of hypersensitivity to the contrast agent, such as dyspnea, nausea, vomiting, sweating, increased heart rate, and numbness of extremities.
- Keep emergency equipment available in case of a hypersensitivity reaction to the contrast agent.
- Measure pulmonary artery pressures. Right ventricular end-diastolic pressure must be less than or equal to 20 mm Hg, and pulmonary artery systolic pressure less than or equal to 70 mm Hg. Pressures greater than this increase the risk of mortality associated with this procedure.

Normal findings

The contrast agent should flow symmetrically and without interruption through the pulmonary circulatory system.

Implications of results

Interruption of blood flow may result from emboli, vascular filling defects, or stenosis.

Post-test care

- Maintain bed rest for about 6 hours.
- Observe the site for bleeding and swelling. If they occur, maintain pressure at the insertion site for 10 minutes and notify the radiologist.
- Check blood pressure, pulse rate, and the procedure site (arm or groin) every 15 minutes for 1 hour, then every hour for 4 hours, then every 4 hours for 16 hours.
- Observe for signs of myocardial perforation or rupture by monitoring vital signs, as ordered.
- Be alert for signs of acute renal failure, such as sudden onset of oliguria, nausea, and vomiting. Check BUN and serum creatinine levels.
- Report symptoms of a delayed hypersensitivity reaction to the contrast agent or local anesthetic (dyspnea, itching, tachycardia, palpitations, hypotension or hypertension, excitation, and euphoria).
- Advise the patient of any activity restrictions, and tell him he may resume his usual diet.
- Encourage the patient to drink fluids, or give him I.V. fluids to help flush the contrast agent from his body.

Interfering factors

None.

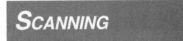

Lung perfusion scan

A lung perfusion scan produces a visual image of pulmonary blood flow after I.V. injection of a radiopharmaceutical — human serum albumin microspheres (particles) or macroaggregated albumin, both of which are bonded to technetium. This test is useful for confirming pulmonary vascular obstruction, such as pulmonary emboli. When performed in addition to a lung ventilation scan, this scan assesses ventilation-perfusion ratios.

Purpose

- To assess arterial perfusion of the lungs
- To detect pulmonary emboli
- To evaluate pulmonary function before lung resection.

Patient preparation

Explain to the patient that this test helps evaluate respiratory function. Inform him that he needn't restrict food or fluids before the test. Tell him who will perform the test and where and that it takes about 30 minutes.

Inform the patient that the radiopharmaceutical will be injected into a vein in his arm and that the amount of radioactivity is minimal. Tell him that he'll either sit in front of the camera or lie under it and that neither the camera nor the uptake probe emits radiation. Assure him that he'll be comfortable during the test and that he doesn't have to remain perfectly still.

On the test request, note such conditions as chronic obstructive pulmonary disease (COPD), vasculitis, pulmonary edema, tumor, sickle cell disease, and parasitic disease.

Equipment

Scintiscanner ✦ radiopharmaceutical.

Procedure

With the patient supine and taking moderately deep breaths, the radiopharmaceutical is injected slowly over 5 to 10 seconds to allow more even distribution of pulmonary blood flow. After the uptake of the radiopharmaceutical, the gamma camera takes a series of single stationary images in the anterior, posterior, oblique, and both lateral chest views. Images projected on an oscilloscope screen show the distribution of radioactive particles.

Precautions

A lung scan is contraindicated in patients who are hypersensitive to the radiopharmaceutical.

Normal findings

Hot spots — areas of high uptake of the radioactive substance — indicate normal blood perfusion; a normal lung shows a uniform uptake pattern.

Implications of results

Cold spots — areas of low radioactive uptake — indicate poor perfusion, suggesting an embolism; however, a ventilation scan is necessary to confirm the diagnosis. Decreased regional blood flow that occurs without vessel obstruction may indicate pneumonitis.

Post-test care

If a hematoma develops at the injection site, apply warm soaks.

Interfering factors

▪ Scheduling the patient for more than one radionuclide test a day (especially if different trace substances are used) can inhibit adequate diffusion of the radioactive substance in the second test.
▪ I.V. injection of the radiopharmaceutical while the patient is sitting can produce abnormal images because a large proportion of the particles settle to the lung bases.
▪ Conditions such as COPD, vasculitis, pulmonary edema, tumor, sickle cell disease, and parasitic disease may cause abnormal perfusion, affecting the accuracy of test results.

Lung ventilation scan

A lung ventilation scan — a nuclear scan performed after inhalation of air mixed with radioactive gas — delineates areas of the lung ventilated during respiration. The scan consists of recording the distribution of the gas during three phases: during the buildup of radioactive gas (wash-in phase), after the patient rebreathes from a bag and the radioactivity reaches a steady level

Comparing normal and abnormal ventilation scans

The normal ventilation scan on the left, taken 30 minutes to 1 hour after the wash-out phase, shows equal gas distribution. The abnormal scan on the right, taken 1½ to 2 hours after the start of the wash-out phase, shows unequal gas distribution represented by the area of poor wash-out on both the left and right sides.

Normal scan　　　　　　　　　**Abnormal scan**

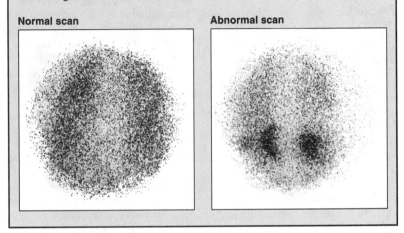

(equilibrium phase), and after removal of the radioactive gas from the lungs (wash-out phase). (See *Comparing normal and abnormal ventilation scans*.) In a patient on mechanical ventilation, krypton gas must be substituted for xenon gas during the test.

Performed in combination with a lung perfusion scan, a lung ventilation scan helps distinguish between parenchymal disease, such as emphysema, sarcoidosis, bronchogenic carcinoma, and tuberculosis, and conditions caused by vascular abnormalities, such as pulmonary emboli.

Purpose

- To help diagnose pulmonary emboli
- To identify areas of the lung that are capable of ventilation
- To help evaluate regional respiratory function before lung resection
- To locate regional hypoventilation, which may indicate atelectasis, obstruct-

ing tumors, or chronic obstructive pulmonary disease.

Patient preparation

Describe the procedure to the patient, and explain that this test helps evaluate respiratory function. Inform him that he needn't restrict food or fluids. Tell him who will perform the test and where and that it takes 15 to 30 minutes.

Instruct the patient to remove all metal objects in the scanning field. Tell him that he'll be asked to hold his breath for a short time after inhaling gas and to remain still while a machine scans his chest. Reassure him that the amount of radioactive gas used in minimized.

Equipment

Breathing mask that fits tightly over the nose and mouth ✦ radioactive gas (xenon 133 or krypton 85) ✦ nuclear scanner.

Procedure

After the patient inhales air mixed with a small amount of radioactive gas through a mask, its distribution in the lungs is monitored on a nuclear scanner. The patient's chest is scanned as the gas is exhaled.

Precautions

 Watch for leaks in the closed system of radioactive gas, such as through the mask. Such leaks can contaminate the surrounding atmosphere.

Normal findings

Gas should be equally distributed in both lungs, and wash-in and wash-out phases should be normal.

Implications of results

Unequal gas distribution in both lungs indicates poor ventilation or airway obstruction in areas with low radioactivity. When compared with a lung perfusion scan, in vascular obstructions such as pulmonary embolism, perfusion to the embolized area is decreased, but ventilation to this area is maintained; in parenchymal diseases such as pneumonia, both ventilation and perfusion are abnormal within the areas of consolidation.

Post-test care

None.

Interfering factors

Failure to remove jewelry and other metal objects in the scanning field during scanning may interfere with accurate test results.

Thoracic computed tomography

Thoracic computed tomography (CT) scanning provides cross-sectional views of the chest by passing an X-ray beam from a computerized scanner through the body at different levels. CT scanning may be done with or without an injected radioiodine contrast agent, which is used primarily to highlight blood vessels and to allow greater visual discrimination.

This test provides a three-dimensional image and is especially useful in detecting small differences in tissue density. Thoracic CT scanning is one of the most accurate and informative diagnostic tests and may replace mediastinoscopy in diagnosis of mediastinal masses and Hodgkin's disease; its clinical application in the evaluation of pulmonary pathology has been proven.

Purpose

- To locate suspected neoplasms (for example, in Hodgkin's disease), especially with mediastinal involvement
- To differentiate coin-sized calcified lesions (indicating tuberculosis) from tumors
- To differentiate empyema or bronchopleural fistula from lung abscess
- To distinguish tumors adjacent to the aorta from aortic aneurysms
- To detect the invasion of a neck mass in the thorax
- To evaluate a primary malignant tumor that may metastasize to the lungs, especially in patients with primary bone tumors, soft-tissue sarcomas, or melanomas
- To evaluate the mediastinal lymph nodes
- To evaluate an aortic aneurysm

- To detect a dissection or leak of an aortic or aortic arch aneurysm
- To plan radiation treatment.

Patient preparation

Explain to the patient that this test provides cross-sectional views of the chest and distinguishes small differences in tissue density. If a contrast agent won't be used, inform him that he needn't restrict food or fluids. If the test will be performed with contrast enhancement, instruct him to fast for 4 hours before the test. Tell him who will perform the test and where, that the procedure usually takes 1 hour, and that it won't cause him discomfort.

Tell the patient that he'll be lying on his back with his arms above his head on an X-ray table that moves into the center of a large, ring-shaped piece of X-ray equipment and that the equipment may be noisy. Inform him that if a radiographic contrast agent is injected into a vein in his arm, he may experience warmth, flushing of the face, and a salty taste. Reassure him that the amount of radiation exposure is minimal. Tell him not to move during the test but to breathe as instructed (usually holding his breath for each image). Instruct him to remove all jewelry and metal in the X-ray field.

Check the patient history for hypersensitivity to iodine or radiographic contrast agents. Start an I.V. saline lock if the patient is to receive a contrast medium.

Equipment

CT scanner ✦ contrast agent for injection, if ordered.

Procedure

After the patient is placed in a supine position on the X-ray table and while the contrast agent is being injected, the machine scans the patient at different levels while the computer calculates small differences in the densities of various tissues, water, fat, bone, and air. This information is displayed as a printout of numerical values and as a projection on an oscilloscope screen. Images may be recorded for further study.

Precautions

 Thoracic CT scanning is contraindicated during pregnancy and, if a contrast agent is used, in people with a history of hypersensitivity reactions to iodine, shellfish, or radiographic contrast agents.

Normal findings

Black and white areas on a thoracic CT scan refer, respectively, to air and bone densities. Shades of gray correspond to fluid, fat, and soft-tissue densities. (See *Comparing normal and abnormal thoracic CT scans,* page 678.)

Implications of results

Abnormal thoracic CT scan findings include tumors, nodules, cysts, aortic aneurysm, enlarged lymph nodes, pleural effusion, and accumulations of blood, fluid, or fat.

Post-test care

Watch for signs of delayed hypersensitivity to the contrast agent, including itching, hypotension or hypertension, and respiratory distress. Encourage fluid intake if a contrast agent was used.

Interfering factors

- Failure to remove all metal objects from the scanning field may interfere with an accurate diagnosis.
- The patient's inability to lie still during scanning may interfere with accurate diagnosis and may require repetition of the test, which increases his exposure to radiation.
- Obese patients may exceed the weight limit of the scanning table.

Comparing normal and abnormal thoracic CT scans

In the abnormal thoracic computed tomography (CT) scan (top), note atelectasis in the right middle lobe and cancer in the right hilum. The normal scan (bottom) shows no such deviations.

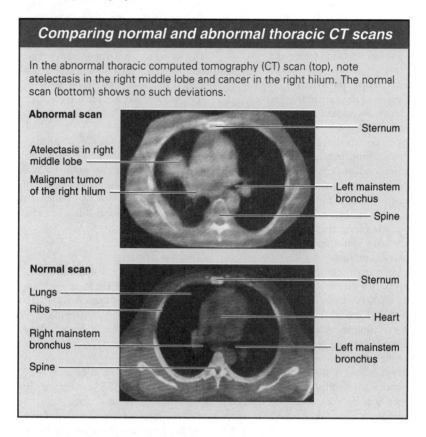

Abnormal scan

Atelectasis in right middle lobe

Malignant tumor of the right hilum

Sternum

Left mainstem bronchus

Spine

Normal scan

Lungs

Ribs

Right mainstem bronchus

Spine

Sternum

Heart

Left mainstem bronchus

Selected Readings

Black, J.M., and Matassarin-Jacobs, E., eds. *Luckmann and Sorensen's Medical-Surgical Nursing: A Psychophysiologic Approach,* 4th ed. Philadelphia: W.B. Saunders Co., 1993.

Diseases, 2nd ed. Springhouse, Pa.: Springhouse Corp., 1996.

Fischbach, F. *A Manual of Laboratory and Diagnostic Tests,* 5th ed. Philadelphia: Lippincott-Raven Pubs., 1996.

George, R.B., et al. *Chest Medicine: Essentials of Pulmonary and Critical Care Medicine,* 3rd ed. Baltimore: Williams & Wilkins Co., 1995.

Henry, J.B., ed. *Clinical Diagnosis and Management by Laboratory Methods,* 19th ed. Philadelphia: W.B. Saunders Co., 1996.

Isselbacher, K.J., et al., eds. *Harrison's Principles of Internal Medicine,* 13th ed. New York: McGraw-Hill Book Co., 1994.

Nursing97 Drug Handbook. Springhouse, Pa.: Springhouse Corp., 1997.

Phipps, W.J., et al. *Medical-Surgical Nursing: Concepts and Clinical Practice,* 5th ed. St. Louis: Mosby–Year Book, Inc., 1995.

Scanlan, C.L., et al. *Egan's Fundamentals of Respiratory Care,* 6th ed. St. Louis: Mosby–Year Book, Inc., 1995.

Tilkian, S.M., et al. *Clinical and Nursing Implications of Laboratory Tests,* 5th ed. St. Louis: Mosby–Year Book, Inc., 1995.

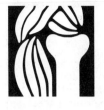

CHAPTER TWENTY-FOUR

Skeletal system

Learning objectives

After completing this chapter, the reader will be able to:
- explain the anatomy and physiology of the skeletal system
- describe the procedure for evaluating skeletal disorders
- identify the types of tests used to evaluate the skeletal system
- state the purpose of each test discussed in the chapter
- prepare the patient physically and psychologically for each test
- describe the procedure for performing each test

- specify appropriate precautions for safe administration of each test
- recognize signs of an adverse reaction and respond appropriately
- implement appropriate post-test care
- provide appropriate patient teaching
- identify the normal findings of each test
- discuss the implications of abnormal test results
- list factors that may interfere with accurate test results.

INTRODUCTION

Diagnostic tests of the skeletal system help evaluate bones and their inner structures as well as the joints and lubricating fluids within them. These tests include a wide range of radiographic, nuclear medicine, and endoscopic techniques as well as joint aspiration, computed tomography scans, and magnetic resonance imaging.

Several skeletal tests combine diagnosis and treatment. For example, arthroscopy permits direct visualization of a joint as well as removal of loose bodies within the joint, meniscectomy, meniscal repair, abrasion arthroplasty, and release of the vastus lateralis muscle. Arthrocentesis provides a fluid sample for laboratory analysis as well as an avenue for local drug therapy.

Structure of bone

Bones are complex structures composed of living cells and nonliving intercellular substance. The intercellular matrix consists of inorganic salts — mostly calcium and phosphate — embedded in collagen fibers. All bones have some basic structures in common. They are covered by the periosteum — a dense layer of connective tissue that contains osteoblasts, blood vessels, nerves, and lymphatics — and have an inner generative membrane called the marrow (medullary) cavity.

Histologically, bone is of two basic types. *Cancellous (spongy) bone* contains many open spaces between thin strands of bone called *trabeculae,* which are oriented along lines of stress or pressure and give the bone extra structural strength. *Compact bone* is strong and dense with many networks of interconnecting canals, each of which is known as a *haversian system.* A haversian canal runs centrally through each system, parallel to the bone's long axis, and contains one or two blood vessels that provide much of the bone's blood supply. The haversian canals are surrounded by concentric cylindrical layers called *lamellae,* which are closely spaced in compact bone. Small cavities called *lacunae* appear between the lamellae; each lacuna contains *osteocytes,* mature bone-forming cells that are suspended in tissue fluid. The lacunae are joined by a network of tiny canals called *canaliculi,* each of which contains one or more capillaries and provides an additional route for tissue fluids.

Red marrow, which produces blood cells, occupies the spaces in cancellous bone. In adults, red marrow appears mainly in the spongy part of cranial bones, in the ribs and sternum, in the vertebrae, and in portions of the femur, humerus, and other long bones. In neonates and children, it appears in many other bones. *Yellow marrow* is present in the shafts of long bones and extends into the haversian system. It is composed of adipose cells and can change to red marrow, if necessary.

Types of bone
Bones are classified by shape.

■ *Long bones* are found in the extremities and consist of a shaft *(diaphysis)* and two bulbous ends *(epiphyses).* The parts of the shaft that flare to join the epiphyses are called *metaphyses;* these contain the bone's growth zones and become continuous with the epiphyses at maturity. Long bones are composed primarily of compact bone and include the humerus, radius, ulna, femur, tibia, fibula, phalanges, and metatarsals.

■ *Short bones* consist mainly of cancellous bone with a thin compact bone shell and include the tarsal and carpal bones.

■ *Flat bones* have a large surface area and provide protection for soft body parts. They have an inner layer of cancellous bone that is surrounded by compact bone. Examples of flat bones are the frontal and parietal bones of the cranium and the ribs, sternum, scapulae, ilium, and pubis.

■ *Irregular bones* are of various shapes and composition and include the spine (vertebrae, sacrum, coccyx) and certain skull bones (sphenoid, ethmoid, and mandible).

Bones not classified by shape include the sesamoid (free-floating) bones — such as the patella — and the wormian bones, small clusters of bones found between some cranial bones.

All bones are covered with a fibrous layer called the *periosteum* — except at joints, where they're covered by articular cartilage.

Types of joints
Joints consist of two bones joined in various ways; like bones, they have varying forms.

■ *Fibrous joints* (synarthroses) have only minute motion and provide stability when tight union is necessary, as in the sutures joining the cranial bones.

■ *Cartilaginous joints* (amphiarthroses) allow limited movement, as between vertebrae.

■ *Synovial joints* (diarthroses), the most common type, allow angular and circular movement. To achieve freedom of movement, synovial joints have special characteristics: The bones' two articulating surfaces have a smooth hyaline covering (articular cartilage) that is resilient to pressure; their opposing surfaces are congruous and glide smoothly on each other; a fibrous capsule holds them together. Lining the joint cavity is the *synovial membrane,* which secretes a clear viscous fluid called synovial fluid. This fluid lubricates the two opposing surfaces during motion and nourishes the articular cartilage. Surrounding each synovial joint are ligaments, muscles, and tendons, which strengthen and stabilize the joint but allow free movement.

In some synovial joints, the synovial membrane forms two additional structures — bursae and tendon sheaths — which reduce friction. *Bursae are* small

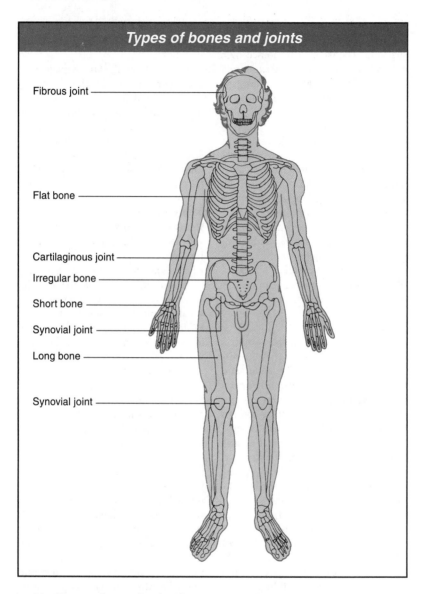

Types of bones and joints

Fibrous joint

Flat bone

Cartilaginous joint

Irregular bone

Short bone

Synovial joint

Long bone

Synovial joint

cushionlike sacs that are lined with synovial membranes and filled with synovial fluid; most are located between tendons and bones, as in the shoulders, knees, and elbows, but others are found between muscles and bones, ligaments and bones, and skin and bones. *Tendon sheaths* are modified bursae that wrap around a tendon to cushion it as it stretches across a joint. (See *Types of bones and joints.*)

Evaluating skeletal disorders

When a patient's chief complaint involves the skeletal system, be sure to obtain an accurate medical and personal history. Ask the patient about general activities that may be affected by skeletal disease or trauma, such as his job, diet, recreation, sexual activity, and elimination habits. Does he have difficulty getting around or performing normal daily activities?

Ask the patient to describe his symptoms. When did they begin? Have they lessened or worsened? Has he previously sought treatment for the problem? If so, what was the result? Did he comply with the prescribed treatment? Ask if he's in pain at the moment. Has he been able to get relief from the pain? Does he require medication? If so, what kind and how much does he take?

Because joint or bone pain symptoms may indicate a systemic disease, a complete physical examination is essential. Observe the patient's general appearance; check for localized edema, reddening of pressure points, point tenderness, and other deformities. Check the joint's range of motion, which may be restricted or painful. Palpate swollen joints to determine the nature of the swelling, which may result from synovial thickening, bone enlargement, or simple fluid effusion.

Pain thought to originate in a major joint may actually come from a minor one. Check the patient's neurovascular status, including motion, sensation, and circulation. Measure and record dissimilarities in muscle circumference or limb length. Compare the size and shape of the affected joint with those of its unaffected opposite.

Diagnostic tests

Radiography is probably the most widely used skeletal test. Because osseous tissue is quite dense, radiography readily demonstrates the skeletal system. A plain X-ray film doesn't require special patient preparation or restrictions but does require patient cooperation in assuming various positions during the procedure. X-rays are usually taken with the patient in the anteroposterior, lateral, or oblique position or in a combination of these. Although the basic views provide valuable diagnostic information, radiography doesn't allow visualization of certain areas.

Bone scan is the examination of bone after I.V. injection of radioisotopes, which have an affinity for bone. Bone scans permit detection of primary and metastatic tumors 3 to 6 months earlier than X-ray films alone, and they help detect infection and trauma.

Arthrography is the radiographic examination of a joint after injection of air, a radiopaque dye, or both into the joint space. By outlining soft-tissue structures and the contours of the joint, it can detect a torn meniscus or the presence of loose bodies, capsular leaks, and other joint abnormalities.

Arthrocentesis is the aspiration of synovial fluid from a joint space (usually the knee) for diagnosis or to relieve pain caused by fluid accumulation.

Arthroscopy, the direct visualization of joint structures (usually the knee) using a fiber-optic endoscope, is particularly useful for detecting knee disorders (such as arthritis, a torn meniscus, cysts, and loose bodies) that aren't readily revealed by radiography or arthrography.

Computed tomography scanning provides cross-sectional images that can show in detail successive layers or a specific plane of involved bone. It identifies the location and extent of fractures in difficult-to-define areas (sometimes using contrast media).

Magnetic resonance imaging, a noninvasive imaging technique, uses magnetic fields, radio waves, and computers to show skeletal and soft-tissue abnormalities.

For a discussion of bone and synovial membrane biopsies commonly performed on patients with skeletal disorders, see Chapter 18.

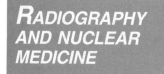

Vertebral radiography

Vertebral radiography visualizes all or part of the vertebral column. A commonly performed test, it's used to evaluate the vertebrae for deformities, fractures, dislocations, tumors, and other abnormalities. Bone films determine bone density, texture, erosion, and changes in bone relationships. X-rays of the cortex of the bone reveal the presence of any widening or narrowing as well as signs of irregularity. Joint X-rays can reveal the presence of fluid, spur formation, narrowing, and changes in joint structure.

In neonates, the vertebral column normally consists of 33 interlocked vertebrae, most of which are separate and movable. Anatomically, the vertebral column is divided in descending order into five segments: cervical, thoracic, lumbar, sacral, and coccygeal. The cervical segment, the most flexible part, includes the 7 vertebrae that form the bony framework of the neck. The thoracic segment, with 12 vertebrae, lies behind the thorax and supports the 12 pairs of ribs. The lumbar segment, with 5 vertebrae, supports the small of the back. The sacral segment, originally 5 separate vertebrae, fuses into a single bone by adulthood. The coccygeal segment begins as 4 or 5 small vertebrae and eventually fuses to form the coccyx. The fusion of the vertebrae in these last two segments reduces the number of vertebrae from 33 at birth to 26 in the adult spine.

All vertebrae are similar in structure but vary in size, shape, and articular surface, according to location. Fibrocar-

tilaginous intervertebral disks allow some movement between the individual vertebrae.

The type and extent of vertebral radiography depend on the patient's condition. For example, a patient with lower back pain requires only study of the lumbar and sacral segments.

Purpose
- To detect vertebral fractures, dislocations, subluxations, and deformities
- To detect vertebral degeneration, infection, and congenital disorders (such as scoliosis)
- To detect disorders of the intervertebral disks
- To determine the vertebral effects of arthritic and metabolic disorders.

Patient preparation
Explain to the patient that this test examines the spine. Inform him that he needn't restrict food or fluids. Tell him that the test requires X-ray films, who will perform the test and where, and that the procedure usually takes 15 to 30 minutes. Advise him that he'll be placed in various positions for the X-ray films and that although some positions may cause slight discomfort, his cooperation ensures accurate results. Stress that he must keep still and hold his breath for film exposure during the procedure.

Procedure
The procedure varies considerably, depending on which vertebral segment is being examined. Initially, the patient is placed in a supine position on the X-ray table for an anteroposterior view. He may be repositioned for lateral or right and left oblique views; specific positioning depends on the vertebral segment or adjacent structures of interest. For example, to obtain a lateral view of C7 (and possibly T1 and T2), the patient's shoulders should be depressed or pulled down and rotated.

Precautions

■ Vertebral radiography is contraindicated during the first trimester of pregnancy unless the benefits outweigh the risk of fetal radiation exposure.

 ■ Exercise extreme caution when handling trauma patients with suspected spinal injuries, particularly of the cervical area. Such patients should be filmed while on the stretcher to avoid further injury during transfer to the X-ray table.

Normal findings

Vertebrae should show no fractures, subluxations, dislocations, curvatures, or other abnormalities. Specific positions and spacing of the vertebrae vary with the patient's age. In the lateral view, adult vertebrae are aligned to form four alternately concave and convex curves. The cervical and lumbar curves are convex anteriorly; the thoracic and sacral curves are concave anteriorly. Although the structure of the coccyx varies, it usually points forward and downward. Neonatal vertebrae form only one curve, which is concave anteriorly.

Implications of results

Vertebral radiography readily shows spondylolisthesis, fractures, subluxations, dislocations, wedging, and such deformities as kyphosis, scoliosis, and lordosis. To confirm other disorders, spinal structures and their spatial relationships on the X-ray must be examined and the patient's history and clinical status must be considered. These disorders include congenital abnormalities, such as torticollis (wry-neck), absence of sacral or lumbar vertebrae, hemivertebrae, and Klippel-Feil syndrome; degenerative processes, such as hypertrophic spurs, osteoarthritis, and narrowed disk spaces; tuberculosis (Pott's disease); benign or malignant intraspinal tumors; ruptured disks and cervical disk syndrome; and systemic disorders, such as rheumatoid arthritis, Charcot's disease, ankylosing spondylitis, osteoporosis, and Paget's disease.

Depending on the results of radiography, a definitive diagnosis may also require additional tests, such as myelography and computed tomography.

Post-test care

None.

Interfering factors

Improper positioning of the patient or movement during radiography may produce inaccurate films.

Arthrography

Arthrography is the radiographic examination of a joint after the injection of a radiopaque dye, air, or both (double-contrast arthrography) to outline soft-tissue structures and the contour of the joint. In this procedure, the joint is put through its range of motion while a series of radiographs are taken. Arthrography is useful for identifying acute or chronic tears of the joint capsule or supporting ligaments of the knee, shoulder, ankle, hips, or wrist. It can also visualize internal joint derangements and synovial cysts. However, magnetic resonance imaging (MRI) is currently the imaging method of choice for demonstrating joint abnormalities.

Indications for arthrography include persistent unexplained joint discomfort or pain. Complications may include persistent joint crepitus, allergic reactions to the contrast medium, and infection.

Purpose

- To identify acute or chronic abnormalities of the joint capsule or supporting ligaments of the knee, shoulder, ankle, hips, or wrist
- To detect internal joint derangements
- To locate synovial cysts.

Patient preparation

Describe the procedure to the patient, and answer any questions he may have. Explain that this test permits examination of a joint. Inform him that he needn't restrict food or fluids. Tell him who will perform the procedure and where. Explain that the fluoroscope allows the doctor to track the contrast medium as it fills the joint space. Inform him that standard X-ray films will also be taken after diffusion of the contrast medium.

Tell the patient that although the joint area will be anesthetized, he may experience a tingling sensation or pressure in the joint when the contrast medium is injected. Instruct him to remain as still as possible during the procedure, except when following instructions to change position. Stress the importance of his cooperation in assuming various positions because films must be taken as quickly as possible to ensure optimum quality.

Check the patient's history for hypersensitivity to local anesthetics, iodine, and the contrast media used for other diagnostic tests.

Equipment

Fluoroscope ✦ skin cleansing solution ✦ local anesthetic ✦ two 2" 20G needles ✦ two 24G needles ✦ three 3-ml syringes ✦ short lumbar puncture needle (3" 22G for arthrography of the shoulder) ✦ water-soluble radiopaque dye (5 to 15 ml), to be used alone or with air ✦ four sterile sponges ✦ elastic knee bandage ✦ sterile towels ✦ sterile specimen container for fluid ✦ culture tube ✦ sterile adhesive bandage ✦ collodion (optional) ✦ shave preparation kit.

Procedure

For knee arthrography: The knee is cleaned with an antiseptic solution, and the area around the puncture site anesthetized. (It's not usually necessary to anesthetize the joint space itself.) A 2" needle is then inserted into the joint space between the patella and the femoral condyle, and fluid is aspirated. While the needle is still in place, the aspirating syringe is removed and replaced with one containing the contrast medium. If fluoroscopic examination demonstrates correct placement of the needle, the contrast medium is injected into the joint space. The aspirated fluid is usually sent to the laboratory for analysis. (See "Synovial fluid analysis" in this chapter.)

After the needle is removed, the site is rubbed with a sterile sponge to prevent air form escaping, and the wound may be sealed with collodion. The patient is asked to walk a few steps or to move his knee through a range of motion, as directed, to distribute the contrast medium in the joint space. A film series is taken quickly — before the contrast medium can be absorbed by the joint tissue — with the knee held in various positions. If the films are clean and demonstrate proper dye placement, the knee is bandaged.

For shoulder arthrography: The skin is prepared, and a local anesthetic is injected subcutaneously, just in front of the acromioclavicular joint. Additional anesthetic is injected directly onto the head of the humerus. The short lumbar puncture needle is then inserted until the point is embedded in the joint cartilage. The stylet is removed, a syringe of contrast medium attached and, using fluoroscopic guidance, about 1 ml of the contrast medium is injected into the joint space as the needle is with-

Comparing normal and abnormal arthrograms

The arthrogram on the left shows a normal medial meniscus. The view on the right shows a torn medial meniscus (indicated by the arrow).

Normal arthrogram of knee

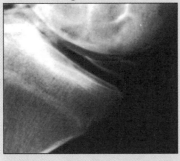

Abnormal arthrogram of knee

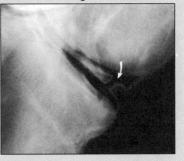

The arthrogram on the left shows a normal shoulder. The arthrogram on the right shows a shoulder with a ruptured rotator cuff. Contrast medium has collected in the subacromial bursa (indicated by the arrows).

Normal arthrogram of shoulder

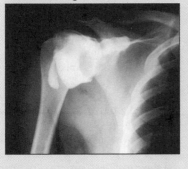

Abnormal arthrogram of shoulder

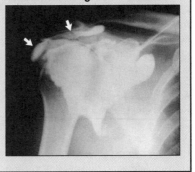

drawn sightly. If fluoroscopic examination demonstrates correct needle placement, the remainder of the contrast medium is injected while the needle is slowly withdrawn, and the site is wiped with a sterile sponge. A film series is then taken quickly to achieve maximum contrast.

Precautions

This procedure is contraindicated during pregnancy or in patients with active arthritis, joint infection, or previous sensitivity to radiopaque media.

Normal findings

A normal knee arthrogram shows a characteristic wedge-shaped shadow pointed toward the interior of the joint, which indicates a normal medial meniscus. A normal shoulder arthrogram shows the bicipital tendon sheath, redundant inferior joint capsule, and subscapular bursa intact. (See *Comparing normal and abnormal arthrograms.*)

Implications of results

Arthrography accurately detects medial meniscal tears and lacerations in 90%

to 95% of cases. Because the entire joint lining is opacified, arthrography can demonstrate extrameniscal lesions, such as osteochondritis dissecans, chondromalacia patellae, osteochondral fractures, cartilaginous abnormalities, synovial abnormalities, tears of the cruciate ligaments, and disruption of the joint capsule and collateral ligaments.

Arthrography can reveal shoulder abnormalities, such as adhesive capsulitis, bicipital tenosynovitis or rupture, and rotator cuff tears. It can also evaluate damage from recurrent dislocations.

Post-test care
■ Tell the patient to rest the joint for 6 to 12 hours. If knee arthrography was performed, wrap the knee in an elastic bandage, if ordered. Tell the patient to keep the bandage in place for several days, and teach him how to rewrap it.
■ Inform the patient that he may experience some swelling or discomfort and hear crepitant noises in the joint after the test but that these symptoms usually disappear after 1 to 2 days; tell him to contact the doctor if symptoms persist. Advise him to apply ice to the joint for swelling and to take a mild analgesic for pain.

Interfering factors
■ Incomplete aspiration of joint effusion dilutes the contrast medium, diminishing the quality of the film.
■ Improper injection technique may cause misplacement of the contrast medium.

Bone scan

A bone scan permits imaging of the skeleton by a scanning camera after I.V. injection of a radioactive tracer compound. The tracer of choice, radioactive technetium diphosphonate, collects in bone tissue in increased concentrations at sites of abnormal metabolism. When scanned, these sites appear as hot spots that are often detectable months before radiography can reveal a lesion.

This test is primarily indicated in patients with symptoms of metastatic bone disease, with bone trauma, or with a known degenerative disorder that requires monitoring for signs of progression. It may be performed with a gallium scan to promote early detection of lesions.

Purpose
■ To detect or rule out malignant bone lesions when radiographic findings are normal but cancer is confirmed or suspected
■ To detect occult bone trauma due to pathologic fractures
■ To monitor degenerative bone disorders
■ To detect infection
■ To evaluate unexplained bone pain
■ To stage cancer.

Patient preparation
Describe the procedure to the patient, and answer any questions he may have. Explain that this test often detects skeletal abnormalities sooner than ordinary X-rays can. In the interval between injection of the tracer and the actual scanning (about 1 to 3 hours), advise the patient to drink lots of fluids to maintain hydration and to reduce the radiation dose to the bladder.

Tell him who will perform the test and where and that he must keep still for the scan. Assure him that the scan itself, which takes about 1 hour, is painless and that the isotope, although radioactive, emits less radiation than a standard X-ray machine.

If a bone scan is ordered to diagnose cancer, evaluate the patient's emotional

Comparing normal and abnormal bone scans

The bone scan of the thorax on the left is normal. The isotope technetium diphosphonate is distributed evenly throughout the skeletal tissue; darker areas indicate the density of bone masses, as in the vertebrae. The scan on the right reveals isotope accumulation in multiple metastases in the ribs and spine.

Normal bone scan

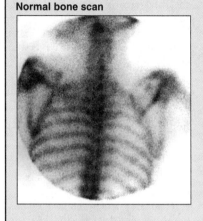

Abnormal bone scan

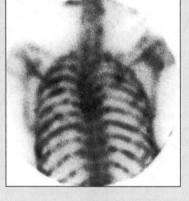

state and offer support, as needed. Administer an analgesic, as ordered.

Equipment

Bone mineral tracer ✦ 3-ml syringe ✦ 21G needle ✦ 70% alcohol or povidone-iodine solution ✦ sterile sponge ✦ tourniquet ✦ scanning camera.

Procedure

After the patient receives an I.V. injection of the tracer and imaging agent, encourage him to increase his intake of fluids for the next 1 to 3 hours to facilitate renal clearance of the circulating free tracer (not being picked up by the bone). Instruct him to urinate immediately before the procedure. (If he can't urinate, a urinary catheter may be inserted to empty the bladder.) Then position him on the scanner table.

As the scanner head moves over the patient's body, it detects low-level radiation emitted by the skeleton and translates this into a film or paper chart, or both, to produce two-dimensional pictures of the area scanned. The scanner takes as many views as needed to cover the specified area; the patient may have to be repositioned several times during the test to obtain adequate views. Children who can't hold still for the scan may need to be sedated.

Precautions

▪ To avoid exposing a fetus or an infant to radiation, a bone scan is contraindicated during pregnancy or lactation.
▪ Allergic reactions to the radionuclide may occur but are rare.

Normal findings

The tracer concentrates on bone tissue at sites of new bone formation or increased metabolism. The epiphyses of growing bone are normal sites of high concentration (hot spots). (See *Comparing normal and abnormal bone scans*.)

Implications of results

Although a bone scan demonstrates hot spots that identify sites of bone formation, it doesn't distinguish between normal and abnormal bone formation. But scan results can identify all types of bone cancer, infection, fracture, and other disorders if viewed in light of the patient's medical and surgical history, radiographic findings, and laboratory test results.

Post-test care

Check the injection site for redness and swelling. Don't schedule any other radionuclide test for 24 to 48 hours. Instruct the patient to drink lots of fluids and to empty his bladder frequently for 24 to 48 hours. Provide analgesics for pain resulting from positioning on the scanning table, as needed.

Interfering factors

▪ A distended bladder may obscure pelvic detail.
▪ Improper injection technique allows the tracer to seep into muscle tissue, producing erroneous hot spots.
▪ Antihypertensives may affect test results.

Bone densitometry

Bone densitometry assesses bone mass quantitatively. This noninvasive technique, also known as dual energy X-ray absorptiometry (DEXA), uses an X-ray tube to measure bone mineral density and exposes the patient to only minimal radiation. The images detected are analyzed by computer to determine bone mineral status. The computer calculates the size and thickness of the bone as well as its volumetric density to determine its potential resistance to mechanical stress.

This test can scan the lumbar spine and the proximal femur, two sites at high risk for fractures. It's precise enough to scan three lumbar vertebrae and the introchanteric area of the hip. Scanning the distal forearm is also useful because research has shown a high correlation between bone mineral density of this area of the forearm and the bone mineral density of the spine and femur.

Bone densitometry may be done in the radiology department of a hospital, a doctor's office, or a clinic. It's usually performed by a technician or a nurse.

Purpose

▪ To determine bone mineral density
▪ To identify people at risk for osteoporosis
▪ To evaluate a patient's clinical response to therapy aimed at reducing the rate of bone loss.

Patient preparation

Reassure the patient that the test is painless and that exposure to radiation is minimal. Tell him that it will take from 10 minutes to 1 hour, depending on the areas to be scanned. Tell him who will perform the test and where it will be done.

Procedure

The patient is instructed to remove all metal objects from the area to be scanned. He is positioned on a table located under the scanning device, with the radiation source below him and the detector above. The detector measures the bone's absorption of the radiation and registers a digital readout. The scan is completed in less than 10 minutes.

Precautions

Bone densitometry is contraindicated during pregnancy.

Normal findings

The results of the scan are analyzed by a computer program according to the patient's age, sex, and height. The patient's rate of bone loss can be tracked over time.

Implications of results

The value and reliability of bone densitometry as a predictor of fractures are under investigation. Controversy exists regarding the scanning site and whether bone loss occurs as a general phenomenon or occurs first in the spine. Also, large-scale studies are being conducted to establish an "at-risk" level of bone density to help predict fractures.

Post-test care

None.

Interfering factors

The accuracy of the test may be influenced by osteoarthritis, fractures, the size of the region to be scanned, and fat tissue distribution.

SCANNING

Skeletal computed tomography

Skeletal computed tomography (CT) scanning provides a series of tomograms, translated by a computer and displayed on a video monitor, that represent cross-sectional images of various layers (or slices) of bone. This technique can reconstruct cross-sectional, horizontal, sagittal, and coronal plane images. Hundreds of thousands of readings of radiation levels absorbed by tissues may be combined to depict anatomic slices of varying thickness. Taking more collimated (parallel) radiographs increases the number of radiation density calculations the computer makes, thereby improving the degree of resolution and thus specificity and accuracy.

Purpose

- To determine the existence and extent of primary bone tumors, skeletal metastases, and soft-tissue tumors
- To diagnose joint abnormalities difficult to detect by other methods.

Patient preparation

Explain to the patient that this procedure allows visualization of bones and joints. Unless a contrast medium has been ordered, tell him that he needn't restrict food or fluids. (If contrast enhancement is ordered, instruct him to fast for 4 hours before the test.) Explain who will perform the procedure and where and that it takes 30 to 60 minutes. Reassure him that the test is painless.

Explain that he'll be positioned on an X-ray table inside a CT scanner and asked to lie still; the computer-controlled scanner will revolve around him, taking multiple scans. Inform him that the scanner makes clicking noises as it rotates. Tell him to lie as still as possible because movement may cause distorted images. If a contrast medium is used, tell him that he may feel flushed and warm and may experience a transient headache and nausea or vomiting after it's injected. Reassure him that these reactions are normal.

Instruct the patient to wear a radiologic examination gown and to remove all metal objects and jewelry that may appear in the X-ray field. Check the patient's history for hypersensitivity reactions to iodine, shellfish, and contrast media. Mark any such reactions on the chart and notify the doctor, who may order prophylactic medications or choose not to use a contrast medium.

If the patient appears restless or apprehensive about the procedure, notify the doctor, who may prescribe a mild sedative.

Equipment
CT scanner ✦ contrast medium, as ordered.

Procedure
The patient is placed in a supine position on an X-ray table and told to lie as still as possible. The table is then moved into the circular opening of the CT scanner. The scanner revolves around the patient, taking scans at preselected intervals.

After the first set of scans is taken, the patient is removed from the scanner and a contrast medium is administered, if ordered. (Most CT scanners use automatic contrast injectors, which inject the medium at a preset rate while the patient is being scanned.) Observe the patient for signs and symptoms of a hypersensitivity reaction (pruritus, rash, and respiratory difficulty) for 30 minutes after the contrast medium has been injected.

After the injection, the patient is moved back into the scanner and another series of scans is taken. The images obtained from the scan are displayed on a video monitor during the procedure and stored on magnetic tape to create a permanent record for subsequent study.

Precautions
■ This procedure is contraindicated during pregnancy.
■ Some patients may experience claustrophobia or anxiety when inside the CT scanner. For such patients, the doctor may order a mild sedative to help reduce anxiety.
■ For patients with significant bone or joint pain, administer analgesics, as ordered, so that the patient can lie still comfortably during the scan.

Normal findings
The scan should reveal no pathology in the bones or joints. It produces crisp images of the structure while blurring or eliminating details of surrounding structures.

Implications of results
Because of its ability to display cross-sectional anatomy, CT scanning is useful for obtaining images of the shoulder, spine, hip, and pelvis. This cross-sectional view eliminates the confusing shadows of superimposed structures that occur with conventional radiographs. The scan can reveal primary bone and soft-tissue tumors as well as skeletal metastases. It can also reveal joint abnormalities that are difficult to detect by other methods.

Post-test care
■ If a contrast medium was used, observe for a delayed allergic reaction and treat it as necessary. (Diphenhydramine is the drug of choice.)
■ Encourage the patient to drink lots of fluids to help his body eliminate the contrast agent.
■ Tell the patient that he may resume his usual activities and diet.
■ Provide comfort measures and pain medication as needed because of prolonged positioning on the table.

Interfering factors
■ Claustrophobia may interfere with the patient's ability to lie in the scanner for long periods.
■ Excessive movement by the patient during the scan may distort the images.
■ Radiopaque objects in the X-ray field may produce unclear images.

Skeletal magnetic resonance imaging

A noninvasive technique, magnetic resonance imaging (MRI) produces clear and sensitive tomographic images of bone and soft tissue. It provides superior contrast of body tissues and allows imaging of multiple planes, including direct sagittal and coronal views in regions that can't be easily visualized with X-rays or computed tomography scans. MRI eliminates the risks associated with exposure to X-ray beams and causes no known harm to cells.

During an MRI scan, the patient is placed on a table that slides into a cylindrical magnet. The magnet causes the body's atomic protons to line up and spin in the same direction. A radio-frequency beam is then introduced into the magnetic field, causing the protons to move out of alignment. When the beam is stopped, the protons realign and release energy. The release of proton energy is detected as a signal. A receiver coil measures the signal, and these measurements provide information about the type of tissue in which the protons lie. A computer uses this information to construct an image on a video monitor, showing the proton distribution of certain atoms.

Magnetic resonance images are most easily generated from the proton of the hydrogen atom. Each water molecule has two hydrogen atoms, but the distribution of water molecules varies according to specific body tissue. For example, bone is considered "dry" because it doesn't contain much hydrogen. Consequently, bone produces a weak signal and can't be visualized. However, normal bone marrow has the brightest signal and can be seen well.

Purpose
- To evaluate bony and soft-tissue tumors
- To identify changes in the bone marrow cavity
- To identify spinal disorders.

Patient preparation
First, make sure the scanner can accommodate the patient's weight and abdominal girth. Explain to the patient that this test assesses bone and soft tissue. Tell him who will perform the test, where it will be done, and that it takes 30 to 90 minutes. Explain that although MRI is painless and involves no exposure to radiation, a contrast medium may be used, depending on the type of tissue being studied.

Inform him that the opening for the patient's head and body is small and deep. Tell him that he'll hear the scanner clicking, whirring, and thumping as it moves inside its housing to obtain different images, so he may receive earplugs. Reassure him that he'll be able to communicate with the technician at all times. Ask if claustrophobia has ever been a problem; if so, sedation may help him to tolerate the scan. ("Open" scanners have been developed for use on patients with extreme claustrophobia or morbid obesity, but tests using such machines take longer.)

Instruct the patient to remove all metallic objects, including jewelry, hairpins, and watch. Ask if he has any surgically implanted joints, pins, clips, valves, pumps, or pacemakers containing metal, which could be attracted to the strong MRI magnet. If he does, he won't be able to have the test. Also, discontinue I.V. infusion pumps, feeding tubes with metal tips, pulmonary artery catheters, and similar devices before the test.

The patient and a family member accompanying him will have to complete a screening sheet before entering the scanner room. If your hospital requires it, have the patient or a responsible family member sign a consent form.

Equipment
MRI scanner and computer ✦ display screen ✦ recorder (film or magnetic tape).

Procedure
At the scanner room door, the patient is checked one last time for metal objects. Then he's placed on a narrow, padded, nonmetallic table that moves into the scanner tunnel. Fans continuously circulate air in the tunnel, and a call bell or intercom is used to maintain verbal contact with the technician. The patient must remain still during the procedure and may need frequent reminders to avoid any movement.

While the patient lies within the strong magnetic field, the area to be studied is stimulated with radio-frequency waves. The MRI computer measures resulting energy changes at these body sections and uses them to generate images. The images look like two-dimensional slices through the tissues, bone, or organs.

Precautions
- Monitor the patient for claustrophobia and anxiety.
- MRI works through a powerful magnetic field, so don't allow any metal objects — including I.V. pumps, ventilators, and other metallic equipment — to enter the testing area. Computer-based equipment also can't enter the MRI area.
- If the patient is unstable, make sure an I.V. line without metal components is in place and that all equipment is compatible with MRI imaging. If necessary, monitor his oxygen saturation, cardiac rhythm, and respiratory status during the test. An anesthesiologist may be needed to monitor a heavily sedated patient.
- A technician should maintain verbal contact with the conscious patient.

Normal findings
MRI should reveal no pathology in bone, muscles, and joints.

Implications of results
MRI is an excellent method for visualizing disease of the spinal canal and cord and for identifying primary and metastatic bone tumors. It's useful in providing anatomic delineation of muscles, ligaments, and bones. The images show superior contrast of body tissues and sharply define healthy, benign, and malignant tissues.

Post-test care
- If the test took a long time, you may need to observe or monitor the patient for postural hypotension.
- Provide comfort measures and pain medication as needed because of prolonged positioning in the scanner.
- Tell the patient he may resume normal activities after the test.
- Provide emotional support to the patient with claustrophobia or anxiety about his diagnosis.

Interfering factors
- Radio music can't be played during the MRI scan because radio waves would interfere with the radio frequency of the scanner.
- Inaccurate imaging can occur if the patient moves during the procedure.
- Overweight patients who don't fit into the scanner tunnel properly can produce inaccurate imaging.

Arthroscopy

Arthroscopy is the visual examination of the interior of a joint with a specially designed fiber-optic endoscope. It is most commonly used to examine the knee. In evaluating a patient with suspected or confirmed joint disease, the initial diagnostic approach consists of a complete history and physical examination and plain X-ray films. Arthroscopy, with about 98% diagnostic accuracy, may prove to be the definitive diagnostic procedure.

Unlike radiographic studies, arthroscopy permits concurrent surgery or biopsy using a technique called triangulation, in which instruments are passed through a separate cannula. Thus, arthroscopy provides a safe, convenient alternative to open surgery (arthrotomy) and separate biopsy. Although arthroscopy is commonly performed under a local anesthetic, it may also be performed under a spinal or general anesthetic, particularly when surgery is anticipated. (See *Knee arthroscopy findings,* page 696.)

Complications associated with arthroscopy seldom occur but may include infection, hematoma, thrombophlebitis, and joint injury.

Purpose

- To detect and diagnose meniscal, patellar, condylar, extrasynovial, and synovial diseases
- To monitor the progression of disease
- To perform joint surgery
- To monitor effectiveness of therapy.

Patient preparation

Describe the procedure to the patient, and answer any questions he may have. Explain that this test permits examination of the interior of the joint and evaluation of joint disease. If appropriate, tell the patient this test monitors his response to therapy. (If surgery or another treatment is anticipated, explain that in many cases, this may be safely and conveniently accomplished through the arthroscope.) Instruct the patient to fast after midnight before the procedure. Tell him who will perform this procedure and where.

If local anesthesia is to be used, tell the patient he may experience transient discomfort from the injection of the local anesthetic and the pressure of the tourniquet on his leg. He'll also feel a thumping sensation as the cannula is inserted in the joint capsule.

Make sure the patient or a responsible family member has signed a consent form. Check the patient's history for hypersensitivity to the anesthetic. Just before the procedure, shave the area 5" (12.5 cm) above and below the joint; then administer a sedative, as ordered.

Equipment

Skin antiseptic (povidone-iodine solution) ✦ arthroscope and accessory equipment ✦ pointed scalpel ✦ sterile gloves ✦ local anesthetic ✦ sterile needle ✦ 12-ml and 60-ml syringes ✦ waterproof stockinette ✦ elastic bandages ✦ pneumatic tourniquet ✦ epinephrine (1:100,000 in 1% lidocaine solution) ✦ 500 ml sterile normal saline solution ✦ continuous drainage system ✦ sponges ✦ sterile 2" x 2" gauze pads ✦ sterile drapes ✦ small adhesive bandages.

Procedure

Arthroscopic techniques vary, depending on the surgeon and the type of arthroscope used. In most cases, as much blood as possible is drained from the leg

Knee arthroscopy findings

With the patient's knee flexed about 40 degrees, the arthroscope is introduced into the joint. The examiner moves the knee into various degrees of flexion, extension, and rotation to obtain different arthroscopic views of the joint space. Counterclockwise from the top, you'll see a normal patellofemoral joint, showing smooth joint surfaces; the articular surface of the patella, showing chondromalacia; and a tear in the anterior cruciate ligament.

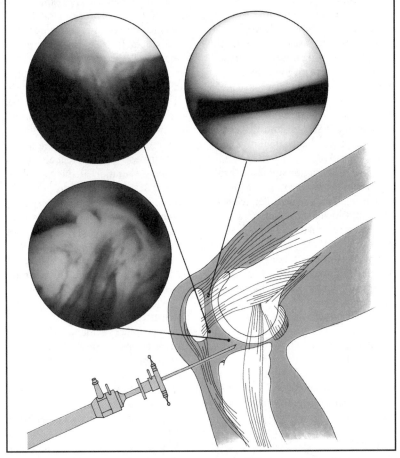

by wrapping it in an elastic bandage and elevating the leg or by instilling a mixture of lidocaine with epinephrine and sterile normal saline solution into the patient's knee to distend the knee and help reduce bleeding. Then the joint is anesthetized, a small incision is made, and a cannula is passed through the incision and positioned in the joint cavity. Next, the arthroscope is inserted through the cannula and the knee structures are visually examined and, if necessary, photographed for further study.

When the examination is complete, a synovial biopsy or appropriate surgery is performed. After the surgery, the arthroscope is removed, the joint is irrigated, and an adhesive strip and compression bandage are applied to the site.

Precautions

Arthroscopy is contraindicated in a patient with fibrous ankylosis with flexion of less than 50 degrees. It's also contraindicated in a patient with local skin or wound infections because of the risk of subsequent joint involvement.

Normal findings

The knee is a typical diarthrodial joint surrounded by muscles, ligaments, cartilage, and tendons and lined with synovial membrane. In children, the menisci are smooth and opaque, with their thick outer edges attached to the joint capsule and their inner edges lying snugly against the condylar surfaces, unattached. Articular cartilage appears smooth and white; ligaments and tendons appear cablelike and silvery. The synovium is smooth and marked by a fine vascular network. Degenerative changes begin during adolescence.

Implications of results

Arthroscopic examination can reveal meniscal disease, such as a torn medial or lateral meniscus or other meniscal injuries; patellar disease, such as chondromalacia, dislocation, subluxation, fracture, and parapatellar synovitis; condylar disease, such as degenerative articular cartilage, osteochondritis dissecans, and loose bodies; extrasynovial disease, such as torn anterior cruciate or tibial collateral ligaments, Baker's cyst, and ganglion cyst; and synovial disease, such as synovitis, rheumatoid and degenerative arthritis, and foreign bodies associated with gout, pseudogout, and osteochondromatosis.

Depending on test findings, appropriate treatment or surgery can follow arthroscopy. If arthroscopic surgery can't be performed, arthrotomy is the procedure of choice.

Post-test care

- Watch for fever and for swelling, increased pain, and localized inflammation at the incision site. If the patient reports discomfort, administer analgesics, as ordered.
- Monitor the patient's circulation and the sensation in his leg.
- Advise the patient to elevate his leg and apply ice for the first 24 hours.
- Instruct him to report any fever or increased swelling or pain in the joint.
- Advise him to bear only partial weight — using crutches, a walker, or a cane — for 48 hours.
- If an immobilizer is ordered, teach the patient how to apply it.
- Tell the patient that he may shower after 48 hours but should avoid a tub bath until after the postoperative visit.
- Tell him that he may resume his usual diet.

Interfering factors

Failure to use the arthroscope properly can result in an incomplete examination of the joint.

Synovial fluid analysis

Synovial fluid is normally a viscid, colorless to pale yellow liquid found in small amounts in the diarthrodial (synovial) joints, bursae, and tendon sheaths. (See *Normal findings in synovial fluid,* page 698.) It's thought to be produced by the dialysis of plasma across the synovial membrane and by the secretion of hyaluronic acid, a mucopolysaccharide. Although its functions aren't clearly understood, synovial fluid probably lubricates the joint space,

Normal findings in synovial fluid

FEATURE	RESULTS
Gross	
Color	Colorless to pale yellow
Clarity	Clear
Quantity (in knee)	0.3 to 3.5 ml
Viscosity	5.7 to 1,160
pH	7.2 to 7.4
Mucin clot	Good
Microscopic	
WBC count	0 to 200/µl
WBC differential:	
▪ Lymphocytes	▪ 0 to 78/µl
▪ Monocytes	▪ 0 to 71/µl
▪ Clasmatocytes	▪ 0 to 26/µl
▪ Polymorphonuclears	▪ 0 to 25/µl
▪ Other phagocytes	▪ 0 to 21/µl
▪ Synovial lining cells	▪ 0 to 12/µl
Microbiological	
Formed elements	Absence of crystals and cartilage debris
Bacteria	None
Serologic	
Complement:	
▪ For 10 mg protein/dl	3.7 to 33.7 U/ml
▪ For 20 mg protein/dl	7.7 to 37.7 U/ml
Rheumatoid arthritis cells	None
Lupus erythematosus cells	None
Chemical	
Total protein	10.7 to 21.3 mg/dl
Fibrinogen	None
Glucose	70 to 100 mg/dl
Uric acid	2 to 8 mg/dl (men), 2 to 6 mg/dl (women)
Hyaluronate	0.3 to 0.4 g/dl
$Paco_2$	40 to 60 mm Hg
Pao_2	40 to 80 mm Hg

nourishes the articular cartilage, and protects the cartilage from mechanical damage while stabilizing the joint.

In synovial fluid aspiration (arthrocentesis), a sterile needle is inserted into a joint space — most commonly the knee — under strict sterile conditions to obtain a fluid specimen for analysis. This procedure is indicated in patients with undiagnosed articular disease and symptomatic joint effusion (excessive accumulation of synovial fluid).

Although rare, complications associated with synovial fluid aspiration include joint infection and hemorrhage leading to hemarthrosis (accumulation of blood within the joint).

Purpose
■ To aid differential diagnosis of arthritis, particularly septic or crystal-induced arthritis (see *Synovial fluid findings in various disorders,* pages 700 and 701)
■ To identify the cause or nature of joint effusion
■ To relieve the pain and distention resulting from joint effusion
■ To administer local drug therapy (usually corticosteroids).

Patient preparation
Describe the procedure to the patient, and answer any questions he may have. Explain that this test helps determine the cause of joint inflammation and swelling and helps relieve the associated pain. If glucose testing of synovial fluid is ordered, instruct him to fast for 6 to 12 hours before the test; otherwise, he needn't restrict food or fluids before the test. Tell him who will perform the test and where. Warn him that although he'll receive a local anesthetic, he may still feel transient pain when the needle penetrates the joint capsule. (Sometimes a sedative is ordered for a young child.)

Make sure the patient or a responsible family member has signed a consent form. Check the patient's history for hypersensitivity to iodine compounds (such as povidone-iodine), procaine, lidocaine, and other local anesthetics. Administer a sedative, as ordered.

Equipment
Surgical detergent ✦ skin antiseptic (usually tincture of povidone-iodine) ✦ alcohol sponges ✦ local anesthetic (procaine or lidocaine, 1% or 2%) ✦ sterile, disposable 1½" 25G needle ✦ sterile, disposable 1½" to 2" 20G needle ✦ sterile 5-ml syringe for injecting anesthetic ✦ sterile 20-ml syringe for aspiration ✦ 3-ml syringe for administering sedative ✦ sterile 2" x 2" gauze pads ✦ sterile dressings ✦ sterile drapes ✦ elastic bandage ✦ tubes for culture, cytologic, clot, and glucose analysis ✦ anticoagulants (heparin, EDTA, and potassium oxalate) ✦ venipuncture equipment, if ordered.

For corticosteroid administration: corticosteroid suspension such as hydrocortisone ✦ 2-ml and 5-ml syringes (or one 10-ml syringe if procaine and steroid are to be injected simultaneously).

Procedure
Position the patient as ordered, and explain that he'll need to maintain this position throughout the procedure. Clean the skin over the puncture site with surgical detergent and alcohol. Paint the site with tincture of povidone-iodine, and allow it to air-dry for 2 minutes. After the local anesthetic is administered, the aspirating needle is quickly inserted through the skin, subcutaneous tissue, and synovial membrane into the joint space. As much fluid as possible is aspirated into the syringe, preferably at least 15 ml. The joint (except for the area around the puncture site) may be wrapped with an elastic bandage to compress the free fluid into this portion of the sac, ensuring maximal collection of fluid.

If a corticosteroid is being injected, prepare the dose as ordered. For instil-

Synovial fluid findings in various disorders

DISEASE	COLOR	CLARITY	VISCOSITY	MUCIN CLOT
Group I noninflammatory				
Traumatic arthritis	Straw to bloody to yellow	Transparent to cloudy	Variable	Good to fair
Osteoarthritis	Yellow	Transparent	Variable	Good to fair
Group II inflammatory				
Systemic lupus erythematosus	Straw	Clear to slightly cloudy	Variable	Good to fair
Rheumatic fever	Yellow	Slightly cloudy	Variable	Good to fair
Pseudogout	Yellow	Slightly cloudy (if acute)	Low (if acute)	Fair to poor
Gout	Yellow to milky	Cloudy	Low	Fair to poor
Rheumatoid arthritis	Yellow to green	Cloudy	Low	Fair to poor
Group III septic				
Tuberculous arthritis	Yellow	Cloudy	Low	Poor
Septic arthritis	Gray or bloody	Turbid, purulent	Low	Poor

lation, the syringe is detached, leaving the needle in the joint, and the syringe containing the steroid is attached to the needle instead. After the steroid is injected and the needle withdrawn, wipe the puncture site with alcohol. Apply pressure to the puncture site for about 2 minutes to prevent bleeding; then apply a sterile dressing.

If synovial fluid glucose is being measured, perform venipuncture to obtain a specimen for blood glucose analysis.

Precautions

■ Wear gloves when handling all specimens.

■ This test should not be performed in areas of skin or wound infections.

■ Use strict sterile technique throughout aspiration to prevent contamination of the joint space or the synovial fluid specimen.

■ Add anticoagulants to the specimen, according to the laboratory tests requested. Gently invert the tube several times to mix the specimen and anticoagulant adequately. *For cultures,* obtain 2 to 5 ml of synovial fluid and, if possible, inoculate the medium immediately. Otherwise, add 1 or 2 drops of heparin to the specimen. *For cytologic analysis,* add 5 mg of EDTA or 1 or 2 drops

WBC COUNT/ % NEUTROPHILS	CARTILAGE DEBRIS	CRYSTALS	RHEUMATOID ARTHRITIS CELLS	BACTERIA
1,000; 25%	None	None	None	None
700; 15%	Usually present	None	None	None
2,000; 30%	None	None	Lupus erythematosus (LE) cells	None
14,000; 50%	None	None	Possibly LE cells	None
15,000; 70%	Usually present	Calcium pyrophosphate	None	None
20,000; 70%	None	Urate	None	None
20,000; 70%	None	Occasionally, cholesterol	Usually present	None
20,000; 60%	None	None	None	Usually present
90,000; 90%	None	None	None	Usually present

of heparin to 2 to 5 ml of synovial fluid. *For glucose analysis,* add potassium oxalate, as specified by the laboratory, to 3 to 5 ml of fluid. *For crystal examination,* add heparin if specified by the laboratory. *For other studies,* such as general appearance and clot evaluation, obtain 2 to 5 ml of synovial fluid, but don't add an anticoagulant.

■ Send the properly labeled specimens to the laboratory immediately — gonococci are particularly labile. If a white blood cell (WBC) count is being performed, clearly label the specimen "Synovial Fluid" and "Caution — Don't use acid diluents."

Normal findings

Routine examination of synovial fluid consists of gross analysis for color, clarity, quantity, viscosity, pH, and the presence of a mucin clot as well as microscopic analysis for WBC count and differential. Special examinations include microbiological analysis for formed elements (including crystals) and bacteria, serologic analysis, and chemical analysis for such components as glucose, protein, and enzymes.

Implications of results

Examination of synovial fluid may reveal various joint disease, including noninflammatory disease (traumatic arthritis and osteoarthritis), inflammatory disease (systemic lupus erythematosus, rheumatic fever, gout, pseudogout, and rheumatoid arthritis), and septic disease (tuberculous and septic arthritis).

Post-test care
■ Apply ice or cold packs to the affected joint for 24 to 36 hours after aspiration to decrease pain and swelling. Use pillows for support. If a large quantity of fluid was aspirated, apply an elastic bandage to prevent fluid reaccumulation.
■ If the patient's condition permits, tell him that he may resume normal activities immediately after the procedure. However, warn him to avoid excessive use of the joint for a few days after the test, even if pain and swelling have subsided. Excessive use may cause transient pain, swelling, and stiffness.
■ Watch for increased pain and fever, which may indicate joint infection.
■ Carefully handle the dressings and linens of patients with drainage from the joint space, especially if septic arthritis is confirmed or suspected.
■ Advise the patient that he may resume his usual diet.

Interfering factors
■ Acid diluents added to the specimen for WBC count alter the cell count.
■ Failure to mix the specimen and the anticoagulant adequately or to send the specimen to the laboratory immediately may cause inaccurate test results.
■ Patient failure to adhere to dietary restrictions can affect glucose levels.
■ Contamination of the specimen can invalidate test results.

SELECTED READINGS

Black, J.M., and Matassarin-Jacobs, E., eds. *Luckmann and Sorensen's Medical-Surgical Nursing: A Psychophysiologic Approach*, 4th ed. Philadelphia: W.B. Saunders Co., 1993.

Diseases, 2nd ed. Springhouse, Pa.: Springhouse Corp., 1996.

Fischbach, F. *A Manual of Laboratory and Diagnostic Tests*, 6th ed. Philadelphia: Lippincott-Raven Pubs., 1996.

Guyton, A.C., and Hall, J.E. *Textbook of Medical Physiology*, 9th ed. Philadelphia: W.B. Saunders Co., 1996.

Henry, J.B., ed. *Clinical Diagnosis and Management by Laboratory Methods*, 19th ed. Philadelphia: W.B. Saunders Co., 1996.

Maher, A.B., et al. *Orthopaedic Nursing*. Philadelphia: W.B. Saunders Co., 1994.

Nursing97 Drug Handbook. Springhouse, Pa.: Springhouse Corp., 1997.

Phipps, W.J., et al. *Medical-Surgical Nursing: Concepts and Clinical Practice*, 5th ed. St. Louis: Mosby–Year Book, Inc., 1995.

Salmon, S., et al. *Core Curriculum for Orthopaedic Nursing*, 3rd ed. Pitman, N.J.: National Association of Orthopaedic Nurses, 1996.

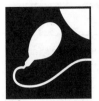

Reproductive system

Learning objectives

After completing this chapter, the reader will be able to:
- explain the anatomy and physiology of the reproductive system
- describe normal fetal development and the three stages of labor
- identify the sequence of tests used to evaluate the reproductive system
- explain how DNA and RNA influence protein synthesis
- discuss how cell division occurs
- discuss chromosomal analysis and its clinical implications
- list the major sex chromosome anomalies
- state the purpose of each test discussed in the chapter
- prepare the patient physically and psychologically for each test
- describe the procedure for performing each test
- specify appropriate precautions for safe administration of each test
- recognize signs of an adverse reaction and respond appropriately
- implement appropriate post-test care
- identify the normal findings and reference values for each test
- discuss the implications of abnormal test results
- list factors that may interfere with accurate test results.

INTRODUCTION

Diagnostic testing of the reproductive system may be performed to assess the organs and associated structures for abnormalities, to detect malignant tumors, or to determine the cause of infertility or sexual dysfunction. Some diagnostic tests are especially useful during pregnancy — first, to confirm pregnancy and, later, to detect genetic defects and monitor the fetus's well-being.

Reproductive organs

The reproductive system consists of essential and accessory organs for procreation. Essential organs are the gonads — the testes and the ovaries. The testes produce the germ cells known as spermatozoa and the hormone testosterone, which induces and maintains secondary sexual characteristics; the ovaries produce ova and the hormones estrogen and progesterone, which also promote and maintain secondary sexual characteristics.

Male accessory organs consist of the scrotum and a transport system of ducts and glands, including the urethra, epididymis, vas deferens, ejaculatory duct, seminal vesicles, prostate, bulbourethral glands, and penis.

Female accessory organs include the fallopian tubes, uterus, and vagina. External structures of female genitalia, collectively called the vulva, include the mons pubis, labia majora, labia minora, clitoris, vestibule, urethral meatus, hymen, Bartholin's glands, Skene's glands, fourchette, and perineum. The mammary glands, whose primary function is lactation, are also generally considered part of the reproductive system. (See *Male reproductive system,* opposite, and *Female reproductive system,* page 706.)

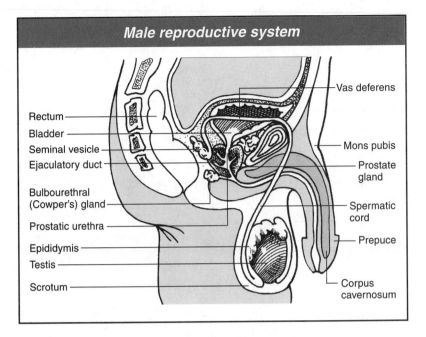

Male reproductive system

Rectum

Bladder

Seminal vesicle

Ejaculatory duct

Bulbourethral (Cowper's) gland

Prostatic urethra

Epididymis

Testis

Scrotum

Vas deferens

Mons pubis

Prostate gland

Spermatic cord

Prepuce

Corpus cavernosum

Fetal development

Normally, the spermatozoon fertilizes the ovum in the upper to middle third of the fallopian tube. At fertilization, the sperm, which contains 22 autosomes and either an X or a Y chromosome, fuses with the ovum, which contains 22 autosomes and an X chromosome, to form a zygote made up of 44 autosomes and 2 sex chromosomes. The 44 autosomes determine genetic characteristics; the sex chromosomes determine sex. Two X chromosomes produce a female zygote; the combination of an X and a Y, a male zygote.

After fertilization, the fertilized ovum develops in two stages over a 40-week gestation period. During the *embryonic stage,* which begins at conception and lasts 8 weeks, the blastocyst develops and is implanted, and primitive chorionic villi start to form. The amnion begins to ensheathe the body stalk, which will become the umbilical cord. Embryonic heart chambers develop, and a primitive cardiovascular system begins to

function. By the end of the embryonic stage, the eyes, ears, nose, and mouth are recognizable; the arms, legs, fingers, and toes are formed; and most organs have begun to develop.

During the *fetal stage,* a period lasting from 8 weeks after conception until delivery, the major structures and organs that are already developed grow and mature. (See *Reviewing fetal growth and development,* pages 707 and 708.)

Stages of labor

- *Stage I* is the time between the beginning of regular contractions and full cervical dilation — usually about 12 hours for a primigravida and about 6 hours for a multigravida.
- *Stage II,* the period lasting from full dilation until delivery, lasts about 1½ hours for a primigravida and 30 minutes for a multigravida.
- *Stage III* lasts from delivery to the expulsion of the placenta — usually 3 to 4 minutes for a primigravida and 4 to 5

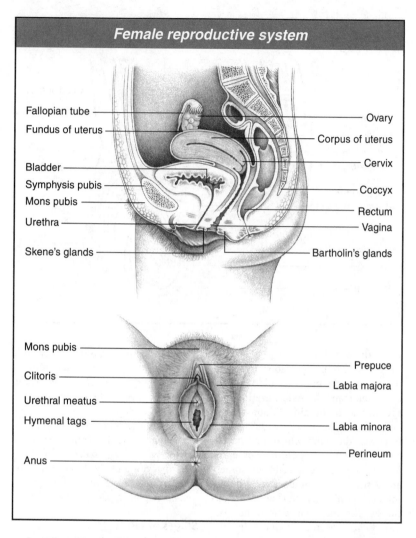

Female reproductive system

Fallopian tube
Fundus of uterus
Bladder
Symphysis pubis
Mons pubis
Urethra
Skene's glands

Ovary
Corpus of uterus
Cervix
Coccyx
Rectum
Vagina
Bartholin's glands

Mons pubis
Clitoris
Urethral meatus
Hymenal tags
Anus

Prepuce
Labia majora
Labia minora
Perineum

minutes for a multigravida (but possibly as long as 1 hour).

Special diagnostic tests

Evaluation of the reproductive system begins with a physical examination and a detailed history to detect abnormalities that may require further testing. Special tests using various techniques include the following:

■ *Papanicolaou (Pap) test,* the cytologic examination of cervical scrapings, allows early detection of cervical cancer.
■ *Colposcopy* provides direct visualization of cervical and vaginal abnormalities, such as benign lesions and invasive carcinoma.
■ *Semen analysis* evaluates male fertility (semen count and motility analysis), validates the effectiveness of a vasectomy, and detects the presence of semen for medicolegal investigations.

Reviewing fetal growth and development

1. At the end of 1 month, the embryo has a definite form. The head and trunk are apparent, and the tiny buds that will become the arms and legs are discernible. The cardiovascular system has begun to function, and the umbilical cord is visible in its most primitive form.

2. In the next month, the embryo — called a fetus from the seventh week on — grows to 1" (2.5 cm) in length and weighs $\frac{1}{30}$ oz. The head and facial features develop as the eyes, ears, nose, lips, tongue, and tooth buds form. The arms and legs also take shape, with the elbows, forearms, hands, fingers, thighs, knees, ankles, and toes becoming visible. Although the gender of the fetus is not yet discernible, all external genitalia are present. Cardiovascular function is complete, and the umbilical cord has a definite form. At the end of 2 months, the fetus resembles a full-term baby except for size.

3. During the third month, the fetus grows to 3" (8 cm) in length and weighs 1 oz (28 g). Teeth and bones begin to appear, and the kidneys start to function. Although the mother can't yet feel activity, the fetus is moving. It opens its mouth to swallow, grasps with its fully developed hands, and — even though its lungs are not functioning — prepares for breathing by inhaling and exhaling. At the end of the first trimester, its gender is distinguishable.

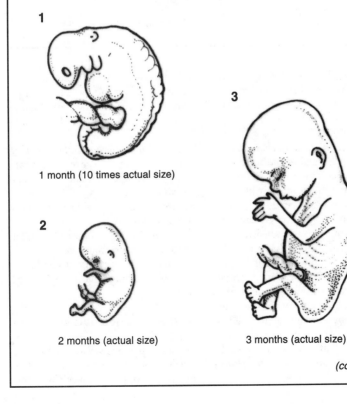

1

1 month (10 times actual size)

2

2 months (actual size)

3

3 months (actual size)

(continued)

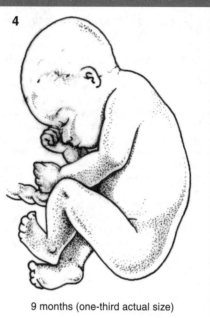

Reviewing fetal growth and development (continued)

4. In the remaining 6 months, fetal growth continues as internal and external structures develop at a rapid rate. In the third trimester, the fetus stores the fats and minerals it will need to live outside the womb. At birth, the average full-term fetus measures 20" (51 cm) and weighs 7 to 7½ lb (3 to 3.5 kg).

4

9 months (one-third actual size)

■ *Sex chromatin tests* screen for abnormalities of the sex chromosomes.

■ *Chromosomal analysis* can evaluate genetic defects in the fetus, thus aiding genetic counseling.

■ *Amniotic fluid analysis, chorionic villi biopsy,* and *pelvic and vaginal ultrasonography* can facilitate early diagnosis of fetal abnormalities, some of which may be successfully treated in utero. (For instance, amniotic fluid analysis can identify Rh isoimmunization before birth, allowing treatment with intrauterine transfusions to prevent stillbirth.)

■ *Laparoscopy* can determine if female infertility results from anatomic defects. It also detects pathology of the ovaries, fallopian tubes, and uterus, through direct visualization, thus allowing early treatment of life-threatening conditions, such as cancers or severe hemorrhage.

■ *Hysteroscopy* can investigate abnormal uterine bleeding and provide visualization of the interior of the uterus for other diagnoses, such as adhesions and fibroids.

■ *Internal* and *external fetal monitoring,* and *Doppler stethoscope testing* can rapidly assess fetal distress during pregnancy, labor, and delivery.

■ *Mammography* can aid assessment of breast lumps.

■ *Hysterosalpingography* provides visualization of malformations, adhesions, and occlusions of the uterus and fallopian tubes through fluoroscopic examination.

Significance of emotional support

For many patients scheduled for diagnostic tests of the reproductive system, emotional support is especially important. For one thing, fertility or ability to deliver a child can be closely related to self-image. Also, the tests themselves may cause anxiety. For example, a patient scheduled for amniocentesis may fear having a deformed or retarded infant, and a patient scheduled for mammography is likely to fear cancer and mastectomy. Therefore, make sure you assess a patient's psychological state before the test so you can deal with the patient appropriately.

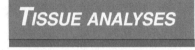

Papanicolaou test

The Papanicolaou (Pap) test, a cytologic test, is widely used for early detection of cervical cancer. To perform this test, a doctor or a specially trained nurse scrapes secretions from the patient's cervix and spreads them on a slide. After the slide is immersed in a fixative, it is sent to the laboratory for cytologic analysis. This test relies on the ready exfoliation of malignant cells from the cervix.

Although cervical scrapings are the most common test specimen, the Pap test also permits cytologic evaluation of the vaginal pool, prostatic secretions, urine, gastric secretion, cavity fluids, bronchial aspirations, sputum, and solid tumor cells obtained by fine-needle aspiration. It also shows cell maturity, metabolic activity, and morphology variations. The Pap test can also detect atypical cells, which may indicate vaginitis. (See *Vaginal smears*, page 710.)

The American Cancer Society recommends a Pap test every 3 years for women between ages 20 and 40 who are not in a high-risk category and who have had negative results from three previous Pap tests. Yearly tests (or tests at doctor-recommended intervals) are advised for women over age 40, for those in a high-risk category, and for those who have had a positive test previously. If a Pap test is positive or suggests malignancy, a cervical biopsy can confirm the diagnosis.

Purpose
- To detect malignant cells
- To detect inflammatory changes in tissue
- To assess response to chemotherapy and radiation therapy
- To detect viral, fungal and, occasionally, parasitic invasion.

Patient preparation
Explain to the patient that the test allows the study of cervical cells. Stress its importance as an aid for detecting cancer at a stage when the disease is often asymptomatic and still curable. The test should not be scheduled during the menstrual period: The best time is midcycle. To prepare for the test, instruct the patient to avoid having intercourse for 24 hours, douching for 48 hours, and using vaginal creams or medications for 1 week because these activities can wash away cellular deposits and change the vaginal pH.

Tell her the test requires that the cervix be scraped, who will perform the procedure and when, and that she may experience slight discomfort but no pain from the speculum. Reassure her that the procedure takes only 5 to 10 minutes to perform (slightly longer if the vagina, pelvic cavity, and rectum are examined bimanually).

Obtain an accurate patient history, and ask the following questions: When did you last have a Pap test? Have you ever had an abnormal Pap test? When was your last menstrual period? Are your periods regular? How many days

Vaginal smears

Although the Papanicolaou (Pap) test was not developed to detect vaginitis, a cytologist can usually identify cells associated with vaginitis while examining the stained cells for cancer. The most reliably detected cells are *Trichomonas vaginalis, Candida,* and herpes progenitalis. If such cells are present, the Pap test indicates atypical cells, but not evidence of malignancy.

The most conventional way to detect vaginitis is the vaginal smear. Using a cotton-tipped applicator or wooden spatula, the examiner collects vaginal secretions and places them at opposite ends of a slide. After adding a drop of normal saline solution to one end of the slide and a drop of 10% to 20% potassium hydroxide (KOH) to the other end (wet mount preparation), he examines the slide immediately. Trichomonads, white cells, epithelial cells, "clue" cells, and bacteria readily appear at the saline-treated end; *Candida,* at the KOH-treated end.

In the vaginal pool smear, secretions are aspirated through a pipette that's attached to a bulb for suction. Part of the secretion is smeared on a slide and fixed.

Scrapings for cytohormonal evaluation can also be taken from the vaginal pool. In this procedure, the lateral vaginal wall is gently scraped, and the scrapings spread on a glass slide and fixed. Using the pyknotic index, the estrogenic effect is assessed by determining the percentage of superficial and intermediate squamous cells with a fatty pyknotic nucleus.

---

do they last? Is bleeding heavy or light? Have you taken or are you presently taking hormones or oral contraceptives? Do you use an intrauterine device? Do you have any vaginal discharge, pain, or itching? What, if any, gynecologic disorders have occurred in your family? Have you ever had gynecologic surgery, chemotherapy, or radiation therapy? If so, describe it fully.

Note any pertinent history information on the laboratory request. If the patient is anxious, be supportive and tell her approximately when test results should be available.

Just before the test, ask the patient to empty her bladder.

Equipment
Gloves ✦ drape ✦ vaginal speculum ✦ collection device, such as a Pap stick (wooden spatula) ✦ endocervical brush or cotton-tipped applicator ✦ saline solution ✦ glass microscopic slides ✦ fixative (commercial spray or 95% ethyl alcohol solution in a jar) for slides.

Procedure
After instructing the patient to disrobe from the waist down and to drape herself, ask her to lie on the examining table and to place her heels in the stirrups. (She may be more comfortable if she keeps on her shoes.) Tell her to slide her buttocks to the edge of the table. Adjust the drape to minimize exposure. To avoid startling the patient, tell her when the examiner will begin the examination.

The examiner puts on gloves and inserts an unlubricated speculum into the vagina. To make insertion easier, he may moisten the speculum with saline solution or warm water. After the examiner locates the cervix, he'll collect secretions from the cervix and material from the endocervical canal. He'll place the endocervical brush or cotton-tipped applicator (for pregnant patients) inside the endocervix and roll it firmly inside the canal. If he's using a Pap stick (wooden spatula), he'll place it against the cervix with the longest protrusion in the cervical canal, then rotate the stick clockwise 360 degrees firmly against the cervix. Then he'll spread the specimen on the slide, according to laboratory policy, and immediately immerse the slide in a fixative or spray it with fixative held 9" to 12" (23 to 30 cm) from the slide. Alternatively, he may collect posterior vaginal pool secretions and pancervical material and smear it on a single slide, then fix it immediately according to laboratory instructions.

Label the specimen appropriately, including the date; the patient's name and age; the date of her last menstrual period; and the collection site and method. A bimanual examination may follow removal of the speculum. When the examination is completed, help the patient up and instruct her to dress.

Precautions

- Make sure the cervical specimen is aspirated and scraped from the cervix.
- Examine the consistency of the specimen. It should be thick enough that it's not transparent. A specimen that is too thin will dry and leave too few cells for adequate screening; if it's too thick, the stain will not penetrate.
- A vaginal pool sample is not recommended for cervical or endometrial cancer screening.
- If vaginal or vulval lesions are present, scrapings taken directly from the lesion are preferred.
- In a patient whose uterus is involuting or atrophying from age, use a small pipette, if necessary, to aspirate cells from the squamocolumnar junction and the

cervical canal. Use two slides to reduce air-drying artifact.

- Preserve the slides immediately.

Normal findings

No malignant cells or abnormalities are present in a normal specimen.

Implications of results

Usually, malignant cells have relatively large nuclei and only small amounts of cytoplasm. They show abnormal nuclear chromatin patterns and marked variation in size, shape, and staining properties, and they may have prominent nucleoli.

A Pap smear may be graded in different ways, so check your laboratory's reporting format. The Bethesda system is the current standardized method. In this system, potentially premalignant squamous lesions fall into three categories: atypical squamous cells of undetermined significance, low-grade squamous intraepithelial lesions, and high-grade squamous intraepithelial lesions. The low-grade squamous intraepithelial lesion category includes mild dysplasia and the changes of the human papillomavirus. The high-grade squamous intraepithelial lesion category includes moderate to severe dysplasia and carcinoma in situ.

To confirm a suggestive or positive cytology report, the test may be repeated or followed by a biopsy (or both).

Post-test care

- If cervical bleeding occurs, supply the patient with a sanitary napkin.
- Tell the patient when to return for her next Pap test.

Interfering factors

- Delay in fixing a specimen allows the cells to dry, destroys the effectiveness of the nuclear stain, and makes cytologic interpretation difficult.

- Excessive use of lubricating jelly on the speculum can alter the specimen.
- Douching within 48 hours or having intercourse within 24 hours of a Pap test can wash away cellular deposits.
- Exclusive use of a specimen collected from the vaginal fornix may yield false-negative test results.
- Collection of the specimen during menstruation may affect the accuracy of test results.

Colposcopy

In colposcopy, the cervix and vagina are visually examined by means of a colposcope — an instrument that contains a magnifying lens and a light. Although originally used as a screening test for cancer, colposcopy is now primarily used to evaluate abnormal cytology or grossly suspicious lesions and to examine the cervix and vagina after a positive Papanicolaou (Pap) test. During the examination, a biopsy may be performed and photographs taken of suspicious lesions with the colposcope and its attachments. Risks of biopsy include bleeding (especially during pregnancy) and infection.

Purpose

- To help confirm cervical intraepithelial neoplasia or invasive carcinoma after a positive Pap test
- To evaluate vaginal or cervical lesions
- To monitor conservatively treated cervical intraepithelial neoplasia
- To monitor patients whose mothers received diethylstilbestrol during pregnancy.

Patient preparation

Explain to the patient that this test magnifies the image of the vagina and cer-

vix, providing more information than routine vaginal examination. Inform her that she needn't restrict food or fluids. Tell her who will perform the examination and where, that it's safe and painless, and that it takes 10 to 15 minutes. Advise her that a biopsy may be performed at the time of examination and that this may cause minimal but easily controlled bleeding and mild cramping.

Equipment

For colposcopy: gloves ✦ colposcope ✦ vaginal speculum ✦ 3% acetic acid solution ✦ swabs.

For biopsy: gloves ✦ biopsy forceps ✦ endocervical curette ✦ forceps for uterine dressing ✦ tenaculum ✦ ring forceps ✦ Monsel's (ferric subsulfate) solution ✦ biopsy bottle and preservative ✦ sterile cotton balls ✦ Pap test equipment (glass slide, wooden spatula, swabs, and fixative).

Procedure

The examiner puts on gloves. With the patient in the lithotomy position, the examiner inserts the speculum and, if indicated, performs a Pap test. (Help the patient relax during insertion by telling her to breathe through her mouth and to relax her abdominal muscles.) Then he swabs the cervix with acetic acid solution to remove mucus. After examining the cervix and vagina, he performs a biopsy on areas that appear abnormal (in blood vessel pattern or tissue color, for example). Finally, he stops bleeding by applying pressure or hemostatic solutions or by cautery.

Precautions

None.

Normal findings

Cervical vessels should show a network and hairpin capillary pattern, with about 100 microns between them. Surface contour should be smooth and pink; columnar epithelium should appear grapelike. Different tissue types should be sharply demarcated.

Implications of results

Abnormal colposcopy findings include white epithelium or punctuation and mosaic patterns, which may indicate underlying cervical intraepithelial neoplasia; keratinization in the transformation zone, which may indicate cervical intraepithelial neoplasia or invasive carcinoma; and atypical vessels, which may indicate invasive carcinoma. Other abnormalities visible during colposcopy include inflammatory changes (usually from infection), atrophic changes (usually from aging or, less often, the use of oral contraceptives), erosion (probably from increased pathogenicity of vaginal flora due to changes in vaginal pH), and papilloma and condyloma (possibly from viruses).

Histologic study of the biopsy specimen confirms colposcopic findings. However, if the results of the examination and biopsy are inconsistent with the results of the Pap test and biopsy of the squamocolumnar junction, conization of the cervix for biopsy may be needed.

Post-test care

After a biopsy, instruct the patient to abstain from intercourse and to avoid inserting anything in her vagina (except a tampon) until healing of the biopsy site is confirmed.

Interfering factors

Failure to clean the cervix of foreign materials, such as creams and medications, may impair visualization.

Semen analysis

Inexpensive, technically simple, and reasonably definitive, semen analysis is usually the first test performed on a male to evaluate fertility. The procedure for analyzing semen for infertility usually includes measuring the volume of seminal fluid, assessing the sperm count, and examining the specimen under a microscope. Sperm are counted in much the same way that red and white blood cells and platelets are counted on an anticoagulated blood sample. Staining and microscopic examination of a drop of semen permits the sperms' motility and morphology to be evaluated.

Abnormal semen may require further testing (such as liver, thyroid, pituitary, and adrenal function tests) to identify the underlying cause and screen for metabolic abnormalities (such as diabetes mellitus). Significantly abnormal semen — such as greatly decreased sperm count or motility, or a marked increase in morphologically abnormal forms — may require a testicular biopsy.

Semen analysis can also be used to detect semen on a rape victim, to identify the blood group of an alleged rapist, or to prove sterility in a paternity suit. (See *Identifying semen for medicolegal purposes,* page 714.) Some laboratories offer specialized semen tests, such as screening for antibodies to spermatozoa.

Purpose
- To evaluate male fertility in an infertile marriage (most common use)
- To determine the effectiveness of vasectomy
- To detect semen on the body or clothing of a suspected rape victim or elsewhere at the crime scene
- To identify blood group substances or

Identifying semen for medicolegal purposes

Spermatozoa (or their fragments) persist in the vagina for more than 72 hours after sexual intercourse. This allows detection and positive identification of semen from vaginal aspirates or smears, or from stains on clothing, other fabrics, skin, or hair, which is commonly necessary for medicolegal purposes, usually in connection with rape or homicide investigations. Spermatozoa taken from the vagina of an exhumed body that has been properly embalmed and remains reasonably intact can also be identified.

To determine which stains or fluids require further investigation, clothing or other fabrics can be scanned with ultraviolet light to detect the typical green-white fluorescence of semen. Soaking appropriate samples of clothing, fabric, or hair in physiologic saline solution elutes the semen and spermatozoa. Deposits of dried semen can be gently sponged from the victim's skin.

The two most common tests to identify semen are the determination of *acid phosphatase concentration* (the more sensitive test) and *microscopic examination* for the presence of spermatozoa. Acid phosphatase appears in semen in significantly greater concentrations than in any other body fluid. In microscopic examination, spermatozoa or head fragments can be identified on stained smears prepared directly from vaginal scrapings or aspirates, or from the concentrated sediment of eluates or lavages.

Like other body fluids, semen contains the soluble A, B, and H blood group substances in the approximately 80% of males who are genetically determined secretors (males who have the dominant secretor gene in a homozygous or heterozygous state). Thus, the male who has group A blood and is a secretor has soluble blood group A substance in his seminal fluid and group A substance on the surface of his red blood cells. This fact can be of considerable medicolegal importance. Semen analysis can demonstrate that the semen of a suspect in a rape or homicide investigation is different from or consistent with semen found in or on the victim's body.

exonerate or incriminate a criminal suspect (rare)
■ To rule out paternity on grounds of complete sterility (rare).

Patient preparation

For evaluation of fertility: Provide written instructions, and inform the patient that the most desirable specimen requires masturbation, ideally in a doctor's office or a laboratory. Instruct him to follow the doctor's orders regarding the period of continence before the test because it may increase his sperm count. Some doctors specify a fixed number of days, usually 2 to 5; others advise a period of continence equal to the usual interval between episodes of sexual intercourse.

If the patient prefers to collect the specimen at home, emphasize the importance of delivering the specimen to the laboratory within 1 hour after collection. Warn him not to expose the specimen to extreme temperatures or to direct sunlight (which can also increase its temperature). Ideally, it should remain at body temperature until liquefaction is complete (about 20 minutes). To deliver a semen specimen to the laboratory during cold weather, suggest that the patient keep the specimen container in a coat pocket on the way to the laboratory to protect it from the cold.

Alternatives to collection by masturbation include coitus interruptus or the use of a condom or special sheath. For collection by coitus interruptus, instruct the patient to withdraw immediately before ejaculation and to deposit the ejaculate in a suitable specimen container. For collection by condom, tell the patient to wash the condom with soap and water, rinse it thoroughly, and allow it to dry completely. (Powders or lubricants applied to the condom may be spermicidal.) Special sheaths that do not contain spermicides are also available for semen collection. After collection, instruct the patient to tie the condom, place it in a glass jar, and deliver it to the laboratory promptly.

Fertility may also be determined by collecting semen postcoitally from the female to assess the ability of the spermatozoa to penetrate the cervical mucus and remain active. The postcoital cervical mucus test should be performed 1 or 2 days before ovulation. After reviewing several months of basal body temperature, the provider will be able to advise the patient when to schedule testing.

A urine luteinizing hormone test may help predict ovulation in patients with irregular cycles. Instruct the couple to abstain from intercourse for 2 days and then to have sex 2 to 8 hours before the examination. Remind them to avoid using lubricants. Explain to the patient scheduled for this test that it takes only a few minutes. Tell her she'll be placed in the lithotomy position and the doctor will insert a speculum in the vagina to collect the specimen. She may feel some pressure but no pain during this procedure.

For semen collection from a rape victim: Explain to the patient that the doc-

tor will try to obtain a semen specimen from her vagina. Prepare her for insertion of the speculum as you would the patient scheduled for postcoital examination. Handle the patient's clothes as little as possible. If her clothes are moist, put them in a paper bag — not a plastic bag (which causes seminal stains and secretions to mold). Label the bag properly, and send it to the laboratory immediately.

Provide emotional support by speaking to the patient calmly and reassuringly. Encourage her to express her fears and anxieties. Listen sympathetically. If the patient is scheduled for vaginal lavage, tell her to expect a cold sensation when saline solution is instilled to wash out the specimen. To help her relax during this procedure, instruct her to breathe deeply and slowly through her mouth. Just before the test, instruct the patient to urinate, but warn her not to wipe the vulva afterward, because this may remove semen.

Equipment

For semen collection by masturbation, by coitus interruptus, or with a condom: clean plastic specimen container (for example, disposable urine or sputum container, with lid).

For semen collection from a rape victim: clean plastic specimen container ✦ vaginal speculum ✦ rubber gloves ✦ cotton-tipped applicators ✦ glass microscopic slides with frosted ends ✦ physiological (0.85%) saline solution ✦ Pap sticks ✦ Coplin jars containing 95% ethanol ✦ large syringe, rubber bulb, or other device suitable for vaginal lavage.

For postcoital specimen collection: clean plastic specimen container ✦ vaginal speculum ✦ rubber gloves ✦ cotton-tipped applicators ✦ glass microscopic slides with frosted ends ✦ 1-ml tuberculin syringe without a cannula or needle.

Procedure

To obtain a semen specimen for a fertility study, ask the patient to collect semen in a clean, plastic specimen container.

The doctor obtains a specimen from the vagina of a rape victim by direct aspiration, saline lavage, or a direct smear of vaginal contents, using a Pap stick or, less desirably, a cotton-tipped applicator. Dried smears are usually collected from the suspected rape victim's skin by gently washing the skin with a small piece of gauze, moistened with physiological saline solution. Prepare direct smears on glass microscopic slides after labeling the frosted end. Immediately place the smeared slides in Coplin jars containing 95% ethanol.

Before a postcoital examination, the examiner wipes any excess mucus from the external cervix and collects the specimen by direct aspiration of the cervical canal, using a 1-ml tuberculin syringe without a cannula or needle.

Precautions

▪ Instruct the male patient who wants to collect a specimen during coitus interruptus to prevent any loss of semen during ejaculation.

▪ Deliver all specimens, regardless of source or collection method, to the laboratory within 1 hour.

▪ Protect semen specimens for fertility studies from extreme temperatures and direct sunlight during delivery to the laboratory.

▪ *Don't lubricate the vaginal speculum.* Both oil and grease hinder examination of spermatozoa by interfering with smear preparation and staining and by inhibiting sperm motility through toxic ingredients. Instead, moisten the speculum with water or physiological saline solution.

▪ Use extreme caution in securing, labeling, and delivering all specimens to be used for medicolegal purposes. You may be asked to testify as to when, where, and from whom the specimen was obtained; the specimen's general appearance and identifying features; steps taken to ensure the specimen's integrity; and when, where, and to whom the specimen was delivered for analysis. If your facility uses routing slips for such specimens, fill them out carefully, and deposit them in the permanent medicolegal file.

Normal findings

Semen volume normally ranges from 0.7 to 6.5 ml. Paradoxically, many males in infertile marriages have increased semen volume. Abstinence for 1 week or more results in progressively increased semen volume. (With abstinence up to 10 days, the sperm count increases, sperm motility progressively decreases, and sperm morphology stays the same.) Liquefied semen is generally highly viscid, translucent, and gray-white, with a musty or acrid odor. After liquefaction, specimens of normal viscosity can be poured in drops. Normally, semen is slightly alkaline, with a pH of 7.3 to 7.9.

Other normal characteristics of semen: It coagulates immediately and liquefies within 20 minutes; the normal sperm count ranges from 20 to 150 million/ml; a least 40% of spermatozoa have normal morphology; and at least 20% of spermatozoa show progressive motility within 4 hours of collection. However, keep in mind that a reference value for the number of motile sperm per high power field has not been established. Some suggest that virtually any number of motile sperm is normal, while others maintain that 10 to 20 sperm per high power field is normal.

A spinnbarkeit (a measurement of the tenacity of the mucus) of at least 4" (10 cm) indicates adequate receptivity of the cervical mucus. Shaking or dead sperm may indicate antisperm antibodies.

Implications of results

Abnormal semen is *not* synonymous with infertility. Only one viable spermatozoon is needed to fertilize an ovum. Although a normal sperm count is more than 20 million/ml, many males with sperm counts below 1 million/ml have fathered normal children. Only males who can't deliver any viable spermatozoa in their ejaculate during sexual intercourse are absolutely sterile. Nevertheless, subnormal sperm counts, decreased sperm motility, and abnormal morphology are usually associated with decreased fertility.

Adding to the difficulty of diagnosing male infertility is the variability in count and motility that can be seen in successive semen specimens from the same individual. Other tests may be necessary to evaluate the patient's general health and metabolic status or the function of specific endocrine systems (pituitary, thyroid, adrenal, or gonadal).

Post-test care

■ Inform a patient who is undergoing infertility studies that test results should be available in 24 hours.

■ Refer a suspected rape victim to appropriate specialists for counseling: a gynecologist, psychiatrist, clinical psychologist, nursing specialist, member of the clergy, or representative of a community support group, such as Women Organized Against Rape.

Interfering factors

■ Delayed delivery of the specimen, exposure of the specimen to extreme temperatures or direct sunlight, or the presence of toxic chemicals in the specimen container or the condom can decrease the number of viable sperm.

■ An incomplete specimen — from faulty collection by coitus interruptus, for example — diminishes the volume of the specimen.

■ The most common cause of an abnormal postcoital test is poor timing within the menstrual cycle.

■ Prior cervical conization or cryotherapy as well as some medications, such as clomiphene citrate, may adversely affect cervical mucus and yield abnormal postcoital test results.

Sex chromatin tests

Although sex chromatin tests can screen for abnormalities in the number of sex chromosomes, they've been largely replaced by the full karyotype (chromosome analysis) test, which is faster, simpler, and more accurate. Sex chromatin tests are usually indicated for abnormal sexual development, ambiguous genitalia, amenorrhea, and suspected chromosomal abnormalities.

Fluorescent-staining techniques have identified the Y chromosome as the most fluorescent chromosome in a karyotype. Such fluorescence is confined to the long arm of the Y chromosome, which is tightly condensed in cells during interphase. When these cells are stained with quinacrine, a bright dot (the Y chromatin mass) appears in the nuclei of cells containing a Y chromosome. The number of such masses is identical to the number of Y chromosomes in the cell. Barr bodies (the X chromatin mass) can be stained with any nuclear stain, usually carbolfuchsin, to reveal the number of X chromatin bodies. (See *Understanding sex chromosome anomalies,* pages 718 and 719.)

Purpose

■ To quickly screen for abnormal sexual development (both X and Y chromatin tests)

Understanding sex chromosome anomalies

DISORDER AND CHROMOSOMAL ANEUPLOIDY	CAUSE AND INCIDENCE	PHENOTYPIC FEATURES
Klinefelter's syndrome ■ 47,XXY ■ 48,XXXY ■ 49,XXXXY ■ 48,XX,YY ■ 49,XXX,YY ■ Mosaics: XXY, XXXY, or XXXXY/XX or XY	Nondisjunction or improper chromatid separation during anaphase I or II of oogenesis or spermatogenesis results in abnormal gamete. 1 in 1,000 male births	■ Syndrome usually inapparent until puberty ■ Small penis and testes ■ Sparse facial and abdominal hair; feminine distribution of pubic hair ■ Somewhat enlarged breasts (gynecomastia) ■ Sexual dysfunction ■ Truncal obesity ■ Sterility ■ Possible mental retardation (greater incidence with increased X chromosomes)
Polysomy Y ■ 47,XYY	Nondisjunction during anaphase II of spermatogenesis causes both Y chromosomes to pass to the same pole and results in a YY sperm. 1 in 1,000 male births	■ Above-average stature (often over 72" [1.8 ml]) ■ Increased incidence of severe acne ■ May display aggressive, psychopathic, or criminal behavior ■ Normal fertility ■ Learning disabilities
Turner's syndrome (ovarian dysgenesis) ■ 45,XO ■ Mosaics: XO/XX or XO/XXX ■ Aberrations of X chromosomes, including deletion of short arm of one X chromosome, presence of a ring chromosome, or presence of an isochromosome on the long arm of an X chromosome	Nondisjunction during anaphase I or II of spermatogenesis results in sperm without any sex chromosomes. 1 in 3,500 female births (most common chromosome complement in first-trimester spontaneous abortions)	■ Short stature (usually under 57" [130 cm]) ■ Webbed neck ■ Low posterior hairline ■ Broad chest with widely spaced nipples ■ Underdeveloped breasts ■ Juvenile external gentalia ■ Primary amenorrhea common ■ Congenital heart disease (30% with coarctation of the aorta) ■ Renal abnormalities ■ Sterility due to underdeveloped internal reproductive organs (ovaries are merely strands of connective tissue) ■ No mental retardation, but possible problems with space perception and orientation
Other X polysomes ■ 47,XXX	Nondisjunction at anaphase I or II of oogenesis 1 in 1,400 female births	■ In many cases, no obvious anatomic abnormalities ■ Normal fertility

Understanding sex chromosome anomalies (continued)		
DISORDER AND CHROMOSOMAL ANEUPLOIDY	**CAUSE AND INCIDENCE**	**PHENOTYPIC FEATURES**
Other X polysomes (continued) ▪ 48,XXXX	Rare	▪ Mental retardation ▪ Ocular hypertelorism ▪ Reduced fertility
▪ 49,XXXXX	Rare	▪ Severe mental retardation ▪ Ocular hypertelorism with uncoordinated eye movement ▪ Abnormal development of sexual organs ▪ Various skeletal anomalies

▪ To aid assessment of an infant with ambiguous genitalia (X chromatin test only)

▪ To determine the number of Y chromosomes in an individual (Y chromatin test only).

Patient preparation

Explain to the patient or to his parents, if appropriate, why the test is being performed. Tell him the test requires that the inside of his cheek be scraped to obtain a specimen and who will perform the test. Inform the patient that the test takes only a few minutes but may require a follow-up chromosome analysis. Tell him that the laboratory generally requires as long as 4 weeks to complete the analysis.

Equipment

Wooden or metal spatula ✦ clean glass slide ✦ cell fixative.

Procedure

Scrape the buccal mucosa firmly with a wooden or metal spatula at least twice to obtain a specimen of healthy cells (vaginal mucosa is occasionally used in young women). Rub the spatula over the glass slide, making sure the cells are evenly distributed. Spray the slide with cell fixative, and send it to the laboratory with a brief patient history and indications for the test.

Precautions

Make sure the buccal mucosa is scraped firmly to ensure a sufficient number of cells. Check that the specimen isn't saliva, which contains no cells.

Normal findings

A normal female (XX) has only one X chromatin mass (the number of X chromatin masses discernible is one less than the number of X chromosomes in the cells examined). An X chromatin mass is ordinarily discernible in only 20% to 50% of the buccal mucosal cells of a normal female.

A normal male (XY) has only one Y chromatin mass (the number of Y chromatin masses equals the number of Y chromosomes in the cells examined).

Implications of results

In most laboratories, if less than 20% of the cells in a buccal smear contain an X chromatin mass, some cells are presumed to contain only one X chromosome, necessitating full karyotyping. Persons with female phenotypes and positive Y chromatin masses run a high risk of developing malignant tumors in their intra-abdominal gonads. In such persons, removal of these gonads is indicated, and should generally be performed before age 5.

Post-test care

After the cause of a chromosomal abnormality has been identified, the patient or his parents require genetic counseling. If a child is phenotypically of one sex and genotypically of the other, a medical team of knowledgeable doctors, psychologists, psychiatrists, and possibly educators must decide the child's sex. This careful evaluation should be made early to prevent developmental problems related to incorrect gender identification.

Interfering factors

■ Obtaining saliva instead of buccal cells provides a false specimen.

■ Failure to apply cell fixative to the slide allows cells to deteriorate.

■ The presence of bacteria or wrinkles in the cell membrane, analysis of degenerative cells, or use of an outdated stain can produce misleading results.

Chromosome analysis

Chromosomes — threadlike bodies in the cellular nucleus — each contain thousands of genes with biochemical programs for cell function that are stored in deoxyribonucleic acid (DNA),

the basic genetic material. (See *DNA, RNA, and protein synthesis.*) Chromosome analysis, an integral facet of cytogenetics, studies the relationship between the microscopic appearance of chromosomes and the person's phenotype — the expression of the genes in physical, biochemical, and physiological traits.

Light microscopy can visualize the chromosomes but is not yet capable of showing individual genes. Ideally, chromosomes should be studied during metaphase, the middle phase of mitosis, when new cell poles appear. (See *Understanding mitosis and meiosis,* pages 723 to 726.) Only rapidly dividing cell lines, such as bone marrow or neoplastic cells, permit direct, immediate study. Most other cell types require stimulation of mitosis by addition of phytohemagglutinin to the culture. Subsequently, the addition of colchicine (a cell poison) arrests the cell division in metaphase. Harvested, stained, and viewed under a microscope, the cells are finally photographed to provide a karyotype, the systematic arrangement of chromosomes in groupings according to size and shape.

Indications for the test determine the type of specimen required (blood, bone marrow, amniotic fluid, skin, or placental tissue) and the procedure. Umbilical cord sampling may also be used to perform chromosome analysis. (See *Percutaneous umbilical blood sampling,* page 727.)

Purpose

■ To identify chromosomal abnormalities, such as hypoploidy or hyperploidy, as the underlying cause of malformation, maldevelopment, or disease.

Patient preparation

Explain to the patient or to his parents, if appropriate, that this test identifies the underlying cause of maldevelopment or

DNA, RNA, and protein synthesis

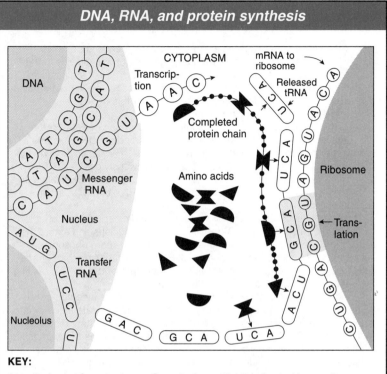

KEY:

A = adenine   G = guanine   C = cytosine   T = thymine   U = uracil

The chromosomes in every body cell are composed of genes, individual units of deoxyribonucleic acid (DNA) that carry genetic information. DNA also synthesizes the proteins that make up the enzymes fundamental to cellular growth and function.

Located primarily in the cell nucleus, the DNA molecule consists of two tightly coiled helical chains. The backbone of each chain consists of alternating units of deoxyribose (a 5-carbon sugar) and phosphate. A mixture of four nitrogenous bases — adenine (A), guanine (G), cytosine (C), and thymine (T) — form the links of each chain. (The sequential arrangement of these four bases represents the inherited genetic code of a particular trait.) From chain to chain, adenine is always paired with thymine and cytosine is always paired with guanine.

Ribonucleic acid (RNA) transmits genetic messages from DNA to the cytoplasmic ribosomes, site of protein formation. Single-stranded, RNA consists of alternating ribose-phosphate units and a mixture of four bases, three of which constitute DNA. The fourth base, uracil, replaces thymine. Various types of RNA are distinguished by the number of the components and the arrangement of their bases.

When a cell needs a specific protein enzyme to carry out a chemical reaction, the cell alerts the appropriate DNA molecule and protein synthesis begins. The double-stranded DNA helix unwinds and separates into individual

(continued)

DNA, RNA, and protein synthesis *(continued)*

chains. The bases of each chain are arranged in sequential triplets (or codons) that eventually determine the arrangement of amino acids in the final protein molecule. (The human body has only 20 types of amino acids available for protein construction. The total number and sequential combinations of these amino acids determine the many protein molecules in the body and their various biological properties.)

Next, the DNA code is transcribed onto a single strand of RNA. Before transcription can occur, however, the individual strands of DNA become a template or blueprint for a matching RNA molecule. The bases of DNA and RNA pair off according to the A-T, C-G pattern previously described. (However, in RNA uracil replaces thymine; therefore, the adenine in DNA takes on a new partner.) When base pairing is complete, the RNA and DNA strands separate.

Carrying a specific DNA code or message for amino acid formation, the newly formed messenger RNA (mRNA) leaves the nucleus and enters the cytoplasm. There, the mRNA attaches itself to one or more ribosomes, spherical bodies of protein and ribosomal RNA (rRNA) running through the cytoplasm. Attached, the ribosome travels the length of the mRNA, reading the genetic message in a process called *translation*.

As the ribosome translates the message, it calls for the insertion of the proper amino acids into the growing protein chain. To facilitate its entry into the protein chain, each amino acid binds with a complementary molecule of transfer RNA (tRNA). While one end of the tRNA molecule is firmly attached to its complementary amino acid, the other end (specific triplet arrangement of bases) joins corresponding triplet bases of mRNA. After the bases of tRNA and mRNA align, the newly formed protein frees itself of the ribosome to produce the enzyme needed for chemical reaction.

disease due to a chromosomal abnormality. Tell him who will perform the test and what kind of specimen will be required. Inform him when results will be available, according to the specimen required. For example, test results on a blood sample are generally available 72 to 96 hours after stimulation; analysis of skin biopsy specimens or amniotic fluid cells may take several weeks.

Procedure

As appropriate, collect a blood sample (in a 5- to 10-ml *green-top* [heparinized] tube), a tissue specimen, 1 ml of bone marrow, or at least 20 ml of amniotic fluid.

Precautions

■ Keep all specimens sterile, especially those requiring a tissue culture.

■ To facilitate interpretation of test results, send the specimen to the laboratory immediately, with a brief patient history and the indication for the test. If transport must be delayed, refrigerate the specimen but don't freeze it.

 ■ Before a skin biopsy, make sure the povidone-iodine solution is thoroughly removed with alcohol. This solution could prevent cell growth in the tissue culture.

(Text continues on page 727.)

Understanding mitosis and meiosis

All living cells arise from existing living cells. During an uninterrupted process of nuclear division known as *mitosis* (figures 1A to 6A), newly formed daughter nuclei receive the same diploid number (2n) of chromosomes as the parent cell.

Meiosis (figures 1B to 10B) — another kind of cell division, which takes place in two sequences — occurs in the gonads and produces ova or spermatozoa. During meiosis, the chromosomes in each sex cell or gamete are reduced to one-half the number (haploid or n) found in somatic cells. Despite this reduction, the diploid number is restored when an ovum and spermatozoon unite to form a new cell, or zygote. Without this reduction in each sex cell, the union of gametes would result in a zygote with twice the number of chromosomes as the parent cells.

MITOSIS

1A: Interphase

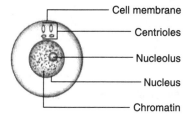

- Cell membrane
- Centrioles
- Nucleolus
- Nucleus
- Chromatin

2A: Late prophase

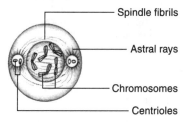

- Spindle fibrils
- Astral rays
- Chromosomes
- Centrioles

During interphase and before mitosis, the nondividing cell must duplicate its genetic material before distributing it to daughter cells. Although the nucleus and one or more nucleoli are visible, the chromosomes are seen only as a chromatinic mass. In this preliminary phase, the cylindrical centrioles migrate from their right angular position and equip themselves for cellular division.

Throughout prophase, the first stage of mitosis, both the nucleus and nucleoli become less distinct and finally disappear. Conversely, the chromosomes take shape and eventually appear as short, rodlike, mobile structures. As the centrioles continue to migrate toward opposite sides of the nucleus, they align thin, projecting fibrils or spindles. (Astral fibrils radiate from each centriole; spindle fibrils link them.) At the end of prophase, each chromosome has moved to the midpoint of one of the spindle fibrils making up the biconical spindle.

(continued)

Understanding mitosis and meiosis (continued)

3A: Metaphase

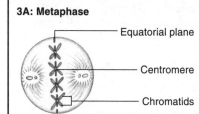

Equatorial plane

Centromere

Chromatids

When metaphase begins, the chromosomes are double-stranded structures consisting of two chromatids united by a single body called a centromere. Each chromosome is attached by its centromere to a fibril in the equatorial plane of the spindle. This brief phase ends when each centromere divides and each chromatid becomes a single-stranded chromosome.

4A: Late anaphase

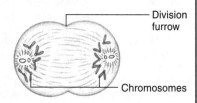

Division furrow

Chromosomes

Anaphase marks the migratory separation of each set of single-stranded chromosomes. By late anaphase, the chromosomes have neared their respective poles, and cytokinesis — division of the cytoplasm — has begun.

5A: Telophase

Nucleus

Nucleolus

Duplicated centrioles

Chromosomes

Telophase, the last stage of mitosis, reverses the processes of prophase. Having reached their respective poles, the two sets of chromosomes become encapsulated in newly developing nuclei that evolve as the spindles disappear. Likewise, the nuclei slowly reappear as the chromosomes become less visible, resembling the thin, intertwined filaments of early prophase. By late telophase, the centriole of each nucleus has replicated and cytokinesis has ended.

6A: Late telophase (interphase)

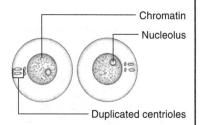

Chromatin

Nucleolus

Duplicated centrioles

When telophase, and hence mitosis, is complete, the newly formed nuclei typify interphase. Furthermore, each new daughter cell has the same number (46) and types of chromosomes (23) as its parent cell and can thus function characteristically.

Understanding mitosis and meiosis (continued)

MEIOSIS

1B: Late prophase I

Spindle — Centriole — Homologous pairs of double-stranded chromosomes

Usually, first meiotic prophase resembles mitotic prophase. Individual chromosomes become more transparent as the nucleoli and nuclear membrane fade, spindles form and centrioles polarize. In meiotic prophase I, paired homologous chromosomes — from the male and female pronuclei — move together toward the spindles' equator.

2B: Metaphase I

Equatorial plane

Because these double-stranded, homologous chromosomes are traveling side by side, each pair occupies a single fibral spindle during first metaphase. (In mitosis, each chromosome travels alone and thus occupies a separate fibral spindle.)

3B: Anaphase I

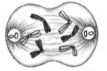

During mitosis, metaphase ends and anaphase begins when the centromeres linking the double-stranded chromosomes divide, leaving single-stranded chromosomes. In meiosis, however, such division does not occur. During anaphase I, therefore, double-stranded chromosomes comprising each homologous pair separate and polarize. Consequently, when cytokinesis occurs, the two daughter nuclei will have one of each type of chromosome or one-half the number of chromosomes as each parent cell.

4B: Telophase I

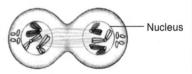

Nucleus

Meiotic and mitotic telophase are essentially alike. As cytokinesis ends, two new nuclei are formed and the spindles disappear. The difference, however, lies in the number of chromosomes per newly formed nuclei. When mitosis is complete, each daughter cell has the same number of chromosomes as the parent cell and is therefore diploid. Following meiosis, each new nucleus has only one of each type of chromosome or one-half the number of each parent cell, and is therefore haploid.

(continued)

Understanding mitosis and meiosis (continued)

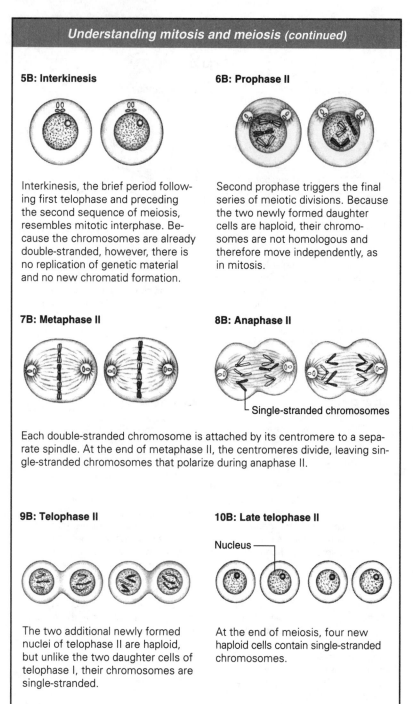

5B: Interkinesis

Interkinesis, the brief period following first telophase and preceding the second sequence of meiosis, resembles mitotic interphase. Because the chromosomes are already double-stranded, however, there is no replication of genetic material and no new chromatid formation.

6B: Prophase II

Second prophase triggers the final series of meiotic divisions. Because the two newly formed daughter cells are haploid, their chromosomes are not homologous and therefore move independently, as in mitosis.

7B: Metaphase II

8B: Anaphase II

Single-stranded chromosomes

Each double-stranded chromosome is attached by its centromere to a separate spindle. At the end of metaphase II, the centromeres divide, leaving single-stranded chromosomes that polarize during anaphase II.

9B: Telophase II

The two additional newly formed nuclei of telophase II are haploid, but unlike the two daughter cells of telophase I, their chromosomes are single-stranded.

10B: Late telophase II

Nucleus

At the end of meiosis, four new haploid cells contain single-stranded chromosomes.

Percutaneous umbilical blood sampling

Useful in chromosomal analysis, percutaneous umbilical blood sampling (PUBS) provides a fetal blood sample for karyotype, direct Coombs' test, or complete blood count. PUBS, sometimes called cordocentesis, can also be used to determine fetal blood type, check blood gas levels and acid-base status, and identify and treat isoimmunization.

To obtain a percutaneous umbilical blood sample, a needle is inserted transabdominally (using ultrasound guidance) into a fetal umbilical vessel. A blood sample is then tested to ensure that fetal and not maternal blood has been drawn. Possible complications include blood leakage at the puncture site, fetal bradycardia, or infection.

Normal findings

The normal cell contains 46 chromosomes: 22 pairs of nonsex chromosomes (autosomes) and 1 pair of sex chromosomes (Y for the male-determining chromosome, X for the female-determining chromosome). On a karyotype, chromosomes are arranged according to size and the location of their primary constrictions, or centromeres. The centromere may be medial (metacentric), slightly to one end of the chromosome (submetacentric), or entirely to one end (acrocentric). The largest chromosomes are displayed first; the others are arranged in order of decreasing size, with the two sex chromosomes traditionally placed last.

By convention, the centromere is always placed at the top in a karyotype. Thus, if the two pairs of chromosomal arms are of unequal length, the arm above the centromere will be shorter. The letter p designates the short arm; the letter q, the long arm.

Special stains identify individual chromosomes and locate and enumerate particular portions of chromosomes. Trypsin, alkali, heat denaturization, and Giemsa stain are used for visible light microscopy; quinacrine stain, for ultraviolet microscopy. These staining techniques produce nonuniform staining of each chromosome in a repetitive, banded pattern. The mechanism of chromosome banding is unknown but seems related to primary DNA sequence and protein composition of the chromosome.

Implications of results

Chromosomal abnormalities may be numerical or structural. Numerical deviation from the norm of 46 chromosomes is called aneuploidy. Less than 46 chromosomes is called hypoploidy; more than 46, hyperploidy. Special designations exist for whole multiples of the haploid number 23: diploidy for the normal somatic number of 46, triploidy for 69, tetraploidy for 92, and so forth. When the deviation occurs within a single pair of chromosomes, the suffix *-somy* is used, as in trisomy for the presence of three chromosomes instead of the usual pair, or monosomy for the presence of only one chromosome.

Aneuploidy most commonly follows failure of the chromosomal pair to separate (nondisjunction) during anaphase, the mitotic stage that follows metaphase. It may also result from anaphase lag, in which one of the normally separated chromosomes fails to move to a pole and is left out of the daughter cells. If nondisjunction or

Chromosome analysis findings

Specimens for chromosome analysis can be obtained from blood, bone marrow, skin, amniotic fluid, placental tissue, and tumor tissue. This chart lists the indications for chromosome analysis, the possible findings, and the implications of such findings.

SPECIMEN AND INDICATION	POSSIBLE FINDINGS	IMPLICATIONS
Blood		
To evaluate abnormal appearance of development suggesting chromosomal irregularity	Abnormal chromosome number (aneuploidy) or arrangement	Identifies specific chromosomal abnormality
To evaluate couple with history of miscarriages, or to identify balanced translocation carriers having unbalanced offspring	Normal chromosomes	Miscarriage unrelated to parenteral chromosomal abnormality
	Parental balanced translocation carrier	Increased risk of repeated abortion or unbalanced offspring indicates need for amniocentesis in future pregnancies
To detect chromosomal rearrangements in rare genetic diseases predisposing patient to malignant neoplasms	Chromosomal rearrangements, gaps, and breaks	Occurs in Bloom syndrome, Fanconi's syndrome, telangiectasia; patient predisposed to malignant neoplasms
Blood and bone marrow		
To identify Philadelphia chromosome and confirm chronic myelogenous leukemia	Translocation of chromosome 22q (long arm) to another chromosome (often chromosome 9)	Aids diagnosis of chronic myelogenous leukemia
	Aneuploidy (usually due to abnormalities in chromosomes 8 and 12)	Occurs in acute myelogenous leukemia
	Trisomy 21	Occasionally occurs in chronic lymphocytic leukemia cells
Skin		
To evaluate abnormal appearance or development suggesting chromosomal irregularity	All chromosomal abnormalities are possible.	Same as chromosomal abnormality in blood; rarely, mosaic individual has normal blood but abnormal skin chromosomes

	Chromosome analysis findings (continued)	

SPECIMEN AND INDICATION	POSSIBLE FINDINGS	IMPLICATIONS
Amniotic fluid		
To evaluate developing fetus with possible chromosomal abnormality	All chromosomal abnormalities are possible.	Same as chromosomal abnormality in blood or fetus
Placental tissue		
To evaluate products of conception after a miscarriage to determine if abnormality is fetal or placental in origin	All chromosomal abnormalities are possible.	Over 50% of aborted tissue is chromosomally abnormal
Tumor tissue		
For research purposes only	Many chromosomal abnormalities are possible.	Although malignant tumors are not associated with specific chromosomal aberrations, most are aneuploid (usually hyperploid).

anaphase lag occurs during meiosis, the cells of the zygote will all be the same. Errors in mitotic division after the formation of the zygote will produce more than one cell line (mosaicism).

Structural chromosomal abnormalities result from chromosome breakage. Intrachromosomal rearrangement occurs within a single chromosome in the following forms:

- *deletion:* loss of an end (terminal) or middle (interstitial) portion of a chromosome
- *inversion:* end-to-end reversal of a chromosome segment, which may be pericentric inversion (including the centromere) or paracentric inversion (occurring in only one arm of the chromosome)
- *ring chromosome formation:* breakage of both ends of a chromosome and reunion of the ends

- *isochromosome formation:* abnormal splitting of the centromere in a transverse rather than longitudinal plane.

Interchromosomal rearrangements (of more than one chromosome, usually two) also occur. The most common rearrangement is translocation, or exchange, of genetic material between two chromosomes. Translocations may be balanced, in which the cell neither loses nor gains genetic material; unbalanced, in which a piece of genetic material is gained or lost from each cell; reciprocal (in children), in which two chromosomes exchange material; or robertsonian, in which two chromosomes join to form one combined chromosome with little or no loss of material.

Implications of chromosome analysis results depend on the type of specimen and the indications for the test. (See *Chromosome analysis findings.*)

Post-test care

■ Provide appropriate post-test care, depending on the procedure used to collect the specimen.

■ Explain the test results and their implications to the patient or to the parents of a child with a chromosomal abnormality.

■ If necessary, recommend appropriate genetic or other counseling and follow-up care, such as an infant stimulation program for a child with Down syndrome.

Interfering factors

■ Chemotherapy may cause abnormal results, such as chromosome breaks.

■ Contamination of tissue with bacteria, fungus, or a virus may inhibit growth of the culture.

■ Inclusion of maternal cells in a specimen obtained by amniocentesis, with subsequent culturing, may cause false results.

Amniotic fluid analysis

Amniocentesis is the transabdominal needle aspiration of 10 to 20 ml of amniotic fluid for laboratory analysis. This test can be performed only when the amniotic fluid level reaches 150 ml, usually after the 16th week of pregnancy. Such analysis can detect several birth defects (especially Down syndrome and spina bifida), detect hemolytic disease of the newborn, detect gender and chromosomal abnormalities (through karyotyping), and determine fetal maturity (especially pulmonary maturity).

Amniotic fluid reflects important metabolic changes in the fetus, the placenta, and the mother. It protects the fetus from external trauma, allows the fetus to move, and provides for the fe-

tus an even body temperature and limited source of protein (10% to 15%). Although the origin of amniotic fluid is uncertain, its original composition is essentially the same as that of interstitial fluid. As the fetus matures, however, the amniotic fluid becomes progressively more diluted with hypotonic fetal urine.

One of the chief differences between amniotic fluid and maternal plasma during intrauterine development is the amniotic fluid's relatively high levels of uric acid, urea, and creatinine. The volume of amniotic fluid steadily rises from 50 ml at the end of the first trimester to an average of 1,000 ml near term; at 40 weeks' gestation, the volume decreases to 700 to 800 ml.

Amniocentesis is indicated when a pregnant woman is over age 35; has a family history of genetic, chromosomal, or neural tube defects; or has had a previous miscarriage. Complications from this test are rare but may include spontaneous abortion, trauma to the fetus or placenta, bleeding, premature labor, infection, and Rh sensitization from fetal bleeding into the maternal circulation. For this reason, amniocentesis is contraindicated as a general screening test. Abnormal test results or failure of the tissue cultures to grow may necessitate repetition of the test.

Purpose

■ To detect fetal abnormalities, particularly chromosomal and neural tube defects

■ To detect hemolytic disease of the newborn

■ To diagnose metabolic disorders, amino acid disorders, and mucopolysaccharidoses

■ To determine fetal age and maturity, especially pulmonary maturity (see *Shake test*)

■ To assess fetal health by detecting the presence of meconium or blood or by

Shake test

Amniotic fluid from mature fetal lungs contains surface-active material (surfactants). In this test (also known as the foam stability test), bubbles should appear on the surface of a test tube of amniotic fluid that is shaken vigorously if adequate amounts of surfactants are present.

Using a chemically clean 13x100 mm glass tube with a Teflon-lined screw cap or a rubber stopper, combine 1 ml of amniotic fluid and 1 ml of 95% ethanol. In another tube, combine 0.5 ml of amniotic fluid, 0.5 ml of normal saline solution, and 1 ml of 95% ethanol. Shake both tubes vigorously for 15 seconds, and place them upright in a rack for 15 minutes.

If a complete ring of bubbles is still evident in both tubes after 15 minutes (as shown), the test is positive and the risk of respiratory distress is low. A positive result in the second tube indicates pulmonary maturity. Negative results indicate a risk of respiratory distress. Blood or meconium in the fluid invalidates the test.

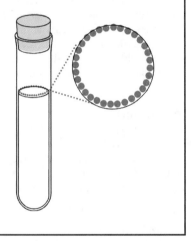

measuring amniotic levels of estriol and fetal thyroid hormone
■ To identify the fetus's gender when one or both parents are carriers of a sex-linked disorder.

Patient preparation

Describe the procedure to the patient, and explain that this test detects fetal abnormalities. Assess her understanding of the test, and answer any questions she may have. Inform her that she needn't restrict food or fluids. Tell her the test requires a specimen of amniotic fluid and who will perform the test. Advise her that normal test results can't guarantee a normal fetus because some fetal disorders are undetectable.

Make sure the patient has signed a consent form. Explain that she'll feel a stinging sensation when the local anesthetic is injected. Provide emotional support before and during the test, and reassure her that complications are rare.

Just before the test, ask her to urinate to minimize the risk of puncturing the bladder and aspirating urine instead of amniotic fluid.

Equipment

70% alcohol or povidone-iodine solution ✦ sponge forceps ✦ 2" x 2" gauze pads ✦ local anesthetic (1% lidocaine) ✦ sterile 25G needle ✦ 3-ml syringe ✦ sterile 20G to 22G spinal needle with stylet ✦ 10-ml syringe ✦ sterile amber or foil-covered 10-ml test tube.

Procedure

After determining fetal and placental position, usually through palpation and ultrasonography, the doctor locates a pool of amniotic fluid. After preparing the skin with an antiseptic and alcohol, he injects 1 ml of 1% lidocaine with a 25G needle, first intradermally and then subcutaneously. Then he inserts the 20G to 22G spinal needle, with a stylet, into the amniotic cavity and withdraws the stylet. After attaching a 10-ml syringe to the needle, he aspirates the fluid and places it in an amber or foil-covered test tube. Approximately 20 to 30 ml of fluid is drawn when cells from amniotic fluid are needed for culturing. After the needle is withdrawn, an adhesive bandage is placed over the needle insertion site.

Precautions

■ Instruct the patient to fold her hands behind her head to prevent her from accidentally touching the sterile field and causing contamination.
■ Send the specimen to the laboratory immediately.

Normal findings

Amniotic fluid should be clear but may contain white flecks of vernix caseosa when the fetus is near term. (See *Amniotic fluid analysis findings.*)

Implications of results

Blood in amniotic fluid is usually of maternal origin and doesn't indicate a fetal abnormality. However, it does inhibit cell growth and changes the level of other amniotic fluid constituents.

Large amounts of *bilirubin,* a breakdown product of red blood cells, may indicate hemolytic disease of the newborn. Normally, the bilirubin level increases from the 14th to the 24th week of pregnancy, then declines as the fetus matures, essentially reaching zero at term. Testing for bilirubin usually isn't performed until the 26th week, the earliest time that successful therapy for Rh sensitization can begin.

Meconium, a semisolid viscous material found in the fetal GI tract, consists of mucopolysaccharides, desquamated cells, vernix, hair, and cholesterol. Meconium passes into the amniotic fluid when hypoxia causes fetal distress and relaxation of the anal sphincter; it's a normal finding in breech presentation. Meconium in the amniotic fluid produces a peak of 410 mµ on the spectrophotometric analysis. However, serial amniocentesis may show a clearing of meconium over a 2- to 3-week period. If meconium is present during labor, the newborn's nose and throat require thorough cleaning to prevent meconium aspiration.

Creatinine, a product of fetal urine, increases in the amniotic fluid as the fetus's kidneys mature. The creatinine level usually exceeds 2 mg/dl in a mature fetus.

Alpha-fetoprotein (AFP) is a fetal alpha globulin produced first in the yolk sac and, later, in the parenchymal cells of the liver and GI tract. Fetal serum levels of AFP are about 150 times more than amniotic fluid levels; maternal serum levels are far less than amniotic fluid levels. High amniotic fluid levels indicate neural tube defects, but levels may remain normal if the defect is small and closed. Elevated AFP levels may occur in multiple pregnancy; in disorders such as omphalocele, congenital nephrosis, esophageal or duodenal atresia, cystic fibrosis, exomphalos, Turner's syndrome, and obstruction of the fetal bladder neck with hydronephrosis; and in impending fetal death.

The amount of *uric acid* in the amniotic fluid increases as the fetus matures, but these levels fluctuate widely and can't accurately predict fetal maturity. Laboratory studies indicate that severe erythroblastosis fetalis, familial hyperuricemia, and Lesch-Nyhan syndrome tend to increase the level of uric acid.

Amniotic fluid analysis findings

TEST	NORMAL FINDINGS	FETAL IMPLICATIONS OF ABNORMAL FINDINGS
Color	Clear, with white flecks of vernix caseosa in a mature fetus	Blood of maternal origin is usually harmless. "Port wine" fluid may indicate abruptio placentae. Fetal blood may indicate damage to the fetal, placental, or umbilical cord vessels.
Bilirubin	Absent at term	High levels indicate hemolytic disease of the newborn in isoimmunized pregnancy.
Meconium	Absent (except in breech presentation)	Presence indicates fetal hypotension or distress.
Creatinine	More than 2 mg/dl in a mature fetus	Decrease may indicate immature fetus (less than 37 weeks).
Lecithin-sphingomyelin ratio	More than 2 generally indicates fetal pulmonary maturity	Less than 2 indicates pulmonary immaturity and subsequent respiratory distress syndrome.
Phosphatidylglycerol	Present	Absence indicates pulmonary immaturity.
Glucose	Less than 45 mg/dl	Excessive increases at term or near term indicate hypertrophied fetal pancreas and subsequent neonatal hypoglycemia.
Alpha-fetoprotein	Variable, depending on gestation age and laboratory technique. Highest concentration (about 18.5 µg/ml) occurs at 13 to 14 weeks.	Inappropriate increases indicate neural tube defects, such as spina bifida or anencephaly, impending fetal death, congenital nephrosis, or contamination of fetal blood.
Bacteria	Absent	Presence indicates chorioamnionitis.
Chromosome	Normal karyotype	Abnormal karyotype may indicate fetal sex and chromosome disorders.
Acetylcholinesterase	Absent	Presence may indicate neural tube defects, exomphalos, or other serious malformations.

The Apt test

Blood in the amniotic fluid can be of maternal or fetal origin. The Apt test, based on the premise that fetal hemoglobin is alkali-resistant and adult hemoglobin changes to alkaline hematin after the addition of alkali, can differentiate between the two. This test may be performed on all bloody amniotic fluid samples.

To perform this test, dilute 1 ml of amniotic fluid with water until it turns pink. Centrifuge for 10 minutes, and decant the supernatant. Add five parts supernatant to one part 0.25 N (1%) sodium hydroxide, and observe for 1 to 2 minutes. Fetal blood appears red; maternal blood, yellow-brown. To confirm results, repeat the test with known maternal blood.

Estrone, estradiol, estriol, and *estriol conjugates* appear in amniotic fluid in varying amounts. Estriol, the most prevalent estrogen, increases from 25.7 ng/ml during the 16th to 20th weeks to almost 1,000 ng/ml at term. Severe erythroblastosis fetalis decreases the estriol level.

Blood in the amniotic fluid, which occurs in about 10% of amniocenteses, results from a faulty tap. If the origin is maternal, the blood generally has no special significance; however, "port wine" fluid may be a sign of abruptio placentae, and blood of fetal origin may indicate damage to the fetal, placental, or umbilical cord vessels by the amniocentesis needle. (See *The Apt test.*)

The Type II cells lining the fetal lung alveoli produce lecithin slowly in early pregnancy and then markedly increase production around the 35th week.

The *sphingomyelin* level parallels that of lecithin until the 35th week, when it gradually decreases. Measuring the lecithin-sphingomyelin (L/S) ratio confirms fetal pulmonary maturity (L/S ratio above 2) or suggests a risk of respiratory distress (L/S ratio below 2). However, fetal respiratory distress may develop in the fetus of a diabetic patient or in a fetus with sepsis even if the L/S ratio is greater than 2.

With pulmonary maturity, *phosphatidylglycerol* is present (indicating that respiratory distress is unlikely) and *phosphatidylinositol* levels decrease. Measuring *glucose* levels in the fluid can aid in assessing glucose control in a diabetic patient, but it isn't done routinely. A level greater than 45 mg/dl indicates poor maternal and fetal control. Insulin levels normally increase slightly from the 27th to the 40th week but increase sharply (up to 27 times normal) in a patient with poorly controlled diabetes.

Laboratory analysis can identify at least 25 different enzymes (usually in low concentrations) in amniotic fluid. The enzymes have few known clinical implications, although elevated *acetylcholinesterase* levels may occur with neural tube defects, exomphalos, and other serious malformations.

When the mother carries an X-linked disorder, determining the fetus's sex is important: A male fetus has a 50% chance of being affected; a female fetus won't be affected but has a 50% chance of being a carrier.

Chorionic villi sampling can detect fetal abnormalities up to 10 weeks sooner than amniocentesis. (See *Chorionic villi sampling.*)

Chorionic villi sampling

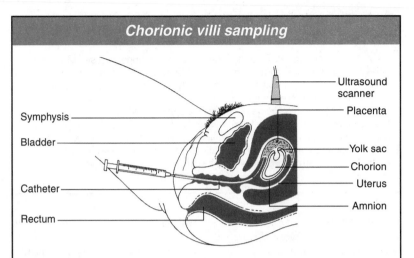

Symphysis

Bladder

Catheter

Rectum

Ultrasound scanner

Placenta

Yolk sac

Chorion

Uterus

Amnion

Chorionic villi sampling (CVS) is a prenatal test for quick detection of fetal chromosomal and biochemical disorders that is performed during the first trimester of pregnancy. Preliminary results may be available within hours; complete results within a few days. In contrast, amniocentesis cannot be performed before the 16th week of pregnancy, and the results aren't available for at least 2 weeks. Thus, CVS can detect fetal abnormalities up to 10 weeks sooner than amniocentesis.

The chorionic villi are fingerlike projections that surround the embryonic membrane and eventually give rise to the placenta. Cells obtained from an appropriate sample are of fetal, rather than maternal, origin and thus can be analyzed for fetal abnormalities. Samples are best obtained between the 8th and 10th weeks of pregnancy. (Before 7 weeks, the villi cover the embryo and make selective sampling difficult. After 10 weeks, maternal cells begin to grow over the villi and the amniotic sac begins to fill the uterine cavity, making the procedure difficult and potentially dangerous.)

Procedure
To collect a chorionic villi sample, place the patient in the lithotomy position. The doctor checks the placement of the patient's uterus bimanually, and then inserts a Graves' speculum and swabs the cervix with an antiseptic solution. If necessary, he may use a tenaculum to straighten an acutely flexed uterus, permitting cannula insertion. Guided by ultrasound and, possibly, endoscopy, he directs the catheter through the cannula to the villi. He applies suction to the catheter to remove about 30 mg of tissue from the villi. Then he withdraws the sample, places it in a petri dish, and examines it with a dissecting microscope. Part of the specimen is then cultured for further testing.

Indications and risks
CVS can be used to detect about 200 diseases prenatally. For example, direct analysis of rapidly dividing fetal cells can detect chromosome disorders; deoxyribonucleic acid analysis can detect hemoglobinopathies; and lysosomal enzyme assays can screen for lysosomal storage disorders, such as Tay-Sachs disease.

(continued)

Chorionic villi sampling (continued)
Unlike amniocentesis, CVS can't detect complications in cases of Rh sensitization, uncover neural tube defects, or determine pulmonary maturity. However, it may prove to be the best way to detect other serious fetal abnormalities early in pregnancy.
This test seems to provide reliable results except when the sample contains too few cells or the cells fail to grow in culture. Possible complications appear to be similar to those for amniocentesis: a small risk of spontaneous abortion, cramps, infection, and bleeding. However, recent studies have found limb malformations in neonates whose mothers underwent CVS.

Post-test care

■ Monitor fetal heart rate and maternal vital signs every 15 minutes for at least 30 minutes.

■ If the patient feels faint or nauseous or sweats profusely, position her on the left side to counteract uterine pressure on the vena cava.

■ Before the patient is discharged, instruct her to notify the doctor immediately if she experiences abdominal pain or cramping, chills, fever, vaginal bleeding or leakage of serous vaginal fluid, or fetal hyperactivity or unusual fetal lethargy.

Interfering factors

■ Failure to place the fluid specimen in an appropriate amber or foil-covered tube may result in abnormally low bilirubin levels.

■ Blood or meconium in the fluid adversely affects the L/S ratio.

■ Maternal blood in the fluid may lower creatinine levels.

■ Fetal blood in the fluid specimen invalidates the AFP results because even small amounts of fetal blood can double AFP concentrations.

■ Several disorders that are not associated with pregnancy (including infectious mononucleosis, cirrhosis, hepatic cancer, teratoma, endodermal sinus tumor, gastric carcinoma, pancreatic carcinoma, and subacute hereditary ty-

rosinemia) can cause increased AFP levels.

■ Plastic disposable syringes can be toxic to amniotic fluid cells.

ENDOSCOPY

Laparoscopy

Laparoscopy permits visualization of the peritoneal cavity by the insertion of a small fiber-optic telescope (laparoscope) through the anterior abdominal wall. This surgical technique may be used diagnostically to detect such abnormalities as cysts, adhesions, fibroids, and infection; it can also be used therapeutically to perform such procedures as lysis of adhesions, ovarian biopsy, tubal sterilization, removal of foreign bodies, and fulguration of endometriotic implants.

Laparoscopy has largely replaced laparotomy because it requires a smaller incision, it can be completed in less time, it's less costly, it causes less physiologic stress and therefore allows faster recovery, and it reduces the risk of postoperative adhesions. Nevertheless, laparotomy is usually preferred when extensive surgery is indicated. Potential risks of laparoscopy include a punctured visceral organ, causing bleeding or spilling of intestinal contents into the peritoneum.

Purpose

- To identify the cause of pelvic pain
- To help detect endometriosis, ectopic pregnancy, or pelvic inflammatory disease (PID)
- To evaluate pelvic masses or the fallopian tubes of infertile patients
- To stage carcinoma.

Patient preparation

Explain the procedure to the patient and tell her that it helps detect abnormalities of the uterus, fallopian tubes, and ovaries. Instruct her to fast after midnight before the test or for at least 8 hours before surgery. Tell her who will perform the procedure and that it takes 15 to 30 minutes.

Inform the patient that she'll receive a local or general anesthetic, and tell her whether the procedure will require an outpatient visit or overnight hospitalization. Warn her that she may experience pain at the puncture site and in the shoulder.

Make sure the patient or a responsible member of the family has signed a consent form. Check the patient's history for hypersensitivity to the anesthetic. Make sure all laboratory work is completed and results reported before the test. Instruct the patient to empty her bladder just before the test.

Equipment

Indwelling urinary or straight catheter ✦ sterile tray with scalpel, hemostats, needle holder, suture, and suture scissors ✦ Verees needle ✦ gas insufflator ✦ laparoscope ✦ fiberoptic light source and cable ✦ laparoscope sheath and trocar ✦ electrosurgical generator ✦ tenaculum and intrauterine manipulator ✦ probes, scissors, or forceps ✦ adhesive bandages.

Procedure

The patient is anesthetized and placed in the lithotomy position. The examiner catheterizes the bladder and then performs a bimanual examination of the pelvic area to detect abnormalities that may contraindicate the test and to ensure that the bladder is empty. After placing the tenaculum on the cervix and inserting a uterine manipulator, he makes an incision at the inferior rim of the umbilicus. He inserts the Verees needle into the peritoneal cavity and insufflates 2 to 3 L (2 to 3 qt) of carbon dioxide or nitrous oxide to distend the abdominal wall and provide an organ-free space for insertion of the trocar. Next, he removes the needle and inserts a trocar and sheath into the peritoneal cavity. After removing the trocar, he inserts the laparoscope through the sheath to examine the pelvis and abdomen. To evaluate tubal patency, the examiner infuses a dye through the cervix and observes the fimbria of the tubes for spillage.

After the examination, minor surgical procedures, such as ovarian biopsy, may be performed. A second trocar may be inserted at the pubic hairline to provide a channel for the insertion of other instruments.

Precautions

- Laparoscopy is contraindicated in patients with advanced abdominal wall cancer, advanced respiratory or cardiovascular disease, an intestinal obstruction, a palpable abdominal mass, a large abdominal hernia, chronic tuberculosis, or a history of peritonitis.
- During the procedure, check for proper drainage of the catheter.

Normal findings

The uterus and fallopian tubes are of normal size and shape, free from adhesions, and mobile. The ovaries are of normal size and shape; cysts and endometriosis are absent. Dye injected through the cervix flows freely from the fimbria.

Implications of results

An ovarian cyst appears as a bubble on the surface of the ovary. The cyst may be clear; filled with follicular fluid or serous or mucous material; or red, blue, or brown if filled with blood. Adhesions appear as sheets or strands of tissue that are almost transparent or thick and fibrous. Endometriosis resembles small, blue powder burns on the peritoneum or the serosa of any pelvic or abdominal structure. Fibroids appear as lumps on the uterus; hydrosalpinx, as an enlarged fallopian tube; ectopic pregnancy, as an enlarged or ruptured fallopian tube. In PID, infection or abscess is evident.

Post-test care

■ Monitor vital signs and urine output. Report sudden changes immediately; they may indicate complications.
■ After administration of a general anesthetic, check for an allergic reaction, and monitor electrolyte balance and hemoglobin and hematocrit levels, as ordered. Help the patient ambulate after recovery, as ordered.
■ Tell the patient he may resume his normal diet, as ordered.
■ Instruct the patient to restrict activity for 2 to 7 days, as ordered.
■ Reassure the patient that some abdominal and shoulder pain is normal and should disappear within 24 to 36 hours. Provide analgesics as ordered.

Interfering factors

■ Adhesions or marked obesity may obstruct the field of vision.

■ If tissue or fluid becomes attached to the lens, the examiner's vision may be obscured.
■ Soft tissues or the inside of a hollow viscus can't be palpated.

Hysteroscopy

In hysteroscopy, a small-diameter endoscope is used to visualize the interior of the uterus. Performed in the doctor's office under local anesthesia, this procedure has become widely used to investigate abnormal uterine bleeding. It also aids in the removal of polyps and in the diagnosis and treatment of other uterine abnormalities. Other investigational uses for hysteroscopy are being studied, including its possible use in sterilization procedures.

Purpose

■ To investigate abnormal uterine bleeding
■ To remove polyps
■ To evaluate infertile patients
■ To direct removal of intrauterine devices
■ To aid in diagnosis and treatment of intrauterine adhesions
■ To diagnose uterine fibroids.

Patient preparation

Explain the procedure to the patient, and tell her that it helps detect abnormalities in the uterus. Tell her that the doctor will perform this procedure in his office, usually using a local anesthetic. (However, if the patient's problems appear extensive, an in-hospital operative hysteroscopy would be indicated.) Inform the patient that the test should take place within the first week after the end of her menstrual cycle. Ask her when her last Papanicolaou test was performed and obtain the results. Tell her that the doctor will perform a complete pelvic examination before the hysteroscopy and that cultures of the vagina and cervix will be taken if necessary. Inform her that she'll be asked to empty her bladder before the test.

Tell the patient that she may have some vaginal bleeding and mild abdominal cramping after the test. Explain that the doctor may inflate her uterus with carbon dioxide (CO_2) gas so that he can see the interior of the uterus better. This gas will be absorbed and dispersed by her body and may cause upper abdominal or shoulder pain lasting 24 to 36 hours after the test. Recommend that she have a friend or relative drive her home.

Make sure the patient or a responsible family member has signed an informed consent form. Check the patient's history for hypersensitivity to the anesthetic. Make sure laboratory work is completed and results reported before the test.

Equipment
Vaginal speculum ✦ gas insufflator ✦ hysteroscope ✦ spinal needle ✦ 1% lidocaine ✦ sanitary pad. Equipment needs may vary, depending on the purpose of the procedure.

Procedure
Place the patient in a modified dorsal lithotomy position with her legs held in the stirrups. The doctor will expose the cervix using the smallest speculum possible, then suffuse the cervix with 1% lidocaine. Depending on the purpose of the procedure, a paracervical block, an anxiolytic, or an analgesic may also be used. In some cases, a regional or general anesthetic may be used.

The doctor will gently sound the endocervical canal and uterine cavity and will dilate the canal, as necessary, to insert the hysteroscope. (Modern hysteroscopes are 10" [25 cm] in length.) Visualization of the uterine cavity begins at the level of the internal os.

The two primary types of hysteroscopy are contact and panoramic. In *contact hysteroscopy*, the uterus isn't distended and only the area in direct contact with the hysteroscope can be viewed. In *panoramic hysteroscopy*, the more common type, an external illumination source and media (such as carbon dioxide gas) for distention are needed. This method allows visualization of the tissue from a distance.

Precautions
■ Hysteroscopy requires experience in topographic interpretation of the uterus and skill in manipulation of the required instruments.
■ During the procedure, monitor the patient's vital signs and discomfort level.

Normal findings
The interior of the uterus is normal in size and shape and free from adhesions and lesions.

Implications of results
Hysteroscopy may detect polyps, uterine wall tumors, and other uterine abnormalities.

Post-test care
■ Monitor vital signs.
■ Most patients have slight vaginal bleeding and lower abdominal cramping. Provide a sanitary pad if needed.
■ Severe cramps, dyspnea, and upper abdominal and right shoulder pain can develop if CO_2 passes into the peritoneal cavity. Reassure the patient that some abdominal and shoulder pain is normal and should disappear within 24 to 36 hours. Recommend that she have a friend or relative drive her home.
■ Provide analgesics as needed.

Interfering factors

- Heavy bleeding may interfere with visualization.
- A distended bladder or improper patient positioning can interfere with visualization.

DIRECT GRAPHIC RECORDING

External fetal monitoring

In external fetal monitoring, a noninvasive test, an electronic transducer and a cardiotachymeter amplify and record the fetal heart rate (FHR) while a pressure-sensitive transducer — the tokodynamometer — simultaneously records uterine contractions. This procedure records the baseline FHR (average FHR over two contraction cycles or 10 minutes), periodic fluctuations in the baseline FHR, and beat-to-beat heart rate variability. Fluctuations in FHR can occur as baseline changes (unrelated to uterine contractions) or as periodic changes (in response to uterine contractions). Such fluctuations are described in terms of amplitude (difference in beats per minute [bpm] between baseline readings and maximum or minimum fluctuation), lag time (difference between the peak of the contraction and the lowest point of deceleration), and recovery time (difference between the end of the contraction and the return to the baseline FHR).

External fetal monitoring is also used for other tests of fetal health — the nonstress test and the contraction stress test (CST). The relationship between FHR and the uterine contraction pattern is described by acceleration (transient rise in FHR lasting longer than 15 seconds and associated with a uterine contraction) and deceleration (transient fall in FHR related to a uterine contraction).

Purpose

- To measure FHR and the frequency of uterine contractions
- To evaluate antepartum and intrapartum fetal health during stress and nonstress situations
- To detect fetal distress
- To determine the necessity for internal fetal monitoring.

Patient preparation

Describe the procedure to the patient and her partner or family, and answer any questions they may have. Explain that the test assesses fetal health. If monitoring is to be performed antepartum, instruct the patient to eat a meal just before the test to increase fetal activity, which decreases the test time. If the patient is still smoking, advise her to abstain for 2 hours before testing because smoking decreases fetal activity.

Assure her that external fetal monitoring is painless and noninvasive, and that it won't hurt the fetus or interfere with labor. Tell her she may have to restrict movement during baseline readings but that she may change position between readings. Make sure the patient has signed a consent form.

Equipment

Tokodynamometer (to measure uterine contractions) ◆ ultrasonic transducer (to amplify FHR) ◆ cardiotachymeter (to record FHR) ◆ mineral oil or ultrasound transmission jelly ◆ elastic band, stockinette, or abdominal strap.

Procedure

Place the patient in the semi-Fowler or left lateral position, with her abdomen exposed. Cover the ultrasonic transducer receiver crystal with ultrasound transmission jelly. After palpating the abdomen to identify the fetal chest area, locate the most distinct fetal heart sounds, and secure the ultrasound transducer over this area with the elastic band, stockinette, or abdominal strap. Check the recordings to ensure an adequate printout, and verify the fetal monitor's alarm boundaries.

During monitoring, periodically check the elastic band, stockinette, or abdominal strap securing the transducer to ensure that it fits tight enough to produce good tracing but is loose enough to be comfortable. As labor progresses, reposition the pressure transducer as needed so that it remains on the fundal portion of the uterus. You may have to reposition the ultrasonic transducer as fetal position changes.

For antepartum monitoring with non-stress test: Tell the patient to hold the pressure transducer in her hand and to push it each time she feels the fetus move. Within a 20-minute period, monitor the baseline FHR until you record two fetal movements that last longer than 15 seconds each and cause heart rate accelerations of more than 15 bpm from the baseline. If you can't obtain two FHR accelerations, wait 30 minutes, shake the patient's abdomen to stimulate the fetus, and repeat the test.

For antepartum monitoring with CST: Induce contractions by oxytocin infusion or nipple stimulation (endogenous oxytocin). If you administer oxytocin, infuse a dilute solution at a rate of 1 mU/minute, and increase the oxytocin rate until the patient experiences three contractions within 10 minutes, each lasting longer than 45 seconds. If nipple stimulation is used, tell the patient to stimulate one nipple by hand until contractions begin. If a second contraction doesn't occur in 2 minutes, have her restimulate the nipple. Stimulate both nipples if contractions don't occur in 15 minutes. Continue the test

until 3 contractions occur in 10 minutes. If no decelerations occur during three contractions, the patient may be discharged. Late decelerations during any of the contractions require notification of the doctor and additional testing. (See *Contraction stress test,* page 742.)

For intrapartum monitoring: Secure the pressure transducer with an elastic band, stockinette, or abdominal strap over the area of greatest uterine electrical activity during contractions (usually the fundus). Adjust the machine to record 0 to 10 mm Hg pressure between palpable contractions. (Readings during contractions vary, depending on the tightness of the bands, the amount of adipose tissue, and the placement of the pressure transducer.) Reposition the ultrasound and pressure transducers, as necessary, to ensure continuous accurate readings. Review the tracing frequently for baseline abnormalities, periodic changes, variability changes, and uterine contraction abnormalities. Record maternal movement, administration of drugs, and procedures performed directly on the tracing so that changes in the tracing can be evaluated in view of these activities. Report any abnormalities immediately.

Precautions
During CST, watch for fetal distress with oxytocin infusion or nipple stimulation.

Reference values
Normally, FHR baseline ranges from 120 to 160 bpm, with 5 to 25 bpm variability.

For antepartum nonstress test: If two fetal movements associated with FHR acceleration of more than 15 bpm from baseline occur within 20 minutes, the fetus is considered healthy and should remain so for another week.

For contraction stress test: If three contractions occur during a 10-minute pe-

Contraction stress test

The contraction stress test measures the fetus's ability to withstand the stress of contractions induced before actual labor begins. Late decelerations in the fetal heart rate in response to uterine contractions during this test may indicate that the placenta can't deliver enough oxygen to the fetus. Placental insufficiency may result from maternal vascular disease associated with diabetes mellitus, preeclampsia, or chronic hypertension. Intrauterine growth retardation, postmaturity syndrome, and Rh isoimmunization may also cause fetal compromise.

Because the contraction stress test mimics labor, it's contraindicated in patients who have had a previous cesarean section or placenta previa and in those likely to have premature labor (as in premature rupture of the membrane, multiple pregnancy, or incompetent cervix).

riod, with no late decelerations, the fetus is considered healthy and should remain so for another week.

Implications of results

Bradycardia — an FHR of less than 120 bpm — may indicate fetal heart block, malposition, or hypoxia. Fetal bradycardia may also be drug-induced.

Tachycardia — an FHR of more than 160 bpm — may result from vagolytic drugs; maternal fever, tachycardia, or hyperthyroidism; early fetal hypoxia; or fetal infection or arrhythmia. Decreased variability — a fluctuation of less than 5 bpm in the FHR — may be due to fetal cardiac arrhythmia or heart block; fetal hypoxia, CNS malformation, or infection; or use of vagolytic drugs.

When FHR patterns indicate fetal distress, fetal oxygenation can often be improved by turning the mother on her side (preferably the left) to alleviate supine hypoxia; by giving oxygen to the mother; or by loading maternal fluids to increase placental perfusion. If the FHR returns to normal, labor may continue. If abnormal FHR patterns persist, cesarean delivery may be required.

Accelerations in FHR may result from early hypoxia. They may precede or follow variable decelerations and may indicate a breech position (See *Comparing decelerated fetal heart rates and uterine contractions.*)

For antepartum nonstress tests: A positive nonstress test result (less than two accelerations of FHR that last longer than 15 seconds each, with a heart rate acceleration over 15 bpm) indicates an exaggerated risk of perinatal morbidity and mortality, and usually necessitates performance of the CST. But CST produces a high rate of false-positive results.

For CST: Persistent late decelerations during two or more contractions may indicate increased risk of fetal morbidity or mortality. Hyperstimulation (long or frequent uterine contractions) or suspicious results require repetition of the test on the following day. If results are still positive, internal fetal monitoring or cesarean birth may be necessary.

Post-test care

Repeat antepartum monitoring weekly as long as indications, such as pregnancy over 42 weeks' gestation or fetal growth retardation, persist.

Interfering factors

▪ Drugs that affect the sympathetic and the parasympathetic nervous systems may depress FHR.

Comparing decelerated fetal heart rates and uterine contractions

Unlike variable decelerations, early and late decelerations in the fetal heart rate (FHR) correspond to uterine contractions.

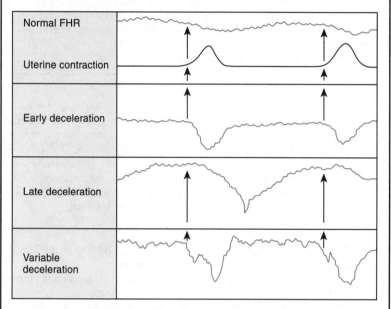

Decelerations in FHR may be affected by uterine contractions. The three types of FHR decelerations — early, late, and variable — occur at different points in the contraction phase.

Early FHR decelerations occur at onset of uterine contraction and reach their lowest point at the peak of the contraction. In early deceleration, FHR returns to the average baseline by the end of the contraction. FHR produces a smooth wave pattern that mirrors the uterine contraction. There is a consistent relationship between the fall in FHR and the uterine contractions. Early deceleration is usually benign and is most commonly caused by compression of the fetal head. This pattern often occurs with advanced dilation (more than 7 cm).

Late decelerations begin about 20 seconds after onset of a contraction and reach their lowest point well after the contraction has peaked. In late deceleration, FHR recovery occurs later than 15 seconds following the contraction. Although the FHR tracing in late deceleration resembles the smooth wave of early deceleration, its implications are far more serious. Late decelerations usually result from uteroplacental insufficiency and may lead to fetal death. When associated with increased variability or with tachycardia and no variability, late decelerations indicate fetal central nervous system depression and myocardial hypoxia.

(continued)

> ### *Comparing decelerated fetal heart rates and uterine contractions (continued)*
>
> Variable decelerations — sudden drops in the FHR — may occur at any time during a contraction. After the decline, baseline FHR recovery may be rapid or prolonged. Because the fall in FHR is unrelated to uterine contractions, wave patterns also vary. Variable decelerations occur in about 50% of all labors and are usually associated with transitory umbilical cord compression. But a severe drop (to less than 70 beats/minute for more than 60 seconds) may indicate fetal acidosis, hypoxia, and low Apgar scores.

■ Maternal position (particularly if supine) may cause artifactual fetal distress.
■ Maternal obesity, or excessive maternal or fetal activity may inhibit recording of uterine contractions or of FHR.
■ Loose or dirty leads or transducer connections may cause artifacts.

Internal fetal monitoring

In internal fetal monitoring, an invasive procedure, an electrode attached directly to the fetal scalp measures the fetal heart rate (FHR) — especially its beat-to-beat variability — and a fluid-filled catheter that has been introduced into the uterine cavity measures the frequency and pressure of uterine contractions. This procedure is performed exclusively during labor, after the membranes have ruptured and the cervix has dilated 1¼" (3 cm), with the fetal head lower than the −2 station.

Internal monitoring is indicated when external monitoring provides inadequate or suspicious data. Because internal monitoring records FHR directly, it supplies more accurate information about fetal health than external monitoring; measuring the pressure of uter-

ine contractions allows better assessment of the progress of labor. Consequently, internal monitoring is especially useful in determining if cesarean delivery is necessary. Risks to the mother (perforated uterus or intrauterine infection) or to the fetus (scalp abscess or hematoma) are minimal.

Purpose
■ To monitor FHR, especially beat-to-beat variability
■ To measure the frequency and pressure of uterine contractions
■ To evaluate intrapartum fetal health
■ To supplement or replace external fetal monitoring.

Patient preparation
Describe the procedure to the patient, and answer any questions she may have. Explain that this test provides an accurate assessment of fetal health. Warn her that she may feel mild discomfort when the uterine catheter and scalp electrode are inserted, but reassure her that this part of the procedure takes only a few minutes. Make sure the patient has signed a consent form.

Equipment
Sterile fetal scalp electrode and guide tube ✦ intrauterine pressure catheter ✦ catheter guide ✦ pressure transducer ✦ fetal heart monitor.

Understanding internal fetal monitoring

In internal fetal monitoring, an electrode is attached to the fetal scalp. The resultant fetal electrocardiograms (FECGs) are transmitted to an amplifier. Subsequently, a cardiotachometer measures the interval between FECGs and plots a continuous fetal heart rate (FHR) graph, which is displayed on a two-channel oscilloscope screen. Intrauterine catheters attached to a transducer in the leg plate measure the frequency and pressure of uterine contractions, which are plotted below the FHR graph.

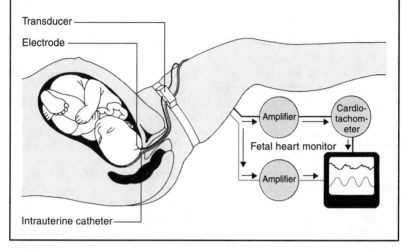

Procedure

For measuring FHR: Place the patient in the dorsal lithotomy position, and prepare her perineal area for a vaginal examination, explaining each step of the procedure as it's performed. As the procedure begins, ask the patient to breathe through her mouth and to relax her abdominal muscles. After the vaginal examination, the fetal scalp is palpated, and an area not over a fontanel is identified. Then the plastic guide tube surrounding the small corkscrew-type electrode is introduced into the cervix, pressed firmly against the fetal scalp, and rotated 180 degrees clockwise to insert the electrode into the scalp. After the electrode wire is tugged slightly to make sure it's attached properly, the tube is withdrawn, leaving the electrode in place.

Next, after a conduction medium is applied to a leg plate, the leg plate is strapped to the mother's thigh. The electrode wires are attached to the leg plate, and a cable from the leg plate is plugged into the fetal monitor. To check proper placement of the scalp electrode, the monitor is turned on and the electrocardiogram button is pressed; an FHR signal indicates proper electrode attachment. (See *Understanding internal fetal monitoring*.)

For measuring uterine contractions: Before inserting the uterine catheter, fill it with sterile normal saline solution to prevent air emboli. Explain each step of the procedure to the patient, and ask her to breathe deeply through her mouth and to relax her abdominal muscles. After the vagina has been examined and the presenting part of the fetus has been palpated, the fluid-filled catheter and catheter guide are inserted $\frac{3}{8}$" to $\frac{3}{4}$" (1 to 2 cm) into the cervix, usually between the fetal head and the posterior cervix. The catheter is then gently inserted into the uterus until the black mark on the catheter is flush with the vulva. (The catheter guide should *never* be passed deeply into the uterus.) Next, the guide is removed and the catheter is connected to a transducer that converts the intrauterine pressure, as measured by the fluid in the catheter, to an electrical signal. To standardize pressure readings, the transducer is exposed to air (it should measure zero pressure). The system is then closed to the air and intrauterine pressure readings are checked.

Precautions

■ Internal fetal monitoring is contraindicated in the presence of uncertainty as to the fetal presenting part, technical inability to attach the lead, or cervical or vaginal herpes lesions.
■ Prevent artifactual pressure readings by flushing the pressure transducer with normal saline solution; to relieve catheter obstruction (by vernix caseosa, for example), inject a small amount of sterile normal saline solution into the catheter (while the transducer is isolated from the system).
■ Make sure a low heart rate is actually the FHR, not the maternal heart rate.
■ Ensure that the fetal scalp electrode and the uterine catheter are removed before cesarean delivery.

Reference values

Normally, FHR ranges from 120 to 160 beats per minute (bpm), with a variability of 5 to 25 bpm from FHR baseline. (See *Normal intrauterine pressure readings during labor.*)

Implications of results

Bradycardia — an FHR of less than 120 bpm — may indicate fetal heart block,

malposition, or hypoxia. Fetal bradycardia may also result from maternal ingestion of certain drugs, such as propranolol or narcotic analgesics.

Tachycardia — an FHR of more than 160 bpm — may result from maternal use of vagolytic drugs; maternal fever, tachycardia, or hyperthyroidism; early fetal hypoxia; fetal infection or arrhythmia; or prematurity.

Decreased variability — fluctuation of less than 5 bpm from FHR baseline — may result from maternal use of vagolytic drugs; fetal cardiac arrhythmia or heart block; or fetal hypoxia, CNS malformation, or infection.

Early decelerations (slowing of FHR at onset of the contraction, with recovery to baseline no greater than 15 seconds after completion of the uterine contraction) are related to fetal head compression and usually mean that the fetus is healthy. Late decelerations (slowing of FHR, with onset after the start of the contraction, a lag time greater than 20 seconds, and a recovery time greater than 15 seconds) may be related to uteroplacental insufficiency, fetal hypoxia, or acidosis. Recurrent and persistent late decelerations with decreased variability usually indicate serious fetal distress, which may result from conduction (spinal, caudal, or epidural) anesthesia or fetal depression. Variable decelerations (sudden precipitous drops in FHR unrelated to uterine contractions) are commonly related to cord compression. A severe drop in FHR (to less than 70 bpm for longer than 60 seconds) with decreased variability indicates fetal distress and may result in a neonate with CNS depression.

When FHR patterns indicate fetal distress, fetal oxygenation can often be improved by loading maternal fluids to increase placental perfusion, turning the mother on her side (preferably the left) to alleviate supine hypotension, and administering oxygen to the mother. If

Normal intrauterine pressure readings during labor

STAGE OF LABOR	CONTRACTIONS PER 10 MINUTES	BASELINE PRESSURE	PRESSURE DURING CONTRACTION
Prelabor	1 to 2	—	25 to 40 mm Hg
First stage	3 to 5	8 to 12 mm Hg	30 to 40 mm Hg (or more)
Second stage	5	10 to 20 mm Hg	50 to 80 mm Hg

these measures return heart rate patterns to normal, labor may continue. If abnormal patterns persist, cesarean delivery may be necessary. Poor beat-to-beat variability without periodic patterns may indicate fetal stress, requiring further evaluation, such as analysis of fetal blood gases.

Decreased intrauterine pressure during labor that's not progressing normally may require oxytocin stimulation. Elevated intrauterine pressure readings may indicate abruptio placentae or overstimulation from oxytocin, possibly resulting in fetal distress due to decreased placental perfusion.

Post-test care
■ After removal of the fetal scalp electrode, apply antiseptic or antibiotic solution to the site of attachment.
■ Watch for signs of fetal scalp abscess or maternal intrauterine infection.

Interfering factors
Drugs that affect the parasympathetic and the sympathetic nervous systems may influence FHR.

RADIOGRAPHY

Mammography

Mammography is a radiographic technique used to detect breast cysts or tumors, especially those not palpable on physical examination. In xeromammography, an electrostatically charged plate records the X-ray images and transfers them to a special paper. Biopsy of suspicious areas may be required to confirm malignancy. Mammography may follow screening procedures such as ultrasonography or thermography. (See *Using ultrasound to detect breast cancer,* page 748.) Although 90% to 95% of malignant breast tumors can be detected by mammography, this test produces many false-positive results.

The American College of Radiologists and the American Cancer Society have established separate guidelines for the use and potential risks of mammography. (See *Guidelines for mammography,* page 749.) Both groups agree that despite low radiation levels (0.1 to 0.3 rad), the test is contraindicated during pregnancy.

Magnetic resonance imaging is becoming a more popular method of breast imaging; it tends to be highly sen-

Using ultrasound to detect breast cancer

Ultrasonography is especially useful for diagnosing tumors less than ¼" in diameter. It's also helpful in distinguishing cysts from solid tumors in dense breast tissue. As in other ultrasound techniques, a transducer is used to focus a beam of high-frequency sound waves through the patient's skin and into the breast. The sound waves then bounce back to the transducer as an echo that varies in strength with the density of the underlying tissues. A comput-er processes these echoes and displays the resulting image on a screen for interpretation.

Ultrasound can show all areas of a breast, including the difficult area close to the chest wall, which is hard to study with radiographs. When used as an adjunct to mammography, ultrasound increases diagnostic accuracy; when used alone, it's more accurate than mammography in examining the denser breast tissue of young patients.

sitive but not very specific, leading to biopsies of many benign lesions.

Purpose
- To screen for malignant breast tumors
- To investigate palpable and unpalpable breast masses, breast pain, or nipple discharge
- To help differentiate between benign breast disease and malignant tumors
- To monitor patients with breast cancer who have been treated with breast-conserving surgery and radiation.

Patient preparation
Assess the patient's understanding of the test, answer her questions, and correct any misconceptions. Tell her who will perform the test and where, and assure her that the test is usually painless. Tell the patient not to use underarm deodorant or powder the day of her examination to avoid having confusing shadows on the film. If she has breast implants, tell her to inform the staff when she schedules the mammogram so that a technologist familiar with imaging breast implants is on duty.

Inform her that although the test takes only about 15 minutes to perform, she may be asked to wait while the films are checked to make sure they're readable. Advise her that the test has a high rate of false-positive results.

Just before the test, give her a gown to wear that opens in the front, and ask her to remove all jewelry and clothing above the waist.

Equipment
Mammograph ✦ X-ray film ✦ plastic compressor.

Procedure
The patient is asked to rest one of her breasts on a table above an X-ray cassette. The compressor is placed on the breast, and the patient is told to hold her breath. Then a radiograph is taken of the craniocaudal view. The machine is rotated, the breast is compressed again, and a radiograph of the lateral view is taken. The procedure is then repeated on the other breast. After the films are developed, they are checked to make sure they're readable.

Precautions
Mammography is never a substitute for biopsy because it may not reveal clinical cancer.

Guidelines for mammography

The American Cancer Society (ACS) recommends that all women have a screening mammogram between ages 35 and 39 as well as a clinical physical examination of the breast every 3 years from age 20 to 39. For women age 40 and older, the ACS recommends a yearly mammogram and a yearly physical examination of the breast.

Normal findings

A normal mammogram reveals normal ducts, glandular tissue, and fat architecture. No abnormal masses or calcifications should be seen.

Implications of results

Well-outlined, regular, and clear spots suggest benign cysts; irregular, poorly outlined, and opaque areas suggest a malignant tumor. Malignant tumors are generally solitary and unilateral, whereas benign cysts tend to occur bilaterally. Findings that suggest cancer require further tests, such as biopsy, for confirmation.

Post-test care

None.

Interfering factors

■ Very glandular breasts (common under age 30) and previous breast surgery can impair readability of the films.

■ Powders or salves on the breast may cause false-positive results.

■ Failure to remove jewelry and clothing from the X-ray field may result in false-positive findings or unsatisfactory films.

■ Breast implants may prevent detection of masses.

Hysterosalpingography

Hysterosalpingography is a radiologic examination that allows visualization of the uterine cavity, the fallopian tubes, and the peritubal area. The procedure consists of taking fluoroscopic X-rays as a contrast medium flows through the uterus and the fallopian tubes. Generally performed as part of an infertility study, this test also helps evaluate the cause of repeated miscarriage and may be used as a follow-up to surgery, especially uterine unification procedures and tubal reanastomosis.

Although ultrasonography has virtually replaced hysterosalpingography in detecting foreign bodies such as a dislodged intrauterine device, it can't evaluate tubal patency, which is the main purpose of hysterosalpingography. Risks of this test include uterine perforation, intravascular injection of the contrast medium, and exposure to potentially harmful radiation.

Purpose

■ To confirm tubal abnormalities, such as adhesions and occlusion

■ To confirm uterine abnormalities, such as the presence of foreign bodies, congenital malformations, and traumatic injuries

- To confirm the presence of fistulas or peritubal adhesions.

Patient preparation

Explain to the patient that this test confirms uterine and fallopian tube abnormalities. Tell her who will perform the test and where and that it takes about 15 minutes. The test should be performed 2 to 5 days after menstruation ends.

Advise the patient that she may experience moderate cramping from the procedure; however, she may receive a mild sedative, such as diazepam, or a nonprescription prostaglandin inhibitor, if ordered, 30 minutes before the procedure.

Equipment

Antiseptic cleansing solution ✦ sterile needle ✦ contrast medium ✦ vaginal speculum ✦ tenaculum ✦ cannula, with acorn tip on one end and luer-lock on the other ✦ X-ray machine with fluoroscopic capabilities.

Procedure

With the patient in the lithotomy position, a scout film is taken. Then a speculum is inserted in the vagina, the tenaculum is placed on the cervix, and the cervix is cleaned. Next, the cannula is inserted into the cervix and anchored to the tenaculum. After the contrast medium is injected through the cannula, the uterus and the fallopian tubes are viewed fluoroscopically, and radiographs are taken. To take oblique views, the X-ray table may be tilted or the patient asked to change position. Films may also be taken later to evaluate spillage of contrast medium into the peritoneal cavity.

Precautions

- Hysterosalpingography is contraindicated in menstruating patients and in those with undiagnosed vaginal bleeding or pelvic inflammatory disease.
- Watch for an allergic reaction to the contrast medium, such as hives, itching, or hypotension.

Normal findings

Films should reveal a symmetrical uterine cavity; the contrast medium should course through fallopian tubes of normal caliber, spill freely into the peritoneal cavity, and not leak from the uterus.

Implications of results

An asymmetrical uterus suggests intrauterine adhesions or masses, such as fibroids or foreign bodies; impaired contrast flow through the fallopian tubes suggests partial or complete blockage due to intraluminal agglutination, extrinsic compression by adhesions, or perifimbrial adhesions. Leakage of contrast medium through the uterine wall suggests fistulas. Laparoscopy with contrast instillation confirms positive or equivocal findings.

Post-test care

- Watch for signs of infection, such as fever, pain, increased pulse rate, malaise, and muscle ache.
- Assure the patient who experiences cramps or a vagal reaction (slow pulse rate, nausea, and dizziness) that these symptoms are transient.

Interfering factors

- Tubal spasm or excessive traction may cause the appearance of a stricture in normal fallopian tubes.
- Excessive traction can displace adhesions, making the fallopian tubes appear normal.

ULTRASONOG-RAPHY

Pelvic ultrasonography

In pelvic ultrasonography, a crystal generates high-frequency sound waves that are reflected to a transducer, which converts sound energy into electrical energy and forms images of the interior pelvic area on a screen. Ultrasound techniques include *A-mode* (amplitude modulation), a one-dimensional system that records only distances between interfaces (recorded as spikes); *B-mode* (brightness modulation), a two-dimensional or cross-sectional image that reflects the intensity of the returning sound wave by the brightness of the dot; *gray scale,* a representation of organ texture in shades of gray on a television screen; and *real-time imaging,* instantaneous images of the tissues in motion, similar to fluoroscopic examination. Selected views may be photographed for later examination and a permanent record of the test. (See *Understanding A-mode ultrasonography,* page 752.)

Pelvic ultrasonography is used most commonly to evaluate symptoms that suggest pelvic disease, to confirm a tentative diagnosis, and to determine fetal growth during pregnancy. It's often required during pregnancy for women with a history or signs of fetal anomalies or multiple pregnancies, a history of bleeding, inconsistency of fetal size and conception date, or indications for amniocentesis.

Purpose
- To detect foreign bodies and distinguish between cysts and solid masses (tumors)
- To measure organ size

- To evaluate fetal viability, position, gestational age, and growth rate
- To detect multiple pregnancy
- To confirm fetal abnormalities (such as molar pregnancy, and abnormalities of the arms and legs, spine, heart, head, kidneys, and abdomen) and maternal abnormalities (such as posterior placenta and placenta previa)
- To guide amniocentesis by determining placental location and fetal position.

Patient preparation
Describe the test to the patient, and tell her the reason it is being performed. Assure her that this procedure is safe, noninvasive, and painless. Because pelvic ultrasonography requires a full bladder as a landmark to define pelvic organs, instruct the patient to drink liquids and to avoid urinating before the test. Tell her who will perform the procedure and where, and inform her that it will take a few minutes to several hours.

Explain that a water enema may be necessary to produce a better outline of the large intestine. Reassure the patient that the test won't harm the fetus, and provide emotional support throughout.

Equipment
Mineral oil or water-soluble jelly ✦ ultrasound machine and transducer ✦ camera and film, or videotape.

Procedure
With the patient in the supine position, the pelvic area is coated with mineral oil or water-soluble jelly to increase sound wave conduction. Then the transducer crystal is guided over the area, images are observed on the oscilloscope screen, and a good image is photographed.

Precautions
None.

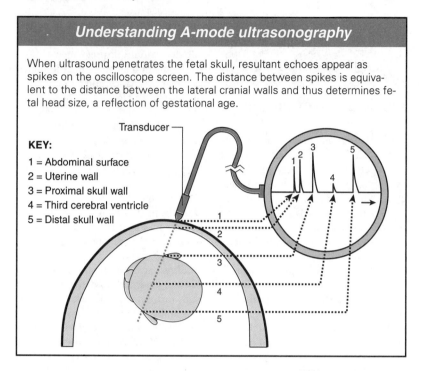

Understanding A-mode ultrasonography

When ultrasound penetrates the fetal skull, resultant echoes appear as spikes on the oscilloscope screen. The distance between spikes is equivalent to the distance between the lateral cranial walls and thus determines fetal head size, a reflection of gestational age.

Transducer

KEY:

1 = Abdominal surface
2 = Uterine wall
3 = Proximal skull wall
4 = Third cerebral ventricle
5 = Distal skull wall

Normal findings

The uterus is normal in size and shape. The ovaries are normal in size, shape, and sonographic density. No other masses are visible. If the patient is pregnant, the gestational sac and fetus are of normal size for date.

Implications of results

Although both cysts and solid masses have homogeneous densities, solid masses (such as fibroids) appear more dense on ultrasonography. Inappropriate fetal size may indicate miscalculation of conception or delivery date, or a dead fetus. Abnormal echo patterns may indicate foreign bodies (such as an intrauterine device), multiple pregnancy, maternal abnormalities (such as placenta previa or abruptio placentae), or fetal abnormalities (such as molar pregnancy, or abnormalities of the arms and legs, spine, heart, head, kidneys, and

abdomen). Ultrasonography can also delineate fetal malpresentation (such as breech [at term] or shoulder presentation) and cephalopelvic disproportion.

Post-test care

Allow the patient to empty her bladder immediately after the test.

Interfering factors

Failure to fill the bladder, obesity, or fetal head positioned deep in the pelvis can render the image uninterpretable.

Vaginal ultrasonography

In vaginal ultrasonography, a probe is inserted into the vagina and high-frequency sound waves are reflected to a transducer, forming an image of the pelvic structures. By bringing the probe closer to the pelvic structures, vaginal ultrasonography shows these structures in greater detail. It also allows better evaluation of pelvic anatomy and diagnosis of pregnancy at an earlier gestational age. This imaging technique eliminates the need for a full bladder and circumvents difficulties encountered with obese patients.

Purpose

- To establish early pregnancy with fetal heart motion as early as the 5th to 6th week of gestation
- To determine ectopic pregnancy
- To monitor follicular growth during infertility treatment
- To evaluate abnormal pregnancy (such as blighted ovum, missed or incomplete abortion, or molar pregnancy)
- To visualize retained products of conception
- To diagnose fetal abnormalities and placental location
- To evaluate adnexal pathology, such as tubo-ovarian abscess, hydrosalpinx, and ovarian masses
- To evaluate the uterine lining (in cases of dysfunctional uterine bleeding and postmenopausal bleeding).

Patient preparation

Describe the procedure to the patient and explain the reason for the test. Assure her that the procedure is safe. Because this technique requires the insertion of a vaginal probe, allowing the patient to introduce the probe may decrease her anxiety. If the sonographer is male, a female assistant should be present during the examination.

Equipment

Water-soluble lubricant ✦ ultrasound machine and vaginal transducer ✦ pro-

tective sheath such as a condom for the transducer.

Procedure

Place the patient in the lithotomy position. Water-soluble gel will be placed on the transducer tip to allow better sound transmission, and a protective sheath will be placed over the transducer. Additional lubricant will be placed on the sheathed transducer tip, which will be gently inserted into the vagina by the patient or the sonographer. The pelvic structures are observed by rotating the probe 90 degrees to one side and then the other.

Precautions

Guard the patient's privacy.

Normal findings

The uterus and ovaries are normal in size and shape. If the patient is pregnant, the gestational sac and fetus are of normal size for dates.

Implications of results

The closer the vaginal probe is to the pelvic organs, the better the visualization of organs. Vaginal ultrasonography may reveal an empty uterus (no fetus or adnexal masses). Free peritoneal fluid may be visible in the pelvic cavity, indicating possible peritonitis. Ectopic pregnancies may also be visible in the pelvic cavity.

Interfering factors

- The bowel may be mistaken for the ovaries, but careful observation for peristalsis easily differentiates the two structures.
- Ectopic pregnancies can be missed when a tubal mass is small.

Selected Readings

Beck, J.S. *Novak's Textbook of Gynecology,* 12th ed. Baltimore: Williams & Wilkins Co., 1996.

Cunningham, F.G., et al. *Williams Obstetrics,* 19th ed. Stamford, Conn.: Appleton & Lange, 1993.

Diseases, 2nd ed. Springhouse, Pa.: Springhouse Corp., 1996.

Glass, R.H. *Office Gynecology,* 4th ed. Baltimore: Williams & Wilkins Co., 1993.

Henry, J.B., ed. *Clinical Diagnosis and Management by Laboratory Methods,* 19th ed. Philadelphia: W.B. Saunders Co., 1996.

Knuppel, R.A., and Drukker, J.E., eds. *High-Risk Pregnancy: A Team Approach,* 2nd ed. Philadelphia: W.B. Saunders Co., 1993.

Nursing97 Drug Handbook. Springhouse, Pa.: Springhouse Corp., 1997.

Olds, S.B., et al. *Maternal-Newborn Nursing: A Family-Centered Approach,* 5th ed. Reading, Mass.: Addison-Wesley Publishing Co., 1996.

Ravel, R.A. *Clinical Laboratory Medicine: Clinical Application of Laboratory Data,* 6th ed. St. Louis: Mosby–Year Book, Inc., 1995.

Rock, J.A., et al. *Advances in Obstetrics and Gynecology,* vol. 3. St. Louis: Mosby–Year Book, Inc., 1996.

Speroff, L., and Glass, R.H. *Clinical Gynecologic Endocrinology and Infertility,* 5th ed. Baltimore: Williams & Wilkins Co., 1994.

Tucker, S.M. *Pocket Guide to Fetal Monitoring and Assessment,* 3rd ed. St. Louis: Mosby–Year Book, Inc., 1996.

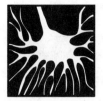

Nervous system

Learning objectives

After completing this chapter, the reader will be able to:

- explain the anatomy and physiology of the nervous system
- describe how to position the patient for a routine skull X-ray series
- discuss the diagnostic applications of magnetic resonance imaging
- explain why computed tomography typically yields better diagnostic information than conventional X-rays
- state the purpose of each test discussed in the chapter
- prepare the patient physically and psychologically for each test

- describe the procedure for performing each test
- specify appropriate precautions for safe administration of each test
- recognize signs of an adverse reaction and respond appropriately
- implement appropriate post-test care
- identify the normal findings of each test
- discuss the implications of abnormal test results
- list factors that may interfere with accurate test results.

INTRODUCTION

The study of the human nervous system — neurology — comes closer than any other discipline to examining the fundamental mystery of life. It seeks to understand how we come to feel, to think, and to be aware of who and what we are. The field of neurodiagnostics faces an equally difficult challenge: to devise safe, effective methods of detecting the diseases and disorders that affect what is one of the most powerful body systems and yet contains some of its most fragile tissues. Sophisticated procedures, such as magnetic resonance imaging, help to meet this challenge.

The tests discussed in this chapter allow diagnosis of the major disorders of the brain and its cavities, vasculature, and coverings; the brain stem and cranial nerves; the spinal cord and spinal roots; as well as the peripheral nerves and the major skeletal muscle groups they innervate. These disorders constitute the substance of clinical neurology, a clear understanding of which is essential to neuroscience nursing practice.

The nervous system

The nervous system has three major divisions: the central nervous system (CNS), peripheral nervous system (PNS), and autonomic nervous system (ANS). The CNS consists of the brain, brain stem, and spinal cord; the PNS consists of cranial and spinal nerves; and the ANS has sympathetic and parasympathetic divisions that automatically modulate the function of the glands, blood vessels, smooth muscle, and internal organs.

Neurons, the basic structural unit of the nervous system, carry electrical impulses along their axons (or major processes) and transmit them electrochemically across junctions called synapses. These impulses are received by the branching dendrites of other neurons. Synaptic transmission is the basis for all cellular transactions within the CNS and in certain parts of the PNS and ANS.

When many neurons are bundled together, the groups of axons created are called nerves or nerve tracts. Nerve tracts contain two types of axons or nerve fibers: afferent and efferent. Afferent nerve fibers bring electrical impulses into the CNS. Sensations are carried in on afferent fibers or received by the CNS via sensory nerves. Efferent nerve fibers carry electrical impulses away from the CNS. Movement depends on efferent fibers or motor neurons that execute commands given by the CNS.

Supporting cells

Within the brain, cells known as glia (from the Greek word for glue) support and help nourish nerve tissue. Glia may also be involved in the biosynthesis of myelin, the insulating material that surrounds certain portions of central and peripheral axons and that assist the conduction of nerve impulses. Glia may undergo malignant metamorphosis, forming glia tumors.

Healthy brain function depends on the integrity of cerebral circulation and metabolism. Blood flows to the brain through two internal carotid arteries and two vertebral arteries. The carotid arteries supply 80% of blood to the brain, mainly to the cerebrum, and the vertebral arteries supply 20% of blood to the brain, mainly to the brain stem and cerebellum. The vertebral arteries unite posteriorly to form the basilar artery. The circle of Willis — consisting of six large vessels supplying the cortex — is situated at the base of the brain.

Venous drainage occurs by way of deep veins and large dural sinuses that empty into the internal jugular veins. Cerebral blood vessels are amply supplied by various kinds of nerve fibers. When a major cerebral artery is occluded, cerebral ischemia occurs distal to the occlusion. Collateral circulation may develop in the presence of gradual occlusion or reduced blood flow through certain areas of the brain, particularly during the aging process.

Blood-brain barrier

The brain has no lymph nodes. Instead, a complex combination of factors and structural elements exists to form a functional blood-brain barrier. This barrier consists mostly of tight endothelial junctions that prohibit passage of many substances through the capillary beds and cellular membranes that must also be traversed by substances leaving the circulation and entering the brain.

A healthy blood-brain barrier helps maintain a sterile, homeostatic environment for brain cells. Because a breakdown in the blood-brain barrier commonly occurs at the site of tumor growth, a tumor can be identified by substances that rapidly penetrate the tumor tissue (such as radioiodine-labeled albumin), allowing it to stand out radiographically. Acquired immunodeficiency syndrome (AIDS) has also been linked to a breakdown in the blood-brain barrier, and neuroscientists are attempting to clarify the role that the blood-brain barrier plays in the immune response.

Protective fluid

Cerebrospinal fluid (CSF) is formed mainly by the choroid plexuses within the brain's four ventricles. The composition of CSF, which depends on filtration and diffusion from the blood, is very similar to that of the brain's extracellular fluid.

Few conditions cause CSF volume and pressure to fall below normal (dehydration might be one), but many conditions can cause it to increase, sometimes under pressure. This may lead to hydrocephalus, in which the flow of CSF form one or more ventricles is blocked, causing CSF buildup and an increase in intracranial pressure. (See *Reviewing CSF circulation*, page 758.)

Reviewing CSF circulation

Cerebrospinal fluid (CSF) is produced from blood in the capillary networks called the choroid plexus. Choroid plexuses are complex structures of vascular folds in the pia mater in the brain's lateral, third, and fourth ventricles. From these sites of origin, CSF passes into the lateral ventricles. It flows through the foramen of Monro into the third ventricle, through the aqueduct of Sylvius into the fourth ventricle, and through the foramina of Luschka and Magendie to the cisterna of the subarachnoid space. The cisterna is continuous with the subarachnoid space, surrounding the entire brain and spinal cord.

   Then the fluid passes under the base of the brain, upward over the brain's upper surface, and down around the spinal cord. When CSF reaches the arachnoid villi, it's absorbed into venous blood at the venous sinuses. Normally, the amount of CSF produced (500 to 800 ml/day) equals the amount absorbed. The average amount circulating at one time is 125 to 175 ml.

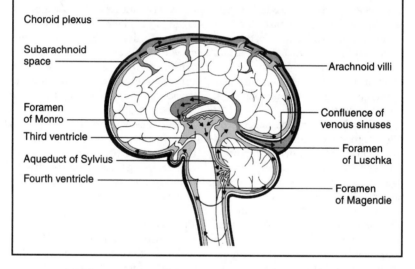

Choroid plexus

Subarachnoid space

Arachnoid villi

Foramen of Monro

Confluence of venous sinuses

Third ventricle

Aqueduct of Sylvius

Foramen of Luschka

Fourth ventricle

Foramen of Magendie

Along with the meninges, CSF protects and supports brain tissue, as evidenced by the pain generated by the withdrawal of spinal fluid. When this cushion of fluid is removed, the brain settles and its weight — combined with traction on pain-sensitive vessels — causes a severe headache.

Neurologic tests

The diagnostic tests in this chapter are used to detect such brain diseases or disorders as congenital defects and anomalies, perinatal defects, ventricular abnormalities, epilepsies, degenerative diseases, and space-occupying lesions. This last category includes neoplasms, infections, and vascular lesions such as arteriovenous malformations.

   These tests can diagnose infectious diseases, including those caused by bacteria (such as meningitis), viruses (such as encephalitis or polioencephalomyelitis), spirochetes (such as neurosyphilis), parasitic infestations (such as toxoplasmosis, common in AIDS patients), and fungal and related infections. Demyelinating diseases (such as multiple sclerosis), cerebrovascular disorders (including stroke, transient ischemic attacks, aneurysms of the blood vessels, and subdural and subarachnoid hemorrhages), and disorders of the skull, vertebral column, and other nonneural tissues may also be diagnosed using the tests in this chapter.

Disorders of the brain stem and cranial nerves that can be detected by these tests include vascular insufficiency due to obstruction to specific regions of the brain stem; cranial nerve syndromes (such as trigeminal neuralgia); headache disorders; and congenital disorders that occur as distortions of normal relationships between the skull and vertebral column or as abnormal formations of the base of the skull.

The spinal cord may be affected by metastasis from non-CNS primary tumors that spread to the vertebrae and meninges, producing extradural tumors that distort the spinal cord or interrupt CSF flow in the spinal subarachnoid spaces. This causes a block in CSF circulation accompanied by spinal cord dysfunction. Both the brain stem and the spinal cord may be affected by Guillain-Barré syndrome, which is typically a myeloradiculopathy.

Because disorders of the PNS are in many cases toxic or metabolic in origin, the tests covered in this chapter are generally not as useful as investigation for exposure to toxins or as a systemic metabolic workup. In addition, diagnosis of peripheral neuropathies commonly depends on nerve biopsy, which allows identification of specific pathologic change in the nerve fibers. Similarly, when attempting to identify myopathies or muscle disorders, muscle biopsy is commonly the preferred diagnostic tool.

The patient's ability to function with neurologic disorders can be evaluated by other tests. (See *Neuropsychological testing*, page 760.)

Noninvasive tests

- *Skull radiography* — X-rays of the skull taken at various planes and from different angles — allows examination of almost all intracranial structures.
- *Computed tomography (CT) scanning* provides a computerized image of a section of the brain or spinal column as if sliced from front to back, in the horizontal plane, or alternatively, in the sagittal or coronal planes. Although generally considered a noninvasive test, CT scanning can become invasive if a radiopaque medium is injected into a peripheral vein, which allows for uptake by an intracranial or spinal lesion.
- *Magnetic resonance imaging (MRI)* relies on the magnetic properties of the body's atoms. It uses radiofrequency energy and a powerful magnetic field to produce computerized multiplanar images of fine detail and resolution. New technology has adapted MRI for new types of diagnostic tests, such as magnetic resonance angiography, diffusion-perfusion imaging, and magnetic resonance spectroscopy.
- *Electroencephalography* detects, records, and amplifies electrical potentials on the scalp that are generated by the brain's neurons, using a noninvasive technique that requires small electrodes to be applied in carefully defined patterns on the scalp. The findings depict the electrical activity of the brain's surface, which reflects — and can be used to interpret — changes in electrical activity of deeper structures.
- *Evoked potential studies* directly evaluate sensory and somatosensory neurologic pathways by recording the electrical response of the brain to external stimuli.
- *Oculoplethysmography* indirectly measures ocular artery pressure and reflects the adequacy of cerebrovascular blood flow of the carotid arteries.
- *Transcranial Doppler studies* measure the velocity of blood flow through the

Neuropsychological testing

Rather than documenting physiologic changes in the nervous system, neuropsychological testing evaluates the effects of neurologic disorders on a patient's ability to function.

Indications

These tests can evaluate cognitive functioning, including general intelligence, attention span, memory, and judgment as well as motor, sensory, and speech ability. Certain tests can assess emotional lability, quality of language production, abstraction, distractibility, persistence, or the ability to sequence learned activities. The neuropsychologist chooses the appropriate test based on the reason for the assessment and the skills being assessed.

Besides determining the type and extent of functional deficits in patients with known neurologic illness, neuropsychological tests can diagnose organic brain dysfunction and dementia. They're also used to determine whether an injured patient can return to a previous occupation or should be declared disabled. What's more, these tests can as-sess the extent of rehabilitation or vocational training required before the patient can fully function again. Neuropsychological tests may be performed before and after a major neurosurgical or radiologic procedure to obtain baseline information for comparison with postprocedural information. A neuropsychologist administers the series of paper-and-pencil tests, possibly in combination with other tests using puzzles, blocks, or word or recall games. The psychologist explains each test prior to administration.

Precautions

Because these tests are mentally demanding and lengthy, they may tire patients. If possible, withdraw medications that affect the patient's ability to concentrate before the test. Patients should be well rested and free of sedatives, if possible, before testing. Any physiologic problem that may interfere with mental function or level of consciousness, such as fever or electrolyte imbalance, should be treated before testing to ensure that test results are as accurate as possible.

cerebral arteries and provide information about the quality and changing nature of circulation to an area of the brain.

Invasive tests

▪ *Cerebral angiography* allows visualization of blood vessels through injection of a substance that is opaque to X-rays and therefore stands out as a white contrast. *Digital subtraction angiography* uses computers and video equipment to eliminate interfering images of bone and soft tissue and further reveal details of the opacified vessels. In addition to

detecting disorders of cerebral blood vessels, angiography may also help detect displacement of blood vessels by other lesions, such as tumors.

▪ *Electromyography* assesses the electrical potential across the muscle membrane through a needle electrode. This procedure yields information on the conduction of the nerve impulse to the muscle as well as the muscle's response to the nerve impulse. The nerve conduction part of this test determines whether the velocity of propagation of the nerve impulse along a particular sensory, motor, or combined sensory-motor nerve is normal. This test also provides general information about the possibility of neuropathy.

■ *Cerebrospinal fluid analysis* provides a general profile of the cellular and chemical composition of CSF at a particular time. Because CSF is secreted and represents a highly refined distillate of the blood, concentrations of certain substances are different in CSF than in serum. The pressure under which CSF is circulating can be determined during lumbar puncture before the CSF specimen is obtained.

■ *Myelography* involves injection of a radiopaque contrast medium into the spinal subarachnoid space. CSF is removed for analysis at the time of myelography — thereby accomplishing two tests with one procedure — and is replaced by the heavier contrast medium, which gravitates toward the head or elsewhere within the spinal canal when the radiographic table is tilted.

■ In the *Tensilon test*, a short-acting potent anticholinesterase drug is administered I.V. to help diagnose myasthenia gravis.

New techniques

A number of techniques have been used by laboratories for many years to conduct fundamental research on the nervous system. One such technique is *positron emission tomography* (PET), which creates an image of a slice of the brain similar to a CT image but is based on different biophysical and radiochemical techniques. (Because it's costly, PET is used mainly for research.) A new clinical application of electroencephalography is *somnography*, the scientific evaluation of sleep and its disorders. These promising new techniques are still essentially investigational and have limited clinical application.

NONINVASIVE TESTS

Skull radiography

Skull radiography is the oldest noninvasive neurologic test and is commonly the second step — after a routine neurologic examination — in a complete neurologic workup. In patients with head injuries, X-rays of the skull offer limited information about skull fractures. However, they're extremely valuable for studying abnormalities of the base of the skull and the cranial vault, congenital and perinatal anomalies, and many systemic diseases that produce bone defects of the skull.

Skull radiography evaluates the three groups of bones that make up the skull — the calvaria (or vault), the mandible (or jaw bone), and the facial bones. The calvaria and the facial bones are closely connected by immovable joints with irregular serrated edges called sutures. The bones of the skull form an anatomic structure so complex that several radiologic views of each area are needed for a complete skull examination.

Purpose

■ To detect fractures in patients with head trauma
■ To aid diagnosis of pituitary tumors
■ To detect congenital anomalies.

Patient preparation

Explain to the patient that this test helps establish a diagnosis and that he needn't restrict food or fluids. Tell him that several X-ray films of his skull will be taken from various angles, and inform him who will perform the test and where. Reassure him that the procedure will cause him no discomfort and that it

Positioning the skull for radiography

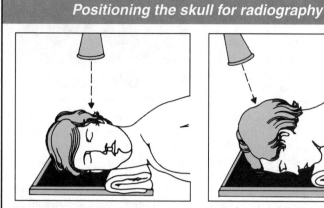

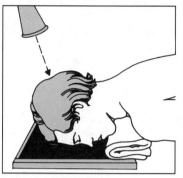

Right lateral and left lateral
The sagittal plane is parallel to the tabletop and the film. A support, such as a folded towel or the patient's clenched fist, is placed under the chin. (Adequate film shows both halves of the mandible directly superimposed.)

Posteroanterior Caldwell
The patient lies prone; his chin may be supported by a folded towel or his fist. The sagittal plane and the canthomeatal line are perpendicular to the tabletop and the film. The X-ray beam is angled 15 degrees toward the feet.

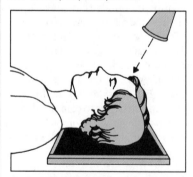

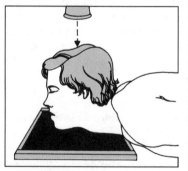

Anteroposterior Towne's
The patient lies supine, with his chin flexed toward the neck; the canthomeatal line is perpendicular to the tabletop and the film. The X-ray beam is angled 30 degrees toward the feet.

Axial (base)
The patient lies prone, with chin fully extended; his head rests in such a way that the line of the face is perpendicular and the canthomeatal line is parallel to the tabletop and the film.

takes about 15 minutes. Instruct him to remove glasses, dentures, jewelry, and any metal objects in the X-ray field.

Equipment
X-ray machine and film.

Procedure
The patient is placed in the supine position on an X-ray table or seated in a chair and is instructed to keep still while X-rays are taken. A head band, foam pads, or sandbags may be used to im-

mobilize the patient's head and increase his comfort. Routinely, five views of the skull are taken: left and right lateral, anteroposterior Towne's, posteroanterior Caldwell, and axial (or base). (See *Positioning the skull for radiography*.) Films are developed and checked for quality before the patient leaves the area.

Precautions
None.

Normal findings
A radiologist interprets the X-rays, evaluating the size, shape, thickness, and position of cranial bones as well as the vascular markings, sinuses, and sutures; all should be normal for the patient's age.

Implications of results
Skull radiography is often diagnostic for fractures of the vault or base, although basilar fractures may not show on the film if the bone is dense. This test may confirm congenital anomalies and may show erosion, enlargement, or decalcification of the sella turcica due to increased intracranial pressure. (A marked rise in pressure may cause the brain to expand and press against the inner bony table of the skull, leaving marks or impressions that have been compared in appearance to beaten silver.)

X-rays of the skull may also show abnormal areas of calcification in conditions such as osteomyelitis (with possible calcification of the skull itself) and chronic subdural hematomas. They can detect neoplasms within the brain substance that contain calcium, such as oligodendrogliomas or meningiomas as well as the midline shifting of a calcified pineal gland caused by a space-occupying lesion. Radiography may also detect other changes in bone structure, for example, those due to metabolic disorders such as acromegaly or Paget's disease.

Post-test care
None.

Interfering factors
Improper positioning of the patient, excessive head movement, or failure to remove radiopaque objects from the X-ray field makes films inadequate for radiologic interpretation.

Intracranial computed tomography

Intracranial computed tomography (CT) provides a series of tomograms, translated by a computer and displayed on an oscilloscope screen, representing cross-sectional images of various layers (or slices) of the brain. This technique can reconstruct cross-sectional, horizontal, sagittal, and coronal-plane images. Hundreds of thousands of readings of radiation levels absorbed by brain tissues may be combined to depict anatomic slices of varying thickness. Specificity and accuracy are enhanced by the degree of resolution, which depends on the number of radiation density calculations made by the computer. This, in turn, depends on the number of collimated (parallel) radiographs taken.

Newer versions of the CT scanner take more radiographs than earlier models, producing more detailed images. These images identify intracranial tumors and other brain lesions as areas of altered density. (See *Comparing normal and abnormal CT scans*, page 764.)

The increasing availability of CT scanners allows faster and safer diagnosis than in the past. In many cases, intracranial CT scanning eliminates the need for painful and hazardous invasive procedures, such as pneumoencephalogra-

Comparing normal and abnormal CT scans

Shown here are two intracranial computed tomography (CT) scans. The scan on the left is normal. The scan on the right shows a large meningioma in the frontal region, represented by the white area.

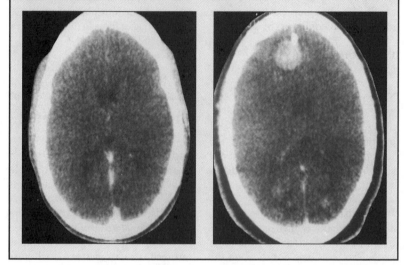

phy and cerebral angiography. CT scans, which often uses contrast enhancement, are especially valuable in assessing a patient with focal neurologic abnormalities and other clinical features that suggest an intracranial mass. In a patient with a suspected head injury, intracranial CT scans may allow diagnosis of a subdural hematoma before characteristic symptoms appear.

Purpose
■ To diagnose intracranial lesions and abnormalities
■ To monitor the effects of surgery, radiotherapy, or chemotherapy on intracranial tumors.

Patient preparation
Explain to the patient that this test permits assessment of the brain. Unless contrast enhancement is scheduled, inform him that he needn't restrict food or fluids. If contrast enhancement is

scheduled, instruct him to fast for 4 hours before the test. Tell him a series of X-ray films will be taken of his brain and that the test takes 15 to 30 minutes. Inform him who will perform the test and where. Reassure him that the test will cause him minimal discomfort from having to lie still.

Tell the patient he'll be positioned on a radiographic table, with his head immobilized and his face uncovered. The head of the table is moved into the scanner, which rotates around his head and makes clacking sounds. If a contrast agent is used, tell the patient he may feel flushed and warm and experience a transient headache, a salty taste, or nausea and vomiting after the dye is injected.

Instruct the patient to wear a hospital gown (outpatients may wear any comfortable clothing) and to remove all metal objects and jewelry in the CT scan field. It the patient is restless or apprehensive, notify the doctor, who may order a sedative.

Check the patient's history for hypersensitivity to shellfish, iodine, or other contrast media, and document such reactions on the patient's chart. Inform the doctor of any sensitivities because he may order prophylactic medications or may choose not to use contrast enhancement.

Equipment

CT scanner ✦ oscilloscope ✦ contrast medium, as ordered (iothalamate meglumine or diatrizoate sodium) ✦ 60-ml syringe ✦ 19G to 21G needle ✦ tourniquet.

Procedure

The patient is placed in a supine position on a radiographic table, with his head immobilized by straps, and is asked to lie still. The head of the table is moved into the scanner, which rotates around the patient's head, taking radiographs at 1-degree intervals in a 180-degree arc.

When this series of radiographs is complete, contrast enhancement is performed, if ordered. Usually, 50 to 100 ml of contrast medium are injected by I.V. infusion or by I.V. drip over 1 to 2 minutes, and the patient is observed for hypersensitivity reactions, such as urticaria, respiratory difficulty, and a rash. Such reactions usually develop within 30 minutes.

After injection of the contrast medium, another series of scans is taken. Information from the scans is stored on magnetic tapes, fed into a computer, and converted into images on an oscilloscope screen. Photographs of selected views are taken for further study.

Precautions

■ Intracranial CT scanning with contrast enhancement is contraindicated in persons who are hypersensitive to iodine or contrast media.

■ Iodine or contrast medium may be harmful or fatal to a fetus, especially during the first trimester.

Normal findings

The density of tissue determines the amount of radiation that passes through it. Tissue densities appear as black, white, or shades of gray on the CT image. Bone, the densest tissue, appears white; brain matter appears in shades of gray; ventricular and subarachnoid CSF — the least dense — appears black. Structures are evaluated according to their density, size, shape, and position.

Implications of results

Areas of altered density (they may be lighter or darker) or displaced vasculature or other structures may indicate intracranial tumor, hematoma, cerebral atrophy, infarction, edema, or congenital anomalies, such as hydrocephalus.

Intracranial tumors vary significantly in appearance and characteristics. Metastatic tumors generally cause extensive edema in early stages and can usually be defined by contrast enhancement. Primary tumors vary in density and in their capacity to cause edema, displace ventricles, and absorb the dye. Astrocytomas, for example, usually have low densities; meningiomas have higher densities and can generally be defined with contrast enhancement; glioblastomas, usually ill-defined, are also enhanced after injection of a contrast medium.

Because the high density of blood contrasts markedly with low-density brain tissue, both subdural and epidural hematomas and other acute hemorrhages are usually easy to detect. Contrast enhancement helps locate subdural hematomas.

Cerebral atrophy customarily appears as enlarged ventricles with large sulci. Cerebral infarction may appear as low-density areas at the obstruction site or

Understanding positron emission tomography

Like computed tomography (CT) scanning and magnetic resonance imaging, positron emission tomography (PET) provides images of the brain through sophisticated computer reconstruction algorithms. However, PET images detail brain *function* as well as structure and thus differ significantly from the images provided by these other advanced techniques.

PET combines elements of both CT scanning and conventional radionuclide imaging. For example, it measures the emissions of injected radioisotopes and converts them to a tomographic image of the brain. But, unlike conventional radionuclide imaging, PET uses radioisotopes of biologically important elements — oxygen, nitrogen, carbon, and fluorine — that emit particles called *positrons.*

Procedure

During PET, pairs of gamma rays are emitted; the PET scanner detects these and relays the information to a computer for reconstruction as an image. Positron-emitters can be chemically "tagged" to biologically active molecules (such as carbon monoxide), neurotransmitters, hormones, and metabolites (particularly glucose), enabling study of their uptake and distribution in brain tissue. For example, blood tagged with

^{11}C-carbon monoxide allows study of hemodynamic patterns in brain tissue, whereas tagged neurotransmitters, hormones, and drugs allow mapping of receptor distribution. Isotope-tagged glucose (which penetrates the blood-brain barrier rapidly) allows dynamic study of brain function because PET can pinpoint the sites of glucose metabolism in the brain under various conditions.

Promising future

This last application is particularly promising: Researchers expect it to prove useful in diagnosing psychiatric disorders, transient ischemic attacks, amyotrophic lateral sclerosis, Parkinson's disease, Wilson's disease, multiple sclerosis, seizure disorders, cerebrovascular disease, and Alzheimer's disease. The reason: All of these disorders may alter the location and patterns of cerebral glucose metabolism.

PET is a costly test because the radioisotopes used have very short half-lives and must be produced at an on-site cyclotron and attached quickly to the desired tracer molecules. So far, this prohibitive cost has limited PET's use, except as a research tool. However, PET has already provided significant information about the brain and may someday have widespread clinical applications.

---

may not be apparent if the infarction is small or doesn't cause edema. With contrast enhancement, the infarcted area may not appear in the acute phase but will show clearly after resolution of the lesion. Cerebral edema usually appears as an area of marked generalized lucency. In children, enlargement of the fourth ventricle usually indicates hydrocephalus.

Normally, the cerebral vessels don't appear on CT images. However, in patients with arteriovenous malformation, cerebral vessels may appear with slightly increased density. Contrast enhancement allows a better view of the abnormal area, but MRI is now the preferred procedure for imaging cerebral vessels.

Another imaging method, positron emission tomography, combines CT technology and radionuclide imaging to detail brain function as well as structure. (See *Understanding positron emission tomography*.)

Post-test care
None, if the test was performed without contrast enhancement. If a contrast agent was used, watch for residual adverse reactions (headache, nausea, and vomiting). Inform the patient that he may resume his usual diet.

Interfering factors
▪ Movement of the patient's head makes CT scan images difficult to interpret.
▪ Failure to remove metal objects from the scanning field may produce unclear images.

Magnetic resonance imaging

Although its full range of clinical applications is still being established, magnetic resonance imaging (MRI) is recognized as a safe, valuable tool for diagnosing neurologic disorders. Like computed tomography, MRI produces cross-sectional images of the brain and spine in multiple planes.

MRI's greatest advantages are its ability to "see through" bone and to delineate fluid-filled soft tissue. It's proven useful in diagnosing cerebral infarction, tumors, abscesses, edema, hemorrhage, nerve fiber demyelination (as in multiple sclerosis), and other disorders that increase the fluid content of affected tissues. It can also show irregularities of the spinal cord with a resolution and detail previously unattainable as well as images of organs and vessels in motion.

MRI relies on the magnetic properties of the atom. (Hydrogen, the most abundant and magnetically sensitive of the body's atoms, is most commonly selected for MRI studies.) The scanner uses a powerful magnetic field and radiofrequency (RF) energy to produce images based on the hydrogen content (primarily water) of body tissues. Exposed to an external magnetic field, positively charged atomic nuclei and their negatively charged electrons align uniformly in the field. RF energy is then directed at the atoms, knocking them out of this magnetic alignment and causing them to precess, or spin. When the RF pulse is discontinued, the atoms realign themselves with the magnetic field, emitting RF energy as a tissue-specific signal based on the relative density of nuclei and the realignment time. These signals are monitored by the MRI computer, which processes them and displays the information on a video monitor as a high-resolution image.

The magnetic fields and RF energy used for MRI are imperceptible to the patient; no harmful effects have been documented. Research is continuing on the optimal magnetic fields and RF waves for each type of tissue.

Several new techniques for monitoring cerebral function and examining aspects of the brain are currently under study. (See *New methods of monitoring cerebral function*, page 768, and *New applications for MRI*, page 769.)

Purpose
▪ To aid diagnosis of intracranial and spinal lesions and soft-tissue abnormalities.

Patient preparation
Explain to the patient that this test assesses bone and soft tissue in the brain and nervous system. Tell him who will perform the test, where it will be done, and that it takes up to 90 minutes. Explain that although MRI is painless and involves no exposure to radiation from

New methods of monitoring cerebral function

Two new diagnostic procedures are giving researchers a better understanding of how the brain functions.

Optical imaging

This technique uses fiber-optic light and a camera to produce visual images of the brain as it responds to stimulation. Optical imaging produces higher-resolution pictures of the brain than either magnetic resonance imaging (MRI) or positron emission tomography (PET) scans. Researchers believe that it may be valuable during neurosurgery to minimize damage to crucial areas of the brain that control speech, movement, and other activities. Because the procedure scans only the brain's surface, it's meant to be used in combination with other diagnostic techniques.

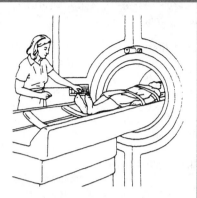

Fast MRI

This technique produces pictures less than a second apart. These images display blood flow through the brain and the changes that occur in blood flow when the patient performs different tasks. Neuroscientists believe that active areas of the brain must consume more oxygen and that areas of the brain that are currently working become laden with oxygen. Fast MRI can distinguish between oxygen-laden blood and oxygen-depleted blood. Thus, it may be used to help identify which areas of the normal brain are involved in certain activities and emotions.

Researchers are finding that preliminary results of these studies confirm those of PET studies. They hope that by pinpointing which areas of the brain are involved in certain feelings and thoughts they will be able to provide a map of the patient's brain. Possible applications for fast MRI include guiding neurosurgeons during surgery and helping researchers better understand epilepsy, brain tumors, and even psychiatric illnesses.

the scanner, a radioactive contrast dye may be used, depending on the type of tissue being studied. Advise him that he'll have to remain still for the entire procedure.

Inform the patient that the opening for the head and body is quite small and deep. He'll hear the scanner clicking, whirring, and thumping as it moves inside its housing to obtain different images (he may receive earplugs). Reassure him that he'll be able to communicate with the technician at all times. Provide emotional support to the patient with claustrophobic anxiety or anxiety over his diagnosis. If claustrophobia is severe, he may not be able to tolerate the scan or he may need sedation.

Instruct the patient to remove all metallic objects, including jewelry, hair pins, and watch, and ask if he has any surgically implanted joints, pins, clips, valves, pumps, or pacemakers containing metal because they could be attracted to the strong MRI magnet. If he does, he won't be able to have the test.

New applications for MRI

New uses for magnetic resonance imaging (MRI) continue to be developed. MRI currently provides clear images of parts of the brain that are difficult to visualize by other methods, such as the brain stem and cerebellum. Now four new MRI techniques are available to examine other aspects of the brain.

■ *Magnetic resonance angiography* produces images of cerebral blood vessels by taking advantage of the movement of blood through them.

■ *Magnetic resonance spectroscopy* provides images over time showing the metabolism of certain chemical markers in an area of the brain. Researchers at Yale University dubbed this test a "metabolic biopsy" because it reveals pathologic neurochemistry over a given time period.

■ *Diffusion-perfusion imaging* requires a stronger magnetic gradient than is usually available in conventional equipment, but it allows you to see an area of focal cerebral ischemia within minutes. This test, currently used in stroke research, may someday be used by diagnosticians to distinguish permanent from reversible ischemia.

■ *Neurograms* provide three-dimensional imaging of nerves. They may be used in the future to find the exact location of nerves that are damaged, crimped, or in disarray.

If required, obtain a signed consent form from the patient or his family.

Equipment
MRI scanner and computer ✦ display screen ✦ recorder (film or magnetic tape).

Procedure
The patient is placed in the supine position on a narrow bed, which then moves him to the desired position inside the scanner. RF energy is directed at his head or spine; the resulting images are displayed on a monitor and recorded on film or magnetic tape for permanent storage. The radiologist may vary RF waves and use the computer to manipulate and enhance the images. The patient must remain still during the entire procedure.

Precautions
■ Because MRI works through a powerful magnetic field, it can't be performed on patients with pacemakers, intracranial aneurysm clips, or other ferrous metal implants or on patients with gunshot wounds to the head.

■ Because of the strong magnetic field, metallic or computer-based equipment (for example, ventilators and I.V. pumps) can't enter the MRI area.

Normal findings
MRI can show normal anatomic details of the central nervous system in any plane, without bone interference. Brain and spinal cord structures should appear distinct and sharply defined. Tissue color and shading will vary, depending on the RF energy, magnetic strength, and degree of computer enhancement.

Implications of results
Because the MRI signal represents the proton density (water content) of tissue, MRI clearly shows structural changes resulting from disorders that increase tissue water content, such as cerebral edema, demyelinating disease (such as multiple sclerosis), and pontine and cerebellar tumors. Edematous fluid, for example, generally appears cloudy or

gray, whereas blood generally appears dark. Lesions of multiple sclerosis appear as areas of demyelination (curdlike gray or gray-white areas) around the edges of ventricles. Tumors appear as changes in normal anatomy, which computer enhancement may further delineate.

Post-test care
- The patient may resume normal activity after the test.
- If the test took a long time, you may need to observe the patient for postural hypotension.

Interfering factors
Excessive movement can blur images.

Electroencephalography

In electroencephalography, electrodes attached to standard areas of the patient's scalp record a portion of the brain's electrical activity. These electrical impulses are transmitted to an electroencephalograph, which magnifies them 1 million times and records them as brain waves on moving strips of paper.

Especially valuable in assessing patients with seizure disorders, electroencephalography is also used to evaluate patients with symptoms of brain tumors, abscesses, or cerebral damage due to other causes. The procedure is usually performed in a room designed to eliminate electrical interference and minimize distractions. However, portable units are available to perform electroencephalography at bedside, which is commonly done to confirm brain death.

Purpose
- To determine the present and type of epilepsy
- To aid diagnosis of intracranial lesions, such as abscesses and tumors
- To evaluate the brain's electrical activity in metabolic disease, head injury, meningitis, encephalitis, mental retardation, and psychological disorders
- To confirm brain death.

Patient preparation
Describe the procedure to the patient or his family, and explain that this test records the brain's electrical activity. Inform him that, except for fluids containing caffeine, he needn't restrict food or fluids before the test. (Skipping the meal before the test can cause relative hypoglycemia and alter brain wave patterns.)

Thoroughly wash and dry the patient's hair to remove hair sprays, creams, or oils. Tell the patient he'll be asked to relax in a reclining chair or lie on a bed and that electrodes will be attached to his scalp with a special paste. Assure him that the electrodes won't shock him. If needle electrodes are used, he'll feel pricking sensations when they're inserted; however, flat electrodes are more commonly used. Do your best to allay the patient's fears because anxiety can affect brain wave patterns.

Check the patient's medication history for drugs that may interfere with test results. As ordered, withhold anticonvulsants, tranquilizers, barbiturates, and other sedatives for 24 to 48 hours before the test. Infants and very young children occasionally require sedation to prevent crying and restlessness during the test.

To evaluate a patient with a seizure disorder, a "sleep electroencephalogram" (EEG) may be ordered. For this test, keep the patient awake the night before the test, and as ordered, administer a sedative (such as chloral hydrate) to help him sleep during the test. If an EEG is being performed to confirm brain death, provide emotional support to the family.

Equipment

Electroencephalograph and recorder ✦ electrodes with leads ✦ electrode paste.

Procedure

The patient is positioned comfortably on a bed or a reclining chair, and electrodes are attached to his scalp. Before the recording procedure begins, the patient is instructed to close his eyes, relax, and remain still. During the recording, the patient is carefully observed through a window in an adjoining room, and blinking, swallowing, talking, or other movements that may cause artifacts on the tracing are noted. The recording may be stopped periodically to allow the patient to reposition himself and get comfortable. This is important because restlessness and fatigue can alter brain wave patterns.

After an initial baseline recording, the patient may be tested in various stress situations to elicit abnormal patterns not obvious in the resting stage. For example, he may be asked to breathe deeply and rapidly for 3 minutes (hyperventilation), which may elicit brain wave patterns typical of seizure disorders or other abnormalities. This technique is commonly used to detect absence seizures. Photic stimulation — another technique — tests central cerebral activity in response to bright light, accentuating abnormal activity in absence or myoclonic seizures. In this procedure, a strobe light placed in front of the patient is flashed 1 to 20 times/second; recordings are made with the patient's eyes opened and closed.

Precautions

Observe the patient carefully for seizure activity. Record seizure patterns, and be prepared to provide assistance in the rare event of a severe seizure. Have suction equipment and diazepam for I.V. injection readily available.

Normal findings

Electroencephalography records a portion of the brain's electrical activity as waves; some are irregular, while others demonstrate common patterns. Among the basic waveforms are the alpha, beta, theta, and delta rhythms.

Alpha waves occur at frequencies of 8 to 12 cycles/second in a regular rhythm. They're present only in the waking state when the patient's eyes are closed but he's mentally alert; they usually disappear with visual activity or mental concentration. *Beta waves* (13 to 30 cycles/second) — generally associated with anxiety, depression, or use of sedatives — are seen most readily in the frontal and central regions of the brain. *Theta waves* (4 to 7 cycles/second) — most common in children and young adults — appear in the frontal and temporal regions. *Delta waves* (0.5 to 3.5 cycles/second) normally occur only in young children and during sleep. (See *Comparing EEG tracings,* page 772.)

Implications of results

Usually, a 100' to 200' (30 to 60-m) strip of the recording is evaluated, with particular attention paid to basic waveforms, symmetry of cerebral activity, transient discharges, and response to stimulation. A specific diagnosis depends on the patient's clinical status.

In patients with epilepsy, EEG patterns may identify the specific disorder. In patients with absence seizures, for example, the EEG shows spikes and waves at a frequency of 3 cycles/second. In generalized tonic-clonic seizures, it generally shows multiple, high-voltage, spiked waves in both hemispheres. In temporal lobe epilepsy, the EEG usually shows spiked waves in the affected temporal

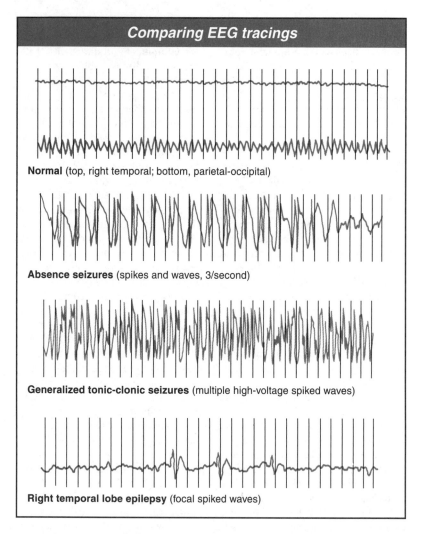

Comparing EEG tracings

Normal (top, right temporal; bottom, parietal-occipital)

Absence seizures (spikes and waves, 3/second)

Generalized tonic-clonic seizures (multiple high-voltage spiked waves)

Right temporal lobe epilepsy (focal spiked waves)

region. In patients with focal seizures, it usually shows localized, spiked discharges.

In patients with intracranial lesions, such as tumors or abscesses, the EEG may show slow waves (usually delta waves, but possibly unilateral beta waves). Vascular lesions, such as cerebral infarcts and intracranial hemorrhages, generally produce focal abnormalities in the injured area.

Generally, any condition that causes a diminishing level of consciousness alters the EEG pattern in proportion to the degree of consciousness lost. For example, in a patient with a metabolic disorder, an inflammatory process (such as meningitis or encephalitis), or increased intracranial pressure, the EEG shows generalized, diffuse, and slow brain waves. The most pathologic finding of all, of course, is an absent EEG pattern — a "flat" tracing (except for artifacts) — which may indicate brain death.

Post-test care

■ Ask the doctor whether anticonvulsants or other drugs withheld before the test can be resumed.

■ Carefully observe the patient for seizures, and provide a safe environment.

■ Help the patient remove electrode paste from his hair.

■ If the patient received a sedative before the test, take safety precautions, such as raising the side rails.

■ If brain death is confirmed, provide emotional support for the family.

Interfering factors

■ Excessive artifact may be caused by extraneous electrical activity; head, body, eye, or tongue movement; and muscle contractions.

■ Anticonvulsants, tranquilizers, barbiturates, and other sedatives interfere with the accuracy of test results.

■ Acute drug intoxication or severe hypothermia resulting in loss of consciousness causes a flat EEG.

Evoked potential studies

These tests evaluate the integrity of visual, somatosensory, and auditory nerve pathways by measuring evoked potentials — the brain's electrical response to stimulation of the sensory organs or peripheral nerves. Evoked potentials are recorded as electronic impulses by surface electrodes attached to the scalp and skin over various peripheral sensory nerves. A computer extracts these low-amplitude impulses from background brain wave activity and averages the signals from repeated stimuli.

Three types of response are measured. *Visual evoked potentials,* produced by exposing the eye to a rapidly reversing checkerboard pattern, help evaluate demyelinating disease (such as multiple sclerosis), traumatic injury, and puzzling visual complaints. *Somatosensory evoked potentials,* produced by electrically stimulating a peripheral sensory nerve, help diagnose peripheral nerve disease and locate brain and spinal cord lesions. *Auditory brain stem evoked potentials,* produced by delivering clicks to the ear, help locate auditory lesions and evaluate brain stem integrity.

Evoked potential studies are also useful for monitoring comatose or anesthetized patients, monitoring spinal cord function during spinal cord surgery, and evaluating neurologic function in infants whose sensory systems normally can't be adequately assessed.

Purpose

■ To aid diagnosis of nervous system lesions and abnormalities

■ To assess neurologic function.

Patient preparation

Explain to the patient that this group of tests measures the electrical activity of his nervous system. Inform him who will perform the procedure and where and that it takes 45 to 60 minutes. Tell the patient that he'll be positioned in a reclining chair or on a bed. If visual evoked potentials will be measured, tell him that electrodes will be attached to his scalp; if somatosensory evoked potentials will be measured, tell him electrodes will be placed on his scalp, neck, lower back, wrist, knee, and ankle.

Assure the patient that the electrodes won't hurt him; encourage him to relax because tension can affect neurologic function and interfere with test results. Have him remove all jewelry.

Equipment

Evoked potential unit ✦ auditory, visual, or tactile stimuli ✦ amplifier ✦ oscilloscope tube face ✦ magnetic tape.

Procedure

The patient is positioned in a reclining chair or on a bed and is instructed to relax and remain still.

For visual evoked potentials: Electrodes are attached to the patient's scalp at occipital, parietal, and vertex locations; a reference electrode is placed on the midfrontal area or on the ear. The patient is positioned 1 m (3') from the pattern-shift stimulator, which displays the pattern on a television screen or uses an array of light-emitting diodes, or a mechanical stimulator, which projects the pattern from a slide projector onto a translucent screen. One eye is occluded, and the patient is instructed to fix his gaze on a dot in the center of the screen. A checkerboard pattern is projected and then rapidly reversed or shifted 100 times, once or twice per second. A computer amplifies and averages the brain's response to each stimulus, and the results are plotted as a waveform. The procedure is then repeated for the other eye.

For somatosensory evoked potentials: Electrodes are attached to the patient's skin over somatosensory pathways (which usually include the wrist, knee, and ankle) to stimulate peripheral nerves. Recording electrodes are placed on the scalp over the sensory cortex of the hemisphere opposite the limb to be stimulated. Additional electrodes may be placed at Erb's point (above the clavicle overlying the brachial plexus) and at the second cervical vertebra for upper-limb stimulation, and over the lower lumbar vertebrae for lower-limb stimulation. Midfrontal or noncephalic electrodes are placed for reference.

A painless electric shock is delivered to the peripheral nerve through the stimulating electrode. The intensity of the shock is adjusted to produce a minor muscle response, such as a thumb twitch upon median nerve stimulation at the wrist. The shock is delivered at least 500 times, at a rate of five per second. A computer measures and averages the time it takes for the electric current to reach the cortex; the results, expressed in milliseconds, are recorded as waveforms. The test is repeated once to verify results; then the electrodes are repositioned and the entire procedure is repeated for the other side.

Normal findings

For visual evoked potentials: On the waveform, the most significant wave is P100, a positive wave appearing about 100 msec after the pattern-shift stimulus is applied. The most clinically significant measurements are absolute P100 latency (the time between stimulus application and peaking of the P100 wave) and the difference between the P100 latencies of each eye. Because many physical and technical factors affect P100 latency, normal results vary greatly between laboratories and patients.

For somatosensory evoked potentials: The waveforms obtained vary, depending on locations of the stimulating and recording electrodes. The positive and negative peaks are labeled in sequence, based on normal time of appearance. For example, N19 is a negative peak normally recorded 19 msec after application of the stimulus. Each wave peak arises from a discrete location: N19 is generated mainly from the thalamus, P22 from the parietal sensory cortex, and so on. Interwave latencies (time between waves), rather than absolute latencies, are used as a basis for clinical interpretation. Latency differences between sides are significant. (See *Normal and abnormal evoked potential waveforms.*)

Implications of results

For visual evoked potentials: Generally, abnormal (extended) P100 latencies confined to one eye indicate a visual

Normal and abnormal evoked potential waveforms

In *pattern-shift potentials,* visual neural impulses are recorded as they travel along the pathway from the eye to the occipital cortex. Wave P100 is the most significant component of the resultant waveform — normal P100 latency occurs approximately 100 msec after the application of a visual stimulus (top diagram). Increased P100 latency (bottom diagram) is an abnormal finding indicating a lesion along the visual pathway — in this case, in a patient with multiple sclerosis (MS).

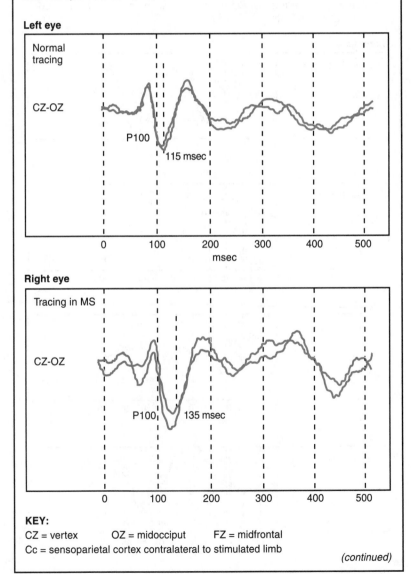

Left eye

Normal tracing

CZ-OZ

P100

115 msec

0 100 200 300 400 500
msec

Right eye

Tracing in MS

CZ-OZ

P100 135 msec

0 100 200 300 400 500

KEY:
CZ = vertex   OZ = midocciput   FZ = midfrontal
Cc = sensoparietal cortex contralateral to stimulated limb

(continued)

Normal and abnormal evoked potential waveforms (continued)

In *somatosensory evoked potentials,* the conduction time of an electrical impulse is measured as it travels along a somatosensory pathway to the cortex. Interwave latency is the most significant component of the resultant waveform. On the set of upper- and lower-limb tracings shown below, the top tracings represent normal interwave latencies; the bottom tracings, typical abnormal latencies found in a patient with multiple sclerosis. Because of the close correlation between waveforms and the anatomy of somatosensory pathways, such tracings allow precise localization of lesions that produce conduction defects.

Upper limb

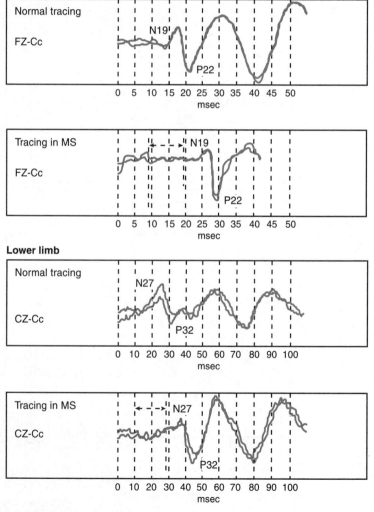

pathway lesion anterior to the optic chiasm. A lesion posterior to the optic chiasm usually doesn't produce abnormal P100 latencies: Because each eye projects to both occipital lobes, the unaffected pathway transmits sufficient impulses to produce a normal latency response.

Bilateral abnormal P100 latencies have been found in patients with multiple sclerosis, optic neuritis, retinopathies, amblyopias (although abnormal latencies don't correlate well with impaired visual acuity), spinocerebellar degeneration, adrenoleukodystrophy, sarcoidosis, Parkinson's disease, and Huntington's disease.

For somatosensory evoked potentials: Because somatosensory evoked potential components are assumed to be linked in series, an abnormal interwave latency indicates a conduction defect between the generators of the two peaks involved. This often allows precise localization of a neurologic lesion.

Abnormal upper-limb interwave latencies may indicate cervical spondylosis, intracerebral lesions, or sensorimotor neuropathies. Abnormalities in the lower limb demonstrate peripheral nerve and root lesions, such as those in Guillain-Barré syndrome, compressive myelopathies, multiple sclerosis, transverse myelitis, and traumatic spinal cord injury.

Information from evoked potential studies is insufficient to confirm a specific diagnosis. Test data must be interpreted in light of clinical information.

Post-test care
None.

Interfering factors
■ Incorrect placement of electrodes or equipment failure can alter test results.
■ Patient tension or failure to cooperate can affect the accuracy of test results.

■ Extremely poor visual acuity can hinder accurate determination of visual evoked potentials.

Computed tomography of the spine

Much more versatile than conventional radiography, computed tomography (CT) scans of the spine provide detailed, high-resolution images in the cross-sectional, longitudinal, sagittal, and lateral planes. In this procedure, multiple X-ray beams from a computerized body scanner are directed at the spine from different angles; they pass through the body and strike radiation detectors, producing electrical impulses. A computer than converts these impulses into digital information, which is displayed as a three-dimensional image on a video monitor. Storage of the digital information allows electronic recreation and manipulation of the image, creating a permanent record that allows reexamination without repeating the procedure.

Two variations of spinal CT scanning further expand the procedure's diagnostic capabilities. Contrast-enhanced CT scanning accentuates spinal vasculature and highlights even subtle differences in tissue density. Air CT scanning, which involves removing a small amount of cerebrospinal fluid (CSF) and injecting air via lumbar puncture, intensifies the contrast between the subarachnoid space and surrounding tissue.

Purpose
■ To diagnose spinal lesions and abnormalities
■ To monitor the effects of spinal surgery or therapy.

Patient preparation

Explain that this procedure allows visualization of the spine. Unless contrast enhancement is ordered, tell the patient that he needn't restrict food or fluids. (If a contrast dye will be used, instruct him to fast for 4 hours before the test.) Tell the patient that a series of scans will be taken of his spine and that the test takes 30 to 60 minutes. Explain who will perform the procedure and where. Reassure him that the procedure is painless but that he'll have to remain still for a prolonged period, which may be uncomfortable.

Explain that he'll be positioned on an X-ray table inside a CT body scanning unit and told to lie still because movement during the procedure may cause distorted images. The computer controlled scanner will revolve around him taking multiple scans. If contrast dye is used, tell him that he may feel flushed and warm and may experience a transient headache, a salty taste, and nausea or vomiting after the contrast dye is injected. Reassure him that these reactions are normal.

Instruct the patient to wear a radiologic examining gown and to remove all metal objects and jewelry from the scanning field. Check the patient's history for hypersensitivity reactions to iodine, shellfish, or contrast media. If such reactions have occurred, note them on the patient's chart and notify the doctor, who may order prophylactic medications or choose not to use contrast enhancement.

If the patient appears restless or apprehensive about the procedure, notify the doctor, who may prescribe a mild sedative.

Equipment

Computerized body scanner ✦ oscilloscope ✦ recording equipment ✦ contrast medium, as ordered (iothalamate meglumine or diatrizoate sodium) ✦ 60-ml syringe ✦ 19G or 20G needle ✦ tourniquet.

Procedure

The patient is placed in the supine position on an X-ray table and is told to lie as still as possible. The table is then slid into the circular opening of the body CT scanner. The scanner revolves around the patient, taking radiographs at preselected intervals.

After the first set of scans is taken, the patient is removed from the scanner and a contrast medium (usually, 50 to 100 ml) is administered. Observe the patient for signs and symptoms of a hypersensitivity reaction — pruritus, rash, and respiratory difficulty — for 30 minutes after the contrast dye has been injected.

After dye injection, the patient is moved back into the scanner, and another series of scans is taken. The images obtained from the scan are displayed on a video monitor during the procedure and stored on magnetic tape to create a permanent record for subsequent study.

Precautions

■ Body CT scanning with contrast enhancement is contraindicated in patients who are hypersensitive to iodine, shellfish, or contrast media used in radiographic studies.

■ Some patients may experience strong feelings of claustrophobia or anxiety inside the body CT scanner. For such patients, the doctor may order a mild sedative to help reduce anxiety.

■ For patients with significant back pain, administer analgesics prior to the scan, if ordered, so the patient can lie still comfortably.

Normal findings

In the CT image, spinal tissue appears black, white, or gray, depending on its density. Vertebrae, the densest tissues, are white; soft tissues appear in shades of gray; CSF is black.

Implications of results

By highlighting areas of altered density and depicting structural malformation, CT scanning can reveal all types of spinal lesions and abnormalities. It's particularly useful in detecting and localizing tumors, which appear as masses of varying density. Measuring this density and noting the configuration and location relative to the spinal cord can often identify the type of tumor. For example, a neurinoma (schwannoma) appears as a spherical mass dorsal to the cord; a darker, wider mass lying more laterally or ventrally to the cord may be a meningioma.

CT scanning also reveals degenerative processes and structural changes in detail. Herniated nucleus pulposus appears as an obvious herniation of disk material with unilateral or bilateral nerve root compression; if the herniation is midline, spinal cord compression will be evident. Cervical spondylosis appears as cervical cord compression due to bony hypertrophy of the cervical spine; lumbar stenosis appears as hypertrophy of the lumbar vertebrae, causing cord compression by decreasing space within the spinal column. Facet disorders appear as soft-tissue changes, bony overgrowth, and spurring of the vertebrae, resulting in nerve root compression.

Fluid-filled arachnoidal and other paraspinal cysts appear as dark masses displacing the spinal cord. Vascular malformations, evident after contrast enhancement, appear as masses or clusters, usually on the dorsal aspect of the spinal cord. Congenital spinal malformations such as meningocele, myelocele, and spina bifida show as abnormally large, dark gaps between the white vertebrae.

Post-test care

None, if the procedure was done without contrast enhancement. After testing with contrast enhancement, observe the patient for residual effects, such as headache, nausea, and vomiting, and inform him that he may resume his usual diet.

Interfering factors

■ Excessive movement by the patient during the scanning procedure may create artifact, making the images difficult to interpret.

■ Failure to remove metal objects from the scanning field may result in unclear images.

Oculoplethysmography

An important cerebrovascular test, oculoplethysmography (OPG) is a noninvasive procedure that indirectly measures blood flow in the ophthalmic artery. Because the ophthalmic artery is the first major branch of the internal carotid artery, its blood flow accurately reflects carotid blood flow and ultimately that of cerebral circulation. Two techniques are used for this test. In OPG, pulse arrival times in the eyes and ears are measured and compared to detect carotid occlusive disease. In ocular pneumoplethysmography (OPG-Gee), ophthalmic artery pressures are measured indirectly and compared with the higher brachial pressure and with each other.

Indications for both of these tests include symptoms of transient ischemic attacks, asymptomatic carotid bruits, and nonhemispheric neurologic symptoms, such as dizziness, ataxia, or syncope. This test may also be performed as a follow-up procedure after carotid endarterectomy or with transcranial

Doppler studies or carotid imaging. If indicated, it may be followed by cerebral angiography. Carotid phonoangiography is often a valuable complement to OPG. (See *Carotid phonoangiography*.)

Purpose

■ To aid detection and evaluation of carotid occlusive disease.

Patient preparation

Explain to the patient that this test evaluates carotid artery function. Inform him that he needn't restrict food or fluids. Tell him who will perform the test and where, and that the procedure takes only a few minutes.

Warn the patient that his eyes may burn slightly after the eyedrops are instilled. If OPG-Gee is scheduled, warn him that he may experience transient loss of vision when suction is applied to the eyes. Instruct him not to blink or move during the procedure. If he wears contact lenses, tell him to remove them before the test. Patients with glaucoma may take their usual medications and eyedrops.

Equipment

Oculoplethysmograph or oculopneumoplethysmograph ✦ anesthetic eyedrops (such as proparacaine 0.5%) ✦ tissues.

Procedure

For OPG: Anesthetic eyedrops are instilled to minimize patient discomfort during the test. Small photoelectric cells are attached to the earlobes; these cells can detect blood flow to the ear through the external carotid artery. Tracings for both ears are taken and compared, but only right ear tracings are compared with the eyes. (Tracings for the ears should be the same; if they're not, this is considered during interpretation of test results.)

Eyecups resembling contact lenses are applied to the corneas and held in place with light suction (40 to 50 mm Hg). Tracings of the pulsations within each eye are compared with each other and with tracings for the right ear.

For OPG-Gee: Anesthetic eyedrops are instilled, and eyecups like those used in OPG are attached to the scleras of the eyes. A vacuum of 300 mm Hg is applied to each eye, corresponding to a mean pressure of 100 mm Hg in the ophthalmic artery, and then is gradually released.

When suction is applied, the pulse in both eyes disappears; when suction is gradually released, both pulses should return simultaneously. Pulse arrival times are converted to ophthalmic artery pressures and then compared. Both brachial pressures are taken. The higher systolic pressure is then compared with the ophthalmic artery pressures. (See *OPG examination and tracings*, page 782.)

Precautions

■ OPG is contraindicated in patients who have had recent eye surgery (within 2 to 6 months), enucleation, or a history of retinal detachment or lens implantation and in those who are hypersensitive to the local anesthetic. Because of the risk of scleral hematoma or erythema, OPG-Gee is contraindicated in patients receiving anticoagulants.

■ To limit the risk of corneal abrasions, both techniques must be performed only by specially trained personnel.

Normal findings

For OPG: All pulses should occur simultaneously.

For OPG-Gee: The difference between ophthalmic artery pressures should be less than 5 mm Hg. Ophthalmic artery pressure divided by the higher brachial systolic pressure should be greater than 0.67.

Carotid phonoangiography

Carotid phonoangiography graphically records the intensity of carotid bruits during systolic and diastolic phases. It thus helps identify the presence, site, and severity of carotid artery occlusive disease.

For this test, the patient assumes a supine position and holds his breath while a transducer is placed at several sites along the carotid artery. Soundings are made directly over the clavicle (common carotid artery), midway up the neck (carotid bifurcation), and directly below the mandible (internal carotid artery). Oscillographic recordings are obtained and stored on Polaroid film and magnetic tape for later study.

Absence of bruits generally indicates an absence of significant carotid artery disease. However, bruits may also be absent when stenosis nears total occlusion. Bruits heard at all three sites, but loudest over the clavicle, usually originate in the aortic arch or in the heart. Blood flow in the carotid artery itself is unobstructed. Bruits heard over the carotid bifurcation and internal carotid sites, but louder over the latter, indicate turbulent blood flow in the internal carotid artery and the probability of more than 40% occlusion.

Carotid phonoangiography is a quick test and relatively simple to perform, but it's less sensitive and less specific than other noninvasive techniques, such as carotid imaging with Doppler ultrasound. Nevertheless, this test is approximately 85% accurate in detecting carotid artery stenosis of more than 40%.

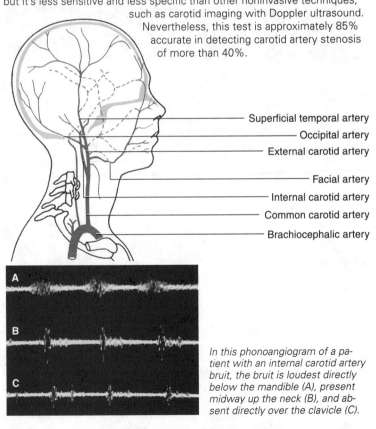

Superficial temporal artery
Occipital artery
External carotid artery

Facial artery
Internal carotid artery
Common carotid artery
Brachiocephalic artery

In this phonoangiogram of a patient with an internal carotid artery bruit, the bruit is loudest directly below the mandible (A), present midway up the neck (B), and absent directly over the clavicle (C).

OPG examination and tracings

The patient shown here is undergoing oculoplethysmography (OPG). The eyecups on her corneas detect ocular pulsations, which are compared with each other and with the blood flow in the ear. Blood flow in the ear is detected by a small photoelectric cell (not shown).

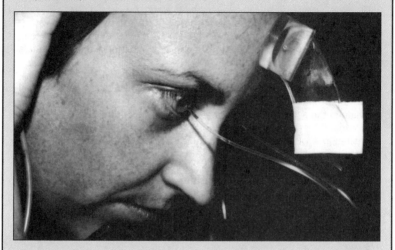

The OPG tracing on the left is normal, showing simultaneous pulsations in the right and left eyes and in the right ear. The differential waveform of ocular pulses (horizontal waveform), which amplifies pulse differences, and the vertical lines drawn on valleys and peaks of pulses to indicate pulse delays confirm simultaneous pulsation. The OPG tracing on the right is abnormal; the left-eye pulsation (vertical lines) arrives later than the other two pulsations, indicating left internal carotid artery stenosis. Note the elevation of the differential waveform.

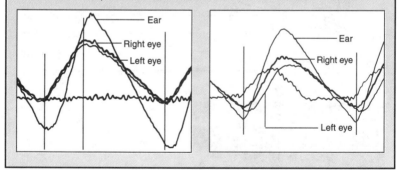

Implications of results

For OPG: Carotid occlusive disease reduces the rate of blood flow during systole and delays the arrival of a pulse in the ipsilateral eye or ear. When all pulses are compared, any delay can be measured and the degree of carotid artery stenosis estimated as mild, moderate, or severe. This test only estimates the extent of stenosis; it can't provide an exact percentage. (See *Understanding carotid imaging.*)

Understanding carotid imaging

Carotid imaging is a diagnostic test that assesses the carotid arteries for occlusive disease. In this test, a pulsed Doppler ultrasonic flow transducer or a real-time imager produces images of the carotid artery and records them.

Real-time imaging (top photo) uses the echo technique to visualize the carotid artery. In this technique, a Doppler signal can be directed to specific points along the vessel. The audio signal is then evaluated.

Pulsed Doppler technique (bottom photos) uses a transducer with a range-gating system that allows alternate transmission and reception of ultrasonic signals. The sound reflected from moving red blood cells within the lumen is then collected and stored in a computer for subsequent image reconstruction.

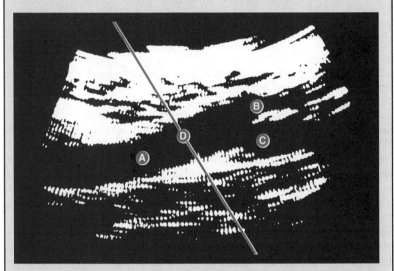

This normal real-time image, taken by echo technique, shows the common carotid artery (A), external carotid artery (B), internal carotid artery (C), and Doppler beam (D).

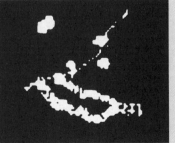

The abnormal pulsed Doppler image at left shows total occlusion (E) of the internal carotid artery. Compare this to the normal pulsed Doppler image at right.

(continued)

Understanding carotid imaging (continued)

Procedure
The patient is placed in the supine position, and the probe is placed on his neck and moved slowly from the vicinity of the common carotid artery to that of the bifurcation, and then to the site of the internal and external carotid arteries.

Advantages and disadvantages
Carotid imaging detects ulcerating plaques that can't be detected by other methods; it can also differentiate between total and near-total arterial occlusion.

Intramural calcification prevents sound penetration and may lead to false-positive results.

For OPG-Gee: A difference between ophthalmic artery pressures of more than 5 mm Hg suggests the presence of carotid occlusive disease on the side with the lower pressure. A ratio between the ophthalmic artery pressure and the higher brachial systolic pressure of less than 0.67 reinforces this finding. In other words, the ratio is related to the degree of stenosis: The lower the ratio, the more severe the stenosis. As with OPG, OPG-Gee only estimates the degree of stenosis present; angiography may be necessary to provide a precise evaluation.

Post-test care
▪ To prevent corneal abrasion, instruct the patient not to rub his eyes for 2 hours after the test. Observe for symptoms of corneal abrasion, such as pain or photophobia, and report them to the doctor.
▪ Advise the patient that mild burning as the eyedrops wear off is normal. Tell him to report severe burning.
▪ If the patient wears contact lenses, instruct him not to reinsert them for about 2 hours after OPG; this will allow the effect of the anesthetic drops to wear off.

Interfering factors
▪ In patients with hypertension, OPG-Gee test results may be more difficult to interpret because of elevated ophthalmic artery pressures.
▪ Constant blinking or nystagmus may cause an artifact, making the tracings difficult to interpret.
▪ Severe cardiac arrhythmias may alter test results.

Transcranial Doppler studies

By measuring the velocity of blood flow through cerebral arteries, transcranial Doppler studies provide information about the presence, quality, and changing nature of circulation to an area of the brain. Narrowed blood vessels produce high velocities, indicating possible stenosis or vasospasm. High velocities may also indicate an arteriovenous malformation due to the accumulated signal from the extra blood flow associated with such lesions.

Purpose
- To measure the velocity of blood flow through certain cerebral vessels
- To detect and monitor the progression of cerebral vasospasm
- To determine whether collateral blood flow exists before surgical ligation or radiologic occlusion of diseased blood vessels.

Patient preparation
Explain the purpose of the study to the patient (or to his family). Tell him that the test will be performed while he lies on a bed or stretcher or sits in a reclining chair. (It can be performed at the bedside if he's too ill to be transported to the laboratory.) Explain that a small amount of gel will be applied to his skin, and then a probe will be used to transmit a signal to the artery being studied.

Inform the patient that the study usually takes less than 1 hour, depending on the number of vessels that will be examined and on any interfering factors. Tell him that he needn't fast before the test.

Equipment
Transcranial Doppler unit ✦ probe ✦ gel.

Procedure
The patient reclines in a chair or on a stretcher or bed. A small amount of gel is applied to the transcranial "window," an area where bone is thin enough to allow the Doppler signal to enter and be detected. The most common approaches are temporal, transorbital, and through the foramen magnum. The technician next directs the signal toward the artery being studied, and then records the velocities detected. In a com-

plete study, the middle cerebral arteries, anterior cerebral arteries, ophthalmic arteries, carotid siphon, vertebral arteries, and basilar artery are studied.

The Doppler signal — measured in millimeters — can be transmitted to varying depths. Waveforms may be printed for later analysis. When the study is completed, wipe the gel away.

Precautions
- Make sure that you remove turban head dressings or thick dressings over the test site.

Normal findings
The type of waveforms and velocities obtained indicate whether or not pathology exists.

Implications of results
Although this test often isn't definitive, it provides diagnostic information in a noninvasive manner. Typically, high velocities are abnormal and suggest that blood flow is too turbulent or the vessel is too narrow.

After the transcranial Doppler study and before surgery, the patient may undergo cerebral angiography to further define cerebral blood flow patterns and to locate the exact vascular abnormality.

Post-test care
Making choices about surgery and undergoing further tests may increase the patient's anxiety. Help the patient cope with anxiety, decisional conflict, and fear by listening to his concerns and encouraging him to ask questions.

Interfering factors
Failure to remove the dressings over the test site may affect the accuracy of the Doppler study.

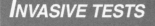

INVASIVE TESTS

Cerebral angiography

Cerebral angiography allows radiographic examination of the cerebral vasculature after injection of a contrast medium. Possible injection sites include the femoral, carotid, and brachial arteries. The femoral artery is used most often because it allows visualization of four vessels (the carotid and vertebral arteries). The usual clinical indication for this test is a suspected abnormality of the cerebral vasculature, often as suggested by intracranial computed tomography, lumbar puncture, magnetic resonance imaging, or magnetic resonance angiography.

Purpose
■ To detect cerebrovascular abnormalities, such as aneurysm or arteriovenous malformation, thrombosis, narrowing, or occlusion
■ To study vascular displacement caused by tumor, hematoma, edema, herniation, vasospasm, increased intracranial pressure (ICP), or hydrocephalus
■ To locate clips applied to blood vessels during surgery and to evaluate the postoperative status of such vessels.

Patient preparation
Explain to the patient that this test shows blood circulation to the brain. Instruct him to fast for 8 to 10 hours before the test. Tell him who will perform the test and where and that it takes 2 to 4 hours, depending on the extent of testing ordered.

Instruct the patient to wear a hospital gown and to remove jewelry, dentures, hairpins, and other metal objects in the X-ray field. If ordered, administer a sedative and an anticholinergic 30 to 45 minutes before the test. Make sure the patient voids before leaving his room.

Tell the patient he'll be positioned on an X-ray table, with his head immobilized, and will be told to lie still. Tell him a local anesthetic will be administered. (Some patients — especially children — may receive a general anesthetic.) Explain that he'll probably feel a transient burning sensation as the contrast medium is injected and may feel flushed and warm and experience a transient headache, a salty taste, or nausea and vomiting after the dye is injected.

Make sure the patient or responsible family member has signed a consent form if required. Check the patient's history for hypersensitivity to iodine, iodine-containing substances (such as shellfish), or other contrast media. Mark any hypersensitivities on the patient's chart, and notify the doctor; he may order prophylactic drugs or may cancel the test.

Equipment
Contrast medium ✦ automatic contrast injector ✦ X-ray machine, with rapid biplane cassette changer ✦ arterial needles: 18G or 19G 2½" needle for adults; 20G 1½" needle for children ✦ femoral arterial catheters for femoral injection.

Procedure
The patient is placed in the supine position on a radiographic table, and the injection site (femoral, carotid, or brachial artery) is shaved. He is then instructed to lie still, with his arms at his sides. The skin is cleaned with alcohol and povidone-iodine, and the local anesthetic is injected.

The artery is then punctured with the appropriate needle and catheterized. If the femoral approach is used, a catheter is threaded up the aortic arch. If the carotid artery is used, the patient's neck is hyperextended, and a rolled-up towel or sandbag is placed under his shoulders. His head is then immobilized with a restraint or tape. If the brachial artery (least common) is used, a blood pressure cuff is placed distal to the puncture site and inflated before injection to prevent the contrast medium from flowing into the forearm and hand.

After placement of the needle (or catheter) is verified by radiography or fluoroscopy, the contrast medium is injected. The patient is observed for a reaction, such as urticaria, flushing, and laryngeal stridor. A first series of lateral and anteroposterior radiographs is taken, developed, and reviewed. Depending on the results of this initial series, more contrast medium may be injected and another series of radiographs taken. Arterial catheter patency is maintained by continuous or periodic flushing with normal saline or heparin solution. Vital and neurologic signs are monitored throughout the test.

When an acceptable series of radiographs have been obtained, the needle (or catheter) is withdrawn, and firm pressure is applied to the pressure site for 15 minutes. The patient is observed for bleeding, distal pulses are checked, and a pressure bandage is applied.

Precautions

- Cerebral angiography is contraindicated in patients with hepatic, renal, or thyroid disease and in those with a hypersensitivity to iodine or contrast media.
- For patients who have been receiving aspirin daily, take extra care to compress the puncture site.

Normal findings

During the arterial phase of perfusion, the contrast medium fills and opacifies superficial and deep arteries and arterioles; it opacifies superficial and deep veins during the venous phase. The finding of apparently normal (symmetrical) cerebral vasculature, however, must be correlated with the patient's history and clinical status. (See *Comparing normal and abnormal angiograms,* page 788.)

Implications of results

Changes in the caliber of vessel lumina suggest vascular disease, possibly due to spasms, plaques, fistulas, arteriovenous malformation, or arteriosclerosis. Diminished blood flow to vessels may be related to increased ICP.

Vessel displacement may reflect the presence and size of a tumor, areas of edema, or obstruction of the CSF pathway. Cerebral angiography may also show circulation within a tumor, often giving precise information on the tumor's position and nature. Meningeal blood supply originating in the external carotid artery may indicate an extracerebral tumor but usually designates a meningioma. Such a tumor may arise outside the brain substance, but it may still be within the cerebral hemisphere.

Post-test care

- Enforce bed rest for 12 to 24 hours, and provide pain medication as ordered. Monitor vital signs and neurologic status for 24 hours — every hour for the first 4 hours, then every 4 hours.
- Check the puncture site for signs of extravasation, such as redness and swelling. To ease the patient's discomfort and minimize swelling, apply an ice bag to the site. If bleeding occurs, apply firm pressure on the puncture site.

 - If the femoral approach was used, keep the affected leg straight for at least 12 hours, and routinely check pulses distal to the site (dorsalis pedis and popliteal). Check the temperature, color, and tactile sensations of the affected leg because thrombosis or hematoma can occlude blood flow. Extravasation can also block blood flow by exerting pressure on the artery.

Comparing normal and abnormal angiograms

The cerebral angiogram on the left is a normal view. The cerebral angiogram on the right shows occluded vasculature caused by a large arteriovenous malformation.

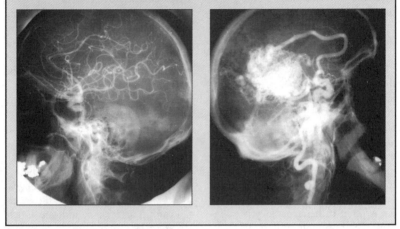

■ If a carotid artery was used as the injection site, watch for dysphagia or respiratory distress, which can result from hematoma or extravasation. Also watch for disorientation and weakness or numbness in the extremities (signs of thrombosis or hematoma) and for arterial spasms, which produce symptoms of transient ischemic attacks. Notify the doctor if abnormal signs develop.

■ If the brachial approach was used, immobilize the arm for at least 6 hours, and routinely check the radial pulse. Place a sign above the patient's bed warning personnel against taking blood pressure readings from the affected arm. Observe the arm and hand, noting any change in color, temperature, or tactile sensations. If it becomes pale, cool, or numb, notify the doctor.

■ Tell the patient he may resume his usual diet.

■ Encourage oral fluids to help pass the contrast dye.

Interfering factors

■ Head movement during the test affects the clarity of the angiographs.

■ Failure to remove metal objects from the X-ray field may yield unclear images.

Digital subtraction angiography

Digital subtraction angiography (DSA) is a sophisticated radiographic technique that uses video equipment and computer-assisted image enhancement to examine the vascular systems. As in conventional angiography, X-ray images are obtained after injection of a contrast medium. However, unlike conventional angiography, in which images of bone and soft tissue often obscure vascular detail, DSA provides a high-contrast view of blood vessels without interfering images or shadows.

This unique view is made possible by digital subtraction, in which fluoroscopic images are taken both before and after injection of a contrast medium. A computer converts these images into digital information and then "subtracts" the first image from the second, eliminating most information (mainly bone and soft tissue) common to both images. The result is a better image of the contrast-enhanced vasculature.

In addition to superior image quality, DSA has other advantages over conventional angiography. Because the digital subtraction process allows I.V., rather than intra-arterial, injection of the contrast medium, DSA avoids one risk of conventional angiography — stroke — and reduces the pain and the discomfort associated with arterial catheterization.

Although DSA has been used to study peripheral and renal vascular disease, it's probably most useful in diagnosing cerebrovascular disorders, such as carotid stenosis and occlusion, arteriovenous malformation, aneurysms, and vascular tumors. It's also useful in visualizing displacement of vasculature by other intracranial abnormalities or traumatic injuries and in detecting lesions often missed by computed tomography scans, such as thrombosis of the superior sagittal sinus.

Purpose

- To visualize extracranial and intracranial cerebral blood flow
- To detect and evaluate cerebrovascular abnormalities
- To aid postoperative evaluation of cerebrovascular surgery, such as arterial grafts and endarterectomies.

Patient preparation

Explain to the patient that this test visualizes cerebral blood vessels. Tell him he'll need to fast for 4 hours before the test but he needn't restrict fluids. Explain that he'll receive an injection of a contrast medium, either by needle or through a venous catheter inserted in his arm, and that a series of X-rays will be taken of his head. Tell him who will perform the test and where and that it takes 30 to 45 minutes.

Inform the patient that he'll be positioned on an X-ray table, with his head immobilized, and will be asked to lie still. (Some patients — especially children — may be given a sedative to prevent movement during the procedure.) Instruct him to remove all jewelry, dentures, and other radiopaque objects from the X-ray field. Tell him that he'll probably feel some transient pain from insertion of the needle or catheter and that he may experience a feeling of warmth, a headache, a metallic taste, and nausea or vomiting after the contrast agent is injected.

Make sure the patient or a responsible family member has signed a consent form if required. Check the patient's history for hypersensitivity to iodine, iodine-containing substances such as shellfish, and contrast media. If he's had such reactions, note them on the chart and inform the doctor. He may order prophylactic medications or choose not to perform the test.

Equipment

X-ray machine with biplane cassette changer ✦ computer and video monitor ✦ video recorder ✦ I.V. equipment and 250 ml normal saline solution ✦ contrast medium ✦ automatic contrast medium injector.

Procedure

The patient is placed in the supine position on an X-ray table and is told to lie still, with his arms at his sides. After an initial series of fluoroscopic pictures (mask images) of his head is taken, the injection site — most commonly the antecubital basilic or cephalic vein — is shaved and cleaned with an antiseptic solution.

If catheterization is ordered, a local anesthetic is administered, a venipuncture is performed, and a catheter is inserted and advanced to the superior vena cava. After placement is verified by X-ray, I.V. lines from a bag of normal saline solution and from an automatic contrast medium injector are connected. While the saline is administered, the injector delivers the contrast medium at a rate of about 14 ml/second. If a simple injection of the contrast medium is ordered, a bolus of 40 to 60 ml is administered I.V. by needle.

The patient's vital signs and neurologic status are monitored, and he's observed for signs of a hypersensitivity reaction, such as urticaria, flushing, and respiratory distress. After allowing time for the contrast medium to clear the pulmonary circulation and enter the cerebral vasculature, a second series of fluoroscopic images (contrast images) is taken. The computer digitizes the information received from both series and compares mask and contrast images, subtracting the information (images of bone and soft tissue) common to both. A detailed image of the contrast medium–filled vessels is displayed on a video monitor; the image may be stored on videotape or a video disc for future reference.

Precautions

DSA may be contraindicated in patients with a hypersensitivity to iodine or contrast media; poor cardiac function; renal, hepatic, or thyroid disease; diabetes; or multiple myeloma.

Normal findings

The contrast medium should fill and opacify all superficial and deep arteries, arterioles, and veins, allowing visualization of normal cerebral vasculature. The digital subtraction process may intensify areas that should receive only contrast medium. However, conventional angiography provides a more detailed image of the carotid arteries than DSA.

Implications of results

Vascular filling defects, seen as areas of increased vascular opacity, may indicate arteriovenous occlusion or stenosis, possibly due to vasospasm, vascular malformation or angiomas, arteriosclerosis, or cerebral embolism or thrombosis. Outpouchings in vessel lumina may reflect cerebral aneurysms; such aneurysms frequently rupture, causing subarachnoid hemorrhage. Vessel displacement or vascular masses may indicate an intracranial tumor. DSA can clearly depict the vascular supply of some tumors, reflecting the tumor's position, size, and nature.

Post-test care

- Because the contrast medium acts as a diuretic, encourage the patient to increase his fluid intake for 24 hours after this test. Advise him that extra fluid intake will also speed excretion of the contrast medium. Monitor intake and output as ordered.
- Check the venipuncture site for signs of extravasation, such as redness or swelling. If bleeding occurs, apply firm pressure to the puncture site. If a hematoma develops, elevate the arm and apply warm soaks.
- Observe the patient for a delayed hypersensitivity reaction to the contrast medium. A delayed reaction can occur up to 18 hours after the procedure.
- Allow the patient to resume his normal diet.

Interfering factors

- Patient movement during the procedure may cause blurred images.
- Radiopaque objects in the fluoroscopic field may impair image clarity.

Electromyography

Electromyography (EMG) is the recording of the electrical activity of selected skeletal muscle groups at rest and during voluntary contraction. In this test, a needle electrode is inserted percutaneously into a muscle. The electrical discharge (or motor unit potential) of the muscle is then displayed and measured on an oscilloscope screen. Nerve conduction time — a separate procedure — is often measured simultaneously. (See *Nerve conduction studies,* page 792.) EMG is a useful diagnostic technique for evaluating muscle disorders.

Purpose

■ To aid differentiation between primary muscle disorders, such as the muscular dystrophies, and those that are secondary

■ To help determine diseases characterized by central neuronal degeneration, such as amyotrophic lateral sclerosis (ALS)

■ To aid diagnosis of neuromuscular disorders such as myasthenia gravis.

Patient preparation

Explain to the patient that this test measures the electrical activity of his muscles. Normally, foods and fluids aren't withheld before this test, but some doctors may forbid cigarettes, coffee, tea, and cola for 2 to 3 hours before the test. Tell the patient who will perform the test and where and that it takes at least 1 hour.

The patient may wear a hospital gown for the test or any comfortable clothing that permits access to the muscles to be tested. Advise him that a needle will be inserted into selected muscles and that he may experience some discomfort. Reassure him that side effects or complications are rare. Make sure the patient or responsible member of the family has signed a consent form if required.

Check the patient's history for medications that may interfere with test results (such as cholinergics, anticholinergics, and skeletal muscle relaxants). If the patient is receiving such medications, note this on the chart, and withhold the medications as ordered.

Equipment

Electromyograph and recorder ✦ needle electrodes ✦ oscilloscope.

Procedure

The patient lies on a stretcher or bed or sits on a chair, depending on the muscles to be tested. The arm or leg is positioned so the muscle to be tested is at rest. The needle electrodes are then quickly inserted into the selected muscle, and a metal plate is placed under the patient to serve as a reference electrode. The muscle's resulting electrical signal (motor unit potential), recorded during rest and contraction, is amplified 1 million times and displayed on an oscilloscope screen. Photographs are taken of the display for a permanent record. The lead wires of the recorder are usually attached to an audio-amplifier so that voltage fluctuations within the muscle can be heard.

Precautions

EMG is contraindicated in patients with bleeding disorders.

Normal findings

At rest, a normal muscle exhibits minimal electrical activity. During voluntary contraction, however, electrical activity increases markedly. A sustained contraction or one of increasing strength produces a rapid "train" of motor unit potentials that can be heard as a crescendo of sounds, similar to the sound of

---

Nerve conduction studies

Nerve conduction studies aid diagnosis of peripheral nerve injuries and diseases affecting the peripheral nervous system, such as peripheral neuropathies. To measure nerve conduction time, a nerve is stimulated electrically through the skin and underlying tissues. The patient experiences a mild electric shock with each stimulation. At a known distance from the point of stimulation, a recording electrode detects the response from the stimulated nerve.

The time between stimulation of the nerve and the detected response is measured on an oscilloscope. The speed of conduction along the nerve is then calculated by dividing the distance between the point of stimulation and the recording electrode by the time between stimulus and response. In peripheral nerve injuries and diseases such as peripheral neuropathies, nerve conduction time is abnormal.

---

an outboard motor, over the audioamplifier.

At the same time, the oscilloscope screen displays a sequence of waveforms that vary in amplitude (height) and frequency. Waveforms that are close together indicate a high frequency; waveforms that are far apart signify a low frequency.

Implications of results

In primary muscle disease, such as the muscular dystrophies, motor unit potentials are short (low amplitude), with frequent, irregular discharges. In disorders such as ALS and in peripheral nerve disorders, motor unit potentials are isolated and irregular but show increased amplitude and duration. In myasthenia gravis, motor unit potentials may be normal initially, but they diminish in amplitude progressively with continuing contractions. The interpreter makes a distinction between waveforms that indicate a muscle disorder and those that indicate denervation.

Findings must be correlated with the patient's history, clinical features, and the results of other neurodiagnostic tests.

Post-test care

■ If the patient experiences residual pain, apply warm compresses and administer analgesics as ordered.

■ Medications or substances that were withheld before the test may be resumed, as ordered.

Interfering factors

■ The patient's inability to comply with instructions during the test may invalidate results.

■ Drugs that affect myoneural junctions, such as cholinergics, anticholinergics, and skeletal muscle relaxants, interfere with test results.

Cerebrospinal fluid analysis

Cerebrospinal fluid (CSF), a clear substance that circulates in the subarachnoid space, has many vital functions. It protects the brain and spinal cord from injury and transports products of neurosecretion, cellular biosynthesis, and cellular metabolism through the central nervous system (CNS). For qualitative analysis, CSF is most commonly obtained by lumbar puncture (usually between the third and fourth lumbar vertebrae); rarely, by cisternal or ventricular puncture. (See *Alternate methods of obtaining CSF,* page 794.) Specimens of CSF for laboratory analysis are commonly obtained during other neurologic tests, such as myelography.

Purpose

■ To measure CSF pressure as an aid in detecting obstruction of CSF circulation
■ To aid diagnosis of viral or bacterial meningitis, and subarachnoid or intracranial hemorrhage, tumors, and brain abscesses
■ To aid diagnosis of neurosyphilis and chronic CNS infections.

Recently, two new tests have become available that use CSF specimens to test for Alzheimer's disease. (See *Two new tests for Alzheimer's disease,* page 795.)

Patient preparation

Describe the procedure to the patient, and explain that this test analyzes the fluid within the spinal cord. Inform him that he needn't restrict food or fluids. Tell him who will perform the procedure and where and that it usually takes at least 15 minutes.

Advise the patient that a headache is the most common side effect of lumbar puncture, but reassure him that his cooperation during the test helps minimize this reaction. Make sure the patient or a responsible family member has signed a consent form if required. If the patient is unusually anxious, assess his vital signs and notify the doctor.

Equipment

Lumbar puncture tray ✦ sterile gloves ✦ local anesthetic (usually 1% lidocaine) ✦ povidone-iodine ✦ small adhesive bandage.

Procedure

Position the patient on his side at the edge of the bed, with his knees drawn up to his abdomen and his chin on his chest. Provide pillows to support the spine on a horizontal plane. This position allows full flexion of the spine and easy access to the lumbar subarachnoid space. Help the patient maintain this position by placing one arm around his knees and the other arm around his neck. If a sitting position is preferred, have the patient sit up and bend his chest and head toward his knees. Help him maintain this position throughout the procedure.

After the skin is prepared for injection, the area is draped. Warn the patient that he'll probably experience a transient burning sensation when the local anesthetic is injected. Tell him that when the spinal needle is inserted, he may feel some transient local pain as the needle transverses the dura mater. Ask him to report any pain or sensations that differ from or continue after this expected discomfort because these may indicate irritation or puncture of a nerve root, requiring repositioning of the needle. Instruct the patient to remain still and breathe normally; movement and hyperventilation can alter pressure readings or cause injury.

The anesthetic is injected, and the spinal needle is inserted in the midline, between the spinous processes of the vertebrae (usually between the third and fourth lumbar vertebrae). When the stylet is removed from the needle, CSF will drip from it if the needle is properly positioned. A stopcock and manometer are attached to the needle to measure initial (or opening) CSF pressure. After the specimen is collected, label the containers in the order in which they were filled, and ask the doctor if he has any specific instructions for the laboratory. A final pressure reading is taken, and the needle is removed. Clean the

Alternate methods of obtaining CSF

Cisternal puncture

When lumbar puncture is contraindicated by infection at the puncture site, lumbar deformity, or some other problem, the doctor may perform a cisternal puncture to obtain cerebrospinal fluid (CSF). A short-beveled, hollow needle is inserted into the cisterna cerebellomedularis, below the occipital bone, between the first cervical vertebra and the rim of the foramen magnum. Adverse reactions are minimal; the severe headaches that often occur after lumbar puncture are uncommon with this procedure. Cisternal puncture is hazardous, however, because the needle is positioned close to the brain stem. Contraindications are the same as for lumbar puncture — infection or deformity at the puncture site; increased intracranial pressure; or a history of thrombocytopenia or anticoagulant therapy because of the potential for hemorrhage into the posterior fossa or cerebellar–brain stem area.

Prepare the patient as for lumbar puncture; a cisternal puncture tray contains the necessary equipment. The patient's neck should be flexed forward so that his chin touches his chest. Hold his head firmly in place to bring the brain stem and spinal cord forward and to allow more space for the cisternal needle to enter. (If the doctor prefers, the patient may assume a sitting position, with his neck flexed forward.)

Post-test care is the same as for lumbar puncture. With an outpatient, instruct a family member to check the puncture site for redness, swelling, and drainage and to watch for signs of complications (neck rigidity, irritability, and decreased level of consciousness).

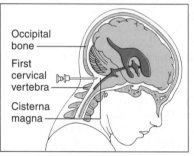

Occipital bone

First cervical vertebra

Cisterna magna

Ventricular puncture

Although rarely performed, a ventricular puncture is the procedure of choice when a spinal puncture may cause brain stem herniation or other complications. A ventricular puncture is usually done in the operating room. The doctor makes a small incision in the parieto-occipital region of the scalp, then drills a hole in the skull. A short-beveled, hollow needle is inserted through the hole and into a lateral ventricle, and CSF is withdrawn. Complications, such as ventriculitis and hemorrhage from ruptured blood vessels, are rare.

Post-test care is the same as for lumbar puncture, but don't elevate the head of the patient's bed more than 15 degrees. Bed rest is usually prescribed for 24 hours.

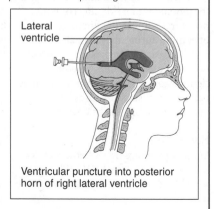

Lateral ventricle

Ventricular puncture into posterior horn of right lateral ventricle

Two new tests for Alzheimer's disease

Two new tests were recently introduced for use in patients with symptoms of dementia. One test determines the levels of tau protein and beta-amyloid in the cerebrospinal fluid (CSF) and requires a lumbar puncture. Elevated levels of tau and reduced levels of beta-amyloid are associated with Alzheimer's disease. The manufacturer claims that this test is 95% accurate in ruling out or confirming Alzheimer's disease in about 60% of symptomatic patients over age 60.

The second test determines apolipoprotein E (ApoE) genotype, which is statistically significant in determining the probability of Alzheimer's. The presence of two copies of the ApoE4 allele may increase the probability to over 90%.

Although these tests may prove helpful in diagnosing Alzheimer's disease, experts caution that further studies are necessary to confirm their reliability.

---

puncture site with a local antiseptic, such as povidone-iodine solution, and apply a small adhesive bandage.

Precautions
▪ Infection at the puncture site contraindicates removal of CSF; in a patient with increased intracranial pressure, CSF should be removed with extreme caution because the rapid reduction in pressure that follows withdrawal of fluid can cause cerebellar tonsillar herniation and medullary compression.

 ▪ During the procedure, observe closely for signs of an adverse reaction, such as elevated pulse rate, pallor, or clammy skin. Alert the doctor immediately to any significant changes.

▪ Record the collection time on the test request. Send the form and labeled specimens to the laboratory immediately.

Normal findings
Normally, the doctor records CSF pressure and checks the appearance of the specimen. Three tubes are collected routinely and are sent to the laboratory for analysis of protein, sugar, and cells as well as for serologic testing, such as the Venereal Disease Research Laboratory test for neurosyphilis. A separate specimen is also sent to the laboratory for culture and sensitivity testing. Electrolyte analysis and Gram stain may be ordered as supplementary tests. CSF electrolyte levels are of special interest in patients with abnormal serum electrolyte levels or CSF infection and in those receiving hyperosmolar agents.

Implications of results
For the implications of abnormal CSF analysis findings, see *Interpreting CSF findings*, pages 796 and 797.

Post-test care
▪ Find out if the patient must lie flat or if the head of his bed may be slightly elevated. In most cases, you'll be instructed to keep the patient lying flat for 8 hours after lumbar puncture, but some doctors allow a 30-degree elevation. Remind the patient that although he must not raise his head, he can turn from side to side.

▪ Encourage the patient to drink fluids. Provide a flexible straw.

▪ Check the puncture site for redness, swelling, and drainage every hour for

Interpreting CSF findings

TEST	NORMAL	ABNORMAL	IMPLICATIONS
Pressure	50 to 180 mm H_2O	Increase	Increased intracranial pressure due to hemorrhage, tumor, or edema caused by trauma
		Decrease	Spinal subarachnoid obstruction above puncture site
Appearance	Clear, colorless	Cloudy	Infection (elevated white blood cell [WBC] count and protein, or many microorganisms)
		Xanthochromic or bloody	Subarachnoid, intracerebral, or intraventricular hemorrhage; spinal cord obstruction; traumatic lumbar puncture (usually noted only in initial specimen)
		Brown, orange	Elevated protein levels, red or yellow blood cell (RBC) breakdown (blood present for at least 3 days)
Protein	15 to 45 mg/dl	Marked increase	Tumors, trauma, hemorrhage, diabetes mellitus, polyneuritis, blood in CSF
		Marked decrease	Rapid CSF production
Gamma globulin	3% to 12% of total protein	Increase	Demyelinating disease (such as multiple sclerosis), neurosyphilis, Guillain-Barré syndrome
Glucose	50 to 80 mg/dl (two-thirds of blood glucose)	Increase	Systemic hyperglycemia
		Decrease	Systemic hypoglycemia, bacterial or fungal infection, meningitis, mumps, postsubarachnoid hemorrhage
Cell count	0 to 5 WBCs	Increase	Active disease: meningitis, acute infection, onset of chronic illness, tumor, abscess, infarction, demyelinating disease
	No RBCs	RBCs	Hemorrhage or traumatic lumbar puncture

Interpreting CSF findings (continued)			
TEST	NORMAL	ABNORMAL	IMPLICATIONS
Venereal Disease Research Laboratories and other serologic tests	Nonreactive	Positive	Neurosyphilis
Chloride	118 to 130 mEq/L	Decrease	Infected meninges (as in tuberculosis or meningitis)
Gram stain	No organisms	Gram-positive or gram-negative organisms	Bacterial meningitis

the first 4 hours, then every 4 hours for the first 24 hours.

▪ If CSF pressure is elevated, assess neurologic status every 15 minutes for 4 hours. If the patient is stable, assess every hour for 2 hours, then every 4 hours or according to pretest schedule.

▪ Watch for complications of lumbar puncture, such as a reaction to the anesthetic, meningitis, bleeding into the spinal canal, and cerebellar tonsillar herniation and medullary compression. Signs of meningitis include fever, neck rigidity, and irritability; signs of herniation include decreased level of consciousness, changes in pupil size and equality, altered vital signs (including widened pulse pressure, decreased pulse rate, and irregular respirations), and respiratory failure.

Interfering factors

▪ The patient's position and activity can alter CSF pressure. Crying, coughing, or straining may increase pressure.
▪ Delay between collection time and laboratory testing can invalidate results, especially cell counts.

Myelography

Myelography combines fluoroscopy and radiography to evaluate the spinal subarachnoid space after injection of a contrast medium. Because the contrast medium is heavier than cerebrospinal fluid (CSF), it will flow through the subarachnoid space to the dependent area when the patient, lying prone on a fluoroscopic table, is tilted up or down. The fluoroscope allows visualization of the flow of the contrast medium and the outline of the subarachnoid space. X-rays are taken for a permanent record.

Myelography can help locate a spinal lesion, a ruptured disk, spinal stenosis, or an abscess. Sometimes it's performed to confirm the need for surgery; in such cases, a neurosurgeon may stand by. If this test confirms a spinal tumor, the patient may be taken directly to the operating room. Immediate surgery may also be necessary when the contrast medium causes a total block of the subarachnoid space.

Purpose

- To demonstrate lesions that partially or totally block the flow of CSF in the subarachnoid space, such as tumors and herniated intervertebral disks
- To help detect arachnoiditis, spinal nerve root injury, or tumors in the posterior fossa of the skull.

Patient preparation

Explain that this test reveals obstructions in the spinal cord. Instruct the patient to restrict food and fluids for 8 hours before the test. If an afternoon test is scheduled and hospital policy permits, the patient may have clear liquids before the test. Tell him who will perform the test and where and that the procedure takes at least 1 hour.

Explain to the patient that he'll probably feel transient burning as the contrast medium is injected and may experience flushing and warmth, a headache, a salty taste, or nausea and vomiting after the contrast dye is injected. Warn him that he may feel some pain during the procedure from the position he'll assume, from insertion of the needle or, in some cases, from removal of the contrast medium.

If required, make sure the consent form is signed. Check the patient's history for hypersensitivity to iodine and iodine-containing substances (such as shellfish), contrast media, and medications associated with the procedure. If metrizamide is used as the contrast medium, discontinue phenothiazines 48 hours before the test. Tell the patient that the head of his bed must be elevated for 6 to 8 hours after the test and that he'll remain on bed rest for an additional 6 to 8 hours. If an oil-based contrast agent is used, inform the patient that it will be manually removed after the test and that he'll need to remain flat in bed for 6 to 24 hours. Notify the radiologist if the patient has a history of epilepsy or phenothiazine use.

Instruct the patient to remove jewelry and metal objects in the X-ray field. Administer pretest medications and perform pretest procedures, as ordered. In the lumbar region, a cleansing enema may be ordered. A sedative and an anticholinergic (such as atropine sulfate) may be ordered to reduce swallowing during the procedure.

Equipment

Alcohol ✦ 1% lidocaine solution ✦ lumbar puncture tray ✦ contrast medium (iophendylate or metrizamide sodium ✦ two 10-ml syringes ✦ spinal needle (18G for iophendylate and 11G for metrizamide) ✦ X-ray machine capable of fluoroscopy ✦ povidone-iodine solution ✦ sterile gloves ✦ small adhesive bandage.

Procedure

The patient is positioned on his side at the edge of the table, with his knees drawn up to his abdomen and his chin on his chest. (If he has a lumbar deformity or an infection at the puncture site, a cisternal puncture may be done.) A lumbar puncture is performed, and the fluoroscope is used to verify proper needle position in the subarachnoid space. Some CSF may be removed for routine laboratory analysis. The patient is then turned to the prone position and is secured with straps across his upper back, under his arms, and across his ankles. His chin is hyperextended to prevent the flow of contrast medium into the cranium; a towel or sponge is placed under his chin for comfort. In this position, the patient may complain of a headache, have trouble swallowing, or feel he's not inhaling enough oxygen. If so, reassure him that he'll have opportunities during the procedure to rest from this uncomfortable position.

With the spinal needle in place, the contrast medium is injected and the table tilted so that the contrast flows through the subarachnoid space. (Rare-

Removing contrast media after myelography

Some contrast media must be removed after a test and some are left to be absorbed by the body, depending on which agent is used.

The contrast medium *iophendylate* must be removed after the procedure because it's not water-soluble and won't be excreted. Left in the body, it could cause inflammation or adhesive arachnoiditis.

Two methods may be used to remove iophendylate: With the patient in the prone position, the contrast agent pools in the lumbar lordosis and can then be aspirated; with the patient on his side (the usual position for lumbar puncture), the dye may be aspirated or allowed to drip from the needle. Removal of iophendylate may produce pain in the buttocks or legs from nerve root irritation. The patient must return to his room on a stretcher and lie flat for 24 hours after myelography.

Metrizamide is water-soluble and doesn't have to be removed. After it's absorbed into the bloodstream, the kidneys excrete it. However, the patient who receives metrizamide must return to his room in a wheelchair or on a stretcher with the head elevated at least 60 degrees. In his room, he must sit in a chair or lie in bed with his head elevated at least 60 degrees. He must *not* lie flat for at least 8 hours because this contrast medium can irritate cervical nerve roots and cranial structures.

ly, air may be injected as a contrast agent [negative contrast], but this is mainly reserved for patients with suspected congenital abnormalities such as syringomyelia.) The flow of the contrast dye is studied on the fluoroscope, and radiographs are taken. If an obstruction in the subarachnoid space blocks the upward flow of the contrast, a cisternal puncture may be performed. When the required radiographs have been obtained, the contrast dye is withdrawn, if necessary, and the needle is removed. The puncture site is cleaned with povidone-iodine solution, and a small adhesive bandage is applied. (See *Removing contrast media after myelography*.)

Precautions

■ Myelography is usually contraindicated in patients with increased intracranial pressure, hypersensitivity to iodine or contrast media, or an infection at the puncture site.

■ Improper positioning after the test may affect recovery.

Normal findings

The contrast medium should flow freely through the subarachnoid space, showing no obstruction or structural abnormalities.

Implications of results

This test can identify and localize lesions within or surrounding the spinal cord or subarachnoid space. Common extradural lesions include herniated intervertebral disks and metastatic tumors. Common lesions within the subarachnoid space include neurofibromas and meningiomas; lesions within the spinal cord, ependymomas and astrocytomas. This test may also detect syringomyelia, a congenital abnormality marked by fluid-filled cavities in the spinal cord and widening of the cord itself. Myelography may also detect arachnoiditis, spinal nerve root injury, and tumors in the posterior fossa of the skull. Test results must be correlated with the patient's history and clinical status.

Post-test care

■ Find out which contrast medium was used for the test, and position the patient accordingly.

■ Monitor vital signs and neurologic status at least every 30 minutes for the first 4 hours, then every 4 hours for 24 hours.

■ Encourage the patient to drink extra fluids. He should void within 8 hours after returning to his room.

■ If no complications or adverse reactions occur, the patient may resume his usual diet and activities the day after the test. If radicular pain, fever, back pain, or signs of meningeal irritation (headache, irritability, or neck stiffness) develop, keep the room quiet and dark, and provide an analgesic or an antipyretic, as ordered.

Interfering factors

Incorrect needle placement or the patient's failure to cooperate may alter results.

Tensilon test

This test involves careful observation of the patient after I.V. administration of Tensilon (edrophonium chloride), a rapid, short-acting anticholinesterase that improves muscle strength by increasing muscle response to nerve impulses. It is especially useful in diagnosing myasthenia gravis, an abnormality of the myoneural junction in which nerve impulses fail to induce normal muscular responses. Patients with myasthenia gravis experience extreme fatigue at the end of the day and after repetitive activity or stress. Results of other procedures, including electromyography, may supplement Tensilon test findings in diagnosing this disease.

Purpose

■ To aid diagnosis of myasthenia gravis
■ To help differentiate between myasthenic and cholinergic crises
■ To monitor oral anticholinesterase therapy.

Patient preparation

Explain to the patient that this test helps determine the cause of muscle weakness. Inform him that he needn't restrict food or fluids. Tell him who will perform the test and where and that it takes 15 to 30 minutes.

Don't describe the exact response that will be evaluated because this knowledge may interfere with the test's objectivity. Simply tell the patient that a small tube will be inserted into a vein in his arm and that a drug will be administered periodically. Tell him he'll then be closely observed as he is asked to make repetitive muscular movements. Advise him that he may feel some unpleasant side effects from the Tensilon, but reassure him that someone will be with him at all times and that such reactions will quickly disappear. To ensure accuracy, the test may be repeated several times.

Check the patient's history for use of medications that affect muscle function and for anticholinesterase therapy, drug hypersensitivities, and respiratory disease. Withhold medications as ordered. If the patient is receiving anticholinesterase therapy, note this on the requisition along with the last dose he received and the time it was administered. Patients with respiratory ailments, such as asthma, should receive atropine during the test to minimize Tensilon's adverse effects.

Equipment

Standard: 10 mg Tensilon ✦ 0.4 mg atropine (as ordered, for patients with respiratory distress) ✦ one tuberculin and one 3-ml syringe ✦ I.V. infusion set ✦ 50-ml bag of I.V. solution (dextrose 5% in water [D$_5$W] or normal saline solution) ✦ tape, tourniquet, alcohol swabs.

Emergency: 0.5 to 1 mg atropine I.V., for cholinergic crisis ✦ 0.5 to 2 mg neostigmine methylsulfate I.V., for myasthenic crisis (may be repeated up to 5 mg) ✦ extra tuberculin and 3-ml syringes (for atropine or neostigmine injections) ✦ resuscitation equipment, including a tracheotomy tray.

Procedure

Begin I.V. infusion of D$_5$W or normal saline solution.

To help diagnose myasthenia gravis: 2 mg of Tensilon is administered initially. Infants and children require a dosage adjustment. Before the rest of the dose is administered, the doctor may want to tire the muscles by asking the patient to perform various exercises, such as looking up until ptosis develops, counting to 100 until his voice diminishes, or holding his arms above his shoulders until they drop. When the muscles are fatigued, the remaining 8 mg of Tensilon is administered over 30 seconds.

Some doctors prefer to begin this test with a placebo injection to evaluate the patient's muscle response more accurately. If so, the placebo is administered and the patient is observed. This placebo isn't necessary when cranial muscles are being tested because cranial strength can't be stimulated voluntarily.

After administration of Tensilon, the patient is asked to perform repetitive muscular movements, such as opening and closing his eyes and crossing and uncrossing his legs. Assist the doctor by closely observing the patient for improved muscle strength. If muscle strength doesn't improve within 3 to 5 minutes, the test may be repeated.

To differentiate between myasthenic crisis and cholinergic crisis: 1 to 2 mg of Tensilon is infused. After infusion, continually monitor the patient's vital signs. Watch closely for respiratory distress, and be prepared to provide respiratory assistance. If muscle strength doesn't improve, more Tensilon is infused cautiously — 1 mg at a time up to a maximum of 5 mg — and the patient is observed for distress. Neostigmine is administered immediately if the test demonstrates myasthenic crisis; atropine is administered for cholinergic crisis.

To evaluate oral anticholinesterase therapy: 2 mg of Tensilon is infused 1 hour after the patient's last dose of the anticholinesterase. The patient is observed carefully for adverse reactions and muscle response. After administration of Tensilon, the I.V. line is kept open at a rate of 20 ml/hour until all the patient's responses have been evaluated. When the test is complete, discontinue the I.V. infusion as ordered, and check the patient's vital signs. Check the puncture site for hematoma, excessive bleeding, and swelling.

Precautions

■ Because of the systemic adverse reactions Tensilon may produce, this test may be contraindicated in patients with hypotension, bradycardia, apnea, or mechanical obstruction of the intestine or urinary tract.

■ Stay with the patient during the test, and observe him closely for adverse reactions.

■ Keep resuscitation equipment handy in case of respiratory failure.

Normal findings

Persons who don't have myasthenia gravis usually develop fasciculations in response to Tensilon. The doctor must interpret the responses carefully to distinguish between a normal person and one with myasthenia gravis.

Implications of results

If the patient has myasthenia gravis, his muscle strength should improve as soon as Tensilon is administered. The degree of improvement depends on the muscle group being tested. Improvement usually becomes obvious within 30 seconds; although the maximum benefit lasts only several minutes, lingering effects may persist (up to 2 hours in a patient receiving prednisone, for example). Although all patients with myasthenia gravis show improved muscle strength in this test, some respond only slightly, and the test may need to be repeated to confirm the diagnosis.

This test provides inconsistent results when myasthenia gravis affects only ocular muscles, as in mild or early forms of the disorder. It may produce a positive response in motor neuron disease and in some neuropathies and myopathies. However, the response is usually less dramatic and less consistent than in myasthenia gravis.

Patients in myasthenic crisis (an exacerbation of the disease requiring increased anticholinesterase therapy) show a brief improvement in muscle strength after Tensilon administration. In patients in cholinergic crisis (anticholinesterase overdose), Tensilon promptly exaggerates muscle weakness. If Tensilon increases muscle strength without increasing adverse reactions, anticholinesterase therapy can be increased. If Tensilon decreases muscle strength in a person with serious adverse reactions, therapy should be reduced. If the test shows no change in muscle strength and produces only mild adverse effects, therapy should remain the same.

Post-test care
As ordered, resume medications.

Interfering factors
■ In patients receiving prednisone, the effect of Tensilon on muscle strength may be delayed.
■ Quinidine and anticholinergics interfere with test results by inhibiting the action of Tensilon.

■ Procainamide and muscle relaxants interfere with test results by inhibiting normal muscle responses.

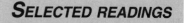

SELECTED READINGS

Fischbach, F. *A Manual of Laboratory and Diagnostic Tests,* 5th ed. Philadelphia: Lippincott-Raven Pubs., 1996.

Guyton, A.C., and Hall, J.E. *Textbook of Medical Physiology,* 9th ed. Philadelphia: W.B. Saunders Co., 1996.

Isselbacher, K.J., et al, eds. *Harrison's Principles of Internal Medicine,* 13th ed. New York: McGraw-Hill Book Co., 1994.

Jordam, K.G. "Neurophysiologic Monitoring in the Neuroscience ICU," *Neurologic Clinics* 13(3):579-626, 1995.

Nettina, S. *The Lippincott Manual of Nursing Practice,* 6th ed. Philadelphia: Lippincott-Raven Pubs., 1996.

Nursing97 Drug Handbook. Springhouse, Pa.: Springhouse Corp., 1997.

Nursing Procedures, 2nd ed. Springhouse, Pa.: Springhouse Corp., 1996.

Pagana, K.D., and Pagana, T.J. *Mosby's Diagnostic and Laboratory Test Reference,* 2nd ed. St. Louis: Mosby–Year Book, Inc., 1995.

Ravel, R.A. *Clinical Laboratory Medicine: Clinical Application of Laboratory Data,* 6th ed. St Louis: Mosby–Year Book Inc., 1995.

Gastrointestinal system

Learning objectives

After completing this chapter, the reader will be able to:

- explain the anatomy and physiology of the digestive system
- identify seven investigative techniques used in gastroenterology
- state the purpose of each test discussed in the chapter
- prepare the patient physically and psychologically for each test
- describe the procedure for performing each test

- specify appropriate precautions for safe administration of each test
- recognize signs of an adverse reaction and respond appropriately
- implement appropriate post-test care
- identify the reference values and normal findings for each test
- discuss the implications of abnormal test results
- list factors that may interfere with accurate test results.

INTRODUCTION

The GI tract and the adjoining liver, gallbladder, and pancreas are responsible for the proper digestion and absorption of food and for the elimination of metabolic waste products. Numerous diagnostic tests evaluate this system to detect diseases, functional disorders, and abnormalities resulting from emotional stress. They range from laboratory analysis of stool and esophageal, gastric, and peritoneal contents to specialized invasive and noninvasive procedures, such as endoscopy, contrast radiography, nuclear imaging, ultrasonography, and computed tomography (CT). (See *Specialized tests in gastroenterology.*) These specialized laboratory procedures are considered the most valuable because they produce results that are usually specific for a particular disease. However, the choice of an appropriate test or test battery always depends on the patient's signs and symptoms and on the results of a physical examination.

Anatomy and physiology

The GI tract includes the mouth, pharynx, esophagus, stomach (fundus, body, antrum), small intestine (duodenum, jejunum, ileum), and large intestine (cecum, colon, rectum, anal canal). Throughout the GI tract, peristalsis propels the ingested material along; sphincters prevents its reflux.

Digestion begins in the mouth through chewing and the action of the enzyme amylase, which is secreted in saliva and breaks down starches. Food is lubricated by the glycoprotein mucin,

Specialized tests in gastroenterology

TEST	PROCEDURE	CLINICAL OBJECTIVES
Endoscopy (direct visualization of the lining of a hollow viscus using an endoscope)	A cablelike cluster of glass fibers within the endoscope transmits light into the viscus, then returns an image to the scope's optical head.	■ To diagnose inflammatory, ulcerative, and infectious diseases; benign and malignant tumors; and other lesions of the esophageal, gastric, and intestinal mucosa
Radiography (passage of X-ray beams through the patient to create a radiograph)	X-ray films depict body structures and air in shades of gray, which reflect their density: Air appears black, fat appears dark gray, soft tissue appears light gray, and bone appears white. Use of contrast media accentuates density.	■ To detect obstructions, strictures, and deviations in the biliary tract ■ To detect inflammatory disease, tumors, ulcers, and other lesions ■ To diagnose hiatal hernia and other structural changes in the GI tract
Cineradiography (rapid-sequence X-ray examination that films motion)	Replay of this film at slow speeds allows close observation of such motion.	■ To detect vascular abnormalities by recording the stages of perfusion ■ To evaluate the condition of the pharynx by recording its muscular contraction
Fluoroscopy (projection of X-ray films into a fluoroscope, or specialized screen, to permit continuous observation of motion)	Spot films record significant findings.	■ To detect obstructions, strictures, and deviations in the biliary tract ■ To detect inflammatory disease, tumors, ulcers, and other lesions ■ To diagnose hiatal hernia and other structural changes in the GI tract ■ To check catheter placement in angiography by observing small injections of dye
Nuclear medicine imaging (use of a gamma camera or rectilinear scanner)	Distribution of a decaying radiopharmaceutical is recorded after I.V. injection	■ To screen for hepatocellular disease and for focal disease in the liver and spleen ■ To detect hepatomegaly and splenomegaly ■ To diagnose liver or spleen hematoma after abdominal trauma ■ To detect site of GI bleeding ■ To evaluate acute cholecystitis

(continued)

Specialized tests in gastroenterology (continued)		
TEST	**PROCEDURE**	**CLINICAL OBJECTIVES**
Ultrasonography (focused beam of high-frequency sound waves)	The sound waves pass through the patient, creating echoes that vary with tissue density. These echoes are converted into electrical energy and amplified by a transducer; then they appear on an oscilloscope screen in shades of gray as spokes or dots.	■ To detect splenomegaly ■ To differentiate between tumors, cysts, and abscesses in the liver ■ To diagnose liver or spleen hematoma after abdominal trauma ■ To differentiate between obstructive and nonobstructive jaundice ■ To diagnose cholelithiasis
Computed tomography (CT) scan (multiple X-ray beams pass through the patient, detectors record tissue attenuation, and a computer then reconstructs this information as a three-dimensional image on an oscilloscope screen)	Attenuation varies with tissue density and appears in shades of gray on the oscilloscope screen. Use of contrast media accentuates density.	■ To differentiate between tumors, cysts, and abscesses in the liver, spleen, and pancreas ■ To detect metastases in the liver ■ To diagnose liver or spleen hematoma after abdominal trauma ■ To evaluate, diagnose, or confirm pancreatitis ■ To distinguish obstructive from nonobstructive jaundice ■ To evaluate retroperitoneal disease

then swallowed as a bolus. While the food is passing through the esophagus, it's also lubricated by mucous secretions. Digestion continues in the stomach through the action of glandular secretions, such as mucus, pepsinogen, hydrochloric acid, gastrin, and intrinsic factor, a glycoprotein essential in vitamin B_{12} absorption. The hormone gastrin, the most potent stimulus of gastric secretion, enhances the release of hydrochloric acid. In turn, hydrochloric acid lowers the pH of gastric contents, promoting the conversion of pepsinogen to pepsin, a proteolytic enzyme. Pepsin begins protein catabolism, breaking down dietary protein into products ranging from large polypeptides to amino acids.

Through a churning motion, the stomach breaks food into tiny particles, mixes them with gastric juices, and pushes the mass toward the pylorus. The liquid portion (chyme) enters the duodenum in small amounts; solid material remains in the stomach until it liquefies (usually in 1 to 6 hours). Although limited amounts of water, alcohol, and certain drugs are absorbed in the stomach, chyme passes unabsorbed into the duodenum.

Digestion and absorption occur primarily in the small intestine, where millions of villi increase the surface area. For digestion, the small intestine relies on the many enzymes produced by the pancreas and by the intestinal lining. Pancreatic enzymes empty into the duodenum through the ampulla of Vater. These enzymes include trypsin, which digests protein to amino acids; lipase, which digests protein to amino acids; lipase, which digests fat to fatty acids and glycerol; and amylase, which digests starches to sugars. Intestinal enzymes include peptidases, which convert protein to amino acids; lactase, maltase, and sucrase, which digest complex sugars like glucose, fructose, and galactose; and enterokinase, which activates trypsin.

Bile also participates in digestion and absorption. After formation in the liver, bile is stored and concentrated in the gallbladder. It's released in response to cholecystokinin, a hormone secreted by the duodenum, and is then emptied into the duodenum through the ampulla of Vater. Bile helps neutralize stomach acid and promotes the emulsification of fats and the absorption of the fat-soluble vitamins A, D, E, and K.

When food reaches the ileocecal valve and enters the large intestine (3 to 10 hours after ingestion), all its nutritional value has been absorbed. The first half of the large intestine absorbs water, sodium, and chloride, reducing bulk; the second half stores and further dehydrates the digestive material until defecation. The second half of the large intestine may also excrete water, potassium, and bicarbonate.

Bacterial action in the colon putrefies undigested foods; synthesizes vitamins K, B_{12}, B_2 (riboflavin), and B_1 (thiamine); and produces gas, which helps propel feces toward the anus. Intestinal gas may also result from swallowed air or diffusion of blood gases. Rectal distention by feces stimulates the defecation reflex, which is assisted by voluntary sphincter relaxation. The passage of feces through the large intestine normally takes 24 to 40 hours.

Analysis of esophageal, gastric, and peritoneal contents

Examination of esophageal and gastric contents reveals the secretory function of the mucosa in each organ; excessive or deficient mucosal secretions or the presence of blood often aids diagnosis. Peritoneal fluid analysis provides a broader assessment of abdominal integrity because this fluid lubricates all organs within the peritoneum.

Esophageal contents consist entirely of mucus, whereas gastric contents (after a 12-hour fast) include water, hydrochloric acid, mucus, electrolytes, and pepsin. The fasting interval normally clears food particles from the stomach into the duodenum, but a small amount of food residue may be present.

Gastric contents may vary, too. For example, if excessive gagging accompanies nasogastric intubation, gastric juice may contain bile that gives it a lemon yellow to cloudy green color. It may contain mucus arising from stomach glandular secretions or from swallowed saliva and nasorespiratory secretions. Although gastric contents may normally contain flecks or streaks of bright red blood after minor trauma during intubation, a large amount of blood is abnormal. Partially digested blood appears as dark, coffee-colored particles and indicates chronic bleeding, as from ulceration or carcinoma.

Peritoneal fluid, normally clear and pale yellow, is removed from the abdominal cavity by needle aspiration. Less than 50 ml of this fluid normally lubricates the peritoneal surfaces; an excessive volume indicates pathology.

Nasogastric intubation

Aspiration of gastric contents through a nasogastric (NG) tube can help diagnose GI disorders by evaluating both the secretory activity of the gastric mucosa and the efficiency of gastric emptying into the duodenum. Although intubation is somewhat unpleasant for the patient, it can be accomplished quickly, safely, and with minimal discomfort. Diagnostic intubation is contraindicated in pregnant patients and in those with aortic aneurysms, myocardial infarction, diverticula, esophageal varices, head trauma, or stenosis; however, it may be performed cautiously in an emergency.

Fecal analysis

The GI tract processes about 10 qt (10 L) of chyme daily, of which 100 to 300 grams are eventually expelled as feces. Normal defecation patterns — influenced by food and fluid intake, medications, exercise, and rate of digestion — vary from two or three times daily to two or three times weekly. Fecal analysis can evaluate digestive efficiency and the integrity of the stomach and intestines.

Feces normally consist of 75% water and 25% solids, such as cellulose and other indigestible fiber, bacteria, unabsorbed minerals, fat and fat derivatives, desquamated epithelial cells, mucus, and small amounts of digestive enzymes and secretions. Fecal analysis begins with gross examination of color, consistency, odor, and other characteristics and concludes with microscopic, chemical, or bacterial analysis.

Feces are usually light to dark brown, soft, and slightly acidic. Their normal brown color stems from the metabolism of bile pigments to stercobilin but may also be affected by diet, drugs, absorption efficiency, and bilirubin concentration. Fecal pH depends on dietary influences: Acidic pH results from a high carbohydrate intake; alkaline pH results from high protein intake. Fecal odor results from the presence of indole and skatole, end products of protein catabolism.

Stool is usually about 1" (2.5 cm) in diameter and has the tubular shape of the colon, but it may be larger or smaller, depending on the condition of the colon. If the colon is partially obstructed or loses its elasticity, the passage of stool often traumatizes the colon and may cause bleeding; blood in the stool may also result from hemorrhoids. A black, tarry stool can result from bleeding high in the intestinal tract. A large, bulky, foul-smelling stool that floats on water may indicate malabsorption of fat (steatorrhea) or a large quantity of air or other gases in the stool.

Diarrhea results from too-rapid passage of food through the GI tract, often spurred by viral infection. Mucus-containing stool can indicate colitis or a mucus-producing tumor. Pus, detected in microscopic analysis, can result from rectal abscess or ulcerative colitis.

Stool specimen collection

Collection of a stool specimen is often required for diagnosis of infectious diseases, GI bleeding, and other GI tract disorders. Because stool specimens can't be obtained on demand, close cooperation between nurse and patient is necessary to secure a suitable specimen. Stool specimens may be collected randomly or for a specified period; for example, a random specimen is required for urobilinogen, and a 72-hour specimen is required for lipids. Three specimens are usually required to test for occult blood.

Before collecting a stool specimen, have ready a clean (preferably sterile), dry bedpan; a specimen container; and tongue blades. Then teach the patient how to collect a random or timed stool specimen. Tell him to notify you when he feels the urge to defecate.

To collect a random specimen: Provide the patient with a bedpan, and instruct him to avoid contaminating the stool with urine or toilet tissue, which would interfere with test results. Using a tongue blade, carefully transfer the stool from the bedpan to the specimen container. Then tightly secure the lid of the container. If the patient passes blood or mucus with the stool, be sure to include these with the specimen. Carefully label the container, and send it to the laboratory immediately because a fresh specimen produces the most accurate results. If the specimen can't be transported immediately, refrigerate it.

To collect a timed specimen: Consider the first stool passed by the patient as the start of the collection period. Prepare this specimen and all other stools passed during the collection period in the same manner as for a random specimen. As ordered, send each specimen to the laboratory immediately, or refrigerate the specimens collected during the test period and send them when collection is completed.

Endoscopy, radiography, and ultrasonography

Accurate diagnosis of GI tract, hepatic, biliary, and pancreatic disorders often requires more than one test. Such tests often proceed in the following logical order:

■ *Fecal occult bleeding test* generally detects GI bleeding.

■ *Barium studies* (upper GI and small-bowel series, and barium enema) visualize GI structures. They may reveal inflammation or ulcers, tumors, strictures, or other lesions.

■ *Endoscopies* (esophagogastroduodenoscopy, colonoscopy, and proctosigmoidoscopy) directly visualize an abnormality, locate sources of bleeding and, if necessary, provide a channel for biopsy.

The selection of a diagnostic test or test battery may depend on hospital resources. If they're available, noninvasive procedures, such as ultrasonography and CT scans, are preferred over invasive procedures, such as endoscopic retrograde cholangiopancreatography, in evaluating pancreatic disorders. Similarly, oral cholecystography and ultrasonography commonly replace percutaneous transhepatic cholangiography in evaluating gallbladder and biliary tract disorders.

Other useful tests

Breath hydrogen analysis, a simple method of detecting lactose intolerance, measures the hydrogen content of breath samples in the fasting state before and after ingestion of lactose. Lactose, a disaccharide composed of glucose and galactose, normally breaks down in the small intestine and is then absorbed. When lactase, the enzyme that breaks down lactose, is deficient, lactose passes unabsorbed into the large intestine. Bacteria then ferment and split lactose, producing hydrogen and other gases that the lungs exhale.

To produce a sample for this test, the patient exhales into an anesthesia balloon. The hydrogen content of the sample is then determined by gas chromatography and a thermistor detector. Increased hydrogen content after lactose ingestion indicates lactose intolerance. Despite this test's widespread use, experts disagree about its specificity and sensitivity. False-negative test results have been reported in patients who take antibiotics or suffer from severe diarrhea.

The *HIDA scan* (technetium-labeled iminodiacetic acid, or ^{99m}Tc HIDA) is a simple procedure for evaluating hepatobiliary function. Because the scan requires only a 2-hour fast, it permits quicker diagnosis than oral cholecystography, particularly in a patient with severe abdominal pain that suggests acute gallbladder disease.

The injected radioisotope, HIDA, is taken up by the liver and excreted into the biliary tree. Serial imaging with a gamma camera then depicts radioactivity in the liver, bile ducts, gallbladder, and duodenum. Adequate visualization of the gallbladder requires normal gallbladder and liver function as well as patency of the biliary tree. Failure to visualize the gallbladder can result from hepatocellular disease, which impairs the uptake of HIDA, or from biliary obstruction, which prevents the release of HIDA into the gallbladder. Abnormally diminished radioactivity in the liver characterizes hepatocellular disease; absence of radioactivity in both the gallbladder and duodenum suggests biliary obstruction.

The *saline-load test,* a rarely used test that measures gastric retention during fasting, requires aspiration of stomach contents before and after instillation of 750 ml of normal saline solution through an NG tube. The amount of saline solution remaining in the stomach after 30 minutes provides an index of intrinsic gastric motility. Excessive retention of saline solution (more than 300 ml) may indicate gastric outlet obstruction stemming from edema, tumor, or stenosis.

The *secretin test* assesses pancreatic exocrine function. It involves insertion of a double-lumen oral tube into the duodenum and aspiration of gastric and duodenal contents before and after I.V. injection of secretin, an intestinal hormone that stimulates liver and pancreatic secretions. After such injection, an abnormal volume of secretions or of bicarbonate or enzymes may indicate pancreatic carcinoma, ductal obstruction, chronic pancreatitis, or advanced pancreatic insufficiency.

ESOPHAGEAL, GASTRIC, AND PERITONEAL CONTENT TESTS

Esophageal acidity

In contrast to the stomach's high acidity (pH 1.1 to 2.4), the esophagus normally maintains a pH over 5.0. Although some reflux of gastric juices into the lower esophagus is common, a sharp increase in such backflow may acidify the intraesophageal pH to as low as 1.5. When repeated reflux occurs, esophageal mucosa becomes inflamed by the acidic gastric juices, resulting in pyrosis (heartburn).

The esophageal acidity test evaluates the competence of the lower esophageal sphincter — the major barrier to reflux — by measuring intraesophageal pH with an electrode attached to a manometric catheter. This test, which is the most sensitive indicator of gastric reflux, is indicated for patients who complain of persistent heartburn with or without regurgitation. Esophageal sphincter pressure can also be measured. (See *Esophageal manometry.*)

Purpose
- To evaluate the competence of the lower esophageal sphincter.

Patient preparation
Explain to the patient that this test evaluates the function of the sphincter between the esophagus and stomach. Instruct him to fast and avoid smoking after midnight before the test. Tell him who will perform the test and where and that it usually takes about 45 minutes.

Inform the patient that a tube will be passed through his mouth into the

Esophageal manometry

Esophageal manometry measures esophageal sphincter pressure and records the duration and sequence of peristaltic contractions to detect motility disorders, such as achalasia, diffuse esophageal spasm, and scleroderma.

Preparation

Cholinergic and anticholinergic drugs are withheld before the test. The patient is told to avoid tobacco and alcohol for 24 hours and to fast for 4 hours before the test. These restrictions help prevent esophageal sphincter pressures from increasing or decreasing, which would interfere with test results.

Procedure

In this test, the patient is asked to swallow a manometric catheter that contains a small pressure transducer along its length. With the catheter placed at various levels in the esophagus, baseline measurements of pressures are made, followed by measurement of pressures in the lower esophageal sphincter immediately before and after swallowing; then peristaltic contractions are recorded. The patient may be asked to take wet swallows as well as swallows with ice water to obtain more specific information.

Normal findings

Normally, baseline sphincter pressure is about 20 mm Hg; relaxation pressure (the pressure immediately before swallowing) is at least 18 mm Hg. Peristalsis usually appears as a series of high-pressure peaks, representing sequential contractions of the esophagus.

Implications of abnormal findings

In *achalasia,* baseline sphincter pressure commonly reaches 50 mm Hg; relaxation pressure, less than 25 mm Hg. Peristalsis is usually weak and nonpropulsive. Food and fluids accumulate in the esophagus until their weight can overcome sphincter resistance.

In *diffuse spasm of the esophagus,* sphincter pressure is usually normal, but peristalsis is disordered. Instead of sequential, orderly contractions, different segments of the esophagus contract simultaneously — often with abnormal force — after swallowing. Contractions may also occur without the stimulus of swallowing, or more than one contraction may follow a single swallow.

In *esophageal scleroderma,* impaired sphincter function and peristalsis result from replacement of smooth muscle by fibrous tissue in the lower two-thirds of the esophagus. Both baseline and relaxation pressures are depressed. Peristalsis is normal in the upper third of the esophagus, where striated muscle predominates, but it's weak or absent in the lower two-thirds.

stomach and that he may experience slight discomfort and may cough or gag. Just before the test, check the patient's pulse rate and blood pressure, and instruct him to void.

Withhold antacids, anticholinergics, cholinergics, adrenergic blockers, alcohol, corticosteroids, cimetidine, and reserpine for 24 hours before the test, as ordered. If these medications must be continued, note this on the laboratory request.

Procedure

After placing the patient in high Fowler's position, introduce the catheter with pH electrode into his mouth, and instruct him to swallow when the electrode reaches the back of his throat. Locate the lower esophageal sphincter manometrically; then raise the catheter ¾" (2 cm). Instruct the patient to perform Valsalva's maneuver or lift his legs, to stimulate reflux. After he does so, determine the intraesophageal pH.

If the pH remains normal, pass the catheter into the patient's stomach. Instill 300 ml of 0.1 N HCl over 3 minutes (100 ml/minute); then raise the catheter ¾" (2 cm) above the sphincter. Again, to stimulate reflux, ask the patient to perform Valsalva's maneuver or lift his legs; after he does so, again determine the intraesophageal pH.

Precautions

■ During insertion, the electrode may enter the trachea instead of the esophagus. If the patient develops cyanosis or paroxysmal coughing, move the electrode immediately.
■ Observe the patient closely during intubation because arrhythmias may develop.
■ Clamp the catheter before removing it to prevent aspiration of fluid into the lungs.

Reference values

Normally, the pH of the esophagus is over 5.0.

Implications of results

An intraesophageal pH of 1.5 to 2.0 indicates gastric acid reflux due to incompetence of the lower esophageal sphincter. Persistent reflux leads to chronic reflux esophagitis. Additional studies, such as barium swallow and esophagogastroduodenoscopy, are necessary to diagnose and determine the extent of esophagitis.

Post-test care

■ As ordered, resume administration of medications withheld before the test, and tell the patient he may resume his usual diet.
■ If the patient complains of a sore throat, provide soothing lozenges.

Interfering factors

■ Failure to adhere to pretest restrictions interferes with accurate testing.
■ Antacids, anticholinergics, and cimetidine may depress intraesophageal pH by decreasing gastric secretions or reducing their acidity; cholinergics, reserpine, alcohol, adrenergic blockers, and corticosteroids may elevate intraesophageal pH by increasing gastric secretions or by promoting reflux by relaxing the lower esophageal sphincter.

Acid perfusion

The lower esophageal sphincter normally prevents gastric reflux. However, if this sphincter is incompetent, the recurrent backflow of acidic juices (and of bile salts, if the pyloric sphincter is also incompetent) into the esophagus inflames the esophageal mucosa. This inflammation (esophagitis) is manifested by burning epigastric or retrosternal pain that radiates to the back or arms.

The acid perfusion test (also known as the Bernstein test) distinguishes such pain from that caused by angina pectoris or other disorders. In this test, normal saline and acidic solutions are perfused separately into the esophagus through a nasogastric (NG) tube.

Purpose

■ To distinguish heartburnlike pains caused by esophagitis from those caused by cardiac disorders.

Patient preparation

Explain to the patient that this test helps determine the cause of heartburn. Instruct him to observe the following pretest restrictions: no antacids for 24 hours, as ordered; no food for 12 hours; and no fluids or smoking for 8 hours before the test. Tell him who will perform the test and where and that it takes about 1 hour.

Inform the patient that the test requires passage of a tube through his nose into the esophagus and that he may experience some discomfort and may cough or gag during tube passage. Tell him that liquid is slowly perfused through the tube into the esophagus; instruct him to report immediately pain or burning during perfusion.

Just before the test, check the patient's pulse rate and blood pressure. Ask him if he's experiencing any heartburn and, if so, to describe it.

Procedure

After seating the patient, insert an NG tube that has been marked 12" (30 cm) from the tip into his stomach. Attach a 20-ml syringe to the tube, and aspirate the stomach contents. Then withdraw the tube into the esophagus (to the 12" mark).

Hang labeled containers of normal saline solution and of 0.1 N HCl solution on an I.V. pole behind the patient; then connect the NG tube to I.V. tubing. Open the line from the normal saline solution, and begin a drip at a rate of 60 to 120 drops/minute. Continue to perfuse this solution for 5 to 10 minutes. Then ask the patient if he's experiencing any discomfort, and record his response.

Without the patient's knowledge, close the line from the saline solution and open the line from the acidic solution. Begin a drip into the esophagus at the same rate as for the saline solution, but continue the perfusion for 30 minutes. Ask the patient if he's experiencing any discomfort, and record his response. If he experiences discomfort, immediately close the line from the acidic solution and open the line from the saline solution. Continue to perfuse saline solution until the discomfort subsides.

If ordered, repeat perfusion of the acidic solution to verify the patient's response. If this is not required, or if the patient experiences no discomfort after perfusion of the acidic solution for 30 minutes, stop the solution and withdraw the NG tube.

Precautions

■ The acid perfusion test is contraindicated in patients with esophageal varices, congestive heart failure, acute myocardial infarction, or other cardiac disorders.

■ During intubation, make sure the tube enters the esophagus, not the trachea. Withdraw the tube immediately if the patient develops cyanosis or paroxysmal coughing.

■ Observe the patient closely for arrhythmias.

■ Clamp the tube before removing it to prevent aspiration of fluid into the lungs.

Normal findings

Absence of pain or burning during perfusion of either solution indicates a healthy esophageal mucosa.

Implications of results

In patients with esophagitis, the acidic solution causes pain or burning, whereas the normal saline solution usually produces no adverse reactions. Occasionally, both solutions cause pain in patients with esophagitis; they may cause no pain in patients with asymptomatic esophagitis.

Post-test care

■ If the patient continues to experience pain or burning, administer an antacid as ordered. If he complains of a sore throat, provide soothing lozenges or obtain an order for an ice collar.

■ As ordered, the patient may resume his usual diet and medications withheld before the test.

Interfering factors

Failure to adhere to pretest restrictions may interfere with the accuracy of test results.

Basal gastric secretion

Although gastric secretion peaks after ingestion of food, small amounts of gastric juices are also secreted between meals. This secretion, known as basal secretion, results from psychoneurogenic influences that are mediated by the vagus nerves and by hormones such as gastrin.

This test measures basal secretion under fasting conditions by aspirating stomach contents through a nasogastric (NG) tube; it's indicated for patients with obscure epigastric pain, anorexia, and weight loss. Because external factors — such as the sight or odor of food — and psychological stress stimulate gastric secretion, accurate testing requires that the patient be relaxed and isolated from all sources of sensory stimulation. Although abnormal basal secretion can suggest various gastric and duodenal disorders, a complete evaluation of secretion requires the gastric acid stimulation test.

In a patient who has had a vagotomy (to reduce gastric acid secretion), an insulin gastric analysis (the Hollander test) can be used to evaluate the surgery's effectiveness. (See *The Hollander test*.)

Purpose

■ To determine gastric output in the fasting state.

Patient preparation

Explain to the patient that this test measures the stomach's secretion of acid. Instruct him to restrict food for 12 hours, and fluids and smoking for 8 hours before the test. Tell him who will perform the test and that it takes approximately $1\frac{1}{2}$ hours (or $2\frac{1}{2}$ hours if followed by the gastric acid stimulation test).

Inform the patient that the test requires insertion of a tube through the nose and into the stomach, and that he may initially experience discomfort and may cough or gag. Withhold antacids, anticholinergics, cholinergics, alcohol, cimetidine, reserpine, adrenergic blockers, and adrenocorticosteroids for 24 hours before the test, as ordered. If these medications must be continued, note this on the laboratory request. Just before the test, check the patient's pulse rate and blood pressure. Then encourage him to relax.

Procedure

After seating the patient comfortably, insert the NG tube. Then attach a 20-ml syringe to it, and aspirate the stomach contents. To ensure complete emptying of the stomach, ask the patient to assume three positions in sequence — supine, and right and left lateral decubitus — while the stomach contents are aspirated. Label the specimen container "Residual Contents." Then connect the NG tube to the suction machine.

Aspirate gastric contents by continuous low suction for 1 hours. (Aspiration can also be performed manually with a syringe.) Collect a specimen every 15 minutes, but discard the first two;

The Hollander test

I.V. injection of insulin in a patient with normal blood glucose levels causes hypoglycemia by promoting cellular absorption of glucose. Hypoglycemia, in turn, affects the vagus nerve, which stimulates acid secretion by the parietal and chief cells. A vagotomy — surgical transection of the vagus nerve — eliminates this neural stimulus for gastric acid secretion.

The Hollander test (insulin gastric analysis) evaluates the effectiveness of vagotomy and is most effective when performed 3 to 6 months after surgery. In this test, gastric contents are aspirated under fasting conditions through a nasogastric tube both before and after a dose of insulin and are then compared; simultaneously, blood glucose levels are determined before and after the insulin injection.

If the acid output after the insulin injection exceeds the preinjection acid output, the vagotomy is likely to be incomplete; if acid output fails to rise after the insulin injection, the vagotomy is considered complete. However, failure to increase acid output is significant only if achlorhydria persists after blood glucose falls below 50 mg/dl.

The Hollander test is contraindicated in patients with coronary artery or cerebrovascular disease, a predisposition to hypoglycemia, or other conditions that prohibit nasogastric intubation. It's not useful in patients with achlorhydria, as demonstrated by the gastric acid stimulation test, because such patients fail to respond to insulin injection.

this eliminates a specimen that could be influenced by the stress of the intubation. Record the color and odor of each specimen, and note the presence of food, mucus, bile, or blood. Label these specimens "Basal Contents," and number them 1 through 4.

If the NG tube is to be left in place, clamp it or attach it to low intermittent suction, as ordered.

Precautions

- This test is contraindicated in patients with conditions that prohibit nasogastric intubation.
- During insertion, make sure the NG tube enters the esophagus, not the trachea; remove it immediately if the patient develops cyanosis or paroxysmal coughing.

- Monitor vital signs during intubation, and watch the patient closely for arrhythmias.
- To prevent contamination of the specimens with saliva, instruct the patient to expectorate excess saliva.
- Send the specimens to the laboratory as soon as the collection is completed.

Reference values

Normally, basal gastric secretion ranges from 1 to 5 mEq/hour in males and from 0.2 to 3.8 mEq/hour in females.

Implications of results

Abnormal basal secretion findings are nonspecific and must be correlated with results of the gastric acid stimulation test. Increased secretion may suggest duodenal or jejunal ulcer (after partial gastrectomy) or, if markedly increased, Zollinger-Ellison syndrome. Decreased secretion may indicate gastric carcinoma or benign gastric ulcer. Absence of secretion may indicate pernicious anemia.

Post-test care

■ Watch for complications — such as nausea, vomiting, and abdominal distention or pain — after removal of the NG tube.

■ If the patient complains of a sore throat, provide soothing lozenges.

■ As ordered, the patient may resume his usual diet and medications withheld before the test unless the gastric acid stimulation test will also be performed.

Interfering factors

■ Failure to adhere to pretest restrictions increases basal secretion.

■ Psychological stress can stimulate excessive basal secretion.

■ Cholinergics, reserpine, alcohol, adrenergic blockers, and adrenocorticosteroids may increase basal secretion; antacids, anticholinergics, and cimetidine may depress it.

Gastric acid stimulation

The gastric acid stimulation test measures the secretion of gastric for 1 hour after subcutaneous injection of pentagastrin or a similar drug that stimulates gastric acid output. It's indicated when the basal secretion test suggests abnormal gastric secretion and is usually performed immediately after that test.

Pentagastrin stimulates the parietal cells to secrete hydrochloric acid. If these cells are damaged or destroyed, acid secretion decreases or is absent; if the cells are hyperactive, acid secretion increases. Although this test detects abnormal gastric secretion, radiographic studies

and endoscopy are necessary to determine the cause.

Purpose

■ To aid diagnosis of duodenal ulcer, Zollinger-Ellison syndrome, pernicious anemia, and gastric carcinoma.

Patient preparation

Explain to the patient that this test determines if the stomach is secreting acid properly. Instruct him to refrain from eating, drinking, and smoking from midnight before the test. Tell him who will perform the test and that it takes 1 hour.

Tell the patient that the test requires passing a tube through the nose and into the stomach and injecting pentagastrin subcutaneously. Describe the possible side effects — abdominal pain, nausea, vomiting, flushing, transitory dizziness, faintness, and numbness of the extremities — and instruct him to report such symptoms immediately.

Check the patient's history for hypersensitivity to pentagastrin. As ordered, withhold antacids, anticholinergics, adrenergic blockers, cimetidine, and reserpine before the test. If these drugs must be continued, note this on the laboratory request. Record baseline vital signs before beginning the procedure.

Procedure

After basal gastric secretions have been collected, keep the nasogastric (NG) tube in place. Pentagastrin is then injected subcutaneously. Wait 15 minutes, and then collect a specimen every 15 minutes for 1 hour.

Record the color and odor of each specimen, and note the presence of food, mucus, bile, or blood. Label all specimens "Stimulated Contents," and number them 1 through 4. If the NG tube is to be left in place, clamp it or attach it to low intermittent suction, as ordered.

Precautions

- The gastric acid stimulation test is contraindicated in patients with hypersensitivity to pentagastrin or with conditions that prohibit NG intubation.
- Observe for adverse effects of pentagastrin.
- To prevent contamination of the specimens with saliva, instruct the patient to expectorate excess saliva.
- Send the specimens to the laboratory as soon as the collection is completed.

Reference values

Normally, gastric secretion following stimulation ranges from 18 to 28 mEq/hour for males and from 11 to 21 mEq/hour for females.

Implications of results

Elevated gastric secretion may indicate duodenal ulcer; markedly elevated secretion suggests Zollinger-Ellison syndrome. Depressed secretion may indicate gastric carcinoma; achlorhydria may indicate pernicious anemia.

Post-test care

- Watch for nausea, vomiting, and abdominal distention and pain after removal of the NG tube.
- If the patient complains of a sore throat, provide soothing lozenges.
- As ordered, the patient may resume his usual diet and medications withheld before the test.

Interfering factors

- Failure to adhere to pretest restrictions may affect the accuracy of test results.
- Gastric acid levels are elevated by cholinergics, adrenergic blockers, and reserpine and depressed by antacids, anticholinergics, and cimetidine.

Peritoneal fluid analysis

The peritoneum is a tough, semipermeable membrane that lines the abdominal and visceral cavities and encloses, supports, and lubricates the organs within these cavities. It also serves an important osmoregulatory function; passive diffusion of water and solute particles (up to a certain size) occurs across this membrane to maintain osmotic and chemical equilibrium with associated blood and lymphatic systems. Accumulation of fluid in the peritoneal space — ascites — can result from such conditions as hepatic, renal, and cardiovascular disorders; inflammation; infection; and neoplasm.

This test assesses a sample of peritoneal fluid obtained by paracentesis, a procedure that entails inserting a trocar and cannula through the abdominal wall with the patient under a local anesthetic. If the sample of fluid is being removed for therapeutic purposes, the trocar can be connected to a drainage system. If only a small amount of fluid is being removed for diagnostic purposes, an 18G needle can be substituted for the trocar and cannula. In a four-quadrant tap, fluid is aspirated from each quadrant of the abdomen to verify abdominal trauma and confirm the need for surgery.

Peritoneal fluid analysis includes examination of gross appearance, erythrocyte and leukocyte counts, cytologic studies, microbiological studies for bacteria and fungi, and determinations of protein, glucose, amylase, ammonia, and alkaline phosphatase levels. Complications associated with this test include shock and hypovolemia, perforation of abdominal organs, hemorrhage, and hepatic coma.

Purpose

- To determine the cause of ascites
- To detect abdominal trauma.

Patient preparation

Explain to the patient that this procedure helps determine the case of ascites or detects abdominal trauma. Inform him that he needn't restrict food or fluids before the test. Tell him that the test requires a peritoneal fluid sample, that he'll receive a local anesthetic to minimize discomfort, and that the procedure may take up to 45 minutes to perform.

Provide psychological support to decrease the patient's anxiety, and assure him that complications are rare. If the patient has severe ascites, inform him that the procedure will relieve his discomfort and allow him to breathe more easily.

Make sure the patient or responsible family member has signed a consent form. Record baseline vital signs and weight for comparison with post-test readings; abdominal girth measurements may also be ordered. Tell the patient a blood sample may be taken for laboratory analysis (hemoglobin level, hematocrit, prothrombin time, activated partial prothrombin time, and platelet count).

Just before the test, tell the patient to urinate. This helps prevent accidental bladder injury during needle insertion.

Procedure

Position the patient on a bed or in a chair, as ordered, with his feet flat on the floor and his back well supported. If he can't tolerate being out of bed, place him in high Fowler's position. Make him as comfortable as you can. Except for the puncture site, keep him covered to prevent chilling. Provide a plastic sheet or absorbent pad to collect spillage and to protect the patient and bed linens.

The puncture site is then shaved, the skin prepared, and the area draped. A local anesthetic is injected, and the needle or trocar and cannula are usually inserted 1" to 2" (2.5 to 5 cm) below the umbilicus. (However, insertion may also be through the flank, the iliac fossa, the border of the rectus, or at each quadrant of the abdomen.) If a trocar and cannula are used, a small incision is made to facilitate insertion. When the needle pierces the peritoneum, it "gives" with an audible sound. The trocar is removed, and a sample of fluid is aspirated with a 50-ml luer-lock syringe.

The paracentesis tray contains specimen tubes for the various tests. If additional fluid is to be drained, assist in attaching one end of an I.V. tube to the cannula and the other end to a collection bag. The fluid is then aspirated (no more than 1,500 ml). If fluid aspiration is difficult, reposition the patient as ordered. After aspiration, the trocar or needle is removed, and a pressure dressing is applied. Occasionally, the wound may be sutured first. Label the specimens in the order that they were drawn. If the patient has received antibiotic therapy, note this on the laboratory request.

Carefully dispose of needles and contaminated articles if the patient has a history of hepatitis; incinerate disposable items and return reusable ones to the central supply area.

Precautions

- Peritoneal fluid analysis should be used cautiously in patients who are pregnant and in those with bleeding tendencies or unstable vital signs.

- Check vital signs every 15 minutes during the procedure. Watch for deviations from baseline findings. Observe for dizziness, pallor, perspiration, and increased anxiety.

▪ If rapid fluid aspiration induces hypovolemia and shock, reduce the distance between the trocar and the collection bag to slow the drainage rate. If necessary, stop drainage by turning the stopcock off or by clamping the tubing.

▪ To ensure the reliability of abdominal X-rays, perform any needed X-rays before peritoneal fluid analysis.

▪ Avoid contaminating the specimens, which alters their bacterial content. Send them to the laboratory immediately.

Reference values

Peritoneal fluid is normally odorless and clear to pale yellow in color. (See *Normal findings in peritoneal fluid analysis,* page 820.)

Implications of results

Milk-colored peritoneal fluid may result from chyle escaping from a thoracic duct that is damaged or blocked by a malignant tumor, lymphoma, tuberculosis, a parasitic infection, an adhesion, or hepatic cirrhosis; a pseudochylous condition may result from the presence of leukocytes or tumor cells.

Differential diagnosis of true chylous ascites depends on the presence of elevated triglyceride levels ($\geq$400 mg/dl) and microscopic fat globules. Cloudy or turbid fluid may indicate peritonitis due to primary bacterial infection, ruptured bowel (after trauma), pancreatitis, strangulated or infarcted intestine, or appendicitis. Bloody fluid may result from a benign or malignant tumor, hemorrhagic pancreatitis, or perforated intestine or duodenal ulcer.

A red blood cell count over 100/μl indicates neoplasm or tuberculosis; a count over 100,000/μl indicates intraabdominal trauma. A white blood cell count over 300/μl, with more than 25% neutrophils, occurs in 90% of patients with spontaneous bacterial peritonitis and in 50% of those with cirrhosis. A high percentage of lymphocytes suggests tuberculous peritonitis or chylous ascites. Numerous mesothelial cells indicate tuberculous peritonitis.

Protein levels rise about 3 g/dl in cancer and above 4 g/dl in tuberculous peritonitis. Peritoneal fluid glucose levels fall below 60 mg/dl in 30% to 50% of patients with tuberculous peritonitis and peritoneal carcinomatosis. Amylase levels rise in about 90% of patients with pancreatic trauma, pancreatic pseudocyst, or acute pancreatitis and may also rise in intestinal necrosis or strangulation. Peritoneal alkaline phosphatase levels rise to more than twice the normal serum levels in about 90% of patients with a ruptured or strangulated small intestine. Peritoneal ammonia levels also exceed twice the normal serum levels in ruptured or strangulated large and small intestines, and in a ruptured ulcer or appendix.

A protein ascitic fluid/serum ratio of 0.5 or greater, a lactate dehydrogenase (LD) ascitic fluid/serum ratio over 0.6, and an LD ascitic fluid level over 400 μ/ml suggest malignant, tuberculous, or pancreatic ascites. Any two of these findings indicates a nonhepatic cause; absence of all three usually suggests uncomplicated hepatic disease. An albumin gradient between ascitic fluid and serum over 1 g/dl indicates chronic hepatic disease; a lesser value suggests malignancy.

Cytologic examination of peritoneal fluid accurately detects malignant cells. Microbiological examination can reveal coliforms, anaerobes, and enterococci, which can enter the peritoneum from a ruptured organ or from infections accompanying appendicitis, pancreatitis, tuberculosis, or ovarian disease. Grampositive cocci commonly indicate primary peritonitis; gram-negative organisms, secondary peritonitis. Fungi may indicate histoplasmosis, candidiasis, or coccidioidomycosis.

Normal findings in peritoneal fluid analysis

ELEMENT	NORMAL FINDINGS
Gross appearance	Sterile, odorless, clear to pale yellow color; scant amount (< 50 ml)
Red blood cells	None
White blood cells	< 300/µl
Protein	0.3 to 4.1 g/dl (albumin, 50% to 70%; globulin, 30% to 45%; fibrinogen, 0.3% to 4.5%)
Glucose	70 to 100 mg/dl
Amylase	138 to 404 amylase U/L
Ammonia	< 50 µg/dl
Alkaline phosphatase	Males over age 18: 90 to 239 U/L Females under age 45: 76 to 196 U/L Females over age 45: 87 to 250 U/L
Lactate dehydrogenase	Equal to serum level
Cytology	No malignant cells present
Bacteria	None
Fungi	None

Post-test care

■ Apply a gauze dressing to the puncture site; make sure it's thick enough to absorb all drainage. Check the dressing frequently, whenever you check vital signs; reinforce or apply a pressure dressing if needed.

■ Position the patient in bed, and monitor his vital signs. Maintain bed rest until vital signs are stable and return to baseline values. If the patient's recovery is poor, check vital signs every 15 minutes, as ordered. Weigh the patient and measure abdominal girth; compare these with baseline measurements.

■ Monitor urine output for at least 24 hours, and watch for hematuria, which may indicate bladder trauma.

■ If a large amount of fluid was aspirated, watch for signs of vascular collapse (color change, elevated pulse rate and respirations, decreased blood pressure and central venous pressure, mental changes, and dizziness). Administer fluids orally if the patient is alert and can accept them.

■ Watch for signs of hemorrhage and shock, and for increasing pain and abdominal tenderness. These may indicate a perforated intestine or, depending on the site of the tap, puncture of the inferior epigastric artery, hematoma of the anterior cecal wall, or rupture of the iliac vein or bladder.

■ Observe the patient with severe hepatic disease for signs of hepatic coma, which may result from loss of sodium and potassium accompanying hypovolemia. Watch for mental changes, drowsiness, and stupor. Such a patient is also prone to uremia, infection, hemorrhage, and protein depletion.

■ Administer I.V. infusions and albumin as ordered. Check the laboratory report for electrolyte (especially sodium) and serum protein levels.

Interfering factors

■ Failure to send the sample to the laboratory immediately or unsterile collection technique will affect the accuracy of test results.

■ Injury to underlying structures during paracentesis may contaminate the sample with bile, blood, urine, or feces.

FECAL CONTENT TESTS

Fecal occult blood

Fecal occult blood, invisible because of its minute quantity, can be detected by microscopic analysis or by chemical tests for hemoglobin, such as the guaiac or orthotolidin test. Because small amounts of blood (2 to 2.5 ml/day) normally appear in the feces, tests for occult blood are designed to detect quantities larger than this. These tests are indicated for patients whose clinical symptoms and preliminary blood studies suggest GI bleeding. However, further tests are required to pinpoint the origin of the bleeding.

Stool color correlates roughly with the site of bleeding — for example, melena usually results from hemorrhage in the esophagus or stomach. Gastric juices act to digest this blood, thereby blackening it. Melena may also result from hemorrhage in the jejunum or ileum, provided that its passage through the intestine is slow. Dark maroon stools result from hemorrhage beyond Treitz's ligament. Stool color can also be affected by ingestion of certain foods. (See *Nonpathologic causes of variant stool color,* page 822.)

Purpose

■ To detect GI bleeding
■ To aid early diagnosis of colorectal cancer.

Patient preparation

Explain to the patient that this test helps detect abnormal GI bleeding. Instruct him to maintain a high-fiber diet and to refrain from eating red meat, poultry, fish, turnips, and horseradish for 48 to 72 hours before the test and throughout the collection period. Tell him the test requires collection of three stool specimens. (Occasionally, only a random specimen is collected.)

As ordered, withhold iron preparations, bromides, iodides, rauwolfia derivatives, indomethacin, colchicine, salicylates, phenylbutazone, steroids, and ascorbic acid for 48 hours before the test and during the collection period. If these medications must be continued, note this on the laboratory request.

Procedure

Collect three stool specimens or a random specimen, as ordered. Be sure to obtain specimens from two different areas of each stool to allow for variation in distribution of blood. Two of the most commonly used screening tests are Hematest and Hemoccult. Hematest uses orthotolidin to detect hemoglobin, and Hemoccult uses guaiac.

For the Hematest reagent tablet test: Use a wooden applicator to smear a bit of the stool specimen on the filter paper supplied with the kit. Or, after performing a digital rectal examination, wipe the finger you used for examination on a square of the filter paper. Place the filter paper with the stool smear on a glass plate.

Remove a reagent tablet from the bot-

Nonpathologic causes of variant stool color

Changes in stool color are not always the result of a disease or disorder. Some benign causes are listed below.

STOOL COLOR	FOOD OR FLUID	DRUG
Red	Carrots, beets, tomatoes, red peppers	Pyrvinium
Black	Licorice, grape juice	Iron salts, phenylbutazone
Brown	Cocoa, high intake of meat protein (dark brown)	Anthraquinone
Green-blue or black	Spinach	Bismuth preparations
Yellow	Rhubarb; high intake of milk (yellow-brown)	Senna
White discoloration or speckling		Antacids containing aluminum hydroxide

tle, and immediately replace the cap tightly. Then place the tablet in the center of the stool smear on the filter paper. Add one drop of water to the tablet, and allow it to soak in for 5 to 10 seconds. Add a second drop, letting it run from the tablet onto the specimen and filter paper. If necessary, tap the plate gently to dislodge any water from the top of the tablet.

After 2 minutes, the filter paper will turn blue if the test is positive. Do not read the color that appears on the tablet itself or develops on the filter paper after the 2-minute period. Note the results, and discard the filter paper. Remove and discard your gloves, and wash your hands thoroughly.

For the Hemoccult slide test: Open the flap on the slide packet, and use a wooden applicator to apply a thin smear of the stool specimen to the guaiac-impregnated filter paper exposed in box A. Or, after performing a digital rectal examination, wipe the finger you used for examination on a square of the filter paper. Apply a second smear from another part of the specimen to the filter paper exposed in box B because some parts of the specimen may not contain blood.

Allow the specimen to dry for 3 to 5 minutes. Open the flap at the rear of the slide package, and place 2 drops of Hemoccult developing solution on the paper over each smear. A blue reaction will appear in 30 to 60 seconds if the test is positive. Record the results and discard the slide package. Remove and discard your gloves, and wash your hands thoroughly.

Precautions
■ Instruct the patient to avoid contaminating the stool specimen with toilet tissue or urine.
■ Send the specimen to the laboratory or perform the test immediately.

Normal findings
Less than 2.5 ml of blood should be present, resulting in a green reaction.

Implications of results
A positive test indicates GI bleeding, which may result from many disorders,

Common sites and causes of GI bleeding

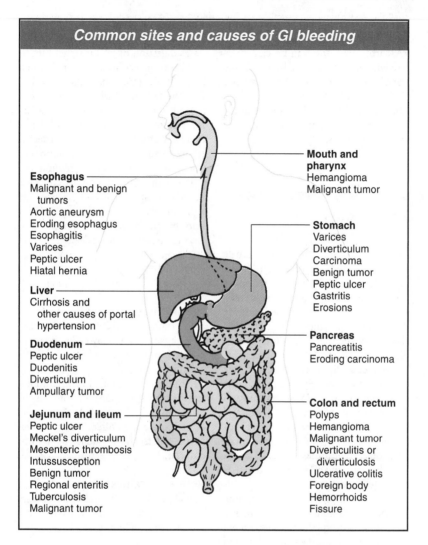

Esophagus
Malignant and benign
   tumors
Aortic aneurysm
Eroding esophagus
Esophagitis
Varices
Peptic ulcer
Hiatal hernia

Liver
Cirrhosis and
   other causes of portal
   hypertension

Duodenum
Peptic ulcer
Duodenitis
Diverticulum
Ampullary tumor

Jejunum and ileum
Peptic ulcer
Meckel's diverticulum
Mesenteric thrombosis
Intussusception
Benign tumor
Regional enteritis
Tuberculosis
Malignant tumor

**Mouth and
pharynx**
Hemangioma
Malignant tumor

Stomach
Varices
Diverticulum
Carcinoma
Benign tumor
Peptic ulcer
Gastritis
Erosions

Pancreas
Pancreatitis
Eroding carcinoma

Colon and rectum
Polyps
Hemangioma
Malignant tumor
Diverticulitis or
   diverticulosis
Ulcerative colitis
Foreign body
Hemorrhoids
Fissure

such as varices, peptic ulcer, carcinoma, ulcerative colitis, dysentery, or hemorrhagic disease. This test is particularly important for early diagnosis of colorectal cancer because 80% of persons with this type of cancer demonstrate positive results. Further tests, such as barium swallow, analyses of gastric contents, and endoscopic procedures, are necessary to define the site and extent of bleeding. (See *Common sites and causes of GI bleeding*.)

Post-test care

As ordered, the patient may resume his usual diet and medications.

Interfering factors

▪ Failure to adhere to dietary or medication restrictions, to test the specimen immediately, or to send it to the laboratory immediately may affect test results.
▪ Bleeding may result from use of iron preparations, bromides, rauwolfia de-

rivatives, indomethacin, colchicine, phenylbutazone, or steroids.

■ Ascorbic acid (vitamin C) can interfere with accurate testing by producing normal test results even in the presence of significant bleeding.

■ Ingestion of 2 to 5 ml of blood (for example, from bleeding gums) can cause abnormal results.

Fecal lipids

Lipids excreted in feces include monoglycerides, diglycerides, triglycerides, phospholipids, glycolipids, soaps (fatty acids and fatty acid salts), sterols, and cholesterol esters. These lipids are derived from sloughed intestinal bacterial cells and epithelial cells, unabsorbed dietary lipids, and GI secretions. Normally, dietary lipids emulsified by bile are almost completely absorbed in the small intestine, provided that biliary and pancreatic secretions are adequate. However, excessive excretion of fecal lipids (steatorrhea) occurs in various malabsorption syndromes.

Both qualitative and quantitative tests can detect excessive excretion of lipids in patients with signs of malabsorption: weight loss, abdominal distention, and scaly skin. In the qualitative test, a specimen from a random stool is stained with Sudan III dye and examined microscopically for evidence of malabsorption — undigested muscle fibers and various fats. In the quantitative test, the entire 72-hour specimen is dried and weighed; the lipids therein are extracted with a solvent, evaporated, and weighed. Only the quantitative test can confirm steatorrhea.

Purpose

■ To confirm steatorrhea.

Patient preparation

Explain to the patient that this test evaluates digestion of fats. Instruct him to abstain from alcohol and to maintain a high-fat diet (100 g/day) for 3 days before the test and during the collection period. Tell him the test requires a 72-hour stool collection. Withhold drugs that may affect test results, as ordered. If these medications must be continued, note this on the laboratory request.

Teach the patient how to collect a timed stool specimen, and provide him with the necessary equipment. Inform him that the laboratory requires 1 or 2 days to complete the analysis.

Procedure

Collect a 72-hour stool specimen.

Precautions

■ Don't use a waxed collection container because the wax may become incorporated in the stool and interfere with accurate testing.

■ Tell the patient to avoid contaminating the stool specimen with toilet tissue or urine.

■ Refrigerate the collection container between defecations, and keep it tightly covered.

Reference values

Fecal lipids normally make up less than 20% of excreted solids, with excretion of less than 7 g/24 hours.

Implications of results

Both digestive and absorptive disorders cause steatorrhea. Digestive disorders may affect the production and release of pancreatic lipase or bile; absorptive disorders may affect the integrity of the intestine. In pancreatic insufficiency, impaired lipid digestion may result from insufficient production of lipase. Pancreatic resection, cystic fibrosis, chronic pancreatitis, or ductal obstruction by stone or tumor may prevent the normal release or action of lipase.

In impaired hepatic function, faulty lipid digestion may result from inadequate production of bile salts. Biliary obstruction, which may accompany gallbladder disease, may prevent the normal release of bile salts into the duodenum. Extensive small-bowel resection or bypass may also interrupt normal enterohepatic circulation of bile salts.

Diseases of the intestinal mucosa affect normal absorption of lipids; regional ileitis and atrophy due to malnutrition cause gross structural changes in the intestinal wall, while celiac disease and tropical sprue produce mucosal abnormalities. Scleroderma, radiation enteritis, fistulas, intestinal tuberculosis, small intestine diverticula, and altered intestinal flora may also cause steatorrhea. Whipple's disease and lymphomas cause lymphatic obstruction that may inhibit fat absorption.

Post-test care

As ordered, tell the patient he may resume his usual diet and medications withheld before the test.

Interfering factors

▪ The following drugs and substances may produce inaccurate test results by inhibiting absorption or affecting chemical digestion: azathioprine, bisacodyl, cholestyramine, kanamycin, neomycin, colchicine, aluminum hydroxide, calcium carbonate, alcohol, potassium chloride, and mineral oil.

▪ Failure to observe pretest restrictions, use of a waxed collection container, contamination of the sample, or incomplete stool specimen collection (total weight less than 300 g) will affect the accuracy of test results.

Fecal urobilinogen

Urobilinogen, the end product of bilirubin metabolism, is a brown pigment formed by bacterial enzymes in the small intestine. It's excreted in feces or reabsorbed into portal blood, where it's returned to the liver and reexcreted in bile; a small amount of urobilinogen is also excreted in urine. Because bilirubin metabolism depends on a properly functioning hepatobiliary system and a normal erythrocyte life span, measurement of fecal urobilinogen is a useful indicator of hepatobiliary and hemolytic disorders. However, this test is rarely performed because serum bilirubin and urine urobilinogen can be measured more easily.

Purpose

▪ To aid diagnosis of hepatobiliary and hemolytic disorders.

Patient preparation

Explain to the patient that this test evaluates the function of the liver and bile ducts or detects red blood cell disorders. Inform him that he needn't restrict food or fluids before the test. Tell him the test requires collection of a random stool specimen.

Withhold broad-spectrum antibiotics, sulfonamides, and salicylates for 2 weeks before the test, as ordered. If these medications must be continued, note this on the laboratory request.

Procedure

Collect a random stool specimen.

Precautions

▪ Tell the patient not to contaminate the stool specimen with toilet tissue or urine.

▪ Use a light-resistant collection container because urobilinogen breaks

down to urobilin on exposure to light.
■ Send the specimen to the laboratory immediately. If transport or testing is delayed more than 30 minutes, refrigerate the specimen; if testing is being performed by an outside laboratory, freeze the specimen.

Reference values
Normally, fecal urobilinogen values range from 50 to 300 mg/24 hours.

Implications of results
Low levels or absence of urobilinogen in the feces indicates obstructed bile flow, which may result from intrahepatic disorders (such as hepatocellular jaundice due to cirrhosis or hepatitis), extrahepatic disorders (such as tumor of the head of the pancreas, the ampulla of Vater, or the bile duct), or choledocholithiasis. Low fecal urobilinogen levels are also characteristic of depressed erythropoiesis, as occurs in aplastic anemia.

Post-test care
Resume administration of medications withheld before the test, as ordered.

Interfering factors
■ Broad-spectrum antibiotics can depress fecal urobilinogen levels by inhibiting bacterial growth in the colon. Sulfonamides, which react with the reagent used by the laboratory in this test, and large doses of salicylates can raise fecal urobilinogen levels.
■ Failure to use a light-resistant collection container or contamination of the specimen will affect the accuracy of test results.

ENDOSCOPY

Esophagogastroduo-denoscopy

Esophagogastroduodenoscopy (EGD) is the visual examination of the lining of the esophagus, the stomach, and the upper duodenum, using a flexible fiberoptic endoscope. It's indicated in patients with hematemesis, melena, or substernal or epigastric pain and in postoperative patients with recurrent or new symptoms. This procedure is generally safe, but it can cause perforation of the esophagus, stomach, or duodenum, especially if the patient is restless or uncooperative.

EGD, which can detect small or surface lesions missed by radiography, eliminates the need for extensive exploratory surgery. It also permits laboratory evaluation of abnormalities first detected by radiography because the scope provides a channel for biopsy forceps or a cytology brush. Similarly, it allows removal of foreign bodies by suction (for small, soft objects) or by electrocautery snare or forceps (for large, hard objects).

Purpose
■ To diagnose inflammatory disease, malignant and benign tumors, ulcers, Mallory-Weiss syndrome, and structural abnormalities
■ To evaluate the stomach and duodenum postoperatively
■ To obtain emergency diagnosis of duodenal ulcer or esophageal injury, such as that caused by ingestion of chemicals.

Patient preparation
Explain to the patient that this procedure permits visual examination of the

lining of the esophagus, the stomach, and the upper duodenum. Instruct him to fast for 6 to 12 hours before the test. Tell him that the test requires that a flexible instrument be passed through his mouth, who will perform this procedure and where, and that it takes about 30 minutes. (If an emergency EGD is to be performed, tell the patient that stomach contents will be aspirated through a nasogastric tube.) Also inform him that a blood sample may be drawn before the procedure.

Inform the patient that a bitter-tasting local anesthetic will be sprayed into his mouth and throat to calm the gag reflex, and that his tongue and throat may feel swollen, making swallowing difficult. Advise him to let the saliva drain from the side of his mouth; a suction machine may be used to remove saliva, if necessary. Tell the patient that an I.V. line will be started to allow infusion of a sedative or I.V. fluids. Tell him that a mouth guard will be inserted to protect his teeth and the endoscope; assure him that the mouth guard won't obstruct his breathing. If the patient wears dentures, instruct him to remove and store them before the test.

Inform him that he'll receive a sedative before the endoscope is inserted to help him relax but that he'll remain conscious. If the procedure is being done on an outpatient basis, advise him to arrange for transportation home because he may feel drowsy from the sedative.

Tell the patient he may experience pressure in the stomach as the endoscope is moved about, and a feeling of fullness when air or carbon dioxide is insufflated. If the patient is apprehensive, administer meperidine or another analgesic I.M. about 30 minutes before the test, as ordered; also administer atropine sulfate subcutaneously at this time, as ordered, to decrease gastric secretions, which would interfere with test results.

Make sure the patient or a responsible family member has signed a consent form. Check the patient's history for hypersensitivity to the medications and anesthetic ordered for the test. Just before the procedure, instruct the patient to remove eyeglasses, necklaces, hairpins, combs, and constricting undergarments.

Procedure

Obtain baseline vital signs, and leave the blood pressure cuff in place for monitoring throughout the procedure. Then ask the patient to hold his breath while his mouth and throat are sprayed with a local anesthetic. The patient is given an emesis basin in which to spit out saliva and is provided with tissues to wipe excess saliva from his mouth. Because the anesthetic spray causes the patient to lose some control of his secretions and increases the risk of aspiration, encourage him to let saliva drain from the side of his mouth.

After the patient is placed in a left lateral position, his head is bent forward and he is asked to open his mouth. The examiner inserts his finger into the mouth and guides the tip of the endoscope alongside his finger to the back of the throat. The rubber tip is deflected downward with the left index finger, and the endoscope is advanced. As the endoscope passes through the posterior pharynx and the cricopharyngeal sphincter, the patient's head is slowly extended to aid advancement of the scope. The patient's chin must be kept at midline. The endoscope is then passed along the esophagus under direct vision. When the endoscope is well into the esophagus (about 12" [30 cm]), the patient's head is positioned with his chin toward the table so that saliva can drain out of his mouth.

Esophageal topography

This diagram of the esophagus and part of the stomach shows the approximate location of the aortic arch and the Z line, an irregular boundary where the smooth esophageal mucosa changes abruptly to the furrowed lining of the stomach.

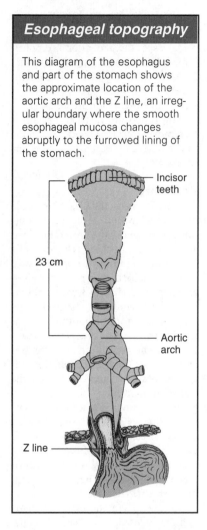

Incisor teeth

23 cm

Aortic arch

Z line

When examination of the esophagus and the cardiac sphincter is completed, the endoscope is rotated clockwise — with the tip angled upward — and is advanced into the stomach. After the lining of the stomach is examined completely, including the gastric side of the cardiac and pyloric sphincters, the endoscope is advanced into the duodenum. Following this examination, the endoscope is slowly withdrawn, and suspicious areas of the gastric and esophageal lining are reexamined.

During the examination, air may be instilled into the GI tract to open the bowel lumen and flatten tissue folds, water may be instilled to rinse material or fluids from the lens, and suction may be applied to remove unnecessary insufflated air or secretions. A camera may be attached to the endoscope to photograph areas for later study, or a measuring tube may be passed through the endoscope to determine the size of a lesion. Biopsy forceps to obtain a tissue specimen or a cytology brush to obtain cells may also be passed through the scope.

Tissue specimens are immediately placed in a specimen bottle containing 10% formaldehyde solution; cell specimens are smeared on glass slides and placed in a Coplin jar containing 95% ethyl alcohol.

Precautions
■ EGD is usually contraindicated in patients with Zenker's diverticulum, a large aortic aneurysm, or a recent ulcer perforation.
■ This procedure should not be performed within 2 days after an upper GI series because barium retention hinders visual examination.
■ Observe closely for medication side effects: respiratory depression, apnea, hypotension, excessive diaphoresis, bradycardia, and laryngospasm. Have available emergency resuscitation equipment and a narcotic antagonist such as naloxone. Be prepared to intervene as necessary.

Normal findings
The smooth mucosa of the esophagus is normally yellow-pink and marked by a fine vascular network. A pulsation on the anterior wall of the esophagus between 8" and 10" (20 and 25 cm) from the incisor teeth represents the aortic arch. The orange-red mucosa of the stomach begins at the Z line, an irregu-

lar transition line slightly above the esophagogastric junction. (See *Esophageal topography*.) Unlike the esophagus, the stomach has rugal folds, and its blood vessels aren't visible beneath the gastric mucosa. The reddish mucosa of the duodenal bulb is marked by a few shallow longitudinal folds. However, the mucosa of the distal duodenum has prominent circular folds, is lined with villi, and appears velvety.

Implications of results

EGD, along with the results of histologic and cytologic tests, may indicate acute or chronic ulcers, benign or malignant tumors, and inflammatory disease, including esophagitis, gastritis, and duodenitis. It may also demonstrate diverticula, varices, Mallory-Weiss syndrome, esophageal rings, esophageal and pyloric stenoses, and esophageal hiatal hernia. Although this procedure can evaluate gross abnormalities of esophageal motility (as in achalasia), manometric studies are more accurate for this purpose.

Post-test care

 ▪ Observe the patient for possible perforation. Perforation in the cervical area of the esophagus produces pain on swallowing and with neck movement; thoracic perforation causes substernal or epigastric pain that increases with breathing or with movement of the trunk; diaphragmatic perforation produces shoulder pain and dyspnea; gastric perforation causes abdominal or back pain, cyanosis, fever, or pleural effusion.

▪ Check vital signs every 15 minutes for 4 hours, every hour for 4 hours, then every 4 hours.

▪ Provide a safe environment for the patient until he has recovered from the sedative. Keep side rails up.

▪ Withhold food and fluids until the gag reflex returns. Test the gag reflex by touching the back of the throat with a tongue blade. When the gag reflex returns — usually within 1 hour — allow fluids and a light meal, as ordered.

▪ Tell the patient he may burp some insufflated air and may have a sore throat for 3 to 4 days. Provide throat lozenges and warm saline gargles to ease his discomfort.

▪ If the patient experiences soreness at the I.V. site, apply warm soaks.

▪ Make sure an outpatient has transportation home because someone who has been sedated shouldn't drive for 12 hours. Instruct him to watch for persistent difficulty swallowing and for pain, fever, black stools, or bloody vomitus. Tell him to notify the doctor immediately if any of these complications develops.

Interfering factors

Failure to adhere to dietary restrictions or to send specimens to the laboratory immediately may affect the accuracy of test results.

Colonoscopy

Colonoscopy is the visual examination of the lining of the large intestine with a flexible fiber-optic endoscope. This test is indicated for patients with a history of constipation and diarrhea, persistent rectal bleeding, or lower abdominal pain when results of proctosigmoidoscopy and a barium enema test prove negative or inconclusive.

The colonoscope is available in 42" to 72" (105- to 180-cm) lengths and contains a bundle of glass fibers that transmit light. It is inserted anally and advanced through the large intestine under direct vision, using the scope's optical system. Fluoroscopy and abdominal palpation may facilitate passage of the endoscope through the bends in the large intestine.

Colonoscopy is usually a safe procedure, but it can cause perforation of the large intestine, excessive bleeding, and retroperitoneal emphysema.

Purpose

■ To detect or evaluate inflammatory and ulcerative bowel disease
■ To locate the origin of lower GI bleeding
■ To aid diagnosis of colonic strictures and benign or malignant lesions
■ To evaluate the colon postoperatively for recurrence of polyps or malignant lesions.

Patient preparation

Explain to the patient that this test permits examination of the lining of the large intestine. Instruct him to maintain a clear liquid diet for 24 to 48 hours before the test and to take nothing by mouth after midnight the evening before the procedure. Tell him the test requires that a flexible instrument be passed through his anus, who will perform the test and where, and that the procedure usually takes 30 to 60 minutes.

Tell the patient that the large intestine must be thoroughly cleansed to be clearly visible. Give him a laxative, such as 10 oz (300 ml) of magnesium citrate, 3 tbs (45 ml) of castor oil, or a gallon of GoLYTELY solution in the evening. Chill the solution to make it more palatable. If you're using GoLYTELY, instruct the patient to drink the preparation quickly (8 oz [240 ml] every 10 minutes until the entire gallon is consumed). This laxative produces watery diarrhea in 30 to 60 minutes and clears the bowel in 4 to 5 hours.

If fecal results are still not clear, the patient will receive a laxative, suppository, or tap-water enema. Don't administer a soapsuds enema because this irritates the mucosa and stimulates mucous secretions that may hinder the examination.

Inform the patient that he may receive a sedative I.M. or I.V. to help him relax. Assure him that the colonoscope is well lubricated to ease its insertion, that it initially feels cool, and that he may feel an urge to defecate when it's inserted and advanced. Instruct him to breathe deeply and slowly through his mouth to relax the abdominal muscles.

Explain to the patient that air may be introduced into the large intestine through the colonoscope to distend the intestinal wall and provide a better view of the lining and to facilitate the instrument's advance. Tell him that flatus normally escapes around the instrument due to air insufflation and that he shouldn't attempt to control it. Tell him that a suction machine may remove any blood or liquid feces that obscure vision but that this won't cause discomfort.

Make sure the patient or responsible member of the family has signed a consent form. Check the patient's vital signs 30 minutes before the test; if they're stable, administer the sedative, as ordered.

Procedure

Place the patient on his left side, with his knees flexed, and drape him. Instruct him to breathe deeply and slowly through his mouth as the doctor inserts his gloved, lubricated index finger into the anus and rectum and palpates the mucosa. After a water-soluble lubricant has been applied to the patient's anus and to the tip of the colonoscope, tell the patient the colonoscope is about to be inserted.

After the colonoscope is inserted through the patient's anus, a small amount of air is insufflated to locate the bowel lumen. The scope is advanced through the rectum into the sigmoid colon under direct vision. When the instrument reaches the descending sigmoid junction, assist the patient to a supine position to aid the scope's advance, if necessary; this position may also be assumed to negotiate the splenic flexure. After the scope has passed the splenic flexure, it's advanced through the transverse colon and hepatic flexure, into the ascending colon and cecum. Abdominal palpation or fluoroscopy may guide the colonoscope through the large intestine. (If the tip of the scope becomes lodged in the colon, fluoroscopy is helpful for locating the tip and adjusting the angle of entry.)

During the examination, suction may be used to remove blood or excessive secretions that obscure vision. Biopsy forceps or a cytology brush may be passed through a channel in the colonoscope to obtain specimens for histologic and cytologic examinations, respectively; an electrocautery snare may be used to remove polyps. If the examiner removes a tissue specimen, immediately place it in a specimen bottle containing 10% formalin; immediately place cytology smears in a Coplin jar containing 95% ethyl alcohol.

Precautions
■ Colonoscopy is contraindicated in pregnant women near term and in patients who have recently had an acute myocardial infarction or abdominal surgery.
■ Colonoscopy is contraindicated in patients who have ischemic bowel disease, acute diverticulitis, peritonitis, fulminant granulomatous colitis, or fulminant ulcerative colitis.

 ■ Watch closely for side effects of the sedative, such as respiratory depression, hypotension, excessive diaphoresis, bradycardia, and confusion. Have available emergency resuscitation equipment and a narcotic antagonist such as naloxone for I.V. use, if necessary.
■ If the doctor has obtained a tissue or cell specimen, send it to the appropriate laboratory immediately.
■ If a polyp is removed but not retrieved during the examination, give the patient enemas and strain stools, as ordered, to retrieve it.

Normal findings
The mucosa of the large intestine beyond the sigmoid colon appears light pink-orange and is marked by semilunar folds and deep tubular pits. Blood vessels are visible beneath the intestinal mucosa, which glistens from mucous secretions. (See *Normal and abnormal colonoscopic views*, page 832.)

Implications of results
Colonoscopy, coupled with histologic and cytologic test results, may indicate proctitis, granulomatous and ulcerative colitis, Crohn's disease, and malignant or benign lesions. Colonoscopy alone can detect diverticular disease or the site of lower GI bleeding.

Post-test care
 ■ Observe the patient closely for signs of bowel perforation: malaise, rectal bleeding, abdominal pain and distention, fever, and mucopurulent drainage. Notify the doctor immediately if such signs develop.
■ Check vital signs until they're stable.
■ Provide a safe environment until the patient has recovered from sedation. Then he may resume his usual diet.
■ Tell the patient he may pass large amounts of flatus, resulting from the air insufflated to distend the colon. Provide privacy in order to minimize embarrassment.
■ If a polyp has been removed, inform the patient that there may be some

Normal and abnormal colonoscopic views

These two views, taken with a fiber-optic colonoscope, show a normal descending colon (left) and a colon with cancer (right).

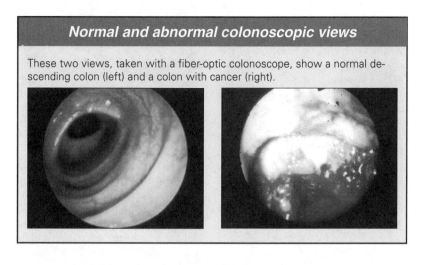

blood in his stool; however, tell him to report excessive bleeding immediately.

Interfering factors

- Barium retained in the intestine from previous diagnostic studies makes accurate visual examination impossible.
- Blood from acute colonic hemorrhage interferes with the examination.
- Fixation of the sigmoid colon from inflammatory bowel disease, surgery, or radiation therapy may inhibit passage of the colonoscope.
- Failure to place histological or cytological specimens in the appropriate preservative or to send the specimens to the laboratory immediately may interfere with test results.

Proctosigmoidoscopy

Proctosigmoidoscopy is the endoscopic examination of the lining of the distal sigmoid colon, the rectum, and the anal canal, using two different instruments: a proctoscope and a sigmoidoscope. It's indicated for patients with recent changes in bowel habits, lower abdominal and perineal pain, prolapse on defecation, anal pruritus, or passage of mucus, blood, or pus in the stool.

This procedure involves three separate steps: a digital examination, sigmoidoscopy, and proctoscopy. During digital examination, the anal sphincters are dilated to detect any obstruction that might hinder the passage of the endoscope. During sigmoidoscopy, a 10" to 12" (25- to 30-cm) rigid sigmoidoscope is inserted into the anus to allow visualization of the distal sigmoid colon and rectum. (Use of a flexible sigmoidoscope also permits visualization of the descending colon.) During proctoscopy, a 2¾" (7-cm) rigid proctoscope is inserted into the anus to aid examination of the lower rectum and anal canal.

At any step in this procedure, specimens may be obtained from suspicious areas of the mucosa by biopsy, lavage or cytology brush, or culture swab. Possible complications of this procedure include rectal bleeding and, rarely, bowel perforation.

Purpose

- To aid diagnosis of inflammatory, infectious, and ulcerative bowel disease

- To diagnose hemorrhoids, hypertrophic anal papilla, polyps, fissures, fistulas, and abscesses within the rectum and anal canal.

Patient preparation

Explain to the patient that this procedure allows visual examination of the lining of the distal sigmoid colon, the rectum, and the anal canal. Tell him the test requires passage of two special instruments through the anus, who will perform this procedure and where, and that it takes 15 to 30 minutes.

Because dietary and bowel preparation for this procedure varies considerably, follow the doctor's orders carefully. As ordered, instruct the patient to maintain a clear liquid diet for 24 to 48 hours before the test, to avoid eating fruits and vegetables before the procedure, and to fast the morning of the procedure. If a special bowel preparation is ordered, explain to the patient that this clears the intestine to provide a better view.

As ordered, administer a warm tapwater or sodium biphosphate enema 3 to 4 hours before the procedure. (The procedure may be started without bowel preparation because enemas can alter intestinal markings and traumatize mucous membranes. For this reason, irritating soapsuds enemas are inappropriate before this test. If the examination is hindered by excessive fecal matter, an enema may be ordered before the examination proceeds.)

Describe to the patient the position he'll be asked to assume (a knee-to-chest or left lateral position), and assure him that he'll be adequately draped to minimize embarrassment. Tell him he may be placed on a tilting table that rotates into horizontal and vertical positions but that he'll be adequately secured to the table.

Tell the patient that the doctor's finger and the instrument are well lubricated, to ease insertion, that the instrument initially feels cool, and that he may experience the urge to defecate when it's inserted and advanced. Inform him that the instrument may stretch the intestinal wall and cause transient muscle spasms or a colicky lower abdominal pain. Instruct him to breathe deeply and slowly through his mouth to relax the abdominal muscles; this reduces the urge to defecate and eases discomfort.

Explain to the patient that air may be introduced through the endoscope into the intestine to distend its walls. Tell him this causes flatus to escape around the endoscope and he shouldn't attempt to control it. Inform him that a suction machine may remove blood, mucus, or liquid feces that obscure vision, but it will cause no discomfort.

Make sure the patient or responsible member of the family has signed a consent form. Check the patient's history for barium tests within the past week because the presence of barium in the colon makes accurate examination impossible. If the patient has rectal inflammation, provide a local anesthetic about 15 to 20 minutes before the procedure, if ordered, to minimize discomfort. Tell him that he may receive a sedative I.M. or I.V. to help him relax.

Procedure

Place the patient in a knee-to-chest or left lateral position, with knees flexed, and drape him. If a left lateral position is used, a sandbag may be placed under the patient's left hip, so the buttocks project over the edge of the table. The right buttock is gently raised, and the anus and perianal region are examined under good lighting. Instruct the patient to breathe deeply and slowly through his mouth as the doctor inserts a well-lubricated, gloved index finger into the anus and carefully palpates the anal canal for induration and tenderness. The doctor advances his finger into the rectum and palpates the rectal mucosa; then he withdraws the finger and checks for the presence of blood, mucus, or fecal matter.

The sigmoidoscope is lubricated, and the patient is told that the instrument is about to be inserted. The right buttock is raised, and the sigmoidoscope is inserted into the anus. As the scope is passed with steady pressure through the anal sphincters, instruct the patient to bear down as though defecating to aid its passage. The sigmoidoscope is advanced through the anal canal into the rectum. At the rectosigmoid junction, a small amount of air may be insufflated to open the bowel lumen. The scope is then gently manipulated backward and forward to negotiate this flexure, and is advanced to its full length into the distal sigmoid colon.

As the sigmoidoscope is slowly withdrawn, air is carefully insufflated, and the intestinal mucosa is thoroughly examined. If fecal matter obscures vision, the eyepiece on the scope is removed, a cotton swab is inserted through the scope, and the bowel lumen is swabbed. (A suction machine may remove blood, excessive secretions, or liquid feces.)

To obtain specimens from a suspicious area of the intestinal mucosa, the magnifying lens of the eyepiece is removed, and a biopsy forceps, a cytology brush, or a culture swab is passed through the sigmoidoscope. Polyps may also be removed for histologic examination by insertion of an electrocautery snare through the sigmoidoscope. After the specimen is obtained, it is immediately placed in a specimen bottle containing 10% formalin; cytology slides are placed in a Coplin jar containing 95% ethyl alcohol; and the culture swab is placed in a culture tube.

After the sigmoidoscope is withdrawn, the proctoscope is lubricated, and the patient is told that the procto-scope is about to be inserted. Assure him that he will experience less discomfort during passage of the proctoscope. The right buttock is raised, and the proctoscope is inserted through the anus and gently advanced to its full length. The obturator is removed, and the light source is inserted through the handle of the proctoscope. As the instrument is slowly withdrawn, the rectal and anal mucosa are carefully examined. To obtain specimens from suspicious areas of the intestinal mucosa, the same steps are followed as during sigmoidoscopy. However, if a biopsy of the anal canal is required, a local anesthetic may be administered first because this area is sensitive to pain. After the examination is completed, the proctoscope is withdrawn.

If the patient has been examined in a knee-to-chest position, instruct him to rest in a supine position for several minutes before standing to prevent postural hypotension.

Precautions

If a tissue specimen or culture swab has been obtained, label it and send it to the appropriate laboratory immediately.

Normal findings

The mucosa of the sigmoid colon appears light pink-orange and is marked by semilunar folds and deep tubular pits. The rectal mucosa appears redder because of its rich vascular network, deepens to a purple hue at the pectinate line (the anatomic division between the rectum and anus), and has three distinct valves. The lower two-thirds of the anus (anoderm) is lined with smooth gray-tan skin and joins with the hair-fringed perianal skin.

Implications of results

Visual examination and palpation demonstrate abnormalities of the anal ca-

Colon abnormalities

These abnormal views of the colon were taken with a proctosigmoidoscope. The view on the left demonstrates familial polyposis — multiple adenomatous growths with high malignancy potential. The view on the right shows diverticular orifices of the colon associated with muscle hypertrophy, which almost obscures the slitlike lumen (far right).

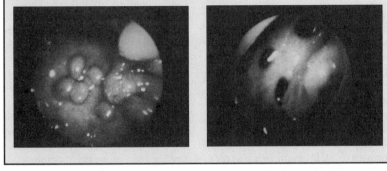

nal and rectum, including internal and external hemorrhoids, hypertrophic anal papilla, anal fissures, anal fistulas, and anorectal abscesses. (See *Colon abnormalities*.) However, biopsy, culture, and other laboratory tests are often necessary to detect various disorders. For example, biopsy can distinguish benign from malignant tumors and can aid diagnosis of ulcerative and ischemic colitis. X-rays after barium enema or colonoscopy can conform Crohn's disease and polyposis. Stool culture and serum agglutination tests demonstrate bacterial infection; culture and serologic tests, such as the Venereal Disease Research Laboratory test, detect syphilis.

Post-test care

 ■ Observe the patient closely for signs of bowel perforation (malaise, rectal bleeding, abdominal distention and pain, mucopurulent drainage, and fever) and for vasovagal attack due to emotional stress (depressed blood pressure, pallor, diaphoresis, and bradycardia). Notify the doctor immediately if such signs develop.

■ Allow the patient nothing by mouth until he is alert.

■ Monitor vital signs every 30 minutes until the patient is alert.

■ Provide a safe environment until the patient is alert.

■ If air was introduced into the intestine, tell the patient that he may pass large amounts of flatus. Provide privacy while he rests after the test.

■ If a biopsy or polypectomy was performed, inform the patient that blood may appear in his stool.

Interfering factors

■ Barium retained in the intestine from previous diagnostic studies makes accurate visual examination impossible.

■ Large amounts of stool in the intestine hinders visual examination and the advancement of the endoscope.

■ Failure to place histologic or cytologic specimens in the appropriate preservative or to send them to the laboratory immediately may interfere with accurate test results.

CONTRAST RADIOGRAPHY

Barium swallow

Barium swallow (also known as esophagography) is the cineradiographic, radiographic, or fluoroscopic examination of the pharynx and the fluoroscopic examination of the esophagus after ingestion of thick and thin mixtures of barium sulfate. This test, most commonly performed as part of the upper GI series, is indicated for patients with a history of dysphagia and regurgitation. Further testing is usually required for a definitive diagnosis. (See *Gastroesophageal reflux scanning*.) However, cholangiography and the barium enema test, if ordered, should precede the barium swallow because ingested barium may obscure anatomic details on the X-rays.

Purpose
▪ To diagnose hiatal hernia, diverticula, and varices
▪ To detect strictures, ulcers, tumors, polyps, and motility disorders.

Patient preparation
Explain to the patient that this test evaluates the function of the pharynx and esophagus. Instruct him to fast after midnight before the test. (If the patient is an infant, delay feeding to ensure complete digestion of barium.) Tell him who will perform the test and where and that it takes approximately 30 minutes.

Describe the milk shake consistency and chalky taste of the barium preparation the patient will ingest; although it's flavored, he may find it unpleasant to swallow. Tell him he'll first receive a thick mixture, then a thin one, and that he must drink 12 to 14 oz (355 to 415 ml) during the examination. Inform

him that he'll be placed in various positions on a tilting X-ray table and that X-rays will be taken. Reassure him that safety precautions will be maintained.

Withhold antacids, as ordered, if gastric reflux is suspected. Just before the procedure, instruct the patient to put on a hospital gown without snap closures and to remove jewelry, dentures, hairpins, and other radiopaque objects from the X-ray field.

Procedure
The patient is placed in an upright position behind the fluoroscopic screen, and his heart, lungs, and abdomen are examined. He's then instructed to take one swallow of the thick barium mixture, and the pharyngeal action is recorded using cineradiography. (This action occurs too rapidly for adequate fluoroscopic evaluation.) The patient is then told to take several swallows of the thin barium mixture. The passage of the barium is examined fluoroscopically, and spot films of the esophageal region are taken from lateral angles and from right and left posteroanterior angles.

Esophageal strictures and obstruction of the esophageal lumen by the lower esophageal ring are best detected when the patient is upright. To accentuate small strictures or demonstrate dysphagia, the patient may be requested to swallow a special "barium marshmallow" (soft white bread that has been soaked in barium).

The patient is then secured to the X-ray table and is rotated to the Trendelenburg position to evaluate esophageal peristalsis or demonstrate hiatal hernia and gastric reflux. Again he's instructed to take several swallows of barium while the esophagus is examined fluoroscopically, and spot films of significant findings are taken when indicated.

After the table is rotated to a horizontal position, the patient is told to take

Gastroesophageal reflux scanning

When results of a barium swallow are inconclusive, gastroesophageal reflux scanning may be done to evaluate esophageal function and detect reflux. This test delivers less radiation than a barium swallow and is a much more sensitive indicator of reflux. It also allows reflux to be measured without insertion of an esophageal tube — an important consideration in testing infants, small children, and other patients for whom intubation is contraindicated.

Procedure
The patient is instructed to fast after midnight before the test to clear stomach contents that impede passage of the imaging agent. As the test begins, the patient is placed in a supine or upright position and is asked to swallow a solution containing a radiopharmaceutical, such as technetium-99m sulfur colloid (^{99m}Tc). A gamma counter placed over the patient's chest records passage of the ^{99m}Tc through the esophagus into the stomach, to determine transit time and to evaluate esophageal function.

If gastroesophageal reflux is suspected, the patient is repositioned as his stomach distends, and continuous recordings visualize reflux and estimate its quantity. (Depending on hospital policy, manual pressure may be applied to the patient's upper abdomen, and recordings may be taken at specific intervals.)

Findings and contraindications
Normally, ^{99m}Tc descends through the esophagus in about 6 seconds; radioactivity is then detected only in the stomach and small bowel. However, diffuse spasm of the esophagus, achalasia, or other esophageal motility disorders may prolong transit time. In gastroesophageal reflux, radioactivity may be detected in the esophagus.

Like other radionuclide studies, this scan is usually contraindicated during pregnancy and lactation. It can be modified for use in infants and children.

---

several swallows of barium so that the esophagogastric junction and peristalsis can be evaluated. The passage of the barium is then fluoroscopically observed, and spot films of significant findings are taken with the patient in supine and prone positions.

During fluoroscopic examination of the esophagus, the cardia and fundus of the patient's stomach are also carefully studied because neoplasms in these areas may invade the esophagus and cause obstruction.

Precautions
Barium swallow is usually contraindicated in a patient with intestinal obstruction.

Normal findings
After the barium sulfate is swallowed, the bolus pours over the base of the tongue into the pharynx. A peristaltic wave propels the bolus through the entire length of the esophagus in about 2 seconds. When the peristaltic wave reaches the base of the esophagus, the cardiac sphincter opens, allowing the bolus to enter the stomach. After passage of the bolus, the cardiac sphincter closes. Normally, the bolus evenly fills and distends the lumen of the pharynx and esophagus, and the mucosa appears smooth and regular.

GI motility study

When intestinal disease is strongly suspected, the GI motility study may follow the upper GI and small-bowel series. This study, which evaluates intestinal motility and the integrity of the mucosal lining, records the passage of barium through the lower digestive tract.

About 6 hours after barium ingestion, the head of the barium column is usually in the hepatic flexure; the tail, in the terminal ileum. The barium completely opacifies the large intestine 24 hours after ingestion. Because the amount of barium passing through the large intestine isn't sufficient to fully extend the lumen, spot films taken 24, 48, or 72 hours after barium ingestion prove inferior to the barium enema. However, when spot films suggest intestinal abnormalities, the barium enema and colonoscopy can provide more specific, confirming diagnostic information.

Implications of results

Barium swallow may reveal hiatal hernia, diverticula, and varices. Although strictures, tumors, polyps, ulcers, and motility disorders (pharyngeal muscular disorders, esophageal spasms, and achalasia) may be detected, a definitive diagnosis commonly requires endoscopic biopsy or, for motility disorders, manometric studies. (See *GI motility study*.)

Post-test care

- Check that additional spot films and repeat fluoroscopic evaluation haven't been ordered before allowing the patient to resume his usual diet.
- Instruct the patient to drink plenty of fluids to help eliminate the barium (unless contraindicated).
- Administer a cathartic, if ordered.
- Inform the patient that his stools will be chalky and light colored for 24 to 72 hours. Record descriptions of all stools that the patient passes in the hospital. Barium retained in the intestine may harden, causing obstruction or fecal impaction. Notify the doctor if the patient hasn't expelled the barium in 2 or 3 days.
- Check the patient for abdominal distention and absent bowel sounds, which are associated with constipation and may suggest barium impaction.

Interfering factors

A poor swallowing reflex allows for aspiration of barium into lungs.

Upper GI and small-bowel series

This test involves the fluoroscopic examination of the esophagus, stomach, and small intestine after the patient ingests barium sulfate, a contrast agent. As the barium passes through the digestive tract, fluoroscopy outlines peristalsis and the mucosal contours of the respective organs, and spot films record significant findings. This test is indicated for patients who have upper GI symptoms (difficulty swallowing, regurgitation, burning or gnawing epigastric pain), signs of small-bowel disease (diarrhea, weight loss), and signs of GI bleeding (hematemesis, melena).

Although this test can detect various mucosal abnormalities, many patients need a biopsy afterward to rule out cancer or distinguish specific inflammatory diseases. Oral cholecystography, barium enema, and routine X-rays should always precede this test because retained barium clouds anatomic detail on X-ray films.

Purpose
- To detect hiatal hernia, diverticula, and varices
- To aid diagnosis of strictures, ulcers, tumors, regional enteritis, and malabsorption syndrome
- To help detect motility disorders.

Patient preparation
Explain to the patient that this procedure examines the esophagus, stomach, and small intestine through X-rays taken after the ingestion of barium. Instruct him to maintain a low-residue diet for 2 or 3 days before the test and then to fast and avoid smoking after midnight before the test. Tell him who will perform the procedure and where. Because the procedure takes up to 6 hours to complete, encourage him to bring reading material to the X-ray department.

Inform the patient that he'll be placed on an X-ray table that rotates into various positions. Assure him that he'll be adequately secured to the table and will be assisted to supine, prone, and side-lying positions. Describe the milk shake consistency and chalky taste of the barium mixture; although it's flavored, he may find its taste unpleasant. Tell him he must drink 16 to 20 oz (500 to 600 ml) for a complete examination. Inform him that his abdomen may be compressed to ensure proper coating of the stomach or intestinal walls with barium or to separate overlapping bowel loops.

As ordered, withhold most oral medications after midnight and anticholinergics and narcotics for 24 hours because these drugs affect small intestine motility. Antacids are also sometimes withheld for several hours if gastric reflux is suspected.

Just before the procedure, instruct the patient to put on a hospital gown without snap closures and to remove jewelry, dentures, hairpins, and other objects that might obscure anatomic detail on the X-rays.

Procedure
After the patient is secured in a supine position on the X-ray table, the table is tilted until the patient is erect, and the heart, lungs, and abdomen are examined fluoroscopically. The patient is then instructed to take several swallows of the barium suspension, and its passage through the esophagus is observed. (Occasionally, the patient is given a thick barium suspension, especially when esophageal pathology is strongly suspected.) During fluoroscopic examination, spot films of the esophagus are taken from lateral angles and from right and left posteroanterior angles.

When barium enters the stomach, the patient's abdomen is palpated or compressed to ensure adequate coating of the gastric mucosa with barium. To perform a double contrast examination, the patient is instructed to sip the barium through a perforated straw. As he does so, a small amount of air is also introduced into the stomach to allow detailed examination of the gastric rugae, and spot films of significant findings are taken. The patient is then instructed to ingest the remaining barium suspension, and the filling of the stomach and emptying into the duodenum are observed fluoroscopically. Two series of spot films of the stomach and duodenum are taken from posteroanterior, anteroposterior, oblique, and lateral angles, with the patient erect and then supine.

The passage of barium into the remainder of the small intestine is then observed fluoroscopically, and spot films are taken at 30- to 60-minute intervals until the barium reaches the ileocecal valve and the region around it. If abnormalities in the small intestine are detected, the area is palpated and compressed to help clarify the defect, and a spot film is taken. When the barium enters the cecum, the examination is ended.

Precautions

The upper GI and small-bowel series is contraindicated in patients with obstruction or perforation of the GI tract because barium may intensify the obstruction or seep into the abdominal cavity. If a perforation is suspected, gastrografin (a water-soluble contrast medium) may be used instead of barium.

Normal findings

After the barium suspension is swallowed, it pours over the base of the tongue into the pharynx, and is propelled by a peristaltic wave through the entire length of the esophagus in about 2 seconds. The bolus evenly fills and distends the lumen of the pharynx and esophagus, and the mucosa appears smooth and regular. When the peristaltic wave reaches the base of the esophagus, the cardiac sphincter opens, allowing the bolus to enter the stomach. Then, the cardiac sphincter closes.

As barium enters the stomach, it outlines the characteristic longitudinal folds called rugae, which are best observed using the double-contrast technique. When the stomach is completely filled with barium, its outer contour appears smooth and regular without evidence of flattened, rigid areas suggesting intrinsic or extrinsic lesions.

After barium enters the stomach, it quickly empties into the duodenal bulb through relaxation of the pyloric sphincter. Although the mucosa of the duodenal bulb is relatively smooth, circular folds become apparent as barium enters the duodenal loop. These folds deepen and become more numerous in the jejunum. Barium temporarily lodges between these folds, producing a speckled pattern on the X-ray film. As barium enters the ileum, the circular folds become less prominent and, except for their broadness, resemble those in the duodenum. The film also shows that the diameter of the small intestine tapers gradually from the duodenum to the ileum.

Implications of results

X-ray studies of the esophagus may reveal strictures, tumors, hiatal hernia, diverticula, varices, and ulcers (particularly in the distal esophagus). Benign strictures usually dilate the esophagus, whereas malignant ones cause erosive changes in the mucosa. Tumors produce filling defects in the column of barium, but only malignant ones change the mucosal contour. Nevertheless, a biopsy is necessary for a definitive diagnosis of esophageal strictures and tumors.

Motility disorders, such as esophageal spasm, are usually difficult to detect because spasms are erratic and transient; manometry, which measures the length and pressure of peristaltic contractions and evaluates the function of the cardiac sphincter, is generally performed to detect such disorders. However, achalasia (cardiospasm) is strongly suggested when the distal esophagus appears to narrow. Gastric reflux appears as a backflow of barium from the stomach into the esophagus.

X-ray studies of the stomach may reveal tumors and ulcers. Malignant tumors, usually adenocarcinomas, appear as filling defects on the X-ray and usually disrupt peristalsis. Benign tumors, such as adenomatous polyps and leiomyomas, appear as outpouchings of the gastric mucosa and generally don't affect peristalsis. Ulcers occur most commonly in the stomach and duodenum (particularly in the duodenal bulb). Benign ulcers usually demonstrate evidence of partial or complete healing and are characterized by radiating folds extending to the edge of the ulcer crater. Malignant ulcers usually have radiating folds that extend beyond the ulcer crater to the edge of the mass. However, a biopsy is necessary for a definitive diagnosis of both tumors and ulcers.

Occasionally, this test detects signs that suggest pancreatitis or pancreatic carcinoma, such as edematous changes in the mucosa of the antrum or duodenal loop, or dilation of the duodenal loop. These findings mandate further studies for pancreatic disease, such as endoscopic retrograde cholangiopancreatography, abdominal ultrasonography, or computed tomography.

X-ray studies of the small intestine may reveal regional enteritis, malabsorption syndrome, and tumors. Although regional enteritis may not be detected in its early stages, small ulcerations and edematous changes develop in the mucosa as the disease progresses. Edematous changes, segmentation of the barium column, and flocculation characterize malabsorption syndrome. Filling defects occur with Hodgkin's disease and lymphosarcoma.

Post-test care

■ Make sure additional X-rays haven't been ordered before allowing the patient food, fluids, and oral medications (if applicable).
■ Tell the patient to drink plenty of fluid (unless contraindicated) to help eliminate the barium.

■ Administer a cathartic or enema to the patient, as ordered. Tell him his stool will be lightly colored for 24 to 72 hours. Record and describe any stool that he passes in the hospital. Because barium retention in the intestine may cause obstruction or fecal impaction, notify the doctor if the patient doesn't pass barium within 2 to 3 days. Also, barium retention may affect scheduling of other GI studies.
■ Tell the patient to advise the doctor of abdominal fullness or pain, or a delay in return to brown stools.

Interfering factors

■ Failure to observe restriction of diet, smoking, and medications may interfere with accurate test results.
■ Excess air in the small bowel or failure to remove radiopaque objects in X-ray field can obscure details on the X-ray films.

Barium enema

Barium enema (also known as a lower GI examination) is the radiographic examination of the large intestine after rectal instillation of barium sulfate (single-contrast technique) or barium sulfate and air (double-contrast technique). This test is indicated for patients with a history of altered bowel habits, lower abdominal pain, or passage of blood, mucus, or pus in the stools. It may also be performed after colostomy or ileostomy; in such patients, barium (or barium and air) is instilled through the stoma.

The single-contrast technique provides a profile view of the large intestine; the double-contrast technique provides profile and frontal views. The latter technique is better for detecting small intraluminal tumors (especially polyps), the early mucosal changes of inflammatory disease, and the subtle intestinal bleeding caused by ulcerated polyps or shallow ulcerations of inflammatory disease.

Although barium enema clearly outlines most of the large intestine, proctosigmoidoscopy provides the best view of the rectosigmoid region. Barium enema should precede barium swallow and the upper GI and small-bowel series because barium retained in the GI tract from the latter tests may interfere with subsequent X-ray studies.

Possible complications of barium enema include perforation of the colon, water intoxication, barium granulomas and, rarely, intraperitoneal and extraperitoneal extravasation of barium and barium embolism.

Purpose
- To aid diagnosis of colorectal cancer and inflammatory disease
- To detect polyps, diverticula, and structural changes in the large intestine.

Patient preparation
Explain to the patient that this test allows the examination of the large intestine through X-rays taken after a barium enema. Tell him who will perform the test and where and that it takes 30 to 45 minutes.

NURSING ALERT Follow the prescribed bowel preparation carefully because residual fecal material in the colon will obscure normal anatomic detail on X-rays. Although various diets, laxatives, and cleansing enemas may be used, remember that certain conditions, such as ulcerative colitis and active GI bleeding, may prohibit the use of laxatives and enemas. Stress to the patient that accurate test results depend on his cooperating with the prescribed dietary restrictions and bowel preparation.

Instruct the patient to restrict dairy products and to follow a liquid diet for 24 hours before the test. Encourage him to drink five 8-oz (240-ml) glasses of water or clear liquids for 12 to 24 hours before the test to ensure adequate hydration. Administer a bowel preparation supplied by the X-ray department. (A GoLYTELY preparation is not recommended because it leaves the bowel too wet and the barium will not coat the walls of the bowel.) An enema or repeat enemas may be ordered until return is clear. Withhold breakfast before the procedure; however, if the test is scheduled for late afternoon (or delayed), clear liquids may be allowed.

Tell the patient that he'll be adequately draped during the test and will be placed on a tilting X-ray table. Assure him that he'll be secured to the table and will be assisted to various positions. Inform him that he may experience cramps or the urge to defecate as the barium or air is introduced into the intestine. Instruct the patient to breathe deeply and slowly through his mouth to ease this discomfort. Tell him to keep his anal sphincter tightly contracted against the rectal tube; this holds the tube in position and helps prevent the barium from leaking.

Stress the importance of retaining the barium enema; if the intestinal walls aren't adequately coated with barium, test results may be inaccurate. Assure the patient that the barium enema is fairly easy to retain because of its cool temperature.

Procedure
After the patient is in a supine position on a tilting X-ray table, spot films of the abdomen are taken. The patient is then assisted to Sims' position, and a well-lubricated rectal tube is inserted through the anus. If the patient has anal sphincter atony or severe mental or physical debilitation, a rectal tube with

a retaining balloon may be inserted. The barium is then administered slowly, and the filling process is monitored fluoroscopically. To aid filling, the table may be tilted or the patient assisted to supine, prone, and lateral decubitus positions.

As the flow of barium is observed, spot films are taken of significant findings. When the intestine is filled with barium, overhead films of the abdomen are taken. The rectal tube is withdrawn, and the patient is escorted to the toilet or provided with a bedpan and instructed to expel as much barium as possible. After evacuation, an additional overhead film is taken to record the mucosal pattern of the intestine and to evaluate the efficiency of colonic emptying.

A double-contrast barium enema may directly follow this examination or may be performed separately. If it's performed immediately, a thin film of barium remains in the patient's intestine, coating the mucosa, and air is carefully injected to distend the bowel lumen. When the double-contrast technique is performed separately, a colloidal barium suspension is instilled, filling the patient's intestine to either the splenic flexure or the middle of the transverse colon. The suspension is then aspirated, and air is forcefully injected into the intestine. The intestine may also be filled to the lower descending colon and then air forcefully injected, without prior aspiration of the suspension.

The patient is then assisted to erect, prone, supine, and lateral decubitus positions in sequence. Barium filling is monitored fluoroscopically, and spot films are taken of significant findings. After the required films are taken, the patient is escorted to the toilet or provided with a bedpan.

Precautions
Barium enema is contraindicated in patients with tachycardia, fulminant ulcerative colitis associated with systemic toxicity and megacolon, toxic megacolon, or suspected perforation. It should be performed cautiously in patients with obstruction, acute inflammatory conditions (such as ulcerative colitis or diverticulitis), acute vascular insufficiency of the bowel, acute fulminant bloody diarrhea, or suspected pneumatosis cystoides intestinalis.

Normal findings
In the single-contrast test: The intestine is uniformly filled with barium, and colonic haustral markings are clearly apparent. The intestinal walls collapse as the barium is expelled, and the mucosa has a regular, feathery appearance on the postevacuation film.

In the double-contrast test: The intestine is uniformly distended with air, with a thin layer of barium providing excellent detail of the mucosal pattern. As the patient is assisted to various positions, the barium collects on the dependent walls of the intestine by the force of gravity.

Implications of results
Although most colon cancers occur in the rectosigmoid region and are best detected by proctosigmoidoscopy, barium enema may reveal adenocarcinoma and, rarely, sarcomas occurring higher in the intestine. Carcinoma usually appears as a localized filling defect, with a sharp transition between the normal and the necrotic mucosa. These characteristics help distinguish carcinoma from the more diffuse lesions of inflammatory disease, but endoscopic biopsy may be necessary to confirm the diagnosis.

Barium enema demonstrates and defines the extent of inflammatory diseases, such as diverticulitis, ulcerative colitis, and granulomatous colitis. Ulcerative colitis usually originates in the anal region and ascends through the intestine; granulomatous colitis usually originates in the cecum and terminal ileum, then descends through the intestine. However, biopsy may be necessary to confirm the diagnosis.

This test may also reveal saccular adenomatous polyps, broad-based villous polyps, structural changes in the intestine (such as intussusception, telescoping of the bowel, sigmoid volvulus [360-degree turn or greater], and sigmoid torsion [up to 180- degree turn]), gastroenteritis, irritable colon, vascular injury due to arterial occlusion, and selected cases of acute appendicitis.

Post-test care

■ Make sure further studies haven't been ordered before allowing the patient food and fluids. Encourage extra fluid intake, as ordered, to prevent dehydration and help eliminate the barium.

■ Encourage rest because this test and the bowel preparation that precedes it exhausts most patients.

■ Because barium retention after this test can cause intestinal obstruction or fecal impaction, administer a mild cathartic or a cleansing enema, as ordered. Tell the patient his stool will be lightly colored for 24 to 72 hours. Record and describe any stools that the patient passes in the hospital.

Interfering factors

■ Inadequate bowel preparation impairs the quality of the X-ray films.

■ Barium swallow performed within a few days of barium enema impairs the quality of subsequent X-ray films.

■ The patient's inability to retain the barium enema will result in an incomplete test.

Hypotonic duodenography

Hypotonic duodenography (also called enterodysis) is the fluoroscopic examination of the duodenum after instillation of barium sulfate and air through an intestinal catheter. This test is indicated for patients with symptoms of a duodenal or pancreatic disorder, such as persistent upper abdominal pain.

After the catheter is passed through the patient's nose into the duodenum, I.V. infusion of glucagon or I.M. injection of propantheline bromide (or another anticholinergic) induces duodenal atony. Instillation of barium and air distends the relaxed duodenum, flattening its deep circular folds; spot films then record the precise delineation of the duodenal anatomy. Although these films readily demonstrate small duodenal lesions and tumors of the head of the pancreas that impinge on the duodenal wall, differential diagnosis requires further studies.

Purpose

■ To detect small postbulbar duodenal lesions, tumors of the head of the pancreas, and tumors of the ampulla of Vater

■ To aid diagnosis of chronic pancreatitis.

Patient preparation

Explain to the patient that this test examines the duodenum and pancreas after the instillation of barium and air. Instruct him to fast from midnight before the test. Tell him who will perform the test and where and that it takes approximately 60 minutes.

Inform the patient that a tube will be passed through his nose into the duodenum to serve as a channel for the barium and air. Tell him he may experience a cramping pain as air enters into the duodenum. Instruct him to breathe deeply and slowly through his mouth if he experiences this pain to help relax the abdominal muscles.

If glucagon or an anticholinergic is to be administered during the procedure, describe the possible adverse effects of glucagon (nausea, vomiting, hives, and flushing) and of anticholinergics (dry mouth, thirst, tachycardia, urine retention [especially in patients with prostatic hypertrophy], and blurred vision). If an anticholinergic is being administered to an outpatient, advise him to have someone accompany him home.

Just before the test, tell the patient to remove dentures, glasses, necklaces, hairpins, combs, and constricting undergarments. Then instruct him to void.

Procedure

While the patient is in a sitting position, a catheter is passed through his nose into the stomach. Then he's placed in a supine position on the X-ray table, and the catheter is advanced into the duodenum under fluoroscopic guidance. To induce duodenal atony for approximately 20 minutes, glucagon is administered I.V. or an anticholinergic is injected I.M. Throughout the procedure, the patient is observed for adverse reactions.

Barium is then instilled through the catheter, and spot films are taken of the duodenum. Some of the barium is then withdrawn and air is instilled; then additional spot films are taken. When the required films have been obtained, the catheter is removed.

Precautions

■ Anticholinergics are contraindicated in patients with severe cardiac disorders or glaucoma.

■ Glucagon is contraindicated in patients with uncontrolled diabetes and should be used cautiously in patients with insulin-dependent diabetes mellitus.

■ Patients with strictures in the upper GI tract, particularly those associated with ulcerations or large masses, shouldn't undergo this procedure.

■ Monitor elderly or very ill patients for gastric reflux.

Normal findings

When barium and air distend the atonic duodenum, the mucosa normally appears smooth and even. The regular contour of the head of the pancreas also appears on the duodenal wall.

Implications of results

Irregular nodules or masses on the duodenal wall could mean duodenal lesions, tumors of the ampulla of Vater, tumors of the head of the pancreas, or chronic pancreatitis. Differential diagnosis requires further tests, such as endoscopic retrograde cholangiopancreatography, serum and urine amylase determinations, pancreatic ultrasonography, and pancreatic computed tomography.

Post-test care

■ Encourage the patient to drink extra fluids (unless contraindicated) to help eliminate the barium.

■ Watch for adverse reactions after administration of glucagon or an anticholinergic. If an anticholinergic was given, make sure the patient voids within a few hours after the test. Advise an outpatient to rest in a waiting area until his vision clears (about 2 hours) unless someone can take him home.

■ Administer a cathartic, as ordered.

■ Inform the patient that he may burp instilled air or pass flatus and that the barium colors the stool chalky white for 24 to 72 hours. Record descriptions of any stools the patient passes in the hospital, and notify the doctor if the patient hasn't expelled the barium after 2 to 3 days.

Interfering factors
None.

Oral cholecystography

Oral cholecystography is the radiographic examination of the gallbladder after administration of a contrast medium. It's indicated for patients with symptoms of biliary tract disease, such as right upper quadrant epigastric pain, fat intolerance, and jaundice, and is most commonly performed to confirm gallbladder disease.

After the contrast medium is ingested, it's absorbed by the small intestine, filtered by the liver, excreted in the bile, and then concentrated and stored in the gallbladder. Full gallbladder opacification usually occurs 12 to 14 hours after ingestion, and a series of X-ray films then records gallbladder appearance. Additional information is obtained by giving the patient a fat stimulus, causing the gallbladder to contract and empty the contrast-laden bile into the common bile duct and small intestine. Films are then taken to record this emptying and to evaluate patency of the common bile duct. Oral cholecystography should precede barium studies because retained barium may cloud subsequent X-ray films.

Purpose
- To detect gallstones
- To aid diagnosis of inflammatory disease and tumors of the gallbladder.

Patient preparation
Explain that this procedure examines the gallbladder through X-rays taken after ingestion of a contrast medium. If ordered, instruct the patient to eat a meal containing fat at noon the day before the test and a fat-free meal in the evening. The former stimulates release of bile from the gallbladder, preparing it to receive the contrast-laden bile; the latter inhibits gallbladder contraction, promoting accumulation of bile. After the evening meal, instruct the patient not to eat or drink, except for water.

Give the patient six tablets (3 g) of iopanoic acid (or another contrast agent) 2 to 3 hours after the evening meal, as ordered. Instruct him to swallow the tablets one at a time, at 5-minute intervals, with one or two mouthfuls of water, for a total of 8 oz (240 ml) of water. Thereafter, withhold water, cigarettes, and gum.

Tell the patient who will perform the procedure and where and that it usually takes 30 to 45 minutes (possibly longer if a fat stimulus is to be given, followed by another series of films). Inform the patient that he'll be placed on an X-ray table and that films will be taken of his gallbladder.

Check the patient's history for hypersensitivity to iodine, seafood, or contrast media used for other diagnostic tests. Inform him that the possible side effects of dye ingestion include diarrhea (common) and, rarely, nausea, vomiting, abdominal cramps, and dysuria. Tell him to report such symptoms immediately if they develop.

 Examine any vomitus or diarrhea for undigested tablets. If any tablets were expelled, notify the doctor and the X-ray department.

Administer a cleansing enema the morning of the test, if ordered. This clears the GI tract of interfering shadows that may obscure the gallbladder.

Procedure

After the patient is in the prone position on the X-ray table, his abdomen is examined fluoroscopically to evaluate gallbladder opacification, and films are taken of significant findings. The patient is then examined in the left lateral decubitus and erect positions to detect layering or mobility of any filling defects, and additional films are taken.

The patient may then be given a fat stimulus, such as a high-fat meal or a synthetic fat-containing agent (for example, Bilevac). Fluoroscopy is used to observe the emptying of the gallbladder in response to the fat stimulus, and spot films are taken at 15 and 30 minutes to visualize the common bile duct. If the gallbladder empties slowly or not at all, films are also taken at 60 minutes.

Precautions

Oral cholecystography is contraindicated in patients with severe renal or hepatic damage and in those with a hypersensitivity to iodine, seafood, or other contrast media.

Normal findings

The gallbladder is normally opacified and appears pear-shaped, with smooth, thin walls. Although its size varies, its basic structure — neck, infundibulum, body, and fundus — is clearly outlined on film.

Implications of results

When the gallbladder is opacified, filling defects (typically appearing within the lumen as negative shadows that show mobility) indicate the presence of gallstones. Fixed defects, on the other hand, may indicate the presence of cholesterol polyps or a benign tumor, such as an adenomyoma.

When the gallbladder fails to opacify or when only faint opacification occurs, inflammatory disease, such as cholecystitis — with or without gallstone formation — may be present. Gallstones may obstruct the cystic duct and prevent the contrast medium from entering the gallbladder; inflammation may impair the concentrating ability of the gallbladder mucosa and prevent or diminish opacification.

When the gallbladder fails to contract following stimulation by a fatty meal, cholecystitis or common bile duct obstruction may be present. If the X-rays are inconclusive, the test will have to be repeated the next day. Repeating the procedure results in opacification of the gallbladder in about two-thirds of patients.

Post-test care

■ If the test results are normal, the patient may resume his usual diet.

■ If gallstones are discovered during opacification, the doctor will order an appropriate diet — usually one that restricts fat intake — to help prevent acute attacks.

■ If oral cholecystography must be repeated, the low-fat diet must be continued until a definitive diagnosis can be made.

Interfering factors

■ Failure to follow dietary restrictions before the test can interfere with accurate results.

■ Failure to ingest the full dose of contrast medium, partial loss of the contrast medium through emesis or diarrhea, inadequate absorption of the contrast medium in the small intestine, or barium retained from previous studies of the biliary tract can affect the accuracy of test results.

■ Impaired hepatic function and moderate jaundice (serum bilirubin levels greater than 3 mg/dl) cause diminished excretion of the contrast medium into the bile, thereby hindering visualization of the biliary tract.

Percutaneous transhepatic cholangiography

Percutaneous transhepatic cholangiography is the fluoroscopic examination of the biliary ducts after injection of an iodinated contrast medium directly into a biliary radicle. This test opacifies the biliary ducts without depending on the gallbladder's concentrating ability. It's therefore especially useful for evaluating patients with persistent upper abdominal pain after cholecystectomy and patients with severe jaundice because impaired hepatic function commonly prevents uptake and excretion of the contrast medium during oral cholecystography or I.V. cholangiography.

Although a computed tomography scan or ultrasonography is usually performed first when obstructive jaundice is suspected, percutaneous transhepatic cholangiography may provide the most detailed view of the obstruction; however, this invasive procedure carries a potential risk of complications, including bleeding, septicemia, bile peritonitis, extravasation of the contrast medium into the peritoneal cavity, and subcapsular injection.

In this test, the patient's liver is punctured with a thin, flexible needle (Chiba needle) under fluoroscopic guidance, and the contrast medium is injected as the needle is slowly withdrawn. When the contrast medium enters a biliary radicle, it begins to outline the biliary tree. As it flows through the biliary ducts, the filling process is visualized by fluoroscopy. Spot films are then taken of any significant findings.

Purpose

■ To determine the cause of upper abdominal pain after cholecystectomy
■ To distinguish between obstructive and nonobstructive jaundice
■ To determine the location, the extent and, in many cases, the cause of mechanical obstruction.

Patient preparation

Explain to the patient that this procedure allows examination of the biliary ducts through X-rays taken after injection of a contrast medium into the liver. Instruct him to fast for 8 hours before the test. Tell him who will perform the test and where and that it takes about 30 minutes. Inform him that he may receive a laxative the night before and a cleansing enema the morning of the test.

Inform the patient that he'll be placed on a tilting X-ray table that rotates into vertical and horizontal positions during the procedure. Assure him that he'll be adequately secured to the table and assisted to various positions throughout the procedure. If appropriate, advise him that a sedative will be administered just before the procedure.

Warn him that injection of the local anesthetic may sting the skin and produce transient pain when it punctures the liver capsule. Also, advise him that injection of the contrast medium may produce a sensation of pressure and epigastric fullness, and may cause transient upper back pain on his right side. Tell him that he'll need to rest for at least 6 hours after the procedure.

Make sure the patient or a responsible member of the family has signed a consent form. Check the patient's history for hypersensitivity to iodine, seafood, the local anesthetic, and contrast media used in other diagnostic tests. Advise him of the possible side effects of contrast agents, such as nausea, vomiting, excessive salivation, flushing, urticaria, sweating and, rarely, anaphylaxis; tachycardia and fever may also accompany intraductal injection. Also check the patient's history for normal

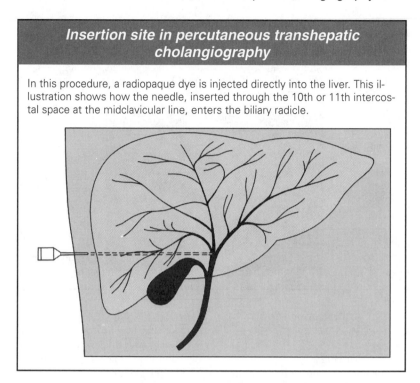

Insertion site in percutaneous transhepatic cholangiography

In this procedure, a radiopaque dye is injected directly into the liver. This illustration shows how the needle, inserted through the 10th or 11th intercostal space at the midclavicular line, enters the biliary radicle.

bleeding, clotting, and prothrombin times and a normal platelet count.

If ordered, administer 1 g of ampicillin I.V. every 4 to 6 hours for 24 hours before the procedure or other broad-spectrum antibiotics to prevent sepsis. Just before the procedure, administer a sedative and pain medication, if ordered.

Procedure

After the patient is placed in the supine position on the X-ray table and is adequately secured, the right upper quadrant of the abdomen is cleaned and draped, and the skin, subcutaneous tissue, and liver capsule are infiltrated with a local anesthetic. While the patient holds his breath at the end of expiration, the flexible needle is inserted under fluoroscopic guidance, through the 10th or 11th intercostal space at the right midclavicular line.

The needle is aimed toward the xiphoid process and is advanced through the liver parenchyma. Then it is slowly withdrawn, injecting the contrast medium to locate a biliary radicle. When fluoroscopy reveals placement in a radicle, the needle is held in position and the remaining contrast dye is injected.

Using a fluoroscope and television monitor, the opacification of the biliary ducts is observed, and spot films of significant findings are taken with the patient in supine and lateral recumbent positions. When the required films have been taken, the needle is removed, and a sterile dressing is applied to the puncture site. (See *Insertion site in percutaneous transhepatic cholangiography*.)

Precautions

This test is contraindicated in patients with cholangitis, massive ascites, uncor-

Abnormal percutaneous cholangiogram

In this percutaneous cholangiogram, the dilated hepatic ducts indicate obstruction of the common bile duct by a tumor. The catheter tip has been passed through the tumor into the duodenum.

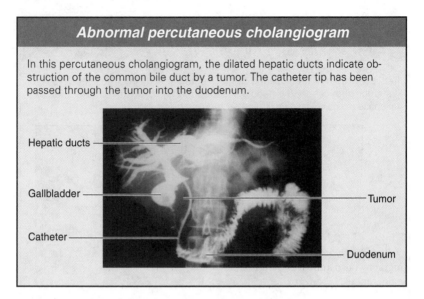

Hepatic ducts

Gallbladder

Catheter

Tumor

Duodenum

rectable coagulopathy, or hypersensitivity to iodine.

Normal findings
The biliary ducts should be of normal diameter and appear as regular channels homogeneously filled with contrast medium.

Implications of results
Distinguishing between obstructive and nonobstructive jaundice hinges on whether biliary ducts are dilated or of normal size. Obstructive jaundice is associated with dilated ducts; nonobstructive jaundice, with normal-sized ducts. When ducts are dilated, the obstruction site may be defined. Obstruction may result from cholelithiasis, biliary tract cancer, or cancer of the pancreas or papilla of Vater that impinges on the common bile duct, causing deviation or stricture.

When ducts are of normal size and intrahepatic cholestasis is indicated, a liver biopsy may be performed to distinguish between hepatitis, cirrhosis, and granulomatous disease. If ducts are dilated as a result of obstruction, a drainage tube may be inserted to allow percutaneous drainage of bile into a collection bag. After a few days, when the dilation and inflammation have diminished, an internal stent may be inserted to allow bile drainage into the bowel. (See *Abnormal percutaneous cholangiogram*.)

Post-test care
■ Check the patient's vital signs until they're stable.
■ Enforce bed rest for at least 6 hours after the test, preferably with the patient lying on his right side, to help prevent hemorrhage.

 ■ Check the injection site for bleeding, swelling, and tenderness. Watch for signs of peritonitis: chills, temperature of 102° to 103° F (38.9° to 39.4° C), and abdominal pain, tenderness, and distention. Notify the doctor immediately if such complications develop.

■ Tell the patient he may resume his usual diet.

Interfering factors

Marked obesity or gas overlying the biliary ducts may affect the clarity of the X-rays.

Postoperative cholangiography

In many cases, a T-shaped rubber tube is inserted into the common bile duct immediately after cholecystectomy or common bile duct exploration to facilitate drainage. Postoperative cholangiography (also known as T-tube cholangiography), performed 7 to 10 days after this surgery, is the radiographic and fluoroscopic examination of the biliary ducts after the injection of a contrast medium through the T tube. The contrast dye flows through the biliary ducts and outlines the size and patency of the ducts, revealing any obstruction overlooked during surgery. Operative cholangiography, an alternative method, may be used to visualize the biliary ducts during surgery. (See *Understanding operative cholangiography,* page 852.)

Purpose

■ To detect calculi, strictures, neoplasms, and fistulae in the biliary ducts.

Patient preparation

Explain to the patient that this procedure permits examination of the biliary ducts through X-rays taken after the injection of a contrast medium through the T tube. Tell him who will perform the test and where and that it takes approximately 15 minutes. Although this procedure isn't painful, warn the patient that he may feel a bloating sensation in the right upper quadrant as the contrast medium is injected.

Clamp the T tube the day before the procedure, if ordered. Bile fills the tube after clamping, which helps prevent air bubbles from entering the ducts. Withhold the meal just before the test, and administer a cleansing enema about 1 hour before the procedure, if ordered.

Make sure the patient or a family member has signed a consent form, if required. Check the patient's history for hypersensitivity to iodine, seafood, or contrast media used in other diagnostic tests. Advise the patient of possible side effects of contrast dye administration, including nausea, vomiting, excessive salivation, flushing, hives, sweating and, rarely, anaphylaxis.

Procedure

After the patient is supine on the X-ray table, the injection area of the T tube is cleaned with povidone-iodine-soaked sponges. The T tube is held in a vertical position, which allows trapped air to surface, and a needle attached to a long transparent catheter is carefully inserted into the end of the T tube. Care must be taken to avoid injecting air into the biliary tree because air bubbles may affect the clarity of the X-ray films.

Approximately 5 ml of contrast medium (usually diatrizoate sodium) is injected under fluoroscopic guidance, and a spot film is taken in the anteroposterior projection. Additional injections are then administered, totaling 20 to 25 ml, and spot films and plain films are taken with the patient in the supine and right lateral decubitus positions. The T tube is then clamped, and the patient is assisted to an erect position for additional films; in this position, air bubbles may be distinguished from calculi and other abnormalities.

A final film is taken 15 minutes after contrast injection to record the emptying of contrast-laden bile into the duodenum. If emptying is delayed, additional films may be taken at 15- or 30-

Understanding operative cholangiography

Operative cholangiography is an alternate method of visualizing the biliary ducts, and is recommended in patients with suspected cholelithiasis or with jaundice resulting from calculus disease of the biliary tree. The test is performed during surgery by the injection of a contrast medium, such as diatrizoate sodium, directly into the common bile duct, the cystic duct, or the gallbladder through a thin needle or catheter. If the gallbladder has been removed before injection, the contrast medium may be administered through a T tube (shown below) inserted after cholecystectomy (operative T-tube cholangiography).

As the contrast agent flows through the biliary ducts, it reveals calculi and small intraluminal neoplasms, permitting the surgeon to remove them before closing the incision. Operative cholangiography can therefore eliminate the need for two surgical procedures because gallbladder disease requiring cholecystectomy is often associated with biliary tract disease. However, this advantage must be weighed against the risks associated with administration of a contrast medium during a simple cholecystectomy.

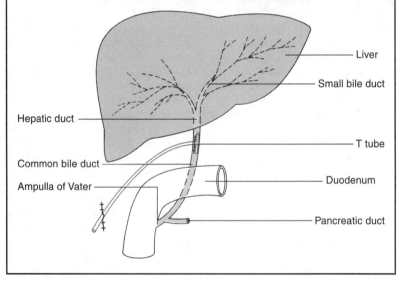

minute intervals until this action is demonstrated.

Precautions

Postoperative cholangiography is contraindicated in patients who are hypersensitive to iodine.

Normal findings

Biliary ducts demonstrate homogeneous filling with contrast medium and are normal in diameter. When the sphincter of Oddi is functioning properly and the ducts are patent, the contrast agent flows unimpeded into the duodenum. (See *Normal T-tube cholangiogram.*)

Implications of results

Negative shadows or filling defects within the biliary ducts associated with dilatation may indicate calculi or neo-

Normal T-tube cholangiogram

This T-tube cholangiogram shows homogeneous filling of biliary ducts. The ducts are of normal diameter, and the presence of contrast medium in the duodenum shows that the ducts are also patent.

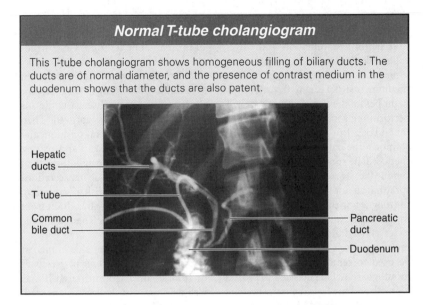

Hepatic ducts

T tube

Common bile duct

Pancreatic duct

Duodenum

plasms overlooked during surgery. Abnormal channels of contrast medium departing from the biliary ducts indicate fistulae.

Post-test care
■ If a sterile dressing is applied after removal of the T tube, observe and record any drainage. Change the dressing as necessary.
■ If the T tube is left in place, attach it to the drainage system, as ordered.

Interfering factors
Marked obesity or gas overlying the biliary ducts may invalidate the X-rays.

Endoscopic retrograde cholangiopancreatography

Endoscopic retrograde cholangiopancreatography (ERCP) is the radiograph-

ic examination of the pancreatic ducts and hepatobiliary tree after injection of a contrast medium into the duodenal papilla. It's indicated in patients with confirmed or suspected pancreatic disease or with obstructive jaundice of unknown etiology.

With the development of smaller, side-viewing endoscopes, ERCP is now being performed more frequently, especially when abdominal ultrasonography, computed tomography scanning, liver scanning, hypotonic duodenography, and biliary tract X-ray studies (including percutaneous transhepatic cholangiography) prove diagnostically inadequate. Complications may include cholangitis and pancreatitis.

Purpose
■ To evaluate obstructive jaundice
■ To diagnose cancer of the duodenal papilla, the pancreas, and the biliary ducts
■ To locate calculi and stenosis in the pancreatic ducts and hepatobiliary tree.

Patient preparation

Explain to the patient that this procedure permits examination of the liver, gallbladder, and pancreas through X-ray films taken after injection of a contrast medium. Instruct him to fast after midnight before the test. Tell him who will perform the procedure and where and that it takes 1 to 2 hours.

Inform the patient that a local anesthetic will be sprayed into his mouth to subdue the gag reflex. Warn him that the spray has an unpleasant taste and makes the tongue and throat feel swollen, causing difficulty swallowing. Instruct him to let saliva drain from the side of his mouth, and tell him that suction may be used to remove saliva. Tell him a mouthguard will be inserted to protect his teeth and the endoscope; assure him that it won't obstruct his breathing.

Advise the patient that he'll receive a sedative before the endoscope is inserted to help him relax, but explain that he'll remain conscious during the procedure. Tell him that he'll also receive an anticholinergic or glucagon I.V. after insertion of the scope. Describe the possible side effects of anticholinergics (dry mouth, thirst, tachycardia, urine retention, and blurred vision) or of glucagon (nausea, vomiting, hives, and flushing). Warn him that he may experience transient flushing as the contrast medium is injected and may have a sore throat for 3 to 4 days after the examination.

Make sure the patient or responsible family member has signed a consent form. Check the patient's history for hypersensitivity to iodine, seafood, or contrast media used for other diagnostic procedures. Just before the test, obtain baseline vital signs. Instruct the patient to remove all metal and other radiopaque objects and constricting undergarments. Then have him void to minimize the discomfort of urine retention, which may follow the test.

Procedure

An I.V. infusion is started with 150 ml of normal saline solution. First, the local anesthetic is administered, as ordered; this usually takes effect in about 10 minutes. If a spray is used, ask the patient to hold his breath while his mouth and throat are sprayed. Then place him in a left lateral position, and give him an emesis basin and tissues. Because the anesthetic causes the patient to lose some control of his secretions and thus increases the risk of aspiration, encourage him to let saliva drain from the side of his mouth. Then insert the mouthguard.

While the patient remains in the left lateral position, 5 to 20 mg of diazepam or midazolam is administered I.V. as well as a narcotic analgesic if needed. When ptosis or dysarthria develops, the patient's head is bent forward, and he is asked to open his mouth. The examiner inserts his left index finger into the patient's mouth and guides the tip of the endoscope along his finger to the back of the patient's throat. The scope is then deflected downward with the left index finger and advanced. As the endoscope passes through the posterior pharynx and cricopharyngeal sphincter, the patient's head is slowly extended to assist the advance of the scope. The patient's chin must be kept midline.

When the endoscope has passed the cricopharyngeal sphincter, it's advanced under direct vision. When it's well into the esophagus (about 12" [30 cm]), the patient's chin is moved toward the table or a continuous suction catheter is placed in his mouth to allow drainage of saliva. The endoscope is advanced through the remainder of the esophagus and into the stomach under direct vision. When the pylorus is located, a small amount of air is insufflated, and the tip of the endoscope is angled upward and passed into the duodenal bulb.

After the endoscope is rotated clockwise to enter the descending duodenum, the patient is assisted to the prone position. An anticholinergic or glucagon I.V. is then administered to induce duodenal atony and to relax the ampullary sphincter. A small amount of air is insufflated, and the endoscope is manipulated until its optic lens lies opposite the duodenal papilla. Then the cannula, filled with contrast medium, is passed through the biopsy channel of the endoscope, the duodenal papilla, and into the ampulla of Vater. The pancreas is visualized first, under fluoroscopic guidance, by injection of 2 to 5 ml of contrast medium.

The cannula is repositioned at a more cephalad angle, and the hepatobiliary tree is visualized by injection of 10 to 15 ml of contrast medium. After each injection, rapid-sequence X-rays are taken. The patient is told to remain prone while the films are developed and reviewed. If necessary, additional films may be taken. When the required films have been obtained, the cannula is removed. Before the endoscope is withdrawn, a tissue specimen may be obtained or fluid aspirated for histologic and cytologic examination, respectively.

Precautions

■ ERCP is contraindicated in patients with infectious disease, pancreatic pseudocysts, stricture or obstruction of the esophagus or duodenum, or acute pancreatitis, cholangitis, or cardiorespiratory disease.

 ■ Vital signs are monitored, and the airway is kept patent throughout the procedure. Oxygen (via nasal cannula) may be administered during the procedure as needed. If you assist with this procedure, watch for signs of respiratory depression, apnea, hypotension, excessive diaphoresis, bradycardia,

and laryngospasm. Be sure to have available emergency resuscitation equipment and a benzodiazepine antagonist such as flumazenil or a narcotic antagonist such as naloxone. A second nurse also assists with the procedure, as ordered.

Normal findings

The duodenal papilla appears as a small red or sometimes pale erosion protruding into the lumen. Its orifice is commonly bordered by a fringe of white mucosa, and a longitudinal fold running perpendicular to the deep circular folds of the duodenum helps mark its location. Although the pancreatic and hepatobiliary ducts usually unite in the ampulla of Vater and empty through the duodenal papilla, separate orifices are sometimes present. The contrast agent uniformly fills the pancreatic duct, the hepatobiliary tree, and the gallbladder.

Implications of results

Obstructive jaundice may result from various abnormalities of the hepatobiliary tree and pancreatic duct. Examination of the hepatobiliary tree may reveal calculi, strictures, or irregular deviations that suggest biliary cirrhosis, primary sclerosing cholangitis, or cancer of the bile ducts. Examination of the pancreatic ducts may also show calculi, strictures, and irregular deviations that may indicate pancreatic cysts and pseudocysts, pancreatic tumor, cancer of the head of the pancreas, chronic pancreatitis, pancreatic fibrosis, carcinoma of the duodenal papilla, or papillary stenosis. (See *Abnormal ERCP,* page 856.)

Depending on test findings, a definitive diagnosis may require further studies. In addition, certain interventions, such as placement of a stent to allow drainage or a papillotomy to decrease scar tissue and allow bile drainage, may be indicated.

Abnormal ERCP

This endoscopic retrograde cholangiopancreatographic (ERCP) view shows a dilated pancreatic duct secondary to stenosis. Stenosis was caused by carcinoma at the head of the pancreas.

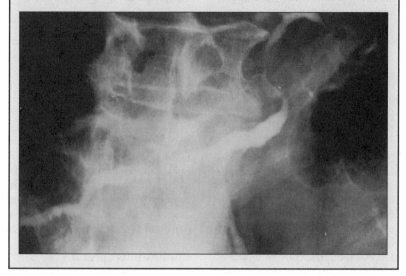

Post-test care

■ Observe the patient closely for signs of cholangitis and pancreatitis. Hyperbilirubinemia, fever, and chills are the immediate signs of cholangitis; hypotension associated with gram-negative septicemia may develop later. Left upper quadrant pain and tenderness, elevated serum amylase levels, and transient hyperbilirubinemia are the usual signs of pancreatitis. Draw blood samples for amylase and bilirubin values, if ordered, but remember that these levels usually rise after ERCP.

■ Observe the patient for signs of perforation, such as abdominal pain, bleeding, and fever.

■ Tell the patient that he may experience a feeling of fullness, some cramping, and passage of flatus several hours after the test.

■ Continue to watch for signs of respiratory depression, apnea, hypotension, excessive diaphoresis, bradycardia, and laryngospasm. Check vital signs every 15 minutes for 4 hours, every hour for 4 hours, then every 4 hours for 48 hours.

■ Withhold food and fluids until the gag reflex returns. Test the gag reflex by touching the back of the throat with a tongue blade. When the gag reflex returns, allow fluids and a light meal.

■ Discontinue or maintain the I.V. infusion, as ordered.

■ Check for signs of urine retention. Notify the doctor if the patient hasn't voided within 8 hours.

■ If the patient has a sore throat, provide soothing lozenges and warm saline gargles to ease discomfort.

■ If a tissue biopsy or polypectomy occurred, a small amount of blood in the patient's first stool is normal. Report excessive bleeding immediately.

Interfering factors
None.

Celiac and mesenteric arteriography

Celiac and mesenteric arteriography is the radiographic examination of the abdominal vasculature after intra-arterial injection of a contrast medium through a catheter. The catheter is usually passed through the femoral artery into the aorta and is then positioned in the celiac, superior mesenteric, or inferior mesenteric artery using fluoroscopy. Injection of a contrast medium into one or more of these arteries provides a map of abdominal vasculature; injection into specific arterial branches, called superselective angiography, permits detailed visualization of a particular area. As the contrast medium flows through the abdominal vasculature, serial radiographs outline abdominal vessels in the arterial, capillary, and venous phases of perfusion.

Celiac and mesenteric arteriography is indicated when endoscopy can't locate the source of GI bleeding or when barium studies, ultrasonography, nuclear medicine, or computed tomography scanning prove inconclusive in evaluating neoplasms. It's also used to evaluate cirrhosis and portal hypertension (especially when a portacaval shunt is being considered); to evaluate vascular damage, particularly in the spleen and liver, after abdominal trauma; and to detect vascular abnormalities. Arteriography can demonstrate the portal vein even when portal venous flow is reversed. It can also be used to help control GI bleeding when other measures fail. (See *Using angiography to control GI bleeding,* page 858.) Complications as-

sociated with this test include hemorrhage, venous and intracardiac thrombosis, cardiac arrhythmia, and emboli caused by dislodging atherosclerotic plaques.

Purpose
- To locate the source of GI bleeding
- To help distinguish between benign and malignant neoplasms
- To evaluate cirrhosis and portal hypertension
- To evaluate vascular damage after abdominal trauma
- To detect vascular abnormalities.

Patient preparation
Explain that this test examines the abdominal blood vessels after injection of a contrast medium. Instruct the patient to fast for 8 hours before the test. Tell him that he'll receive I.V. conscious sedation and a local anesthetic. Explain that he may feel a brief, stinging sensation as the anesthetic is injected. He may also feel pressure when the femoral artery is palpated, but the anesthetic will minimize the pain when the needle is introduced into the artery. Tell him he may feel a transient burning as the contrast medium is injected.

Inform the patient that the X-ray equipment makes a clicking sound as the films are taken. Instruct him to lie still during the test to avoid blurring the films, and inform him that restraints may be used to help him remain still. Warn him that he may feel temporary stiffness after the test from lying still on the hard X-ray table. Tell him who will perform the test and where and that it takes 30 minutes to 3 hours, depending on the number of vessels studied.

Make sure the patient or a responsible member of the family has signed a consent form, if required. Check the patient's history for hypersensitivity to iodine, shellfish, or the contrast medium. Make sure blood studies (hemoglo-

Using angiography to control GI bleeding

When conservative measures, such as blood transfusion, fail to control GI bleeding, angiography can provide a safe, effective alternative. Once the site of bleeding is identified, vasopressin infusion or arterial embolization can usually control bleeding.

Vasopressin infusion

In vasopressin infusion, the angiographic catheter is positioned in the appropriate artery, and vasopressin is infused slowly. After 20 minutes, a radiograph shows the effectiveness of vasopressin, and the rate of infusion may then be changed, as appropriate, to curtail bleeding. Selective vasopressin infusion is generally effective in controlling hemorrhagic gastritis, most intestinal bleeding, and bleeding from Mallory-Weiss lacerations and stress ulcers. It is less consistently effective in controlling bleeding from gastric ulcers and rarely effective in control-

ling bleeding from duodenal ulcers. This technique should be used cautiously in patients with coronary artery disease, since its adverse effects include arrhythmias and fluid retention.

Arterial embolization

If vasopressin infusion fails to control GI bleeding, or if bleeding results from gastric or duodenal ulcers, arterial embolization may prove effective. In this technique, the angiographic catheter is positioned in the appropriate artery and embolic material, such as an epsilon-aminocaproic acid (Amicar) clot or absorbable gelatin sponge (Gelfoam) is injected through the catheter. X-ray films are taken to assess the placement of embolization. Additional material may be injected, if necessary. This technique shouldn't be used after gastric or intestinal surgery because it exaggerates the risk of infection.

---

bin level, hematocrit, clotting time, prothrombin time, activated partial thromboplastin time, and platelet count) have been completed. Just before the procedure, instruct the patient to put on a hospital gown and to remove jewelry and other objects that might obscure anatomic detail on the X-rays. Tell him to void; then record baseline vital signs. Administer a sedative, if ordered.

Procedure

After the patient is placed in the supine position on the X-ray table, an I.V. infusion is started to maintain hydration, to provide I.V. sedation, and to permit emergency administration of medication. Scout films of the patient's abdomen are taken, and the peripheral pulses are palpated and marked. The punc-

ture site — usually the right groin at the femoral vein — is cleaned with soap and water; the area is shaved, cleaned with povidone-iodine, and surrounded by sterile drapes. Then the local anesthetic is injected.

The femoral artery is located by palpation, and the needle is gently inserted until a pulsing blood flow is obtained. A guide wire is passed through the needle into the artery; then the needle is removed, leaving the guide wire in place. After the angiographic catheter is inserted over the guide wire, the guide wire is withdrawn to inject contrast dye to check for catheter placement. The guide wire is again inserted into the selected artery for fluoroscopic guidance. When the wire is in position, the catheter is advanced over it into the artery. The wire is then removed and placement verified by hand injection of contrast medium. The automatic injector is then attached to the catheter. As the contrast dye is injected, a series of films are taken in rapid sequence.

After injections into one or more major arteries, superselective catheterization may be performed. Using fluoroscopy, the catheter is repositioned in a specific branch of a major artery, contrast medium is injected, and rapid-sequence films are taken. If necessary, several specific branches may be catheterized.

After filming, the catheter is withdrawn, and firm pressure is applied to the puncture site for about 15 minutes. The site is observed for hematoma formation and peripheral pulses are checked.

Precautions

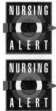 ■ Celiac and mesenteric arteriography should be performed cautiously in patients with coagulopathy.

■ Most reactions to the contrast medium occur within 30 minutes. Watch carefully for cardiovascular shock or arrest, flushing, laryngeal stridor, and urticaria.

Normal findings

X-ray films show the three phases of perfusion: arterial, capillary, and venous. The arteries normally taper regularly, becoming gradually smaller with subsequent divisions. The contrast medium then spreads evenly within the sinusoids. The portal vein appears 10 to 20 seconds after the injection, as the contrast medium empties from the spleen into the splenic vein or from the intestine into the superior mesenteric vein, and further into the portal vein.

Implications of results

GI hemorrhage appears on the angiogram as the extravasation of contrast medium from the damaged vessels. Upper GI hemorrhage can result from such conditions as Mallory-Weiss syndrome, gastric or peptic ulcer, hemorrhagic gastritis, and eroded hiatal hernia. Esophageal hemorrhage rarely appears on the angiogram because the contrast medium usually fails to fill the esophageal vein. Lower GI hemorrhage can result from such conditions as bleeding diverticula and angiodysplasia.

Abdominal neoplasms — carcinoid tumors, adenomas, leiomyomas, angiomas, and adenocarcinomas — can disrupt the normal vasculature in several ways. Neoplasms can invade or encase nearby arteries and veins, distorting their regular channel-like appearance and, in late stages, displacing them. Vessels within the neoplasm, known as neovasculature, appear as abnormal vascular areas. Areas of necrosis appear as puddles of contrast medium.

Contrast medium may also remain in the neoplasm longer during capillary perfusion, producing a tumor blush or stain on the angiogram. Arteriovenous shunting may also be present, depending on the size and location of the tumor. Because these characteristics aren't uniformly present in all neoplasms, combinations of theses characteristics can in many cases help to distinguish between benign and malignant neoplasms. (See *Types of arterial encasement*, page 860.)

In early or mild cirrhosis, portal venous flow to the liver remains relatively unaffected, and the hepatic artery and its branches appear normal. As the disease progresses, portal venous flow diminishes, the hepatic artery and its branches become dilated and tortuous, and collateral veins develop. In advanced cirrhosis, portal venous flow reverses. However, the portal vein still ap-

Types of arterial encasement

When a tumor invades or encases nearby arteries, it distorts their regular channel-like appearance into serrated, serpiginous, or smooth forms, as shown below.

Serrated encasement

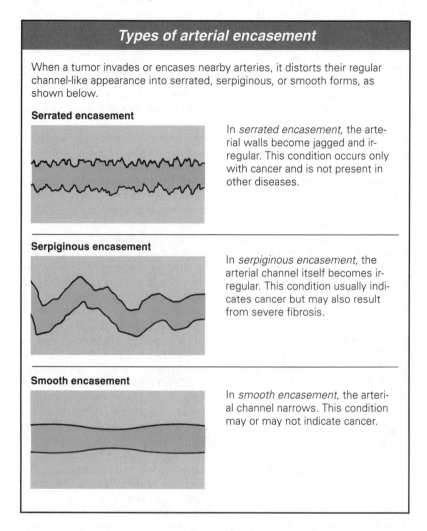

In *serrated encasement,* the arterial walls become jagged and irregular. This condition occurs only with cancer and is not present in other diseases.

Serpiginous encasement

In *serpiginous encasement,* the arterial channel itself becomes irregular. This condition usually indicates cancer but may also result from severe fibrosis.

Smooth encasement

In *smooth encasement,* the arterial channel narrows. This condition may or may not indicate cancer.

pears on the X-ray film, which may also show thrombi.

Abdominal trauma commonly causes splenic injury (less commonly, hepatic injury). In many cases, splenic rupture displaces intrasplenic arterial branches, and contrast medium leaks from splenic arteries into the splenic pulp. When rupture occurs without subcapsular hematoma, the spleen usually maintains its normal size. However, in subcapsular hematoma, the spleen enlarges to displace the splenic artery and

vein; the subcapsular hematoma itself appears as a large, avascular mass that stretches intrasplenic arteries and compresses the splenic pulp away from the capsule.

Hepatic injury causes similar vascular distortion, such as displacement of the common hepatic artery and extrahepatic branches. Intrahepatic and subcapsular hematomas displace and stretch intrahepatic arteries. As the hepatic vascular supply is disrupted, arteriovenous fistula may develop between the hepatic artery and the portal vein.

Various abnormalities affecting the diameter and course of an artery may appear on the angiogram. Atherosclerotic plaques or atheromas — lipid deposits on the intima — narrow the arterial lumen and may even occlude it, resulting in formation of collaterals. Other identifiable vascular abnormalities include aneurysms, thrombi, and emboli.

Post-test care

■ Inform the patient that he'll be on bed rest for 4 to 6 hours and must keep the leg with the puncture site straight. The bed may be raised no more than 30 degrees. The patient will be able to logroll and may use the unaffected leg to reposition himself to use the bedpan.

■ Monitor vital signs, as ordered, until stable, and check peripheral pulses. Note the color and temperature of the leg that was used for the test. If the leg is pulseless, cold, and blue, notify the doctor immediately.

■ Check the puncture site for bleeding and hematoma. If bleeding develops, apply pressure to the site; if it continues or is excessive, notify the doctor. If a hematoma develops, apply warm soaks.

■ Ask the doctor if the patient can resume his usual diet. If the patient isn't receiving I.V. infusions, encourage him to drink fluids to speed excretion of the contrast medium.

Interfering factors

■ The patient's failure to remain still during the procedure can invalidate the test.

■ The presence of gas, feces, or barium from a previous procedure can affect the accuracy of test results.

■ An atherosclerotic lesion in the vessel to be cannulated prevents entry and passage of the catheter.

Enteroclysis

Enteroclysis (also called a small-bowel enema) is the fluoroscopic examination of the small bowel using a contrast medium. In this procedure, a small-lumen catheter is inserted through the nose or mouth and is passed through the stomach into the distal duodenum or the jejunum. A small balloon at the tip of the catheter may be inflated to prevent reflux of the contrast medium into the stomach. Barium is instilled by infusion; then methylcellulose may be infused to obtain a double-contrast study of the small bowel.

The contrast media distend and opacify the bowel loops to allow evaluation and diagnosis. Metoclopramide may also be administered to facilitate peristalsis (which helps pass the catheter into the small bowel). Fluoroscopy and spot films are used to demonstrate and evaluate the small bowel.

Purpose

■ To diagnose and evaluate Crohn's disease

■ To diagnose Meckel's diverticulum

■ To aid in the diagnosis of small-bowel obstruction

■ To detect tumors.

Patient preparation

Explain to the patient that this test evaluates the small bowel. Tell him that contrast media will be instilled into his bowel and that X-ray films will then be taken to track the flow of the media and allow evaluation of small-bowel function. Inform him that he'll receive a laxative (such as Dulcolax) the afternoon before the examination and then he'll receive nothing by mouth until the test. (If the test is being done on an emergency basis, no preparation is required.)

Inform him that he should not take peristalsis-inhibiting drugs (such as Demerol or Percodan) on the day of the test. Tell him the examination will take about 45 minutes and that just before the test, he'll be asked to change into a patient gown, remove underwear and jewelry, and empty his bladder.

Inform the patient that an I.V. line will be inserted for medication administration. Inform him that he may receive an I.V. sedative, if needed, and that a local anesthetic will be injected inside his nose to make the catheter insertion more comfortable. A GI stimulant (such as metoclopramide) will be administered to aid passage of the tube and to speed the flow of barium by increasing peristalsis.

Tell the patient that he'll be asked to turn from side to side and sometimes onto his abdomen during the procedure. Inform him that his cooperation will help the test proceed smoothly. After the study, he'll go to a recovery area until he's ready for discharge. If the patient is having the procedure as an outpatient, tell him he'll need someone to drive him home if he receives I.V. sedation.

Procedure

Place the patient in the supine position on the X-ray table with his neck slightly extended. Administer I.V. medication to help relax the patient and to aid in passage of the tube, as ordered. The local anesthetic is administered nasally; instruct the patient to swallow if he feels it at the back of his throat. The tube is passed through the nose into the nasopharynx, and the patient's chin is brought down to the chest; the tube is advanced into the stomach and duodenum and, if possible, into the jejunum. A small balloon is inflated at the tip of the catheter to prevent reflux of the contrast agent into the patient's stomach.

The barium contrast is administered by infusion pump. Methylcellulose is then administered to help propel the barium into the distal bowel. This double-contrast administration distends the bowel walls and opacifies the bowel loops, allowing clearer evaluation. Then spot films and overhead films are taken. The flow of the barium is followed on fluoroscopy. The doctor examines individual loops of bowel as they are opacified, and compresses the abdomen to better evaluate the loops. The patient is asked to turn from side to side during the examination.

After the examination, the balloon is deflated and the catheter is removed. Assist the patient to the bathroom to expel the barium through defecation.

Precautions

The patient may experience discomfort with the passage of the catheter. Provide reassurance as well as the prescribed anesthetic and sedative when needed.

Normal findings

The bowel loops and walls are visible and are free of tumors, ulcers, and constrictions.

Implications of results

Anatomy of the bowel loops can be evaluated by observing Kerckring's folds, lumen diameters, and wall thickness. Abnormalities may indicate Crohn's disease, tumors, partial or complete bowel obstruction, Meckel's diverticula, or congenital disorders.

Post-test care

■ Observe the patient in the recovery area until he's ready for discharge.
■ Monitor vital signs until the patient is alert.
■ Help the patient to the bathroom to expel the contrast medium, as needed.

Interfering factors

Complete gastric or duodenal obstruction may interfere with accurate testing.

Liver-spleen scanning

In this test, a gamma camera records the distribution of radioactivity within the liver and spleen after I.V. injection of a radioactive colloid. The colloid most commonly used, technetium-99m (^{99m}Tc) concentrates in the reticuloendothelial cells through phagocytosis. About 80% to 90% of the injected colloid is taken up by Kupffer's cells in the liver, 5% to 10% by the spleen, and 3% to 5% by bone marrow. The gamma camera images either organ instantaneously without moving.

Liver-spleen scanning is indicated for patients with palpable abdominal masses to demonstrate hepatomegaly or splenomegaly and in those with suspected hematoma after abdominal trauma. It's usually the most reliable screening test for detecting hepatocellular disease, hepatic metastasis, and focal disease, such as tumors, cysts, and abscesses. However, this test demonstrates focal disease nonspecifically as a cold spot (a defect that fails to take up the colloid) and may fail to detect focal lesions smaller than $\frac{3}{4}$" (2 cm) in diameter.

Although clinical signs and symptoms may aid diagnosis, liver-spleen scanning commonly requires confirmation by ultrasonography, computed tomography (CT) scanning, gallium scanning, or biopsy. Flow studies may help distinguish between metastases, tumors, cysts,

and abscesses. (See *Flow studies,* page 864.)

Purpose

- To screen for hepatic metastases and hepatocellular disease, such as cirrhosis and hepatitis
- To detect focal disease, such as tumors, cysts, and abscesses, in the liver and spleen
- To demonstrate hepatomegaly, splenomegaly, and splenic infarcts
- To assess the condition of the liver and spleen after abdominal trauma.

Patient preparation

Explain to the patient that this procedure permits examination of the liver and spleen through scans taken after I.V. injection of a radioactive substance. Inform him that he needn't restrict food or fluids before the test. Tell him who will perform the test and where, that he may experience transient discomfort from the needle puncture, and that the test takes about 1 hour.

 Make sure the patient isn't scheduled for more than one radionuclide scan on the same day.

Assure him that the injection isn't dangerous because the test substance contains only trace amounts of radioactivity, and that allergic reactions to it are rare. Tell him the detector head of the gamma camera may touch his abdomen (if appropriate), and reassure him that this isn't dangerous. Advise him that he'll be asked to lie still and breathe quietly during the procedure to ensure images of good quality; he may also be asked to hold his breath briefly. Explain that this technique helps to evaluate liver mobility and pliability.

Procedure

The ^{99m}Tc is injected I.V., and after 10 to 15 minutes, the patient's abdomen is scanned with the patient in the supine,

Flow studies

In contrast to liver-spleen scanning, which provides static nuclear images, flow studies (dynamic scintigraphy) record in rapid sequence the stages of perfusion after I.V. injection of a radionuclide, such as technetium sulfide-99m. Because flow studies demonstrate the vascularity of a nonspecific focal defect, they sometimes help distinguish between metastases, tumors, cysts, and abscesses.

In flow studies, a hot defect demonstrates early, increased uptake of the radionuclide when compared to the surrounding parenchyma and then appears as a filling defect — or cold spot — on later routine images. Cysts and abscesses, which are avascular, fail to take up the radionuclide; hemangiomas appear characteristically hot because of their enlarged vessels.

Tumors and metastases are generally more difficult to evaluate because their vascularity is more variable. Although vascular metastases may appear hot, most metastases demonstrate poor uptake of the radionuclide. Hepatomas can also appear hot or can show perfusion similar to normal parenchyma.

---

left and right lateral, left and right anterior oblique, and prone positions to ensure optimal visualization of the liver and spleen. The left anterior oblique position provides the best view of the spleen, separate from the left lobe of the liver. With the patient supine, liver mobility and pliability may be evaluated by marking the costal margin and scanning as the patient breathes deeply. Because the liver normally moves and changes shape with deep breathing, fixation suggests pathology.

After the required scintigraphs have been taken, they're reviewed for clarity before the patient is allowed to leave. If necessary, additional views are obtained.

Precautions

Liver-spleen scanning is usually contraindicated in children and in pregnant or breast-feeding women.

Normal findings

Because the liver and spleen contain equal numbers of reticuloendothelial cells, both organs normally appear equally bright on the image. However, distribution of the radioactive colloid is generally more uniform and homogeneous in the spleen than in the liver. The liver has various normal indentations and impressions, such as the gallbladder fossa and falciform ligament, that may mimic focal disease. (See *Identifying liver indentations.*)

Implications of results

Although liver-spleen scanning may fail to detect early hepatocellular disease, it shows characteristic, distinct patterns as such disease progresses. The most prominent sign of hepatocellular disease is a shift of the radioactive colloid caused by reduced hepatic blood flow and impaired function of Kupffer's cells. This inhibits distribution of the colloid in the liver, causing it to appear uniformly decreased or patchy. The spleen and bone marrow then take up the abnormally large amounts of the colloid unabsorbed by the liver, thus concentrating more radioactivity than the liver, and appear brighter on the scan. This same distribution pattern (colloid shift) also accompanies portal hypertension due to extrahepatic causes.

Identifying liver indentations

In nuclear imaging, normal indentations and impressions may be mistaken for focal lesions. These drawings of the liver — anterior view and posterior view — identify the contours and impressions that may be misread.

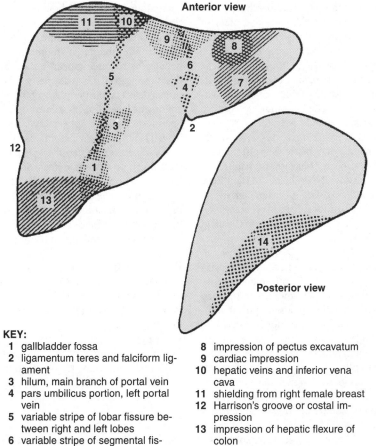

Anterior view

Posterior view

KEY:
1 gallbladder fossa
2 ligamentum teres and falciform ligament
3 hilum, main branch of portal vein
4 pars umbilicus portion, left portal vein
5 variable stripe of lobar fissure between right and left lobes
6 variable stripe of segmental fissure, left lobe
7 thinning of left lobe
8 impression of pectus excavatum
9 cardiac impression
10 hepatic veins and inferior vena cava
11 shielding from right female breast
12 Harrison's groove or costal impression
13 impression of hepatic flexure of colon
14 right renal impression

Hepatitis and cirrhosis are both associated with hepatomegaly and a colloid shift, but certain characteristics help distinguish them. In hepatitis, distribution of the colloid is usually uniformly decreased; in cirrhosis, it's patchy. Splenomegaly is typical in cirrhosis but not in hepatitis.

Metastasis to the liver or spleen may appear on the scan as a focal defect and requires a biopsy to confirm the diagnosis. Liver metastasis usually originates in the GI or genitourinary tract, the breast, or the lung; metastasis to the spleen is less common. After metastasis is confirmed, serial liver-spleen studies are useful to evaluate the effectiveness of therapy.

Because cysts, abscesses, and tumors fail to take up the radioactive colloid, they appear on the scan as solitary or multiple focal defects. Hepatic cysts may appear as solitary defects; polycystic hepatic disease, as multiple defects. Splenic cysts are rarer than hepatic cysts and may have a parasitic or nonparasitic origin. Ultrasonography can confirm hepatic or splenic cysts.

Intrahepatic abscesses are usually pyogenic or amebic. Subphrenic abscesses, located beneath the diaphragm, may distort the dome of the right lobe. Splenic abscesses are characteristic in bacterial endocarditis. All abscesses require CT scanning to confirm the diagnosis.

Benign hepatic tumors, such as hemangiomas, adenomas, and hamartomas, require a confirming biopsy or flow studies. Primary malignant tumors, such as hepatomas, also require a biopsy. Benign splenic tumors are rare and include hemangiomas, fibromas, myomas, and hamartomas. Primary malignant splenic tumors are also rare, except in lymphoreticular malignancies such as Hodgkin's disease. Splenic tumors also require a biopsy to confirm the diagnosis. Although focal disease usually inhibits uptake of radioactive colloid, both obstruction of the superior vena cava and Budd-Chiari syndrome cause markedly increased uptake.

Liver-spleen scanning can verify palpable abdominal masses and differentiate between splenomegaly and hepatomegaly. A left upper quadrant mass may result from splenomegaly, or from hepatomegaly if the liver is grossly extended across the abdomen. A right up-

per quadrant mass may result from hepatomegaly; a right lower quadrant mass may be a Riedel's lobe or a large dependent gallbladder. Splenic infarcts, commonly associated with bacterial endocarditis and massive splenomegaly, appear as peripheral defects, with decreased and irregular colloid distribution.

Scanning can assess hepatic or splenic injury after abdominal trauma. Intrahepatic hematoma appears as a focal defect; subcapsular hematoma, as a lentiform defect on the periphery of the liver; hepatic laceration, as a linear defect. Splenic hematoma appears as a focal defect; subcapsular hematoma, as a lentiform defect on the periphery; hepatic laceration, as a linear defect. Splenic hematoma appears as a focal defect in or next to the spleen and may transect it. CT scanning is the fastest and preferred method of evaluating liver and splenic injury in abdominal trauma.

Post-test care

- Watch for anaphylactoid or pyrogenic reactions that may result from a stabilizer, such as dextran or gelatin, added to ^{99m}Tc.
- Inform the patient that the radioactive substance is eliminated from the body within 6 to 24 hours. Urge him to increase his fluid intake (unless contraindicated) to encourage this process.

Interfering factors

- Radionuclides administered in other studies on the same day can interfere with the accuracy of liver-spleen imaging.
- The patient's inability to remain still during the procedure can hinder accurate testing.

Computed tomography of the biliary tract and liver

In computed tomography (CT) of the biliary tract and liver, multiple X-rays pass through the upper abdomen and are measured while detectors record differences in tissue attenuation. A computer reconstructs this data as a two-dimensional image on a television screen. Because soft-tissue appearance varies with tissue attenuation, CT scanning accurately distinguishes the biliary tract and the liver if the ducts are large. Use of an I.V. contrast medium during the procedure can accentuate differences in tissue density.

CT images can specify focal defects detected by liver-spleen scanning as solid, cystic, inflammatory, and vascular lesions; however, biopsy may be necessary to rule out malignancy or to distinguish between metastatic and primary tumors. CT-guided liver biopsies and liver cyst or abscess drainage can be performed easily in the medical imaging department. CT scanning can also detect suspected hematoma after abdominal trauma and can determine the type of jaundice.

Although CT scanning and ultrasonography both detect biliary tract and liver disease equally well, the latter technique is performed more often. That's because CT scans are more expensive than ultrasonography and expose the patient to moderate amounts of radiation. However, CT scanning is the test of choice in patients who are obese and in those whose liver is positioned high under the rib cage because bone and excessive fat hinder ultrasound transmission.

Barium studies should precede this test by at least 4 days or should be performed after CT scan because barium may hinder visualization.

Purpose

- To detect intrahepatic tumors and abscesses, subphrenic and subhepatic abscesses, cysts, and hematomas
- To distinguish between obstructive and nonobstructive jaundice.

Patient preparation

Explain to the patient that this test helps detect biliary tract and liver disease. Tell him that he'll be given a contrast medium to drink and then he should fast until after the examination. If contrast won't be used, fasting isn't necessary. Tell him who will perform the test and where and that it takes approximately 1 hour.

Inform the patient that he'll be placed on an adjustable table, which is positioned inside a scanning gantry. Assure him that the test will be painless. Tell him he'll be asked to remain still during the test because movement can cause artifacts, thereby prolonging the test and limiting its accuracy. If an I.V. contrast medium is being used, inform the patient that he may feel transient discomfort from the needle puncture and a localized feeling of warmth on injection. He may also experience a salty or metallic taste and nausea. Inform him that these sensations usually last for about 2 minutes. Tell the patient to report immediately nausea, vomiting, dizziness, headache, or hives.

Check the patient's history for hypersensitivity to iodine or the contrast media used in other diagnostic tests. If ordered, give him the oral contrast agent supplied by the radiology department. This contrast helps define and demarcate the intestinal tract.

Procedure

The patient is placed in the supine position on an X-ray table, and the table is positioned in the opening of the scanning gantry. A series of transverse X-rays are taken and recorded on magnetic tape. This information is reconstructed by a computer and appears as images on a television screen. These images are studied, and selected ones are photographed.

When the first series of films is completed, the images are reviewed. Then I.V. contrast enhancement may be ordered. After the contrast medium is injected, a second series of films is taken, and the patient is carefully observed for an allergic reaction.

Precautions

This test is usually contraindicated during pregnancy; if I.V. contrast medium is used, it's also contraindicated in patients with hypersensitivity to iodine or with severe renal or hepatic disease.

Normal findings

The liver has a uniform density that's slightly greater than that of the pancreas, kidneys, and spleen. Linear and circular areas of slightly lower density, representing hepatic vascular structures, may interrupt this uniform appearance. The portal vein is usually visible; the hepatic artery usually isn't. I.V. contrast medium enhances both vascular structures and the liver parenchyma, and they become dense.

Intrahepatic biliary radicles are normally not visible, but the common hepatic and bile ducts are occasionally visible as low-density structures. Because bile has the same density as water, use of I.V. contrast aids visualization of the biliary tract by enhancing surrounding parenchyma and vascular structures.

Like the biliary ducts, the gallbladder is visible as a round or elliptic low-density structure. A contracted gallbladder may be impossible to visualize.

Implications of results

Most focal hepatic defects appear less dense than the normal parenchyma, and CT scans can detect small lesions. Use of rapid-sequence scanning with I.V. contrast medium helps distinguish between the two because the normal parenchyma shows greater enhancement than focal defects. Primary and metastatic neoplasms may appear as well-circumscribed or poorly defined areas of slightly lower density than the normal parenchyma. However, some lesions have the same density as the liver parenchyma and may thus prove undetectable. Neoplasms that are especially large may distort the liver's contour. Hepatic abscesses appear as relatively low-density, homogeneous areas, usually with well-defined borders. Hepatic cysts appear as sharply defined round or oval structures, and have a density lower than abscesses and neoplasms.

The density of a hepatic hematoma varies with its age. A fresh clot is as dense or slightly denser than the normal parenchyma; a resolving clot is of slightly lower density than the normal parenchyma. Intrahepatic hematomas vary in shape; subcapsular hematomas are usually crescent-shaped and compress the liver away from the capsule.

In distinguishing between obstructive and nonobstructive jaundice, dilatation of the biliary ducts indicates the former; absence of dilatation, the latter. Dilated intrahepatic bile ducts appear as low-density linear and circular branching structures. Dilatation of the common hepatic duct, common bile duct, and gallbladder may also be apparent, depending on the site and severity of obstruction. Use of an I.V. contrast medium helps detect biliary dilatation, especially when the ducts are only slightly dilated.

CT scans can usually identify the cause of obstruction, such as calculi or pancreatic carcinoma. However, when the site of obstruction must be located before surgery, percutaneous transhepatic cholangiography or, less commonly, endoscopic retrograde cholangiopancreatography may also be performed.

Post-test care

- The patient may resume his normal diet and activities unless otherwise indicated.
- Observe for delayed signs and symptoms of an allergic reaction to the dye (urticaria, headache, and vomiting). An oral antihistamine may be ordered for a mild reaction.

Interfering factors

- Use of oral or I.V. contrast media that were excreted in the bile in previous diagnostic studies can interfere with detection of biliary dilatation because they may cause the biliary tract to appear as dense as the surrounding parenchyma.
- Barium studies performed within 4 days before a CT scan may obscure the image.

Computed tomography of the pancreas

In computed tomography (CT) of the pancreas, multiple X-rays penetrate the upper abdomen and are measured, while a detector records the differences in tissue attenuation. A computer then reconstructs this data as a two-dimensional image on a television screen. A series of cross-sectional views can provide a detailed look at the pancreas. Because attenuation varies with tissue density, CT scanning accurately distinguishes the pancreas and surrounding organs and vessels if enough fat is present between the structures. Use of an I.V. or oral contrast medium can accentuate differences in tissue density.

CT scanning of the pancreas is indicated for patients with signs and symptoms of pancreatic cancer (weight loss, jaundice, gnawing epigastric pain radiating to the back), for patients with pancreatitis to detect and evaluate its complications, and for patients with suspected pancreatitis, when radiologic and biochemical tests prove inconclusive. CT scans can't detect tumors too small to alter pancreatic size and shape and may fail to distinguish between carcinoma and pancreatitis.

CT scanning is replacing ultrasonography as the test of choice for examining the pancreas. Although ultrasonography costs less and involves less risk for the patient, it is also somewhat less accurate. In retroperitoneal disorders — specifically when pancreatitis is suspected — CT scanning goes beyond ultrasonography by showing the general swelling that accompanies acute inflammation of the gland. In chronic cases, CT scanning easily detects calcium deposits commonly missed by simple radiography, particularly in patients who are obese.

Besides detecting tumors, cysts, and abscesses, CT scanning can also distinguish between benign and malignant tumors because of its unique sensitivity to variations in tissue density. Although less reliable in the early detection of pancreatic carcinomas, CT scanning can spot presymptomatic warning signs, such as localized swelling in the head, body, or tail of the gland.

Purpose

- To detect pancreatic carcinoma or pseudocysts
- To detect or evaluate pancreatitis

■ To distinguish between pancreatic disorders and disorders of the retroperitoneum.

Patient preparation

Explain to the patient that this test helps detect disorders of the pancreas. Instruct him to fast after administration of the oral contrast medium. Tell him who will perform the test and where and that it takes about 1½ hours.

Inform the patient that he'll be placed on an adjustable table that is positioned inside a scanning gantry. Assure him that, although the test equipment looks formidable, the procedure is painless. Tell him he'll be asked to remain still during the test and to hold his breath at certain times. Inform him that he may be given a contrast medium I.V. or orally to aid visualization of the pancreas. Describe the possible adverse effects of the contrast agent — nausea, flushing, dizziness, and sweating — and tell the patient to report them if they develop.

Check the patient's history for recent barium studies and for hypersensitivity to iodine, seafood, or the contrast media used in other diagnostic tests. Give him the oral contrast agent, as ordered, to clearly define and demarcate the stomach and intestines.

Procedure

The patient is placed in the supine position on an X-ray table, and the table is positioned in the opening of the scanning gantry. A series of transverse X-rays is taken and recorded on magnetic tape. The varying tissue absorption is calculated by a computer, and the information is reconstructed as images on a television screen. These images are studied, and selected ones are photographed. After the first series of films is completed, the images are reviewed. Then contrast enhancement may be ordered. After the contrast medium is administered, another series of films is taken,

and the patient is observed for an allergic reaction (itching, hypotension, hypertension, diaphoresis, dyspnea, tachycardia, or urticaria).

Precautions

CT scanning of the pancreas is contraindicated during pregnancy and, if a contrast medium is used, in patients with hypersensitivity to iodine or with severe renal or hepatic disease.

Normal findings

The pancreas generally lies obliquely across the upper abdomen, and its parenchyma demonstrates a uniform density (particularly if an I.V. contrast medium is used). The gland normally thickens from tail to head and generally has a smooth surface. A contrast medium administered orally opacifies the adjacent stomach and duodenum, and helps outline the pancreas, particularly in persons with little peripancreatic fat, such as children and very thin adults. (See *Normal CT scan of the pancreas.*)

Implications of results

Because the tissue density of pancreatic carcinoma resembles that of the normal parenchyma, changes in pancreas size and shape help demonstrate carcinoma and pseudocysts. Carcinoma usually first appears as a localized swelling of the head, body, or tail of the pancreas and may spread to obliterate the fat plane, dilate the main pancreatic duct and common bile duct by obstructing them, and produce low-density focal lesions in the liver from metastasis. Use of an I.V. contrast medium helps detect metastases by opacifying the pancreatic and hepatic parenchyma.

Adenocarcinoma and islet cell tumor are the most common types of pancreatic cancer. Cystadenomas and cystadenocarcinomas, usually multilocular, occur most often in the body and tail of the pancreas and appear as low-density

Normal CT scan of the pancreas

This normal computed tomography (CT) scan shows the pancreas opacified by contrast medium.

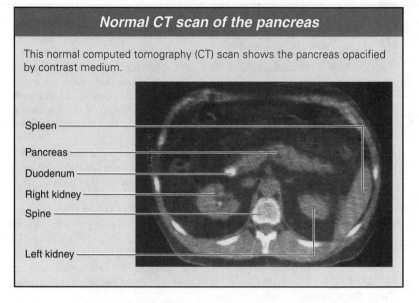

Spleen

Pancreas

Duodenum

Right kidney

Spine

Left kidney

focal lesions marked by internal septa. An oral contrast medium helps distinguish between bowel loops and tumors in the tail of the pancreas.

Acute pancreatitis, either edematous (interstitial) or necrotizing (hemorrhagic), produces diffuse enlargement of the pancreas. In acute edematous pancreatitis, the density of the parenchyma is uniformly decreased. In acute necrotizing pancreatitis, the density is not uniform because of the presence of both necrosis and hemorrhage. The areas of tissue necrosis have diminished density. In acute pancreatitis, inflammation commonly spreads into the peripancreatic fat and blurs the margin of the gland.

Abscesses, phlegmons, and pseudocysts may occur as complications of acute pancreatitis. Abscesses, either within or outside the pancreas, appear as low-density areas and are most readily detected when they contain gas. Pseudocysts, which may be unilocular or multilocular, appear as sharply circumscribed, low-density areas that may contain debris. Ascites and pleural ef-

fusion may also be apparent in acute pancreatitis.

In chronic pancreatitis, the pancreas may appear normal, enlarged (localized or generalized), or atrophic, depending on the severity of the disease. Calcification of the ducts and dilatation of the main pancreatic duct are characteristic. Pseudocysts, obliteration of the fat plane, and secondary complications (such as biliary obstruction) may occur.

Post-test care
- The patient may resume his usual diet and activity.
- Observe for a delayed allergic reaction to the contrast dye (urticaria, headache, and vomiting).

Interfering factors
- Barium retained in the GI tract from an earlier test may obscure visualization.
- Excessive movement by the patient or excessive peristalsis during scanning may produce artifacts.

ULTRASONOG-RAPHY

Ultrasonography of the gallbladder and biliary system

In ultrasonography of the gallbladder and the biliary system, a focused beam of high-frequency sound waves passes into the right upper quadrant of the abdomen, creating echoes that vary with changes in tissue density. When these echoes are converted to electrical energy and amplified by a transducer, they're displayed as real-time images on a screen. These images can reveal the size, shape, structure, and position of the gallbladder and biliary system.

Ultrasonography of the biliary system has largely replaced oral cholecystography because it doesn't expose the patient to radiation and doesn't require contrast enhancement. (However, oral cholecystography is performed when ultrasonography is inconclusive.) Ultrasound of the gallbladder is the procedure of choice for evaluating jaundice (because it readily distinguishes between obstructive and nonobstructive types) and for emergency diagnosis of patients with signs of acute cholecystitis, such as right upper quadrant pain, with or without local tenderness.

Purpose
- To confirm diagnosis of cholelithiasis
- To diagnose acute cholecystitis
- To distinguish between obstructive and nonobstructive jaundice.

Patient preparation
Explain to the patient that this procedure allows examination of the gallbladder and the biliary system. Instruct him to eat a fat-free meal in the evening and then to fast for 8 to 12 hours before the procedure, if possible; this promotes accumulation of bile in the gallbladder and enhances ultrasonic visualization. Tell him who will perform the procedure and where, that the room may be darkened slightly to aid visualization on the screen, and that the test takes 15 to 30 minutes.

Tell the patient that a transducer will pass smoothly over his abdomen, in direct contact with his skin, but assure him that he'll feel only mild pressure. Instruct him to remain as still as possible during the procedure and to hold his breath when requested; this ensures that the gallbladder is in the same position for each scan. Just before the procedure, have the patient put on a hospital gown.

Procedure
The patient is placed in the supine position. A water-soluble lubricant is applied to the face of the transducer, and transverse scans of the gallbladder are taken at $\frac{3}{8}$" (1-cm) intervals, starting at the level of the xiphoid and moving laterally to the right subcostal area. Longitudinal oblique scans are taken at 5-mm intervals parallel to the long axis of the gallbladder marked on the patient's skin, beginning medial to the gallbladder and continuing through to its lateral border. During each scan, the patient is asked to exhale deeply and hold his breath. If the gallbladder is positioned deeply under the right costal margin, a scan may be taken through the intercostal spaces, while the patient inhales deeply and holds his breath.

The patient is then placed in a left lateral decubitus position and is scanned beneath the right costal margin. This position and scanning angle are particularly useful for displacing stones lodged in the cystic duct region, which may escape detection when the patient is supine. Scanning with the patient erect helps demonstrate mobility or fixation of suspicious echogenic areas. When good oscilloscopic views are obtained, they are photographed for later study.

Precautions
The patient must remain in a fasting state to prevent the excretion of bile in the gallbladder. Even *smelling* greasy foods such as popcorn can cause the gallbladder to empty.

Normal findings
The normal gallbladder is sonolucent; it appears circular on transverse scans and pear-shaped on longitudinal scans. Although the gallbladder's size varies, its outer walls normally appear sharp and smooth. Intrahepatic radicles seldom appear, because the flow of sonolucent bile is very fine. The cystic duct may also be indistinct — the result of folds known as Heister's valves that line the cystic duct lumen. When visualized, the cystic duct has a serpentine appearance. The common bile duct, in contrast, has a linear appearance but is sometimes obscured by overlying bowel gas.

Implications of results
Gallstones within the gallbladder lumen or the biliary system typically appear as mobile, echogenic areas, usually associated with an acoustic shadow. The size of gallstones generally parallels the size of their shadows; gallstones 5 mm or larger usually produce shadows. However, if the gallbladder is distended with bile, gallstones as small as 1 cm can be detected. Sonolucent bile provides the ideal background for demonstrating stones because of the great acoustic contrast between fluid bile and solid gallstones; this explains why it's sometimes difficult to detect stones in the biliary ducts, which contain much less bile.

When the gallbladder is shrunken or fully impacted with gallstones, inadequate bile may again make gallstone detection difficult, and the gallbladder itself may fail to be visualized. In this case, the presence of an acoustic shadow in the gallbladder fossa indicates cholelithiasis, even though gallstones can't be seen; the presence of such a shadow in the cystic and common bile ducts can also indicate cholelithiasis.

Polyps and carcinoma within the gallbladder lumen are distinguished from gallstones by their fixity. Polyps usually appear as sharply defined, echogenic areas; carcinoma appears as a poorly defined mass, commonly associated with a thickened gallbladder wall.

Biliary sludge within the gallbladder lumen appears as a fine layer of echoes that slowly gravitates to the dependent portion of the gallbladder as the patient changes position. Although biliary sludge may arise without accompanying pathology, it may also result from obstruction and can predispose to gallstone formation.

Acute cholecystitis is indicated by an enlarged gallbladder with thickened, double-rimmed walls that's usually accompanied by gallstones within the lumen. In chronic cholecystitis, the walls of the gallbladder also appear thickened, but the organ itself is usually contracted. In obstructive jaundice, ultrasonography demonstrates a dilated biliary system and, usually, a dilated gallbladder. Dilated intrahepatic radicles appear tortuous and irregular; a dilated gallbladder usually loses its characteristic pear shape, becoming spherical.

Biliary obstruction may result from intrinsic factors, such as a gallstone or small carcinoma within the biliary system. (Ultrasonography can't distinguish between these two echogenic masses.) Or it may result from extrinsic factors, such as a mass in the hepatic portal that compresses the cystic duct and interferes with bile drainage from the intrahepatic radicles, or from pathology in the head of the pancreas that obstructs the common bile duct; such pathology includes carcinoma and pancreatitis, although ultrasonography can't distinguish between the two. When ultrasonography fails to clearly define the site of biliary obstruction, percutaneous transhepatic cholangiography or endoscopic retrograde cholangiopancreatography should be performed.

Post-test care

▪ Make sure the lubricating jelly is removed from the patient's skin. Many brands of lubricating jelly moisturize the skin, but some dry and flake on the skin.

▪ As ordered, the patient may resume his usual diet.

Interfering factors

▪ The patient's failure to observe pretest dietary restrictions interferes with accurate testing.

▪ Overlying bowel gas or retention of barium from a preceding test hinders ultrasound transmission.

▪ In a patient who is dehydrated, ultrasonography can fail to demonstrate the boundaries between organs and tissue structures because of deficiency of body fluids.

Ultrasonography of the liver

This ultrasound examination produces cross-sectional images of the liver by channeling high-frequency sound waves into the right upper quadrant of the abdomen. The resultant echoes are converted to electrical energy, amplified by a transducer, and displayed on a monitor. Different shades of gray depict various tissue densities. Ultrasound can show intrahepatic structures as well as organ size, shape, and position.

Liver ultrasonography is indicated for patients with jaundice of unknown etiology, with unexplained hepatomegaly and abnormal biochemical test results, with suspected metastatic tumors and elevated serum alkaline phosphatase levels, and with recent abdominal trauma. When used to complement liver-spleen scanning, ultrasonography can define cold spots — focal defects that fail to pick up the radionuclide — as tumors, abscesses, or cysts; it also provides better views of the periportal and perihepatic spaces than liver-spleen scanning. If ultrasonography fails to provide a definitive diagnosis, computed tomography, gallium scanning, or liver biopsy may provide more specific information.

Purpose

▪ To distinguish between obstructive and nonobstructive jaundice

▪ To screen for hepatocellular disease

▪ To detect hepatic metastases and hematoma

▪ To define cold spots as tumors, abscesses, or cysts.

Patient preparation

Explain to the patient that this procedure allows examination of the liver. Instruct him to fast for 8 to 12 hours before the test. Tell him who will perform the test and where, that the room will be darkened slightly to aid visualization on the screen, and that the test takes 15 to 30 minutes.

Tell the patient a transducer will pass smoothly over his abdomen, channeling sound waves into the liver. Assure him that the test isn't harmful or painful, although he may feel mild pressure as the transducer presses against his skin. Instruct him to remain as still as possible during the procedure and to hold his breath when requested; this technique aids visualization. Just before the procedure, instruct the patient to put on a hospital gown.

Procedure

The patient is placed in the supine position. A water-soluble lubricant is applied to the face of the transducer, and transverse scans are taken at ⅜" (1-cm) intervals, using a single-sweep technique between the costal margins. Although this technique easily demonstrates the left lobe of the liver and part of the right lobe, sector scans are taken through the intercostal spaces to view the remainder of the right lobe.

Scans are taken longitudinally, from the right border of the liver to the left. For better demonstration of the right lateral dome, oblique cephalad-angled scans may be taken beneath the right costal margin. Scans are then taken parallel to the hepatic portal, at a 45-degree angle toward the superior right lateral dome, to examine the peripheral anatomy, portal venous system, common bile duct, and biliary tree. During each scan, the patient is asked to hold his breath briefly in deep inspiration. When clear images are obtained, they're photographed for later study.

Precautions

None.

Normal findings

The liver demonstrates a homogeneous, low-level echo pattern, interrupted only by the different echo patterns of its vascular channels. Although intrahepatic biliary radicles and hepatic arteries aren't apparent, portal and hepatic veins, the aorta, and the inferior vena cava do appear. Hepatic veins appear completely sonolucent, whereas portal veins have margins that are highly echogenic.

Implications of results

In obstructive jaundice, ultrasonography shows dilated intrahepatic biliary radicles and extrahepatic ducts. Conversely, in nonobstructive jaundice, ultrasonography shows a biliary tree of normal diameter.

Ultrasound characteristics of hepatocellular disease are generally nonspecific, and budding disorders can escape detection; liver-spleen scanning, which assesses hepatic function by evaluating the uptake of a radionuclide, is a more sensitive diagnostic tool. In cirrhosis, ultrasonography may demonstrate variable liver size; dilated, tortuous portal branches associated with portal hypertension; and an irregular echo pattern with increased echo amplitude, causing overall increased attenuation. Demonstration of splenomegaly — also associated with portal hypertension — by spleen ultrasonography or liver-spleen scanning aids diagnosis. In fatty infiltration of the liver, ultrasonography may show hepatomegaly and a regular echo pattern that, although greater in echo amplitude than that of normal parenchyma, doesn't alter attenuation.

Ultrasound characteristics of metastases in the liver, the most common intrahepatic neoplasm, vary widely; metastases may appear either hypoechoic or echogenic, and either poorly defined or well defined. For example, metastatic lymphomas and sarcomas are generally hypoechoic, whereas mucin-secreting adenocarcinoma of the colon is highly echogenic. Liver biopsy is necessary to confirm tumor type, but after the tumor is identified and treatment begun, serial ultrasonography can be used to monitor the effectiveness of therapy.

Primary hepatic tumors also present a varied appearance and may mimic metastases, requiring angiography and liver biopsy for definitive diagnosis. Hepatomas are the most common malignant tumors in adults; hepatoblastomas are most common in children. Benign tumors are far less common than malignant ones.

Abscesses usually appear as sonolucent masses with ill-defined, slightly thickened borders, and accentuated posterior wall transmission; scattered internal echoes, caused by necrotic debris, may also be present. Intrahepatic abscesses are occasionally mistaken for hematomas, necrotic metastases, or hemorrhagic cysts because they produce similar echo patterns. Gas-containing intrahepatic abscesses, which may be echogenic, are sometimes confused with solid intrahepatic lesions. Subphrenic abscesses occur between the diaphragm and the liver, whereas subhepatic abscesses appear inferior to the liver and anterior to the upper pole of the right kidney. The presence of ascitic fluid may stimulate a subhepatic abscess, but such fluid lacks internal echoes and has a more regular border.

Cysts usually appear as spherical, sonolucent areas with well-defined borders and accentuated posterior wall transmission. When a cyst can't be distinguished from an abscess or necrotic metastases, gallium scanning, computed tomography, and angiography should be performed.

Hematomas — either intrahepatic or subcapsular — usually result from trauma. Intrahepatic hematomas appear as poorly defined, relatively sonolucent masses, and may have scattered internal echoes due to clotting; serial ultrasonography can differentiate between a hematoma and a cyst or tumor as the hematoma becomes smaller. Subcapsular hematoma may appear as a focal, sonolucent mass on the periphery of the liver or as a diffuse, sonolucent area surrounding part of the liver.

Post-test care

■ Make sure the lubricating jelly is removed from the patient's skin. Many brands of lubricating jelly moisturize the skin, but some dry and flake on the skin.
■ The patient may resume his usual diet.

Interfering factors

■ Overlying ribs and gas or residual barium in the stomach or colon hinder transmission of ultrasound.
■ Dehydration may prevent accurate demonstration of the boundaries between organs and tissue structures because of the lack of body fluids.

Ultrasonography of the spleen

In this procedure, a focused beam of high-frequency sound waves passes into the left upper quadrant of the abdomen, creating echoes that vary with changes in tissue density. These echoes, when converted to electrical energy and amplified by a transducer, are displayed on a monitor as a series of real-time images representing the size, shape, and position of the spleen and surrounding viscera.

Ultrasonography is indicated for patients with a left upper quadrant mass of unknown origin; with known splenomegaly to evaluate changes in the spleen's size; with left upper quadrant pain and local tenderness; and with recent abdominal trauma. Although ultrasonography can show splenomegaly, it usually doesn't identify the cause; computed tomography (CT) scanning can provide more specific information. However, as a supplementary diagnostic procedure after liver-spleen scanning, ultrasonography can clarify the nature of cold spots or detect focal defects not infiltrated by tracer radioisotopes.

Purpose

- To demonstrate splenomegaly
- To monitor progression of primary and secondary splenic disease, and to evaluate effectiveness of therapy
- To evaluate the spleen after abdominal trauma
- To help detect splenic cysts and subphrenic abscess.

Patient preparation

Explain to the patient that this procedure allows examination of the spleen. Instruct him to fast for 8 to 12 hours before the procedure, if possible. Tell him who will perform this test and where, that the room may be darkened slightly to aid visualization on the monitor screen, and that this procedure takes approximately 15 to 30 minutes.

Tell the patient a transducer will pass smoothly over his abdomen, in direct contact with his skin, but assure him that he'll feel only mild pressure. Instruct him to remain as still as possible during the procedure and to hold his breath when requested; this technique aids visualization.

Just before the procedure, instruct the patient to put on a hospital gown.

Procedure

Because the procedure for ultrasonography varies, depending on the size of the spleen or the patient's physique, the patient is usually repositioned several times; the transducer scanning angle or path is also changed. Generally, the patient is first placed in the supine position, with his chest uncovered. A water-soluble lubricant is applied to the face of the transducer, and transverse scans of the spleen are taken at $\frac{3}{8}$" to $\frac{3}{4}$" (1- to 2-cm) intervals, beginning at the level of the diaphragm and moving posteri-

orly while the transducer is angled anteromedially.

After the patient is placed in right lateral decubitus position, additional transverse scans are taken through the intercostal spaces, using a sectoring motion. A pillow may be placed under the patient's right side to help separate the intercostal spaces, making it easier to position the transducer face between them. For longitudinal scans, the patient remains in the right lateral decubitus position, and scans are taken from the axilla toward the iliac crest. To prevent rib artifacts, oblique scans are taken by passing the transducer face along the intercostal spaces; this scan provides the best view of the splenic parenchyma.

During each scan, the patient may be asked to hold his breath briefly at varying stages of inspiration. When good views are obtained, they are photographed for later study.

Precautions

None.

Normal findings

The splenic parenchyma normally demonstrates a homogeneous, low-level echo pattern; its individual vascular channels aren't usually apparent. The superior and lateral splenic borders are clearly defined, each having a convex margin. The undersurface and medial borders, in contrast, show indentations from surrounding organs (stomach, left kidney, and pancreas).

The hilar region, where the vascular pedicle enters the spleen, commonly produces an area of highly reflected echoes. The medial surface is generally concave, a characteristic particularly useful when differentiating between left upper quadrant masses and an enlarged spleen. Even when splenomegaly is present, the spleen usually remains concave medially, unless a space-occupying lesion distorts this contour.

Implications of results

Splenomegaly is generally characterized by increased echogenicity. Enlarged vascular channels are commonly visible, especially in the hilar region. If space-occupying lesions distort the splenic contour, liver-spleen scanning should be performed to confirm splenomegaly. However, CT scanning can demonstrate the extent of enlargement most accurately.

Abdominal trauma may result in splenic rupture or subcapsular hematoma. In splenic rupture, ultrasonography demonstrates splenomegaly and an irregular, sonolucent area (the presence of free intraperitoneal fluid); however, these findings must be confirmed by arteriography. In subcapsular hematoma, ultrasonography shows splenomegaly as well as the presence of a double contour, altered splenic position, and a relatively sonolucent area on the periphery of the spleen. The double contour results from blood accumulation between the splenic parenchyma and the intact splenic capsule. As the spleen enlarges, a transverse section shows its anterior margin extending more anteriorly than the aorta.

Ultrasonography may prove difficult and painful after abdominal trauma because the transducer may have to pass across fractured ribs and contusions. If so, CT scanning should be performed instead. This technique offers the advantage of differentiating between blood and fluid in the peritoneal space.

In subphrenic abscess, ultrasonography shows a sonolucent area beneath the diaphragm, and the patient's clinical symptoms help differentiate between abscess and blood or fluid accumulation.

As a complement to liver-spleen scanning, ultrasonography differentiates cold spots as cystic or solid lesions. It shows cysts as spherical, sonolucent areas with well-defined, regular margins, with acoustic enhancement behind them. When ultrasonography fails to identify a cyst as splenic or extrasplenic — especially if the cyst is located in the upper pole of the left kidney and the adrenal gland or in the tail of the pancreas — CT arteriography is appropriate. Ultrasonography can readily clarify cystic cold spots, but CT scanning with a contrast medium is superior for evaluating primary and metastatic tumors.

Ultrasonography usually fails to identify tumors associated with lymphoma or chronic leukemia because they resemble tumors of the splenic parenchyma.

Post-test care

- Make sure the lubricating jelly is removed from the patient's skin. Many brands of lubricating jelly moisturize the skin, but some dry and flake on the skin.
- Tell the patient that he may resume his usual diet.

Interfering factors

- Overlying ribs, an aerated left lung, or gas or residual barium in the colon or stomach may prevent visualization of the spleen.
- In a dehydrated patient, ultrasonography may fail to show the boundaries between organs and tissue structures because of the lack of body fluids.
- Body physique affecting the spleen's shape or adjacent masses that displace the spleen may be confused with splenomegaly.
- The patient with splenic trauma may be unable to tolerate the procedure because of pain caused by the transducer moving across his abdomen.

Ultrasonography of the pancreas

In this noninvasive test, cross-sectional images of the pancreas are produced by channeling high-frequency sound waves into the epigastric region, converting the resultant echoes to electrical impulses, and then displaying them as real-time images on a monitor. The pattern varies with tissue density and so represents the size, shape, and position of the pancreas and surrounding viscera.

Although ultrasonography cannot provide a sensitive measure of pancreatic function, it can help detect anatomic abnormalities, such as pancreatic carcinoma and pseudocysts, and can guide the insertion of biopsy needles. Because ultrasonography doesn't expose the patient to radiation, it has largely replaced hypotonic duodenography, endoscopic retrograde cholangiopancreatography, radioisotope studies, and arteriography.

Purpose

■ To aid diagnosis of pancreatitis, pseudocysts, and pancreatic carcinoma.

Patient preparation

Explain to the patient that this procedure permits examination of the pancreas. Instruct him to fast for 8 to 12 hours before the test to reduce bowel gas, which hinders transmission of ultrasound. Tell him who will perform the procedure and where, that the room is darkened slightly to aid visualization on the screen, and that this test takes 30 minutes. If the patient is a smoker, ask him to abstain before the test; this eliminates the risk of swallowing air while inhaling, which interferes with test results.

Tell the patient a transducer will pass smoothly over his epigastric region, channeling sound waves into the pancreas. Assure him that this procedure isn't harmful or painful, although he may experience mild pressure. Tell him he'll be asked to inhale deeply during scanning, and instruct him to remain as still as possible during the procedure. Just before the procedure, instruct the patient to put on a hospital gown.

Procedure

The patient is placed in the supine position. (See *Positioning the patient for ultrasonography of the pancreas,* page 880.) A water-soluble lubricant or mineral oil is applied to the abdomen and, with the patient at full inspiration, transverse scans are taken at 1-cm intervals, starting from the xiphoid and moving caudally.

Other scanning techniques include the longitudinal scan to view the head, body, and tail of the pancreas in sequence; the right anterior oblique view for the head and body of the pancreas; the oblique sagittal view for the portal vein; and the sagittal view for the vena cava. When good oscilloscopic views are obtained, they're photographed for later study.

Precautions

None.

Normal findings

The pancreas demonstrates a coarse, uniform echo pattern (reflecting tissue density) and usually appears more echogenic than the adjacent liver. (See *Normal and abnormal images of the pancreas,* page 881.)

Implications of results

Ultrasonography can detect alterations in the size, contour, and parenchymal texture of the pancreas — changes that characterize pancreatic disease. An enlarged pancreas with decreased echogenicity and distinct borders suggests pancreatitis; a well-defined mass with an

Positioning the patient for ultrasonography of the pancreas

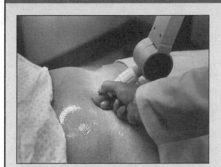

For ultrasonography of the pancreas, the patient is placed in the supine position (at left). A water-soluble lubricant is applied to the patient's abdomen, and the transducer is passed over the epigastric region near the xiphoid. To visualize the pancreas at other angles, the patient may need to change his position (below).

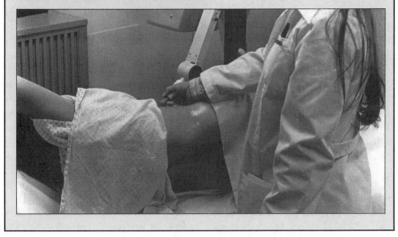

essentially echo-free interior indicates pseudocyst; an ill-defined mass with scattered internal echoes, or a mass in the head of the pancreas (obstructing the common bile duct) and a large noncontracting gallbladder suggest pancreatic carcinoma.

Subsequent CT scanning and biopsy of the pancreas may be necessary to confirm the diagnosis suggested by ultrasonography.

Post-test care

■ Make sure the lubricating jelly is removed from the patient's skin. Many brands of lubricating jelly moisturize the skin, but some dry and flake on the skin.

■ Tell the patient he may resume his usual diet.

Interfering factors

■ Gas or residual barium in the stomach and intestine hinders ultrasound transmission.

■ In a dehydrated patient, ultrasound may fail to demonstrate the boundaries between organs and tissue structures because of the lack of body fluids.

Normal and abnormal images of the pancreas

The ultrasound view on the top shows a normal pancreas (outlined in color). The ultrasound view on the bottom shows a diffusely enlarged pancreas due to pancreatitis. The color outline indicates the extent of enlargement.

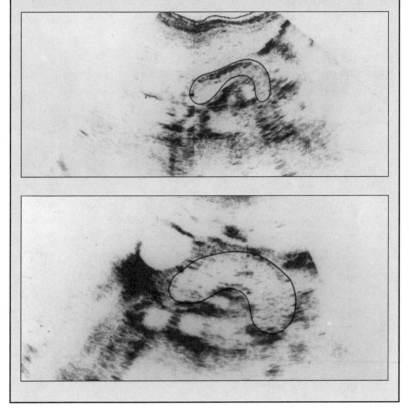

■ Obesity interferes with ultrasound transmission, and fatty infiltration of the gland makes it difficult to distinguish the pancreas from surrounding tissue.

SELECTED READINGS

Black, J.M., and Matassarin-Jacobs, E., eds. *Luckmann and Sorensen's Medical-Surgical Nursing: A Psychophysiologic Approach,* 4th ed. Philadelphia: W.B. Saunders Co., 1993.

Fischbach, F. *A Manual of Laboratory and Diagnostic Tests,* 5th ed. Philadelphia: Lippincott-Raven Pubs., 1996.

Henry, J.B., ed. *Clinical Diagnosis and Management by Laboratory Methods,* 19th ed. Philadelphia: W.B. Saunders Co., 1996.

Isselbacher, K.J., et al, eds. *Harrison's Principles of Internal Medicine,* 13th ed. New York: McGraw-Hill Book Co., 1994.

Nursing97 Drug Handbook. Springhouse, Pa.: Springhouse Corp., 1997.

Nursing Procedures, 2nd ed. Springhouse, Pa.: Springhouse Corp., 1996.

Pagana, K.D., and Pagana, T.J. *Mosby's diagnostic and Laboratory Test Reference,* 2nd ed. St. Louis: Mosby–Year Book, Inc., 1995.

Ravel, R.A. *Clinical Laboratory Medicine: Clinical Application of Laboratory Data,* 6th ed. St. Louis: Mosby–Year Book, Inc., 1995.

Smeltzer, S.C., and Bare, B.G. *Brunner and Suddharth's Textbook of Medical-Surgical Nursing,* 8th ed. Philadelphia: Lippincott-Raven Pubs., 1996.

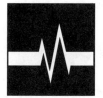

CHAPTER TWENTY-EIGHT

Cardiovascular system

Learning objectives

After completing this chapter, the reader will be able to:
- explain the anatomy and physiology of the cardiovascular system
- understand how the heart's conduction system works
- state the major test groups that identify cardiovascular dysfunction
- discuss the importance of the cardiac series
- identify electrocardiogram tracings of three pathologic changes that occur during myocardial infarction
- compare the treadmill and bicycle ergometer tests
- describe electrode placement for exercise electrocardiography
- state the purpose of each test discussed in the chapter
- prepare the patient physically and psychologically for each test
- describe the procedure for performing each test
- specify appropriate precautions for safe administration of each test
- recognize signs of an adverse reaction and respond appropriately
- implement appropriate post-test care
- identify the normal findings of each test
- discuss the implications of abnormal test results
- list factors that may interfere with accurate test results.

INTRODUCTION

According to the American Heart Association, disorders of the cardiovascular system afflict nearly 70 million people in North America. Because a wide range of diagnostic tests can detect many such disorders, it's important to understand the indications for each test and its clinical implications in order to prepare the patient physically and psychologically before the test, assist the doctor during the test, and implement proper care after the test.

The tests for cardiovascular dysfunction fall into six major groups: cardiac enzyme analysis, radiography, graphic recording, ultrasonography, nuclear medicine, and catheterization. *Cardiac enzyme analysis* (covered in Chapter 4) proves most useful in detecting acute myocardial infarction (MI). *Radiography,* including X-rays of the heart, is one of the first diagnostic tests used to assess myocardial or vascular dysfunction. *Graphic recording,* such as electrocardiography, is a noninvasive technique for evaluating cardiac electrical activity performed by specially trained personnel. *Ultrasonography,* another noninvasive technique, now holds an important place in cardiovascular testing; for example, echocardiography has superseded cardiac series fluoroscopy for most diagnostic applications. *Nuclear medicine imaging* is one of the most rapidly changing areas of diagnostic testing, partly because of the development of new radiopharmaceuticals. *Catheterization* is an effective invasive method for evaluating cardiac and vascular dysfunction.

The choice of a specific diagnostic test depends on the doctor's clinical suspicions, the kind of information needed, and the risk to the patient. As a rule, noninvasive tests precede invasive tests because the latter are usually more hazardous and more costly. However, invasive tests are often necessary to obtain the most diagnostic information.

The pump

The heart is the mechanism and the arteries, veins, and capillaries are the pathway by which blood circulates throughout the body. Together they act to deliver oxygen and vital nutrients to the body cells and to remove carbon dioxide and other waste products.

The heart is a hollow, muscular organ located in the mediastinum between the lungs. It is enclosed by a membranous sac called the *pericardium,* which consists of two layers, one inside the other: an external fibrous (parietal) layer attached to the great vessels leaving the heart, and an internal serous (visceral) sac that envelops the heart and lines the fibrous portion. Space between these layers is filled with 10 to 50 ml of pericardial fluid, which lubricates the layers as they glide over each other during heart movement.

The heart pump consists of four chambers. The *atria* — the two smaller upper chambers — receive blood from the systemic and the pulmonary circulation. The two larger, thicker lower chambers — the *ventricles* — receive blood from the atria. The interventricular septum divides the heart into right and left halves. Two valves separate the atria from the ventricles: the tricuspid valve in the right side and the mitral valve in the left side of the heart. The mitral valve has two movable leaflets; the tricuspid has three. Two semilunar valves, each with three fibrous cusps, guard the entrances to the aortic and pulmonary arteries. (See *The conduction system,* page 886.)

The vascular system

The vascular system consists of the arteries, arterioles, capillaries, venules, and veins. Both arteries and veins have three layers: the tunica intima (inner coat), consisting of endothelial, connective, and elastic tissues; the tunica media (middle coat), consisting of smooth-muscle fibers and elastic and collagenous tissue; and the tunica adventitia (external coat), consisting of connective, smooth muscle, and elastic tissue. *Capillaries* consist of endothelial tissues one cell thick, whereas venules and arterioles have a variable composition, depending on their size.

Arteries, which contain 15% of circulating blood volume, carry blood away from the heart. Normally, the aorta (the largest artery) and its branches can withstand significant changes in cardiac pressure that distend them during ventricular contraction; these pressure changes are detectable as a palpable wave (pulse) in certain arteries near the skin. The aorta and other large arteries add little to total peripheral vascular resistance because they don't ordinarily impede blood flow. By their ability to dilate and contract, the *arterioles* largely control the degree of total peripheral resistance and, consequently, the amount of blood flow to and in the tissues.

The *veins* carry blood toward the heart and contain 50% of total circulating blood volume. The superior and inferior venae cavae, which empty into the right atrium, are the body's largest veins. In the venous system, pressure changes only slightly with vessel dilation or constriction. However, total circulating blood volume, heart and lung function, venomotor tone, and the condition of the one-way venous valves in the limbs may affect the capacitance and pressure of the venous system. (See *The heart's blood supply,* page 887, and *The cardiac cycle,* page 888.)

In the coronary circulation, blood flow occurs mainly during diastole and depends directly on the perfusion pressure (the pressure gradient between the coronary arteries and the right atrium).

The conduction system

The heart's conduction system contains specialized muscle fibers that generate and conduct their own electrical impulses.

SA node
The sinoatrial (SA) node — located in the right atrium, beneath the orifice of the superior vena cava — normally controls heart rate and is called the *pacemaker*. The SA node sends an impulse through the internodal pathways and atrial muscle to the atrioventricular (AV) node, in the lower posterior part of the right atrium, near the lumen of the coronary sinus. As an impulse passes through the atrial muscles, the atria contract.

After a short delay in the AV node, the impulse continues down the His bundle — which divides into right and left bundle branches — and finally, into the subendothelial Purkinje fibers, which transmit the impulse into the ventricular myocardium, causing it to contract.

Repolarization
After this contraction, the myocardium repolarizes, while the ventricles relax and begin to fill with blood, in preparation for the next impulse from the SA node. Evidence of this conduction of electric currents through the heart may be picked up on the skin surface and graphically recorded by an electrocardiogram.

Automaticity
The SA node discharges 60 to 100 impulses/minute. If it fails to generate the expected impulses, the AV node can also discharge, but at a slower rate of 40 to 60 impulses/minute. If both nodes fail to discharge, the Purkinje fibers can discharge at a rate of 15 to 40 impulses/minute. The ability of the heart to spontaneously generate and maintain its own impulse rate is known as *automaticity*.

When any part of the heart other than the SA node takes over to pace the heart, this part is known as an *ectopic pacemaker*. If the electrical impulse is too weak, it won't excite the muscle fiber at all; if it's strong enough to cause the fiber to reach its electrical threshold potential, excitation occurs. The current then spreads to neighboring fibers by virtue of the low resistance of their cell walls, and the entire muscle mass reacts as a unit. This response is known as the "all-or-nothing" principle.

(See *Stroke volume and Starling's law*, page 889.) Coronary blood flow may diminish if aortic pressure decreases or right-sided heart pressure increases. It may also be influenced by tachycardias, which reduce diastolic flow time, and by conditions that reduce diastolic perfusion pressure such as hypotension.

Coronary circulation, which constitutes 5% of total cardiac output in the resting heart, uses 70% of the arterial oxygen. Increased oxygen demand requires increased coronary blood flow because the heart extracts virtually all oxygen from the blood, even at rest.

Radiographic tests
Cardiac radiography permits visualization of the position, size, and contour of the heart and great vessels of the circulatory system. Chest X-rays can show enlargement of the heart, interstitial and alveolar edema, aortic dilation, left-sided heart failure, and intracardiac calcification.

The heart's blood supply

The heart's blood supply system is shown in these schematic anterior and posterior views. Coronary angiography — a cardiac catheterization procedure — evaluates coronary artery function. Coronary artery disease results mainly from atherosclerosis, which impedes blood flow and thus interferes with the supply of oxygen and nutrients to the myocardium.

ANTERIOR

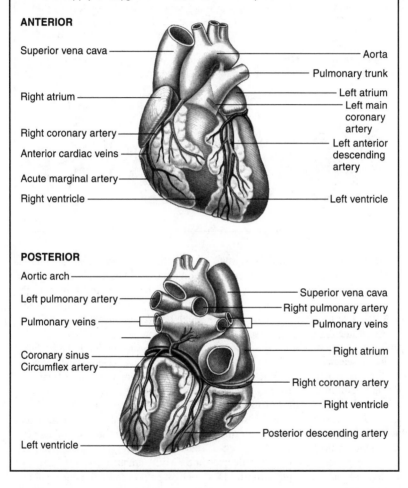

Superior vena cava

Right atrium

Right coronary artery

Anterior cardiac veins

Acute marginal artery

Right ventricle

Aorta

Pulmonary trunk

Left atrium

Left main coronary artery

Left anterior descending artery

Left ventricle

POSTERIOR

Aortic arch

Left pulmonary artery

Pulmonary veins

Coronary sinus

Circumflex artery

Left ventricle

Superior vena cava

Right pulmonary artery

Pulmonary veins

Right atrium

Right coronary artery

Right ventricle

Posterior descending artery

Cardiac series (chest fluoroscopy) shows the heart's motion and the pulsations of the heart and great vessels during systole and diastole; it also helps detect and confirm malfunctioning prosthetic heart valves. Although largely replaced by echocardiography, the cardiac series is used in some cases for placing temporary pacemakers or pulmonary artery catheters.

By injecting a contrast medium into the veins for filming, *lower limb venography* may confirm deep vein thrombosis (DVT), identify the causes of edema,

The cardiac cycle

These schematic drawings show events during a single cardiac cycle.
- *Period of rapid ventricular filling* (1): Unoxygenated blood returning from the tissues enters the right atrium at the same time that oxygenated blood from the lungs enters the left atrium. The atria and ventricles are passively filled.
- *Atrial kick* (2): About 70% of incoming blood flows through the atria directly into the ventricles before the atria contract; when they do, they force an additional 30% of blood into the ventricles — the atrial kick.
- *Period of isovolumic contraction* (3): The ventricles begin contracting before emptying.
- *Period of ejection* (4): The ventricles contract, pushing the unoxygenated blood into pulmonary arteries and the oxygenated blood into the aorta.

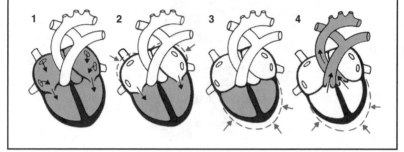

and assess preoperative vascular status. The benefits of the test must outweigh the risks of radiation exposure.

Graphic recording

Electrocardiography (ECG) records the conduction, magnitude, and duration of the heart's electrical activity to identify rhythm disturbances, conduction abnormalities, and electrolyte imbalances. It reveals the size of the heart's chambers and the heart's relative position in the chest. ECG is used to diagnose and document the progression of MI, ischemia, and pericarditis and to evaluate artificial pacemakers and cardiotonic drug therapy.

Exercise ECG measures the cardiovascular effects of controlled physical stress (bike riding or treadmill walking). An ergometer (a push wheel with handlebars) is used for exercise stress testing for patients who can't physically walk or ride a bike. The exercise ECG may re-

veal ischemia, arrhythmias, or conduction abnormalities. It can also find the cause of chest pain and thus help the staff plan appropriate therapy. A thorough clinical workup must precede exercise ECG.

Holter monitoring (ambulatory ECG) records the heart's electrical activity for 24 hours or longer as the patient performs his usual activities and encounters normal physical and emotional stress. This portable ECG can detect intermittent arrhythmias, evaluate antiarrhythmic drugs, and assess recovery after MI. It can also detect the cause of vertigo, palpitations, and chest pain. A thorough clinical workup must precede Holter monitoring.

Impedance plethysmography evaluates changes in blood volume in the limbs. Less reliable than venography in detecting small thrombi, it can confirm a diagnosis of DVT.

Stroke volume and Starling's law

Total ventricular volume in each cardiac cycle reaches 120 to 130 ml during diastolic filling (end-diastolic volume) and falls to 50 to 60 mg as the ventricles empty during contraction; this 70-ml difference represents the *stroke volume*. The stroke volume multiplied by heart rate per minute equals *cardiac output*, or the volume of blood pumped in 1 minute. Normally, the cardiac output for a resting person is about 5 L, but this amount varies with body size, heart rate, and stroke volume.

The heart's remarkable ability to deliver equal volumes of blood each minute, even when the right and left ventricles deliver very different volumes of blood per stroke, is explained by *Starling's law:* The force of contraction of each heartbeat depends on the length of the muscle fibers of the walls of the heart. Thus, if right ventricular output exceeds left ventricular output, the fibers of the left ventricle lengthen at end-diastole to increase the force of contraction.

In the diagrams on the left (A), normal diastolic filling during diastole causes normal fiber stretch, normal contractile force, and normal stroke volume. In the diagrams on the right (B), increased filling during diastole increases fiber stretch, force of contraction, and stroke volume.

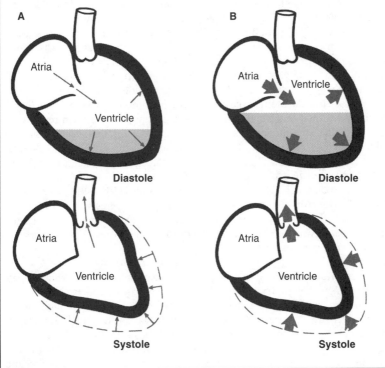

Ultrasonography

Echocardiography directs ultra-high-frequency sound waves into the heart, which reflects these waves at various frequencies, depending on the density of cardiac tissue. By assessing cardiac structure and function, this test can reveal valve deformities, tumors, septal defects, and pericardial effusion. It can also assess left ventricular function after an MI, prosthetic valve functioning, and hypertrophic cardiomyopathy (also known as idiopathic hypertrophic subaortic stenosis).

Transesophageal echocardiography uses ultrasonography and endoscopy to view the heart posteriorly. This test helps diagnose thoracic aortic pathology, valvular disease, congenital heart disease, cardiac tumors, and intracardiac thrombi.

Doppler ultrasonography — in which sound waves are reflected from moving blood cells in underlying blood vessels — evaluates the major vascular network of the arms and legs and the extracranial cerebrovascular system. This test helps detect DVT, peripheral arterial aneurysms, congenital defects, and carotid arterial occlusive disease, and can be used to assess valve function.

Ultrasonography of the abdominal aorta is used to detect and monitor the progression of abdominal aortic aneurysms, to evaluate the inferior vena cava, and to locate visceral arteries.

Nuclear medicine imaging

Positron emission tomography images the extent of myocardial contractility to help distinguish viable tissue from infarcted tissue. After the appropriate positron emitter is injected, a scan is obtained.

Magnetic resonance imaging uses a strong magnetic field to image cardiac anatomic structures and their functions noninvasively. This test is rarely used to diagnose cardiac disease because of its high cost.

Technetium Tc 99m pyrophosphate scanning reveals damaged myocardial tissue as hot spots — areas where the radioisotope accumulates. This test helps

to detect acute MI and define its location and size.

Thallium imaging evaluates myocardial blood flow and the status of myocardial cells after I.V. injection of the radioisotope thallium-201; healthy myocardial tissue absorbs this radioisotope, but ischemic or necrotic tissue does not. This test can detect abnormalities from perfusion defects in the coronary arteries and myocardium. *Stress testing* after thallium injection can reveal areas of ischemia.

Radiopharmaceutical myocardial perfusion imaging (also called chemical stress imaging and persantine-thallium scanning) is an alternative to exercise ECG. A persantine injection may stimulate an ischemic event; then a thallium injection helps record cardiac vessels' response to this event.

Cardiac blood pool imaging, in which a radioisotope is tagged to red blood cells or albumin and injected I.V., outlines the heart cavities to detect left ventricular regional wall motion abnormalities (commonly seen after MI). In this test, a scintillation camera records the first pass of the radioisotope through the heart; then, in subsequent gated or timed imaging, the camera records two or more points in the cardiac cycle, allowing study of left ventricular function. Blood pool imaging also aids diagnosis of left ventricular aneurysm, cardiomyopathies, and intracardiac shunts.

Catheterization

Cardiac catheterization permits visualization of cardiac contraction and coronary artery anatomy through the insertion of a catheter into the right or left side of the heart and the injection of a contrast medium. *Left-sided heart catheterization* helps evaluate aortic and mitral valve function, cardiac output, and coronary artery patency. It also helps assess candidates for coronary artery bypass surgery or interventional procedures, such as percutaneous trans-luminal coronary angioplasty, stent placement, and directional coronary atherectomy.

Right-sided heart catheterization permits evaluation of pulmonic and tricuspid valve function, cardiac output, right-sided heart pressures, and pulmonary artery wedge pressure (PAWP). It can demonstrate valvular efficiency or defects, assess the causes of chest pain, and detect congenital heart defects.

In *electrophysiology studies,* an electrode-tipped catheter is passed into the right atrium and ventricle to record and study the activity of the heart's electrical conduction system. These studies allow precise location of bundle-branch blocks, detection of arrhythmias, and evaluation of the effects of antiarrhythmic drugs. Electrophysiology studies are contraindicated in patients with severe coagulopathy or acute pulmonary embolism.

Pulmonary artery catheterization permits measurement of PAWP after passage of a balloon-tipped, flow-directed catheter into a small branch of the pulmonary artery; PAWP reflects both left atrial and left ventricular end-diastolic pressure. This test, performed primarily in patients who have suffered an acute MI, helps assess left-sided heart failure and monitors the effects of therapy after complications develop. It should be performed cautiously in patients with left bundle- branch block because the catheter could cause right bundle-branch block, resulting in complete heart block.

Miscellaneous tests

The *cold stimulation test for Raynaud's syndrome,* performed by immersing a patient's hand in ice water and checking digital temperatures after removing the hand from the water, can verify Raynaud's syndrome in patients who do not exhibit arterial-tree occlusion.

Pericardial fluid analysis, performed after needle aspiration of fluid from the pericardial sac, helps detect the cause of pericardial effusion. After aspiration, the fluid specimen is sent to the laboratory for biochemical analysis and bacterial culture.

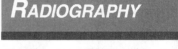

Cardiac radiography

Among the most commonly used tests for evaluating cardiac disease and its effects on the pulmonary vasculature, cardiac radiography provides images of the thorax, mediastinum, heart, and lungs. In a routine evaluation, posteroanterior and left lateral views are taken. The posteroanterior view is preferable to the anteroposterior view because it places the heart slightly closer to the plane of the film, providing a sharper, less distorted image. Portable equipment can take X-rays of patients who are bedridden but provides only anteroposterior views.

Another form of cardiac radiography, the cardiac series, provides a constant image of the heart in motion. (See *The cardiac series,* page 892.)

Purpose
- To help detect cardiac disease and abnormalities that change the size, shape, or appearance of the heart and lungs
- To ensure correct positioning of pulmonary artery and cardiac catheters and of pacemaker wires.

Patient preparation
Explain to the patient that this test reveals the size and shape of the heart. Tell him who will perform the test and

The cardiac series

Now superseded by echocardiography for most diagnostic purposes, the cardiac series remains useful for comprehensive examination of heart action. Using X-rays, this test provides a constant image of the heart in motion on a fluoroscope.

By examining the beating heart from four directions, the test permits observation of cardiac pulsations, assessment of heart chamber structural abnormalities (such as aneurysm and congenital heart disease), detection of aortic and mitral valve calcification, and evaluation of prosthetic valve function. When performed with a barium swallow, the cardiac series highlights abnormal deviation of esophageal contours (possibly caused by left atrial enlargement) or makes abnormalities of the aortic arch more visible. Views may be preserved for later study on spot films or motion pictures.

Because the cardiac series entails exposure to 15 to 20 times more radiation than standard cardiac radiography, it may be contraindicated in some patients, especially pregnant women. If this test is necessary during pregnancy, the patient's pelvic and abdominal areas must be adequately shielded during the test.

where. Reassure him that the test uses little radiation and is harmless.

Instruct the patient to remove all metal objects and all clothing above his waist and to put on a hospital gown with ties instead of metal snaps.

Procedure

Posteroanterior view: The patient stands erect about 6' (2 m) from the X-ray machine, with his back to the machine and his chin resting on top of the film cassette holder. The holder is adjusted to slightly hyperextend the patient's neck. The patient places his hands on his hips, with his shoulders touching the holder, and centers his chest against it. Then he's asked to take a deep breath and hold it during the X-ray film exposure.

Left lateral view: The patient is positioned with his arms extended over his head and his left torso flush against the cassette and centered. Then he is asked to take a deep breath and hold it during the X-ray film exposure.

Anteroposterior view of a bedridden patient: The head of the bed is elevated

as much as possible, and the patient is assisted to an upright position to reduce visceral pressure on the diaphragm and other thoracic structures. The film cassette is centered under the patient's back. Although the distance between the patient and the X-ray machine may vary, the path between the two should be clear. The patient is instructed to take a deep breath and hold it while the X-ray film is being exposed.

Precautions

■ Cardiac radiography is usually contraindicated during the first trimester of pregnancy. If it is performed during pregnancy, a lead shield or apron should cover the abdomen and pelvic area during the X-ray exposure.

■ When testing an ambulatory patient, make sure the radiographic order stipulates a posteroanterior view and not an anteroposterior view. Include on the order the indication for the test and any pertinent findings from previous cardiac radiography.

■ When testing a bedridden patient, make sure anyone else in the room is protected from X-rays by a lead shield, a room divider, or sufficient distance.

Normal findings

In the posteroanterior view, the thoracic cage appears at least twice as wide as the heart. However, in the anteroposterior view, relative heart size and position may look different, and the cardiac silhouette and vascular markings may increase.

If cardiac radiography is performed to evaluate the position of cardiac catheters and pacemakers, the films should confirm accurate placement.

Implications of results

Cardiac X-rays must be evaluated in light of the patient's history, physical examination findings, electrocardiography results, and results of previous radiographic tests for cardiac abnormalities.

An abnormal cardiac silhouette usually reflects enlargement of the left or right ventricle or the left atrium. In left ventricular enlargement, the posteroanterior view shows a rounded, convex left-sided heart border, with lateral extension of the lower left border; the lateral view shows posterior bulging of the left ventricle. In right ventricular enlargement, the posteroanterior view shows secondary prominence of the pulmonary artery segment at the left-sided heart border; the lateral view shows anterior bulging in the region of the right ventricular outflow tract.

In left atrial enlargement, the posteroanterior view shows double density of the enlarged left atrium, straightening of the left-sided heart border, elevation of the left main bronchus and, rarely, lateral extension of the right-sided heart border superior to the right ventricle; the lateral view shows a posterior bulge at the level of the left atrium.

In the posteroanterior view, dilation of pulmonary venous shadows in the superior lateral aspect of the hilus and vascular shadows horizontally and inferiorly along the margin of the right side of the heart may be the first signs of pulmonary vascular congestion. Chronic pulmonary venous hypertension produces an antler pattern caused by dilated superior pulmonary veins and normal or constricted inferior pulmonary veins. Acute alveolar edema may produce a butterfly appearance, with increased densities in central lung fields; interstitial pulmonary edema may produce a cloudy or cotton-puff appearance.

Post-test care

▪ None.

Interfering factors

▪ Patient failure to maintain inspiration or to remain motionless during the test interferes with image clarity.
▪ If the patient's chest isn't centered on the film cassette, the costophrenic angle may not be visible on the X-ray.
▪ Thoracic deformity such as scoliosis affects the interpretation of X-rays.
▪ Overexposed or underexposed X-ray films can invalidate the test.

Lower-limb venography

Venography (also known as ascending contrast phlebography), the radiographic examination of a vein, is commonly used to assess the condition of the deep leg veins after injection of a contrast medium. It's the definitive test for deep vein thrombosis (DVT), an acute condition marked by inflammation and thrombus formation in the deep veins of the legs. Such thrombi usually develop in valve pockets — venous junctions or sinuses of the calf muscle — then travel to the deep calf veins; if untreated, they may occlude the popliteal, femoral, and iliac vein systems, which may lead to pulmonary embolism, a potentially lethal complication. Predisposing factors to DVT include vein wall injury, prolonged bed rest, coagulation abnormalities, surgery, childbirth, and use of oral contraceptives.

Venography shouldn't be used for routine screening because it exposes the patient to relatively high doses of radiation and can cause complications, such as phlebitis, local tissue damage and, occasionally, DVT itself. It's also expensive and isn't easily repeated. A combination of three noninvasive tests — Doppler ultrasonography, impedance plethysmography, and ^{125}I fibrinogen scanning — provides an acceptable though less accurate alternative to venography. Radionuclide tests, such as the ^{125}I fibrinogen scan, are also used to detect DVT in a patient who is too ill for venography or is hypersensitive to the contrast medium.

Purpose

■ To confirm diagnosis of DVT
■ To distinguish clot formation from venous obstruction (such as a large tumor of the pelvis impinging on the venous system)
■ To evaluate congenital venous abnormalities
■ To assess deep vein valvular competence (especially helpful in identifying underlying causes of leg edema)
■ To locate a suitable vein for arterial bypass grafting.

Patient preparation

Explain that this test helps detect abnormal conditions in the leg veins. Instruct the patient to restrict food and to drink only clear liquids for 4 hours before the test. Tell him who will perform the test and where and that it takes 30 to 45

minutes. Warn him that he may feel a burning sensation in his leg when the contrast medium is injected and some discomfort during the procedure.

Make sure the patient or a responsible family member has signed a consent form. Check the patient's history for hypersensitivity to iodine, iodine-containing foods, or contrast media. Mark any sensitivities on the chart and notify the doctor. Reassure the patient that contrast media complications are rare, but tell him to report nausea, severe burning or itching, constriction in the throat or chest, or dyspnea at once. If ordered, restrict anticoagulant therapy.

Just before the test, instruct the patient to void, to remove all clothing below the waist, and to put on a hospital gown. If ordered, give an anxious or uncooperative patient a mild sedative.

Procedure

The patient is positioned on a tilting X-ray table so that the leg being tested doesn't bear any weight. (See *Patient positioning for lower-limb venography.*) He is instructed to relax this leg and keep it still; a tourniquet may be tied around the ankle to expedite venous filling. Then normal saline solution is injected into a superficial vein in the dorsum of the patient's foot. Once correct needle placement is achieved, 100 to 150 ml of contrast medium is slowly injected (90 seconds to 3 minutes), and the presence of extravasation is checked. (If a suitable superficial vein can't be found because of edema, a surgical cutdown of the vein may be performed). Using a fluoroscope, the distribution of the contrast medium is monitored, and spot films of the thigh and femoroiliac regions are taken from the anteroposterior and oblique views. Then overhead films are taken of the calf, knee, thigh, and femoral area.

After filming, the patient is repositioned horizontally, the leg being tested

Patient positioning for lower-limb venography

In lower-limb venography, the patient lies on an X-ray table that's inclined 40 to 60 degrees, while keeping his weight off the leg being tested. Fluoroscopy monitors the progress of the contrast medium, and spot films are taken as the contrast circulates through the venous system of the leg.

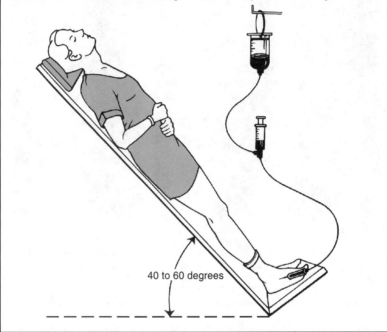

40 to 60 degrees

is quickly elevated, and normal saline solution is infused to flush the contrast medium from the veins. The fluoroscope is checked to confirm complete emptying. Then the needle is removed, and an adhesive bandage is applied to the injection site.

Precautions

 NURSING ALERT Because most allergic reactions to the contrast medium occur within 30 minutes of injection, carefully observe the patient for signs of anaphylaxis: flushing, urticaria, and laryngeal stridor.

Normal findings

A normal venogram shows steady opacification of the superficial and deep vasculature with no filling defects.

Implications of results

A venogram that shows consistent filling defects on repeat views, abrupt termination of a column of contrast material, unfilled major deep veins, or diversion of flow (through collaterals, for example) is diagnostic of DVT. (See *Abnormal venograms,* page 896.)

Post-test care

■ Monitor vital signs until stable; check the pulse rate on the dorsalis pedis, popliteal, and femoral arteries.

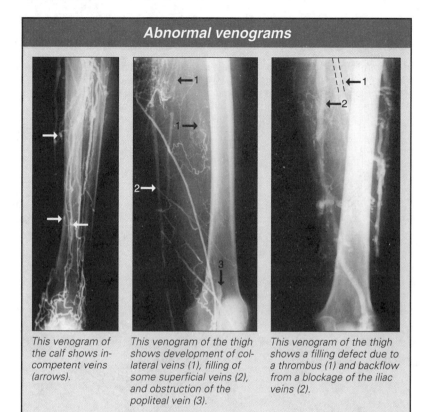

Abnormal venograms

This venogram of the calf shows incompetent veins (arrows).

This venogram of the thigh shows development of collateral veins (1), filling of some superficial veins (2), and obstruction of the popliteal vein (3).

This venogram of the thigh shows a filling defect due to a thrombus (1) and backflow from a blockage of the iliac veins (2).

■ Administer analgesics, as ordered, to counteract the irritating effects of the contrast medium.

■ Watch for hematoma, redness, bleeding, or infection (especially if a cutdown of the vein was performed) at the puncture site, and replace the dressing when necessary. Notify the doctor if complications develop.

■ If the venogram indicates DVT, initiate therapy (heparin infusion, bed rest, leg elevation or support, blood chemistry tests), as ordered.

■ As ordered, the patient may resume his usual diet and medications.

Interfering factors

■ If the patient places weight on the leg being tested, the contrast medium may fail to fill the leg veins.

■ Movement of the leg being tested, excessive tourniquet constriction, insufficient injection of contrast medium, or delay between injection and radiography affect the accuracy of test results.

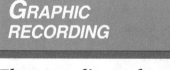

GRAPHIC RECORDING

Electrocardiography

Electrocardiography, the most commonly used test for evaluating cardiac status, graphically records the electrical current (electrical potential) generated by the heart. This current radiates from the heart in all directions and, on reaching the skin, is measured by electrodes connected to an amplifier and strip chart recorder. The standard resting (scalar) electrocardiogram (ECG) uses 5 electrodes to measure the electrical potential from 12 different leads: the standard limb leads (I, II, III), the augmented limb leads (aV_F, aV_L, and aV_R), and the precordial, or chest, leads (V$_1$ through V$_6$).

ECG tracings normally consist of three identifiable waveforms: the P wave, the QRS complex, and the T wave. The P wave depicts atrial depolarization; the QRS complex, ventricular depolarization; and the T wave, ventricular repolarization. Although the ECG records only about 50 to 100 of the more than 100,000 cardiac cycles that occur in 24 hours, it's useful for detecting the presence and location of myocardial infarction (MI), ischemia, conduction delays, chamber enlargement, arrhythmias, and myocardial necrosis.

New, computerized ECG machines do not routinely use gel and suction bulbs. The electrodes are small tabs that peel off a sheet and adhere to the patient's skin. The leads coming from the ECG machine are clearly marked (LA, RA, LL, RL, V$_1$ through V$_6$) and are applied to the electrodes with alligator clamps. The entire ECG tracing is displayed on a screen so that abnormalities (loose leads or artifacts) can be corrected before printing; then it's printed on one sheet of paper. The electrode tabs can remain on the patient's chest, arms, and legs to provide continuous lead placements for serial ECG studies.

Purpose
■ To help identify primary conduction abnormalities, cardiac arrhythmias, cardiac hypertrophy, pericarditis, electrolyte imbalance, myocardial ischemia, and the site and extent of MI (see *Right ventricular MI,* page 898)
■ To monitor recovery from MI
■ To evaluate the effectiveness of cardiac medication (digitalis glycosides, antiarrhythmics, antihypertensives, and vasodilators)
■ To observe pacemaker performance
■ To determine the effectiveness of thrombolytic therapy and the resolution of ST-segment depression or elevation and T-wave changes.

Patient preparation
Explain to the patient that this test evaluates the heart's function by recording its electrical activity. Inform him that he needn't restrict food or fluids before the test. Tell him who will perform the test and where, that the test is painless, and that it takes 5 to 10 minutes.

Inform the patient that electrodes will be attached to his arms, legs, and chest. Tell him he'll be asked to lie still, to relax, and to breathe normally during the procedure. Advise him not to talk during the test because the sound of his voice may distort the ECG tracing.

Check the patient's history for use of cardiac drugs, and note any current therapy on the test request form.

Equipment
ECG machine ✦ recording paper ✦ pregelled disposable electrodes ✦ shaving supplies (if necessary) ✦ marking pen ✦ moist towel (for cleanup).

Procedure
Place the patient in the supine position. If he can't tolerate lying flat, help him to semi-Fowler's position. Instruct him to expose his chest, both ankles, and both wrists for electrode placement. Drape the female patient's chest until chest leads are applied. Check the paper supply.

For multichannel ECG: Place electrodes on the inner aspect of the wrists,

Right ventricular MI

Effective treatment for a patient with an acute inferior wall myocardial infarction (MI) depends on an accurate assessment of the right side of the heart. To obtain an electrocardiogram of the right side, reverse the precordial lead placement to provide a better picture of the electrical activity on the right side of the heart. This illustration shows correct placement of the six precordial leads.

Treatment for a right ventricular MI differs from that for a left ventricular MI. A patient with a right ventricular MI requires volume expansion to increase right ventricular end-diastolic volume; one with a left ventricular MI usually requires conventional diuretic therapy.

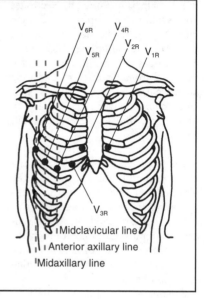

the medial aspect of the lower legs, and on the chest. (For the proper chest positions, see *Standard 12-lead ECG*.) If you're using disposable electrodes, remove the paper backing before positioning them. Then connect the leadwires after all electrodes are in place.

If frequent ECGs will be necessary, indicate lead positions on the patient's chest with a marking pen to ensure consistent placement. Press the START button and input any required information (for example, patient's name and room number). The machine will produce a printout showing all 12 leads simultaneously on thermal or pressure-sensitive recording paper.

As the machine records the ECG, make sure that all leads are represented in the tracing. If not, determine which one has come loose, reattach it, and restart the tracing. Also make sure that the wave doesn't peak beyond the top edge of the recording grid. If it does, adjust

the machine to bring the wave inside the boundaries. When the machine finishes the tracing, remove the electrodes and reposition the patient's gown and bed covers.

For single-channel ECG: Apply either disposable or standard electrodes to the inner aspects of the wrists and medial aspects of the lower legs. Connect each leadwire to the corresponding electrode by inserting the wire prong into the terminal post and tightening the screw.

Set the paper speed to 25 mm/second or as ordered. Calibrate the machine by adjusting the sensitivity to normal and checking the quality and baseline position of the tracing. Recalibrate the machine after running each lead to provide a consistent test standard. Turn the lead selector to I. Then mark the lead by writing "I" on the paper strip or by depressing the marking button on the machine. (Some machines do this automatically.) Record for 3 to 6 seconds, and then re-

Standard 12-lead ECG

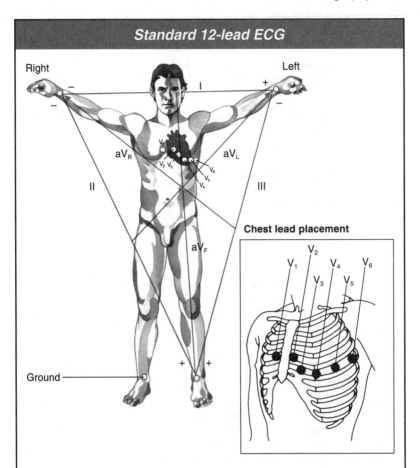

In a standard 12-lead electrocardiogram (ECG), 10 electrodes (4 limb, 6 chest) record the heart's electrical potential from 12 different views, or leads. Standard bipolar limb leads (I, II, III) detect variations in electrical potential at two points (the negative pole and the positive pole) and record the difference. When current flows toward the positive pole, the ECG wave deflects upward; when it flows toward the negative pole, the wave inverts. (The arrows, called Einthoven's reference lines, form a triangle indicating the direction in which electrical current moves to produce a positive [upward] deflection.)

Lead I connects the left and the right arms, and the ECG tracing shows an upward deflection because the left arm is positive and the right arm, negative. Lead II connects the left leg and right arm, and the tracing deflects upward because the left leg is positive and the right arm, negative. Lead III connects the left leg and left arm, and the tracing deflects upward because the left leg is positive and the left arm, negative.

The unipolar augmented limb leads (aV_F, aV_L, and aV_R), which use the same electrode placement as standard limb leads, measure electrical potential be-

(continued)

Standard 12-lead ECG (continued)

tween one augmented limb lead and the electrical midpoint of the remaining two leads (determined electronically by the ECG machine). Both standard and augmented leads measure electrical potential while viewing the heart from the front, in a vertical plane.

The six unipolar chest leads (V_1 through V_6), shown in the inset on page 899, view the electrical potential from a horizontal plane that helps locate disorders in the lateral, anterior, and posterior walls of the heart. The ECG machine averages the electrical potentials of all three limb lead electrodes. Recordings made with the V connection show electrical potential variations that occur under the chest electrode as its position is changed.

---

turn the machine to the standby mode. Repeat this procedure for leads II, III, aV_F, aV_L, and aV_R.

Determine the proper placement for the chest electrodes. If frequent ECGs are necessary, indicate lead positions on the patient's chest with a marking pen to ensure consistent placement. Connect the chest leadwire to the suction bulb in the same manner that you connect the limb electrodes. Apply gel to each of the six chest positions; then firmly press the suction bulb to attach the chest lead to the V_1 position. Mark the strips as before. Then turn the lead selector to V and record V_1 for 3 to 6 seconds. Return the lead selector to standby. Reposition the electrode and repeat the procedure for V_2 to V_6.

After completing V_6, run a rhythm strip on lead II for at least 6 seconds. Assess the quality of the tracings, and repeat any that are unclear. Disconnect the equipment, remove the electrodes, and wipe the gel from the patient with a moist cloth towel. Wash the gel from the electrodes and dry them well.

Each ECG strip should be labeled with the patient's name and room number (if applicable), the date and time of the procedure, and the doctor's name. Note whether the ECG was performed during or upon resolution of a chest pain episode.

Precautions

■ All recording and other nearby electrical equipment should be properly grounded to prevent electrical interference, which distorts ECG recording.

■ Double-check color codes and lead markings to make sure that connectors match.

■ Ensure that electrodes are firmly attached; reattach them if you suspect loose skin contact.

■ Make sure the patient is quiet and motionless during the test because talking or movement distorts the recordings.

■ If the patient has a pacemaker in place, the ECG may be performed with or without a magnet. Indicate on the laboratory request and the patient's record that a pacemaker is present and whether or not a magnet is used. (Many pacemakers function only when the heartbeat falls below a preset rate; a magnet makes the pacemaker fire regularly, which permits evaluation of pacemaker performance.)

Normal findings

The lead II waveform, known as the rhythm strip, depicts the heart's rhythm more clearly than any other waveform. (See *Normal ECG waveforms.*) In lead II, the normal P wave does not exceed 2.5 mm (0.25 mV) in height or last longer than 0.11 second. The PR interval,

Normal ECG waveforms

Because each lead takes a different view of heart activity, it generates its own characteristic tracing. The traces shown here represent each of the 12 leads. Leads aV_R, V_1, V_2, and V_3 normally show strong negative deflections below the baseline. Negative deflections indicate that the electrical current is flowing away from the positive electrode; positive deflections, that the current is flowing toward the positive electrode.

Lead I

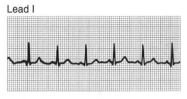

Lead II

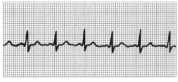

Lead III

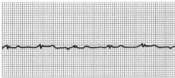

Lead aV_R

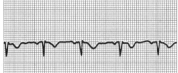

Lead aV_L

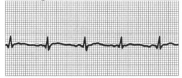

Lead aV_F

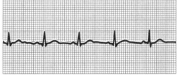

Lead V_1

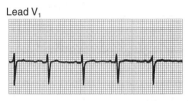

Lead V_2

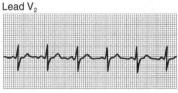

Lead V_3

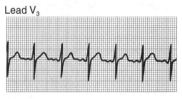

Lead V_4

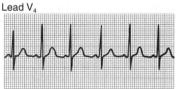

Lead V_5

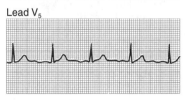

Lead V_6

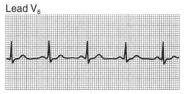

ST-segment monitoring

ST-segment monitoring, a useful tool for bedside monitoring of myocardial ischemia and infarction, helps provide a more accurate and timely diagnosis of the patient's problem. The technology consists of a software package that can be added to current hardware monitoring systems.

During monitoring, a computer stores the baseline ST-segment data and compares it with the electrical activity being generated by the patient and transmitted to the computer. The method of analysis varies, depending on the hardware and software used.

Tracking ST changes
The computer can track ST-segment changes and trends to help identify ischemic and other ST-related changes as they occur. This allows you to gauge a patient's ability to tolerate activity and procedures. For instance, if you note ST-segment elevation during activity, you can immediately alter, interrupt, or postpone the activity to reverse the ischemic event or initiate treatment. If necessary, ST-related changes can also be compared with a 12-lead electrocardiogram so that appropriate interventions can be started quickly.

Indications
Continuous ST-segment monitoring is useful in patients with known coronary artery disease and after cardiac surgery, thrombolytic therapy, transluminal coronary angioplasty, chest trauma, head injury, and major surgery requiring massive transfusion. It also helps diagnose and monitor patients with episodes of "silent" ischemia by determining precipitating events.

which includes the P wave and the PR segment, persists for 0.12 to 0.2 second for cardiac rates over 60 beats/minute. The QT interval varies with the cardiac rate and lasts 0.4 to 0.52 second for rates above 60; the voltage of the R wave in the V_1 through V_6 leads doesn't exceed 27 mm. The total QRS interval lasts 0.06 to 0.1 second.

ST-segment data is also useful for assessing myocardial ischemia. (See *ST-segment monitoring.*)

Implications of results

An abnormal ECG may show MI, right or left ventricular hypertrophy, arrhythmias, right or left bundle-branch block, ischemia, conduction defects or pericarditis, electrolyte abnormalities such as hypokalemia, or the effects of cardioactive drugs. Sometimes an ECG may reveal abnormal waveforms only during episodes of angina or during exercise. (See *Some abnormal ECG waveforms.*)

Post-test care

Disconnect the equipment. The electrode patches are usually left in place if the patient is having recurrent chest pain or if serial ECGs are ordered, as with the use of thrombolytics.

Interfering factors

■ Mechanical difficulties, such as ECG machine malfunction, electrode patches that don't adhere well (for example, from diaphoresis), or electromagnetic interference, can produce artifacts.
■ Improper placement of electrodes, patient movement or muscle tremor, strenuous exercise before the test, or

Some abnormal ECG waveforms

Premature ventricular contractions (lead V₁)

Premature ventricular contractions (PVCs) originate in an ectopic focus of the ventricular wall. They can be unifocal (having the same single focus), as shown in this tracing from lead V₁, or multifocal, arising from more than one ectopic focus. In PVCs, the P wave is absent, and the QRS complex shows 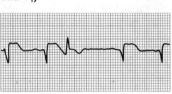 considerable distortion, usually deflecting in the opposite direction from the patient's normal QRS. The T wave also deflects in the opposite direction from the QRS complex, and the PVC usually precedes a compensatory pause. Some causes of PVCs include electrolyte imbalance (especially hypokalemia), a previous myocardial infarction, hypoxia, and drug toxicity (digitalis glycosides or beta-adrenergics).

First-degree heart block (lead V₁)

First-degree heart block — the most common conduction disturbance — occurs in healthy hearts as well as in diseased hearts and is usually clinically insignificant. It's often characteristic in elderly patients with 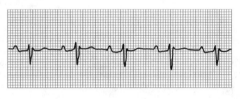 chronic degeneration of the cardiac conduction system, and it occasionally occurs in patients receiving digitalis glycosides or antiarrhythmics (such as procainamide or quinidine). In children, first-degree heart block may be the earliest sign of acute rheumatic fever. In this lead V₁ tracing, the interval between the P wave and QRS complex (the PR interval) exceeds 0.20 second.

Hypokalemia (lead V₁)

A common type of electrolyte imbalance caused by low blood potassium levels, hypokalemia affects the electrical activity of the myocardium. Mild hypokalemia may cause only 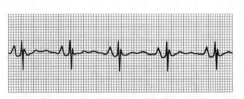 muscle weakness and fatigue, and possibly atrial or ventricular irritability; a severe deficiency causes pronounced muscle weakness, paralysis, atrial tachycardia with varying degrees of block, and PVCs that may progress to ventricular tachycardia and fibrillation.

Early electrocardiogram (ECG) indicators of hypokalemia, as shown on this V₁ tracing, include prominent U waves, a prolonged QU interval, and flat or inverted T waves. T waves do not usually flatten or invert until potassium depletion becomes severe.

(continued)

Some abnormal ECG waveforms *(continued)*

Stages of MI

Myocardial infarction (MI) produces typical ECG changes in several leads at once, enabling the doctor to determine the exact location and extent of tissue damage. MI causes three changes: an inner zone of tissue necrosis, a surrounding zone of inflamed tissue, and an outer zone of ischemia (as shown below). As the infarction progresses, the first ECG change is an elevated ST segment, which indicates formation of an ischemic zone. Then the T wave begins to flatten and finally inverts, and enlarged Q waves appear, indicating developing necrosis — a true infarction. (Abnormal Q waves should be larger than one small square on the chart — 0.04 second by 0.1 mV.) The T wave may stay inverted for the rest of the patient's life, or it can revert to normal, while the deep Q wave remains as a permanent indicator of necrosis. The infarction can be located by studying the characteristic ST-, T-, and Q-wave changes in various lead combinations.

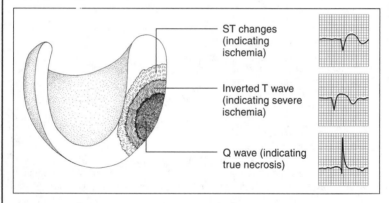

ST changes (indicating ischemia)

Inverted T wave (indicating severe ischemia)

Q wave (indicating true necrosis)

ECG changes in an inferior MI

In the three tracings shown below, the ST segments elevated in leads I, II, and aV$_F$ indicate an infarction in the inferior (diaphragmatic) area of the heart.

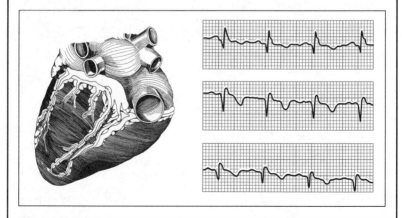

medication reactions can produce inaccurate test results.

Exercise electrocardiography

Exercise electrocardiography (commonly known as a stress test) evaluates heart action during physical stress — when the demand for oxygen increases — and thus provides important diagnostic information that can't be obtained from a resting electrocardiogram (ECG) alone.

In this test, ECG and blood pressure readings are taken while the patient walks on a treadmill or pedals a stationary bicycle, and his response to a constant or an increasing workload is observed. Unless complications develop, the test continues until the patient reaches the target heart rate (determined by an established protocol) or experiences chest pain or fatigue. The patient with recent myocardial infarction (MI) or coronary artery surgery may walk the treadmill at a slow pace to determine his activity tolerance before discharge from the hospital.

The risk of MI during exercise ECG is less than 1 in 500; the risk of death, less than 1 in 10,000.

Purpose
■ To help diagnose the cause of chest pain or other possible cardiac pain
■ To determine the functional capacity of the heart after surgery or MI
■ To screen for asymptomatic coronary artery disease (CAD), particularly in men over age 35
■ To help set limitations for an exercise program
■ To identify cardiac arrhythmias that develop during physical exercise
■ To evaluate the effectiveness of antiarrhythmic or antianginal therapy.

Patient preparation
Explain to the patient that this test records the heart's electrical activity and performance under stress. Instruct him not to eat, smoke, or drink alcoholic or caffeinated beverages for 3 hours before the test, but to continue any drug regimen unless the doctor directs otherwise. Tell him who will perform the test and where.

Inform the patient that the test will cause him to feel fatigued, slightly breathless, and sweaty, but inform him that it has few risks and that he may stop the test if he experiences fatigue or chest pain. Advise him to wear comfortable socks and shoes, and loose, lightweight shorts or slacks during the procedure; men usually don't wear a shirt during the test, and women generally wear a bra and a lightweight short-sleeved blouse or a patient gown with a front closure.

Inform the patient that several areas on his chest and, possibly, on his back will be cleaned and abraded to prepare the skin for the electrodes. Tell him that he won't feel any current from the electrodes but that the electrode sites may itch slightly. Mention that his blood pressure will be checked periodically throughout the procedure, and reassure him that his heart rate will be monitored continuously.

If the patient is scheduled for a multistage *treadmill test,* explain that the speed and incline of the treadmill increase at predetermined intervals and that he'll be informed of each adjustment. If he's scheduled for a *bicycle ergometer test,* explain that the resistance he experiences in pedaling increases gradually as he tries to maintain a spe-

Comparing treadmill and bicycle ergometer tests

Treadmill test

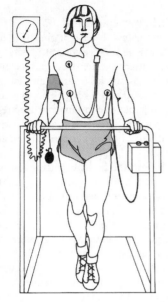

Advantages
- Standardized and most reproducible
- Walking is a familiar activity
- Constant work rate
- Attains highest maximum oxygen uptake
- Involves muscles commonly used (less chance of fatigue)

Disadvantages
- Possibility of patient losing balance and falling off
- Workload depends on weight (as weight increases, workload increases)
- Harder to obtain blood pressure readings and electrocardiogram (ECG) recordings because upper body is in motion
- Expensive
- Noisy, making communication with patient more difficult

Bicycle ergometer test

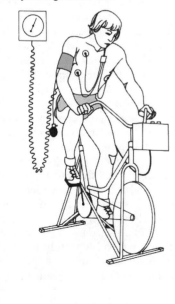

Advantages
- Workload doesn't depend on weight
- Easy to obtain blood pressure readings and ECG recordings because upper body remains relatively still
- Less expensive

Disadvantages
- Constant rate of pedaling required to maintain power
- Frequent calibration necessary
- Induces more stress
- Attains lower maximum oxygen uptake
- Involves muscles less commonly used (more chance of fatigue)

cific speed. (See *Comparing treadmill and bicycle ergometer tests.*) Encourage the patient to report his feelings during the test. Tell him his blood pressure and ECG will be monitored for 10 to 15 minutes after the test.

Check the patient's history for a recent physical examination (within 1 week) and for baseline 12-lead ECG results. Make sure the patient or a responsible family member has signed a consent form.

Procedure

The electrode sites are thoroughly cleaned with an alcohol pad. The superficial epidermal cell layer and excess skin oils are removed with a gauze pad, fine sandpaper, or dental burr. After thorough cleaning and abrading, adequately prepared sites will appear slightly red.

Chest electrodes are placed according to the lead system selected and are secured with adhesive tape or a rubber belt. The leadwire cable is placed over the patient's shoulder, and the leadwire box is placed on his chest. The cable is secured by pinning it to the patient's clothing or taping it to his shoulder or back. Then the leadwires are connected to the chest electrodes. (See *Electrode placement for exercise ECG,* page 908.)

The monitor is started, and a stable baseline tracing is obtained. A baseline rhythm strip is checked for arrhythmias. Then a blood pressure reading is taken, and the patient is auscultated for S_3 or S_4 gallops and crackles.

For the treadmill test: The treadmill is turned on to a slow speed, and the patient is shown how to step onto it and how to use the support railings to maintain balance but not to support weight. Then the treadmill is turned off. The patient is instructed to step onto the treadmill, and it is turned on to a slow speed until the patient gets used to walking on it.

For the bicycle ergometer test: The patient is instructed to sit on the bicycle. The seat and handlebars are adjusted, if necessary, so that he can pedal the bike comfortably. The patient is instructed not to grip the handlebars tightly, but to use them only for maintaining balance, and to pedal until he reaches the desired speed, as shown on the speedometer.

In both tests, a monitor is observed continuously for changes in the heart's electrical activity. The rhythm strip is checked at preset intervals for arrhythmias, premature ventricular contractions (PVCs), ST-segment changes, and T-wave changes. The test level and the amount of time it took to reach that level are marked on each strip. Blood pressure is monitored at predetermined intervals — usually at the end of each test level — and changes in systolic readings are noted. Some common responses to maximal exercise are dizziness, lightheadedness, leg fatigue, dyspnea, diaphoresis, and a slightly ataxic gait.

If symptoms become severe, the test is stopped. Usually, testing stops when the patient reaches the target heart rate. As the treadmill speed slows, he may be instructed to continue walking for several minutes to prevent nausea or dizziness. Then the treadmill is turned off, the patient is helped to a chair, and his blood pressure and ECG are monitored for 10 to 15 minutes.

Precautions

■ Because exercise ECG places considerable stress on the heart, it may be contraindicated in patients with ventricular or dissecting aortic aneurysm, uncontrolled arrhythmias, pericarditis, myocarditis, severe anemia, uncontrolled hypertension, unstable angina, or congestive heart failure.

■ Stop the test immediately if the ECG shows three consecutive PVCs or any

Electrode placement for exercise ECG

If you're working with a three-electrode monitor, you can establish the three standard leads (I, II, III) and the three augmented limb leads (aV_F, aV_L, aV_R). However, if you want to obtain readings similar to the V_1 and V_6 chest leads, you can use modified chest leads (MCL_1, MCL_6). If you're using a five-electrode monitor, the most sensitive of these recording devices, you can record standard and augmented leads as well as the six chest leads.

TYPE	LEAD	ELECTRODE PLACEMENT	
Three-electrode monitor	Lead II	Positive (+): left side of chest, lowest palpable rib, mid-clavicular line Negative (-): right shoulder, below clavicular hollow Ground (G): left shoulder, below clavicular hollow	
	MCL_1	Positive (+): right sternal border, lowest palpable rib Negative (-): left shoulder, below clavicular hollow Ground (G): right shoulder, below clavicular hollow	
	MCL_6	Positive (+): left side of chest, lowest palpable rib, mid-clavicular line Negative (-): left shoulder, below clavicular hollow Ground (G): right shoulder, below clavicular hollow	
Five-electrode monitor	V_1 through V_6	Positive (+): left side of chest, just below lowest palpable rib Negative (-): right shoulder, midclavicular line Ground (G): right side of chest, just below lowest palpable rib Inactive (I): left shoulder, midclavicular line Chest V_1: fourth intercostal space to right of sternum Chest V_2: fourth intercostal space to left of sternum Chest V_3: halfway between V_2 and V_4 Chest V_4: fifth intercostal space, midclavicular line, left side Chest V_5: halfway between V_4 and V_6 Chest V_6: same line as V_5 at midaxillary line	

significant increase in ectopy, if systolic blood pressure falls below resting level, if the heart rate falls 10 beats/minute below resting level, or if the patient becomes exhausted. Depending on the patient's condition, the test may be stopped if the ECG shows bundle-branch block, ST-segment depression exceeding 1.5 to 2 mm, or frequent or complicated PVCs; if blood pressure fails to rise above resting level; if systolic pressure exceeds 220 mm Hg; or if the patient experiences angina. The test will also be stopped if the examiner suspects that persistent ST-segment elevation may indicate transmural myocardial ischemia.

Normal findings

In a normal exercise ECG, the P, QRS, and T waves and the ST segment change slightly; a slight ST-segment depression occurs in some patients, especially women. The heart rate rises in direct proportion to the workload and metabolic oxygen demand; systolic blood pressure also rises as workload increases. The normal patient attains the endurance levels appropriate for his age and the exercise protocol.

Implications of results

Although criteria for judging test results vary, two findings strongly suggest an abnormality: a flat or downsloping ST-segment depression of 1 mm or more for at least 0.08 second after the junction of the QRS and ST segments (J point); and a markedly depressed J point, with an upsloping, but depressed, ST segment of 1.5 mm below the baseline 0.08 second after the J point. T-wave inversion also signifies ischemia. Initial ST-segment depression on the resting ECG must be further depressed by 1 mm during exercise to be considered abnormal.

Hypotension resulting from exercise, ST depression of 3 mm or more, downsloping ST segments, and ischemic ST segments appearing within the first 3 minutes of exercise and lasting 8 minutes into the post-test recovery period may indicate multivessel or left CAD. ST-segment elevation may indicate dyskinetic left ventricular wall motion or severe transmural ischemia. (See *Abnormal exercise ECG tracings,* page 910.)

The predictive value of this test for CAD varies with the patient's history and sex; however, false-negative and false-positive test results are common. To detect CAD accurately, thallium imaging and stress testing, exercise multiple-gated acquisition scanning, or coronary angiography may be necessary.

Post-test care

- Assist the patient to a chair, and continue monitoring heart rate and blood pressure for 10 to 15 minutes or until the ECG returns to baseline.
- Auscultate for S_3 or S_4 gallops. In many patients, an S_4 gallop develops after exercise because of increased blood flow volume and turbulence. However, an S_3 gallop — indicating transient left ventricular dysfunction — is more significant than an S_4 gallop.
- Tell the patient that he may resume any activites discontinued before the test.
- Remove the electrodes and clean the electrode sites before the patient leaves.

Interfering factors

- The patient's failure to observe pretest restrictions hinders the heart's ability to respond to stress.
- Use of beta blockers may make test results difficult to interpret.
- Inability to exercise to the target heart rate because of fatigue or failure to cooperate interferes with accurate testing.
- Wolff-Parkinson-White syndrome (anomalous atrioventricular excitation), electrolyte imbalance, or use of a digi-

Abnormal exercise ECG tracings

The abnormal exercise electrocardiogram (ECG) tracings shown below were obtained during a treadmill test performed on a patient who had just undergone a triple coronary artery bypass graft. The first tracing shows the heart at rest with blood pressure of 124/80 mm Hg. In the second tracing, the patient worked up to a 10% grade at 1.7 mph before experiencing angina at 2 minutes, 25 seconds. The tracing shows a depressed ST segment; heart rate was 85 beats/minute, and blood pressure was 140/70 mm Hg. The third tracing shows the heart at rest 6 minutes after the test; blood pressure was 140/90 mm Hg.

Resting

Angina

Recovery

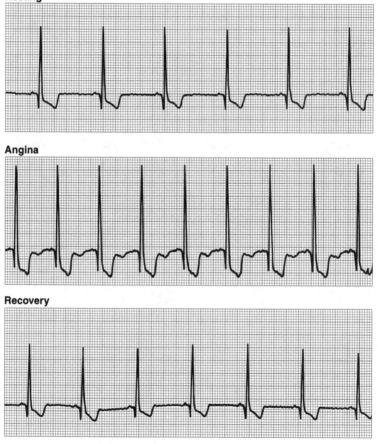

talis glycoside may cause false-positive results.

■ Conditions that cause left ventricular hypertrophy (congenital abnormalities, hypertension) may interfere with testing for ischemia.

Holter monitoring

Holter monitoring (also known as ambulatory electrocardiography [ECG] monitoring) is the continuous recording of heart activity as the patient follows his normal routine, usually for 24 hours or about 100,000 cardiac cycles. In this test (named for the scientist who developed it), the patient wears a small cassette tape recorder connected to electrodes placed on his chest and keeps a diary of his activities and any associated symptoms. At the end of the recording period, the tape is analyzed by a microcomputer and a report is printed, permitting correlation of cardiac irregularities, such as arrhythmias and ST-segment changes, with the activities in the patient's diary.

Although Holter monitoring is not a substitute for coronary care unit surveillance, it can detect sporadic arrhythmias missed by an exercise or resting ECG. It can also evaluate the status of a patient recuperating from an acute myocardial infarction (MI); in such a patient, monitoring may uncover electrical instability or ischemia that delays hospital discharge or requires a change in therapy, additional therapy, or a revised rehabilitation plan.

Patient-activated monitors can be worn for 5 to 7 days. With these devices, the patient manually initiates recording of heart activity only when he experiences symptoms. Intermittent monitoring, triggered only by an unusual heart rhythm, is used in cardiac research.

Purpose
- To detect cardiac arrhythmias
- To evaluate chest pain
- To evaluate cardiac status after acute MI or pacemaker implantation
- To evaluate effectiveness of antiarrhythmic drug therapy
- To assess and correlate dyspnea, central nervous system symptoms (such as syncope and light-headedness), and palpitations with actual cardiac events and the patient's activities.

Patient preparation
Explain to the patient that this test helps determine how his heart responds to normal activity or, if appropriate, to cardioactive medication. Inform him that electrodes will be attached to his chest, that his chest may be shaved, and that he may experience some discomfort during preparation of the electrode sites. Tell him that he'll need to wear a small tape recorder for 24 hours (or for 5 to 7 days if a patient-activated monitor is being used). Mention that a shoulder strap or a special belt will be provided to carry the recorder, which weighs about 2 lb (1 kg). Show him how to position the recorder when he lies down.

Encourage the patient to continue his routine activities during the monitoring period. Stress the importance of logging these activities (including walking, stair climbing, urinating, sleeping, and sexual activity) as well as emotional upsets, physical symptoms (dizziness, palpitations, fatigue, chest pain, and syncope), and ingestion of medication; show the patient a sample diary. Demonstrate how to mark the tape at the onset of symptoms, if applicable. (If a patient-activated monitor is being used, show the patient how to press the EVENT button to activate the monitor if he experiences any unusual sensations.)

Advise the patient to wear loose-fitting clothing with front-buttoning tops during monitoring. Instruct him not to tamper with the monitor or to disconnect the leadwires or electrodes. Bathing instructions depend on the type of recorder being worn because certain equipment must not get wet. Tell him to avoid magnets, metal detectors, high-voltage areas, and electric blankets. Show him how to check the recorder to make sure it's working properly. Explain that if the monitor light flashes, one of the electrodes may be loose and he should depress the center of each one. Tell him to notify you if one comes off.

If the patient won't be returning to the office or hospital immediately after the monitoring period, show him how to remove and store the equipment. Remind him to bring the diary when he returns.

Procedure

The electrode sites are cleaned with an alcohol pad and gently abraded until they redden. After the backings are peeled off, the electrodes are applied to the correct sites; the sides and bottom of each electrode are pressed firmly to ensure that the adhesive portion of the electrode is securely fastened to the skin. Then the center of the electrode is pressed lightly to promote good contact between the jelly and the patient's skin. The electrode cable should be securely attached to the monitor. The monitor (and case) is positioned as the patient will wear it; then the leadwires are attached to the electrodes. There shouldn't be too much slack or pull on the wires.

After a new or fully charged battery is installed in the recorder, the tape is inserted and the recorder is turned on. The electrode attachment circuit is tested by connecting the recorder to a standard ECG machine. Watch for artifacts while the patient moves normally (stands and sits).

Precautions

■ To eliminate muscle artifacts, make sure that the lead cable is firmly plugged in. Also make sure that the electrodes aren't placed over large muscle masses such as the pectorals.

Normal findings

When compared with the patient's diary, a normal ECG pattern shows no significant arrhythmias or ST-segment changes. Changes in heart rate normally occur during various activities.

Implications of results

Cardiac abnormalities detected by Holter monitoring include premature ventricular contractions (PVCs), conduction defects, tachyarrhythmias, bradyarrhythmias, and bradycardia-tachycardia syndrome. Arrhythmias may be associated with dyspnea and central nervous system symptoms, such as dizziness and syncope. During recovery from an MI, this test can monitor for PVCs to help determine the prognosis and the effectiveness of drug therapy.

ST-T wave changes associated with ischemia may coincide with chest pain or increased patient activity. ST-segment changes associated with an acute MI require careful study because smoking, eating, postural changes, use of certain drugs, Wolff-Parkinson-White syndrome, bundle-branch block, myocarditis, myocardial hypertrophy, anemia, hypoxemia, and abnormal hemoglobin binding can produce a similar tracing on the ECG. Monitoring the MI patient 1 to 3 days before discharge and again 4 to 6 weeks after discharge may detect ST-T wave changes associated with ischemia or arrhythmias; such information helps determine appropriate therapy and rehabilitation and clarifies the prognosis. Monitoring a patient with an artificial pacemaker may detect an arrhythmia that the pacemaker fails to override such as bradycardia.

Although Holter monitoring correlates the patient's symptoms and ECG changes, it doesn't always identify their causes. If initial monitoring proves inconclusive, the test may be repeated.

Post-test care
Remove all chest electrodes, and clean the electrode sites.

Interfering factors
- Failure to apply the electrodes correctly can cause muscle or movement artifact.
- The patient's failure to record daily activities and symptoms carefully or to maintain his normal routine interferes with accurate testing.
- If a patient-activated monitor is used, the patient's failure to turn on the monitor during symptoms interferes with accurate testing.
- Physiologic variation in frequency and severity of arrhythmias may cause an arrhythmia to be missed during 24-hour Holter monitoring.

Impedance plethysmography

Impedance plethysmography — a reliable, widely used, noninvasive test for measuring venous flow in the limbs — aims principally to detect deep vein thrombosis (DVT) in the leg. In this test (also known as occlusive impedance phlebography), electrodes from a plethysmograph are applied to the patient's leg to record changes in electrical resistance (impedance) caused by blood volume variations — the result of normal respiration or venous occlusion. If a pressure cuff applied to the thigh is inflated to temporarily occlude venous return without interfering with arterial blood flow, blood volume in the calf distal to the cuff normally increases. However, in DVT, blood volume increases less than expected because the veins are

already at capacity and cuff release causes an abnormally slow return of blood volume to physiologic levels.

This test is especially sensitive for DVT in the popliteal and iliofemoral venous systems. It's less sensitive for calf vein clots or partially occlusive thrombi, which are less likely to cause detectable obstruction in veins below the knee.

Purpose
- To detect DVT in the proximal deep veins of the leg
- To screen patients at high risk for thrombophlebitis
- To evaluate patients with suspected pulmonary embolism (because most pulmonary emboli are complications of DVT in the leg).

Patient preparation
Explain to the patient that this test helps detect DVT. Inform him that he needn't restrict food, fluids, or medications before the test. Tell him the test requires that both legs be tested and that three to five tracings may be made for each leg, who will perform the test and where, and that it takes 30 to 45 minutes. Assure him that the test is painless and safe.

Emphasize that he'll need to relax his leg muscles and breathe normally to ensure accurate testing. Reassure him that if he experiences pain that interferes with leg relaxation, he'll receive a mild analgesic if ordered. Just before the test, instruct the patient to urinate and to put on a hospital gown.

Procedure
The patient is placed in the supine position with the leg being tested elevated 30 to 35 degrees to promote venous drainage (the calf should be above the heart level). He is asked to flex his knee slightly and to rotate his hips by shifting weight to the same side as the leg being tested.

After the electrodes (connected to the plethysmograph) have been loosely attached to the calf, about 3" to 4" (7.5 to 10 cm) apart, the pressure cuff (connected to an air pressure system) is wrapped snugly around the thigh — about 2" (5 cm) above the knee. Then the pressure cuff is inflated with 45 to 60 cm of water, allowing full venous distention without interfering with arterial blood flow. Pressure is maintained for 45 seconds or until the tracing stabilizes. (In a patient with reduced arterial blood flow, pressure is maintained for 2 minutes or longer to permit complete venous filling; then the cuff pressure is rapidly deflated.)

The strip chart tracing, which records the increase in venous volume after cuff inflation and the decrease in venous volume 3 seconds after deflation, is checked. The test is repeated for the other leg. If necessary, three to five tracings for each leg are obtained to confirm full venous filling and outflow; the tracing showing the greatest rise and fall in venous volume is used as the test result. If the result is ambiguous, the position of the patient's leg and cuff and electrode placement are checked.

Precautions
None.

Normal findings
Temporary venous occlusion normally produces a sharp rise in venous volume; release of the occlusion produces rapid venous outflow.

Implications of results
When clots in a major deep vein obstruct venous outflow, the pressure in the distal leg (calf) veins rises, and these veins become distended. Such veins are unable to expand further when additional pressure is applied with an occlusive thigh cuff. Blockage of major deep veins also decreases the rate at which blood flows from the leg. If significant thrombi are present in a major deep vein of the lower leg (popliteal, femoral, or iliac), both calf vein filling and venous outflow rate are reduced. In such cases. the doctor will evaluate the need for further treatment such as anticoagulant therapy, taking the patient's overall condition into consideration.

Post-test care
Make sure the conductive jelly is removed from the patient's skin.

Interfering factors
■ Decreased peripheral arterial blood flow due to shock, increased vasoconstriction, low cardiac output, or arterial occlusive disease may interfere with test results.
■ Extrinsic venous compression, as from pelvic tumors, large hematomas, or constricting clothing or bandages, may alter test results.
■ The patient's failure to relax leg muscles completely or to breathe normally may affect the accuracy of test results.
■ Cold extremities from environmental factors can alter test results.

ULTRASONOGRAPHY

Echocardiography

This widely used, noninvasive test examines the size, shape, and motion of cardiac structures and is useful for evaluating patients with chest pain, enlarged cardiac silhouettes on X-rays, electrocardiographic changes, or abnormal heart sounds on auscultation. In echocardiography, a special transducer placed at an acoustic window (an area where bone and lung tissue are absent) on the patient's chest directs ultra-high-frequency sound waves toward cardiac structures, which reflect these waves. The transducer picks up the echoes, converts them to electrical impulses, and relays them to an echocardiography machine for display on an oscilloscope screen and for recording on a strip chart or videotape. Electrocardiography (ECG) and phonocardiography may be performed simultaneously to time events in the cardiac cycle.

The most commonly used echocardiographic techniques are M-mode (motion-mode) and two-dimensional (cross-sectional). In *M-mode echocardiography,* a single, pencil-like ultrasound beam strikes the heart, producing an "ice pick," or vertical, view of cardiac structures; this method is especially useful for precisely recording the motion and dimensions of intracardiac structures. In *two-dimensional echocardiography,* the ultrasound beam rapidly sweeps through an arc, producing a cross-sectional (or fan-shaped) view of cardiac structures; this technique is useful for recording lateral motion and providing the correct spatial relationship between cardiac structures. In many cases, both techniques are performed to complement each other. (See *Comparing two types of echocardiography,* page 916.)

Unlike highly standardized tests, such as ECG and cardiac radiography, special skill is needed to perform this test and to interpret the results.

Purpose
- To diagnose and evaluate valvular abnormalities
- To measure the size of the heart's chambers
- To evaluate chambers and valves in congenital heart disorders
- To aid diagnosis of hypertrophic and related cardiomyopathies
- To detect atrial tumors
- To evaluate cardiac function or wall motion after myocardial infarction
- To detect pericardial effusion.

Patient preparation
Explain to the patient that this test evaluates the size, shape, and motion of various cardiac structures. Inform him that he needn't restrict food or fluids before the test. Tell him who will perform the test and where and that it usually takes 15 to 30 minutes. Reassure him that the test is safe and painless. Explain that the room may be darkened slightly to aid visualization on the oscilloscope screen and that other procedures (ECG and phonocardiography) may be performed simultaneously.

Tell the patient that conductive jelly will be applied to his chest and a quarter-sized transducer will be placed directly over it. Because pressure is exerted to keep the transducer in contact with the skin, warn the patient that he may feel minor discomfort. Explain that the transducer is angled to observe different parts of the heart and that he may be repositioned on his left side during the procedure.

Inform the patient that he may be asked to breathe in and out slowly, to hold his breath, or to inhale a gas with a slightly sweet odor (amyl nitrite) while changes in heart function are recorded. Describe the possible adverse effects of amyl nitrite (dizziness, flushing, and tachycardia), but reassure the patient that such signs and symptoms quickly subside. Advise him to remain still during the test because movement may distort results.

Procedure
The patient is placed in the supine position. Conductive jelly is applied to the third or fourth intercostal space to the left of the sternum, and the transducer is placed directly over it. The transduc-

Comparing two types of echocardiography

This illustration shows how M-mode and two-dimensional echocardiography differ. The shaded areas beneath the transducer identify the cardiac structures that intercept and reflect the transducer's ultrasonic waves. In M-mode echocardiography, this area is columnar, and echo tracings are plotted against time. In two-dimensional echocardiography, the scanning area comprises an arc of 30 degrees and appears as a real-time TV display.

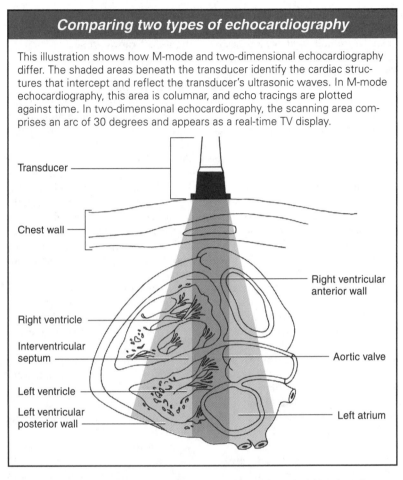

er is systematically angled to direct ultrasonic waves at specific parts of the patient's heart. During the test, the oscilloscope screen, which displays the returning echoes, is observed; significant findings are recorded on a strip chart recorder (M-mode echocardiography) or on a videotape recorder (two-dimensional echocardiography).

For a different view of the heart, the transducer is placed beneath the xiphoid process or directly above the sternum; for a left lateral view, the patient may be positioned on his left side. To record heart function under various conditions, the patient is asked to inhale and

exhale slowly, to hold his breath, or to inhale amyl nitrite.

Doppler echocardiography may also be used in this examination. In this procedure, the speed and direction of blood flow are assessed with color-flow, continuous-wave, and pulsed-wave Doppler ultrasound. The color flow simulates red blood cell flow through the heart valves and is electronically superimposed on the black-and-white echo image. The sound of the blood flow may also be heard as the continuous-wave and pulsed-wave Doppler sampling of cardiac valves is performed. This technique is used primarily to assess heart sounds and murmurs as they relate to cardiac hemodynamics.

Precautions
None.

Normal findings
An echocardiogram can reveal both the motion pattern and structure of the four cardiac valves. Anterior and posterior mitral valve leaflets normally separate in early diastole, with the anterior leaflet moving toward the chest wall and the posterior leaflet moving away from it. The leaflets attain maximum excursion rapidly, then move toward each other during ventricular diastole; after atrial contraction, they come together and remain so during ventricular systole. On an M-mode echocardiogram, the leaflets appear as two fine lines within the echo-free, blood-filled left ventricular cavity.

The aortic valve cusps lie between the parallel walls of the aortic root, which move anteriorly during systole and posteriorly during diastole. During ventricular systole, these cusps separate and appear as a boxlike configuration on an M-mode echocardiogram. They remain open throughout systole and normally demonstrate a characteristic fine, fluttering motion. During diastole, the cusps come together and appear as a single or double line within the aortic root on an M-mode echocardiogram.

An echocardiogram can also show the tricuspid and pulmonic valves. The motion of the tricuspid valve resembles that of the mitral valve; the motion of the pulmonic valve — particularly the posterior cusp — is quite different. During diastole, this cusp gradually moves posteriorly; during atrial systole, it's displaced posteriorly; and during ventricular systole, it quickly moves posteriorly. During right ventricular ejection, the cusp moves anteriorly, attaining its most anterior position during diastole.

An echocardiogram can also help evaluate both the left and right ventricles. The left ventricular cavity normally appears as an echo-free space between the interventricular septum and the posterior left ventricular wall. Echoes produced by the chordae tendineae and the mitral leaflet appear within this cavity. The right ventricular cavity normally appears as an echo-free space between the anterior chest wall and the interventricular septum. (See *Real-time echocardiograms,* pages 918 and 919, and *M-mode echocardiograms,* page 920.)

Implications of results
Valvular abnormalities readily appear on the echocardiogram. In mitral stenosis, the valve narrows abnormally because of the leaflets' thickening and disordered motion. Instead of moving in opposite directions during diastole, both mitral valve leaflets move anteriorly. In mitral valve prolapse, one or both leaflets balloon into the left atrium during systole.

Aortic valve abnormalities — especially aortic insufficiency — can also affect the mitral valve because the anterior mitral leaflet is just below the aortic cusps. When blood regurgitates through the aortic valve during diastole, it strikes this leaflet, causing the flutter seen in M-mode. Although the aortic valve may appear normal, this characteristic fluttering confirms aortic insufficiency. In stenosis due to such conditions as rheumatic fever or bacterial endocarditis, the aortic valve thickens and thus generates more echoes. However, in rheumatic fever, the valve may thicken slightly and allow normal motion during systole, or it may thicken severely and curtail motion. In bacterial endocarditis, valve motion is disrupted, and shaggy or fuzzy echoes usually appear on or near the valve.

Other chamber or valvular abnormalities may indicate a congenital heart dis-

Real-time echocardiograms

The real-time (showing motion) echocardiograms shown below are short-axis, cross-sectional views of the mitral valve from a normal patient (top) and a patient with mitral stenosis (bottom). In the latter, note the greatly reduced mitral valve orifice due to stenotic, calcified valve leaflets.

Normal

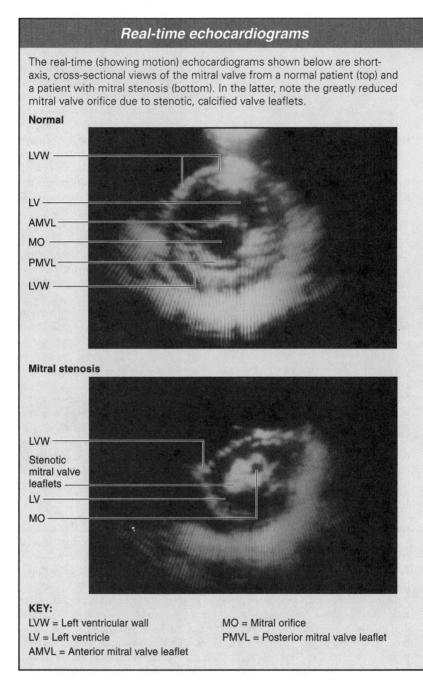

Mitral stenosis

KEY:

LVW = Left ventricular wall
LV = Left ventricle
AMVL = Anterior mitral valve leaflet

MO = Mitral orifice
PMVL = Posterior mitral valve leaflet

order such as aortic stenosis, which may require further tests. A large chamber size may indicate cardiomyopathy, valvular disorders, or congestive heart failure; a small chamber, restrictive pericarditis.

The echocardiograms shown below are long-axis, cross-sectional views of the mitral valve from a normal patient (top) and a patient with hypertrophic cardiomyopathy, also known as idiopathic hypertrophic subaortic stenosis (bottom). Note the markedly thickened left ventricular wall in the latter.

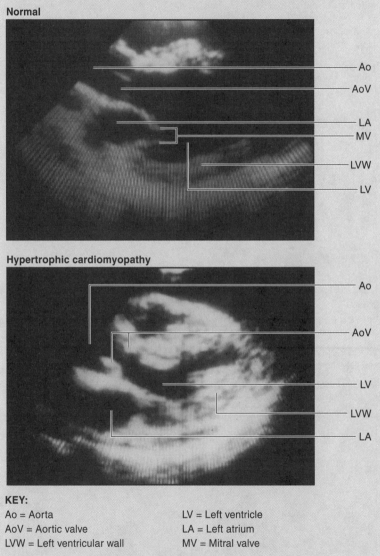

Normal

Ao
AoV
LA
MV
LVW
LV

Hypertrophic cardiomyopathy

Ao
AoV
LV
LVW
LA

KEY:
Ao = Aorta
AoV = Aortic valve
LVW = Left ventricular wall
LV = Left ventricle
LA = Left atrium
MV = Mitral valve

Hypertrophic cardiomyopathy (also known as idiopathic hypertrophic subaortic stenosis) can also be identified by the echocardiogram, with systolic anterior motion of the mitral valve and asymmetrical septal hypertrophy.

M-mode echocardiograms

In this normal motion-mode (M-mode) echocardiogram of the mitral valve, valve movement appears as a characteristic lopsided M-shaped tracing. The anterior and posterior mitral valve leaflets separate (D) in early diastole, quickly reach maximum separation (E), then close during rapid ventricular filling (E-F). Leaflet separation varies during middiastole, and the valve opens widely again (A) following atrial contraction. The valve starts to close with atrial relaxation (A-B) and is completely closed during the start of ventricular systole (C). The steepness of the E-F slope indirectly shows the speed of ventricular filling, which is normally rapid.

Normal

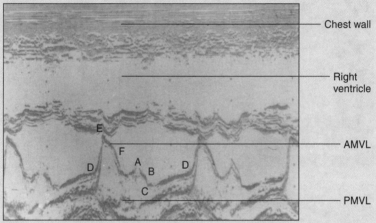

KEY:
AMVL = Anterior mitral valve leaflet   PMVL = Posterior mitral valve leaflet

Mitral stenosis is evident in this abnormal echocardiogram. The E-F slope (dashed line) is very shallow, indicating slowed left ventricular filling.

Mitral stenosis

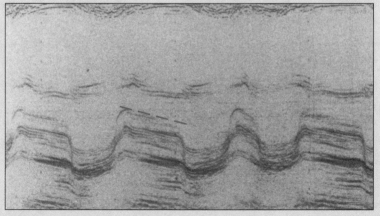

A left atrial tumor is usually located on a pedicle and can thus shift in and out of the mitral opening. During diastole, the tumor appears as a mass of echoes against the anterior mitral valve leaflet; during ventricular systole, these echoes shift back into the body of the atrium.

In coronary artery disease, ischemia or infarction may cause absent or paradoxical motion in ventricular walls that normally move together and thicken during systole. These affected areas may also fail to thicken or they may become thinner, particularly if scar tissue is present.

The echocardiogram is especially sensitive in detecting pericardial effusion. Normally, the epicardium and pericardium are continuous membranes and thus produce a single or near-single echo. However, when fluid accumulates between these membranes, it causes an abnormal echo-free space to appear. In large effusions, pressure exerted by excess fluid can restrict pericardial motion.

An echocardiogram should be correlated with the patient's history, physical examination findings, and results of additional tests.

Post-test care
Remove conductive jelly from the skin.

Interfering factors
■ Incorrect transducer placement and excess movement affect the accuracy of test results.
■ Patients with thick chests, chronic obstructive pulmonary disease, or chest wall abnormalities may be difficult to test.

Transesophageal echocardiography

In this test, ultrasonography is combined with endoscopy to provide a better view of the heart's structures. A small transducer is attached to the end of a gastroscope and inserted into the esophagus, allowing images to be taken from the posterior aspect of the heart. This causes less tissue penetration and interference from chest wall structures and produces high-quality images of the thoracic aorta, except for the superior ascending aorta, which is shadowed by the trachea.

Transesophageal echocardiography is appropriate for inpatients and outpatients, for patients under general anesthesia, and for critically ill intubated patients.

Purpose
To visualize and evaluate:
■ thoracic and aortic disorders, such as dissection and aneurysm
■ valvular disease (especially of the mitral valve) and problems with prosthetic devices
■ endocarditis
■ congenital heart disease
■ intracardiac thrombi
■ cardiac tumors
■ valvular repairs.

Patient preparation
Explain to the patient that this test allows visual examination of heart function and structures through insertion of a special tube. Tell him who will perform the test, when it's scheduled, and that he'll need to fast for 6 hours beforehand. Review the patient's medical history for possible contraindications to the test, such as esophageal obstruction or varices, GI bleeding, previous mediastinal

radiation therapy, or severe cervical arthritis. Ask the patient about any allergies, and note them on the chart.

Before the test, have the patient remove any dentures or oral prostheses, and note any loose teeth. Explain that his throat will be sprayed with a topical anesthetic and that he may gag when the tube is inserted. Tell him that he'll receive an I.V. sedative before the procedure and that he may feel some discomfort from the needle puncture and the pressure of the tourniquet. Reassure him that he'll be made as comfortable as possible during the procedure and that his blood pressure and heart rate will be monitored continuously. Make sure the patient or a responsible family member signs a consent form, if required.

Equipment

Cardiac monitor ✦ sedative ✦ topical anesthetic ✦ bite block ✦ gastroscope ✦ ultrasound equipment ✦ suction equipment ✦ resuscitation equipment.

Procedure

The patient is connected to monitors so that his blood pressure, heart rate, and pulse oximetry values can be assessed during the procedure. He is helped to lie down on his left side, and the ordered sedative is administered. Then the back of his throat is sprayed with a topical anesthetic. A bite block is placed in his mouth, and he's instructed to close his lips around it. The doctor then introduces the gastroscope and advances it 12" to 14" (30 to 35 cm) to the level of the right atrium. To visualize the left ventricle, he advances the scope 16" to 18" (40 to 45 cm). Ultrasound images are recorded and then reviewed after the procedure.

Precautions

■ Keep resuscitation equipment available.

■ Have suction equipment nearby to avoid aspiration if vomiting occurs.

■ Observe the cardiac monitor closely for a vasovagal response, which may occur with gagging.

■ Use pulse oximetry to detect hypoxia.

■ If bleeding occurs, stop the procedure immediately.

■ Laryngospasm, arrhythmias, or bleeding increases the risk of complications. If any of these occurs, postpone the test.

Normal findings

This test should reveal no cardiac problems.

Implications of results

Transesophageal echocardiography can reveal thoracic and aortic disorders, endocarditis, congenital heart disease, intracardiac thrombi, and tumors; it can also evaluate valvular disease or repairs. Findings may include aortic dissection or aneurysm, mitral valve disease, or congenital defects such as patent ductus arteriosus.

Post-test care

■ Monitor the patient's vital signs and oxygenation for any changes.

■ Keep the patient supine until the sedative wears off.

■ Encourage the patient to cough after the procedure, either while lying on his side or sitting upright.

■ Don't give the patient food or water until his gag reflex returns.

■ If the procedure is done on an outpatient basis, advise the patient to have someone else drive him home.

■ Treat a sore throat symptomatically.

Interfering factors

■ Poor imaging can result if the patient doesn't cooperate fully.

■ The transthoracic approach doesn't allow unobstructed visualization of the left atrial appendage and the ascending or descending aorta.

■ Patients with chronic obstructive pulmonary disease and those receiving mechanical ventilation aren't good candidates for this test because excessive air captured in the lungs impedes the movement of ultrasound waves.

Doppler ultrasonography

Doppler ultrasonography is a noninvasive test that evaluates blood flow in the major veins and arteries of the arms and legs and in the extracranial cerebrovascular system. Developed as an alternative to arteriography and venography, Doppler ultrasonography is safer, less costly, and requires a shorter test period than invasive tests. Although this test has a 95% accuracy rate in detecting arteriovenous disease that significantly impairs blood flow (at least 50%), it may fail to detect mild arteriosclerotic plaques and smaller thrombi, and it usually fails to detect major calf vein thrombosis.

In Doppler ultrasonography, a handheld transducer directs high-frequency sound waves to the artery or vein being tested. The sound waves strike moving red blood cells and are reflected back to the transducer at frequencies that correspond to the velocity of blood flow through the vessel. The transducer then amplifies the sound waves to permit direct listening and graphic recording of blood flow. (See *How the Doppler probe works*, page 924.)

Measurement of systolic pressure during this test helps detect the presence, location, and extent of peripheral arterial occlusive disease. Normally, venous blood flow fluctuates with respiration, so observing changes in sound wave frequency during respiration helps detect venous occlusive disease. Compression maneuvers can also help detect occlusion of the veins as well as occlusion or stenosis of carotid arteries.

Pulse volume recorder testing may be performed along with Doppler ultrasonography to yield a quantitative recording of changes in blood volume or flow in an extremity or organ.

Purpose
■ To aid diagnosis of venous insufficiency and superficial and deep vein thromboses (popliteal, femoral, iliac)
■ To aid diagnosis of peripheral artery disease and arterial occlusion
■ To monitor patients who have had arterial reconstruction and bypass grafts
■ To detect abnormalities of carotid artery blood flow associated with such conditions as aortic stenosis
■ To evaluate possible arterial trauma.

Patient preparation
Explain that this test helps evaluate blood flow in the arms and legs or neck. Tell the patient who will perform the test and that it takes about 20 minutes.

Reassure the patient that the test doesn't involve risk or discomfort. Tell him he'll be asked to move his arms to different positions and to perform breathing exercises as measurements are taken to vary blood flow during the exam. Explain that a small ultrasonic probe resembling a microphone is placed at various sites along specific veins and arteries and that blood pressure is checked at several sites. Check with the vascular laboratory to determine if special equipment will be used and if special instructions are necessary.

Procedure
Water-soluble conductive jelly is applied to the tip of the transducer to provide coupling between the skin and the transducer.

How the Doppler probe works

The Doppler ultrasonic probe directs high-frequency sound waves through layers of tissue. When these waves strike red blood cells (RBCs) moving through the bloodstream, their frequency changes in proportion to the flow velocity of the RBCs. Recording of these waves permits detection of arterial and venous obstruction but not quantitative measurement of blood flow.

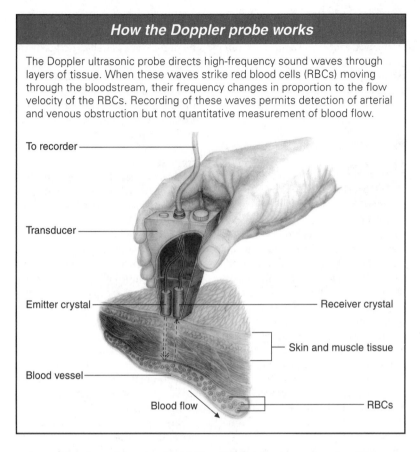

To recorder

Transducer

Emitter crystal

Receiver crystal

Skin and muscle tissue

Blood vessel

Blood flow

RBCs

For peripheral arterial evaluation: This test is always performed bilaterally. The usual test sites in the leg include the common femoral, superficial femoral, popliteal, posterior tibial, and dorsalis pedis arteries; in the arm, the subclavian, brachial, radial, ulnar and, occasionally, the palmar arch and digital arteries.

The patient is instructed to remove all clothing above or below the waist, depending on the test site. After he is placed in the supine position on the examining table or bed, with his arms at his sides, brachial blood pressure is measured, and the transducer is placed at various points along the test arteries.

The signals are monitored and the waveforms recorded for later analysis.

Segmental limb blood pressure is obtained to localize arterial occlusive disease. For lower-extremity tests, a blood pressure cuff is wrapped around the calf, pressure readings are obtained, and waveforms are recorded from the dorsalis pedis and posterior tibial arteries. Then the cuff is wrapped around the thigh, and waveforms are recorded at the popliteal artery. For upper-extremity tests, a blood pressure cuff is wrapped around the forearm, pressure readings are taken, and waveforms are recorded over both the radial and the ulnar arteries. Then the cuff is wrapped around the upper arm, pressure readings are taken, and waveforms are recorded with the transducer over the brachial artery.

Blood pressure readings and waveform recordings are repeated with the arm in extreme hyperextension and hyperabduction to check for possible compression factors that may interfere with arterial blood flow. The upper extremity examination is performed on one arm, with the patient first supine, then sitting; it's then repeated on the other arm.

For peripheral venous evaluation: The usual test sites in the leg include the popliteal, superficial femoral, and common femoral veins and the posterior tibial vein at the ankle; in the arm, the brachial, axillary, subclavian, and jugular veins and, occasionally, the inferior and superior venae cavae.

The patient is instructed to remove all clothing above or below the waist, depending on the test site. He is placed in the supine position and instructed to breathe normally. The transducer is placed over the appropriate vein, waveforms are recorded, and respiratory modulations noted.

Proximal limb compression maneuvers are performed and augmentation noted after release of compression, to evaluate venous valve competency. Changes in respiration are monitored. For lower-extremity tests, the patient is asked to perform Valsalva's maneuver, and venous blood flow is recorded. The procedure is repeated for the other arm or leg.

For extracranial cerebrovascular evaluation: The usual test sites include the supraorbital, common carotid, external carotid, internal carotid, and vertebral arteries. The patient is placed in the supine position on the examining table or bed, with a pillow beneath his head for support. Brachial blood pressure is then recorded, using the Doppler probe. Next, the transducer is positioned over the test artery, and blood flow velocity

is monitored and recorded. The influence of compression maneuvers on blood flow velocity is measured, and the procedure is repeated on the opposite side. (See *Detecting thrombi with a Doppler probe,* page 926.)

Precautions

Don't place the Doppler probe over an open or draining lesion.

Normal findings

Arterial waveforms of the arms and legs are multiphasic, with a prominent systolic component and one or more diastolic sounds. The ankle-arm pressure index — the ratio between ankle systolic pressure and brachial systolic pressure — is normally equal to or greater than 1. (The ankle-arm pressure index is also known as the arterial ischemia index, the ankle-brachial index, and the pedal- brachial index.) Proximal thigh pressure is normally 20 to 30 mm Hg higher than arm pressure, but pressure measurements at adjacent sites are similar. In the arms, pressure readings should remain unchanged despite postural changes.

Venous blood flow velocity is normally phasic with respiration, and is of a lower pitch than arterial flow. Distal compression or release of proximal limb compression increases blood flow velocity. In the legs, abdominal compression eliminates respiratory variations, but release increases blood flow; Valsalva's maneuver also interrupts venous flow velocity.

In cerebrovascular testing, a strong velocity signal is present. In the common carotid artery, blood flow velocity increases during diastole, due to low peripheral vascular resistance of the brain. The direction of periorbital arterial flow is normally anterograde out of the orbit.

Detecting thrombi with a Doppler probe

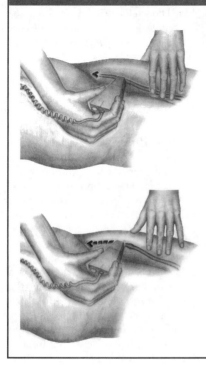

The Doppler probe is typically used to detect venous thrombi by first positioning the transducer and then occluding the blood vessel by compression (as shown in the normal leg at left). Water-soluble conductive jelly is applied to the tip of the transducer to provide coupling between the skin and the transducer.

When pressure is released, allowing blood flow to resume, the transducer picks up the sudden augmentation of the flow sound and permits graphic recording of blood blow. If a thrombus is present, a compression maneuver fails to produce the augmented flow sound because the blood flow (as shown at left in the femoral vein) is significantly impaired.

Implications of results

Arterial stenosis or occlusion diminishes the blood flow velocity signal, with no diastolic sound and a less prominent systolic component distal to the lesion. At the lesion, the signal is high-pitched and, occasionally, turbulent. If complete occlusion is present and collateral circulation has not taken over, the velocity signal may be absent.

A pressure gradient exceeding 20 to 30 mm Hg at adjacent sites of measurement in the leg may indicate occlusive disease. Specifically, low proximal thigh pressure signifies common femoral or aortoiliac occlusive disease. An abnormal gradient between the proximal thigh and the above- or below-knee cuffs indicates superficial femoral or popliteal artery occlusive disease; an abnormal gradient between the below-knee and ankle cuffs, tibiofibular disease. Abnormal gradients of arm and forearm pressure readings may indicate brachial artery occlusion.

An abnormal ankle-arm pressure index is directly proportional to the degree of circulatory impairment: mild ischemia, 1 to 0.75; claudication, 0.75 to 0.50; pain at rest, 0.50 to 0.25; and pregangrene, 0.25 to 0.

If venous blood flow velocity is unchanged by respirations, doesn't increase in response to compression or Valsalva's maneuver, or is absent, venous thrombosis is indicated. In chronic venous insufficiency and varicose veins, the flow velocity signal may be reversed. Confirmation of results may require venography.

Inability to identify Doppler signals during cerebrovascular examination implies total arterial occlusion. Reversed periorbital arterial flow indicates significant arterial occlusive disease of the extracranial internal carotid artery; in addition, the audible signal may take on the acoustic characteristics of a normal peripheral artery. Stenosis of the internal carotid artery causes turbulent signals. Collateral circulation can be assessed by compression maneuvers.

Oculoplethysmography, carotid phonoangiography, or carotid imaging can further evaluate cerebrovascular disease. Retrograde blood velocity in the vertebral artery can indicate subclavian steal syndrome. Weak velocity signal on comparison of contralateral vertebral arteries can indicate diffuse vertebral artery disease.

Post-test care
Remove the conductive jelly from the patient's skin.

Interfering factors
Failure of the patient to cooperate may invalidate test results.

Ultrasonography of the abdominal aorta

In this safe, noninvasive test, a transducer directs high-frequency sound waves into the abdomen over a wide area from the xiphoid process to the umbilical region. The sound waves, echoing to the transducer from tissue of different densities, are transmitted as electrical impulses and displayed on a monitor, to reveal internal organs, the vertebral column, and, most important, the size and course of the abdominal aorta and other major vessels.

Ultrasonography helps confirm a suspected aortic aneurysm and is the method of choice for determining its diameter. Several scans may be performed to detect expansion of a known aneurysm because the risk of rupture is highest when aneurysmal diameter is 7 cm or greater. However, angiography is indicated preoperatively to visualize the extent of atherosclerotic changes and to discover anatomic anomalies such as three renal arteries. It's also indicated when the diagnosis is unclear. After an aneurysm is detected, ultrasonography is used every 6 months to monitor changes in patient status.

Purpose
▪ To detect and measure a suspected abdominal aortic aneurysm
▪ To measure and detect expansion of a known abdominal aortic aneurysm.

Patient preparation
Explain to the patient that this test allows examination of the abdominal aorta. Instruct him to fast for 12 hours before the test to minimize bowel gas and motility. Tell him who will perform the test and where, that the lights may be lowered, and that the test takes 30 to 45 minutes.

Tell the patient that mineral oil or a gel, which may feel cool, will be applied to his abdomen. Explain that a transducer will pass over his skin, from the costal margins to the umbilicus or slightly below, directing safe, painless, and inaudible sound waves into the abdominal vessels and organs. He will feel slight pressure. Reassure the patient with a known aneurysm that the sound waves will not cause a rupture. Instruct him to remain still during scanning and to hold his breath when requested.

If ordered, give simethicone to reduce bowel gas. Just before the test, instruct the patient to put on a hospital gown.

Procedure

The patient is placed in the supine position, and acoustic coupling gel or mineral oil is applied to his abdomen. Longitudinal scans are then made at 0.5- to 1-cm intervals to the left and right of midline until the entire abdominal aorta is outlined. Transverse scans are made at 1- to 2-cm intervals from the xiphoid to the bifurcation at the common iliac arteries. The patient may be placed in right and left lateral positions. Appropriate views are photographed or videotaped.

Precautions

None.

Normal findings

In adults, the normal abdominal aorta tapers from about 2.5 to 1.5 cm in diameter along its length from the diaphragm to the bifurcation. It descends through the retroperitoneal space, anterior to the vertebral column and slightly left of the midline. Four of its major branches are usually well visualized: the celiac trunk, the renal arteries, the superior mesenteric artery, and the common iliac arteries.

Implications of results

Luminal diameter of the abdominal aorta greater than 4 cm indicates the presence of an aneurysm; over 7 cm, indicates an aneurysm with a high risk of rupture.

Post-test care

■ Wipe off the acoustic coupling gel.
■ Instruct the patient to resume his usual diet and medications.

 ■ Aneurysms may expand and dissect rapidly, so check the patient's vital signs frequently. Remember that sudden onset of constant abdominal or back pain accompanies rapid expansion of the aneurysm; sudden,

excruciating pain with weakness, sweating, tachycardia, and hypotension signals rupture.

Interfering factors

The following factors may hinder imaging:
■ bowel gas and motility, excessive body movement, surgical wounds, and severe dyspnea
■ residual barium from GI contrast studies within the past 24 hours and air introduced during endoscopy within the past 12 to 24 hours
■ in obese patients, mesenteric fat.

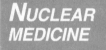

Cardiac positron emission tomography

Positron emission tomography (PET) scanning combines elements of both computed tomography scanning and conventional radionuclide imaging. In this test, positron emitters are injected into the patient and an attenuation scan is obtained and evaluated to determine the extent of myocardial contractility and to distinguish viable from infarcted tissue.

The test works by measuring the emissions of injected radioisotopes and converting them to tomographic images. Unlike conventional radionuclide imaging, PET scanning uses radioisotopes of biologically important elements — oxygen, nitrogen, carbon, and fluorine — that emit particles called positrons. During positron emission, pairs of gamma rays are emitted; the PET scanner detects them and relays the information to a computer for reconstruction as an image. Positron emitters can be chemically "tagged" to biologically active molecules, such as carbon monoxide, neurotransmitters, hormones, and metabolites (particularly glucose), allowing study of their uptake and distribution in tissue.

PET scanning is a costly test because the radioisotopes used have short half-lives and must be produced at an on-site cyclotron and attached quickly to the desired tracer molecules. This prohibitive cost has limited the test's use.

Purpose
- To detect coronary artery disease
- To evaluate myocardial metabolism
- To distinguish viable from infarcted cardiac tissue, especially during early stages of myocardial infarction.

Patient preparation
How you prepare the patient depends on the test's purpose. If you're assessing myocardial contractility, explain that the test distinguishes viable tissue from tissue injured by infarction. Tell the patient that the test may also be used to assess mitochondrial impairment, which is associated with ischemia, and to evaluate coronary artery obstruction.

Inform him that he'll be given a gradually decaying radioactive substance and that a special camera records the amount of radioactive decay and transmits this data to a computer, which converts it to a visual image for interpretation. If the radioisotope is to be given by I.V. infusion, tell the patient who will insert the I.V. line, when it will be done, and that he may feel some discomfort from the needle puncture and the tourniquet. Otherwise, the test is painless. If the radioisotope will be inhaled, explain this painless procedure to him.

Inform the patient if the doctor wants him to fast before the scan. (Whether or not fasting is necessary is still under investigation.) Caution him to remain still during the procedure, and tell him that it takes 1 to 1½ hours. If your hospital requires it, make sure the patient or a responsible family member signs a consent form.

Equipment
PET scanner ✦ cyclotron ✦ appropriate radioisotope.

Procedure
While lying in the supine position with his arms above his head, the patient undergoes an attenuation scan that lasts about 30 minutes. Then he's injected with the appropriate positron emitter and undergoes scanning. If comparative studies are needed, the patient may receive an additional injection of a different positron emitter.

Precautions
The radioisotope may be harmful to a fetus, so female patients of childbearing age should be screened carefully before undergoing this procedure.

Normal findings
A normal PET scan reveals no areas of ischemic tissue. If the patient receives two injections, the flow and distribution of the two tracers should match, indicating normal tissue.

Implications of results
A scan that reveals reduced blood flow but increased glucose use indicates ischemia. Decreased blood flow and glucose use indicate necrotic, scarred tissue.

Post-test care
- Instruct the patient to move slowly immediately after the procedure to avoid postural hypotension.
- Encourage him to drink plenty of fluids to help flush the radioisotope from the bladder.

Interfering factors

Failure of the patient to cooperate can hinder accurate imaging.

Cardiac magnetic resonance imaging

A great asset in the diagnosis of cardiac disorders, magnetic resonance imaging (MRI) has the ability to "see through" bone and to delineate fluid-filled soft tissue in great detail as well as produce images of organs and vessels in motion. In this noninvasive procedure, the patient is placed in a magnetic field and cross-sectional images of the anatomy are viewed in multiple planes and recorded for permanent record.

MRI relies on the magnetic properties of the atom. (Hydrogen, the most abundant and magnetically sensitive of the body's atoms, is most commonly selected for MRI studies.) The scanner uses a powerful magnetic field and radio-frequency (RF) energy to produce images based on the hydrogen (primarily water) content of body tissues. Exposed to an external magnetic field, positively charged electrons align uniformly in the field. RF energy is directed at the atoms, knocking them out of this magnetic alignment and causing them to precess, or spin. When the RF pulse is discontinued, the atoms realign themselves with the magnetic field, emitting RF energy as a tissue specific signal based on the relative density of nuclei and the realignment time. These signals are monitored by the MRI computer, which processes them and displays information as a high-resolution video image.

The magnetic fields and RF energy used for MRI are imperceptible to the patient; no harmful effects have been documented. Research is continuing on the optimal magnetic fields and RF waves for each type of tissue.

Purpose
- To identify anatomic sequelae related to myocardial infarction, such as formation of ventricular aneurysm, ventricular wall thinning, and mural thrombus
- To detect and evaluate cardiomyopathy
- To detect and evaluate pericardial disease
- To identify paracardiac or intracardiac masses
- To detect congenital heart disease, such as atrial or ventricular septal defects and the degree of malposition of the great vessel
- To identify vascular disease, such as thoracic aneurysm and thoracic dissection
- To assess the structure of the pulmonary vasculature.

Patient preparation
Explain to the patient that this test assesses the heart's function and structure. Tell him who will perform the test, where it will be done, and that it takes up to 90 minutes. Explain that although MRI is painless, he may feel uncomfortable because he must remain still inside a small space throughout the test. Ask if he suffers from claustrophobia; if so, he might not be able to tolerate the procedure or might need sedation.

Inform the patient that he'll be positioned on a narrow bed, which slides into a large cylinder that houses the MRI magnets. Tell him that the scanner will make clicking, whirring, and thumping noises as it moves inside its housing to obtain different images and that he may receive earplugs. Reassure him that he'll be able to communicate with the technician at all times and that the procedure will be stopped if he feels claustrophobic.

Immediately before the test, have the patient remove all metal objects. Make sure he doesn't have a pacemaker or any surgically implanted joints, pins, clips, valves, or pumps containing metal because such objects could be attracted to the strong MRI magnet. Ask if the patient has ever worked with metals or has any metal in his eyes. (Some facilities may have a checklist that covers all pertinent questions regarding metals, clips, pins, pacemakers, and other devices.) If he does have such devices, he won't be able to undergo the test.

If your hospital requires it, have the patient or a responsible family member sign a consent form. Administer sedation if ordered.

Equipment
MRI scanner ✦ computer ✦ recorder (film or magnetic tape).

Procedure
At the scanner room door, the patient is checked one last time for metal objects. Then he's placed supine on a narrow, padded, nonmetallic bed that slides to the desired position inside the scanner. RF energy is directed at the chest. The resulting images are displayed on a monitor and recorded on film or magnetic tape for permanent storage. The radiologist may vary RF waves and use the computer to manipulate and enhance the images. During the procedure, the patient must remain still.

Precautions
■ Because claustrophobic patients may experience anxiety, monitor the cardiac patient for signs of an ischemic event, chest pressure, shortness of breath, and changes in hemodynamic status.
■ Because MRI works through a powerful magnetic field, no metal can enter the testing area. Ask patients to remove watches, hairpins, and jewelry. MRI can't be performed on patients with pacemakers, intracranial aneurysm clips, or other ferrous metal implants. Ventilators, I.V. infusion pumps, and other metallic or computer-based equipment also can't enter the MRI area.
■ If the patient is unstable, make sure an I.V. line with no metal components is in place and that all equipment is compatible with MRI imaging. If necessary, monitor the patient's oxygen saturation, cardiac rhythm, and respiratory status during the test. An anesthesiologist may be needed to monitor a heavily sedated patient.
■ A nurse or radiology technician should maintain verbal contact with the conscious patient.

Normal findings
MRI should reveal no anatomic or structural dysfunctions in cardiovascular tissue.

Implications of results
MRI can detect cardiomyopathy and pericardial disease as well as atrial or ventricular septal defects and other congenital defects. The test is also useful for identifying paracardiac or intracardiac masses and evaluating the extent of pericardiac or vascular disease.

Post-test care
■ Assess how the patient responded to the enclosed environment. Provide reassurance if necessary.
■ Monitor the sedated patient's hemodynamic, cardiac, respiratory, and mental status until the effects of the sedative have worn off.

Interfering factors
Excessive patient movement can blur images.

Technetium Tc 99m pyrophosphate scanning

Technetium Tc 99m pyrophosphate scanning (also known as hot spot myocardial imaging and infarct avid imaging) is used to detect recent myocardial infarction (MI) and to determine its extent. In this test, an I.V. tracer isotope (technetium-99m pyrophosphate) is injected into a vein. The isotope accumulates in damaged myocardial tissue (possibly by combining with calcium in the damaged myocardial cells), where it forms a hot spot on a scan made with a scintillation camera. Such hot spots first appear within 12 hours of infarction, are most apparent after 48 to 72 hours, and usually disappear after 1 week. Hot spots that persist longer than 1 week usually suggest ongoing myocardial damage.

This test is most useful for confirming recent MI when serum enzyme tests are unreliable or when patients suffer from obscure cardiac pain (postoperative cardiac patients) or have equivocal electrocardiograms (ECGs), as in left bundle-branch block or old myocardial scars, for example.

Purpose
- To confirm recent MI
- To define the size and location of a recent MI
- To assess the prognosis after acute MI.

Patient preparation
Explain that this test helps determine whether the heart muscle is injured. Inform the patient that he needn't restrict food or fluids. Tell him who will perform the 30- to 60-minute test and where.

Inform the patient that he'll receive a tracer isotope I.V. 2 to 3 hours before the procedure and that multiple images of his heart will be made. Reassure him that the injection causes only transient discomfort, that the scan itself is painless, and that the test involves less exposure to radiation than chest X-rays. Instruct him to remain quiet and motionless while he's being scanned. Make sure the patient or responsible family member has signed a consent form.

Procedure
Usually, 20 mCi of technetium Tc 99m pyrophosphate is injected into the antecubital vein. After 2 to 3 hours, the patient is placed in the supine position, and ECG electrodes are attached for continuous monitoring during the test. Scans are usually taken with the patient in several positions, including anterior, left anterior oblique, right anterior oblique, and left lateral. Each scan takes 10 minutes.

Precautions
None.

Normal findings
A normal technetium scan shows no isotope in the myocardium.

Implications of results
The isotope is taken up by the sternum and ribs, and their activity is compared with the heart's; 2^+, 3^+, and 4^+ activity (equal to or greater than bone) indicate a positive myocardial scan. The technetium scan can reveal areas of isotope accumulation, or hot spots, in damaged myocardium, particularly 48 to 72 hours after the onset of acute MI; however, hot spots are apparent as early as 12 hours after acute MI. In most patients with MI, hot spots disappear after 1 week; in some, they persist for several months if necrosis continues in the area of infarction.

Knowing where the infarct is makes it possible to anticipate complications and to plan patient care. About one-fourth of patients with unstable angina pectoris show hot spots due to subclinical myocardial necrosis and may require coronary arteriography and bypass grafting.

Post-test care
None.

Interfering factors
In about 10% of patients who undergo this test, isotope accumulation may result from ventricular aneurysm associated with dystrophic calcification, pulmonary neoplasm, recent cardioversion, or valvular heart disease associated with severe calcification.

Thallium imaging

This test (also known as cold spot myocardial imaging and thallium scintigraphy) evaluates myocardial blood flow after I.V. injection of the radioisotope thallium-201. Because thallium, the physiologic analogue of potassium, concentrates in healthy myocardial tissue but not in necrotic or ischemic tissue, areas of the heart with normal blood supply and intact cells take it up rapidly. Areas with poor blood flow and ischemic cells fail to take up the isotope and appear as cold spots on a scan.

This test is performed in a resting state or after stress. Resting imaging can detect acute myocardial infarction (MI) within the first few hours of symptoms but does not distinguish an old from a new infarct. Stress imaging, performed after the patient exercises on a treadmill until he experiences angina or rate-limiting fatigue, can assess known or suspected coronary artery disease (CAD) and can evaluate the effectiveness of antianginal therapy or balloon angioplasty and the patency of grafts after coronary artery bypass surgery. Complications of stress testing include arrhythmias, angina pectoris, and MI.

Purpose
■ To assess myocardial scarring and perfusion
■ To demonstrate the location and extent of acute or chronic MI, including transmural and postoperative infarction (resting imaging)
■ To diagnose CAD (stress imaging)
■ To evaluate the patency of grafts after coronary artery bypass surgery
■ To evaluate the effectiveness of antianginal therapy or balloon angioplasty (stress imaging).

Patient preparation
Explain to the patient that this test helps determine if any areas of the heart muscle aren't receiving an adequate supply of blood. For stress imaging, instruct him to restrict alcohol, tobacco, and nonprescription medications for 24 hours before the test and to have nothing by mouth after midnight the night before the test. Tell him who will perform the test and where, that initial testing takes 45 to 90 minutes, and that additional scans may be required.

Tell the patient that he'll receive a radioactive tracer I.V. and that multiple images of his heart will be scanned. Warn him that he may experience discomfort from skin abrasion during preparation for electrode placement. Assure him that the test poses no known radiation danger.

Make sure that the patient or a responsible family member has signed a consent form. For stress imaging, instruct the patient to wear walking shoes during the treadmill exercise and to report fatigue, pain, or shortness of breath immediately.

Procedure

For stress imaging: The patient, wired with electrodes, walks on a treadmill at a regulated pace that's gradually increased while his electrocardiogram (ECG), blood pressure, and heart rate are monitored. When the patient reaches peak stress, the examiner injects 1.5 to 3 mCi of thallium into the antecubital vein and flushes it with 10 to 15 ml of normal saline solution. The patient exercises an additional 45 to 60 seconds to permit circulation and uptake of the isotope and then lies on his back under the scintillation camera. If the patient is asymptomatic, the precordial leads are removed. Scanning begins after 10 minutes with the patient in anterior, left anterior oblique, and left lateral positions. Additional scans may be taken after the patient rests and occasionally after 24 hours.

For resting imaging: Within the first few hours of MI symptoms, the patient receives an injection of thallium I.V. Scanning begins after 10 minutes, with the patient positioned as above.

Precautions

■ This test is contraindicated in pregnant women and in patients with impaired neuromuscular function, locomotor disturbances, acute MI or myocarditis, aortic stenosis, acute infection, unstable metabolic conditions (like diabetes), digitalis toxicity, or recent pulmonary infarction.

 ■ Stress imaging is stopped at once if the patient develops chest pain, dyspnea, fatigue, syncope, hypotension, ischemic ECG changes, significant arrhythmias, or critical signs or symptoms (confusion, staggering, or pale, clammy skin).

Normal findings

Thallium imaging should show normal distribution of the isotope throughout the left ventricle and no defects (cold spots).

Implications of results

Persistent defects indicate MI; transient defects (those that disappear after a 3- to 6-hour rest) indicate ischemia due to CAD. After coronary artery bypass surgery, improved regional perfusion suggests patency of the graft. Increased perfusion after ingestion of antianginal drugs can show that the drugs relieve ischemia. Improved perfusion after balloon angioplasty suggests increased coronary flow.

Post-test care

If further scanning is required, have the patient rest and restrict food and fluids (except water).

Interfering factors

■ Cold spots may be from sarcoidosis, myocardial fibrosis, cardiac contusion, attenuation due to soft tissue and artifacts (for example, diaphragm, implants, breast, electrodes), apical cleft, or coronary spasm.

■ Absence of cold spots in the presence of CAD may result from an insignificant obstruction, inadequate stress, delayed imaging, single-vessel disease (particularly the right or left circumflex coronary arteries), or collateral circulation.

Radiopharmaceutical myocardial perfusion imaging

This imaging test (also known as chemical stress imaging) is an alternative method of assessing coronary vessel function for patients who can't tolerate exercise or treadmill electrocardiography (ECG). The drugs used to chemically stress the patient include adenosine, dobutamine, and dipyridamole. I.V. infusion of the selected drug simulates the effects of exercise by increasing blood flow in the coronary arteries. Next, a radiopharmaceutical is injected I.V. to allow imaging, which assists in evaluating the cardiac vessels' response to the drug-induced stress. Both resting and stress images are obtained to evaluate coronary perfusion.

Purpose
■ To assess the presence and degree of coronary artery disease
■ To evaluate therapeutic procedures, such as bypass surgery or coronary angioplasty.

Patient preparation
For adenosine or dipyridamole: Instruct the patient to avoid taking all theophylline medications for 24 to 36 hours before the examination (theophylline is an antagonist to both these drugs and may result in a false-negative test result) and to avoid all caffeine-containing products (including coffee, tea, cola, chocolate, and medications containing caffeine) for 12 hours before testing.

For dobutamine: Instruct the patient to withhold beta blockers for 48 hours before the test. Also tell him not to eat for 3 to 4 hours before the test, though he may have water. Instruct him to take his other medications as ordered with sips of water.

 NURSING ALERT The patient must continue to take antihypertensive medications. If his systolic blood pressure is higher than 200 mm Hg, the dobutamine stress test cannot be done until his blood pressure is under control. Confirm that female patients are not pregnant before performing this test.

The patient will need to arrive at the test location about 1 hour before examination time. Tell him that an I.V. line will be initiated before the test so that the medication can be administered and that it will be removed after the scan. Tell him that a cardiologist, a nurse, an ECG technician, and a nuclear medicine technologist will be present for the medication infusion. Inform him that he may experience flushing, shortness of breath, dizziness, headache, chest pain, and an increase in heart rate during the infusion, but reassure him that these signs and symptoms will stop as soon as the infusion ends and that emergency equipment will be available if needed. Inform him how long the infusion will take (for adenosine, 6 minutes; for dipyridamole, 4 minutes; and for dobutamine, up to 18 minutes).

Screen the patient for bronchospastic lung disease or asthma. Adenosine and dipyridamole are contraindicated in these patients; dobutamine will be used instead. Weigh the patient to determine the appropriate dosage. Make sure the patient or a responsible family member has signed a consent form.

Equipment
ECG equipment ✦ emergency code chart with cardiac monitor ✦ defibrillator ✦ medication (adenosine, dipyridamole, or dobutamine) ✦ radiopharmaceutical ✦ infusion pump ✦ blood pressure monitor or cuff ✦ I.V. equipment ✦ aminophylline and esmolol.

Procedure
In the medical imaging or ECG department, the patient is placed on a bed or an examination table and I.V. access is obtained. Twelve-lead ECG leadwires are applied, and baseline ECG and blood pressure readings are obtained. The chosen chemical stress medication is infused. During the infusion, blood pressure, pulse, and cardiac rhythm are monitored continuously. The patient will need to tell the doctor or nurse what

symptoms he is feeling. At the appropriate time, the radiopharmaceutical is injected.

Depending on which radiopharmaceutical is used, the patient either undergoes imaging immediately or is instructed to return for imaging 45 minutes to 2 hours later. Resting imaging may be done before stress imaging or 3 to 4 hours after stress imaging, depending on the radiopharmaceutical used. The patient is told whether he needs to remain fasting and when he needs to return. After the images are completed, the I.V. access is removed. When all scans are completed, the patient may resume his regular diet and fluids.

Precautions
■ Keep resuscitation equipment available in case the patient experiences arrhythmias, angina, ST-segment depression, or bronchospasm.
■ Adenosine and dipyridamole are contraindicated for patients with asthma because irreversible bronchospasm can occur. Dobutamine should be administered to these patients.
■ Aminophylline, the reversal agent for adenosine and dipyridamole, can be administered to reverse severe adverse effects.
■ Because dobutamine can cause ventricular fibrillation, esmolol and a defibrillator should be available if needed for treatment.

Normal findings
Imaging should reveal characteristic distribution of the radiopharmaceutical throughout the left ventricle and no visible defects.

Cold spots are usually due to CAD but may result from myocardial fibrosis, attenuation due to soft tissue (for example, breast and diaphragm), or coronary spasm. The absence of cold spots in the presence of CAD may result from insig-

nificant obstruction, single-vessel disease, or collateral circulation.

Post-test care
If the patient must return for further scanning, tell him to rest; he may also need to restrict food and fluids in the interim.

Interfering factors
■ Cold spots may result from artifacts, such as implants and electrodes.
■ Absence of cold spots in the presence of CAD may result from delayed imaging.

Cardiac blood pool imaging

Cardiac blood pool imaging evaluates regional and global ventricular performance after I.V. injection of human serum albumin or red blood cells (RBCs) tagged with the isotope technetium Tc 99m pertechnetate. In first-pass imaging, a scintillation camera records the radioactivity emitted by the isotope in its initial pass through the left ventricle. Higher counts of radioactivity occur during diastole because the ventricle contains more blood; lower counts occur during systole as the blood is ejected. The portion of isotope that's ejected during each heartbeat can then be calculated to determine the ejection fraction; the presence and size of intracardiac shunts can also be determined.

Gated cardiac blood pool imaging, performed after first-pass imaging or as a separate test, has several forms; however, most forms use signals from an electrocardiogram (ECG) to trigger the scintillation camera. In *two-frame gated imaging*, the camera records left ventricular end-systole and end-diastole for 500 to 1,000 cardiac cycles; superimposition of these gated images allows assessment of left ventricular contraction to find areas of dyskinesia or akinesia.

In *multiple-gated acquisition (MUGA) scanning,* the camera records 14 to 64 points of a single cardiac cycle, yielding sequential images that can be studied like motion picture films to evaluate regional wall motion and determine the ejection fraction and other indices of cardiac function. In the *stress MUGA test,* the same test is performed at rest and after exercise to detect changes in ejection fraction and cardiac output. In the *nitro MUGA test,* the scintillation camera records points in the cardiac cycle after the sublingual administration of nitroglycerin to assess the drug's effect on ventricular function.

Blood pool imaging is more accurate and involves less risk to the patient than left ventriculography in assessing cardiac function.

Purpose
- To evaluate left ventricular function
- To detect aneurysms of the left ventricle and other myocardial wall-motion abnormalities (areas of akinesia or dyskinesia)
- To detect intracardiac shunting.

Patient preparation
Explain to the patient that this test permits assessment of the heart's left ventricle. Tell him who will perform the test and where and that he needn't restrict food or fluids. Inform him that he'll receive an I.V. injection of a radioactive tracer and that a detector positioned above his chest will record the circulation of this tracer through the heart. Reassure him that the tracer poses no radiation hazard and rarely produces adverse effects.

Inform him that he may experience transient discomfort from the needle puncture but that the imaging procedure itself is painless. Instruct him to remain silent and motionless during imaging, unless otherwise instructed. Make sure the patient or a responsible family member has signed a consent form.

Procedure
The patient is placed in the supine position beneath the detector of a scintillation camera, and 15 to 20 mCi of albumin or RBCs tagged with technetium Tc 99m pertechnetate are injected. For the next minute, the scintillation camera records the first pass of the isotope through the heart so that the aortic and mitral valves can be located. Then, using an ECG, the camera is gated for selected 60-msec intervals, representing end-systole and end-diastole, and 500 to 1,000 cardiac cycles are recorded on X-ray or Polaroid film.

To observe septal and posterior wall motion, the patient may be assisted to a modified left anterior oblique position; or he may be assisted to a right anterior oblique position and given 0.4 mg of nitroglycerin sublingually. The scintillation camera then records additional gated images to evaluate abnormal contraction in the left ventricle. The patient may be instructed to exercise as the scintillation camera records gated images.

Precautions
Cardiac blood pool imaging is contraindicated during pregnancy.

Normal findings
The left ventricle contracts symmetrically, and the isotope appears evenly distributed in the scans. The normal ejection fraction is 55% to 65%.

Implications of results

Patients with coronary artery disease usually have asymptomatic blood distribution to the myocardium, which produces segmental abnormalities of ventricular wall motion; such abnormalities may also result from preexisting conditions such as myocarditis. In contrast, patients with cardiomyopathy exhibit globally reduced ejection fractions.

In patients with left-to-right shunts, the recirculating radioisotope prolongs the downslope of the curve of scintigraphic data; early arrival of activity in the left ventricle or aorta signifies a right-to-left shunt.

Post-test care

Usually none is necessary. If the patient is elderly or physically compromised, assist him to a sitting position. Make sure he is not dizzy. Then assist him from the examination table.

Interfering factors

None.

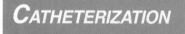

CATHETERIZATION

Cardiac catheterization

Simply stated, cardiac catheterization is the passing of a catheter into the right or left side of the heart (or both). This procedure can determine blood pressure and blood flow in the chambers of the heart, permit collection of blood samples, and record films of the heart's ventricles (contrast ventriculography) and arteries (coronary arteriography or angiography).

In *left-sided heart catheterization,* the catheter is inserted into the brachial or femoral artery through a puncture or cutdown procedure and, guided by fluoroscopy, is advanced retrograde through the aorta into the coronary artery ostium or the left ventricle (or both). Then a contrast medium is injected into the ventricle, permitting radiographic visualization of the ventricle and the coronary arteries as well as filming (cineangiography) of heart activity.

Left-sided heart catheterization assesses the patency of the coronary arteries, mitral and aortic valve function, and left ventricular function. It aids diagnosis of left ventricular enlargement, aortic stenosis and insufficiency, aortic root enlargement, mitral insufficiency, aneurysm, and intracardiac shunt.

In *right-sided heart catheterization,* the catheter is inserted into an antecubital vein or into the femoral vein and advanced through the inferior vena cava or right atrium into the right side of the heart and into the pulmonary artery. Right-sided heart catheterization assesses tricuspid and pulmonic valve function and pulmonary artery pressures. (See *Right- and left-sided heart catheterization.*)

Catheterization permits blood pressure measurement in the heart chambers to determine valve competence and cardiac wall contractility and to detect intracardiac shunts. Use of thermodilution catheters allows calculation of cardiac output.

Purpose

■ To evaluate valvular insufficiency or stenosis, septal defects, congenital anomalies, myocardial function and blood supply, and cardiac wall motion.

Patient preparation

Explain to the patient that this test evaluates the function of the heart and its vessels. Instruct him to restrict food and fluids for at least 6 hours before the test.

Right- and left-sided heart catheterization

For right-sided heart catheterization (below left), the catheter is inserted through veins to the inferior vena cava and to the right atrium and ventricle. For left-sided heart catheterization (below right), the catheter is inserted through arteries to the aorta and into the coronary artery orifices or left ventricle (or both). Note that both approaches use the antecubital and femoral vessels.

Right-sided catheterization   **Left-sided catheterization**

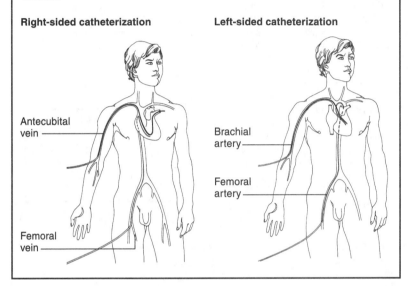

Tell him who will perform the test and where and that it takes 1 to 2 hours. Inform him that he may receive a mild sedative but will remain conscious during the procedure.

Advise the patient that he'll lie on a padded table as the camera rotates so that his heart can be examined from different angles. Tell him that the catheterization team will wear gloves, masks, and gowns to protect him from infection. Inform him that an I.V. needle will be inserted in his arm to allow administration of medication. Assure him that the electrodes attached to his chest during the procedure will cause no discomfort.

Tell the patient that the catheter is inserted into an artery or vein in his arm or leg; if the skin above the vessel is hairy, it will be shaved and cleaned with an antiseptic. Tell him he'll experience a transient stinging sensation when a local anesthetic is injected to numb the incision site for catheter insertion. Assure him that this sensation is normal.

Inform him that injection of the contrast medium through the catheter may produce a hot, flushing sensation or nausea that quickly passes; instruct him to follow directions to cough or breathe deeply. Tell him that he'll be given medication if he experiences chest pain during the procedure and may also receive nitroglycerin periodically to dilate coronary vessels and aid visualization. Reassure him that complications, such as myocardial infarction (MI) or thromboemboli, are rare.

Normal pressure curves

Right heart chambers

Two pressure complexes are represented for each chamber. Complexes at the far right in this diagram represent simultaneous recordings of pressures from the right atrium, right ventricle, and pulmonary artery. The numbered tracings are: 1, RV peak systolic pressure; 2, RV end-diastolic pressure; 3, PA peak systolic pressure; 4, PA dicrotic notch; 5, PA diastolic pressure.

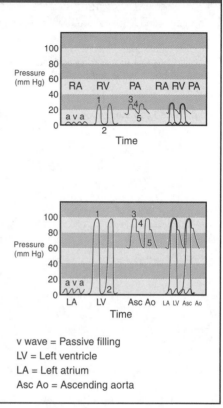

Left heart chambers

Overall pressure configurations are similar to those of the right side of the heart, but left-sided heart pressures are significantly higher because systemic flow resistance is much greater than pulmonary resistance.

KEY:

PA = Pulmonary artery
RV = Right ventricle
RA = Right atrium
a wave = Contraction

v wave = Passive filling
LV = Left ventricle
LA = Left atrium
Asc Ao = Ascending aorta

Make sure that the patient or a responsible member of the family has signed a consent form. Check for patient hypersensitivity to shellfish, iodine, or contrast media used in other diagnostic tests; notify the doctor if such hypersensitivities exist. Discontinue any anticoagulant therapy, as ordered, to reduce the risk of complications from bleeding. Just before the procedure, tell the patient to urinate and to put on a hospital gown.

Procedure

The patient is placed in the supine position on a padded table. Electrocardiogram (ECG) leads are applied for continuous monitoring and an I.V. line is started (if not already in place) with dextrose 5% in water or normal saline solution at a keep-vein-open rate. After the local anesthetic is injected at the catheterization site, a small incision or percutaneous puncture is made into the artery or vein, depending on whether left-side or right-side studies are to be performed, and the catheter is passed through the sheath into the vessel. The catheter is guided to the cardiac chambers or coronary arteries using fluoroscopy. When the catheter is in place, the contrast medium is injected through it to visualize the cardiac vessels and structures.

The patient may be asked to cough or breathe deeply. Coughing helps coun-

Maximum normal cardiac pressures

This chart shows the upper limits of normal pressure in the cardiac chambers and great vessels of recumbent adults.

CHAMBER OR VESSEL	PRESSURE
Right atrium	6 mm Hg (mean)
Right ventricle	30/6 mm Hg*
Pulmonary artery	30/12 mm Hg* (mean, 18)
Left atrium	12 mm Hg (mean)
Left ventricle	140/12 mm Hg*
Ascending aorta	140/90 mm Hg* (mean, 105)
Pulmonary artery wedge	Almost identical to left atrial mean pressure (±1 to 2 mm Hg)

*Peak systolic and end-diastolic

teract nausea or light-headedness caused by the contrast medium and can correct arrhythmias produced by its depressant effect on the myocardium; deep breathing can ease catheter placement into the pulmonary artery or the wedge position and moves the diaphragm downward, making the heart easier to visualize. During the procedure, the patient may be given nitroglycerin to eliminate catheter-induced spasm or measure its effect on the coronary arteries.

Heart rate and rhythm, respiratory and pulse rates, and blood pressure are monitored frequently during the procedure. After the procedure, the catheter is removed, and direct pressure is applied to the incision site for 30 minutes; a dressing is applied when hemostasis is achieved. Pressure can be applied manually (which can tire the health care provider) or by a device known as a C-clamp.

Precautions

■ Coagulopathy, poor renal function, or debilitation usually contraindicates both left- and right-sided heart catheterization. Unless a temporary pace-

maker is inserted to counteract induced ventricular asystole, left bundle-branch block contraindicates right-sided heart catheterization. Acute MI once contraindicated left-sided heart catheterization; however, many doctors perform catheterization and surgically bypass blocked vessels during acute ischemic episodes to prevent myocardial necrosis.

■ If the patient has valvular heart disease, prophylactic antimicrobial therapy may be indicated to guard against subacute bacterial endocarditis.

Normal findings

Cardiac catheterization should reveal no abnormalities of heart chamber size or configuration, wall motion or thickness, or direction of blood flow or valve motion; the coronary arteries should have a smooth and regular outline. (For more information on normal findings, see *Normal pressure curves* and *Maximum normal cardiac pressures*.)

Implications of results

Common abnormalities and defects that can be confirmed by cardiac catheterization include coronary artery dis-

Abnormal coronary arteriogram

This arteriogram taken from the right anterior oblique position shows occlusion of the left anterior descending artery.

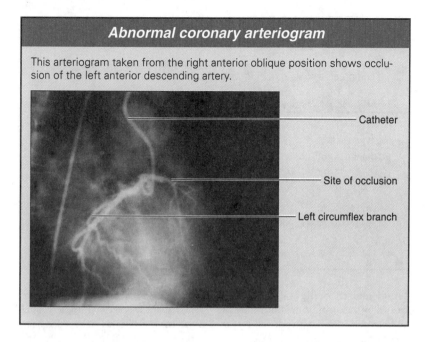

Catheter

Site of occlusion

Left circumflex branch

ease (CAD), myocardial incompetence, valvular heart disease, and septal defects.

In *CAD,* catheterization shows constriction of the lumen of the coronary arteries. Constriction greater than 70% is especially significant, particularly in proximal lesions. Narrowing of the left main coronary artery and occlusion or narrowing high in the left anterior descending artery is often an indication for revascularization surgery. This lesion responds best to coronary artery bypass grafting. (See *Abnormal coronary arteriogram.*)

Impaired wall motion can indicate *myocardial incompetence* from CAD, aneurysm, cardiomyopathy, or congenital anomalies. Comparing the size of the left ventricle in systole and diastole helps assess the efficiency of cardiac muscular contraction, segmental wall motion, chamber size, and ejection fraction (comparison of the amount of blood pumped out of the left ventricle during systole with the amount of blood remaining at end diastole). A normal ejection fraction (60% to 70%) is a good indicator for successful cardiac surgery. An ejection fraction under 35% generally increases the risk of complications from surgery.

Valvular heart disease is indicated by a gradient, or difference in pressures above and below a heart valve. For example, systolic pressure measurements on both sides of a stenotic aortic valve show a gradient across the valve. The higher the gradient, the greater the degree of stenosis. If left ventricular systolic pressure measures 200 mm Hg and aortic systolic pressure is 120 mm Hg, the gradient across the valve is 80 mm Hg. Because these pressures should normally be equal during systole when the aortic valve is open, a gradient of this magnitude indicates the need for corrective surgery (valve replacement or valve repair). Incompetent valves can be visualized in ventriculography by watching retrograde flow of

(Text continues on page 946.)

Complications of cardiac catheterization

Because cardiac catheterization is an invasive test that's usually done on high-risk patients, it poses a greater risk than most other diagnostic tests. Although complications are rare, they are potentially life-threatening and require careful observation during the procedure.

Keep in mind that some complications are common to *both* left-sided and right-sided heart catheterization; others result only from catheterization of one side. In either case, complications require that you notify the doctor and carefully document the complication and its treatment.

Left- or right-sided catheterization

COMPLICATION AND POSSIBLE CAUSES	SIGNS AND SYMPTOMS	NURSING CONSIDERATIONS
Myocardial infarction ■ Emotional stress induced by procedure ■ Blood clot dislodged by catheter tip travels to a coronary artery (left-sided heart catheterization only) ■ Air embolism	■ Chest pain, possibly radiating to left arm, back, or jaw ■ Cardiac arrhythmias ■ Diaphoresis, restlessness, or anxiety ■ Thready pulse ■ Fever ■ Peripheral cyanosis, causing cool skin	■ Keep resuscitation equipment available. ■ Give oxygen or other drugs, as ordered. ■ Monitor patient continuously, as ordered.
Arrhythmias ■ Cardiac tissue irritated by catheter	■ Irregular heart beat ■ Irregular apical pulse ■ Palpitations	■ Monitor patient continuously, as ordered. ■ Administer antiarrhythmic drugs, if ordered.
Cardiac tamponade ■ Perforation of heart wall by catheter	■ Sudden shock ■ Arrhythmias ■ Increased heart rate ■ Decreased blood pressure ■ Chest pain ■ Diaphoresis and cyanosis ■ Distant heart sounds	■ Give oxygen, if ordered. ■ Prepare patient for emergency surgery, if ordered. ■ Monitor patient continuously, as ordered. ■ Keep emergency equipment available.
Infection (systemic) ■ Poor aseptic technique ■ Catheter contaminated during manufacture, storage, or use	■ Fever ■ Increased pulse rate ■ Chills and tremors ■ Unstable blood pressure	■ Collect urine, sputum, and blood samples for culture, as ordered. ■ Monitor vital signs.

(continued)

Complications of cardiac catheterization *(continued)*

Left- or right-sided catheterization *(continued)*

COMPLICATION AND POSSIBLE CAUSES	SIGNS AND SYMPTOMS	NURSING CONSIDERATIONS
Hypovolemia ■ Diuresis from contrast medium used in angiography	■ Increased urine output ■ Hypotension	■ Replace fluids by giving patient 1 or 2 glasses of water every hour, or maintain I.V. infusion of 150 to 200 ml/hr, as ordered. ■ Monitor fluid intake and output closely. ■ Monitor vital signs.
Hematoma or blood loss at insertion site ■ Bleeding at insertion site from vein or artery damage	■ Bloody dressing ■ Limb swelling ■ Decreased blood pressure ■ Increased heart rate	■ Apply direct manual pressure. ■ When the bleeding has stopped, apply a pressure bandage. ■ If bleeding continues, or if vital signs are unstable, notify doctor.
Reaction to contrast medium ■ Allergy to iodine	■ Fever ■ Agitation ■ Hives ■ Itching ■ Decreased urine output, indicating kidney failure	■ Administer antihistamines to relieve itching, as ordered. ■ Administer diuretics to treat kidney failure, as ordered. ■ Monitor fluid intake and output closely.
Pulmonary edema ■ Excessive fluid administration	■ *Early stage:* tachycardia, tachypnea, dependent crackles, diastolic (S_3) gallop ■ *Acute stage:* dyspnea; rapid, noisy respirations; cough with frothy, blood-tinged sputum; cyanosis with cold, clammy skin; tachycardia; hypertension	■ Administer oxygen, as ordered. ■ Monitor vital signs and pulse oximetry, as ordered. ■ Give medication (digitalis glycosides, nitroglycerin, diuretics, morphine), as ordered. ■ Restrict fluids and insert an indwelling urinary catheter. ■ Monitor the patient continuously, as ordered. ■ Maintain the patient's airway, and keep him in semi-Fowler's position. ■ Keep resuscitation equipment available. ■ Monitor potassium level and replace if depleted.

Complications of cardiac catheterization (continued)

Left- or right-sided catheterization *(continued)*

COMPLICATION AND POSSIBLE CAUSES	SIGNS AND SYMPTOMS	NURSING CONSIDERATIONS
Infection at insertion site ■ Poor aseptic technique	■ Swelling, warmth, redness, and soreness at site ■ Purulent discharge at site	■ Obtain drainage sample for culture. ■ Clean site, and apply antimicrobial ointment, if ordered. Cover with sterile gauze pad. ■ Review and improve aseptic technique.

Left-sided catheterization

Arterial embolus or thrombus in limb ■ Injury to artery during catheter insertion, causing blood clot ■ Plaque dislodged from artery wall by catheter	■ Slow or faint pulse distal to insertion site ■ Loss of warmth, sensation, and color in arm or leg distal to insertion site	■ Notify doctor. He may perform an arteriotomy and Fogarty catheterization to remove embolus or thrombus. ■ Protect affected arm or leg from pressure. Keep it at room temperature, and maintain at a level or slightly dependent position. ■ Administer a vasodilator, such as papaverine, to relieve painful vasospasm, if ordered.
Cerebrovascular accident ■ Blood clot or plaque dislodged by catheter tip travels to brain	■ Hemiplegia ■ Aphasia ■ Lethargy confusion, decreased level of consciousness	■ Monitor vital signs closely. ■ Keep suctioning equipment nearby. ■ Administer oxygen, as ordered.

Right-sided catheterization

Thrombophlebitis ■ Vein damaged during catheter insertion	■ Hard, sore, cordlike, warm vein; may look like a red line above catheter insertion site ■ Swelling at site	■ Elevate arm or leg, and apply warm, wet compresses. ■ Administer anticoagulant or fibrinolytic drugs, if ordered.
Pulmonary embolism ■ Blood clot or plaque dislodged by catheter tip travels to lungs	■ Shortness of breath ■ Tachypnea ■ Increased heart rate ■ Chest pain	■ Place patient in high Fowler's position. ■ Give oxygen, if ordered. ■ Monitor vital signs. ■ Monitor pulse oximetry.

(continued)

Complications of cardiac catheterization (continued)

Right-sided catheterization *(continued)*

COMPLICATION AND POSSIBLE CAUSES	SIGNS AND SYMPTOMS	NURSING CONSIDERATIONS
Vagal response ■ Vagus nerve endings irritated in sinoatrial node, atrial muscle tissue, or atrioventricular junction ■ Complete heart block	■ Hypotension ■ Decreased heart rate ■ Nausea	■ Monitor heart rate closely. ■ Administer atropine, if ordered. ■ Keep patient supine and quiet. ■ Give liquids.

the contrast medium across the valve during systole.

Septal defects (both atrial and ventricular) can be confirmed by measuring blood oxygen content in both sides of the heart. Elevated blood oxygen on the right side indicates a left-to-right atrial or ventricular shunt; decreased oxygen on the left side indicates a right-to-left shunt.

Cardiac output can be measured by analyzing blood oxygen levels in the cardiac chambers, by injecting contrast medium into the venous circulation and measuring its concentration as it moves past a thermodilution catheter, or by drawing blood from cardiac chambers.

Post-test care
■ Monitor vital signs every 15 minutes for 2 hours, then every 30 minutes for the next 2 hours, and then every hour for 2 hours. If no hematoma or other problems arise, check every 4 hours. If signs are unstable, check every 5 minutes and notify the doctor. (See *Complications of cardiac catheterization*, pages 943 to 946.)
■ Observe the insertion site for a hematoma or blood loss, and reinforce the pressure dressing as needed.

■ Check the patient's color, skin temperature, and peripheral pulse below the puncture site.
■ Enforce bed rest for 8 hours. If the femoral route was used for catheter insertion, keep the patient's leg extended for 6 to 8 hours; if the antecubital fossa was used, keep the arm extended for at least 3 hours.
■ Consult the doctor about when to resume medications withheld before the test. Administer analgesics as ordered.
■ Unless the patient is scheduled for surgery, encourage intake of fluids high in potassium, such as orange juice, to counteract the diuretic effect of the contrast medium.
■ Make sure a post-test ECG is scheduled to check for possible myocardial damage.

Interfering factors
■ Improperly functioning equipment and poor technique interfere with accurate testing.
■ Patient anxiety increases the heart rate and cardiac chamber pressures.

Electrophysiology studies

Electrophysiology studies (also known as His bundle electrography) permit measurement of discrete conduction intervals by recording electrical conduction during the slow withdrawal of a bipolar or tripolar electrode catheter from the right ventricle through the His bundle to the sinoatrial node. The catheter is introduced into the femoral vein, passing through the right atrium and across the septal leaflet of the tricuspid valve.

These studies can localize disturbances within the atrioventricular conduction system. When an ectopic site takes over as pacemaker of the heart, the tests can help pinpoint its origin. The tests also aid diagnosis of syncope, evaluate a candidate for permanent pacemaker implantation, and help select or evaluate antiarrhythmic drugs.

Possible complications of these tests include arrhythmias, phlebitis, pulmonary emboli, thromboemboli, and catheter-site hemorrhage.

Purpose

■ To diagnose arrhythmias and conduction anomalies
■ To determine the need for an implanted pacemaker, an automatic internal cardioverter-defibrillator, and cardioactive drugs and to evaluate their effects on the conduction system and ectopic rhythms
■ To locate the site of a bundle-branch block, especially in asymptomatic patients with conduction disturbances
■ To determine the presence and location of accessory conducting structures.

Patient preparation

Explain to the patient that electrophysiology studies evaluate the heart's conduction system. Instruct him to restrict food and fluids for at least 6 hours before the test. Tell him who will perform the test and where and that it takes 1 to 3 hours.

Inform the patient that after the groin area is shaved, a catheter will be inserted into the femoral vein and an I.V. line may be started. Tell him although he'll receive a local anesthetic, he may still feel some pressure upon catheter insertion. Inform him that he'll be conscious during the test, and urge him to report any discomfort or pain.

Make sure the patient or responsible member of the family has signed a consent form. Check the patient's history, and inform the doctor of any ongoing drug therapy. Just before the test, advise the patient to void.

Procedure

The patient is placed in the supine position on a special X-ray table. Limb electrodes and precordial leads are applied for electrocardiogram (ECG) recording, and the insertion site is shaved, scrubbed, and sterilized. The local anesthetic is injected, and a J-tip electrode is introduced I.V. into the femoral vein (occasionally, into a vein in the antecubital fossa). Guided by fluoroscopy, the catheter is advanced until it crosses the tricuspid valve and enters the right ventricle. Then the catheter is slowly withdrawn from the tricuspid area, and recordings of conduction intervals are made from each pole of the catheter, either simultaneously or sequentially. After recordings and measurements are completed, the catheter is removed and a pressure dressing is applied to the site. (See *Catheter placement in electrophysiology studies,* page 948.)

Precautions

■ Electrophysiology studies are contraindicated in patients with severe co-

Catheter placement in electrophysiology studies

In this schematic view, a multipolar electrode catheter is inserted through the superior vena cava, right atrium, and tricuspid valve. When the catheter is withdrawn, the tip moves downward along the ventricle wall; as it passes the His bundle — located in the septum — a characteristic spike appears on the electrogram.

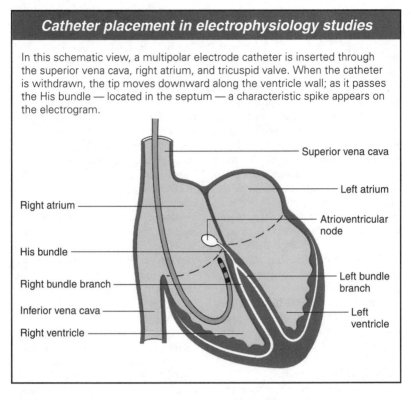

agulopathy, recent thrombophlebitis, or acute pulmonary embolism.

■ Make sure emergency medication is available in case the patient develops arrhythmias during the test.

■ Have resuscitation equipment at hand.

Reference values

Normal conduction intervals in adults are as follows: HV interval, 35 to 55 msec; AH interval, 45 to 150 msec; and PA interval, 20 to 40 msec. (See *Normal His bundle electrogram.*)

Implications of results

A prolonged HV interval (the conduction time from the His bundle to the Purkinje fibers) can result from acute or chronic disease. Atrioventricular nodal (AH interval) delays can stem from atrial pacing, chronic conduction

system disease, carotid sinus pressure, recent myocardial infarction, and use of certain drugs. Intra-atrial (PA interval) delays can result from acquired, surgically induced, or congenital atrial disease and atrial pacing.

Post-test care

■ Monitor the patient's vital signs, as ordered — usually every 15 minutes for 1 hour, and then every hour for 4 hours. If they're unstable, check every 15 minutes and alert the doctor. Observe for shortness of breath, chest pain, pallor, or changes in pulse rate or blood pressure. Enforce bed rest for 4 to 6 hours.

■ Check the catheter insertion site for bleeding, as ordered — usually every 30 minutes for 8 hours; apply a pressure bandage until the bleeding stops.

Normal His bundle electrogram

In a normal His bundle electrogram (shown at right), atrial activation appears as a sharp diphasic or triphasic wave (A) during the P wave, followed by His bundle deflection (H) and ventricular activation (V). By measuring the interval between the beginning of the P wave and His bundle activation (PH interval), or the interval between the beginning of the atrial wave and His bundle activation (AH interval), abnormally prolonged AV nodal conduction can be detected.

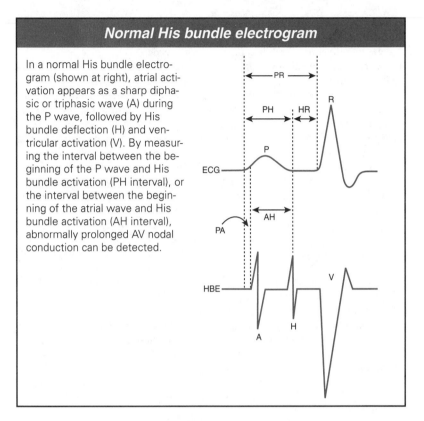

■ Advise the patient that he may resume his usual diet.

■ Make sure a 12-lead resting ECG is scheduled to assess for changes.

Interfering factors

Malfunctioning recording equipment and improper catheter positioning interfere with accurate testing.

Pulmonary artery catheterization

Pulmonary artery catheterization (also known as Swan-Ganz catheterization, balloon flotation catheterization of the pulmonary artery, and right-sided heart catheterization) uses a balloon-tipped, flow-directed catheter to provide intermittent occlusion of the pulmonary artery. Once the catheter is in place, this procedure permits measurement of both pulmonary artery pressure (PAP) and pulmonary artery wedge pressure (PAWP) — also known as pulmonary capillary wedge pressure.

The PAWP reading accurately reflects left atrial pressure and left ventricular end-diastolic pressure, although the catheter itself never enters the left side of the heart. Such a reading is possible because the heart momentarily relaxes during diastole as it fills with blood from the pulmonary veins; at this instant, the pulmonary vasculature, left atrium, and left ventricle act as a single chamber, and all have identical pressures. Thus, changes in PAP and PAWP reflect changes in left ventricular filling pressure, permitting detection of left ventricular impairment.

In this procedure, which is usually performed at bedside in the intensive care unit, the catheter is inserted through the subclavian vein. (The external jugular may be used instead of the femoral site to reduce the risk of cross-contamination from the genitourinary system.) The catheter is threaded into the right atrium, the balloon is inflated, and the catheter follows the blood flow through the tricuspid valve into the right ventricle and out into the pulmonary artery.

In addition to measuring atrial and pulmonary arterial pressures, this procedure evaluates pulmonary vascular resistance and tissue oxygenation, as indicated by mixed venous oxygen content. It should be performed cautiously in patients with left bundle-branch block or an implanted pacemaker.

Purpose

■ To help assess right and left ventricular failure
■ To monitor therapy for complications of acute myocardial infarction (MI), such as cardiogenic shock, pulmonary edema, fluid-related hypovolemia and hypotension, systolic murmur, and various cardiac arrhythmias
■ To monitor fluid status in patients with serious burns, renal disease, noncardiogenic pulmonary edema, or adult respiratory distress syndrome
■ To establish baseline pressures preoperatively in patients with existing cardiac disease (especially aortic stenosis, repeated episodes of heart failure, or multiple MIs) and then adjust I.V. medications (such as nitroglycerin, dopamine, or dobutamine) for optimal surgical success

■ To monitor the effects of cardiovascular drugs, such as nitroglycerin and nitroprusside.

Patient preparation

Explain to the patient that this test evaluates heart pressures and provides information that helps determine appropriate therapy or manage fluid status. Advise him that he needn't restrict food or fluids before the test. Tell him who will perform the test and where.

Inform the patient that he'll be conscious during catheterization and may feel transient local discomfort from administration of the local anesthetic. Tell him catheter insertion takes about 30 minutes, but the catheter will remain in place, causing little or no discomfort, for 48 to 72 hours. Instruct him to report any discomfort immediately. Explain that after insertion, he'll need to have a portable chest X-ray to confirm proper placement of the pulmonary artery (PA) catheter.

Make sure the patient or a responsible family member has signed a consent form.

Equipment

Pressure cuff ✦ balloon-tipped, flow-directed PA catheter ✦ bag of heparin flush solution (usually 500 ml of normal saline solution with 500 to 1,000 U of heparin) ✦ alcohol sponges ✦ medication-added label ✦ pressure tubing with flush device and disposable transducer ✦ monitor and monitor cable ✦ I.V. pole with transducer mount ✦ emergency resuscitation equipment ✦ ECG monitor ✦ ECG electrodes ✦ arm board (for antecubital insertion) ✦ lead aprons (if fluoroscope is used during insertion) ✦ sutures ✦ 4" x 4" gauze pads or other dry occlusive dressing material ✦ prepackaged introducer kit ✦ optional: dextrose 5% in water, shaving materials (if a femoral insertion site is used).

If a prepackaged introducer kit is unavailable, obtain the following: an introducer (one size larger than the catheter) ✦ sterile tray containing instruments for procedure ✦ masks ✦ sterile gowns and gloves ✦ povidone-iodine ointment ✦ sutures ✦ two 10-ml syringes ✦ local anesthetic (1% to 2% lidocaine) ✦ one 5-ml syringe ✦ 25G ½" needle ✦ 1" and 3" tape.

Procedure

The flexible catheter used in this test comes in two-lumen, three-lumen, and four-lumen (thermodilution) modes and in various lengths. In the two-lumen catheter, one lumen contains the balloon, 1 mm behind the catheter tip; the other lumen, which opens at the tip, measures pressure in front of the balloon. The two-lumen catheter measures PAP and PAWP and can be used to sample mixed venous blood and to infuse I.V. solutions. The three-lumen catheter has an additional proximal lumen that opens 12" (30 cm) behind the tip; when the tip is in the main pulmonary artery, the proximal lumen lies in the right atrium, permitting administration of fluids or monitoring of right atrial pressure (central venous pressure).

The four-lumen type includes a transistorized thermistor for monitoring blood temperature, and allows measurement of cardiac output. (See *Measuring cardiac output and cardiac index,* page 952.) Two- and three-lumen catheters are not routinely used in critical care settings. Usually, a four-lumen catheter with thermodilution and pacer port mode is used to allow for pacing if necessary. The introducer part of the system may also be used to infuse large amounts of fluids.

Before catheterization, the equipment is set up according to the manufacturer's directions and the hospital's procedure. The patient is placed in the supine position. For subclavian insertion, he's positioned with his head and shoulders slightly lower than his trunk to make the vein more accessible; for antecubital insertion, his arm is abducted with palm upward on an overbed table for support. If the patient can't tolerate the supine position, he's assisted to semi-Fowler's position. During the test, all pressures are monitored with the patient in the same position.

After the patient is positioned, the catheter balloon is checked for defects using sterile technique, and all ports are flushed to ensure patency. Then the catheter is introduced into the vein percutaneously. The catheter is directed to the right atrium, and the catheter balloon is partially inflated so that venous flow carries the catheter tip through the right atrium and tricuspid valve into the right ventricle and into the pulmonary artery. While the catheter is being directed, the monitor screen is observed for characteristic waveform changes, and the location of the catheter tip is found. A printout of each stage of catheter insertion is obtained for baseline information. (See *PA catheterization: Insertion sites and associated waveforms,* page 953.)

 As the catheter is passed into the chambers on the right side of heart, the monitor screen is observed for frequent premature ventricular contractions, ventricular tachycardia, and other arrhythmias — the result of right ventricular catheter irritation. If irritation occurs, the catheter may be partially withdrawn or medication administered to suppress the arrhythmias or right bundle-branch block.

To record PAWP, the catheter balloon is carefully inflated with the specified amount of air (no more than 1.5 cc); the catheter tip should float into the wedge position, as indicated by an altered waveform on the monitor screen. If a PAWP waveform occurs with less than

Measuring cardiac output and cardiac index

Cardiac output — the amount of blood ejected from the right and left ventricles every 60 seconds — can be measured by a four-lumen thermodilution catheter that's inserted for pulmonary artery catheterization. One catheter lumen houses a thermistor — a pair of wires that terminate in a small bead located about 1½" (4 cm) behind the catheter tip. The thermistor detects changes in blood temperature and transmits this information to a monitoring computer that calculates and displays cardiac output.

Procedure and reference values

To measure cardiac output, 5 to 10 ml of normal saline solution or dextrose 5% in water is injected into the proximal lumen over a period of no more than 4 seconds. The fluid travels quickly through the right atrium and ventricle and into the pulmonary artery, where the thermistor bead records the temperature change.

Normal cardiac output is 4 to 8 L/minute, with a mean of 5 L/minute.

Cardiac index relates to body surface area, which is determined from the patient's height and weight using a nomogram. (The cardiac output divided by the figure obtained from the nomogram equals the *cardiac index*.) A normal cardiac index is 2.5 to 5 L/minute/m^2.

Implications of results

Decreased cardiac output and cardiac index may indicate impaired myocardial contractility due to myocardial infarction or use of certain drugs (negative inotropics, such as procainamide, quinidine, or propranolol); acidosis or hypoxia; decreased left ventricular filling pressure caused by fluid depletion; increased systemic vascular resistance (SVR) from arteriosclerosis or hypertension; or valvular heart disease causing decreased blood flow from the ventricles.

Increased cardiac output and cardiac index (high-output syndrome) with a decreased SVR may indicate septic shock.

---

the recommended inflation volume, the balloon should not be inflated further. After the balloon is inflated, the wedge pressure is recorded. Then the air from the balloon is allowed to return to the syringe, which is then deflated. This allows the catheter to float back into the pulmonary artery. The monitor screen is observed for a PA waveform. Then the system is flushed and recalibrated.

The 1.5-ml syringe that comes in the introducer kit has an indentation along the barrel that won't allow you to inject more than 1.5 cc of air. This is to prevent overinflation of the balloon tip and possible rupture of the pulmonary artery. The port to measure PAWP also has

a stopcock. After obtaining PAWP, the balloon should be deflated and the stopcock should be turned so that it's perpendicular to the insertion port. This extra measure prevents air from the syringe from accidentally inflating the balloon.

 The balloon catheter should not be overinflated. Overinflation could distend the pulmonary artery, causing vessel rupture. If the balloon can't be fully deflated after recording the PAWP, it shouldn't be reinflated unless the doctor is present; balloon rupture could cause a life-threatening air embolism. All connections should be

PA catheterization: Insertion sites and associated waveforms

As the pulmonary artery (PA) catheter is directed through the chambers on the right side of the heart to its wedge position, it produces distinctive waveforms on the oscilloscope screen that are important indicators of the catheter's position in the heart.

Right atrial pressure

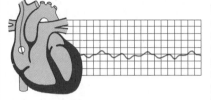

When the catheter tip reaches the right atrium from the superior vena cava, the waveform on the oscilloscope screen or readout strip looks like this. When this waveform appears, the doctor inflates the catheter balloon, which floats the tip through the tricuspid valve into the right ventricle.

Right ventricular pressure

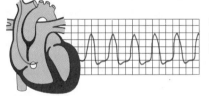

When the catheter tip reaches the right ventricle, the waveform looks like this.

Pulmonary artery pressure

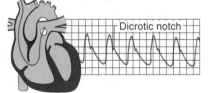

Dicrotic notch

A waveform like the one at left indicates that the balloon has floated the catheter tip through the pulmonic valve into the pulmonary artery. A dicrotic notch should be visible in the waveform, indicating the closing of the pulmonic valve.

Pulmonary artery wedge pressure

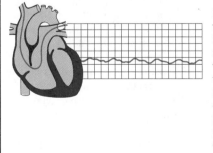

Blood flow in the pulmonary artery then carries the catheter balloon into one of the pulmonary artery's many smaller branches. When the vessel becomes too narrow for the balloon to pass through, the balloon wedges in the vessel, occluding it. The monitor then displays a pulmonary artery wedge pressure waveform such as the one shown at left.

checked for air leaks that may have prevented balloon inflation, particularly if the patient is confused or uncooperative.

When the catheter's correct positioning and function have been established, the catheter is sutured to the skin and antimicrobial ointment and an airtight dressing are applied to the insertion site. A chest X-ray is obtained, as ordered, to verify catheter placement. (The radiology department is notified before the procedure that a catheter is to be inserted.) Alarms are set on the electrocardiograph (ECG) and pressure monitors. Vital signs are monitored, as ordered. PAP waveforms are documented at the beginning of each shift and monitored frequently (as ordered) throughout each shift and whenever changes in treatment are made. PAWP and cardiac output are checked, as ordered (usually every 6 hours). Routine aseptic precautions are taken to prevent infection.

When the catheter is no longer needed, the balloon is deflated, the dressing is removed, and the catheter is slowly withdrawn. The ECG is monitored for arrhythmias. If any difficulty is encountered in removing the catheter, the procedure is stopped and the doctor is notified immediately. In some institutions, the doctor is required to remove the catheter.

After the catheter is withdrawn, pressure and a sterile dressing are applied to the insertion site.

Precautions

■ After each PAWP reading, flush and recalibrate the monitoring system and make sure the balloon is completely deflated; if you encounter difficulty in flushing the system, notify the doctor. Maintain 300 mm Hg of pressure in the pressure bag to permit fluid flow of 3 to 6 ml/hour. Instruct the patient to extend the appropriate arm (or leg, if the catheter is inserted into femoral vein).

NURSING ALERT ■ If a damped waveform occurs, the catheter may need to be withdrawn slightly. Pulmonary infarct may occur if the catheter is allowed to remain in a wedged position.

■ Make sure stopcocks are properly positioned and connections are secure. Loose connections may introduce air into the system or cause blood backup, leakage of deoxygenated blood, or inaccurate pressure readings. (See *Resolving pulmonary artery line problems.*)

■ Make sure the lumen hubs are properly identified to serve the appropriate catheter ports. Don't add or remove fluids from the distal PA port; this could cause pulmonary extravasation or damage the artery.

■ If the catheter has not been sutured to the skin, tape it securely to prevent dislodgment.

■ If the patient shows signs of sepsis, treat the catheter as the source of infection; remove it and send it to the laboratory for culture.

Reference values

Normal pressures are as follows:
■ *right atrial:* 1 to 6 mm Hg
■ *systolic right ventricular:* 20 to 30 mm Hg
■ *end-diastolic right ventricular:* < 5 mm Hg
■ *systolic PAP:* 20 to 30 mm Hg
■ *diastolic PAP:* about 10 mm Hg
■ *mean PAP:* < 20 mm Hg
■ *PAWP:* 6 to 12 mm Hg
■ *left atrial:* about 10 mm Hg.

Implications of results

An abnormally high right atrial pressure can indicate pulmonary disease, right-sided heart failure, fluid overload, cardiac tamponade, tricuspid stenosis and insufficiency, or pulmonary hypertension.

Elevated right ventricular pressure can result from pulmonary hyperten-

Resolving pulmonary artery line problems

PROBLEM	POSSIBLE CAUSES	NURSING CONSIDERATIONS
Damped pressures	▪ Air in system	▪ Check intraflow valves, stopcock, and transducer for bubbles.
	▪ Clot in system	▪ Aspirate blood until it thins; notify doctor.
	▪ Catheter kinked	▪ Instruct patient to cough or extend his arm to 90-degree angle from his body, and gently flush catheter. If problem, obtain X-ray.
	▪ Loose connection	▪ Check connections for security.
	▪ Incorrect stopcock position	▪ Correct stopcock position.
	▪ Pressure tubing too long	▪ Shorten distance between patient and transducer.
	▪ Catheter wedged in pulmonary artery	▪ Withdraw catheter slightly.
Transducer imbalance	▪ Damaged transducer	▪ Try another transducer.
	▪ Wrong amplifier	▪ Check transducer connection to amplifier.
	▪ Broken amplifier	▪ Change the amplifier.
	▪ Set at wrong level (mid-chest)	▪ Readjust the transducer.
False-low reading	▪ Damped waveform	▪ See damped pressures above.
	▪ Transducer imbalance	▪ Place transducer at heart level.
	▪ Wrong calibration	▪ Recalibrate the monitor.
False-high reading	▪ Transducer imbalance	▪ Rebalance the transducer.
	▪ Flush solution administered too quickly	▪ Pour slow continual flush (3 to 6 ml/hour).
Configuration	▪ Improper catheter placement	▪ Try to wedge catheter. Obtain pulmonary artery wedge pressure (PAWP). If problem, obtain X-ray.
	▪ Transducer needs to be calibrated	▪ Recalibrate the transducer.
	▪ Transducer not at right atrial level	▪ Reposition and recalibrate the transducer.
	▪ Transducer loosely connected to catheter	▪ Secure the transducer.
Drifting wedge pressure (with inflated balloon)	▪ Balloon overinflation	▪ Watch monitor while inflating balloon. When waveform changes from a pulmonary artery to a wedge shape, stop inflating.
	▪ Air in system	▪ Remove air from tubing or transducer.
PAWP tracing unobtainable	▪ Incorrect amount of balloon air	▪ Deflate and start again slowly. Check for air to refill syringe during balloon deflation.
	▪ Ruptured balloon	▪ With no resistance to inflation, stop inflation. Notify doctor.
	▪ Catheter inadvertently withdrawn	▪ Catheter may need to be advanced.

sion, pulmonary valvular stenosis, right-sided heart failure, pericardial effusion, constrictive pericarditis, chronic congestive heart failure, or ventricular septal defects.

An abnormally high PAP is characteristic of increased pulmonary blood flow, as in a left-to-right shunt secondary to atrial or ventricular septal defect; increased pulmonary arteriolar resistance, as in pulmonary hypertension or mitral stenosis; chronic obstructive pulmonary disease; pulmonary edema or embolus; and left-sided heart failure from any cause.

Pulmonary artery systolic pressure is the same as right ventricular systolic pressure. Pulmonary artery diastolic pressure is the same as left atrial pressure, except in patients with severe pulmonary disease causing pulmonary hypertension; in such patients, catheterization is still important diagnostically.

Elevated PAWP can result from left-sided heart failure, mitral stenosis and insufficiency, cardiac tamponade, or cardiac insufficiency; depressed PAWP, from hypovolemia.

Post-test care
■ Observe the catheter insertion site for signs of infection — redness, swelling, and discharge.
■ Watch for complications, such as pulmonary emboli, pulmonary artery perforation, heart murmurs, thrombi, and arrhythmias.

Interfering factors
■ Malfunctioning monitoring and recording devices, loose connections, clot formation at the catheter tip, air in the fluid column, or a ruptured balloon will interfere with accurate testing.
■ Incorrect catheter placement causes catheter fling — excessive movement that produces a damped pressure tracing.

■ Migration of the catheter against a vessel wall may cause constant occlusion (wedging) of the pulmonary artery.
■ Mechanical ventilators with positive pressure cause increased intrathoracic pressure, raising catheter pressure.
■ A reading is difficult to obtain with an extremely agitated patient.

MISCELLANEOUS TESTS

Cold stimulation test for Raynaud's syndrome

The cold stimulation test demonstrates Raynaud's syndrome by recording temperature changes in the patient's fingers before and after they're submerged in an ice-water bath. However, digital blood pressure recording or examination of the arteries in the arm and palmar arch should precede this test to rule out arterial occlusive disease.

Raynaud's syndrome is an arteriospastic disorder characterized by intense episodic constriction (vasospasm) of the small cutaneous arteries and arterioles of the hands or, less commonly, the feet after exposure to cold or stress. In this syndrome, the skin on the fingers typically blanches and becomes cyanotic and hyperemic after such exposure; in some patients, color changes are variable.

If this disorder is primary, it's called *Raynaud's disease;* if it's secondary to connective tissue disorders, such as scleroderma or systemic lupus erythematosus (SLE), it's called *Raynaud's phenomenon.* Although the cause of Raynaud's disease is unknown, various theories attribute reduced digital blood flow to intrinsic vascular wall hypersensitivity to cold, to increased vasomotor tone due to sympathetic stimulation, or to an antigen-antibody immune response.

Purpose
■ To detect Raynaud's syndrome.

Patient preparation
Explain to the patient that this test detects a particular vascular disorder. Inform him that he needn't restrict food or fluids before the test. Tell him who will perform the procedure and when, that the test takes 20 to 40 minutes, and that he may experience discomfort when his hands are briefly immersed in ice water. Suggest that he remove his watch and other jewelry, and encourage him to relax.

Procedure
To minimize extraneous environmental stimuli, the test room should be neither too warm nor too cold. A thermistor is taped to each of the patient's fingers (but not so tightly as to restrict circulation), and the temperature is recorded. The patient's hands are submerged in an ice-water bath for 20 seconds. Then he is instructed to remove his hands from the water, and the temperature of his fingers is recorded immediately and every 5 minutes thereafter until it returns to the prebath level.

Precautions
The cold stimulation test is contraindicated in patients with gangrenous fingers or open, infected wounds.

Normal findings
Normally, digital temperature returns to the prebath level within 15 minutes.

Implications of results
If digital temperature takes longer than 20 minutes to return to the prebath level, Raynaud's syndrome is indicated. Its benign form, Raynaud's disease, requires no specific treatment and has no serious sequelae. Its more serious form, Raynaud's phenomenon, is associated with connective tissue disorders — scleroderma, SLE, and rheumatoid arthritis — which may not be clinically apparent for several years. However, distinction between Raynaud's phenomenon and Raynaud's disease is difficult.

Post-test care
None.

Interfering factors
An excessively warm or cold test environment may cause inaccurate results.

Pericardial fluid analysis

Pericardial fluid analysis involves the needle aspiration (pericardiocentesis) and analysis of pericardial fluid. This procedure has both therapeutic and diagnostic purposes. It's most useful as an emergency measure to relieve cardiac tamponade, but it can also provide a fluid sample to confirm and identify the cause of pericardial effusion (excess pericardial fluid).

Normally, small amounts of plasma-derived fluid within the pericardium lubricate the heart, reducing friction during expansions and contractions. Excess pericardial fluid may accumulate after inflammation, rupture, or penetrating trauma (gunshot or stab wounds) of the pericardium. Rapidly forming effusions such as those that develop after penetrating trauma may induce cardiac tamponade, a potentially lethal syndrome — marked by increased intrapericardial pressure — that prevents complete ventricular filling and thus reduces cardiac output. Slowly forming effusions such as those in pericarditis typically pose less immediate danger because they allow the pericardium more time to adapt to the accumulating fluid.

Pericardiocentesis should be performed cautiously because of the risk of potentially fatal complications, such as laceration of a coronary artery or of the myocardium; other possible complications include ventricular fibrillation or vasovagal arrest, pleural infection, and accidental puncture of the lung, liver, or stomach. To minimize the risk of complications, echocardiography should be performed before pericardiocentesis to determine the effusion site. Generally, surgical drainage and biopsy are safer than pericardiocentesis.

Purpose

■ To help identify the cause of pericardial effusion and to help determine appropriate therapy.

Patient preparation

Explain to the patient that this test detects the presence and cause of excessive fluid around the heart, and helps determine appropriate therapy. Inform him that he needn't restrict food or fluids before the test. Tell him who will perform the test and where and that it takes 10 to 20 minutes.

Inform the patient that a local anesthetic will be injected before the aspiration needle is inserted. Although fluid aspiration isn't painful, warn him that he may experience pressure when the needle is inserted into the pericardial sac. Advise him that he may be asked to briefly hold his breath to aid needle insertion and placement.

Tell the patient that an I.V. line will be started just before the procedure and that he'll receive I.V. sedation as ordered. Assure him that someone will remain with him during the test and that his pulse and blood pressure will be monitored after the procedure.

Check the patient's history for current use of antimicrobial drugs, and record such use on the laboratory request. Make sure that the patient or a responsible family member has signed a consent form. If pericardiocentesis is performed to relieve cardiac tamponade and the patient is in shock, explain the test to the family.

Equipment

Prepackaged pericardiocentesis tray. If such a tray is not available, obtain the following: 70% alcohol or povidone-iodine solution ✦ 1% procaine or 1% lidocaine for local anesthetic ✦ sterile needles (25G for anesthetic and 14G, 16G, and 18G 4" or 5" cardiac needles) ✦ 50-ml syringe with luer-lock tip ✦ 7-ml sterile test tubes (one red-top, one green-top [heparin], and one lavender-top [EDTA]) ✦ sterile specimen container for culture ✦ 4" x 4" gauze pads ✦ vial of heparin 1:1,000 ✦ bandage ✦ three-way stopcock ✦ electrocardiograph or bedside monitor ✦ Kelly clamp ✦ alligator clips ✦ defibrillator and emergency drugs.

Procedure

The patient is placed in the supine position with the thorax elevated 60 degrees. When he's positioned comfortably and well supported, he's instructed to remain still during the procedure. After the skin is prepared with povidone-iodine solution from the left costal margin to the xiphoid process, the local anesthetic is administered at the insertion site.

With the three-way stopcock open, a 50-ml syringe is aseptically attached to

Aspirating pericardial fluid

In pericardiocentesis, a needle and syringe assembly is inserted through the chest wall into the pericardial sac (as illustrated below). Electrocardiographic (ECG) monitoring, with a leadwire attached to the needle and electrodes placed on the limbs (right arm [RA], right leg [RL], left arm [LA], and left leg [LL]), helps ensure proper needle placement and avoids damage to the heart.

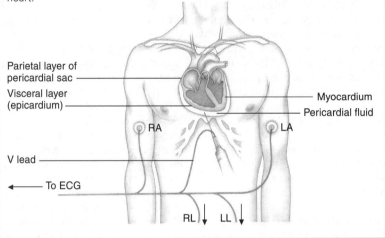

Parietal layer of pericardial sac

Visceral layer (epicardium)

RA

LA

Myocardium

Pericardial fluid

V lead

To ECG

RL   LL

one end and the cardiac needle to the other end. The patient is connected to a bedside monitor, which is set to read lead V. (Make sure a crash cart is nearby.) The needle is inserted through the chest wall into the pericardial sac, maintaining gentle aspiration until fluid appears in the syringe. The needle is angled 35 to 45 degrees toward the tip of the right scapula between the left costal margin and the xiphoid process; this subxiphoid approach minimizes the risk of lacerating the coronary vessels or the pleura.

Once the needle is properly positioned, a Kelly clamp is attached to it at the skin surface so it won't advance further. While the fluid is being aspirated, the specimen tubes are labeled and numbered. When the needle is withdrawn, pressure is applied to the site *immediately* with sterile gauze pads for 3

to 5 minutes. Then a bandage is applied. (See *Aspirating pericardial fluid.*)

Precautions

 ■ Carefully observe the ECG tracing when the cardiac needle is being inserted; ST-segment elevation indicates that the needle has reached the epicardial surface and should be retracted slightly; an abnormally shaped QRS complex may indicate perforation of the myocardium. Premature ventricular contractions usually indicate that the needle has touched the ventricular wall.

■ Watch for grossly bloody aspirate — a sign of inadvertent puncture of a cardiac chamber.

■ Be sure to use specimen tubes with the proper additives. Although fibrin isn't a normal component of pericardial fluid, it does appear in fluid in some pericardial diseases and in carcinoma, and clotting is possible.

■ Clean the top of the culture and sensitivity tube with povidone-iodine solution to reduce the risk of extrinsic contamination.

■ If bacterial culture and sensitivity tests are scheduled, record on the laboratory request any antimicrobial drugs that the patient is receiving. If anaerobic organisms are suspected, consult the laboratory about the proper collection technique to avoid exposing the aspirate to air. The aspirate may be placed in an anaerobic collection tube or the syringe may be filled completely, displacing all air, and the collection tube capped tightly with a sterile rubber tip.

■ Send all specimens to the laboratory immediately.

■ Have resuscitation equipment on hand.

Normal findings

The pericardium normally contains 10 to 50 ml of sterile fluid. Pericardial fluid is clear and straw-colored, without evidence of pathogens, blood, or malignant cells. The white blood cell (WBC) count in the fluid is usually less than 1,000/µl. Its glucose concentration should approximate the glucose levels in whole blood.

Implications of results

Pericardial effusions are typically classified as transudates or exudates. *Transudates* are protein-poor effusions that usually arise from mechanical factors altering fluid formation or resorption, such as increased hydrostatic pressure, decreased plasma oncotic pressure, or obstruction of the pericardial lymphatic drainage system by a tumor.

Most *exudates* result from inflammation and contain large amounts of protein. In these effusions, inflammation damages the capillary membrane, allowing protein molecules to leak into the pericardial fluid. Both types of effusion are characteristic in pericarditis, neoplasms, acute myocardial infarction, tuberculosis, rheumatoid disease, and systemic lupus erythematosus.

An elevated WBC count or neutrophil fraction may accompany inflammatory conditions such as bacterial pericarditis; a high lymphocyte fraction may indicate fungal or tuberculous pericarditis.

Turbid or milky effusions may result from the accumulation of lymph or pus in the pericardial sac or from tuberculosis or rheumatoid disease.

Bloody pericardial fluid may indicate hemopericardium, hemorrhagic pericarditis, or a traumatic tap. Hemopericardium, the accumulation of blood in the pericardium, may result from myocardial rupture after infarction or from aortic rupture secondary to dissecting aortic aneurysm or thoracic trauma. In hemopericardium, the fluid has hematocrit (HCT) similar to that of whole blood; in hemorrhagic pericarditis, it has a relatively low HCT and doesn't clot on standing. Hemorrhagic effusions may indicate cancer, Dressler's syndrome, closed chest trauma, or postcardiotomy syndrome. A traumatic tap is easily distinguished from hemopericardium or hemorrhagic pericarditis because the fluid becomes progressively clearer.

Glucose concentrations below whole blood levels may reflect increased local metabolism due to cancer, inflammation, or infection. Bacterial pericarditis may be caused by *Staphylococcus aureus, Haemophilus influenzae,* and various gram-negative organisms; granulomatous pericarditis, by *Mycobacterium tuberculosis* and various fungal agents; and viral pericarditis, by coxsackieviruses, echoviruses, and others.

Other tests are also useful in detecting effusions. (See *Diagnosing pericardial effusion.*)

Diagnosing pericardial effusion

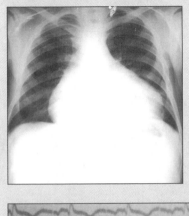

Various tests, such as chest radiography and M-mode echocardiography, aid diagnosis of pericardial effusion. In the chest X-ray shown at left, the bulging white area in the center represents an enlarged pericardial sac, resulting from pericardial effusion.

In the M-mode echocardiogram shown below, the wide light area at the bottom indicates accumulation of pericardial effusion. Pericardiocentesis followed by pericardial fluid analysis can determine the cause of such accumulation.

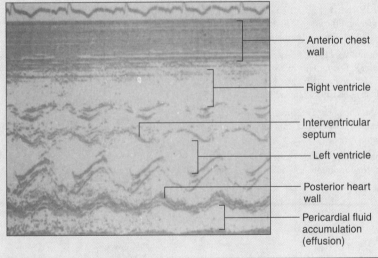

Anterior chest wall

Right ventricle

Interventricular septum

Left ventricle

Posterior heart wall

Pericardial fluid accumulation (effusion)

Post-test care

■ Check blood pressure readings, pulse and respiratory rates, and heart sounds every 15 minutes until stable, then every half hour for 2 hours, every hour for 4 hours, and every 4 hours thereafter. Reassure the patient such monitoring is routine.

■ Be alert for respiratory or cardiac distress. Watch especially for signs of cardiac tamponade, including muffled and distant heart sounds, distended neck veins, paradoxical pulse, and shock. Cardiac tamponade may result from rapid reaccumulation of pericardial fluid or puncture of a coronary vessel, causing bleeding into the pericardial sac.

Interfering factors

■ Failure to use aseptic technique can impair microbiological analysis of the sample because skin contaminants may be isolated and mistaken for the causative organisms. Antimicrobial therapy can prevent isolation of the causative organism.

■ Failure to use the proper additives in test tubes affects the accuracy of test results.

SELECTED READINGS

Conover, M.H. *Understanding Electrocardiography: Arrhythmias and the 12-Lead ECG,* 7th ed. St. Louis: Mosby–Year Book, Inc., 1995.

Guyton, A.C., and Hall, J.E. *Textbook of Medical Physiology,* 9th ed. Philadelphia: W.B. Saunders Co., 1996.

Isselbacher, K.J., et al., eds. *Harrison's Principles of Internal Medicine,* 13th ed. New York: McGraw-Hill Book Co., 1994.

Kinney, M., et al. *Comprehensive Cardiac Care: A Text for Nurses, Physicians and Other Health Practitioners,* 8th ed. St. Louis: Mosby–Year Book, Inc., 1996.

Olbrych, D.D. "Interpreting CPK & LDH Results," *Nursing93* 23(1):48-49, January 1993.

Schlant, R.C., et al. *Hurst's The Heart,* 8th ed. New York: McGraw-Hill Book Co., 1994.

CHAPTER TWENTY-NINE

Urinary system

Learning objectives

After completing this chapter, the reader will be able to:
- name two groups of diagnostic tests used to detect and evaluate urologic abnormalities
- explain the anatomy and physiology of the urinary system
- state the characteristics of cysts and tumors that permit differentiation by nephrotomography
- state the purpose of each test discussed in the chapter
- prepare the patient physically and psychologically for each test
- describe the procedure for performing each test
- specify appropriate precautions for safe administration of each test
- recognize signs of an adverse reaction and respond appropriately
- implement appropriate post-test care
- state the normal findings for each test
- discuss the implications of abnormal test results
- list factors that may interfere with accurate test results.

INTRODUCTION

Two groups of diagnostic tests exist for the detection and evaluation of urologic abnormalities in the urinary system. One group of tests analyzes the properties of urine, the end product of the urinary system; these tests, which include the invaluable routine urinalysis, are discussed in Chapters 12 and 15. The other group of tests — which is detailed in this chapter — is used to study the structures and functions of the components of the urinary system.

Structure of the kidneys

The urinary system consists of the kidneys, ureters, bladder, and urethra. The kidneys are reddish brown, bean-shaped organs situated in the back of the abdomen, flanking the vertebral column. Each kidney is about 4" to 5" (10 to 12.5 cm) long, 3" (7.5 cm) wide, a little more than 1" (2.5 cm) thick, and weighs 4 to 6 oz (113 to 170 g). It has an upper and a lower pole, anterior and posterior surfaces, convex lateral margins, and concave medial margins (or *hila*) that open

into a fat-filled pocket called the *renal sinus,* through which pass the renal blood vessels, nerves, and pelvis. A fibrous capsule encloses the kidney and is continuous with internal connective tissues, which also line the sinus and calyces of the renal pelvis.

The kidneys consist of the *cortex* and the *medulla.* The outer cortical substance is light and granular, while the inner medullary substance is dark and striated. Both the cortex and the medulla contain uriniferous tubules — *nephrons* — and collecting tubules. Each nephron is made up of a renal corpuscle and a renal tubule. Each kidney contains about a million of these functional units.

The cortex, containing vascular glomeruli and convoluted tubules, forms a series of arches, supported on renal columns extending toward the central sinus. The arches and columns enclose the medulla, forming *renal pyramids* (8 to 12 per kidney). The bases of these pyramids project toward the cortex and their apices, ending in *papillae* toward the sinus. The minor *calyces* cap these papillae, collecting the urine that oozes through them. Urine drains from the minor calyces into three major calyces, which empty into the renal pelvis and from there into the ureter. (See *The urinary system,* pages 966 and 967.)

Renal blood supply

Blood flows from the aorta into the two renal arteries, each of which divides into two main branches. Just outside the sinus these main branches subdivide into more branches to supply blood to the entire kidney. These branches are end arteries without anastomoses, so if one of them is obstructed, the result is infarction of the segment it supplies. Straight *interlobular arteries,* too small to be seen with the unaided eye, supply blood to the renal columns and cortical arches. Each of these tiny arteries, in turn, supplies a group of lobules with a series of fine, twiglike *afferent arterioles.*

These minute arterioles enter the renal corpuscle, break into capillary tufts or glomeruli, and emerge as *efferent arterioles,* each of which ends in a *capillary intertubular plexus* along the convoluted tubules of its own nephron. The arterial and venous sets of capillaries are called *vasa recta* because they run parallel to the straight tubules. Venous blood from the cortex and the medulla returns to the interlobular veins and retraces the course of the arterial branches back to the sinus, ending in the *renal vein.*

Ureters and bladder

The *ureters* are narrow, muscular tubes that transport urine from the kidneys to the bladder. They are 10" to 11" (25 to 27.5 cm) long and nearly ¼" (5 mm) in diameter. The *renal pelvis* narrows to form the top of the ureters; the tubes terminate at the posterior aspect of the bladder. The ureters enter the bladder wall obliquely, so that the ureteral openings in the bladder are normally only about 1" (2.5 cm) apart.

An expansile, muscular sac, the *bladder* lies in the space between the pubic bones and the rectum, and serves as a reservoir for urine. When empty, the bladder has an apex (behind the symphysis pubis), a base, a superior aspect, and two inferolateral aspects. The base of the bladder faces downward and backward in both sexes. In males, the ampullae of the vas deferens, the seminal vesicles, and the rectovesical fascia separate the base from the rectum. In females, the uterus and vagina intervene. Superiorly, the peritoneum loosely covers the bladder, with loops of intestine above it in males and the uterus over it in females. Inferolaterally, in both males and females, the bladder abuts the pubic bones, and the internal obturator and levator ani muscles.

The bladder consists of two basic parts: the *trigone* and the *detrusor muscle.* The trigone occupies the space between the internal urethral orifice and the two ureteral openings. The detrusor muscle — a meshwork of muscular fibers — forms most of the bladder wall, encircling the neck of the bladder and running inferiorly adjacent to the proximal urethra.

Urethra

In an adult male, the *urethra* is an S-shaped tube about 9" (23 cm) long, extending from the internal urethral orifice through the prostate gland, the deep perineal pouch, and the corpus spongiosum of the penis. The urethra is anatomically divided into three sections: the prostatic urethra (about 2½" [6.5 cm] long), the membranous urethra (½" to ¾" [1.3 to 2 cm] long), and the spongy (or cavernous) urethra (about 6" [15 cm] long). The first two sections, which easily become infected because of their vascularity and lymph drainage, are clinically considered to be one part — the *prostatic urethra.* The membranous

(Text continues on page 968.)

The urinary system

The urinary system consists of the kidneys, ureters, bladder, and urethra. The kidneys house over 2 million uriniferous tubules (nephrons and collecting tubules), which perform these vital renal functions: cleaning the blood of metabolic wastes and regulating the retention of substances required to preserve the body's fluid, electrolyte, and acid-base balances.

The glomeruli, tufts of capillaries within each nephron's renal corpuscle, accomplish the actual filtration of fluids and solutes from the blood, and the renal tubules reabsorb needed fluids and secrete excess electrolytes. The end product that reaches the collecting tubule is urine.

Overview

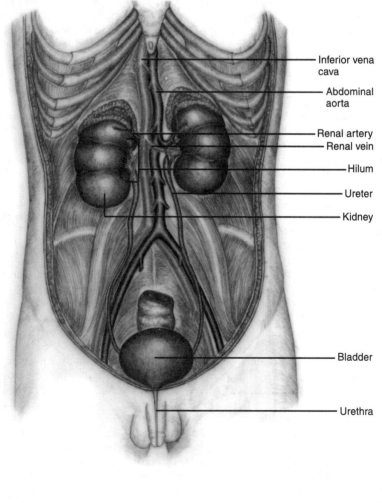

- Inferior vena cava
- Abdominal aorta
- Renal artery
- Renal vein
- Hilum
- Ureter
- Kidney
- Bladder
- Urethra

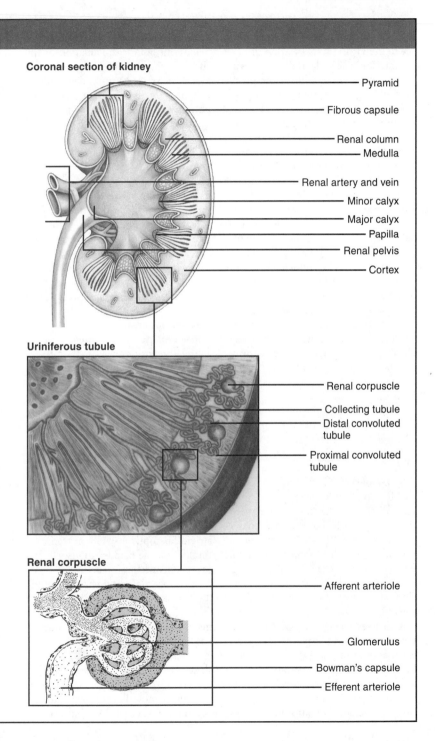

Coronal section of kidney

Pyramid

Fibrous capsule

Renal column

Medulla

Renal artery and vein

Minor calyx

Major calyx

Papilla

Renal pelvis

Cortex

Uriniferous tubule

Renal corpuscle

Collecting tubule

Distal convoluted tubule

Proximal convoluted tubule

Renal corpuscle

Afferent arteriole

Glomerulus

Bowman's capsule

Efferent arteriole

segment — the thin-walled, least mobile part of the urethra — is susceptible to injury on catheterization or pelvic fracture. The male urethra serves as a conduit for urine and for the products of the genital system.

In an adult female, the urethra serves one function: to conduct urine out of the body. The female urethra is only 1½" (4 cm) long and can dilate to a diameter of ¼" (5 mm). It runs downward and forward, from the neck of the bladder to the pudendal cleft, with a slight anterior concavity behind the symphysis pubis. The lower fibers of the urethral sphincter muscle bind the urethra tightly to the anterior vaginal wall, in which it is embedded. The epithelial lining of the urethra, subject to diverse hormonal activity, undergoes postmenopausal attrition along with adjacent structures. Adventitious organisms commonly colonize the external meatus because it's so close to the vagina and the rectum, which largely accounts for the higher incidence of urinary tract infections in females.

Diagnostic applications

The diagnostic tests discussed in this chapter are recommended after a complete history and physical examination have established the presence of clinical abnormalities associated with urologic disease. For example, the patient may complain of hematuria or flank pain, and the history may reveal urinary urgency or frequency, dysuria, nocturia, enuresis, or incontinence. The physical examination may detect fever, hypertension, and weight gain related to fluid retention.

Associated changes in skin color and texture may include pallor, jaundice, excoriation, redness, pitting edema, easy bruising, and urate crystals. Ocular changes may reflect hemorrhage, exudates, and papilledema. Abnormal oral findings include stomatitis and a fetid breath odor. Fluid retention may also cause edema in the eyelids, face, abdomen, arms, and legs. Palpation of the abdomen may reveal tender or enlarged kidney masses or a distended bladder. Examination of the genitalia may reveal phimosis, paraphimosis, or testicular masses; a rectal examination may reveal prostatic hypertrophy.

Urologic tests

Diagnostic testing of a patient with urinary symptoms generally begins with *kidney-ureter-bladder radiography,* which supplies information on the urinary tract, including kidney structure, size, and position.

Nephrotomography allows examination of a single slice or plane of renal tissue. Levels anterior and posterior to the selected plane are blurred, highlighting a specific area.

Renal computed tomography supplies a three-dimensional view of the kidneys that has greater detail than any other urologic test.

Renal ultrasonography, often used with excretory urography, is especially helpful in differentiating between a solid tumor and a simple, fluid-filled cyst.

Lesions, such as urethral strictures and calculi, as well as prostatic urethral disease and bladder disease may be confirmed by *cystourethroscopy.* This procedure, performed under a local or general anesthetic, involves the passage of a rigid fiberoptic instrument transurethrally into the bladder to visually inspect vesicourethral structures.

In *retrograde urethrography,* an indwelling urinary catheter is inserted just far enough to permit contrast medium instillation into the urethra, to outline its structure.

In *retrograde cystography,* bladder structure is evaluated by the instillation of a contrast medium into the bladder, through an indwelling urinary catheter. Several urologic tests use contrast media to outline organ structure and help identify abnormalities, such as calculi and cysts.

When disease severely affects renal function, *retrograde ureteropyelography* may be indicated for more accurate assessment. In this test, contrast medium is introduced into the renal pelvis in retrograde fashion, which allows intense opacification of the collecting system and ureters.

Antegrade pyelography examines the kidney by assessing the pressure and composition of urine drawn directly from it. Then contrast medium is injected into the kidney to detect obstructions.

Magnetic resonance imaging of the urinary tract is sometimes used when other structural tests (computed tomography scans or ultrasonography) produce unsatisfactory images.

Excretory urography, commonly referred to as I.V. pyelography, is the radiographic examination of the kidneys, ureters, and bladder after I.V. administration of a contrast medium. The effectiveness of this procedure depends on the kidneys' capacity to concentrate and excrete the contrast medium.

In *radionuclide renal imaging,* radionuclides are administered by I.V. filter through the kidneys at a specific rate and concentration, providing valuable information about the effectiveness of renal perfusion and function.

Renal angiography evaluates the efficiency of renal circulation and perfusion, and clearly outlines the renal parenchyma to help determine the cause of renovascular hypertension.

Renal venography can detect abnormalities of the renal veins and tributaries such as thrombosis.

A simple noninvasive test, *uroflowmetry* evaluates urine flow to detect lower urinary tract dysfunction or obstruction.

Cystometry evaluates bladder function after instillation of normal saline solution or water, or insufflation of a gas.

Voiding cystourethrography involves injection of a contrast medium, to evaluate urethral function during voiding and to diagnose vesicoureteral reflux.

The *Whitaker test* detects obstructions and determines the need for surgery by measuring urine pressure and flow in the kidneys, ureters, and bladder.

To determine how well the bladder or sphincter muscle interact, *external sphincter electromyography* can measure their activity with electrodes.

Nursing considerations

When caring for a patient who is scheduled for or has undergone urologic testing, remember these points:

■ Make sure the fluid intake of a patient with a suspected urinary tract lesion is adequate (except when underlying medical conditions dictate fluid restriction). Adequate hydration is also necessary to help flush out contrast media.

■ Administer a laxative, as ordered, to a patient scheduled for radiographic tests because overlying gas or feces in the lumen of the GI tract may interfere with the quality of X-ray films.

■ After an invasive procedure such as retrograde cystography, monitor fluid intake and output. Inability to void may necessitate catheterization. Notify the doctor if hematuria persists after the third voiding.

■ Watch for signs of urinary sepsis (such as fever, chills, or hypotension) after any test that involves urinary system instrumentation (such as cystourethroscopy).

■ Because many urologic tests are embarrassing to the patient, minimize his anxiety by clearly describing the procedures he'll undergo.

STRUCTURAL TESTS

Kidney-ureter-bladder radiography

Usually the first step in diagnostic testing of the urinary system, kidney-ureter-bladder (KUB) radiography surveys the abdomen to determine the position of the kidneys, ureters, and bladder, and to detect gross abnormalities. This test (also known as scout film or flat plate of the abdomen) does not require intact renal function and may aid differential diagnosis of urologic and GI diseases, which often produce similar signs and symptoms. However, a KUB test has many limitations and nearly always must be followed by more elaborate tests, such as excretory urography or renal computed tomography. KUB radiography should not follow recent instillation of barium, which obscures the urinary system.

Purpose

■ To evaluate the size, structure, and position of the kidneys
■ To screen for abnormalities such as calcifications in the region of the kidneys, ureters, and bladder.

Patient preparation

Explain to the patient that this test shows the position of the urinary system organs and helps detect abnormalities in them. Inform him that he needn't restrict food or fluids. Tell him who will perform the test and where, and that it takes only a few minutes.

Procedure

The patient is placed on an X-ray table in the supine position and in correct body alignment. His arms are extended overhead, and the iliac crests are checked for symmetrical positioning. If the patient can't extend his arms or stand, he may lie on his left side with his right arm up. A single radiograph is taken. (See *Positioning the patient for KUB radiography.*)

Precautions

The male patient should have gonadal shielding to prevent irradiation of the testes. The female patient's ovaries can't be shielded because they're too close to the kidneys, ureters, and bladder.

Normal findings

The shadows of the kidneys appear bilaterally, the right slightly lower than the left. Both kidneys should be approximately the same size, with the superior poles tilted slightly toward the vertebral column, paralleling the shadows (or stripes) produced by the psoas muscles. The ureters are only visible when an abnormality such as calcification is present. Visualization of the bladder depends on the density of its muscular wall and on the amount of urine in it. Generally, the bladder's shadow can be seen but not as clearly as the kidneys'.

Implications of results

Bilateral renal enlargement may result from polycystic disease, multiple myeloma, lymphoma, amyloidosis, hydronephrosis, or compensatory hypertrophy. A tumor, a cyst, or hydronephrosis may cause unilateral enlargement. Abnormally small kidneys may suggest end-stage glomerulonephritis or bilateral atrophic pyelonephritis. An apparent decrease in the size of one kidney suggests possible congenital hypoplasia, atrophic pyelonephritis, or ischemia. Renal displacement may be due to a retroperitoneal tumor such as an adrenal tumor. Obliteration or bulging of a portion of the psoas muscle stripe may result from tumor, abscess, or hematoma.

Positioning the patient for KUB radiography

For kidney-ureter-bladder (KUB) radiography, the patient is instructed to lie in a supine position with his arms extended over his head. To prevent motion and ensure films of good quality, he is asked to lie still for the few seconds it takes to make the exposure. An obese patient may be asked to exhale and then hold his breath during the brief procedure. As an added precaution, the gonads of male patients should be shielded.

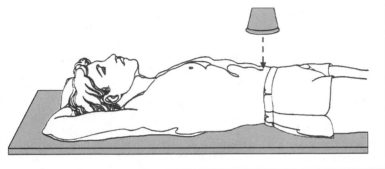

Congenital anomalies, such as abnormal location or absence of a kidney, may be suggested by renal axes that parallel the vertebral column, especially if the inferior poles of the kidneys cannot be clearly distinguished. A lobulated edge or border may indicate polycystic kidney disease or patchy atrophic pyelonephritis.

Opaque bodies may reflect calculi or vascular calcification due to aneurysm or atheroma; opacification may also suggest cystic tumors, fecaliths, foreign bodies, or abnormal fluid collection. Calcifications may appear anywhere in the urinary system, but positive identification requires further testing. The lone exception is a staghorn calculus, which forms a perfect cast of the renal pelvis and calyces.

Post-test care
None.

Interfering factors
■ Gas, feces, contrast medium, or foreign bodies in the intestine may obscure the urinary system.

■ Calcified uterine fibromas or ovarian lesions may prevent clear visualization of the kidneys, ureters, and bladder.

■ Obesity or ascites may result in a radiograph of poor quality.

Nephrotomography

In nephrotomography, special films are exposed before and after opacification of the renal arterial network and parenchyma with contrast medium. The resulting tomographic slices clearly delineate various linear layers of the kidneys, while blurring structures in front of and behind these selected planes.

Nephrotomography can be performed as a separate procedure or as an adjunct to excretory urography. This test is particularly helpful in visualizing space-occupying lesions suggested by excretory urography or retrograde ureteropyelography. Additional films are exposed to define the thickness of the wall of the mass and its interior. Other tests that may resolve nephrotomographic findings include renal angiography and radionuclide renal imaging.

Purpose

■ To differentiate between a simple renal cyst and a solid neoplasm
■ To assess renal lacerations as well as posttraumatic nonperfused areas of the kidneys
■ To localize adrenal tumors when laboratory tests indicate their presence.

Patient preparation

Explain to the patient that this test provides images of sections or layers of the kidney tissues and blood vessels. Instruct him to fast for 8 hours before the test. Tell him who will perform the test and where and that it takes less than 1 hour.

Tell the patient that he'll be positioned on an X-ray table and that he may hear loud, clacking sounds as the films are exposed. Tell him that he may experience transient side effects from the injection of the contrast medium — usually a burning or stinging sensation at the injection site, flushing, and a metallic taste.

Make sure that the patient or responsible member of the family has signed a consent form if required. Check the patient's history for hypersensitivity to iodine or iodine-containing foods or to contrast media used in other diagnostic tests. If the patient has a history of sensitivity, inform the doctor so he can provide antiallergenic prophylaxis (such as diphenhydramine) or use a noniodic contrast medium.

Elderly or dehydrated patients are at increased risk for contrast-induced renal failure. Check serum creatinine levels, and inform the doctor if they exceed 1.5 mg/dl. I.V. fluids may be ordered prior to the test to ensure hydration and decrease nephrotoxic potential.

Equipment

X-ray table ✦ X-ray and tomographic equipment ✦ contrast medium ✦ infusion set and equipment.

Procedure

The test may be performed using either the infusion method or the bolus method. The former is currently the method of choice because it allows for repeating poorly defined tomograms without additional infusion of contrast medium. Complications resulting from either technique are minor and occur infrequently. Regardless of the technique used, first a plain film of the kidneys is exposed, to provide general information about position, size, and shape, and preliminary anteroposterior tomograms are made to determine tomographic levels. Posterior oblique tomograms are made to rule out the presence of radiopaque renal calculi, which would be masked by the contrast medium.

For the infusion method: After test tomograms are reviewed, five vertical slices of renal parenchyma 1 cm apart are selected for filming. Contrast medium is then administered through the antecubital vein — the first half in 4 to 5 minutes (rapid phase) and the second half in the following 8 to 10 minutes (slow phase). Serial tomograms are made as soon as the slow phase begins.

For the bolus method: After test tomograms are reviewed, circulation time from arm to tongue is determined by injecting a bolus of bitter-tasting agent (dehydrocholic acid or sodium dehydrocholate) into the antecubital vein. Arm-to-tongue circulation time is close to arm-to-kidney circulation time (10 to 14 seconds). With the needle still in place, a loading dose of a conventional

Distinguishing between simple cysts and solid tumors

FEATURE	CYST	TUMORS
Consistency	Homogeneous	Irregular
Contact with healthy renal tissue	Sharply distinct	Poorly resolved
Density	Radiolucent	Variable radiolucent patches (or same as normal renal parenchyma)
Shape	Spherical	Variable
Wall of lesion	Thin and well defined	Thick and irregular

urographic contrast medium is injected to perform excretory urography.

Five minutes after this injection, a loading dose of a contrast medium (such as Renografin-76 or Hypaque-M 75%) is quickly injected (within 2 seconds) to ensure a high concentration of the contrast agent in the kidneys. A multifilm tomographic cassette, exposed at the predetermined arm-to-kidney circulation time, visualizes the main renal vessels and possible vessels within tumors. A series of individual tomograms measuring 1 cm are then made in rapid succession (less than 2 minutes) through the opacified kidneys.

Although the bolus method produces exposures comparable to those obtained by the infusion technique, it requires almost perfect timing. If the exposures are poor, a second infusion of contrast medium is required because normal kidneys quickly clear the substance.

Precautions

Although not strictly contraindicated, nephrotomography should be performed with extreme caution in patients with hypersensitivity to iodine-based compounds, cardiovascular disease, or multiple myeloma and in elderly and dehydrated patients with impaired renal function, as evidenced by serum creatinine levels greater than 1.5 mg/dl.

Normal findings

The size, shape, and position of the kidneys appear within normal range, with no space-occupying lesions or other abnormalities.

Implications of results

Among the abnormalities detectable through nephrotomography are simple cysts and solid tumors, ectopic renal lobes, renal sinus-related lesions, adrenal tumors, areas of nonperfusion, and renal lacerations following trauma. (See *Distinguishing between simple cysts and solid tumors*.)

Post-test care

■ If a hematoma develops at the injection site, apply warm soaks.

■ Monitor vital signs and urine output for 24 hours after the test.

■ Ensure adequate hydration (unless contraindicated) and monitor serum creatinine levels because of risk of contrast-induced renal failure.

■ Observe for signs and symptoms of a post-test allergic reaction (flushing, nausea, urticaria, and sneezing). Have epinephrine (1:1,000) and an antihistamine available.

Interfering factors

Residual barium from a recent enema for upper or lower GI series may obscure the kidneys.

Renal computed tomography

Renal computed tomography (CT) scanning provides a useful image of the kidneys made from a series of tomograms (cross-sectional slices), which are then translated by a computer and displayed on an oscilloscope screen. The image density reflects the amount of radiation absorbed by renal tissue and permits identification of masses and other lesions. An I.V. contrast medium may be injected to accentuate the renal parenchyma's density and help differentiate renal masses.

This highly accurate test is usually performed to investigate diseases found by other diagnostic procedures such as excretory urography. It may also precede percutaneous biopsy (to guide needle placement) or follow a kidney transplant (to determine the kidney's size and location in relation to the bladder). In addition, it can localize renal or perinephric abscesses for drainage. Because of this procedure's ability to distinguish subtle differences in density, it has an advantage over ultrasonography.

Purpose

■ To detect and evaluate renal pathology, such as tumor, obstruction, calculi, polycystic kidney disease, congenital anomalies, and abnormal fluid accumulation around the kidneys
■ To evaluate the retroperitoneum.

Patient preparation

Explain to the patient that this test permits examination of the kidneys. If contrast enhancement is not scheduled, inform him that he needn't restrict food or fluids. If a contrast medium will be used, instruct him to fast for 4 hours before the test. Tell him who will perform the test and where and that it takes about an hour.

Inform the patient that he'll be positioned on an X-ray table and that a scanner will take films of his kidneys. Warn him that he may hear loud, clacking sounds as the scanner rotates around his body and that he may experience transient flushing, metallic taste, and headache after the contrast dye is injected.

Make sure that the patient or responsible member of the family has signed a consent form if required. Check the patient's history for hypersensitivity to shellfish, iodine, or contrast media. Mark any sensitivities clearly on the patient's chart and inform the doctor.

Just before the procedure, instruct the patient to put on a hospital gown and to remove any metallic objects that could interfere with the scan. Administer a pretest sedative, if ordered.

Equipment

Total body CT scanner ✦ contrast medium ✦ I.V. infusion setup ✦ syringes and needles.

Procedure

The patient is placed in the supine position on the scanning table and secured with straps. The table is moved into the scanner, and the patient is instructed to lie still. The scanner is operated from an adjacent room, where a technician can hear and see the patient. When the scanner is turned on, it rotates around the patient, taking multiple images at different angles within each cross-sectional slice.

Abnormal renal CT scan

This photograph of a renal computed tomography (CT) scan reveals a renal adenocarcinoma that has displaced and distorted the right kidney and that now exceeds it in size. The left kidney appears normal, the spine is sharp and white in the center of the photograph, and the stomach is equally clear at the top.

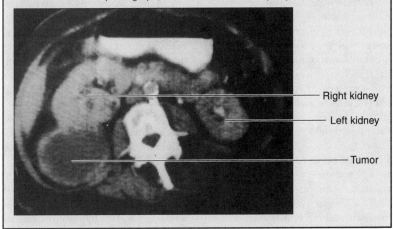

Right kidney

Left kidney

Tumor

When one series of tomograms is complete, contrast enhancement may be performed. An I.V. contrast medium is administered, and the patient is observed for allergic reactions, such as respiratory difficulty and urticaria or other skin eruption. Another series of tomograms is then taken. Information from the scan is stored on a disk or on magnetic tape, fed into a computer, and converted into an image for display on an oscilloscope screen. Radiographs and photographs are taken of selected views.

Precautions
If a contrast medium is used, watch for signs of hypersensitivity.

Normal findings
The normal renal parenchyma is slightly more dense than the liver, but less dense than bone, which appears white on a CT scan. The collecting system usually exhibits low (black) density, unless contrast medium is used to enhance it to a higher (whiter) density. The position of the kidneys is evaluated according to the surrounding structures; the size and shape of the kidneys are determined by counting cuts between the superior and inferior poles and following the contour of the renal outline.

Implications of results
Renal masses appear as areas of different density than normal parenchyma, possibly altering the kidneys' shape or projecting beyond their margins. Renal cysts, for example, appear as smooth, sharply defined masses, with thin walls and a lower density than normal parenchyma. Tumors such as renal cell carcinoma are usually not as well delineated; they tend to have thick walls and nonuniform density. (See *Abnormal renal CT scan.*) With contrast enhancement, solid tumors show a higher density than renal cysts but lower density than normal parenchyma. Tumors with hemorrhage, calcification, or necrosis

show higher densities. Vascular tumors are more clearly defined with contrast enhancement. Adrenal tumors are confined masses, usually detached from the kidneys and from other retroperitoneal organs.

Renal CT scans may also identify other abnormalities, including obstructions, calculi, polycystic kidney disease, congenital anomalies, and abnormal accumulations of fluid around the kidneys, such as hematomas, lymphoceles, and abscesses. After nephrectomy, CT scans can detect abnormal masses — such as recurrent tumors — in a renal fossa that should be empty.

Post-test care
If the procedure was performed with contrast enhancement, observe the patient for hypersensitivity to the contrast medium, and tell him he may resume his usual diet.

Interfering factors
■ Patient failure to lie still during the scan results in blurred images.
■ Artifacts may be caused by many factors, such as recent contrast studies, foreign bodies, catheters, and surgical clips.

Renal ultrasonography

In this test, high-frequency sound waves (usually 1 to 5 million cycles/second) are transmitted from a transducer through the kidneys and perirenal structures. The resulting echoes, amplified and converted into electrical impulses, are displayed on an oscilloscope screen as anatomic images.

Usually performed with other urologic tests, renal ultrasonography can detect abnormalities or provide more information about those detected by other tests. A safe, painless procedure, it's especially valuable when excretory urography is ruled out — for example, because of hypersensitivity to the contrast medium or the need for serial examinations.

Unlike excretory urography, this test does not require adequate renal function and therefore can be useful in patients with renal failure. Evaluation of urologic disorders may also include ultrasonography of the ureter, bladder, and gonads.

Purpose
■ To determine the size, shape, and position of the kidneys, their internal structures, and perirenal tissues
■ To evaluate and localize urinary obstruction and abnormal accumulation of fluid
■ To assess and diagnose complications following kidney transplantation
■ To detect renal or perirenal masses
■ To differentiate between renal cysts and solid masses.

Patient preparation
Explain to the patient that this test helps detect abnormalities in the kidneys. Inform him that he needn't restrict food or fluids. Tell him who will perform the test and where and that it takes about 30 minutes. Reassure him that the test is safe and painless; in fact, it may feel like a back rub. Just before the procedure, instruct the patient to put on a hospital gown.

Equipment
Ultrasound transducer and jelly ◆ cathode ray tube and amplifier ◆ oscilloscope ◆ Polaroid camera ◆ dynamic or real-time imaging equipment.

Procedure
The patient is placed in the prone position, and the area to be scanned is exposed. Ultrasound jelly is applied to the

area before the scanning begins. First, the longitudinal axis of the kidneys is located, using measurements from excretory urography or by performing transverse scans through the upper and lower renal poles. These points are marked on the skin and connected with straight lines. Sectional images (1 to 2 cm apart) can then be obtained by moving the transducer longitudinally and transversely or at any other angle required. During the test, the patient may be asked to breathe deeply to visualize upper ports of kidney.

Precautions
None.

Normal findings
The kidneys are located between the superior iliac crests and the diaphragm. The renal capsule should be outlined sharply; the cortex should produce more echoes than the medulla. In the center of each kidney, the renal collecting systems appear as irregular areas of higher density than surrounding tissue. The renal veins and, depending on the scanner, some internal structures can be visualized. If the bladder is also being evaluated, its size, shape, position, and urine content can be determined.

Implications of results
Cysts are usually fluid-filled, circular structures that don't reflect sound waves. Tumors produce multiple echoes and appear as irregular shapes. Abscesses found within or around the kidneys usually echo sound waves poorly; their boundaries are slightly more irregular than those of cysts. A perirenal abscess may displace the kidney anteriorly.

As a rule, acute pyelonephritis and glomerulonephritis aren't detectable unless the renal parenchyma is significantly scarred and atrophied. In such patients, the renal capsule appears irregular and the kidney may appear smaller than normal; also, an increased number of echoes may arise from the parenchyma because of fibrosis.

In hydronephrosis, renal ultrasonography may show a large, echo-free, central mass that compresses the renal cortex. Calyceal echoes are usually circularly diffused and the pelvis significantly enlarged. This test can also detect congenital anomalies, such as horseshoe, ectopic, or duplicated kidneys. Ultrasonography clearly detects renal hypertrophy.

After kidney transplantation, compensatory hypertrophy of the transplanted kidney is normal but an acute increase in size indicates rejection of the transplant.

This test allows identification of abnormal accumulations of fluid within or around the kidneys that sometimes arise from an obstruction. It also allows evaluation of perirenal structures and can identify abnormalities of the adrenal glands, such as tumors, cysts, and adrenal dysfunction. However, a normal adrenal gland is difficult to define by ultrasonography because of its small size.

Renal ultrasonography can detect changes in the shape of the bladder that result from masses and can assess urine volume. Increased urine volume or residual urine postvoiding may indicate bladder dysfunction.

Post-test care
Remove ultrasound jelly from the patient's skin.

Interfering factors
▪ Retained barium from X-ray studies may cause poor results.
▪ Obesity adversely affects tissue visualization.

Cystourethroscopy

Cystourethroscopy, a test that combines two endoscopic techniques, allows visual examination of the bladder and the urethra. One of the instruments used in this test is the cystoscope, which has a fiber-optic light source, a magnification system, a right-angled telescopic lens, and an angled beak for smooth passage into the bladder. The other instrument, the urethroscope (or panendoscope), is similar but has a straight-ahead lens and is used for examination of the bladder neck and the urethra. The cystoscope and urethroscope pass through a common sheath inserted into the urethra to obtain the desired view.

Other invasive procedures, such as biopsies, lesion resection, removal of calculi, dilatation of a constricted urethra, and catheterization of the renal pelvis for pyelography, may also be performed through this sheath.

Kidney-ureter-bladder radiography and excretory urography usually precede this test.

Purpose
■ To diagnose and evaluate urinary tract disorders by directly visualizing urinary structures.

Patient preparation
Explain to the patient that this test permits examination of the bladder and the urethra. Unless a general anesthetic has been ordered, inform the patient that he needn't restrict food or fluids. If a general anesthetic will be administered, instruct the patient to fast for 8 hours before the test. Tell him who will perform the test and where and that it takes about 20 to 30 minutes. Inform him that he may experience some discomfort after the procedure, including a slight burning when he urinates.

Make sure the patient or responsible family member has signed a consent form. Before the procedure, administer a sedative, if ordered, and instruct the patient to urinate.

Equipment
Cystourethroscope (components include sheath, cystoscope, and urethroscope) ✦ light source ✦ bougies á boule (for urethral calibration) ✦ sounds (for urethral dilatation) ✦ filiforms and followers (for severe stricture) ✦ preparatory tray ✦ local anesthetic set ✦ irrigating solution and administration set ✦ sterile gloves, gown, and drape ✦ sterile specimen containers.

Procedure
After general or regional anesthetic (as required) has been administered, the patient is placed in lithotomy position on a cystoscopic table. The genitalia are cleaned with an antiseptic solution, and the patient is draped. (Local anesthetic is instilled at this point.)

As the first step in cystourethroscopy, most urologists prefer to visually examine the urethra as they move the instrument toward the bladder. To do this, a urethroscope is inserted into the well-lubricated sheath (instead of an obturator), and both are passed gently through the urethra into the bladder. The urethroscope is then removed, and a cystoscope inserted through the sheath into the bladder. After the bladder is filled with irrigating solution, the scope is rotated to inspect the entire surface of the bladder wall and ureteral orifices with the right-angled telescopic lens. The cystoscope is then removed, the urethroscope reinserted, and both the urethroscope and the sheath are slowly withdrawn, permitting examination of the bladder neck and the various portions of the urethra, including the internal and external sphincters. (See *Using a cystourethroscope.*)

Using a cystourethroscope

This cross-sectional illustration shows how a urologic examination is performed with a cystourethroscope, a device that allows direct visualization of the tissues of the lower urinary tract. The sheath of the cystourethroscope permits passage of a cystoscope and a urethroscope for illuminating the urethra, bladder, and ureters. This instrument also provides a channel for minor surgical procedures, such as biopsies, excision of small lesions, and removal of calculi.

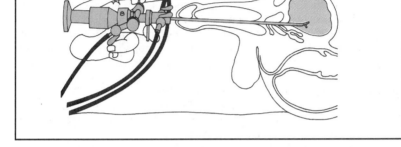

During cystourethroscopy, a urine specimen is routinely taken from the bladder for culture and sensitivity testing, and residual urine is measured. If a tumor is suspected, a urine specimen is sent to the laboratory for cytologic examination; if a tumor is found, biopsy may be performed. If a urethral stricture is present, urethral dilatation may be necessary before cystourethroscopy.

If the patient has received only a local anesthetic, he may complain of a burning sensation when the instrument is passed through the urethra. He may also feel an urgent need to urinate as the bladder fills with irrigating solution. Reassure the patient that these sensations are common and generally transient.

Precautions

■ Cystourethroscopy is contraindicated in patients with acute forms of urethritis, prostatitis, or cystitis because instrumentation can lead to sepsis.

■ The test is also contraindicated in patients with bleeding disorders because instrumentation can lead to increased bleeding.

Normal findings

The urethra, bladder, and ureteral orifices appear normal in size, shape, and position. The mucosa lining the lower urinary tract should appear smooth and shiny, with no evidence of erythema, cysts, or other abnormalities. The bladder should be free from obstructions, tumors, and calculi.

Implications of results

One of the most common abnormal findings detected in cystourethroscopy is an enlarged prostate gland in older men. In both males and females, urethral stricture, calculi, tumors, diverticula, ulcers, and polyps are also common findings. In addition, this test may detect bladder wall trabeculation and various congenital anomalies, such as ureteroceles, duplicate ureteral orifices, or urethral valves in children.

Post-test care

■ Care and assessment measures are similar to those for any postoperative patient who has undergone general anesthesia.

■ Monitor vital signs for 15 minutes for the first hour after the test, then every hour until they stabilize.

■ If local anesthesia was used, keep the patient supine for several minutes; then help him to sit or stand. Watch for orthostatic hypotension.

■ Instruct the patient to drink lots of fluids (or increase I.V. fluids if ordered) and to take the prescribed analgesic. Reassure him that burning and frequency will soon subside.

■ Administer antibiotics, as ordered, to prevent bacterial sepsis due to urethral tissue trauma.

■ Report flank or abdominal pain, chills, fever, an elevated white blood cell count, or low urine output to the doctor immediately.

■ Record intake and output for 24 hours, and observe the patient for distention. If the patient doesn't void within 8 hours after the test, or if bright red blood continues to appear after three voidings, notify the doctor.

■ Instruct the patient to abstain from alcohol for 48 hours.

■ Apply heat to the lower abdomen to relieve pain and muscle spasm (if ordered). A warm sitz bath may be ordered.

Interfering factors

None.

Retrograde urethrography

Used almost exclusively in males, this radiographic study is performed during instillation or injection of a contrast medium into the urethra, permitting visualization of its membranous, bulbar, and penile portions.

Indications for retrograde urethrography include outlet obstructions, congenital anomalies, and urethral lacerations or other trauma. This test may also be performed as a follow-up examination after surgical repair of the urethra. Although visualization of the anterior portion of the urethra is excellent with this test alone, the posterior portion is outlined more effectively by retrograde urethrography in conjunction with voiding cystourethrography.

Purpose

■ To diagnose urethral strictures, lacerations, diverticula, and congenital anomalies.

Patient preparation

Explain to the patient that this test helps diagnose urethral structural problems. Inform him that he needn't restrict food or fluids. Tell him who will perform the test and where and that it takes about 30 minutes.

Inform the patient that he may experience some discomfort when the catheter is inserted and when the contrast medium is instilled through the catheter. Tell him he'll hear loud, clacking sounds as the X-ray films are made.

Make sure the patient or responsible member of the family has signed a consent form. Check the patient's history for hypersensitivity to iodine-based contrast media or iodine-containing foods such as shellfish. Inform the doctor of any sensitivities. Because the contrast medium is injected directly into the lower urinary tract and does not enter the bloodstream, the patient is at decreased risk for contrast-induced acute renal failure or an allergic response.

Just before the procedure, administer a sedative, as ordered, and instruct the patient to urinate before leaving the unit.

Equipment
X-ray machine and table ✦ penile clamp ✦ 50-ml syringe with tapered universal adapter ✦ indwelling urinary catheter ✦ 1" roller gauze ✦ contrast medium (half-strength preparation).

Procedure
The patient (usually male) is placed in a recumbent position on the examining table. Anteroposterior exposures of the bladder and urethra are made, and the resulting films are studied for radiopaque densities, foreign bodies, and stones. The glans and meatus are cleaned with an antiseptic solution. The catheter is filled with the contrast medium before insertion to eliminate air bubbles. Although no lubricant should be used, the tip of the catheter may be dipped in sterile water to facilitate insertion.

The catheter is inserted until the balloon portion is inside the meatus; the balloon is then inflated with 1 to 2 ml of water, which prevents the catheter from slipping during the procedure.

The patient then assumes the right posterior oblique position, with his right thigh drawn up to a 90-degree angle and the penis placed along its axis. The left thigh is extended. The contrast medium is then injected through the catheter. After three-fourths of the contrast agent has been injected, the first X-ray film is exposed, while the rest of the contrast is injected. Left lateral oblique views may also be taken. Fluoroscopic control may be helpful, especially for evaluating urethral injury.

This test may be used in females when urethral diverticula are suspected. A double-balloon catheter occludes the bladder neck from above and the external meatus from below. In children, the procedure is the same as for adults, except that a smaller catheter is used.

Precautions
Retrograde urethrography should be performed cautiously in patients with a urinary tract infection.

Normal findings
The membranous, bulbar, and penile portions of the urethra — and occasionally the prostatic portion — appear normal in size, shape, and course.

Implications of results
Radiographs obtained during retrograde urethrography may show urethral diverticula, fistulas, strictures, false passages, calculi, and lacerations; congenital anomalies, such as urethral valves and perineal hypospadias; and rarely, tumors (in fewer than 1% of patients).

Post-test care
Watch for chills and fever related to extravasation of contrast medium into the general circulation for 12 to 24 hours after retrograde urethrography. Also observe for signs of sepsis and an allergic reaction.

Interfering factors
None.

Retrograde cystography

Retrograde cystography involves the instillation of contrast medium into the bladder, followed by radiographic examination. This procedure is used to diagnose bladder rupture without urethral involvement because it can determine the location and extent of the rupture.

Other indications for retrograde cystography include neurogenic bladder, recurrent urinary tract infections (especially in children), suspected vesicoureteral reflux, vesical fistulas, diverticula, and tumors. This test is also performed when cystoscopic examination is impractical, as in male infants, or when excretory urography has not adequately visualized the bladder. Voiding cystourethrography is often performed concomitantly.

Purpose
- To evaluate the structure and integrity of the bladder.

Patient preparation
Explain to the patient that this test permits X-ray examination of the bladder. Inform him that he needn't restrict food or fluids. Tell him who will perform the test and where and that it takes about 30 to 60 minutes.

Inform the patient that he may experience some discomfort when the catheter is inserted and when the contrast medium is instilled through the catheter. Tell him that he may hear loud, clacking sounds as the X-rays are made.

Make sure the patient or responsible family member has signed a consent form if required. Check the patient's history for hypersensitivity to contrast media, iodine, or shellfish; mark it on the chart, and inform the doctor.

Equipment
X-ray equipment ♦ drip infusion set or syringes ♦ standard contrast medium ♦ indwelling urinary catheters.

Procedure
The patient is placed in supine position on the examining table, and a preliminary kidney-ureter-bladder radiograph is taken. This radiograph is developed immediately and scrutinized for renal shadows, calcifications, contours of the bone and psoas muscles, and gas patterns in the lumen of the GI tract.

The bladder is then catheterized, and 200 to 300 ml of contrast medium (50 to 100 ml in an infant) is instilled, by gravity or gently by syringe injection. The catheter is then clamped.

With the patient supine, an anteroposterior film is taken. The patient is then tilted to one side, then the other, and two posterior oblique (and sometimes lateral) views are taken. If the patient's condition permits, he is placed in the jackknife position, and a posteroanterior film is taken. A space-occupying vesical lesion may require additional exposures. Rarely, to enhance visualization, 100 to 300 ml of air may be insufflated into the bladder by syringe after removal of the contrast medium (double-contrast technique).

The catheter is then unclamped, the bladder fluid allowed to drain, and a radiograph obtained to detect urethral diverticula, fistulous tracts into the vagina, or intraperitoneal or extraperitoneal extravasation of the contrast dye.

Precautions
- Retrograde cystography is contraindicated during exacerbation of an acute urinary tract infection or if an obstruction prevents passage of a urinary catheter.
- This test should not be performed on a patient with urethral evulsion or transection unless catheter passage and flow of contrast medium are monitored fluoroscopically.

Normal findings
Retrograde cystography shows a bladder with normal contours, capacity, integrity, and urethrovesical angle, with no evidence of tumor, diverticula, or rupture. Viscoureteral reflux should be absent. The bladder should not be displaced or externally compressed; the bladder wall should be smooth, not

Normal and abnormal retrograde cystograms

A normal retrograde cystogram (left) contrasts sharply with one showing a ruptured bladder (right). In the photograph on the right, the bladder, usually smooth and rounded when filled, has collapsed downward on itself, against the pelvic floor, and contrast material has extravasated upward into the peritoneal cavity from the tear in the bladder wall.

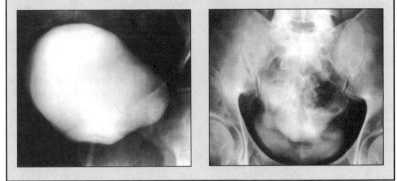

thick. (See *Normal and abnormal retrograde cystograms*.)

Implications of results

Retrograde cystography can identify vesical trabeculae or diverticula, space-occupying lesions (tumors), calculi or gravel, blood clots, high- or low-pressure vesicoureteral reflux, and hypotonic or hypertonic bladder.

Post-test care

■ Monitor vital signs every 15 minutes for the first hour, every 30 minutes during the second hour, then every 2 hours for up to 24 hours.
■ Record the time of the patient's voidings, and the color and volume of the urine. Observe for hematuria. If it persists after the third voiding, notify the doctor.
■ Watch for signs and symptoms of urinary sepsis from urinary tract infection (chills, fever, elevated pulse and respiration rates, hypotension) or similar signs related to extravasation of contrast medium into the general circulation.

Interfering factors

Residual barium from recent diagnostic tests or the presence of feces or gas in the bowel may produce cloudy images and interfere with test results.

Retrograde ureteropyelography

Retrograde ureteropyelography allows radiographic examination of the renal collecting system after injection of a contrast medium through a ureteral catheter during cystoscopy. The contrast medium is usually iodine-based, and although some of it may be absorbed through the mucous membranes, this test is preferred for patients with hypersensitivity to iodine (in whom I.V. administration of an iodine-based contrast medium, as in excretory urography, is contraindicated). This test is also indicated when visualization of the renal collecting system by excretory urography is inadequate because of inferior films or marked renal insufficiency (retrograde ureteropyelography is not influenced by impaired renal function).

Purpose

■ To assess the structure and integrity of the renal collecting system (calyces, renal pelvis, and ureter).

Patient preparation

Explain to the patient that this test permits visualization of the urinary collecting system. If a general anesthetic is ordered, instruct him to fast for 8 hours before the test. See that he's well hydrated to ensure adequate urine flow. Tell him who will perform the test and where and that it takes about 1 hour.

Inform the patient that he'll be positioned on an examining table, with his legs in stirrups, and that the position may be tiring. If he'll be awake throughout the procedure, tell him he may feel pressure as the instrument is passed and a pressure sensation in the kidney area when the contrast medium is introduced. He also may feel an urge to void.

Make sure that the patient or responsible family member has signed a consent form. Just before the procedure, administer premedication, if ordered.

Equipment

Cystoscopy setup ✦ ureteral catheters ✦ 10-ml syringes, with ureteral adapters ✦ X-ray equipment ✦ contrast medium ✦ tilt table with stirrups.

Procedure

The patient is placed in the lithotomy position. (Take care to avoid pressure points or impairment to circulation while his legs are in the stirrups.) After the patient is anesthetized, the urologist first performs a cystoscopic examination. After visual inspection of the bladder, one or both ureters are catheterized with opaque catheters, depending on

the condition or abnormality suspected. Radiographic monitoring allows correct positioning of the catheter tip in the renal pelvis.

The renal pelvis is emptied by gravity drainage or aspiration. About 5 ml of contrast medium (half-strength preparation) is then injected slowly through the catheter, using the syringe fitted with a special adapter. When adequate filling and opacification have occurred, anteroposterior films are taken and immediately developed. Lateral and oblique films can be taken, as needed, after the injection of more contrast dye.

After the radiographs of the renal pelvis are examined, a few more milliliters of contrast medium are injected to outline the ureters, as the catheter is slowly withdrawn. Delayed films (10 to 15 minutes after complete catheter removal) are then taken to check for retention of the contrast medium, indicating urinary stasis. If ureteral obstruction is present, the ureteral catheter may be kept in place and, together with an indwelling urinary catheter, connected to a gravity drainage system until post-test urinary flow is corrected or returns to normal.

Precautions

■ This test is contraindicated in pregnant women unless the benefits of the procedure outweigh the risks to the fetus.
■ Retrograde ureteropyelography must be done carefully if the patient has urinary stasis caused by ureteral obstruction, to prevent further injury to the ureter.

Normal findings

Following a normal cystoscopic examination, ureteral catheterization, and injection of contrast medium through the catheters, opacification of the renal pelvis and calyces should occur immediately. Normal structures should be outlined clearly and should appear symmetrical in bilateral testing. The ureters should fill uniformly and appear normal in size and course. Inspiratory and expiratory exposures, when superimposed, normally create two outlines of the renal pelvis 2 cm apart.

Implications of results

Incomplete or delayed drainage reflects an obstruction, usually at the ureteropelvic junction. Enlargement of the components of the collecting system or delayed emptying of the contrast medium may indicate obstruction due to tumor, blood clot, stricture, or calculi.

Perinephric inflammation or suppuration often causes fixation of the kidney on the same side, resulting in a single sharp radiographic outline of the collecting system when inspiratory and expiratory exposures are superimposed. Upward, downward, or lateral renal displacement can result from renal abscess or tumor or from perinephric abscess. Neoplasms can cause displacement of either pole or of the entire kidney. (See *What ureteropyelography reveals.*)

Post-test care

■ Check vital signs every 15 minutes for the first 4 hours, every hour for the next 4 hours, then every 4 hours for 24 hours.
■ Monitor fluid intake and urine output for 24 hours, and observe each specimen for hematuria. Report gross hematuria or hematuria after the third voiding, which is abnormal. Notify the doctor if the patient doesn't void for 8 hours after the procedure, or immediately if the patient feels distress and his bladder is distended. Urethral catheterization may be necessary.
■ Be especially attentive to catheter output if ureteral catheters have been left in place because inadequate output may reflect catheter obstruction, requiring irrigation by the doctor. Protect ureteral catheters from dislodgment. Note output amounts for each catheter (in-

What ureteropyelography reveals

Ureteropyelography may detect obstruction of urine flow in the calyces, pelvis, or ureter of the renal collecting system. Such obstruction may result from stricture, neoplasm, blood clot, or calculi, as shown below. Small calculi may remain in the calyces and pelvis, or they may pass down the ureter. A staghorn calculus (a cast of the calyceal and pelvic collecting system) may form from a stone that stays in the kidney.

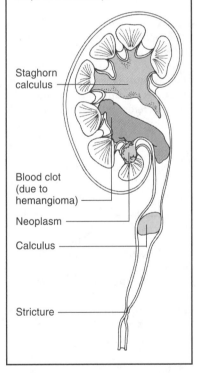

Staghorn calculus

Blood clot (due to hemangioma)

Neoplasm

Calculus

Stricture

dwelling urinary, ureteral) separately; this helps determine the location of an obstruction that's causing reduced output.
■ Administer ordered analgesics, tub baths, and increased fluids for dysuria, which commonly occurs after retrograde ureteropyelography.

■ Watch for and report severe pain in the area of the kidneys as well as any signs or symptoms of sepsis (such as chills, fever, and hypotension).

Interfering factors
Previous contrast studies or the presence of feces or gas in the bowel affects the quality of the radiograph and hinders accurate interpretation.

Antegrade pyelography

This radiographic procedure allows examination of the upper collecting system when ureteral obstruction rules out retrograde ureteropyelography or when cystoscopy is contraindicated. Antegrade pyelography also is indicated when excretory urography or renal ultrasonography demonstrates hydronephrosis and the need for therapeutic nephrostomy.

In this procedure, contrast medium is injected into the renal pelvis or calyces through percutaneous needle puncture. After completion of radiographic studies, a nephrostomy tube can be inserted to provide temporary drainage or access for other therapeutic or diagnostic procedures.

Renal pressure can be measured during the procedure. Also, urine can be collected for cultures and cytologic studies and for evaluation of renal functional reserve before surgery.

Purpose
■ To evaluate obstruction of the upper collecting system by stricture, calculus, clot, or tumor
■ To evaluate hydronephrosis revealed during excretory urography or ultrasonography and to allow placement of a percutaneous nephrostomy tube

■ To evaluate the function of the upper collecting system after ureteral surgery or urinary diversion
■ To assess renal functional reserve before surgery.

Patient preparation
Explain to the patient that this test allows radiographic examination of the kidney. Tell him that he may be required to fast for 6 to 8 hours before the test and may receive antimicrobials before and after the procedure. Tell him who will perform the test and where and that it takes 1 to 2 hours.

Inform the patient that a needle will be inserted into the kidney after he is given a sedative and a local anesthetic. Explain that urine may be collected from the kidney for testing and that, if necessary, a tube will be left in the kidney for drainage. Tell him that he may feel mild discomfort during injection of the local anesthetic and contrast medium and that he may also feel transient burning and flushing from the contrast medium. Warn him that the X-ray machine makes loud clacking sounds as it takes films.

Check the patient's history for hypersensitivity reactions to contrast media, iodine, or shellfish. Mark any sensitivities clearly on the chart and report them to the doctor. Also check the history and recent coagulation studies for indications of bleeding disorders.

Make sure that the patient or a responsible family member has signed an appropriate consent form if required. Just before the procedure, administer a sedative, if ordered.

Equipment
X-ray equipment, including a fluoroscope and possibly ultrasound equipment ✦ percutaneous nephrostomy tray ✦ manometer ✦ preparatory tray ✦ gloves and sterile containers for specimens ✦ syringes and needles ✦ contrast medium

✦ local anesthetic ✦ emergency resuscitation equipment.

Procedure

The patient is placed prone on the X-ray table, the skin over the kidney is cleaned with antiseptic solution, and a local anesthetic is injected. Previous urographic films or ultrasound recordings are studied for anatomic landmarks. (It's important to determine if the kidney to be studied is in normal position. If not, the angle of the needle entry must be adjusted during percutaneous puncture.)

Under guidance of fluoroscopy or ultrasound, the percutaneous needle is inserted below the 12th rib at the level of the transverse process of the second lumbar vertebra. Aspiration of urine confirms that the needle has reached the dilated collecting system (usually 7 to 8 cm below the skin surface in adults). Flexible tubing is connected to the needle to prevent displacement during the procedure. If intrarenal pressure is to be measured, the manometer is connected to the tubing as soon as it's in place. Urine specimens are then collected if needed.

An amount of urine equal to the amount of contrast medium to be injected is withdrawn to prevent overdistention of the collecting system. The contrast medium is injected under fluoroscopic guidance. Posteroanterior, oblique, and anteroposterior radiographs are taken. Ureteral peristalsis is observed on the fluoroscope screen to evaluate obstruction. A percutaneous nephrostomy tube is inserted at this time if drainage is needed because of increased renal pressure, dilation, or intrarenal reflux. If drainage is not needed, the catheter is withdrawn and a sterile dressing is applied.

Precautions

▪ Antegrade pyelography is contraindicated in bleeding disorders.
▪ This procedure is contraindicated in pregnancy unless the results outweigh the risk of harm to the fetus.
▪ Watch for signs of hypersensitivity to the contrast medium.

Normal findings

After injection of the contrast medium, the upper collecting system should fill uniformly and appear normal in size and course. Normal structures should be clearly outlined.

Implications of results

Enlargements of the upper collecting system and parts of the ureteropelvic junction indicate obstruction. Antegrade pyelography shows the degree of dilation, clearly defines obstructions, and demonstrates intrarenal reflux. In hydronephrosis, the ureteropelvic junction shows marked distention. Results of recent surgery or urinary diversion will be obvious; for example, a ureteral stent or a dilated stenotic area will be clearly visualized.

Intrarenal pressures that exceed 20 cm H_2O indicate obstruction. Cultures or cytologic studies of urine specimens taken during antegrade pyelography can confirm antegrade pyelonephrosis or malignant tumor.

Post-test care

▪ Check vital signs every 15 minutes for the first hour, every 30 minutes for the second hour, and every 2 hours for the next 24 hours.
▪ During each check of vital signs, inspect dressings for bleeding, hematoma, or urine leakage at the puncture site. For bleeding, apply pressure. For a hematoma, apply warm soaks. Report urine leakage to the doctor.
▪ Monitor fluid intake and urine output for 24 hours. Notify the doctor if the

patient doesn't void within 8 hours. Observe each specimen for hematuria. Report hematuria if it persists after the third voiding.

 ■ Watch for and report signs and symptoms of sepsis or extravasation of the contrast medium (chills, fever, rapid pulse or respiratory rate, hypotension).

■ Also watch for and report signs and symptoms that adjacent organs have been punctured: pain in the abdomen or flank, or pneumothorax (sudden onset of pleuritic chest pain, dyspnea, tachypnea, decreased breath sounds on the affected side, tachycardia).

■ If a nephrostomy tube is inserted, ensure that it's patent and draining well.

■ Administer antibiotics for several days after the procedure, as ordered, to prevent infection. Administer analgesics as ordered.

Interfering factors

■ Recently performed barium procedures or the presence of feces or gas in the bowel can impair the visualization of the kidney, hindering accurate results.

■ Obesity may hinder needle placement.

Magnetic resonance imaging of the urinary tract

Magnetic resonance imaging (MRI) is just coming into use for diagnosing urinary tract disorders. It is unclear at present whether MRI is better than computed tomography or ultrasound for imaging of the urinary system. In most cases, MRI is used when these alternative tests fail to produce a clear image. MRI uses radiofrequency waves and magnetic fields to visualize specific structures (kidney or prostate), which are then converted to computer-generated images.

Purpose

■ To evaluate genitourinary tumors and abdominal or pelvic masses
■ To distinguish betwen benign and malignant growths in the prostate
■ To detect cancer invasion into seminal vesicles and pelvic lymph nodes.

Patient preparation

Explain to the patient that this test helps evaluate abnormalities in the urinary system. Advise him to avoid alcohol, caffeine-containing beverages, and smoking for at least 2 hours and food for at least 1 hour before the test.

Tell him who will perform the test and where and that it takes about 30 to 90 minutes. He can continue taking medications, except for iron, which interferes with the imaging. Tell him he'll need to remove all clothing, jewelry, and metallic objects before the test and will wear a special hospital gown without snaps or closures. Inform the patient that he won't feel pain but may feel claustrophobic while lying supine in the tubular MRI chamber. If so, the doctor may order an antianxiety medication.

Tell the patient that he'll hear loud, crushing noises throughout the test. However, he'll probably receive a headset with choice of music to decrease the loud noise.

If contrast media will be used, obtain a history of allergies or hypersensitivity to these agents. Mark any sensitivities on the chart and notify the doctor. Ask the patient if he has any implanted metal devices or prostheses, such as vascular clips, shrapnel, pacemakers, joint implants, filters, and intrauterine devices. If so, he may not be able to have the test. If required, obtain a signed consent form from the patient or a responsible family member. Just before the procedure, have the patient urinate.

Equipment

MRI machine (which contains a circular magnet and a radiofrequency coil) ✦ headset with music.

Procedure

If a contrast medium is used, an I.V. line is started and the medium is administered prior to the procedure. The patient is placed in the supine position on a narrow, flat table, and the table is then moved into the enclosed cylindrical scanner. Varying radiofrequency waves are directed at the area being scanned. The patient is told to lie very still in the scanner while the images are being produced.

Although his face remains uncovered to allow him to see out, the patient is advised to keep his eyes closed to promote relaxation and prevent a closed-in feeling. If nausea occurs because of claustrophobia, the patient is encouraged to take deep breaths.

Precautions

■ This test is contraindicated in patients with metal implants, rods, or screws, or prosthetic devices.
■ This test is contraindicated in pregnant patients unless its benefits greatly outweigh the possible risks to the fetus.
■ The scanner cannot be used with patients who are extremely obese.
■ All metal objects, such as jewelry, hairpins, and dentures, are removed prior to the test.

Normal findings

In visualizing the soft-tissue structures of the kidneys, MRI can determine blood vessel size, anatomy, and hemodynamics. However, this test has not proved useful for detecting calculi or calcified tumors.

Implications of results

MRI can reveal tumors, strictures, stenosis, thrombosis, malformations, abscess, inflammation, edema, fluid collection, bleeding, hemorrhage, and organ atrophy.

Post-test care

■ If sedatives were given, monitor vital signs until the patient is awake and responsive.
■ Advise the patient to resume his usual diet, fluids, and medications, if applicable.
■ Monitor the patient for adverse reactions to the contrast medium (flushing, nausea, urticaria, and sneezing).
■ Watch the I.V. site for hematoma, if applicable. If hematoma occurs, apply warm soaks.

Interfering factors

■ Uncooperative behavior, unstable medical conditions (confusion, combativeness), or inability to remain still during the procedure interferes with accurate testing.
■ Use of I.V. pumps or assistive life-support equipment also interferes with accurate testing.

STRUCTURAL AND FUNCTIONAL TESTS

Excretory urography

The cornerstone of a urologic workup, excretory urography allows visualization of the renal parenchyma, calyces, and pelvis as well as the ureters, bladder and, in some cases, the urethra after I.V. administration of a contrast medium. Also known as intravenous pyelography, this common and extremely useful procedure shows the entire urinary tract — not just the renal pelvis, as the prefix *pyelo* implies.

Clinical indications for this test include suspected renal or urinary tract disease, renal calculi, space-occupying lesions, congenital anomalies, or trauma to the urinary system.

Purpose

- To evaluate the structure and excretory function of the kidneys, ureters, and bladder
- To support a differential diagnosis of renovascular hypertension.

Patient preparation

Explain to the patient that this test helps to evaluate the structure and function of the urinary tract. After ensuring that the patient is well hydrated, instruct him to fast for 8 hours before the test. Tell him who will perform the test and where.

Inform the patient that he may experience a transient burning sensation and metallic taste when the contrast agent is injected. Tell him to report any other sensations he may experience. Warn him that the X-ray machine makes loud, clacking sounds during the test.

Make sure that the patient or responsible family member has signed a consent form. Check the patient's history for hypersensitivity to iodine, iodine-containing foods, or contrast media containing iodine. Mark any sensitivities on the chart and notify the doctor. Administer a laxative, if ordered, the night before the test to minimize poor resolution of X-ray films due to feces or gas in the GI tract.

Equipment

Contrast medium (diatrizoate sodium, iothalamate sodium, diatrizoate meglumine, or iothalamate meglumine) ✦ 50-ml syringe (or I.V. container and tubing) ✦ 19G to 21G needle, catheter, or butterfly needle ✦ venipuncture equipment (tourniquet, antiseptic, adhesive bandage) ✦ X-ray table ✦ X-ray and tomographic equipment ✦ emergency resuscitation equipment.

Procedure

The patient is placed in the supine position on the X-ray table. A kidney-ureter-bladder radiograph is performed to detect gross abnormalities of the urinary system. If no such abnormalities are found, the contrast medium is injected (dosage varies according to age), and the patient is observed for signs and symptoms of hypersensitivity (flushing, nausea, vomiting, urticaria, or dyspnea). The first radiograph, visualizing the renal parenchyma, is obtained about 1 minute after the injection. (This may be supplemented by tomography if small, space-occupying masses — such as cysts or tumors — are suspected.) Films are then exposed at regular intervals — usually 5, 10, and 15 or 20 minutes after the injection.

Ureteral compression is performed after the 5-minute film is exposed. This can be accomplished through inflation of two small rubber bladders placed on the abdomen on both sides of the midline, secured by a fastener wrapped around the patient's torso. The inflated bladders occlude the ureters, without causing the patient discomfort, and facilitate retention of the contrast medium by the upper urinary tract. (Ureteral compression is contraindicated in ureteral calculi, aortic aneurysm, pregnancy, or recent abdominal trauma or surgical procedure.) After the 10-minute film is exposed, ureteral compression is released. As the contrast flows into the lower urinary tract, another film is taken of the lower halves of both ureters and then, finally, one is taken of the bladder.

At the end of the procedure, the patient voids, and another film is taken

Abnormal excretory urogram

In a patient with suspected renovascular hypertension (shown below), an excretory urogram taken 8 minutes after injection of a contrast medium shows normal filling of the right kidney but delayed opacification of the left renal calyces, pelvis, and ureter. This impaired excretion of the contrast material commonly results from narrowing of the renal artery feeding the subject kidney. Constriction hinders blood flow to the glomerulus and leads to increased renal absorption of water and decreased urine output. Demonstration of delayed calyceal opacification can differentiate between unilateral renovascular hypertension and essential hypertension.

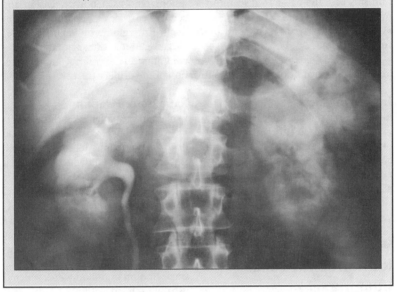

immediately to visualize residual bladder contents or mucosal abnormalities of the bladder or urethra.

Precautions

■ Premedication with corticosteroids may be indicated for patients with severe asthma or a history of sensitivity to the contrast medium.

■ The test may be contraindicated in patients with abnormal renal function (as evidenced by increased creatinine and blood urea nitrogen greater than 40 mg/dl) and in children or elderly patients with actual or potential dehydration.

Normal findings

The kidneys, ureters, and bladder show no gross evidence of soft- or hard-tissue lesions. Prompt visualization of the contrast medium in the kidneys demonstrates bilateral renal parenchyma and pelvicalyceal systems of normal conformity. The ureters and bladder should be outlined, and the postvoiding should show no mucosal abnormalities and little residual urine.

Implications of results

Excretory urography can demonstrate many urinary system abnormalities, including renovascular hypertension (see *Abnormal excretory urogram*), renal and ureteral calculi; abnormal size, shape, or structure of the kidneys, ureters, or bladder; supernumerary or absent kidney; polycystic kidney disease associated with renal hypertrophy; redundant pelvis or ureter; space-occupying lesions; pyelonephritis; renal tuberculosis; and hydronephrosis.

Post-test care

- If a hematoma develops at the injection site, ease the patient's discomfort by applying warm soaks.
- Observe for delayed reactions to the contrast medium.
- Continue I.V. fluids or provide oral fluids to increase hydration.

Interfering factors

End-stage renal disease, fecal matter or gas in the colon, insufficient injection of contrast medium, or a recent barium enema or GI or gallbladder series may produce films of poor quality that cannot be interpreted accurately.

Radionuclide renal imaging

This test, involving I.V. injection of a radionuclide, followed by scintiphotography, can provide a wealth of information for evaluating the kidneys. Observing the uptake concentration and transit of the radionuclide during this test allows assessment of renal blood flow, nephron and collecting system function, and renal structure. Depending on the patient's clinical signs and symptoms, this procedure may include dynamic scans to assess renal perfusion and function or static scans to assess structure.

The radioisotope injected depends on the specific information required and the examiner's preference. However, this procedure often includes double-isotope technique to obtain a sequence of perfusion and function studies, followed by static images. This test may also be substituted for excretory urography in patients with a hypersensitivity to contrast agents.

Purpose

- To detect and assess functional and structural renal abnormalities such as lesions, renovascular hypertension, and acute or chronic disease, such as pyelonephritis or glomerulonephritis
- To assess renal transplantation or renal injury due to trauma and obstruction of the urinary tract.

Patient preparation

Explain to the patient that this test permits evaluation of renal structure, blood flow, and function. Tell him who will perform the test and where and that it takes about 1½ hours. (If static scans are ordered, there will be a delay of several hours before the images are taken.)

Inform the patient that he'll receive an injection of a radionuclide and may experience transient flushing and nausea. Emphasize that he'll receive only a small amount of radionuclide, which is usually excreted within 24 hours. Tell him several series of films will be taken of his bladder.

Make sure the patient or responsible member of the family has signed a consent form and that the patient isn't scheduled for other radionuclide scans on the same day as the test. If the patient takes an antihypertensive, ask the doctor if it should be withheld before the test. Pregnant women and young children may receive supersaturated solution of potassium iodide 1 to 3 hours before the test to block thyroid uptake of iodine.

Equipment

Computerized gamma scintillation camera ✦ technetium Tc 99m pentetate for perfusion study ✦ iodohippurate sodium I 131 (Hippuran) for function study ✦ oscilloscope ✦ magnetic tape ✦ I.V. equipment.

Procedure

The patient is commonly placed in the prone position so that posterior views may be obtained. If the test is being performed to evaluate transplantation, the patient is positioned supine for anterior views. The exact position isn't critical, but the patient should be instructed not to change his position.

A perfusion study (radionuclide angiography) is performed first to evaluate renal blood flow. Technetium is administered I.V., and rapid-sequence photographs (one per second) are taken for 1 minute. Next, a function study is performed to measure the transit time of the radionuclide through the kidneys' functional units. After Hippuran is administered I.V., images are obtained at a rate of one per minute for 20 minutes. This entire procedure can be recorded on computer-compatible magnetic tape. Renogram curves may be plotted concurrently. Finally, static images are obtained 4 or more hours later, after the radionuclide has drained through the pelvicalyceal system. No additional contrast is needed.

Precautions

This test is contraindicated in pregnant women unless the benefits to the mother outweigh the risk to fetus.

Normal findings

Because 25% of cardiac output goes directly to the kidneys, renal perfusion should be evident immediately after uptake of technetium in the abdominal aorta. A normal pattern of renal circulation should appear within 1 to 2 min-

utes. The radionuclide should delineate the kidneys simultaneously, symmetrically, and with equal intensity.

Hippuran, administered for the function study, rapidly outlines the kidneys, which should be normal in size, shape, and position, and defines the collecting system and bladder. Maximum counts of the radionuclide in the kidneys occur within 5 minutes after injection (and within 1 minute of each other), and should fall to approximately one-third or less of the maximum counts of the same kidney within 25 minutes. Within this time, the function of both kidneys can be compared as the concentration of radionuclide shifts from the cortex to the pelvis and, finally, to the bladder.

Renal function is best evaluated by comparing these images to the renogram curves. (See *Radionuclide renography,* page 994.) Total function is considered normal when the effective renal plasma flow is 420 ml/minute or greater and the percentage of the dose excreted in urine at 30 to 35 minutes is greater than 66%.

Implications of results

Images from the perfusion study can identify impeded renal circulation, such as that arising from trauma or renal artery stenosis or renal infarction. These conditions may occur in patients with renovascular hypertension or abdominal aortic disease. Because malignant renal tumors are usually vascular, these images can help differentiate tumors from cysts. In evaluating a transplanted kidney, abnormal perfusion may indicate obstruction of the vascular grafts.

The function study can detect abnormalities of the collecting system and extravasation of the urine. Markedly decreased tubular function causes reduced radionuclide activity in the collecting system; outflow obstruction causes decrease in radionuclide activity

Radionuclide renography

Commonly performed with the kidney function study after I.V. administration of iodohippurate sodium I 131, this test provides a curve illustrating renal activity. Known as a renogram, this curve represents uptake, transit, and excretion time of the radionuclide by each kidney.

After the kidneys are located by a plain film of the kidney region or by kidney-ureter-bladder radiography, detectors placed posteriorly at each kidney record radiation counts, which when plotted, form a curve over minute integrals. The amount of radiation detected over certain periods of time and the shape of the curve have diagnostic significance.

The illustration below shows a normal absorption and excretion curve for one normal kidney (string of red markers) as well as examples of curves associated with renal pathology (solid lines). For example, an obstructed kidney absorbs but fails to excrete the radionuclide; a kidney with a constricted renal artery takes up the radionuclide more slowly and to a lesser degree than normal, and excretes it more slowly; a nonfunctioning kidney fails to absorb the radionuclide, so the radiation counter detects only background radiation.

Renal uptake is represented by an initial sharp rise in the curve. Known as the *vascular phase,* this filling of the renal and perirenal space usually occurs within 30 to 45 seconds after radionuclide administration. Renal transit time, the *tubular phase,* occurs next and is seen as a slower rise in the curve that last for 2 to 5 minutes. Finally, the *excretory phase* represents drainage of the radionuclide from the kidneys.

Although certain curves are characteristic of specific disorders, the curve represents activity of the entire kidney and doesn't distinguish between its different areas. Consequently, renographic findings must be correlated with the patient's clinical status and the results of other urologic tests.

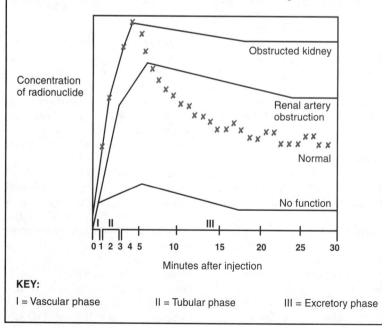

Concentration of radionuclide

Obstructed kidney

Renal artery obstruction

Normal

No function

I II III

0 1 2 3 4 5 10 15 20 25 30

Minutes after injection

KEY:

I = Vascular phase   II = Tubular phase   III = Excretory phase

in the tubules, with increased activity in the collecting system. This test can also define the level of ureteral obstruction.

Static images can demonstrate lesions, congenital abnormalities, and traumatic injury. These images also detect space-occupying lesions within or surrounding the kidney, such as tumors, infarcts, and inflammatory masses (abscesses, for example); they can also identify congenital disorders, such as horseshoe kidney and polycystic kidney disease. They can define regions of infarction, rupture, or hemorrhage after trauma.

A lower-than-normal total concentration of the radionuclide, as opposed to focal defects, suggests a diffuse renal disorder, such as acute tubular necrosis, severe infection, or ischemia. In a kidney transplant patient, decreased radionuclide uptake usually indicates organ rejection. Failure of visualization may indicate congenital ectopia or aplasia.

A definitive diagnosis usually requires the combined analysis of static images, perfusion studies, and function studies.

Post-test care

■ Instruct the patient to flush the toilet immediately every time he urinates for 24 hours as a radiation precaution.
■ If the patient is incontinent, change bed linens promptly and wear gloves to maintain standard precautions and prevent unnecessary skin contact.
■ Monitor the infection site for signs of hematoma, infection, and discomfort. Apply warm compresses for comfort.

Interfering factors

■ The patient's use of antihypertensives may interfere with test results by masking the cause of abnormalities.
■ Scans of different organs performed on the same day may interfere with one another.

Renal angiography

Renal angiography permits radiographic examination of the renal vasculature and parenchyma after arterial injection of a contrast medium. As the contrast agent pervades the renal vasculature, rapid-sequence radiographs show the vessels during three phases of filling: arterial, nephrographic, and venous. This procedure virtually always follows standard bolus aortography, which shows individual variations in the number, size, and condition of the main renal arteries and the aberrant vessels as well as the relationship of the renal arteries to the aorta.

Clinical indications for renal angiography include renal masses, pseudotumors, unilateral or bilateral kidney enlargement, nonfunctioning kidneys in patients with acute renal failure, positive urograms in patients with renovascular hypertension, vascular malformations, and intrarenal calcifications of unexplained etiology.

Purpose

■ To demonstrate the configuration of total renal vasculature before surgical procedures
■ To determine the cause of renovascular hypertension (stenosis, thrombotic occlusion, embolus, or aneurysm)
■ To evaluate chronic renal disease or renal failure
■ To investigate renal masses and renal trauma
■ To detect complications after a kidney transplant, such as a nonfunctioning shunt or rejection of the donor organ.

Patient preparation

Explain to the patient that this test permits visualization of the kidneys, blood vessels, and nephrons and aids in diagnosing renal disease and masses. Instruct him to fast for 8 hours before the test and to drink extra fluids the day before the test and after the test to maintain adequate hydration. (Or start an I.V. line, if needed.) Continue oral medications (a special order is needed for diabetic patients). Tell the patient who will perform the test and where, that it takes about 1 hour, and that he may receive a laxative or cleansing enema the evening before the test.

Describe the procedure to the patient, and inform him that he may experience transient flushing, burning, and nausea during injection of the contrast medium. Check the patient's history for hypersensitivity to iodine-based contrast media or iodine-containing foods such as shellfish. Mark sensitivities on the chart and inform the doctor so he can prescribe prophylactic antiallergenics (diphenhydramine or steroids) or have them available during the procedure.

Make sure the patient or a responsible family member has signed a consent form. Administer medication, if ordered (usually a sedative and a narcotic analgesic), before the test. Instruct the patient to put on a hospital gown and to remove all metallic objects that may interfere with test results. Have him urinate before leaving the unit.

Record baseline vital signs. Ensure that recent laboratory test results (blood urea nitrogen, serum creatinine, bleeding studies) are documented on the patient's chart. Verifying adequate renal functioning and adequate clotting ability is vital. Evaluate peripheral pulse sites, and mark them for easy access in postprocedure assessment.

Equipment

Image-intensified fluoroscope, with television monitor ✦ high-powered X-ray equipment ✦ pressure-injection device ✦ rapid cassette changer ✦ polyethylene radiopaque vascular catheters ✦ flexible guide wire ✦ contrast material (such as Hypaque, Renografin, or Isopaque) ✦ preparation tray, with 70% alcohol or povidone-iodine solution ✦ emergency resuscitation equipment.

Procedure

The patient is placed in the supine position, and a peripheral I.V. infusion is started. The skin over the arterial puncture site is cleaned with antiseptic solution, and a local anesthetic is injected.

Using the Seldinger technique, the femoral artery is punctured and, under fluoroscopic visualization, cannulated. (If a femoral pulse is absent or the artery is convoluted or plaque-ridden, percutaneous transaxillary, transbrachial, or translumbar catheterization may be performed instead.) After passing the flexible guide wire through the artery, the cannula is withdrawn, leaving several inches of wire in the lumen.

Next, a polyethylene catheter is passed over the wire and advanced, under fluoroscopic guidance, up the femoroiliac vessels to the aorta. The guide wire is removed, and the catheter is flushed with heparin flush solution to prevent clotting in the catheter tip. At this juncture, the contrast medium is injected, and screening aortograms are taken before proceeding. On completion of the aortographic study, a renal catheter is exchanged for the former one.

To determine the position of the renal arteries and ensure that the tip of the catheter is in the lumen, a test bolus (3 to 5 ml) of contrast dye is injected immediately. This prevents subintimal injection or arterial spasm that may mimic a renal artery lesion. If the patient has no adverse reaction, 20 to 25 ml of contrast dye is injected just below the origin of the renal arteries so that it doesn't reach the mesenteric vessels first, obscuring the renal arteries. After this injection, a series of rapid-sequence X-ray films of the filling of the renal vascular tree is exposed.

If further selective studies are needed, the catheter remains in place while the films are examined. If the films are satisfactory, the catheter is removed, and a sterile sponge is firmly applied to the puncture site for 15 minutes. Before the patient returns to his room, the puncture site is observed for hematoma.

Precautions

Renal angiography is contraindicated during pregnancy and in patients with bleeding tendencies, an allergy to contrast media, or renal failure due to end-stage renal disease.

Normal findings

Renal arteriographs show normal arborization of the vascular tree and normal architecture of renal parenchyma.

Implications of results

Renal tumors usually show hypervascularity; renal cysts typically appear as clearly delineated, radiolucent masses. Renal artery stenosis due to arteriosclerosis produces a noticeable constriction in the blood vessel, usually within the proximal portion of its length; this is a crucial finding in confirming renovascular hypertension. Renal artery dysplasia, unlike renal artery stenosis, usually affects the middle and distal portions of the vessel. Alternating aneurysms and stenotic regions give this rare disorder a characteristic beads-on-a-string appearance.

In renal infarction, blood vessels may appear to be absent or cut off, the normal tissue replaced by scar tissue. Another typical finding is the appearance of triangular areas of infarcted tissue near the periphery of the affected kidney. The kidney itself may appear shrunken because of tissue scarring.

Renal angiography may also detect renal artery aneurysms (saccular or fusiform), renal arteriovenous fistula with abnormal widening of and direct passage between the renal artery and renal vein. Destruction, distortion, and fibrosis of renal tissue with areas of reduced and tortuous vascularity may be noted in severe or chronic pyelonephritis, and an increase in capsular vessels with abnormal intrarenal circulation may indicate renal abscesses or inflammatory masses.

When angiography is used to evaluate renal trauma, it may detect intrarenal hematoma, parenchymal laceration, shattered kidney, and areas of infarction. This test may also be useful in distinguishing pseudotumors from tumors or cysts, in evaluating the volume of residual functioning renal tissue in hydronephrosis, and in evaluating donors and recipients before and after kidney transplantation.

Post-test care

- Keep the patient flat in bed; keep the leg on the affected side straight for at least 6 hours or as ordered.
- Check vital signs every 15 minutes for 1 hour, every 30 minutes for 2 hours, then every hour until they stabilize. Monitor popliteal and dorsalis pedis pulses for adequate perfusion at least every hour for 4 hours. Note the color and temperature of the involved extremity, and compare them with those of the uninvolved extremity.
- Watch for bleeding or hematomas at the injection site. Keep the pressure dressing in place, and check for bleeding when you check all vital signs. If bleeding occurs, notify the doctor promptly, and apply direct pressure or a weighted sandbag to the site.
- Apply cold compresses to the puncture site to lessen edema and pain.
- Provide extra fluids to prevent nephrotoxicity from the contrast medium.

Interfering factors

- Recent contrast studies (such as a barium enema or an upper GI series) may produce a cloudy radiographic image, thus interfering with accurate interpretation of test results.

- Patient movement during the test may impair the quality of the radiographs.
- The presence of feces or gas in the GI tract may impair the clarity of the films and hinder accurate interpretation.

Renal venography

This relatively simple procedure allows radiographic examination of the main renal veins and their tributaries. In this test, contrast medium is injected by percutaneous catheter passed through the femoral vein and inferior vena cava into the renal vein.

Indications for renal venography include renal vein thrombosis, tumor, and venous anomalies. This test helps distinguish renal parenchymal disease and aneurysms from pressure exerted by an adjacent mass. When other diagnostic tests yield ambiguous results, renal venography can definitively differentiate renal agenesis from a small kidney.

This procedure is also useful in assessing renovascular hypertension. Blood samples can be collected from renal veins during the procedure, and renin assays of the samples can differentiate essential renovascular hypertension from hypertension due to unilateral renal lesions.

Purpose

- To detect renal vein thrombosis
- To evaluate renal vein compression due to extrinsic tumors or retroperitoneal fibrosis
- To assess renal tumors and detect invasion of the renal vein or inferior vena cava
- To detect venous anomalies and defects

- To differentiate renal agenesis from a small kidney
- To collect renal vein blood samples for evaluation of renovascular hypertension.

Patient preparation

Explain to the patient that this test permits radiographic study of the renal veins. If ordered, instruct him to fast for 4 hours before the test. Tell him who will perform the test and where and that it takes about 1 hour.

Inform the patient that a catheter will be inserted into a vein in the groin area after he receives a sedative and a local anesthetic. Tell him that he may feel mild discomfort during injection of these substances and that he may feel transient burning and flushing from the contrast medium. Warn him that the X-ray equipment makes loud, clacking noises as the films are taken.

Check the patient's history for hypersensitivity to contrast media, iodine, or iodine-containing foods such as shellfish. Mark sensitivities on the chart, and report them to the doctor. Check the patient's history and any coagulation studies for indications of bleeding disorders.

If renin assays will be done, check the patient's diet and medications, and consult with the doctor. As ordered, restrict the patient's salt intake and discontinue antihypertensive drugs, diuretics, estrogen, and oral contraceptives.

Make sure that the patient or a responsible family member has signed a consent form. Just before the procedure, administer a sedative, if ordered.

Record baseline vital signs. Make sure that pretest blood urea nitrogen and urine creatinine levels are adequate because the kidneys clear contrast media.

Equipment

X-ray equipment ✦ renal venography tray with flexible guide wires, polyethylene radiopaque vascular catheters, needle and cannula or 18G needle, three-way stopcock, and flexible tubing ✦ preparatory tray ✦ syringes and needles ✦ contrast medium ✦ local anesthetic ✦ emergency resuscitation equipment.

Procedure

The patient is placed in the supine position on the X-ray table, with his abdomen centered over the film. The skin over the right femoral vein near the groin is cleaned with antiseptic solution and draped. (Left femoral vein or jugular veins may be used.)

A local anesthetic is injected, and the femoral vein is cannulated. Under fluoroscopic guidance, a guide wire is threaded a short distance through the cannula, which is then removed. A catheter is passed over the wire into the inferior vena cava. When catheterization of the femoral vein is contraindicated, the right antecubital vein is punctured, and the catheter is inserted and advanced through the right atrium of the heart into the inferior vena cava.

A test bolus of contrast medium is injected to ensure that the vena cava is patent. If so, the catheter is advanced into the right renal vein and contrast medium (usually 20 to 40 ml) is injected. When studies of the right renal vasculature are completed, the catheter is withdrawn into the vena cava, rotated, and guided into the left renal vein.

If visualization of the renal venous tributaries is indicated, epinephrine can be injected into the ipsilateral renal artery by catheter before contrast medium is injected into the renal vein. Epinephrine temporarily blocks arterial flow and allows filling of distal intrarenal veins. Obstructing the artery briefly with a balloon catheter is an alternative method that produces the same effect.

After anteroposterior films are made, the patient lies prone for posteroanterior films. For renin assays, blood samples are withdrawn under fluoroscopy within 15 minutes after venography. After catheter removal, apply pressure to the site for 15 minutes and put on a dressing.

Precautions

▪ Renal venography is contraindicated in severe thrombosis of the inferior vena cava.
▪ The guide wire and catheter should be advanced carefully if severe renal vein thrombosis is suspected.
▪ Watch for signs of hypersensitivity to the contrast medium.

Normal findings

Opacification of the renal vein and tributaries should occur as soon as the contrast agent is injected. The normal renin content of venous blood in a supine adult is 1.5 to 1.6 ng/ml/hour.

Implications of results

Occlusion of the renal vein near the inferior vena cava or the kidney indicates renal vein thrombosis. If the clot is outlined by contrast medium, it may look like a filling defect. However, a clot can usually be identified because it is within the lumen and less sharply outlined than a filling defect. Collateral venous channels, which opacify with retrograde filling during contrast injection, often surround the occlusion. Complete occlusion prolongs transit of the contrast medium through the renal veins.

A filling defect of the renal vein may indicate obstruction or compression by an extrinsic tumor or retroperitoneal fibrosis. A renal tumor that invades the renal vein or inferior vena cava usually produces a filling defect with a sharply defined border.

Venous anomalies are indicated by opacification of abnormally positioned or clustered vessels. Absence of a renal vein differentiates renal agenesis from a small kidney.

Elevated renin content in renal venous blood usually indicates essential renovascular hypertension when assay results correspond for both kidneys. Elevated renin levels in one kidney indicate a unilateral lesion and usually require further evaluation by arteriography.

Post-test care

■ Check vital signs and distal pulses every 15 minutes for the first hour, every 30 minutes for the second hour, then every 2 hours for 24 hours. Keep the patient on bed rest for 2 hours.

■ Observe the puncture site for bleeding or hematoma when checking vital signs; if bleeding occurs, apply pressure and notify the doctor.

 ■ Report signs and symptoms of vein perforation, embolism, and extravasation of contrast medium (chills, fever, rapid pulse and respiration, hypotension, dyspnea, and chest, abdominal, or flank pain). Also report complaints of paresthesia or pain in the catheterized limb — symptoms of nerve irritation or vascular compromise.

■ Administer a sedative and antimicrobials, as ordered.

■ Instruct the patient to increase fluid intake (unless contraindicated) to help clear contrast media.

■ Tell the patient to resume his normal diet and any medications discontinued before the test.

Interfering factors

■ Recent contrast studies or the presence of feces or gas in the bowel impairs visualization of the renal veins.

■ Failure to restrict salt, antihypertensive drugs, diuretics, estrogen, and oral contraceptives can interfere with renin assay results.

Uroflowmetry

This simple noninvasive test uses a uroflowmeter to detect and evaluate dysfunctional voiding patterns. The uroflowmeter, contained in a funnel into which the patient voids, measures flow rate (volume of urine voided per second), continuous flow (time of measurable flow), and intermittent flow (total voiding time, including interruptions).

Several types of uroflowmeters are available: rotary disc, electromagnetic, spectrophotometric, and gravimetric systems. The gravimetric system, which weighs urine as it's voided and plots the weight against time, is the simplest to use and is widely available.

Purpose

■ To evaluate lower urinary tract function

■ To demonstrate bladder outlet obstruction.

Patient preparation

Explain to the patient that this test evaluates his pattern of urination. Advise him not to urinate for several hours before the test and to increase fluid intake so he'll have a full bladder and a strong urge to void. Tell him who will perform the test and where and that it will take 10 to 15 minutes. Instruct him to remain still while voiding during the test to help ensure accurate results.

Assure the patient that he'll have complete privacy during the test; many people have difficulty voiding in the presence of others. As ordered, discontinue drugs that may affect bladder and sphincter tone.

Normal flow rate values

Normal values are listed below for minimum volumes needed to obtain adequate recordings.

AGE	MINIMUM VOLUME (ml)	MALE (ml/sec)	FEMALE (ml/sec)
4 to 7	100	10	10
8 to 13	100	12	15
14 to 45	200	21	18
45 to 65	200	12	15
66 to 80	200	9	10

Equipment

Commode chair with funnel containing a uroflowmeter ✦ beaker to hold urine ✦ transducer ✦ start and flow cables ✦ data recording module.

Procedure

The test procedure is the same with all types of equipment. A male patient is asked to void while standing; a female patient, while sitting. The patient is asked to avoid straining to empty the bladder. Cable connections are checked, and the patient is left alone.

The patient pushes the start button on the commode chair, counts for 5 seconds (one 1,000; two 1,000; and so on), and voids. When finished, he counts for 5 seconds and pushes the button again. The volume of urine voided is then recorded and plotted as a curve over the time of voiding. The patient's position and the route of fluid intake (oral or I.V.) are noted.

Precautions

■ The transducer must be level, and the beaker must be centered beneath the funnel.
■ The beaker must be large enough to hold all urine; overflow can invalidate results and damage the transducer.

Reference values

Flow rate varies by age and sex and the volume of urine voided. (See *Normal flow rate values.*)

Implications of results

An increased flow rate indicates reduced urethral resistance, which may be associated with external sphincter dysfunction. A high peak on the curve plotted over the voiding time indicates decreased outflow resistance, which may be due to stress incontinence. A decreased flow rate indicates outflow obstruction or hypotonia of the detrusor muscle. More than one distinct peak in a normal curve indicates abdominal straining, which may result from pushing against an obstruction to empty the bladder.

Post-test care

Instruct the patient to resume any medications withheld before the test.

Interfering factors

■ Drugs that affect bladder and sphincter tone, such as urinary spasmolytics and anticholinergics, alter test results.
■ Strong drafts can affect transducer function.

▪ If the patient moves while seated on the commode chair, flow recording may be inaccurate.

▪ The presence of toilet tissue in the beaker invalidates test results.

▪ Straining to void will alter test results.

Cystometry

Cystometry assesses the bladder's neuromuscular function by measuring the efficiency of the detrusor muscle reflex, intravesical pressure and capacity, and the bladder's reaction to thermal stimulation. It's especially useful for detecting the cause of involuntary bladder contractions in an unstable bladder. Because cystometry alone can provide ambiguous results, results of this test should always be supported by results of other urologic tests, such as cystourethrography and excretory urography.

Cystometry can be performed by instilling physiologic saline solution or sterile water or by insufflating a gas. In either method, characteristics of the urinary stream and the bladder's reaction to thermal stimulation may furnish accurate pathophysiologic information.

Purpose

▪ To evaluate detrusor muscle function and tonicity

▪ To help determine the cause of bladder dysfunction.

Patient preparation

Explain to the patient that this test evaluates bladder function. Inform him that he needn't restrict food or fluids. Tell him who will perform the test and where and that it takes about 40 minutes, unless additional testing is required.

Describe the procedure to the patient.

Inform him that he'll feel a strong urge to urinate during the test and that the procedure may be embarrassing and uncomfortable. Make sure the patient or a responsible family member has signed a consent form. Also, check the patient's medication history for drugs that may affect test results (such as antihistamines). Just before the procedure, ask the patient to urinate.

Equipment

Four-channel gas cystometer ♦ set of catheters.

Procedure

The patient is placed in the supine position on an examining table, and a catheter is passed into the bladder to measure residual urine. (Any difficulty with catheter insertion may reflect meatal or urethral obstruction.)

To test the patient's response to thermal sensation, 30 ml of room-temperature physiologic saline solution or sterile water is instilled into the bladder. Next, an equal volume of warm fluid (110° to 115° F [43° to 46° C]) is instilled in the patient's bladder. The patient is asked to report his sensations, such as the need to urinate, nausea, flushing, discomfort, and a feeling of warmth.

After the fluid is drained from the patient's bladder, the catheter is connected to the cystometer, and normal saline solution, sterile water, or gas (usually carbon dioxide) is slowly introduced into the bladder. The flow of gas is controlled automatically to the desired reading (100 ml/minute) by a four-channel cystometer. The patient is asked to indicate when he *first* feels an urge to void, then when he feels he *must* urinate. The related pressure and volume are automatically plotted on the graph.

When the bladder reaches its full capacity, the patient is asked to urinate to permit the maximal intravesical voiding pressure to be recorded. The pa-

Supplemental cystometric tests

TEST	PURPOSE	DESCRIPTION	NORMAL RESPONSE
Ice water test	Tests integrity of vesical reflex arc	After deflation of balloon catheter, 60 to 100 ml of sterile ice water is instilled into bladder.	Rapid expulsion of catheter and water through urethra
Bulbocavernosus reflex test	Determines integrity of sacral portion of spinal cord	Insertion of gloved finger into rectum is followed by squeezing of glans penis or clitoris.	Constriction of anal sphincter
Saddle sensation test	Tests reflex activity of conus medullaris	Anocutaneous line of perineum is pricked or stroked with pin.	Visible constriction of anal sphincter
Bethanechol sensitivity test	Defines patient with uninhibited or reflex type neurogenic bladder	Bethanechol chloride (2.5 mg/68 kg body weight) is administered subcutaneously and followed by cystometric measurement at 10, 20, and 30 minutes.	Manometric pressure >15 cm H_2O
Stress incontinence	Tests loss of voluntary control of vesicourethral sphincters	After filling of bladder, catheter is withdrawn and patient is asked to cough, bend over, or lift a heavy object.	No dribbling of urine from urethra (dribbling indicates stress incontinence)

tient's bladder is then drained and, if no additional tests are required, the catheter is removed; otherwise, the catheter is left in place to measure urethral pressure profile or to provide supplemental findings. (See *Supplemental cystometric tests*.)

If abnormal bladder function is caused by muscle incompetence or disrupted innervation, an anticholinergic (atropine) or cholinergic medication (bethanechol) may be injected and the study repeated in 20 to 30 minutes.

Precautions

▪ Cystometry is contraindicated in patients with acute UTIs because uninhibited contractions may cause erroneous readings and the test may lead to pyelonephritis and septic shock.

▪ Tell the patient not to strain when urinating because this could cause ambiguous cystometric readings.

▪ If the patient has a spinal cord injury that has caused motor impairment, transport him on a stretcher so the test can be performed without transferring him to the examining table.

Normal findings and implications of results

See *Cystometry: Normal and abnormal findings,* pages 1004 to 1007, for a summary of typical cystometric test results.

(Text continues on page 1008.)

Cystometry: Normal and abnormal findings

Because cystometry assesses micturition and vesical function, it can aid diagnosis of neurogenic bladder dysfunction. The five main types of neurogenic bladder (presented on the following pages) result from lesions of the central or peripheral nervous systems.

Uninhibited neurogenic bladder (opposite page, left) results from a lesion to the upper motor neuron and causes frequent, often uncontrollable micturition in the presence of even a small amount of urine. *Reflex neurogenic bladder* (opposite page, right) results from a complete upper motor neuron lesion and causes total loss of conscious sensation and vesical control.

Normal bladder function

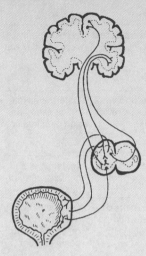

FEATURE OR RESPONSE	
Micturition	
Start	+
Stop	+
Residual urine	0
Vesical sensation	+
First urge to void	150 to 200 ml
Bladder capacity	400 to 500 ml
Bladder contractions	0
Intravesical pressure	L
Bulbocavernosus reflex	+
Saddle sensation test	+
Bethanechol sensitivity test (exaggerated response)	0
Ice water test	+
Anal reflex	+
Heat sensation and pain	+

KEY:

+ Present or positive	**↑** Increased	**V** Variable	**D** Delayed
0 Absent or negative	**↓** Decreased	**E** Early	**L** Low

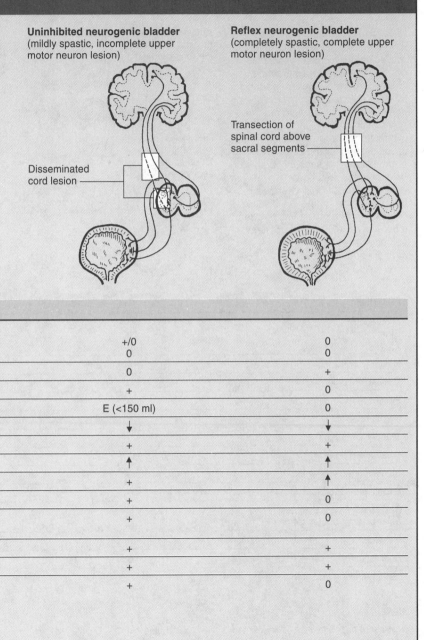

Uninhibited neurogenic bladder
(mildly spastic, incomplete upper
motor neuron lesion)

Reflex neurogenic bladder
(completely spastic, complete upper
motor neuron lesion)

Transection of
spinal cord above
sacral segments

Disseminated
cord lesion

+/0	0
0	0
0	+
+	0
E (<150 ml)	0
↓	↓
+	+
↑	↑
+	↑
+	0
+	0
+	+
+	+
+	0

(continued)

Cystometry: Normal and abnormal findings (continued)

In *autonomous neurogenic bladder* (at right), a lower motor neuron lesion produces a flaccid bladder that fills without contracting. The patient can't perceive bladder fullness or initiate and maintain urination without applying external pressure.

Lower motor neuron lesions can cause sensory or motor paralysis of the bladder. In *sensory paralytic bladder* (opposite page, left), the patient incurs chronic retention because he can't perceive bladder fullness. In *motor paralytic bladder* (opposite page, right), the patient perceives fullness but can't initiate or control urination.

Autonomous neurogenic bladder (flaccid, incomplete lower motor neuron lesion)

Destruction of second, third, and fourth sacral segments

FEATURE OR RESPONSE	
Micturition	
Start	0
Stop	0
Residual urine	+
Vesical sensation	0
First urge to void	0
Bladder capacity	↑
Bladder contractions	0
Intravesical pressure	↓
Bulbocavernosus reflex	0
Saddle sensation test	0
Bethanechol sensitivity test (exaggerated response)	+
Ice water test	0
Anal reflex	0
Heat sensation and pain	0

KEY:

+ Present or positive	↑ Increased	V Variable	D Delayed
0 Absent or negative	↓ Decreased	E Early	L Low

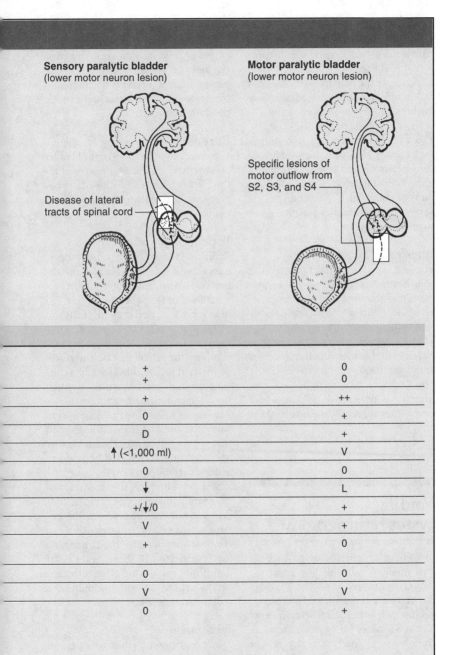

Sensory paralytic bladder
(lower motor neuron lesion)

Motor paralytic bladder
(lower motor neuron lesion)

Specific lesions of
motor outflow from
S2, S3, and S4

Disease of lateral
tracts of spinal cord

+	0
+	0
+	++
0	+
D	+
↑ (<1,000 ml)	V
0	0
↓	L
+/↓/0	+
V	+
+	0
0	0
V	V
0	+

Post-test care

■ Administer a sitz bath or warm rub bath if the patient experiences discomfort after the test.

■ Encourage the patient to drink lots of fluids (unless contraindicated) to relieve burning on urination, a common adverse effect of the procedure.

■ Measure fluid intake and urine output for 24 hours. Notify the doctor if hematuria persists after the third voiding or if the patient develops signs and symptoms of sepsis (such as fever or chills).

■ Short-term antibiotics are often given to prevent infection.

Interfering factors

■ Failure to follow instructions because of a misunderstanding or embarrassment may interfere with test results.

■ Inability to urinate in the supine position will interfere with test results.

■ Concurrent use of drugs that may interfere with bladder function (such as antihistamines) will alter test results.

■ Inconclusive results are likely if cystometry is performed within 6 to 8 weeks after surgery for spinal cord injury.

Voiding cystourethrography

In voiding cystourethrography, a contrast medium is instilled by gentle syringe or gravity into the bladder through a urethral catheter. Fluoroscopic films or overhead radiographs demonstrate bladder filling, then show excretion of the contrast as the patient voids.

This test may be performed to investigate possible causes of chronic urinary tract infection. Other indications for voiding cystourethrography include a suspected congenital anomaly of the lower urinary tract, abnormal bladder emptying, and incontinence. In males, this test can assess hypertrophy of the prostatic lobes, urethral stricture, and the degree of compromise of a stenotic prostatic urethra.

Purpose

■ To detect abnormalities of the bladder and urethra, such as vesicoureteral reflux, neurogenic bladder, prostatic hyperplasia, urethral strictures, or diverticula.

Patient preparation

Explain to the patient that this test permits assessment of the bladder and the urethra. Inform him that he needn't restrict food or fluids before the test. Tell him who will perform the test and where and that it takes 30 to 45 minutes.

Inform the patient that a catheter will be inserted into his bladder and a contrast medium will be instilled through the catheter. Tell him he may experience a feeling of fullness and an urge to void when the contrast is instilled. Explain that X-rays will be taken of his bladder and urethra and that he'll be asked to assume various positions.

Make sure that the patient or responsible family member has signed a consent form if required. Check the patient's history for hypersensitivity to contrast media or iodine-containing foods such as shellfish; mark the chart and notify the doctor of sensitivities. Just before the procedure, administer a sedative, if ordered.

Equipment

X-ray equipment (fluoroscope and screen, and accessories for spot-film radiography) ✦ indwelling urinary catheter ✦ standard urographic contrast medium (up to 1,000 ml of 15% solution)

Normal and abnormal cystourethrograms

In the oblique view of a normal cystourethrogram (left), the clear outline of the bladder and urethra shows normal structure. The oblique view of an abnormal cystourethrogram (right) shows abscesses in the prostate and proximal urethra.

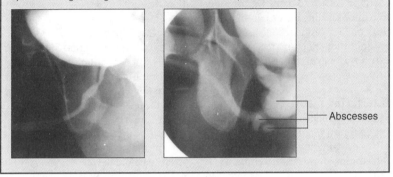

Abscesses

◆ 50-ml syringe (for infants) or gravity-feed apparatus.

Procedure
The patient is placed in the supine position, and an indwelling urinary catheter is inserted into the bladder. The contrast medium is instilled through the catheter until the bladder is full. The catheter is clamped and X-ray films are exposed, with the patient in supine, oblique, and lateral positions. Then the catheter is removed, and the patient assumes the right oblique position — right leg flexed to 90 degrees, left leg extended, penis parallel to right leg — and begins to void.

Four high-speed exposures of the bladder and urethra, coned down to reduce radiation exposure, are usually made on one film during voiding. (Male patients should wear a lead shield over their testes to prevent irradiation of the gonads; female patients can't be shielded without blocking the urinary bladder.) If the right oblique view does not delineate both ureters, the patient is asked to stop urinating and to begin again in left oblique position.

The most reliable voiding cystourethrograms are obtained with the patient recumbent. Patients who can't urinate in this position may do so standing (not sitting). Young children who can't void on command may need to undergo expression cystourethrography under general anesthesia.

Precautions
Voiding cystourethrography is contraindicated in patients with an acute or exacerbated urethral injury. Hypersensitivity to contrast medium may also contraindicate this test.

Normal findings
Delineation of the bladder and urethra shows normal structure and function, with no regurgitation of contrast medium into the ureters.

Implications of results
Voiding cystourethrography may show urethral stricture or valves, vesical or urethral diverticula, ureteroceles, prostatic enlargement, vesicoureteral reflux, or neurogenic bladder. The severity and location of such abnormalities are then evaluated to determine whether surgery is necessary. (See *Normal and abnormal cystourethrograms*.)

Post-test care

- Observe and record the time, color, and volume of the patient's voidings. If hematuria is present after the third voiding, notify the doctor.
- Tell the patient to drink lots of fluids to reduce burning on urination and to flush out any residual contrast dye.
- Monitor for chills and fever related to extravasation of contrast material or urinary sepsis.

Interfering factors

- Embarrassment may inhibit the patient's ability to void on command.
- Pain on voiding resulting from urethral trauma during catheterization may cause an interrupted or less vigorous stream, muscle spasm, or incomplete sphincter relaxation.
- Previous radiographic testing using contrast media or the presence of feces or gas in the bowel may obscure visualization of the urinary tract.

Whitaker test

This study of the upper urinary tract correlates radiographic findings with measurements of pressure and flow in the kidneys and ureters. It assess the upper tract's efficiency in emptying. Radiographs are taken after urethral catheterization, I.V. administration of contrast medium, percutaneous cannulation of the kidney, and renal perfusion of the contrast medium. Intrarenal and bladder pressures are then measured.

The Whitaker test (also known as a pressure-flow study) may be performed as a primary study to detect intrarenal obstruction and to help determine if surgery is needed. It may also follow other procedures, such as percutaneous nephrostomy, for further evaluation of obstruction.

Purpose

- To identify and evaluate renal obstruction.

Patient preparation

Explain to the patient that this test evaluates kidney function. Instruct him to avoid food and fluids for at least 4 hours before the test. Tell him who will perform the test and where and that it takes about 1 hour.

Describe the procedure to the patient. Inform him that he'll be given a mild sedative before the test, that he may feel some discomfort during insertion of the urethral catheter and injection of the local anesthetic, and that he may sense transient burning and flushing after injection of the contrast medium. Warn him that the X-ray machine makes loud clacking sounds as films are exposed.

Ensure that the patient or a responsible family member has signed a consent form if required. Check the patient's history and recent coagulation studies for bleeding disorders. Also check for hypersensitivity reactions to iodine, iodine-containing foods such as shellfish, and contrast media. Document any sensitivities on the chart and inform the doctor.

Just before the procedure, instruct the patient to void, and administer a sedative as ordered. Administer prophylactic antimicrobials, as ordered, to prevent infection from instrumentation.

Equipment

X-ray equipment ✦ perfusion pump with 50 ml luer-lock syringe ✦ transducer and recorder ✦ manometer ✦ three-way and four-way stopcocks ✦ I.V. extension set ✦ manometer lines ✦ one double-male connector to connect urethral catheter and stopcock ✦ sterile water and normal saline solution ✦ contrast medium ✦ local anesthetic ✦ percutaneous puncture tray with 4" to 6" 18G Longdwel cannula ✦ gloves ✦ preparatory tray ✦ emergency resuscitation equipment.

Procedure

The patient is placed in the supine position on the X-ray table. The table is horizontal and must remain at the same height throughout the test. To prepare for measurement of bladder pressure, a urethral catheter is placed in the bladder, which may or may not be emptied. (If an obstruction is suspected, the patient will be asked to void before the test. If a condition such as bladder hypertonia is the suspected cause of inefficient emptying, he should not void.) A plain film of the urinary tract is taken to obtain anatomic landmarks. The catheter is then connected to a three-way stopcock on a manometer line linked to the transducer and recorder. The line is filled with sterile water.

Contrast medium is injected I.V., and the patient is placed prone and made comfortable pillows. The side to be examined is closest to the doctor. When urography demonstrates contrast medium in the kidney, the skin is cleaned with antiseptic solution and draped. Pressure recording equipment is calibrated. The renal perfusion tubing is filled with sterile water or saline solution and held at the level of the kidney.

A local anesthetic is injected, and an incision is made through the flank for cannulation of the kidney. The patient is asked to hold his breath while the needle is inserted into the renal pelvis. Aspiration of urine confirms that the needle is in position. The cannula is then connected by a four-way stopcock to the perfusion tubing and the manometer line.

Perfusion of the contrast medium is begun, serial X-rays are taken, and intrarenal pressure is measured. Bladder pressure is then measured. Perfusion continues at the steady rate of 10 ml/minute until bladder pressure is constant. When pressure holds steady for a few minutes and adequate films have been taken, perfusion is discontinued. Residual fluid is aspirated from the kidney, the cannula is removed, and the wound is dressed. (See *Assessing renal obstruction with the Whitaker test,* page 1012.)

Precautions

The Whitaker test is contraindicated in bleeding disorders and severe infection.

Normal findings

Visualization of the kidney after gradual perfusion of contrast medium shows normal outlines of the renal pelvis and calyces. The ureter should fill uniformly and appear normal in size and course. Normal intrarenal pressure is 15 cm H_2O; normal bladder pressure, 5 to 10 cm H_2O.

Implications of results

Enlargement of the renal pelvis, calyces, or ureteropelvic junction may indicate obstruction. Subtraction of bladder pressure from intrarenal pressure results in a differential that aids diagnosis. A differential of 12 to 15 cm H_2O indicates obstruction. A differential of less than 10 cm H_2O indicates a bladder abnormality, such as hypertonia or neurogenic bladder.

Post-test care

■ Keep the patient supine for 12 hours after the test.

■ Check vital signs every 15 minutes for the first hour, every 30 minutes for the next hour, and then every 2 hours for 24 hours.

■ Check the puncture site for bleeding, hematoma, or urine leakage each time vital signs are checked. If bleeding occurs, apply pressure. If a hematoma de-

Assessing renal obstruction with the Whitaker test

In the Whitaker test, serial X-rays of the upper urinary tract are correlated with measurements of intrarenal and bladder pressure.

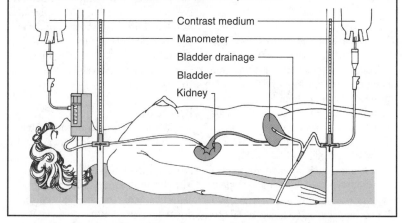

Contrast medium
Manometer
Bladder drainage
Bladder
Kidney

velops, apply warm soaks. If urine leakage occurs, report this to the doctor.

■ Monitor fluid intake and urine output for 24 hours. If hematuria persists after the third voiding, notify the doctor.

■ Watch for signs and symptoms of sepsis or of extravasation of the contrast medium (chills, fever, tachycardia, tachypnea, hypotension).

■ Inform the patient that colicky pains are transient. Administer analgesics as ordered.

■ Administer antibiotics for several days after the test, as ordered, to prevent infection.

Interfering factors
■ Recent barium studies or the presence of feces or gas in the bowel hinders accurate needle placement and visualization of the upper urinary tract.

■ Patient movement interferes with accurate needle placement.

External sphincter electromyography

This procedure measures electrical activity of the external urinary sphincter. The electrical activity can be measured in three ways: by skin electrodes (most commonly used), by needle electrodes inserted in perineal or periurethral tissues, or by electrodes in an anal plug.

The primary indication for external sphincter electromyography is incontinence. Often, this test is done with cystometry and voiding urethrography as part of a full urodynamic study.

Purpose
■ To assess neuromuscular function of the external urinary sphincter

■ To assess functional balance between bladder and sphincter muscle activity.

Patient preparation
Explain to the patient that this test will determine how well his bladder and sphincter muscles work together. Tell

him who will perform the test and where and that it takes 30 to 60 minutes. If skin electrodes are to be used, tell the patient where they'll be placed. Explain the preparatory procedure, which may include shaving a small area.

If needle electrodes will be used, tell the patient where they'll be placed and that the discomfort is equivalent to an intramuscular injection. Assure him that he'll feel discomfort only during insertion. Advise him that the needles are connected to wires leading to the recorder but that there is no danger of electric shock. Explain to the female patient that she may notice slight bleeding the first time she urinates.

If an anal plug will be used, inform the patient that only the tip of the plug will be inserted into the rectum, that he may feel fullness but no discomfort, and that a bowel movement is rare but easily managed.

Check the patient's medications. If he's taking cholinergic or anticholinergic drugs, notify the doctor. Discontinue medications as ordered.

Equipment

Electromyograph and recorder ✦ skin, needle, or anal plug electrodes ✦ ground plate ✦ electrode paste ✦ tape ✦ antiseptic solution such as povidone-iodine ✦ preparatory tray, if shaving is necessary.

Procedure

The patient is placed in the lithotomy position for electrode placement, then may lie supine. Record his position, the type of electrode and measuring equipment used, and any other tests done at the same time. (To obtain comparable results, subsequent studies must be done the same way.)

Electrode paste is applied to the ground plate, which is taped to the thigh and grounded. The electrodes are then applied, as described below, and connected to electrode adaptors.

To place skin electrodes: The skin is cleaned with antiseptic solution and dried. A small area may be shaved for optimum electrode contact. Electrode paste is applied and the electrodes are taped in place: for females, in the periurethral area; for males, in the perineal area beneath the scrotum.

To place needle electrodes: For a male patient, a gloved finger is inserted into the rectum. The needles and wires are inserted 1½" through the perineal skin toward the apex of the prostate. Needle positions are 3:00 and 9:00. While the needles are withdrawn, the wires are held in place and then taped to the thigh.

For a female patient, the labia are spread, and the needles and wires are inserted periurethrally at 2:00 and 10:00. The needles are withdrawn and the wires taped to the thigh.

To place anal plug electrodes: The plug is lubricated, and the patient is informed that only the tip will be inserted into the rectum. The patient is asked to relax by breathing slowly and deeply. He is asked to relax the anal sphincter to accommodate the plug by bearing down as if for a bowel movement.

After the appropriate electrodes are placed and connected to adapters, the adapters are inserted into the preamplifier and recording begins. The patient is asked to alternately relax and tighten the sphincter. When sufficient data have been recorded, he is asked to bear down and exhale while the anal plug and needle electrodes are removed. Remove the electrodes gently to avoid pulling hair and injuring tender skin. Clean and dry the area before the patient dresses.

In some urodynamic laboratories, cystometrography is done with electromyography for a thorough evaluation of detrusor and sphincter coordination.

Precautions

■ Insert the needles quickly to minimize discomfort.

■ The ground plate should be properly applied and anchored; wires should be taped securely to prevent artifact.

Normal findings

The electromyogram shows increased muscle activity when the patient tightens the external urinary sphincter and decreased muscle activity when he relaxes it. (The International Continence Society doesn't specify normal findings for sphincter electromyography.)

If electromyography and cystometrography are done together, a comparison of results shows that muscle activity of the normal sphincter increases as the bladder fills. During voiding and with bladder contraction, muscle activity decreases as the sphincter relaxes. This comparison is important in assessing external sphincter efficiency and functional balance between bladder and sphincter muscle activity.

Implications of results

Failure of the sphincter to relax or increased muscle activity during voiding demonstrates detrusor-sphincter dyssynergia. Confirmation of such muscle activity by electromyography may indicate neurogenic bladder, spinal cord injury, multiple sclerosis, Parkinson's disease, or stress incontinence.

Post-test care

■ Watch for and report hematuria after the first voiding in the female patient tested with needle electrodes.

■ Watch for and report signs and symptoms of mild urethral irritation: dysuria, hematuria, and urinary frequency.

■ Advise the patient to take a warm sitz bath and to drink lots of fluids (2 to 3 L/day) unless contraindicated.

Interfering factors

■ Patient movement during electromyography may distort recordings.

■ Anticholinergic or cholinergic drugs affect detrusor and sphincter activity.

■ Improperly placed and anchored electrodes will cause inaccurate recordings.

SELECTED READINGS

Bennett, J.C., and Plum, F., eds. *Cecil Textbook of Medicine,* 20th ed. Philadelphia: W.B. Saunders Co., 1996.

Diseases, 2nd ed. Springhouse, Pa.: Springhouse Corp., 1996.

Fischbach, F. *A Manual of Laboratory and Diagnostic Tests,* 5th ed. Philadelphia: Lippincott-Raven Pubs., 1996.

Henry, J.B., ed. *Clinical Diagnosis and Management by Laboratory Methods,* 19th ed. Philadelphia: W.B. Saunders Co., 1996.

Isselbacher, K.J., et al., eds. *Harrison's Principles of Internal Medicine,* 13th ed. New York: McGraw-Hill Book Co., 1994.

Kee, J.L. *Laboratory and Diagnostic Tests,* 4th ed. Stamford, Conn.: Appleton & Lange, 1995.

Malarkey, L., and McMorrow, M. *Nurse's Manual of Laboratory Tests and Diagnostic Procedures.* Philadelphia: W.B. Saunders Co., 1996.

Ravel, R.A. *Clinical Laboratory Medicine: Clinical Application of Laboratory Data,* 6th ed. St. Louis: Mosby–Year Book, Inc., 1995.

Watson, J., and Jaffe, M. *Nurse's Manual of Laboratory and Diagnostic Tests,* 2nd ed. Philadelphia: F.A. Davis Co., 1995.

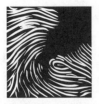

CHAPTER THIRTY

Miscellaneous tests

INTRODUCTION

Some important diagnostic tests resist easy classification. For example, skin tests evaluate the immune response using different procedures from other immunologic tests. The contrast radiography and nuclear medicine tests found elsewhere in this book apply specifically to certain organs or body systems; but others, such as lymphangiography and gallium scanning, apply more widely. D-xylose absorption is the only diagnostic test that uses both serum and urine samples to detect the cause of malabsorption syndrome. And the dexamethasone suppression test is the standard screening test for Cushing's syndrome.

Skin tests

Skin tests evaluate cellular immunity by determining patient response to the intradermal injection or topical application of one or more antigens. In tuberculin skin tests, one antigen assesses the immune response to a specific infectious disease; in delayed hypersensitivity skin tests, a panel of antigens assesses general immunocompetence. In each test, if the patient has an intact secondary immune response (effective recall antigens), erythema and induration develop at the injection or application site within 24 hours, peak at 48 hours, and then begin to resolve thereafter.

Anergy — the ability to react to a battery of common antigens — suggests immunodeficiency. The anergic patient may require additional tests using greater concentrations of the same antigens or using a test antigen that the patient hasn't encountered, such as dinitrochlorobenzene.

Radiology and nuclear medicine

Lymphangiography is the most important test for detecting obstruction, disease, and neoplasm in the lymphatic system. This system transports lymph — derived from tissue fluids — throughout the body and eventually empties it into the veins. The lymphatic system can spread inflammation and disease throughout the body.

In gallium scanning, a gamma camera or rectilinear scanner records distribution of radioactivity after I.V. injection of gallium Ga 67 citrate. Because gallium concentrates at sites of abscesses and carcinomas, it can help detect them or determine the extent of metastases and can also help evaluate the effectiveness of treatment.

The red blood cell (RBC) survival time test measures the life span of RBCs tagged with radioactive chromium 51 to help evaluate unexplained anemia. Serial blood tests and gamma camera scans help identify the type and site of RBC destruction.

Malabsorption test

The D-xylose absorption test distinguishes intestinal disease from other disorders that cause malabsorption. Blood and urine samples are analyzed after ingestion of a standard dose of D-xylose. In malabsorption due to intestinal disease, D-xylose absorption decreases; in malabsorption due to pancreatic insufficiency, cystic fibrosis, or liver disease, absorption remains normal.

Dexamethasone suppression test

The dexamethasone suppression test helps to diagnose Cushing's syndrome. It also helps detect and monitor major depression by measuring the body's level of adrenal steroid hormones.

SKIN TESTS

Tuberculin skin tests

These skin tests are used to screen patients for previous infection by the tubercle bacillus. They are routinely performed in children, young adults, and people with radiographic findings that suggest this infection.

In both the old tuberculin (OT) and the purified protein derivative (PPD)

tests, intradermal injection of the tuberculin antigen causes a delayed hypersensitivity reaction in patients with active or dormant tuberculosis; sensitized lymphocytes gather at the injection site, causing erythema, vesiculation, and induration that peaks within 24 to 48 hours and persists for at least 72 hours.

The most accurate tuberculin test method, the Mantoux test, uses a single-needle intradermal injection of PPD, which permits precise measurement of dosage. Multipuncture tests — such as the tine test, Mono-Vacc test, and Aplitest — involve intradermal injections using tines impregnated with OT or PPD. Because multipuncture tests require less skill and are more rapidly administered than the Mantoux test, they're generally used for screening. However, a positive multipuncture test usually requires a Mantoux test for confirmation.

Another test, the Schick test, can determine susceptibility or immunity to diphtheria. (See *Schick test,* page 1018.)

Purpose

■ To distinguish tuberculosis from blastomycosis, coccidioidomycosis, and histoplasmosis
■ To identify persons who need diagnostic investigation for tuberculosis.

Patient preparation

Explain to the patient that this test helps detect tuberculosis. Tell him the test requires an intradermal injection, which may cause him transient discomfort.

 NURSING ALERT Check the patient's history for active tuberculosis, the results of previous skin tests, and hypersensitivities. If the patient has had tuberculosis, don't perform a skin test; if he's had a positive reaction to previous skin tests, consult the doctor or follow hospital policy; if he's had an allergic reaction to aca-

---

Schick test

Although not performed routinely in the United States, the Schick test determines susceptibility or immunity to diphtheria — an acute, highly contagious bacterial infection. In this skin test, 0.1 ml of purified diphtheria toxin dissolved in buffered human serum albumin is injected intradermally into one forearm, and 0.1 ml of purified diphtheria toxin alone is injected into the other forearm, as a control. Both sites are examined after 24 and 48 hours and again 4 to 7 days after the injection.

Patients who are susceptible to diphtheria — those who have slight amounts of or no circulating antitoxin — demonstrate inflammation and induration at the site of toxin injection within 24 hours and a peak reaction within 7 days. This reaction generally has a dark red center and may reach 1¼" (3 cm) in diameter. Conversely, the site of toxoid injection shows no reaction.

In patients immune to diphtheria (antitoxin levels between 1/30 and 1/100 U), neither site shows a reaction.

---

cia, don't perform an OT test because this product contains acacia.

If you're performing a tuberculin test on an outpatient, instruct him to return at the specified time so that test results can be read. Inform him that a positive reaction to a skin test appears as a red, hard, raised area at the injection site. Although the area may itch, instruct him not to scratch it. Stress that a positive reaction doesn't always indicate active tuberculosis.

Equipment

Alcohol swabs ✦ vial of PPD (intermediate strength) — 5 tuberculin units (TU) per 0.1 ml and 1-ml tuberculin syringe with ½" or ⅝" 25G or 26G needle for the Mantoux test ✦ commercially available device (tine, Mono-Vacc, or Aplitest) for multipuncture tests ✦ epinephrine (1:1,000) and 3-ml syringe (for emergency use).

Procedure

The patient is placed in a sitting position, with his arm extended and supported on a flat surface. Clean the volar surface of the upper forearm with alcohol, and let the area dry completely.

For Mantoux test: Perform an intradermal injection. (See *Giving intradermal injections.*)

For multipuncture tests: Remove the protective cap on the injection device to expose the four tines. Hold the patient's forearm in one hand, stretching the skin of the forearm tightly. Then, with your other hand, firmly depress the device into the patient's skin (without twisting it). Hold the device in place for at least 1 second before removing it. If you've applied sufficient pressure, you'll see four puncture sites and a circular depression made by the device on the patient's skin.

Record where the test was given, the date and time, and when it's to be read. Tuberculin skin tests are generally read 48 to 72 hours after injection; however, the Mono-Vacc test can be read 48 to 96 hours after the test. (See *Reading tuberculin test results,* page 1021.)

Precautions

■ Tuberculin skin tests are contraindicated in patients with active tuberculosis,

Giving intradermal injections

1 Begin by assembling your equipment. You'll need the medication, a 1-cc tuberculin syringe, a 25G ⅝" needle, and several alcohol pads. Attach the needle to the syringe. Check the medication to make sure it's not outdated or contaminated. If not, draw it up into the syringe, expelling any air in the needle. Then cap the syringe and bring all the equipment to the patient's bedside. Explain the procedure to the patient. Position him sitting or lying down, with his ventral forearm exposed and supported on a flat surface and his elbow flexed.

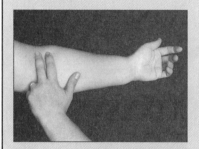

2 Next, locate the patient's antecubital space. Then measure several fingerwidths away from it in the direction of the hand (as shown). Avoid any areas covered with hair or blemishes. These could make reading the test results difficult.

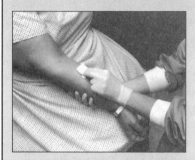

3 Prepare the skin with an alcohol pad, beginning at the center of the site and moving outward in a circular motion (as shown). Never use a disinfectant such as povidone-iodine, which discolors the skin, and don't rub so hard that you cause irritation. This action could hinder the reading of the test.

Let the skin dry thoroughly. Injecting the patient while the skin is wet could introduce alcohol into the dermis.

4 Hold the patient's forearm in one hand, and stretch his skin taut (as shown.)

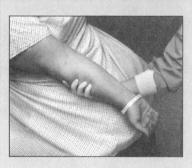

(continued)

a current reaction to smallpox vaccinations, any type of rash, or a skin disorder.

■ Don't perform a skin test in areas with excess hair, acne, or insufficient subcutaneous tissue, such as over a tendon or bone. If the patient is known to be hypersensitive to skin tests, use a first-strength dose in the Mantoux test to avoid necrosis at the puncture site.

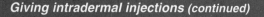

Giving intradermal injections *(continued)*

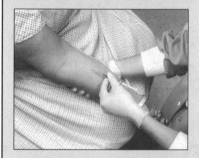

5 Position the syringe so that the needle is almost flat against the patient's skin (as shown). Make sure that the bevel of the needle is up.

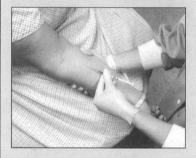

6 Insert the needle by pressing it against the skin until you meet resistance. Then advance the needle through the epidermis so that the point of the needle is visible through the skin (as shown). Stop when it's resting $\frac{1}{8}$" (3 mm) below the skin's surface, between the epidermis and the dermal layers.

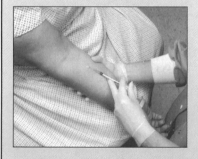

7 Now, inject the medication as slowly and gently as possible. Expect to feel some resistance, which indicates that the needle is properly placed. If the needle moves freely, you've inserted it too deeply; withdraw it slightly and try again. When you've finished injecting the medication, leave the needle in place momentarily. Watch for a small white blister or wheal — about $\frac{1}{4}$" (6 mm) in diameter — to form (as shown).

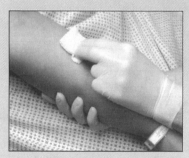

8 When the wheal appears, withdraw the needle and apply gentle pressure to the site (as shown). Don't massage it because doing so could interfere with test results.

Document the name of the medication and the amount given. If the patient has an allergic reaction to the injection within 30 minutes, notify the doctor. Such reactions generally develop within 48 to 72 hours.

Reading tuberculin test results

You should read the Mantoux, tine, and Aplitest skin tests 48 to 72 hours after injection; the Mono-Vacc test, 48 to 96 hours afterward.

In a well-lighted room, flex the patient's forearm slightly. Observe the injection site for erythema and vesiculation; then gently rub your finger over the site to detect induration. If induration is present, measure the diameter in millimeters, preferably using a plastic ruler marked in concentric circles of specific diameter.

In multipuncture tests, you may find separate areas of induration around individual punctures or induration involving more than one puncture site. If so, measure the diameter of the largest single area of induration or coalesced induration.

■ Have epinephrine available to treat an anaphylactic or acute hypersensitivity reaction.

Normal findings

For Mantoux test: induration less than 5 mm in diameter or no induration

For tine test and Aplitest: no vesiculation; no induration or induration less than 2 mm diameter

For Mono-Vacc test: no induration.

Implications of results

A positive tuberculin reaction indicates previous infection by tubercle bacilli. It does not distinguish between an active and dormant infection, nor does it provide a definitive diagnosis. If a positive reaction occurs, sputum smear and culture and chest X-rays are necessary to provide more information.

In the Mantoux test, induration of 5 to 9 mm in diameter indicates a borderline reaction; larger induration, a positive reaction. Because patients infected with atypical mycobacteria other than tubercle bacilli may have borderline reactions, repeat testing is necessary.

In the tine test or Aplitest, vesiculation indicates a positive reaction; induration of 2 mm in diameter without vesiculation requires confirmation by the Mantoux test. Any induration in the Mono-Vacc test indicates a positive reaction but requires confirmation by the Mantoux test.

Post-test care

If ulceration or necrosis develops at the injection site, apply cold soaks or a topical steroid, as ordered.

Interfering factors

■ Subcutaneous injection, usually indicated by erythema greater than 10 mm in diameter without induration, invalidates the test.

■ Corticosteroids, other immunosuppressants, or live vaccine viruses (measles, mumps, rubella, or polio) given within the past 4 to 6 weeks may suppress skin reactions.

■ Elderly people and patients with viral infection, malnutrition, febrile illness, uremia, immunosuppressive disorders, or miliary tuberculosis may have suppressed skin reactions.

■ If less than 10 weeks has elapsed since infection with tuberculosis, the skin reaction may be suppressed.

■ Improper dilution, dosage, or storage of the tuberculin interferes with accurate testing.

Delayed hypersensitivity skin tests

Skin testing is one of the most important methods for evaluating the cell-mediated immune response in a patient with severe recurrent infection, infection caused by unusual organisms, or suspected disorders associated with delayed hypersensitivity. Because diminished delayed hypersensitivity may be associated with a poor prognosis in patients with certain types of cancer, this test may also be useful in determining the prognosis in such patients. A positive test reaction shows that the afferent, central, and efferent limbs of the immune response are intact and that the patient can maintain a nonspecific inflammatory response to infection.

These skin tests use new and recall antigens. *New antigens* — those not previously encountered by the patient, such as dinitrochlorobenzene (DNCB) — evaluate the patient's primary immune response when a sensitizing dose is given, followed by a challenge dose. *Recall antigens* — those to which a patient has had or may have had previous exposure or sensitization — evaluate the secondary immune response; these antigens include candidin, trichophytin, streptokinase-streptodornase, purified protein derivative, staphage lysate, mumps, and mixed respiratory vaccine, among others. The specific antigens chosen for this test are those to which exposure is common and which will usually provoke an immune response.

In these tests, a small amount of antigen (or group of antigens) is injected intradermally or applied topically, and the test site is later examined for a visible reaction. (See *Administering test antigens.*) Skin tests have only limited value in infants because their immune systems are immature and inadequately sensitized.

Another type of skin test, the patch test, is used to confirm allergic contact sensitization and to determine its cause. (See *Performing a patch test,* page 1024.)

Purpose

- To evaluate primary and secondary immune responses
- To assess effectiveness of immunotherapy, when the patient's immune response is augmented by adjuvants (such as bacille Calmette-Guérin [BCG] vaccine) or other means (transfer factor, levamisole)
- To diagnose fungal diseases (coccidioidomycosis, histoplasmosis), bacterial diseases (tuberculosis, brucellosis, leprosy), and viral diseases (infectious mononucleosis)
- To monitor the course of certain diseases, such as Hodgkin's disease and coccidioidomycosis.

Patient preparation

Explain to the patient that this test evaluates the immune system after application or injection of small doses of antigens. Inform him that he needn't restrict food or fluids before the test. Tell him who will perform the test and where, that it takes about 10 minutes for each antigen to be administered, and that reactions should appear in 48 to 72 hours. Explain that some antigens (such as DNCB) are readministered after 2 weeks and, if the test is negative, that a stronger dose of antigen may be given.

Check the patient's history for hypersensitivity to any of the test antigens; if not listed in his history, ask the patient if he's had a skin test previously and, if so, what his reactions were. Check for a history of tuberculosis or previous BCG vaccination. If the patient's history reveals no sensitivity or hypersensitivity, intermediate-strength antigens are typically used.

Because many antigens are approved by the Food and Drug Administration (FDA) for use as vaccines but not for skin testing, check with the pharmacy about FDA approval for this purpose. If the tests require the patient's informed consent such as for use of DNCB in research studies, check with the appropriate hospital committee for guidelines.

Equipment

For DNCB test: DNCB ✦ sterile gauze pad and tape ✦ gloves ✦ surgical mask ✦ alcohol swabs ✦ acetone ✦ cotton swabs.

For recall antigen test: 1-ml tuberculin syringes ✦ 25G ⅝" needles ✦ alcohol swabs ✦ antigens ✦ syringe filled with diluted epinephrine (1:1,000) ✦ extra needle and syringe containing allergy test diluent ✦ pen.

Procedure

For DNCB test: Wear gloves and a mask to avoid sensitizing yourself to DNCB. Dissolve DNCB in acetone, as ordered. Position the patient's forearm comfortably, ventral side up, with his elbow slightly flexed. Clean a small, hairless area midway between the wrist and elbow with an alcohol swab, allow it to dry, and apply the prescribed amount of DNCB (sensitizing dose) with a cotton swab. Allow this to dry, then cover the area with a sterile gauze pad for 24 to 48 hours.

Instruct the patient to watch for a spontaneous flare reaction 10 to 14 days after application of DNCB. (If a reaction occurs, a lower dose of the test solution can be used for the challenge dose.) After 14 days, apply a challenge dose of DNCB to the same spot and in the same manner. Inspect the site 48 to 96 hours after application of DNCB for reactivity. The challenge dose can be repeated 2 weeks later (1 month after the

Administering test antigens

The illustration below shows the arm of a patient who is undergoing a recall antigen test, which determines whether he has previously been exposed to certain antigens. A sample panel of six test antigens has been injected into his forearm, and the test site has been marked and labeled for each antigen.

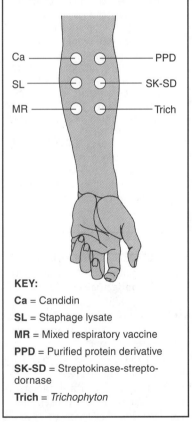

KEY:

Ca = Candidin

SL = Staphage lysate

MR = Mixed respiratory vaccine

PPD = Purified protein derivative

SK-SD = Streptokinase-streptodornase

Trich = *Trichophyton*

sensitizing dose) when test results are negative.

For recall antigen test: Inject each antigen being tested intradermally, using a separate tuberculin syringe, on the

Performing a patch test

A patch test confirms allergic contact sensitivity and can help identify its cause. In this test, a sample series of common allergens (antigens) is applied to the skin in the hope that one or more will produce a positive reaction. A positive patch test proves that the patient has a contact sensitivity but doesn't necessarily confirm that the test substance caused the clinical eruption.

If the patient has an acute inflammation, the patch test should be postponed until the inflammation subsides to avoid exacerbating the inflammation.

Keep the following points in mind when performing a patch test:
- Use only *potentially* irritating substances for a patch test. Testing with primary irritants is not possible.
- To avoid skin irritation, dilute substances that may be irritating to 1% to 2% in petroleum jelly, mineral oil or, as a last choice, water. When there are no clues to a likely allergen in a person with possible contact dermatitis, use a series of common allergens available in standard patch tests.
- Apply the allergens to normal, hairless skin on the back or on the ventral surface of the forearm. First, apply them to a small disk of filter paper attached to aluminum and coated with plastic. Tape the paper to the skin, or use a small square of soft cotton and cover it with occlusive tape. Apply liquids and ointments to the disk or cotton. Apply volatile liquids to the skin and allow the areas to dry before covering. Before application, powder solids and moisten powders and fabrics.
- Patches should remain in place for 48 hours. However, remove the patch immediately if pain, pruritus, or irritation develops. Positive reactions may take time to develop, so check findings 20 to 30 minutes after removing the patch and again 96 hours (4 days) after the application.
- To relieve the effects of a positive reaction, tell the patient to apply topical corticosteroids, as ordered.

---

patient's forearm. Circle each injection site with a pen, and label each according to the antigen given. Instruct the patient to avoid washing off the circles until the test is completed. Then inject the control allergy diluent on the other forearm.

Inspect injection sites for reactivity after 48 and 72 hours. Record induration and erythema in millimeters. A negative test at the first concentration of antigen should be confirmed using a higher concentration.

Precautions
- Store antigens in lyophilized (freeze-dried) form at 39.2° F (4° C), protected from light. Reconstitute them shortly before use, and check their expiration dates. If the patient is suspected of being hypersensitive to the antigens, apply them first in low concentrations.
- Because excess DNCB can burn the patient's skin, apply only the prescribed amount.
- If the forearms are not free from disease (for example, if the patient has atopic dermatitis), use other sites such as the back.

- Observe the patient carefully for signs of anaphylactic shock — urticaria, respiratory distress, and hypotension. If such signs develop, administer epinephrine, as ordered, and notify the doctor immediately.

Normal findings

In the DNCB test, a positive reaction (erythema, edema, induration) appears 48 to 96 hours after the second (challenge) dose; 95% of the population reacts positively to DNCB. In the recall antigen test, a positive response (5 mm or more of induration at the test site) appears 48 hours after injection.

Implications of results

In the DNCB test, failure to react to the challenge dose indicates diminished delayed hypersensitivity. In the recall antigen test, a positive response to less than two of the six test antigens, a persistent unresponsiveness to intradermal injection of higher-strength antigens, or a generalized diminished reaction (causing less than 10 mm combined induration) indicates diminished delayed hypersensitivity.

Diminished delayed hypersensitivity can result from Hodgkin's disease (common); sarcoidosis; liver disease; congenital immunodeficiency disease, such as ataxia-telangiectasia, DiGeorge syndrome, and Wiskott-Aldrich syndrome; uremia; acute leukemia; viral diseases, such as influenza, infectious mononucleosis, measles, mumps, and rubella; fungal diseases, such as coccidioidomycosis and cryptococcosis; bacterial diseases, such as leprosy and tuberculosis; and terminal cancer. Diminished delayed hypersensitivity can also result from immunosuppressive or steroid therapy or viral vaccination.

Post-test care

■ Watch the patient closely for severe local reactions that may occur at the test site, such as pain, blistering, swelling, induration, itching, and ulceration. Scarring or hyperpigmentation also may result. Also observe for swelling and

tenderness in the lymph nodes at the elbow or axillary region. Check for tachycardia and fever, although these rarely occur. Symptoms typically appear in 15 to 30 minutes.

■ Tell the patient experiencing hypersensitivity that steroids will control the reaction but that skin lesions may persist for 10 to 14 days. Instruct him to avoid scratching or otherwise disturbing the affected area.

Interfering factors

■ Use of antigens that have expired or that have been exposed to heat and light or to bacterial contamination interferes with accurate testing.
■ Poor injection technique (subcutaneous instead of intradermal injection) may produce false-negative results.
■ Inaccurate dilution of antigens or an error in reading or timing test results causes inaccurate test results.
■ A strong immediate reaction to the antigen at the injection site may cause a false-negative delayed reaction.
■ Oral contraceptives may cause false-negative results by inhibiting lymphocyte mitosis.

RADIOLOGY AND NUCLEAR MEDICINE

Lymphangiography

Lymphangiography (also known as lymphography) is the radiographic examination of the lymphatic system after the injection of an oil-based contrast medium into a lymphatic vessel in each foot or, less commonly, in each hand. Injection into the foot allows visualization of the lymphatics of the leg, inguinal and iliac regions, and the retro-

The lymphatic system

The lymphatic system plays an important role in the transport of fluids and proteins to the veins, in the functioning of the immune system, and in the reabsorption of fats from the small intestine. It consists of the lymphatic vessels, lymph nodes, lymphoid tissue, lymphocytes, and reticuloendothelial cells.

Lymphatic vessels, which tend to parallel veins, eventually converge into one of two main ducts — thoracic or right lymphatic. The thoracic duct drains the lower extremities, the pelvis, the abdominal cavity, and the left arm (white area of diagram) as well as the left side of the head, neck, and chest. The right lymphatic duct drains the right side of the head, neck, and chest and the right arm (shaded area of diagram). The thoracic and right lymphatic ducts then empty into the venous system at the junction of the left and right subclavian and internal jugular veins, respectively.

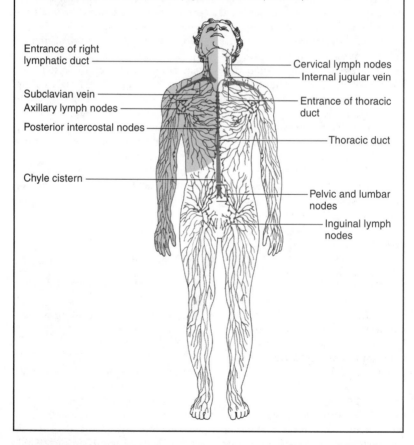

Entrance of right lymphatic duct

Cervical lymph nodes

Internal jugular vein

Subclavian vein

Axillary lymph nodes

Entrance of thoracic duct

Posterior intercostal nodes

Thoracic duct

Chyle cistern

Pelvic and lumbar nodes

Inguinal lymph nodes

peritoneum up to the thoracic duct. Injection into the hand allows visualization of the axillary and supraclavicular nodes. (See *The lymphatic system.*) Lymphangiography may also be used to study the cervical region (retroauricular area), but this is less useful and done less often.

In this procedure, X-rays are taken immediately after injection of the contrast agent to demonstrate the filling of the lymphatic system, and then again 24 hours later to visualize the lymph nodes. Because the contrast remains in the nodes for up to 2 years, subsequent X-rays can assess progression of disease and monitor the effectiveness of treatment.

Lymphangiography is usually performed to stage disease in patients with an established diagnosis of lymphoma or cancer. It may also be performed for patients with enlarged lymph nodes detected by computed tomography (CT) scan or ultrasonography.

Purpose
▪ To detect and stage lymphomas and to identify metastatic involvement of the lymph nodes
▪ To distinguish primary from secondary lymphedema
▪ To suggest surgical treatment or evaluate the effectiveness of chemotherapy or radiation therapy in controlling malignant tumors.

Patient preparation
Explain to the patient that this test permits examination of the lymphatic system through X-rays taken after the injection of a contrast medium. Inform him that he needn't restrict food or fluids before the test. Tell him who will perform this procedure and where and that it takes about 3 hours. Mention that additional X-rays are taken the following day but that these take less than 30 minutes.

Inform the patient that blue contrast dye will be injected into each foot to outline the lymphatic vessels, that the injection causes transient discomfort, and that the contrast discolors urine and stool for 48 hours and may give his skin

and vision a bluish tinge for 48 hours. Tell him a local anesthetic will be injected before a small incision is made in each foot. Inform him that the contrast medium is then injected for the next $1\frac{1}{2}$ hours, using a cannula inserted into a lymphatic vessel. Advise the patient to remain as still as possible during injection of the contrast medium; tell him he may experience some discomfort in the popliteal or inguinal areas when the dye is first injected. If this test is performed on an outpatient basis, advise the patient to be accompanied by a friend or relative. Warn him that the incision site may be sore for several days afterward.

Make sure the patient or responsible member of the family has signed a consent form. Check the patient history for hypersensitivity to iodine, seafood, or the contrast media used in other diagnostic tests such as excretory urography.

Just before the procedure, instruct the patient to void, and check his vital signs for a baseline. If ordered, administer a sedative and an oral antihistamine (if hypersensitivity to the contrast medium is suspected.)

Procedure
A preliminary X-ray of the chest is taken with the patient in an erect or supine position. Then the skin over the dorsum of each foot is cleaned with an antiseptic, and blue contrast is injected intradermally into the area between the toes (usually into the first and fourth toe webs). The contrast infiltrates the lymphatic system and, within 15 to 30 minutes, the lymphatic vessels appear as small blue lines on the upper surface of the instep of each foot. A local anesthetic is then injected into the dorsum of each foot, and a 1" (2.5-cm) transverse incision is made to expose the lymphatic vessel.

Each vessel is cannulated with a 30G needle attached to polyethylene tubing

Staging malignant lymphoma

Stage I: Involvement of a single lymph node region or of a single extralymphatic organ or site

Stage II: Involvement of two or more lymph node regions on the same side of the diaphragm, or localized involvement of an extralymphatic organ or site of one or more lymph node regions on the same side of the diaphragm

Stage III: Involvement of lymph node regions on both sides of the diaphragm, which may also be accompanied by localized involvement of an extralymphatic organ or site or of the spleen (or both)

Stage IV: Diffuse or disseminated involvement of one or more extralymphatic organs or tissue with or without associated lymph node enlargement

and a syringe filled with ethiodized oil. Once the needles are positioned, the patient is instructed to remain still throughout the injection period to avoid dislodging the needles. The syringe is then placed within an infusion pump that injects the contrast medium at a rate of 0.1 to 0.2 ml/minute for about 1½ hours to avoid injuring delicate lymphatic vessels.

Fluoroscopy may be used to monitor filling of the lymphatic system. If so, the infusion is stopped when the contrast reaches the level of the third and fourth lumbar vertebrae. At this point — or when the injection is completed — the needles are removed, the incisions sutured, and sterile dressings applied. X-rays of the legs, pelvis, abdomen, and chest are taken. The patient is then taken to his room but must return 24 hours later for additional films.

Precautions

Lymphangiography is contraindicated in patients with a hypersensitivity to iodine, pulmonary insufficiency, cardiac disease, or severe renal or hepatic disease.

Normal findings

The lymphatic system normally demonstrates homogeneous and complete filling with contrast medium on the initial films. On the 24-hour films, the lymph nodes are fully opacified and well circumscribed; the lymphatic channels are emptied a few hours after injection of the contrast agent.

Implications of results

Enlarged, foamy-looking nodes indicate lymphoma, classified as Hodgkin's or non-Hodgkin's. Filling defects or lack of opacification indicates metastatic involvement of the lymph nodes. The number of nodes affected, unilateral or bilateral involvement, and the extent of extranodal involvement help determine staging of lymphoma. However, definitive staging may require additional diagnostic tests, such as a CT scan, ultrasonography, elective biopsy, and laparotomy. (See *Staging malignant lymphoma.*)

In differential diagnosis of primary or secondary lymphedema, shortened lymphatic vessels and a deficient number of vessels indicate primary lymphedema. Abruptly terminating lymphatic vessels, caused by retroperitoneal tumors impinging on the vessels, inflammation, filariasis, or trauma due to surgery or radiation therapy, indicate secondary lymphedema.

Post-test care

■ Check the patient's vital signs every 4 hours for 48 hours.

■ Watch for pulmonary complications due to embolization of contrast medium, such as shortness of breath, pleuritic pain, hypotension, low-grade fever, and cyanosis.

■ Enforce bed rest for 24 hours, with the patient's feet elevated to help reduce swelling, as ordered.

■ Apply ice packs to the incision sites to help reduce swelling, and administer an analgesic as ordered.

■ Check the incision sites for infection, and leave the dressings in place for 2 days, making sure the wounds remain dry. Tell the patient the sutures will be removed in 7 to 10 days.

■ Prepare the patient for follow-up X-rays, as ordered.

Interfering factors

Inability to cannulate the lymphatic vessels would make this test impossible to perform.

Gallium scanning

This test, a total body scan, is usually performed 24 to 48 hours after I.V. injection of radioactive gallium GA 67 citrate. (Occasionally, it's performed 72 hours after the injection or, in acute inflammatory disease, after 4 to 6 hours.) Although the liver, spleen, bones, and large bowel normally take up gallium, certain neoplasms and inflammatory lesions also attract it. However, many neoplasms and a few inflammatory lesions may fail to demonstrate abnormal gallium activity. Because gallium has an affinity for both benign and malignant neoplasms and inflammatory lesions, exact diagnosis requires additional con-

firming tests, such as ultrasonography and computerized tomography scans.

Gallium scanning is usually indicated when the site of the disease (usually malignancy) hasn't been clearly defined and when the patient's condition won't be jeopardized by the time required for the procedure. It can also clarify focal hepatic defects when liver-spleen scanning and ultrasonography prove inconclusive and can evaluate suspected bronchogenic carcinoma when sputum culture proves positive for malignancy but other tests are normal, or when hydrothorax is present and bronchoscopy is contraindicated.

Purpose

■ To detect primary or metastatic neoplasms and inflammatory lesions

■ To evaluate malignant lymphoma and identify recurrent tumors following chemotherapy or radiation therapy

■ To clarify focal defects in the liver and evaluate bronchogenic carcinoma.

Patient preparation

Explain to the patient that this test helps detect abnormal or inflammatory tissue. Inform him that he needn't restrict food or fluids. Tell him the test requires a total body scan (usually performed 24 to 48 hours after I.V. injection of radioactive gallium), who will perform the test and where, and that it takes 30 to 60 minutes. Warn him that he may experience transient discomfort from the needle puncture when the gallium is injected. Reassure him, however, that the dosage is only slightly radioactive and isn't harmful.

If a gamma scintillation camera is to be used, reassure the patient that although the equipment may touch his skin, he'll experience no discomfort. If a rectilinear scanner is to be used, mention that it makes a soft, irregular clicking noise as it registers the radiation emissions.

Make sure the patient or responsible member of the family has signed a consent form. Administer a laxative or cleansing enema (or both), as ordered.

Procedure

The patient may be positioned erect or recumbent — or in a combination of these positions — depending on his physical condition. Scans or scintigraphs of the patient are taken 24 to 48 hours after injection of gallium from anterior and posterior views and, occasionally, lateral views.

Precautions

■ This test should precede barium studies because barium retention may hinder visualization of gallium activity in the bowel.

■ Gallium scanning is usually contraindicated in children and in pregnant or lactating women; however, it may be performed if the potential diagnostic benefit outweighs the risks of exposure to radiation.

Normal findings

Gallium activity is normally demonstrated in the liver, spleen, bones, and large bowel. Activity in the bowel results from mucosal uptake and fecal excretion of gallium.

Implications of results

Gallium scanning may reveal inflammatory lesions — discrete abscesses or diffuse infiltration. In pancreatic or perinephric abscess, gallium activity is relatively localized; in bacterial peritonitis, gallium activity is spread diffusely within the abdomen.

Abnormally high gallium accumulation is characteristic in inflammatory bowel diseases, such as ulcerative colitis and Crohn's disease, and in colon cancer. However, because gallium normally accumulates in the colon, detection

of inflammatory and neoplastic diseases is sometimes difficult.

Abnormal gallium activity may be present in various sarcomas, Wilms' tumor, and neuroblastomas; cancer of the kidney, uterus, vagina, and stomach; and testicular tumors, such as seminoma, embryonal carcinoma, choriocarcinoma, and teratocarcinoma, which often metastasize via the lymphatic system. In Hodgkin's and non-Hodgkin's lymphoma, gallium scanning can demonstrate abnormal activity in one or more lymph nodes or in extranodal locations. However, gallium scanning supported by results of lymphangiography can gauge the extent of metastasis more accurately than either test alone because neither test consistently identifies all neoplastic nodes.

After chemotherapy or radiation therapy, gallium scanning may be used to detect new or recurrent tumors. However, these forms of therapy tend to diminish tumor affinity for gallium without necessarily eliminating the tumor.

In the differential diagnosis of focal hepatic defects, abnormal gallium activity may help narrow the diagnostic possibilities. Gallium localizes in hepatomas, but not in pseudotumors; in abscesses, but not in pleural effusions; and in tumors, but not in cysts or hematomas. In examining patients with suspected bronchogenic carcinoma, abnormal activity confirms the presence of a tumor. However, because gallium also localizes in inflammatory pulmonary diseases, such as pneumonia and sarcoidosis, chest X-rays should be performed to distinguish between a tumor and an inflammatory lesion.

Post-test care

If the initial gallium scan suggests bowel disease and additional scans are necessary, give the patient a cleansing enema, as ordered, before continuing the test.

Interfering factors

■ Hepatic and splenic uptake may obscure the detection of abnormal para-aortic nodes in Hodgkin's disease, causing false-negative scans.
■ Fecal accumulation can hinder visualization of the retroperitoneal space.
■ Barium studies within 1 week before this scan can interfere with visualization of gallium activity in the bowel.

Red blood cell survival time

Normally, red blood cells (RBCs) are destroyed only when they reach senility. However, in hemolytic diseases, RBCs of all ages are randomly destroyed, resulting in anemia. This test measures the survival time of circulating RBCs and detects sites of abnormal RBC sequestration and destruction, aiding evaluation of unexplained anemia.

Survival time is measured by labeling a random sample of RBCs with radioactive sodium chromate Cr 51 (^{51}Cr). The ^{51}Cr quickly crosses RBC membranes, reduces to chromium ion, and binds to hemoglobin. This labeled group of RBCs is then injected back into the patient. Serial blood samples measure the percentage of labeled cells per unit volume over 3 to 4 weeks, until 50% of the cells disappear (disappearance rate corresponds to destruction of a random cell population).

A normal RBC survives about 120 days (half-life of 60 days); the ^{51}Cr-labeled RBCs have a shorter half-life (25 to 30 days) because about 1% of senescent RBCs are removed from the circulation each day and about 1% of ^{51}Cr is spontaneously eluted from the labeled RBCs each day.

During the test period, a gamma camera scans the body for sites of abnormally high radioactivity, which indicate sites of excessive RBC sequestration and destruction. Other tests performed with the RBC survival time test may include spot checks of the stool to detect GI blood loss; hematocrit; blood volume studies; and radionuclide iron uptake and clearance tests to aid differential diagnosis of anemia.

Purpose

■ To help evaluate unexplained anemia, particularly hemolytic anemia
■ To identify sites of abnormal RBC sequestration and destruction.

Patient preparation

Explain to the patient that this test helps identify the cause of his anemia. Advise him that he needn't restrict food or fluids. Inform him that the test involves labeling a blood sample with a radioactive substance and requires regular blood samples at 3-day intervals for 3 to 4 weeks.

Tell him who will perform the procedures and when and that he may experience slight discomfort from the needle punctures. Reassure him that collecting each sample takes less than 3 minutes and that the small amount of radioactive substance used is harmless. If the doctor orders a stool collection to test for GI bleeding, teach the patient the proper collection technique.

Procedure

A 30-ml blood sample is drawn and mixed with 100 microcuries of ^{51}Cr for an adult (less for a child). After an incubation period, the mixture is injected I.V. into the patient. A blood sample is drawn 30 minutes after injection to determine blood and RBC volumes.

A 6-ml sample is collected in a *green-top* tube after 24 hours; follow-up samples are collected at 3-day intervals for

3 to 4 weeks. (The interval between samples may vary, depending on the laboratory.) To avoid error from physical decay of the ^{51}Cr, each sample is measured with a scintillation well counter on the day it's drawn. Radioactivity per milliliter of RBCs is calculated; these values are then plotted to determine mean RBC survival time. Simultaneous gamma camera scans of the precordium, sacrum, liver, and spleen detect radioactivity at sites of excess RBC sequestration. A hematocrit is done on a small portion of each blood sample to check for blood loss.

At the end of the study, a sample is drawn to compare ending blood and RBC volumes with beginning volumes.

Precautions
■ This test is contraindicated during pregnancy because it exposes the fetus to radiation.
■ Because excess blood loss can invalidate test results, this test is usually contraindicated in patients with active bleeding or poor clotting function. However, if the test is necessary for a patient with poor clotting function, observe the venipuncture sites carefully for signs of hemorrhage.
■ The patient should not receive blood transfusions during the test period and should not have blood samples drawn for other tests.

Normal findings
The normal half-life for RBCs labeled with ^{51}Cr is 25 to 35 days. Normal gamma camera scans reveal slight radioactivity in the spleen, liver, and sometimes the bone marrow.

Implications of results
Decreased RBC survival time indicates a hemolytic disease, such as chronic lymphocytic leukemia, congenital nonspherocytic hemolytic anemia, hemoglobin C–thalassemia disease, heredi-

tary spherocytosis, idiopathic acquired hemolytic anemia, paroxysmal nocturnal hemoglobinuria, elliptocytosis, pernicious anemia, sickle cell anemia, sickle cell–hemoglobin C disease, or hemolytic-uremic syndrome. If hemolytic anemia is diagnosed, additional tests using cross-transfusion of labeled RBCs can determine whether anemia results from an intrinsic RBC defect or an extrinsic factor.

A gamma camera scan that detects a site of excess RBC sequestration provides a direction for treatment. For example, abnormally high RBC sequestration in the spleen may require a splenectomy.

Post-test care
If a hematoma develops at the venipuncture site, apply warm soaks.

Interfering factors
■ Dehydration, overhydration, or blood loss (from hemorrhage or other blood samples) can alter the circulating RBC volume and invalidate test results.
■ Blood transfusions during the test period alter the proportion of labeled RBCs to total RBCs, thus affecting the accuracy of test results.

MISCELLANEOUS TESTS

D-xylose absorption

One of the most important tests for malabsorption, D-xylose absorption evaluates patients with symptoms of malabsorption, such as weight loss and generalized malnutrition, weakness, and diarrhea. In this test, the patient ingests a standard dose of D-xylose — a pentose sugar that's absorbed in the small intestine without the aid of pancreatic enzymes, passed through the liver without being metabolized, and excreted in the urine. Because of its absorption in the small intestine without digestion, measurement of D-xylose in the urine and blood indicates the absorptive capacity of the small intestine. Normally, blood levels of D-xylose peak 2 hours after ingestion, and 80% to 95% of the dose is excreted in 5 hours; the remaining dose, in 24 hours.

To ensure accurate results, the test requires the patient to fast, to remain in bed during the specimen collection period, and to have adequate renal function for the absorption and excretion of D-xylose.

Purpose

■ To aid differential diagnosis of malabsorption
■ To determine the cause of malabsorption syndrome.

Patient preparation

Explain to the patient that this test helps evaluate digestive function by analyzing blood and urine specimens after ingestion of a sugar solution. Advise him to fast overnight before the test. Instruct him to abstain from all food and fluids and to remain in bed during the entire test period because activity affects test results.

Tell him that the test requires several blood samples, who will perform the venipunctures and when, and that he may experience some discomfort from the needle punctures and the pressure of the tourniquet. Reassure him that collecting each blood sample takes less than 3 minutes. Inform him that all his urine will be collected for 5 or 24 hours, as ordered.

As ordered, withhold aspirin and indomethacin, which alter test results, and record any medications the patient is taking on the laboratory request.

Equipment

Tourniquet ✦ venipuncture equipment ✦ 10-ml red-top tube ✦ sterile urine specimen container ✦ specimen labels ✦ gloves ✦ biohazard transport bags.

Procedure

Perform a venipuncture to obtain a fasting blood sample, and collect the sample in a 10 ml *red-top* tube. Then collect a first-voided morning urine specimen. Label these specimens and send them to the laboratory immediately to serve as a baseline.

Give the patient 25 g of D-xylose dissolved in 8 oz (240 ml) of water, followed by an additional 8 oz of water. If the patient is a child, administer 0.5 g of D-xylose per pound of body weight, up to 25 g. Record the time of D-xylose ingestion.

In an adult, draw a blood sample 2 hours after D-xylose ingestion; in a child, 1 hour. Collect the sample in a 10 ml *red-top* tube (or a 10 ml *gray-top* tube if the sample won't be tested immediately). Occasionally, a 5-hour sample may be drawn to support the findings of the 1- or 2-hour sample. Collect and pool all urine during the 5 or 24 hours following D-xylose ingestion, as ordered.

Precautions

■ Handle the blood collection tubes gently to prevent hemolysis.
■ Tell the patient not to contaminate the urine specimens with toilet tissue or stool.
■ Be sure to collect all urine and refrigerate the specimen during the collection period.
■ Check with the doctor to determine how long the collection period should be because patients age 65 and older and those with borderline or elevated creatinine levels tend to have low 5-hour

urine levels but normal 24-hour levels. At the end of the collection period, send the urine specimen to the laboratory immediately.

■ Keep the patient on bed rest and withhold food and fluids (other than D-xylose and water) throughout the test period.

Reference values

The following are normal values for the D-xylose absorption test:

For adults: blood concentration, 25 to 40 mg/dl in 2 hours; urine, more than 3.5 g excreted in 5 hours (age 65 or older, more than 5 g in 24 hours)

For children: blood concentration, more than 30 mg/dl in 1 hour; urine, 16% to 33% of ingested D-xylose excreted in 5 hours

Implications of results

Depressed blood and urine D-xylose levels most commonly result from malabsorptive disorders that affect the proximal small intestine, such as sprue and celiac disease. However, depressed D-xylose levels may also result from regional enteritis involving the jejunum, Whipple's disease, multiple jejunal diverticula, myxedema, diabetic neuropathic diarrhea, rheumatoid arthritis, alcoholism, severe congestive heart failure, and ascites.

Post-test care

■ If a hematoma develops at the venipuncture site, ease discomfort by applying warm soaks.

■ Observe the patient for abdominal discomfort or mild diarrhea caused by D-xylose ingestion.

■ As ordered, resume administration of medications discontinued before the test.

■ Tell the patient that he may resume his normal diet.

Interfering factors

■ Failure to adhere to dietary and activity restrictions affects absorption of D-xylose.

■ Aspirin decreases D-xylose excretion by the kidneys; indomethacin depresses its intestinal absorption.

■ Failure to obtain a complete urine specimen or to collect blood samples at designated times interferes with accurate testing.

■ Intestinal overgrowth of bacteria, renal insufficiency, or renal retention of urine may decrease urine levels.

Dexamethasone suppression

A standard screening test for Cushing's syndrome, the dexamethasone suppression test also helps diagnose major depression and monitor its treatment. That's because certain patients with major depression have high levels of circulating adrenal steroid hormones in their blood. Administration of an oral steroid such as dexamethasone suppresses these levels in normal people but fails to suppress them in patients with Cushing's syndrome and some forms of depression.

Purpose

■ To diagnose Cushing's syndrome
■ To aid diagnosis of clinical depression.

Patient preparation

Explain the purpose of the test. Inform the patient that the test requires two blood samples drawn after administration of dexamethasone. Tell him who will perform the venipuncture and when and that he may experience transient discomfort from the needle puncture and the pressure of the tourniquet. Restrict food and fluids for 10 to 12 hours before the test.

Equipment
Dexamethasone ✦ syringe and needle ✦ tourniquet.

Procedure
Give the patient 1 mg of dexamethasone at 11 p.m. On the following day, collect blood samples at 4 p.m. and 11 p.m. More frequent sampling may increase the likelihood of measuring a nonsuppressed cortisol peak.

Precautions
Many medications — including corticosteroids, oral contraceptives, lithium, methadone, aspirin, diuretics, morphine, and monoamine oxidase (MAO) inhibitors — may affect the accuracy of test results. If possible, don't administer any of these medications after midnight the night before the test.

Reference values
A cortisol level of 5 g/dl (140 nmol/L) or more indicates failure of dexamethasone suppression.

Implications of results
A normal test result doesn't rule out major depression, but an abnormal result strengthens a clinically based diagnosis. Failure of suppression occurs in patients with Cushing's syndrome, severe stress, and depression that's likely to respond to treatment with antidepressants.

The dexamethasone suppression test has proved disappointing in differentiating dysthymic disorder (neurotic depression) from major affective illness (psychotic depression), but it may be useful in patients with other psychiatric disorders (such as schizoaffective disorder) to establish the need for treatment of coexisting depression.

Post-test care
If a hematoma develops at the venipuncture site, apply warm soaks to ease discomfort.

Interfering factors
■ False-positive results can occur in diabetes mellitus, pregnancy, and severe stress (such as trauma, severe weight loss, dehydration, and acute alcohol withdrawal).

■ False-positive results can follow the use of certain drugs, particularly barbiturates or phenytoin, within 3 weeks of the test.

■ False-positive results can occur if caffeine was ingested after midnight the night before the test.

■ Failure to withhold corticosteroids, oral contraceptives, lithium, methadone, aspirin, diuretics, morphine, or MAO inhibitors before the test may interfere with test results.

SELECTED READINGS

Black, J.M., and Matassarin-Jacobs, E., eds. *Luckmann and Sorensen's Medical-Surgical Nursing: A Psychophysiologic Approach,* 4th ed. Philadelphia: W.B. Saunders Co., 1993.

Diseases, 2nd ed. Springhouse, Pa.: Springhouse Corp., 1996.

Fischbach, F. *A Manual of Laboratory and Diagnostic Tests,* 5th ed. Philadelphia: Lippincott-Raven Pubs., 1996.

Guyton, A.C., and Hall, J.E. *Textbook of Medical Physiology,* 9th ed. Philadelphia: W.B. Saunders Co., 1996.

Henry, J.B., ed. *Clinical Diagnosis and Management by Laboratory Methods,* 19th ed. Philadelphia: W.B. Saunders Co., 1996.

Isselbacher, K.J., et al., eds. *Harrison's Principles of Internal Medicine,* 13th ed. New York: McGraw-Hill Book Co., 1994.

Mayo Medical Laboratories 1996 Test Catalog. Rochester, Minn.: Mayo Medical Laboratories, 1996.

Nursing97 Drug Handbook. Springhouse, Pa.: Springhouse Corp., 1997.

Ravel, R.A. *Clinical Laboratory Medicine: Clinical Application of Laboratory Data,* 6th ed. St. Louis: Mosby–Year Book, Inc., 1995.

Tilkian, S.M., et al. *Clinical and Nursing Implications of Laboratory Tests,* 5th ed. St. Louis: Mosby–Year Book, Inc., 1995.

Treseler, K.M. *Clinical Laboratory and Diagnostic Tests: Significance and Nursing Implications,* 3rd ed. Stamford, Conn.: Appleton & Lange, 1995.

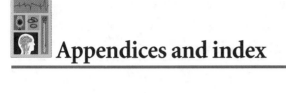

Appendices and index

Guide to abbreviations

<	less than	HLA	human leukocyte antigen
>	greater than		
ABGs	arterial blood gases	IU	international unit
ACTH	adrenocorticotropic hormone	K	potassium
ADH	antidiuretic hormone	kg	kilogram
AFP	alpha-fetoprotein		
ALT	alanine aminotransferase	L	liter
		LD	lactate dehydrogenase
ANA	antinuclear antibodies		
ASO	antistreptolysin-0	LH	luteinizing hormone
AST	aspartate aminotransferase		
		m²	square meter
		mcg, μg	microgram
BUN	blood urea nitrogen	mEq	milliequivalent
		Mg	magnesium
Ca	calcium	mg	milligram
CBC	complete blood count	MHC	major histocompatibility complex
CEA	carcinoembryonic antigen		
		mIU	milli-international unit
CK	creatine kinase	ml	milliliter
Cl	chloride	mm	millimeter
cm³	cubic centimeter	mm³	cubic millimeter
		mm Hg	millimeter of mercury
dl	deciliter	mmol	millimole
		mOsm	milliosmole
EBV	Epstein-Barr virus	mμ	millimicron
ELISA	enzyme-linked immunosorbent assay	mU	milliunut
		μ	micron
ESR	erythrocyte sedimentation rate	μg	microgram
		μIU	micro-international unit
FSH	follicle-stimulating hormone	μl	microliter
		μmol	micromole
FSP	fibrin split products	μU	microunit
g	gram	ng	nanogram
GFR	glomerular filtration rate	nmol	nanomole
GH	growth hormone	pg	picogram
		PT	prothrombin time
Hb	hemoglobin	PTH	parathyroid hormone
hCG	human chorionic gonadotropin	PTT	partial thromboplastin time
Hct, HCT	hematocrit		
HIV	human immunodeficiency virus	RAST	radioallergosorbent test

Guide to abbreviations *(continued)*

RBC	red blood cell
RF	rheumatoid factor
RPR	rapid plasma reagin (test)
sec	second
SI	Système International d'Unités (units)
T$_3$	triiodothyronine
T$_4$	thyroxine
TBG	thyroxine-binding globulin
TSH	thyroid-stimulating hormone
U	unit
VDRL	Venereal Disease Research Laboratory (test)
WBC	white blood cell

Units of measure

Metric measures: weight and volume

PREFIX SYMBOL	FACTOR	WEIGHT	VOLUME
k	1 x 1,000 1	kilogram (kg) gram (g)	kiloliter (kl) liter (L)
d	1 ÷ 10	decigram (dg)	deciliter (dl)
c	1 ÷ 100	centigram (cg)	centiliter (cl)
m	1 ÷ 1,000	milligram (mg)	milliliter (ml)
μ (mc)	1 ÷ 1 million	microgram (μg, mcg)	microliter (μl, mcl)
n	1 ÷ 1 billion	nanogram (ng)	nanoliter (nl)
p	1 ÷ 1 trillion	picogram (pg)	picoliter (pl)
f	1 ÷ 1 quadrillion	femtogram (fg)	femtoliter (fl)

Conversion of metric to customary units

WEIGHT	VOLUME
grams x 0.035 = ounces	milliliters x 0.03 = fluidounces
kilograms x 2.2 = pounds	liters x 2.1 = pints liters x 1.06 = quarts liters x 0.26 = gallons

Units of measure *(continued)*

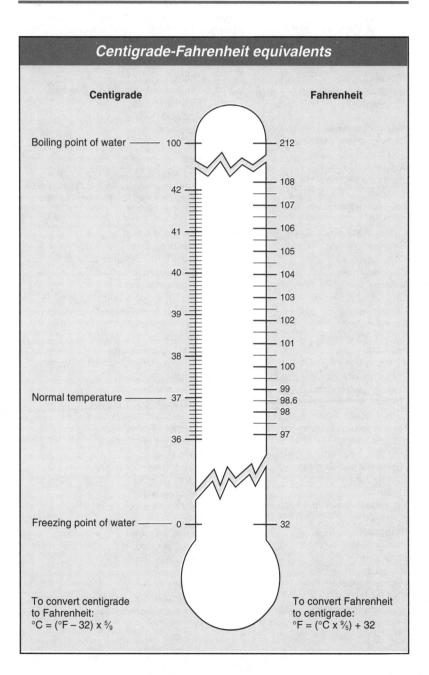

Centigrade-Fahrenheit equivalents

Centigrade   **Fahrenheit**

Boiling point of water ——— 100 — — 212

42 — — 108

— 107

41 — — 106

— 105

40 — — 104

— 103

39 — — 102

— 101

38 — — 100

— 99
Normal temperature ——— 37 — — 98.6
— 98

36 — — 97

Freezing point of water ——— 0 — — 32

To convert centigrade
to Fahrenheit:
$°C = (°F − 32) \times \frac{5}{9}$

To convert Fahrenheit
to centigrade:
$°F = (°C \times \frac{9}{5}) + 32$

Guide to color-top collection tubes

The colors of collection tubes can vary from laboratory to laboratory. This guide lists the most commonly used collection tubes. Consult your laboratory for its specific collection tube requirements.

Marble

Marble-top *tubes contain a silicone gel to separate serum from cells.*

Acid phosphatase
Alanine aminotransferase
Alkaline phosphatase
Amylase
Aspartate aminotransferase
Bilirubin
Blood urea nitrogen
Calcium
Carcinoembryonic antigen
Chloride
Cholesterol, total
Cholinesterase
Creatine
Creatine kinase
Creatinine
Cryoglobulins
Digitalis glycosides
Folic acid
Follicle-stimulating hormone
Free thyroxine and free triiodothyronine
Gamma-glutamyltransferase
Gastrin
Growth hormone/somatotropic hormone
Growth hormone suppression test (glucose loading)
Hepatitis B surface antigen
Hydroxybutyric dehydrogenase
Lactate dehydrogenase
Lipase
Lipoprotein-cholesterol fractionation
Magnesium
Phosphates
Phospholipids
Potassium
Prolactin
Protein electrophoresis
Sodium
Triiodothyronine resin uptake
Testosterone
Thyroid-stimulating hormone

Triglycerides
Tubular reabsorption of phosphate
Urea clearance
Uric acid
Vitamin B_{12}

Red

Red-top *tubes contain no additives. Draw volume may be 2 to 20 ml. These tubes are used for tests performed on serum samples.*

ABO blood typing
Acetaminophen
Acetylcholine receptor antibodies
Alpha-fetoprotein
Androstenedione
Angiotensin-converting enzyme
Antibody screening test
Anticonvulsants
Antidepressants, plasma
Antidiuretic hormone
Antideoxyribonucleic acid antibodies
Antiglobulin, direct
Antimicrobials
Antimitochondrial antibodies
Anti–smooth-muscle antibodies
Antistreptolysin-O test
Antithyroid antibodies
Arginine test
Barbiturates
Bronchodilators
Ceruloplasmin
Cold agglutinins
Complement assays
C-reactive protein
Crossmatching
D-xylose absorption
Estrogens
Ethanol, blood
Extractable nuclear antigen antibodies
Febrile agglutination tests
Ferritin

Guide to color-top collection tubes *(continued)*

Fluorescent treponemal antibody absorption test
Fungal serology
Haptoglobin
Heterophil agglutination tests
Hexosaminidase A and B
Human chorionic gonadotropin
Human placental lactogen
Hypnotics
Immunoglobulins A, G, and M
Immune complex assays
Insulin
Iron and total iron-binding capacity
Isocitrate dehydrogenase
Isopropanol
Leucine aminopeptidase
Leukoagglutinins
Long-acting thyroid stimulator
Lupus erythematosus cell preparation
Luteinizing hormone, plasma
Lyme test
Methanol
Myoglobin
5'-Nucleotidase
Ornithine carbamoyltransferase
Parathyroid hormone (parathormone)
Phenothiazines
Prothrombin consumption
Radioallergosorbent test
Rh typing
Rheumatoid factor
Rubella antibodies
Salicylates
Thyroid-stimulating hormone, neonatal
Thyroxine
Thyroxine-binding globulin
Tranquilizers
Transferrin
Triiodothyronine
Venereal Disease Research Laboratory test
Vitamin A and carotene
Vitamin B_2
Vitamin D_3

Lavender

Lavender-top *tubes contain EDTA. Draw volume may be 2 to 10 ml. These tubes are used for tests performed on whole blood samples.*

ABO blood typing
Adrenocorticotropic hormone
Antidiuretic hormone
Coombs' direct
Erythrocyte sedimentation rate
Glucagon
Glucose-6-phosphate dehydrogenase
Heinz bodies
Hematocrit
Hemoglobin, glycosylated
Hemoglobin, total
Hemoglobins, unstable
Hemoglobin electrophoresis
Lead
Lipoprotein phenotyping
Plasma renin activity
Platelet count
Platelet survival
Pyruvate kinase
Red blood cell count
Red cell indices
Reticulocyte count
Rh typing
Sickle cell test (hemoglobin S)
White blood cell count
White blood cell differential

Green

Green-top *tubes contain heparin (sodium, lithium, or ammonium). Draw volume may be 2 to 15 ml. These tubes are used for tests performed on plasma samples.*

Amino acid scan
Ammonia
Androstenedione
Angiotensin-converting enzyme
Calcitonin (thyrocalcitonin)
Catecholamines
Chromosomal analysis

Guide to color-top collection tubes *(continued)*

Erythropoietic porphyrins
Galactose 1-phosphate uridyltransferase
Insulin tolerance test
Inulin clearance
Lymphocyte transformation tests
Osmotic fragility
Para-aminohippuric acid excretion
Rapid adrenocorticotropic hormone
Red blood cell survival time
Terminal deoxynucleotidyl transferase
Uroporphyrinogen I synthase

Blue

Blue-top *tubes contain sodium citrate and citric acid. Draw volume may be 2.7 or 4.5 ml. These tubes are used for coagulation studies requiring plasma samples.*

Activated partial thromboplastin time
Euglobulin lysis time
Fibrinogen
Hemoglobin derivatives
One-stage assay: Extrinsic coagulation
  system
One-stage assay: Intrinsic coagulation
  system
Plasminogen
Platelet aggregation
Protein C
Protein S
Prothrombin time
Thrombin time
Tissue thromboplastin inhibitor study
  (lupus anticoagulation)

Black

Black-top *tubes contain sodium oxalate. Draw volume may be 2.7 or 4.5 ml. These tubes are used for coagulation studies performed on plasma samples.*

Plasma vitamin C
Fibrin split products

Gray

Gray-top *tubes contain a glycolytic inhibitor (such as sodium fluoride, powdered oxalate, or glycolytic/microbial inhibitor). Draw volume may be 3 to 10 ml. These tubes are used most often for glucose determinations in serum or plasma samples.*

Serum glucose levels (all types)
Insulin tolerance test
Lactic acid and pyruvic acid
Tolbutamide tolerance test

Guide to selected reagent strip tests

Reagent strips	Substance detected							
	Bilirubin	Blood	Glucose	Ketones	Nitrite	pH	Protein	Urobilin-ogen
Albustix							x	
Bili-Labstix	x	x	x	x		x	x	
Chemstrip GK			x	x				
Chemstrip GP			x				x	
Chemstrip 5		x	x	x		x	x	
Chemstrip 6	x	x	x	x		x	x	
Chemstrip 7	x	x	x	x		x	x	x
Chemstrip 8	x	x	x	x	x	x	x	x
Clinistix			x					
Combistix			x			x	x	
Dextrostix (use fingerstick or venous blood)			x					
Diastix			x					
Hema-Combistix		x	x			x	x	
Hemastix (may also test fecal matter)		x						
Hemoccult		x						
Keto-Diastix			x	x				
Ketostix				x				
Labstix		x	x	x		x	x	
Microstix-Nitrite					x			
Multistix	x	x	x	x		x	x	x
Nitrazine paper						x		
N-Multistix	x	x	x	x	x	x	x	x
N-Uristix			x		x		x	
Tes-Tape			x					
Uristix			x				x	
Urobilistix								x

Drug interference with test results

Drugs can interfere with the results of laboratory tests in two ways. A drug in a blood or urine specimen may interact with the chemicals used in the laboratory test, causing a false result. Or a drug may cause a physiologic change in the patient, resulting in an actual increased or decreased blood or urine level of the substance being tested. This chart identifies drugs that can cause these two types of interference in some common blood and urine tests.

TEST	CHEMICAL REACTION	PHYSIOLOGIC CHANGE	
		Increased test values	Decreased test values
alkaline phosphatase	▪ albumin ▪ fluorides	▪ anticonvulsants ▪ hepatotoxic drugs	▪ clofibrate
ammonia, blood		▪ acetazolamide ▪ alcohol ▪ ammonium chloride ▪ asparaginase ▪ barbiturates ▪ diuretics, loop and thiazide	▪ kanamycin, oral ▪ lactulose ▪ neomycin, oral ▪ potassium salts
amylase, serum	▪ chloride salts ▪ fluorides	▪ asparaginase ▪ cholinergic agents ▪ contraceptives, oral ▪ contrast media with iodine ▪ drugs inducing acute pancreatitis: azathioprine, corticosteroids, loop and thiazide diuretics ▪ methyldopa ▪ narcotics	
aspartate aminotransferase	▪ erythromycin ▪ methyldopa	▪ cholinergic agents ▪ hepatotoxic drugs ▪ opium alkaloids	
bilirubin, serum	▪ ascorbic acid ▪ dextran ▪ epinephrine ▪ pindolol	▪ hemolytic agents ▪ hepatotoxic drugs ▪ methyldopa ▪ rifampin	▪ barbiturates
blood urea nitrogen	▪ chloral hydrate ▪ chloramphenicol ▪ streptomycin	▪ anabolic steroids ▪ nephrotoxic drugs	▪ tetracyclines
calcium, serum	▪ aspirin ▪ heparin	▪ asparaginase ▪ calcium salts	▪ acetazolamide ▪ anticonvulsants

Drug interference with test results *(continued)*

TEST	CHEMICAL REACTION	PHYSIOLOGIC CHANGE	
		Increased test values	Decreased test values
calcium, serum *(continued)*	■ hydralazine ■ sulfisoxazole	■ diuretics, loop and thiazide ■ lithium ■ thyroid hormones ■ vitamin D	■ calcitonin ■ cisplatin ■ contraceptives, oral ■ corticosteroids ■ laxatives ■ magnesium salts ■ plicamycin
chloride, serum		■ acetazolamide ■ androgens ■ estrogens ■ nonsteroidal anti-inflammatory drugs	■ corticosteroids ■ diuretics, loop and thiazide
cholesterol, serum	■ androgens ■ aspirin ■ corticosteroids ■ nitrates ■ phenothiazines ■ vitamin D	■ beta-adrenergic blocking agents ■ contraceptives, oral ■ corticosteroids ■ diuretics, thiazide ■ phenothiazines ■ sulfonamides	■ androgens ■ captopril ■ chlorpropamide ■ cholestyramine ■ clofibrate ■ colestipol ■ haloperidol ■ neomycin, oral
creatine kinase (CK)		■ aminocaproic acid ■ amphotericin B ■ chlorthalidone ■ clofibrate ■ ethanol, chronic use	
creatinine, serum	■ cefoxitin (Jaffe method) ■ cephalothin ■ flucytosine	■ cimetidine ■ nephrotoxic drugs	
glucose, serum	■ acetaminophen ■ ascorbic acid (urine) ■ cephalosporins (urine)	■ antidepressants, tricyclic ■ beta-adrenergic blocking agents ■ corticosteroids ■ dextrothyroxine ■ diazoxide ■ diuretics, loop and thiazide ■ epinephrine ■ estrogens ■ isoniazid ■ lithium ■ phenothiazines ■ phenytoin	■ acetaminophen ■ alcohol ■ anabolic steroids ■ clofibrate ■ disopyramide ■ gemfibrozil ■ monoamine oxidase (MAO) inhibitors ■ pentamidine

(continued)

Drug interference with test results *(continued)*

TEST	CHEMICAL REACTION	PHYSIOLOGIC CHANGE	
		Increased test values	Decreased test values
glucose, serum *(continued)*		■ salicylates, toxic levels ■ thiabendazole	
magnesium, serum		■ lithium ■ magnesium salts	■ alcohol ■ aminoglycosides ■ amphotericin B ■ calcium salts ■ cisplatin ■ digitalis glycosides, toxic levels ■ diuretics, loop and thiazide
phosphates, serum		■ vitamin D, excessive amounts	■ antacids, phosphate-binding (such as aluminum phosphate gel) ■ mannitol
potassium, serum		■ aminocaproic acid ■ angiotensin-converting enzyme (ACE) inhibitors ■ antineoplastic agents ■ diuretics, potassium-sparing ■ isoniazid ■ lithium ■ mannitol ■ nephrotoxic drugs ■ succinylcholine	■ ammonium chloride ■ amphotericin B ■ corticosteroids ■ diuretics, potassium-wasting ■ glucose ■ insulin ■ laxatives ■ penicillins, extended-spectrum ■ salicylates
protein, serum		■ anabolic steroids ■ corticosteroids ■ phenazopyridine	■ contraceptives, oral ■ estrogens ■ hepatotoxic drugs
protein, urine	■ aminoglycosides ■ cephalosporins ■ contrast media with iodine ■ magnesium sulfate, large doses ■ miconazole ■ nafcillin ■ phenazopyridine ■ sulfonamides ■ tolbutamide ■ tolmetin	■ cephalosporins ■ contrast media with iodine ■ corticosteroids ■ nafcillin ■ nephrotoxic drugs ■ sulfonamides	

Drug interference with test results *(continued)*

TEST	CHEMICAL REACTION	PHYSIOLOGIC CHANGE	
		Increased test values	**Decreased test values**
prothrombin time		■ anticoagulants ■ asparaginase ■ aspirin ■ azathioprine ■ cefamandole ■ cefoperazone ■ cephalothin ■ chloramphenicol ■ cholestyramine ■ colestipol ■ cyclophosphamide ■ hepatotoxic drugs ■ moxalactam ■ propylthiouracil ■ quinidine ■ quinine ■ sulfonamides ■ tetracyclines	■ anabolic steroids ■ contraceptives, oral ■ estrogens ■ vitamin K
sodium, serum		■ anabolic steroids ■ clonidine ■ contraceptives, oral ■ corticosteroids ■ diazoxide ■ estrogens ■ guanabenz ■ guanadrel ■ guanethidine ■ methyldopa ■ nonsteroidal anti-inflammatory drugs ■ sulfonylureas	■ ammonium chloride ■ carbamazepine ■ desmopressin ■ diuretics ■ lypressin ■ vasopressin
uric acid, serum	■ ascorbic acid ■ caffeine ■ levodopa ■ theophylline	■ acetazolamide ■ alcohol ■ cisplatin ■ diazoxide ■ diuretics ■ epinephrine ■ ethambutol ■ levodopa ■ niacin	■ acetohexamide ■ allopurinol ■ clofibrate ■ contrast media with iodine ■ diflunisal ■ glucose infusions ■ guaifenesin ■ phenothiazines ■ phenylbutazone ■ salicylates, small doses ■ uricosuric agents

Quick-reference guide to laboratory test results

A

Acetylcholine receptor antibodies, serum
Negative or ≤0.03 nmol/L

Acid mucopolysaccharides, urine
Adults: <13.3 µg glucuronic acid/mg creatinine
age 2: 8 to 30 µg glucuronic acid/mg creatinine
age 4: 7 to 27
age 6: 6 to 24
age 8: 4 to 22
age 10: 2 to 18
age 12: 0 to 15
age 14: 0 to 12

Acid phosphatase, serum
0.5 to 1.9 U/L

Activated partial thromboplastin time
25 to 36 seconds

Adrenocorticotropic hormone, plasma
<60 pg/ml

Adrenocorticotropic hormone, rapid, plasma
Cortisol rises 7 to 18 µg/dl above baseline 60 minutes after injection

Alanine aminotransferase
Males: 10 to 35 U/L
Females: 9 to 24 U/L

Albumin, peritoneal fluid
50% to 70% of total protein

Albumin, serum
3.3 to 4.5 g/dl

Aldosterone, serum
0 to 3 weeks: 16.5 to 154 ng/dl
1 to 11 months: 6.5 to 86 ng/dl
1 to 10 years (supine): 3 to 39.5 ng/dl
1 to 10 years (standing): 3.5 to 124 ng/dl
≥11 years: 1 to 21 ng/dl

Aldosterone, urine
2 to 16 µg/24 hours

Alkaline phosphatase, peritoneal fluid
Males >18 years: 90 to 239 U/L
Females <45 years: 76 to 196 U/L;
≥45 years: 87 to 250 U/L

Alkaline phosphatase, serum
Males 0 to 3 years: not established
4 years: 324 to 803 U/L
5 years: 389 to 904 U/L
6 years: 390 to 906 U/L
7 years: 374 to 881 U/L
8 years: 367 to 871 U/L
9 years: 381 to 893 U/L
10 years: 415 to 945 U/L
11 years: 402 to 1,103 U/L
12 years: 403 to 1,222 U/L
13 years: 395 to 1,276 U/L
14 years: 361 to 1,241 U/L
15 years: 299 to 1,110 U/L
16 years: 221 to 906 U/L
17 years: 151 to 677 U/L
18 years: 113 to 482 U/L
≥19 years: 98 to 251 U/L
Females 0 to 3 years: not established
4 years: 368 to 809 U/L
5 years: 352 to 772 U/L
6 years: 367 to 805 U/L
7 years: 398 to 875 U/L
8 years: 433 to 956 U/L
9 years: 461 to 1,018 U/L
10 years: 468 to 1,034 U/L
11 years: 388 to 1,144 U/L
12 years: 290 to 1,055 U/L
13 years: 260 to 976 U/L
14 years: 333 to 787 U/L
15 years: 163 to 595 U/L
16 years: 133 to 573 U/L
17 to 23 years: 114 to 312 U/L
24 to 45 years: 81 to 213 U/L
46 to 50 years: 84 to 218 U/L
51 to 55 years: 90 to 234 U/L
56 to 60 years: 99 to 257 U/L
61 to 65 years: 108 to 282 U/L
≥65 years: 119 to 309 U/L

Alpha-fetoprotein, amniotic fluid
≤18.5 µg/ml at 13 to 14 weeks

Alpha-fetoprotein, serum
Males and nonpregnant females: 0 to 6.4 IU/ml

Ammonia, peritoneal fluid
<50 µg/dl

Ammonia, plasma
<50 µg/dl

Amniotic fluid analysis
Lecithin-sphingomyelin ratio: >2
Meconium: absent
Phosphatidylglycerol: present

Amylase, peritoneal fluid
138 to 404 U/L

Amylase, serum
0 to 23 months: 0 to 265 U/L
2 to 3 years: 31 to 203 U/L
4 to 5 years: 11 to 259 U/L
6 to 7 years: 22 to 150 U/L
8 to 9 years: 14 to 198 U/L
10 to 11 years: 11 to 119 U/L
12 to 13 years: 36 to 160 U/L
14 to 15 years: 29 to 173 U/L
16 to 17 years: 12 to 188 U/L
≥18 years: 35 to 115 U/L

Amylase, urine
10 to 80 amylase units/hour

Androstenedione (radioimmunoassay)
Males 0 to 7 years: 0.1 to 0.2 ng/ml
8 to 9 years: 0.1 to 0.3 ng/ml
10 to 11 years: 0.3 to 0.7 ng/ml
12 to 13 years: 0.4 to 1.0 ng/ml
14 to 17 years: 0.5 to 1.4 ng/ml
≥18 years: 0.3 to 3.1 ng/ml
Females 0 to 7 years: 0.1 to 0.3 ng/ml
8 to 9 years: 0.2 to 0.5 ng/ml
10 to 11 years: 0.4 to 1.0 ng/ml
12 to 13 years: 0.8 to 1.9 ng/ml
14 to 17 years: 0.7 to 2.2 ng/ml
≥18 years: 0.2 to 3.1 ng/ml

Angiotensin-converting enzyme
<1 year: 10.9 to 42.1 U/L
1 to 2 years: 9.4 to 36.0 U/L
3 to 4 years: 7.9 to 29.8 U/L
5 to 9 years: 9.6 to 35.4 U/L
10 to 12 years: 10 to 37 U/L
13 to 16 years: 9 to 33.4 U/L
17 to 19 years: 7.2 to 26.6 U/L
≥20 years: 6.1 to 21.1 U/L

Anion gap
8 to 14 mEq/L

Antibodies to extractable nuclear antigens
Negative

Antibody screening, serum
Negative

Antideoxyribonucleic acid antibodies, serum
<7 IU/ml

Antidiuretic hormone, serum
1 to 5 pg/ml

Antiglobulin test, direct
Negative

Antimitochondrial antibodies, serum
Negative at titer <20

Antinuclear antibodies, serum (Hep-2 substrate)
Negative at ≤1:40

Anti-Smith antibodies
Negative

Anti–smooth-muscle antibodies, serum
Normal titer <1:20

Antistreptolysin-O, serum
<120 Todd units/ml

Antithrombin III
>50% of normal control values

Antithyroid antibodies, serum
Normal titer <1:100

Arginine test
Human growth hormone levels increase to >10 ng/ml in men, to >15 ng/ml in women

Arterial blood gases
pH: 7.35 to 7.45
Pao_2: 75 to 100 mm Hg
$Paco_2$: 35 to 45 mm Hg
O_2Ct: 15% to 23%
Sao_2: 94% to 100%
HCO_3^-: 22 to 26 mEq/L

Arylsulfatase A, urine
Males: 1.4 to 19.3 U/L
Females: 1.4 to 11 U/L

Aspartate aminotransferase
Males: 8 to 20 U/L
Females: 5 to 40 U/L
Children 0 to 5 days: 35 to 140 U/L
6 days to 3 years: 20 to 60 U/L
3 to 6 years: 15 to 50 U/L
6 to 12 years: 10 to 50 U/L
13 to 18 years: 10 to 40 U/L

Aspergillosis antibody, serum
Normal titer <1:8

Atrial natriuretic factor, plasma
20 to 77 pg/ml

Quick-reference guide to laboratory test results *(continued)*

B

Bacterial meningitis antigen
Negative

Bence Jones protein, urine
Negative

Beta-hydroxybutyrate
<0.4 mmol/L

Bilirubin, amniotic fluid
Absent at term

Bilirubin, serum
Adults: direct, <0.5 mg/dl; indirect,
≤1.1 mg/dl
Neonates: total, 1 to 12 mg/dl

Bilirubin, urine
Negative

Blastomycosis antibody, serum
Normal titer <1:8

Bleeding time
Template: 2 to 8 minutes
Modified template: 2 to 10 minutes
Ivy: 1 to 7 minutes
Duke: 1 to 3 minutes

Blood urea nitrogen
8 to 20 mg/dl

B-lymphocyte count
270 to 640/µl

C

Calcitonin, plasma
Baseline: males, ≤40 pg/ml; females,
≤20 pg/ml
Calcium infusion: males, ≤190 pg/ml;
females, ≤130 pg/ml
Pentagastrin infusion: males, ≤110 pg/
ml; females, ≤30 pg/ml

Calcium, serum (atomic absorption)
Males 0 to 11 months: not established
1 to 14 years: 9.6 to 10.6 mg/dl
15 to 16 years: 9.5 to 10.5 mg/dl
17 to 18 years: 9.5 to 10.4 mg/dl
19 to 21 years: 9.3 to 10.3 mg/dl
≥22 years: 8.9 to 10.1 mg/dl
Females 0 to 11 months: not established
1 to 11 years: 9.6 to 10.6 mg/dl
12 to 14 years: 9.5 to 10.4 mg/dl
15 to 18 years: 9.1 to 10.3 mg/dl
≥19 years: 8.9 to 10.1 mg/dl

Calcium, urine
Males: <275 mg/24 hours
Females: <250 mg/24 hours

Calculi, urine
None

***Candida* antibodies, serum**
Negative

Capillary fragility

Petechiae per 5 cm:	Score:
0 to 10	1 +
10 to 20	2 +
20 to 50	3 +
50	4 +

Carbon dioxide, total, blood
22 to 34 mEq/L

Carcinoembryonic antigen, serum
<5 ng/ml

Cardiolipin antibodies
1:2 titer: negative
1:4 titer: borderline
1:8 titer: positive

Carotene, serum
48 to 200 µg/dl

Catecholamines, plasma
Supine: epinephrine, 0 to 110 pg/ml;
norepinephrine, 70 to 750 pg/ml;
dopamine, 0 to 30 pg/ml
Standing: epinephrine, 0 to 140 pg/ml;
norepinephrine, 200 to 1,700 pg/
ml; dopamine, 0 to 30 pg/ml

Catecholamines, urine
Epinephrine
<1 year: 0 to 2.5 µg/24 hours
1 year: 0 to 3.5 µg/24 hours
2 to 3 years: 0 to 6 µg/24 hours
4 to 9 years: 0.2 to 10 µg/24 hours
10 to 15 years: 0.5 to 20 µg/24 hours
≥16 years: 0 to 20 µg/24 hours
Norepinephrine
<1 year: 0 to 10 µg/24 hours
1 year: 1 to 17 µg/24 hours
2 to 3 years: 4 to 29 µg/24 hours
4 to 6 years: 8 to 45 µg/24 hours
7 to 9 years: 13 to 65 µg/24 hours
≥10 years: 15 to 80 µg/24 hours
Dopamine
<1 year: 0 to 85 µg/24 hours
1 year: 10 to 140 µg/24 hours

2 to 3 years: 40 to 260 µg/24 hours
≥4 years: 65 to 400 µg/24 hours

Cerebrospinal fluid
Pressure: 50 to 180 mm H_2O
Appearance: clear, colorless
Gram stain: no organisms

Ceruloplasmin, serum
Males 0 to 11 months: not established
1 to 3 years: 24 to 46 mg/dl
4 to 6 years: 24 to 42 mg/dl
7 to 9 years: 24 to 40 mg/dl
10 to 13 years: 22 to 36 mg/dl
14 to 18 years: 14 to 34 mg/dl
≥19 years: 22.9 to 43.1 mg/dl
Females 0 to 11 months: not established
1 to 3 years: 24 to 46 mg/dl
4 to 6 years: 24 to 42 mg/dl
7 to 9 years: 24 to 40 mg/dl
10 to 13 years: 23 to 43 mg/dl
14 to 18 years: 20 to 45 mg/dl
≥19 years: 22.9 to 43.1 mg/dl

Chloride, cerebrospinal fluid
118 to 130 mEq/L

Chloride, serum
100 to 108 mEq/L

Chloride, sweat
10 to 35 mEq/L

Chloride, urine
110 to 250 mEq/24 hours

Cholesterol, total, serum
170 to 240 mg/dl

Cholinesterase (pseudocholinesterase)
8 to 18 U/ml

Clot retraction
50%

Coccidioidomycosis antibody, serum
Normal titer <1:2

Cold agglutinins, serum
Normal titer <1:32

Complement, serum
Total: 25 to 110 U
CI esterase inhibitor: 8 to 24 mg/dl
C3: 70 to 150 mg/dl
C4: 14 to 40 mg/dl

Complement, synovial fluid
10 mg protein/dl: 3.7 to 33.7 U/ml
20 mg protein/dl: 7.7 to 37.7 U/ml

Copper, urine
15 to 60 µg/24 hours

Copper reduction test, urine
Negative

Coproporphyrin, urine
Males: 0 to 96 µg/24 hours
Females: 1 to 57 µg/24 hours

Cortisol, free, urine
24 to 108 µg/24 hours

Cortisol, plasma
Morning: 7 to 28 µg/dl
Afternoon: 2 to 18 µg/dl

C-reactive protein, serum
Negative

Creatine, serum
Males: 0.2 to 0.6 mg/dl
Females: 0.6 to 1 mg/dl

Creatine kinase
Total
Males 0 to 5 years: not established
6 to 11 years: 150 to 499 U/L
12 to 17 years: 94 to 499 U/L
≥18 years: 52 to 336 U/L
Females 0 to 5 years: not established
6 to 7 years: 134 to 391 U/L
8 to 14 years: 91 to 391 U/L
15 to 17 years: 53 to 269 U/L
≥18 years: 38 to 176 U/L
Isoenzymes
CK-BB: undetectable
CK-MB: 0 to 7 U/L
CK-MM: 5 to 70 U/L
$CK-MB_2$: <1 U/L
$CK-MB_2/CK-MB_1$ ratio: <1.5

Creatinine, serum
Males: 0.8 to 1.2 mg/dl
Females: 0.6 to 0.9 mg/dl

Creatinine, urine
Males: 0 to 40 mg/24 hours
Females: 0 to 80 mg/24 hours

Creatinine clearance
Males (age 20): 85 to 146 ml/min/ 1.73 m^2
Females (age 20): 81 to 134 ml/min/ 1.73 m^2

Cryoglobulins, serum
Negative

Cryptococcosis antigen, serum
Negative

Quick-reference guide to laboratory test results *(continued)*

Cyclic adenosine monophosphate, urine
Parathyroid hormone infusion: 3.6- to 4-µmol increase
Cytomegalovirus antibodies, serum
Negative

D

Delta-aminolevulinic acid, urine
1.5 to 7.5 mg/dl/24 hours
D-xylose absorption
Blood: adults, 25 to 40 mg/dl in 2 hours; children, >30 mg/dl in 1 hour
Urine: adults, >3.5 g excreted in 5 hours; children, 16% to 33% excreted in 5 hours

E

Epstein-Barr virus antibodies
Negative
Erythrocyte distribution, fetal-maternal
No fetal red blood cells
Erythrocyte sedimentation rate
Males: 0 to 10 mm/hour
Females: 0 to 20 mm/hour
Esophageal acidity
pH >5.0
Estriol, amniotic fluid
16 to 20 weeks: 25.7 ng/ml
Term: <1,000 ng/ml
Estrogens, serum
Menstruating women: days 1 to 10 of menstrual cycle, 24 to 68 pg/ml; days 11 to 20, 50 to 186 pg/ml; days 21 to 30, 73 to 149 pg/ml
Males: 12 to 34 pg/ml
Estrogens, total urine
Menstruating women: follicular phase, 5 to 25 µg/24 hours; ovulatory phase, 24 to 100 µg/24 hours; luteal phase, 12 to 80 µg/24 hours
Postmenopausal women: <10 µg/24 hours
Males: 4 to 25 µg/24 hours
Euglobulin lysis time
2 to 4 hours

F

Factor assay, one-stage
50% to 150% of normal activity
Febrile agglutination, serum
Salmonella antibody: <1:80
Brucellosis antibody: <1:80
Tularemia antibody: <1:40
Rickettsial antibody: <1:40
Ferritin, serum
Males: 20 to 300 ng/ml
Females: 20 to 120 ng/ml
Neonates: 25 to 200 ng/ml
1 month: 200 to 600 ng/ml
2 to 5 months: 50 to 200 ng/ml
6 months to 15 years: 7 to 140 ng/ml
Fibrinogen, peritoneal fluid
0.3% to 4.5% of total protein
Fibrinogen, plasma
195 to 365 mg/dl
Fibrinogen, pleural fluid
Transudate: absent
Exudate: present
Fibrin split products
Screening assay: <10 µg/ml
Quantitative assay: <3 µg/ml
Fluorescent treponemal antibody absorption, serum
Negative
Folic acid, serum
3 to 16 ng/ml
Follicle-stimulating hormone, serum
Menstruating women: follicular phase, 5 to 20 mIU/ml; ovulatory phase, 15 to 30 mIU/ml; luteal phase, 5 to 15 mIU/ml
Menopausal women: 5 to 100 mIU/ml
Males: 5 to 20 mIU/ml
Free thyroxine, serum
0.8 to 3.3 ng/dl
Free triiodothyronine
0.2 to 0.6 ng/dl

G

Galactose 1-phosphate uridyltransferase
Qualitative: negative
Quantitative: 18.5 to 28.5 mU/g of hemoglobin

Gamma-glutamyltransferase
Males: 8 to 37 U/L
Females <45 years: 5 to 27 U/L;
    ≥45 years: 6 to 37 U/L
Gastric acid stimulation
Males: 18 to 28 mEq/hour
Females: 11 to 21 mEq/hour
Gastric secretion, basal
Males: 1 to 5 mEq/hour
Females: 0.2 to 3.8 mEq/hour
Gastrin, serum
<300 pg/ml
Globulin, peritoneal fluid
30% to 45% of total protein
Globulin, serum
Alpha$_1$: 0.1 to 0.4 g/dl
Alpha$_2$: 0.5 to 1.0 g/dl
Beta: 0.7 to 1.2 g/dl
Gamma: 0.5 to 1.6 g/dl
Glucagon, fasting, plasma
<250 pg/ml
Glucose, amniotic fluid
<45 mg/dl
Glucose, cerebrospinal fluid
50 to 80 mg/dl
Glucose, peritoneal fluid
70 to 100 mg/dl
Glucose, plasma, fasting
70 to 100 mg/dl
Glucose, plasma, 2-hour postprandial
<145 mg/dl
Glucose, synovial fluid
70 to 100 mg/dl
Glucose, urine
Negative
Glucose-6-phosphate dehydrogenase
8.6 to 18.6 U/g of hemoglobin
Glucose tolerance, oral
Peak at 160 to 180 mg/dl 30 to 60 minutes after challenge dose
Glutathione reductase activity index
0.9 to 1.3
Growth hormone suppression
0 to 3 ng/ml after 30 minutes to 2 hours

H

Ham test
Negative red blood cell hemolysis
Haptoglobin, serum
38 to 270 mg/dl
Heinz bodies
Negative
Hematocrit
Males: 42% to 54%
Females: 38% to 46%
Neonates: 55% to 68%
1 week: 47% to 65%
1 month: 37% to 49%
3 months: 30% to 36%
1 year: 29% to 41%
10 years: 36% to 40%
Hemoglobin (Hb), glycosylated
Total: 5.5% to 9%
Hb A$_{1a}$: 1.6% of total Hb
Hb A$_{1b}$: 0.8% of total Hb
Hb A$_{1c}$: 5% of total Hb
Hemoglobin, total
Males: 14 to 18 g/dl
Males after middle age: 12.4 to 14.9 g/dl
Females: 12 to 16 g/dl
Females after middle age: 11.7 to 13.8 g/dl
Neonates: 17 to 22 g/dl
1 week: 15 to 20 g/dl
1 month: 11 to 15 g/dl
Children: 11 to 13 g/dl
Hemoglobin, unstable
Heat stability: negative
Isopropanol: stable
Hemoglobin, urine
Negative
Hemoglobin (Hb) electrophoresis
Hb A: >95%
Hb A$_2$: 2% to 3%
Hb F: <1%
Hemosiderin, urine
Negative
Hepatitis B surface antigen, serum
Negative
Herpes simplex antibodies, serum
Negative
Heterophil agglutination, serum
Normal titer <1:56

Quick-reference guide to laboratory test results *(continued)*

Hexosaminidase A and B, serum
Total: 5 to 12.9 U/L; hexosaminidase A constitutes 55% to 76% of total
Histoplasmosis antibody, serum
Normal titer <1:8
Homovanillic acid, urine
<8 mg/24 hours
Human chorionic gonadotropin, serum
<4 IU/L
Human chorionic gonadotropin, urine
Pregnant women: first trimester, ≤500,000 IU/24 hours; second trimester, 10,000 to 25,000 IU/24 hours; third trimester, 5,000 to 15,000 IU/24 hours
Human growth hormone, serum
Males: 0 to 5 ng/ml
Females: 0 to 10 ng/ml
Human immunodeficiency virus antibody, serum
Negative
Human placental lactogen, serum
Pregnant women 5 to 27 weeks: <4.6 µg/ml
28 to 31 weeks: 2.4 to 6.1 µg/ml
32 to 35 weeks: 3.7 to 7.7 µg/ml
36 weeks to term: 5 to 8.6 µg/ml
Hydroxybutyric dehydrogenase (HBD)
Serum HBD: 114 to 290 U/ml
Lactate dehydrogenase–HBD ratio: 1.2 to 1.6:1
17-Hydroxycorticosteroids, urine
Males: 4.5 to 12 mg/24 hours
Females: 2.5 to 10 mg/24 hours
5-Hydroxyindoleacetic acid, urine
<6 mg/24 hours
Hydroxyproline, total, urine
14 to 45 mg/24 hours

I J
Immune complex, serum
Negative
Immunoglobulins (Ig), serum
IgG
  Males and females: 700 to 1,500 mg/dl
  0 to 4 months: 141 to 930 mg/dl

5 to 8 months: 250 to 1,190 mg/dl
9 to 11 months: 320 to 1,250 mg/dl
1 to 3 years: 400 to 1,200 mg/dl
4 to 6 years: 560 to 1,307 mg/dl
7 to 9 years: 598 to 1,379 mg/dl
10 to 12 years: 638 to 1,453 mg/dl
13 to 15 years: 680 to 1,531 mg/dl
16 to 17 years: 724 to 1,611 mg/dl
IgA
  Males and females: 60 to 400 mg/dl
  0 to 4 months: 5 to 64 mg/dl
  5 to 8 months: 10 to 87 mg/dl
  9 to 14 months: 17 to 94 mg/dl
  15 to 23 months: 22 to 178 mg/dl
  2 to 3 years: 24 to 192 mg/dl
  4 to 6 years: 26 to 232 mg/dl
  7 to 9 years: 33 to 258 mg/dl
  10 to 12 years: 45 to 285 mg/dl
  13 to 15 years: 47 to 317 mg/dl
  16 to 17 years: 55 to 377 mg/dl
IgM
  Males 0 to 4 months: 14 to 142 mg/dl
  5 to 8 months: 24 to 167 mg/dl
  9 to 23 months: 35 to 200 mg/dl
  2 to 3 years: 41 to 200 mg/dl
  4 to 17 years: 47 to 200 mg/dl
  ≥18 years: 60 to 300 mg/dl
  Females 0 to 4 months: 14 to 142 mg/dl
  5 to 8 months: 24 to 167 mg/dl
  9 to 23 months: 35 to 242 mg/dl
  2 to 3 years: 41 to 242 mg/dl
  4 to 17 years: 56 to 242 mg/dl
  ≥18 years: 60 to 300 mg/dl
Insulin, serum
0 to 25 µU/ml
Insulin tolerance test
10- to 20-ng/dl increase over baseline levels of human growth hormone and adrenocorticotropic hormone
Iron, serum
Males: 70 to 150 µg/dl
Females: 80 to 150 µg/dl
Iron, total binding capacity, serum
Males: 300 to 400 µg/dl
Females: 300 to 450 µg/dl
Isocitrate dehydrogenase
1.2 to 7 U/L

K

17-Ketogenic steroids, urine
Males: 4 to 14 mg/24 hours
Females: 2 to 12 mg/24 hours
Infants to 11 years: 0.4 to 4 mg/24 hours
11 to 14 years: 2 to 9 mg/24 hours

Ketones, urine
Negative

17-Ketosteroids, urine
Males: 6 to 21 mg/24 hours
Females: 4 to 17 mg/24 hours
Infants to 11 years: 0.1 to 3 mg/24 hours
11 to 14 years: 2 to 7 mg/24 hours

L

Lactate dehydrogenase (LD)
Total: 48 to 115 IU/L
LD_1: 14% to 26%
LD_2: 29% to 39%
LD_3: 20% to 26%
LD_4: 8% to 16%
LD_5: 6% to 16%

Lactic acid, blood
0.93 to 1.65 mEq/L

Leucine aminopeptidase
<50 U/L

Leukoagglutinins
Negative

Lipase, serum
<300 U/L

Lipids, amniotic fluid
>20% of lipid-coated cells stain orange

Lipids, fecal
Constitute <20% of excreted solids; <7 g excreted in 24 hours

Lipoproteins, serum
High-density lipoprotein cholesterol: 29 to 77 mg/dl
Low-density lipoprotein cholesterol: 62 to 185 mg/dl

Long-acting thyroid stimulator, serum
Negative

Lupus erythematosus cell preparation
Negative

Luteinizing hormone, serum
Menstruating women: follicular phase, 5 to 15 mIU/ml; ovulatory phase, 30 to 60 mIU/ml; luteal phase, 5 to 15 mIU/ml
Postmenopausal women: 50 to 100 mIU/ml
Males: 5 to 20 mIU/ml
Children: 4 to 20 mIU/ml

Lyme disease serology
Nonreactive

Lysozyme, urine
<3 mg/24 hours

M

Magnesium, serum
1.5 to 2.5 mEq/L
Atomic absorption: 1.7 to 2.1 mg/dl

Magnesium, urine
<150 mg/24 hours

Manganese, serum
0.04 to 1.4 µg/dl

Melanin, urine
Negative

Myoglobin, urine
Negative

N

5'-Nucleotidase
2 to 17 U/L

O

Occult blood, fecal
<2.5 ml/24 hours

Ornithine carbamoyltransferase, serum
0 to 500 sigma U/ml

Oxalate, urine
≤40 mg/24 hours

P Q

Parathyroid hormone, serum
Intact: 210 to 310 pg/ml
N-terminal fraction: 230 to 630 pg/ml
C-terminal fraction: 410 to 1,760 pg/ml

Quick-reference guide to laboratory test results *(continued)*

Pericardial fluid
Amount: 10 to 50 ml
Appearance: clear, straw-colored
White blood cell count: <1,000/µl
Glucose: approximately whole blood level

Peritoneal fluid
Amount: ≤50 ml
Appearance: clear, straw-colored

Phenylalanine, serum
<2 mg/dl

Phosphate, tubular reabsorption, urine and plasma
80% reabsorption

Phosphates, serum
1.8 to 2.6 mEq/L; in children, up to 4.1 mEq/L
Atomic absorption: 2.5 to 4.5 mg/dl; in children, up to 7 mg/dl

Phosphates, urine
<1,000 mg/24 hours

Phospholipids, plasma
180 to 320 mg/dl

Plasma renin activity
Sodium-depleted, peripheral vein (upright position)
  18 to 39 years: 2.9 to 24 ng/ml/hour (range); 10.8 ng/ml/hour (mean)
  ≥40 years: 2.9 to 10.8 ng/ml/hour (range); 5.9 ng/ml/hour (mean)
Sodium-replete, peripheral vein (upright position)
  0 to 2 years: 4.6 ng/ml/hour (mean, standing)
  3 to 5 years: 2.5 ng/ml/hour (mean, standing)
  6 to 8 years: 1.4 ng/ml/hour (mean, standing)
  9 to 11 years: 1.9 ng/ml/hour (mean, standing)
  12 to 17 years: 1.8 ng/ml/hour (mean, standing)
  18 to 39 years: ≤0.6 to 4.3 ng/ml/hour (range); 1.9 ng/ml/hour (mean)
  ≥40 years: ≤0.6 to 3 ng/ml/hour (range); 1 ng/ml/hour (mean)

Plasminogen, plasma
Immunologic method: 10 to 20 ng/ml
Functional method: 80 to 120 U/ml

Platelet aggregation
3 to 5 minutes

Platelet count
Adults: 140,000 to 400,000/µl
Children: 150,000 to 450,000/µl

Platelet survival
50% tagged platelets disappear within 84 to 116 hours; 100% disappear within 8 to 10 days

Porphobilinogen, urine
≤1.5 mg/24 hours

Porphyrins, total
16 to 60 mg/dl of packed red blood cells

Potassium, serum
3.8 to 5.5 mEq/L

Potassium, urine
25 to 125 mEq/24 hours

Pregnanediol, urine
Males: 1.5 mg/24 hours
Nonpregnant females: 0.5 to 1.5 mg/ 24 hours
Postmenopausal women: 0.2 to 1 mg/ 24 hours

Pregnanetriol, urine
Males 0 to 5 years: <0.1 mg/24 hours
  6 to 9 years: <0.3 mg/24 hours
  10 to 15 years: 0.2 to 0.6 mg/24 hours
  ≥16 years: 0.2 to 2 mg/24 hours
Females 0 to 5 years: <0.1 mg/24 hours
  6 to 9 years: <0.3 mg/24 hours
  10 to 15 years: 0.1 to 0.6 mg/24 hours
  ≥16 years: 0 to 1.4 mg/hours

Progesterone, plasma
Menstruating women: follicular phase, <150 ng/dl; luteal phase, 300 ng/ dl; midluteal phase, 2,000 ng/dl
Pregnant women: first trimester, 1,500 to 5,000 ng/dl; second and third trimesters, 8,000 to 20,000 ng/dl

Prolactin, serum
0 to 23 ng/ml

Prostate-specific antigen
40 to 50 years: 2 to 2.8 ng/ml
51 to 60 years: 2.9 to 3.8 ng/ml

61 to 70 years: 4 to 5.3 ng/ml
≥71 years: 5.6 to 7.2 ng/ml
Protein, cerebrospinal fluid
15 to 45 mg/dl
Protein, pleural fluid
Transudate: <3 g/dl
Exudate: >3 g/dl
Protein, serum
Total: 6.6 to 7.9 g/dl
Albumin: 3.3 to 4.5 g/dl
Alpha$_1$-globulin, 0.1 to 0.4 g/dl
Alpha$_2$-globulin: 0.5 to 1 g/dl
Beta globulin: 0.7 to 1.2 g/dl
Gamma globulin: 0.5 to 1.6 g/dl
Protein, total, peritoneal fluid
0.3 to 4.1 g/dl
Protein, total, synovial fluid
<10.7 to 21.3 mg/dl
Protein, urine
≤150 mg/24 hours
Protein C, plasma
70% to 140%
Prothrombin consumption
20 seconds
Prothrombin time
10 to 14 seconds; International Normalized Ratio for patients on warfarin therapy, 2.0 to 3.0 (those with prosthetic heart valves, 2.5 to 3.5)
Protoporphyrins
16 to 60 mg/dl
Pulmonary artery pressures
Right atrial: 1 to 6 mm Hg
Left atrial: approximately 10 mm Hg
Systolic: 20 to 30 mm Hg
Systolic right ventricular: 20 to 30 mm Hg
Diastolic: approximately 10 mm Hg
End-diastolic right ventricular: <5 mm Hg
Mean: <20 mm Hg
Pulmonary artery wedge pressure: 6 to 12 mm Hg
Pyruvate kinase
Ultraviolet: 9 to 22 U/g of hemoglobin
Low substrate assay: 1.7 to 6.8 U/g of hemoglobin

Pyruvic acid, blood
0.08 to 0.16 mEq/L

R

Red blood cell count
Males: 4.5 to 6.2 million/µl venous blood
Females: 4.2 to 5.4 million/µl venous blood
Neonates: 4.4 to 5.8 million/µl venous blood
2 months: 3 to 3.8 million/µl venous blood (increasing slowly)
Children: 4.6 to 4.8 million/µl venous blood
Red blood cell survival time
25 to 35 days
Red blood cells, pleural fluid
Transudate: few
Exudate: variable
Red blood cells, urine
0 to 3 per high-power field
Red cell indices
Mean corpuscular volume: 84 to 99 fl
Mean corpuscular hemoglobin: 26 to 32 fl
Mean corpuscular hemoglobin concentration: 30 to 36 g/dl
Respiratory syncytial virus antibodies, serum
Negative
Reticulocyte count
Adults: 0.5% to 2% of total red blood cell count
Infants (at birth): 2% to 6%, decreasing to adult levels in 1 to 2 weeks
Rheumatoid factor, serum
Negative or titer <1:20
Ribonucleoprotein antibodies
Negative
Rubella antibodies, serum
Titer of 1:8 or less indicates little or no immunity

S

Semen analysis
Volume: 0.7 to 6.5 ml
pH: 7.3 to 7.9

Quick-reference guide to laboratory test results *(continued)*

Liquefaction: within 20 minutes
Sperm: 20 million to 150 million/ml
Sickle cell test
Negative
Sjögren's antibodies
Negative
Sodium, serum
135 to 145 mEq/L
Sodium, sweat
10 to 30 mEq/L
Sodium, urine
30 to 280 mEq/24 hours
Sodium chloride, urine
5 to 20 g/24 hours
Sporotrichosis antibody, serum
Normal titers <1:40
Synovial fluid
Color: colorless to pale yellow
Clarity: clear
Quantity (in knee): 0.3 to 3.5 ml
Viscosity: 5.7 to 1,160
pH: 7.2 to 7.4
Mucin clot: good
Pao$_2$: 40 to 80 mm Hg
Paco$_2$: 40 to 60 mm Hg

T

Terminal deoxynucleotidyl transferase, serum
<2% in bone marrow; undetectable in blood
Testosterone, plasma or serum
Males: 300 to 1,200 ng/dl
Females: 30 to 95 ng/dl
Prepubertal boys: <100 ng/dl
Girls: <40 ng/dl
Thrombin time, plasma
10 to 15 seconds
Thyroid-stimulating hormone, neonatal
≤2 days: 25 to 30 µIU/ml
>2 days: <25 µIU/ml
Thyroid-stimulating hormone, serum
0 to 15 µIU/ml
Thyroid-stimulating immunoglobulin, serum
Negative

Thyroxine, total, serum
5 to 13.5 µg/dl
Thyroxine-binding globulin, serum
Electrophoresis: 10 to 26 µg thyroxine (binding capacity)/dl
Immunoassay: 12 to 25 mg/L (males); 14 to 30 mg/L (females)
T-lymphocyte count
1,400 to 2,700/µl
Tolbutamide tolerance
Plasma glucose drops to one-half fasting level for 30 minutes and recovers in 1 to 3 hours
Transferrin, serum
200 to 400 mg/dl
Triglycerides, serum
Males: 40 to 160 mg/dl
Females: 35 to 135 mg/dl
Triiodothyronine, serum
90 to 230 ng/dl

U

Urea clearance
Maximal clearance: 64 to 99 ml/minute
Uric acid, serum
Males: 4.3 to 8 mg/dl
Females: 2.3 to 6 mg/dl
Uric acid, synovial fluid
Males: 2 to 8 mg/dl
Females: 2 to 6 mg/dl
Uric acid, urine
250 to 750 mg/24 hours
Urinalysis, routine
Color: straw to dark yellow
Appearance: clear
Specific gravity: 1.005 to 1.035
pH: 4.5 to 8.0
Epithelial cells: 0 to 5/high-power field
Casts: occasional hyaline casts
Crystals: present
Urine osmolality
24-hour urine: 300 to 900 mOsm/kg
Random urine: 50 to 1,400 mOsm/kg
Urobilinogen, fecal
50 to 300 mg/24 hours
Urobilinogen, urine
Males: 0.3 to 2.1 Ehrlich units/2 hours
Females: 0.1 to 1.1 Ehrlich units/2 hours

Uroporphyrin, urine
Males: 0 to 42 µg/24 hours
Females: 1 to 22 µg/24 hours
Uroporphyrinogen I synthase
≥7 nmol/second/L

V

Vanillylmandelic acid, urine
0.7 to 6.8 mg/24 hours
Venereal Disease Research Laboratory test, cerebrospinal fluid
Negative
Venereal Disease Research Laboratory test, serum
Negative
Vitamin A, serum
Adults: 30 to 95 µg/dl
Children 1 to 6 years: 20 to 43 µg/dl
7 to 12 years: 26 to 50 µg/dl
13 to 19 years: 26 to 72 µg/dl
Vitamin B$_1$, urine
100 to 200 µg/24 hours
Vitamin B$_2$, urine
0.9 to 1.3 activity index
Vitamin B$_6$ (tryptophan), urine
<50 µg/24 hours
Vitamin B$_{12}$, serum
Adults: 200 to 900 pg/ml
Neonates: 160 to 1,200 pg/ml
Vitamin C, plasma
≥0.3 mg/dl
Vitamin C, urine
30 mg/24 hours
Vitamin D$_3$, serum
10 to 55 ng/ml

W X Y

White blood cell count, blood
4,000 to 10,000/µl
White blood cell count, cerebrospinal fluid
0 to 5/µl
White blood cell count, peritoneal fluid
<300/µl
White blood cell count, pleural fluid
Transudate: few
Exudate: many (may be purulent)

White blood cell count, synovial fluid
0 to 200/µl
White blood cell count, urine
0 to 4 per high-power field
White blood cell differential, blood
Adults
Neutrophils: 47.6% to 76.8%
Lymphocytes: 16.2% to 43%
Monocytes: 0.6% to 9.6%
Eosinophils: 0.3% to 7%
Basophils: 0.3% to 2%
Males age 6 to 18
Neutrophils: 38.5% to 71.5%
Lymphocytes: 19.4% to 51.4%
Monocytes: 1.1% to 11.6%
Eosinophils: 1% to 8.1%
Basophils: 0.25% to 1.3%
Females age 6 to 18
Neutrophils: 41.9% to 76.5%
Lymphocytes: 16.3% to 46.7%
Monocytes: 0.9% to 9.9%
Eosinophils: 0.8% to 8.3%
Basophils: 0.3% to 1.4%
White blood cell differential, synovial fluid
Lymphocytes: 0 to 78/µl
Monocytes: 0 to 71/µl
Clasmatocytes: 0 to 26/µl
Polymorphonuclears: 0 to 25/µl
Other phagocytes: 0 to 21/µl
Synovial lining cells: 0 to 12/µl
Whole blood clotting time
5 to 15 minutes

Z

Zinc, serum
60 to 150 µg/dl

Patient guide to test preparation

The experience of having a diagnostic test may be new to your patient. Even if he has had tests before, your teaching can help reassure him. If he knows what to expect, he'll be more cooperative and relaxed, which may help the procedure go more smoothly.

The following pages include teaching aids for some of the most common tests. They explain what the patient needs to know before, during, and after his test.

You'll find a diet to prepare the patient for an oral glucose tolerance test as well as preparation guides for imaging tests, such as cardiac catheterization, computed tomography (CT) scans, breast ultrasonography, barium enema, and endoscopic retrograde cholangio-pancreatography. Also included are pointers for undergoing a stress test, cystoscopy, needle aspiration of the breast, liver biopsy, and pulmonary function tests.

When you review the test with your patient, be sure to:
- name the test and describe what the patient may see, hear, smell, feel, or taste (be honest about any discomfort he may experience)
- define any unfamiliar terms
- outline any home preparation that's required, such as fasting, bowel preparation, or fluid restriction
- tell the patient where the test will be performed (doctor's office, hospital, or other medical facility) and who will perform it
- inform him if he'll have an I.V. line or receive an anesthetic or a sedative
- suggest that he practice what he'll be asked to do during the test — for example, lying perfectly still for a CT scan
- tell him how long the procedure will take and whether he'll need help getting home
- review possible adverse reactions, if any, including which ones require him to call the doctor
- discuss recommendations for follow-up visits, if applicable
- tell him when to expect test results.

If your patient feels anxious and overwhelmed with information, he may have difficulty remembering everything he's been taught. By giving him an easy-to-read teaching aid, you reinforce your teaching and provide your patient with a handy reference.

Getting ready for an oral glucose tolerance test

Dear Patient:
To prepare for an oral glucose tolerance test and to ensure accurate results, you need to follow a high-carbohydrate diet for 3 days before the test. Below you'll find a sample diet you can use. If you find it too restrictive, follow your regular diet, but eat 12 additional slices of bread each day.

Breakfast
1 serving fruit
Eggs, as desired
5 bread exchanges
1 cup milk
Butter or margarine
Coffee or tea, if desired

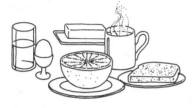

Lunch and dinner
Meat, as desired
5 bread exchanges
2 vegetables
1 serving fruit
1 cup milk
Butter or margarine
Coffee or tea, if desired

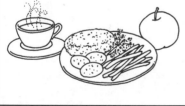

What are bread exchanges?
One of the following equals one bread exchange:
1 slice bread, white or whole wheat
1½-inch cube of corn bread
½ hamburger or hotdog roll
½ cup cooked cereal
¾ cup dry cereal (avoid sugar-coated varieties)
½ cup noodles, spaghetti, or macaroni
½ cup cooked dried beans or peas
⅓ cup corn or ½ small ear of corn
1 biscuit
½ corn muffin
1 roll
5 saltine crackers
2 graham crackers
½ cup grits or rice
1 small white potato
½ cup mashed potato
¼ cup sweet potato
¼ cup baked beans
¼ cup pork and beans

Following a clear liquid diet

Dear Patient:

Your doctor has ordered a clear liquid diet to prepare you for certain intestinal tests that you'll be having. A clear liquid diet consists of foods that are transparent and liquid or that liquefy at room temperature. This type of diet reduces the amount of stools in your bowels, which helps the doctor to better see the inside of your bowels.

The foods listed below are the *only* foods you should eat or drink on a clear liquid diet:

- water
- ice chips
- clear tea (no milk or lemon)
- strained and clear fruit juices, such as apple, grape, and cranberry (no pulp)
- decaffeinated coffee (may vary with institution)
- clear carbonated beverages
- plain fruit gelatin (no fruit added)
- chicken or beef broth (fat-free only)
- chicken or beef bouillon
- frozen ice pops (no fruit or pulp)
- clear, fruit-flavored drink mixes.

Following a low-sodium diet for renin testing

Dear Patient:

Before undergoing renin testing, you must drastically restrict your intake of sodium for 3 days to ensure accurate
test results. If you are following this diet at home, ob-
serve these precautions: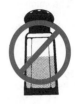

■ Eat only the foods included in the meal plan provided
by the doctor. You may delete foods from the diet, but
you may not add foods.

■ Measure all portions using standard measuring cups
and spoons.

■ Use 4 oz (112 g) *unsalted* beefsteak or ground beef for
lunch and 4 oz *unsalted* chicken for dinner. (Amount refers to weight before
cooking.)

■ You may eat the following *unsalted* (fresh or frozen) vegetables: asparagus,
green or wax beans, cabbage, cauliflower, lettuce, and tomatoes.

■ Use only the specified amount of coffee.

■ If you're thirsty between meals, drink distilled water (but no other food or beverages).

■ Prepare all foods without salt; don't use salt at the table.

Breakfast

1 egg, poached or boiled, or fried in *unsalted* fat
2 slices *unsalted* toast
1 shredded wheat biscuit or ⅔ cup *unsalted* cooked cereal
4 oz (120 ml) milk
8 oz (240 ml) coffee
1 cup orange juice
Sugar, jam or jelly, and *unsalted* butter, as desired

Lunch

4 oz (120 ml) *unsalted* tomato juice
4 oz (112 g) *unsalted* beefsteak or ground beef; may be broiled or fried in
    unsalted fat
½ cup *unsalted* potato
½ cup *unsalted* green beans or other allowed vegetable
1 serving fruit
8 oz (240 ml) coffee
1 slice *unsalted* bread
Sugar, jam or jelly, and *unsalted* butter, as desired

Dinner

4 oz (112 g) *unsalted* chicken; may be baked or broiled, or fried in *unsalted* fat
½ cup *unsalted* potato
Lettuce salad (vinegar and oil dressing)
½ cup *unsalted* green beans or other allowed vegetable
1 serving fruit
8 oz (240 ml) coffee
1 slice *unsalted* bread
Sugar, jam or jelly, and *unsalted* butter, as desired

Learning about a stress test

Dear Patient:
Don't be intimidated by the name *stress test*. The only stress involved is some carefully controlled physical exercise.

What the test does
A stress test tells your doctor how your heart functions while you're exercising. It may be combined with another test, called a thallium scan, to evaluate blood flow through your coronary arteries to the heart muscle itself.

What happens during the test
After not eating or drinking (except for normal medications) for at least 2 hours before the test, you'll go to the cardiology lab. There, a nurse will attach electrocardiogram (ECG) monitors to your chest and arms, along with a blood pressure cuff. Then, you'll either ride a stationary bike or walk on a treadmill at gradually increasing speeds and slopes. While you're exercising, your blood pressure will be checked frequently and an ECG will be run continuously. Be sure to inform the doctor as soon as you feel tired, short of breath, or dizzy, or experience chest pain.

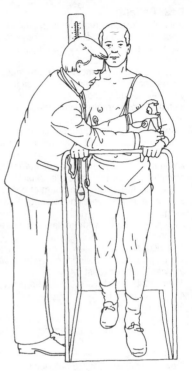

Thallium scan
If the test includes a thallium scan, the doctor will inject thallium into a vein in your arm while you're exercising (see illustration). Then, he'll ask you to continue exercising for several minutes.

Next, you'll be taken to the scanner room, where the doctor will take pictures of your heart with a special scanner. These pictures will show how well your coronary arteries supply blood to your heart during exercise.

About 4 hours after you finish exercising, the doctor may take more pictures of your heart. They'll show how well your coronary arteries supply blood to your heart after a rest period.

Preparing for cardiac catheterization

Dear Patient:

Your doctor has scheduled you for cardiac catheterization, a procedure that allows him to look at the inside of your heart. He does this by first making a small incision in a blood vessel near your elbow or groin and then inserting a long, thin, flexible tube called a catheter into the vessel.

After inserting the catheter, the doctor will slowly thread it through your bloodstream into your heart. When the catheter is in place, the doctor will perform certain tests that may include injection of a special dye. What the doctor sees will help him to decide what additional treatment might improve your heart's functioning.

Catheter route from elbow area

Catheter route from groin area

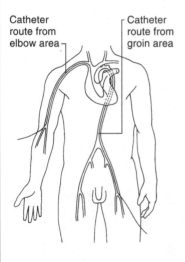

Before the procedure

If your catheterization is scheduled for early morning, you probably won't be allowed to eat or drink anything after midnight the day before the test.

To protect against infection, the nurse will shave the area where the incision will be made. Before you go to the catheterization lab, she'll ask you to urinate, then help you into a hospital gown. Depending on the doctor's orders, she also may start an I.V. line in your arm.

When you reach the catheterization lab, you'll be placed on a padded table and probably be strapped to it. During the test, the doctor will tilt the table to view your heart from different angles. The straps will keep you from slipping out of position. Special foam pads, called leads, may be put on your chest so that your heartbeat can be monitored.

Cardiac catheterization usually takes 1 to 2 hours. You'll be awake throughout the procedure, although the doctor may order medication to help you relax. (Some patients even doze off.) You may feel pain in your chest, flushing, or nausea during catheterization, but these sensations should pass quickly.

During the procedure

First, the doctor will inject a local anesthetic at the catheter insertion site to numb the area before he puts in the catheter. When the catheter is going in, you should feel a little pressure but no pain. You may receive nitroglycerin during the test to enlarge your heart's blood vessels and help the doctor get a better view.

If the catheter's passage is blocked — because of a narrowed blood vessel, for example — the doctor will pull back the catheter and start from another insertion area.

When the catheter enters your heart, you may feel a fluttering sensation. Tell the doctor if you do, but don't worry; this is a normal reaction. You're also likely to feel a warm sensation, some nausea, or the urge to urinate if dye is injected, but these feelings will quickly pass. Throughout the catheterization, remember to let the doctor or the nurse know if you have chest pain.

During the test, your doctor may give you oxygen and ask you to cough or to breathe deeply.

When the test is finished, the doc-

(continued)

Preparing for cardiac catheterization (continued)

tor will slowly remove the catheter and put a special bandage on your arm or groin. You may need a few stitches at the insertion site. Because the anesthetic will still be working, you shouldn't feel anything.

After the procedure

When you're back in your room, the nurse will probably do an electrocardiogram if you're not already on a cardiac monitor. She'll check your bandage and your temperature, pulse, breathing, and blood pressure frequently.

Your bandaged arm or leg must stay completely still for up to 8 hours.

To help keep you from moving, the nurse may splint your arm or leg or weigh it down with a sandbag. She'll check the site frequently for swelling as well as check the blood flow in your arm or leg. She'll probably ask you to wiggle your toes or fingers once an hour or more.

As your anesthetic wears off, you'll probably feel some pain at the insertion site. Let the nurse know so she can give you pain medication.

As soon as the test results are available, the doctor will talk to you and your family about them. Don't hesitate to ask him or the nurse any questions you may have.

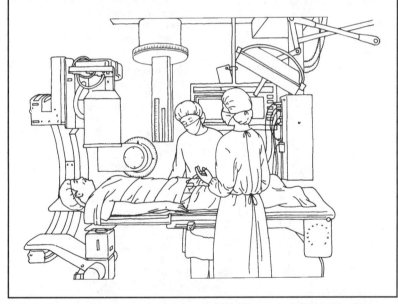

Preparing for pulmonary function tests

Dear Patient:
Your doctor has ordered pulmonary (or lung) function tests for you. These tests measure how well your lungs work. Here's what to expect.

How the tests work
You'll be asked to breathe as deeply as possible into a mouthpiece that's connected to a machine called a spirometer. This device measures and records the rate and amount of air that you inhale and exhale. Or you may sit in a small, boothlike enclosure for a test called body plethysmography. Again, you'll be asked to breathe in and out, and the measurements will be recorded.

Before the tests
Avoid smoking for at least 4 hours before the tests. Eat lightly and drink only a small amount of fluid. Wear loose, comfortable clothing, and urinate before the tests.

To make the tests go quickly, you'll need to cooperate fully. Tell the technician if you don't understand the instructions. If you wear dentures, keep them in — they'll help you keep a tight seal around the spirometer's mouthpiece.

During the tests
During spirometry, you'll sit upright and you'll wear a noseclip to make sure you breathe only through your mouth. During body plethysmography, you won't need a noseclip.

If you feel too confined in the small chamber, keep in mind that you can't suffocate. And you can talk to the nurse or technician through a window.

The tests have several parts. For each test, you'll be asked to breathe a certain way — for example, to inhale deeply and exhale completely or to inhale quickly. You may need to repeat some tests after inhaling a medication to expand the airways in your lungs. Also, the nurse may take a sample of blood from an artery in your arm. This sample will be used to measure how well your body uses the air you breathe.

How will you feel?
During the tests, you may feel tired or short of breath. However, you'll be able to rest between measurements. Tell the technician right away if you feel dizzy, begin wheezing, or have chest pain, a racing or pounding heart, an upset stomach, or severe shortness of breath. Also tell him if your arm swells, if you're bleeding from the spot where the blood sample was taken, or if you experience weakness or pain in that arm.

After the tests
When the tests are over, rest if you feel like it. You may resume your usual activities when you regain your energy.

Preparing for magnetic resonance imaging

Dear Patient:

Your doctor wants you to have a painless test called magnetic resonance imaging — MRI for short. Unlike an X-ray, this test produces images of your body's organs and tissues without exposing you to radiation. Instead, MRI uses a powerful magnetic field and radio-frequency energy to produce computerized pictures. Here's how to prepare for it.

Before the test

You may eat, drink, and take your usual medicines. Try to use the bathroom just before the test because MRI may take up to 90 minutes.

Take off any metal objects you may be carrying or wearing, such as a watch, rings, eyeglasses, and a hearing aid. Metal can be damaged by the strong magnetic field. Also empty your pockets of any coins and plastic card keys or charge cards with metallic strips. The scanner will erase the strips.

Let the doctor know if you have any metal objects inside your body, such as a pacemaker, an aneurysm clip, a joint prosthesis, a metal pin, or bullet fragments, so the scanner can be adjusted.

During the test

You'll lie on a narrow, padded table throughout the test. The technician will tell you to stay still to prevent blurred images. To help you stay still, your head, chest, and arms may be secured with straps. Remember that MRI is painless and involves no exposure to radiation.

The table on which you're lying will slowly glide into the scanner's narrow tunnel. You'll notice the walls are just a few inches from your body. Inside, you'll hear fans and feel air circulating around you, and you may hear thumping noises made by the machine. The technician will probably offer you earphones, or you may request earplugs before the test.

The technician, located in an adjacent room, can see and hear you. And mirrors above your head will enable you to see the technician.

After the test

You may resume your usual activities. If you've been lying down for a long time, however, don't get up too quickly or you may feel slightly dizzy. Rise slowly to give your body a chance to adjust.

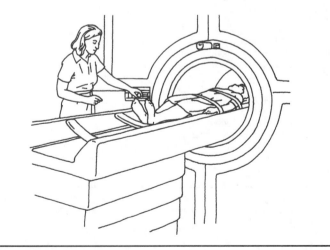

Preparing for a CT scan

Dear Patient:

The doctor has scheduled you for a computed tomography (CT) scan. This test uses X-rays and a computer to create detailed images of the body part being scanned. It involves the use of a large machine called a CT scanner. The test is painless and takes between 30 and 60 minutes.

Before the test

You may receive an injection of a contrast dye in your arm. This substance highlights certain areas of your body. If the test requires this dye, don't eat or drink anything for 4 hours before the test.

Tell your doctor if you've ever had an allergic reaction to X-ray contrast material or if you're allergic or sensitive to shellfish or iodine-containing solutions. Let him know if you have other allergies, too.

Remove all metal objects and jewelry, such as a watch, hairpins, and earrings. Also remember to remove objects that might obstruct the X-ray beam, such as glasses, dentures, and a hearing aid. Wear loose, comfortable clothing or a hospital gown. You may be given a mild sedative to help you relax.

During the test

A technician will position you on an X-ray table. Then the table will slide into the tubelike scanner, which looks like a giant thermos bottle lying on its side. Every few seconds, the table will move a small distance and an X-ray image will be taken. You'll hear clicking or buzzing noises from the scanner as it revolves, obtaining images from many angles.

Remember to lie still. To prevent blurring of the X-ray images, your body will be steadied with straps or a support. You'll be alone in the scanner room during the test, but you can talk to the technician through a two-way intercom.

If you received contrast material, you may develop a headache, have a salty taste in your mouth, or feel warm or flushed and nauseous. These reactions usually subside rapidly, but be sure to mention them to the technician.

After the test

You may resume your usual activities and diet. If you received a contrast dye, drink plenty of fluids for the rest of the day to help flush it from your system. Tell your doctor or nurse if you feel sick, vomit, or have a headache after the test.

Within 1 to 2 days, your doctor will have the full test results. He'll review the scan and discuss the results with you.

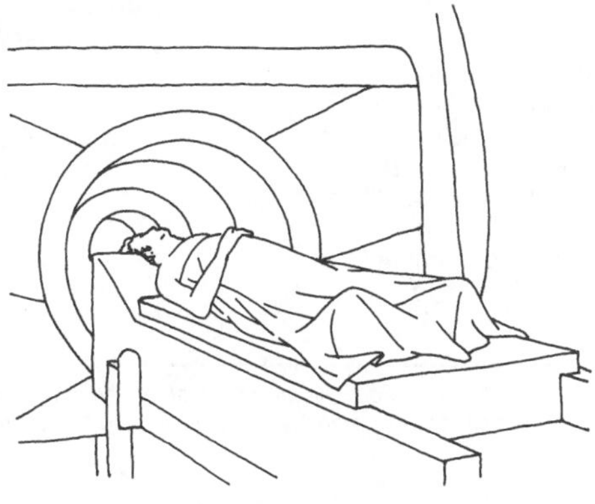

Preparing for breast ultrasonography

Dear Patient:

Your doctor wants you to undergo breast ultrasonography — commonly called ultrasound. This test provides an image of the inside of your breasts and is helpful for detecting and evaluating breast lumps. It can usually determine whether a lump is fluid-filled or solid, but it can't distinguish whether a lump is cancerous.

How the test works

This test uses a small instrument called a transducer that sends a beam of high-frequency sound waves toward your breast. When the sound waves bounce back from breast tissue, they are picked up again by the transducer. This information is then processed by a computer and displayed as an image of the inner breast on a TV screen.

Ultrasound is painless and poses no known health risk. It's also safe if you're pregnant because it uses no radiation.

Before the test

You'll be asked to remove your clothes from the waist up and to put on a hospital gown. In most cases, you won't need to restrict your diet, medications, or activities. If you have questions, ask them now. During the test, you'll need to rest quietly so the operator can concentrate on the images.

During the test

The procedure varies at different hospitals and clinics, so check with your doctor about how the test will be performed at the facility where you'll be examined. Either a doctor or an ultrasonographer will perform the test.

In most places, you'll be asked to lie on your back, with a pillow placed under the shoulder on the same side as the breast to be examined. Then a water-soluble gel will be applied to your breast. The test operator will glide the handheld transducer back and forth over your breast. Unless your breasts are very tender, the test should be painless and feel like a light massage.

In some hospitals and clinics, you'll be asked to lie on your back while a water-filled chamber is lowered over your breasts. Or you may be asked to lie on your stomach with your breasts submerged in a warm-water bath. In these methods, the sound waves are sent through water. You should feel no discomfort, although if you're asked to immerse your breasts in a water bath, the water may feel a bit cool.

During the test, don't expect to hear the high-frequency sound waves, which are inaudible to the human ear.

You'll probably be able to see images of your breast on the TV screen, but they'll look obscure, something like a satellite weather map.

After the test

You may resume your normal activities immediately. To find out your test results, you'll typically wait a day or two until a report is sent to the doctor who referred you for the test.

Preparing for a barium enema test

Dear Patient:

Your doctor has ordered a barium enema test to help find the cause of your gastrointestinal (GI) symptoms. This test, which is also called a lower GI exam, involves taking an X-ray of your large intestine (colon).

To make the intestine visible on an X-ray, liquid barium will be inserted through your anus to fill your colon. The barium makes your colon appear as a white shadow on the X-ray.

Getting ready

For the test to be accurate, your large intestine must be empty, so you'll need to follow a special diet for 1 to 3 days before the test. You'll also need to drink plenty of water or clear liquids for 12 to 24 hours beforehand.

The afternoon before the test, you'll receive a laxative and possibly a suppository. Then the night before or the morning of the test, you'll receive a cleansing enema.

Don't take oral medications after midnight on the day of the test unless your doctor tells you otherwise.

During the test

The test will be done in the X-ray department and will take about 1 hour. You'll be asked to lie on an X-ray table that tilts while holding you secured. First, the radiologist will take an X-ray to make sure your intestine is completely empty.

Then, as you lie on your side, he'll insert a well-lubricated tube gently into your rectum. The barium, stored in a bag, will flow slowly through the tube into your intestine, along with some air. The air and the barium make your intestine more visible on the X-ray.

As the barium and air enter your intestine, you may experience slight cramps or feel as though you need to move your bowels. To ease this discomfort, try to breathe deeply and slowly through your mouth. Tell the radiologist if the cramping increases.

Tighten your anal sphincter muscle against the tube. This will help to hold the tube in place and prevent the barium from leaking out. If too much liquid barium leaks out of the tube, your intestine won't be well coated, and the test will be inaccurate.

After the test

Once the enema tube is removed, you'll be allowed to empty your bowels in the toilet or a bedpan. You should drink lots of fluids, and you may be given a mild laxative or an enema to help you rid your intestine of the extra barium. You may resume your normal diet and medications.

Plan to rest because the test may be tiring. Expect your stools to look chalky for the next 24 to 72 hours. If you have trouble having a bowel movement after the test, call your doctor.

Preparing for ERCP

Dear Patient:

You're about to undergo endoscopic retrograde cholangiopancreatography — called ERCP for short. This procedure uses a dyelike substance, a flexible tube called an endoscope, and X-rays to outline your gallbladder and pancreatic structures.

Performed in the radiology department, ERCP may take up to 1 hour to complete. Read the information below to help you prepare.

Before the test

The day before ERCP, you can eat and drink as usual. Then after midnight before the procedure, don't eat or drink anything unless your doctor directs otherwise. (He may tell you to continue taking certain medications.) Before you enter the test room, be sure to urinate because ERCP can cause you to retain urine.

During the test

You'll lie on an X-ray table for this test. The nurse will take your temperature, blood pressure, and pulse rate. Then she'll insert an I.V. line into your hand or arm to administer medication. You'll receive a sedative to relax you and to ease the procedure. You may be aware of noises around you but you won't be fully awake.

The doctor will spray your throat with a bitter-tasting anesthetic, which will make your mouth and throat feel swollen and numb. Because you'll have difficulty swallowing, the doctor may give you a device to suction your saliva, or may tell you to let it drain from your mouth.

Next, the nurse will give you a mouthguard to keep your mouth open and to protect your teeth during ERCP. Though you'll be unable to talk, you'll have no trouble breathing.

When the doctor passes the endoscope down your throat, you may gag a little, but this reflex is normal.

As the tube reaches the duodenum (small intestine), the doctor may inject some air through it. You'll also receive medication through your I.V. line to relax the duodenum. Next, the doctor will insert a thinner tube through the endoscope to the biliary structures and the duodenum.

When the second tube is in place, the doctor will inject dye and quickly take X-ray images from several angles. After the doctor views the images, he may obtain a tissue sample. Then he'll gently remove the endoscope, tube, and mouthpiece.

After the test

The nurse will check your blood pressure, pulse rate, and temperature frequently for several hours.

When you regain feeling in your throat and your gag reflex returns, you'll be allowed to have a light meal and liquids. You can resume your regular diet the next day.

Expect to have a sore throat for a few days. Call the doctor if you can't urinate or if you experience chills, abdominal pain, nausea, or vomiting.

Learning about cystoscopy

Dear Patient:
Your doctor has scheduled you for cystoscopy. During this procedure, he can look inside your bladder through an instrument called a cystoscope. He'll insert the cystoscope through your urethra (the opening through which you urinate).

Cystoscopy allows the doctor to diagnose and, sometimes, treat your urinary disorder. The test may be done in a hospital or the doctor's office and takes 15 to 45 minutes.

What to expect before the test
You may receive a local anesthetic before the procedure. This means that the doctor will numb the area around the urethra before inserting the cystoscope. Or you may have general anesthesia. In this case, don't eat or drink anything after midnight on the night before the procedure. If the doctor plans to take X-rays of your bladder during the cystoscopy, he may prescribe medication that will clean your bowels to ensure sharper, clearer images.

Just before the procedure begins, an intravenous line will be inserted in your arm to deliver fluids and medications if you need them. You'll also receive a sedative to help you relax.

What to expect during the test
After the anesthetic takes effect, you'll be positioned on your back. Then the doctor will insert the cystoscope. Remember to take deep breaths and try to relax. This will allow the test to proceed smoothly.

If you received a local anesthetic, you may feel a strong urge to urinate as the instrument is inserted and removed. If the doctor instills an irrigant into your bladder, you may feel some pressure. Again, try to relax. If you experience any pain or feel your heart beating irregularly, let your doctor know.

What to expect after the test
Your condition will be monitored until you're fully alert. If you received a local anesthetic, you'll be awake but you may feel weak; so don't chance walking by yourself. Wait for someone to assist you.

For several days after the procedure, your urine may be tinged with blood. You may also have bladder spasms, a feeling that your bladder is full, or a burning sensation when you urinate. Take aspirin or acetaminophen (Tylenol), drink plenty of fluids, and lie in a tub of warm water to help relieve these side effects.

When to call the doctor
Call your doctor if you have heavy bleeding or blood clots in your urine, bladder pain or spasms that aren't relieved by medication, or burning and a frequent urge to urinate that persists for more than 24 hours. Also notify your doctor at once if you can't urinate within 8 hours after the test.

Preparing for a liver biopsy

Dear Patient:

Your doctor wants you to have a liver biopsy, which helps diagnose cirrhosis and other liver disorders. The test involves removing a small sample of liver tissue and studying it under a microscope. Usually, it takes about 15 minutes and results are available within a day.

Before the test

Don't eat or drink anything for 4 to 8 hours before the test, as your doctor orders. You'll probably have a blood test to measure your blood's clotting ability and other factors. Just before the test, be sure to empty your bladder.

During the test

You'll lie on your back with your right hand under your head. You'll need to remain in this position and keep as still as you can. The doctor will drape and clean an area on your abdomen. Then he'll inject a local anesthetic, which may sting and cause brief discomfort.

You'll be told to hold your breath and lie still as the doctor inserts the biopsy needle into the liver (as shown below). The needle will remain in your liver for only about 1 second, but it may cause a sensation of pressure and some discomfort in your right upper back.

After the needle is withdrawn, resume normal breathing. The doctor will apply pressure to the biopsy site to stop any bleeding. Then he'll apply a pressure bandage.

After the test

You'll be told to lie on your right side for 2 hours, with a small pillow tucked under your side. For the next 24 hours, you should rest in bed. Your vital signs will be checked periodically.

Tell your doctor or nurse right away if you experience any problems, such as chest pain, persistent shoulder pain, or difficulty breathing. You can resume your normal diet.

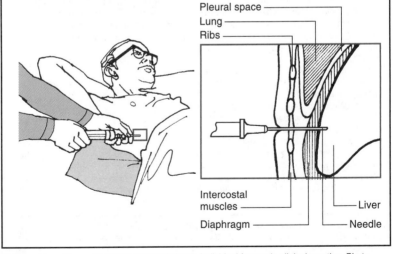

Pleural space
Lung
Ribs
Intercostal muscles
Diaphragm
Liver
Needle

Illustrated guide to home testing

In recent years, the number of diagnostic tests that people can perform themselves at home has greatly increased. The teaching aids on the following pages describe how to accurately perform many of the newest and most common home tests, including tests for blood cholesterol levels, pacemaker function, and the presence of human immunodeficiency virus.

When you review these tests with your patient, be sure to:
- stress the need to follow the manufacturer's instructions precisely
- explain unfamiliar terms
- review any special forms that the patient must complete, such as the diary needed when using a Holter monitor
- discuss how to follow up on test results.

Testing your blood glucose levels

Dear Patient:

Testing blood glucose levels daily will tell you whether your diabetes is under control. Follow these steps to learn how to obtain blood for testing and how to perform the test.

Getting ready

1. Begin by assembling the necessary equipment: your glucose meter, a lancet, and a vial with reagent strips.

2. Remove a reagent strip from the vial. Then replace the cap, making sure it's tight.

3. Turn on the glucose meter and insert the reagent strip according to the manufacturer's instructions. Wait for the display window to show that the meter is ready for the blood sample.

Obtaining blood

1. Wash your hands thoroughly and dry them. Choose a site on the end or side of any fingertip. To enhance blood flow, hold your finger under warm water for a minute or two.

2. Hold your hand below your heart, and milk the blood toward the fingertip you plan to pierce. Squeeze that fingertip with the thumb of the same hand. Then place your fingertip (with your thumb still pressed against it) on a firm surface such as a table.

3. Twist off the lancet's cap. Then grasp the lancet and quickly pierce your fingertip just to the side of the finger pad, where you have more blood

vessels and fewer nerve endings (as shown below).

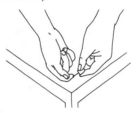

4. Remove your thumb from your fingertip to permit blood flow. Then milk your finger gently until you get a large, hanging drop of blood (as shown below).

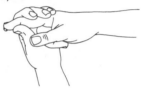

Testing blood

1. When the display window indicates that the meter is ready, touch the drop of blood to the reagent strip at the indicated spot. The drop of blood will automatically start the meter's timer.

2. After the meter has finished the test, you can read the results from the display window. The meter will automatically store the date, time, and results of the test.

Collecting a urine specimen: For males

Dear Patient:
Your doctor wants you to have your urine tested. A urine test can tell whether you have a infection or whether you have too much or too little of certain substances in your body. To make sure that the test results are accurate, your urine shouldn't contain "outside germs" from your hands or your penis.

Follow these directions carefully. Read them through to the end before collecting the specimen.

1. Wash your hands thoroughly. Open the package of disposable wipes that the nurse gave you, and place it on a clean, dry surface nearby.

2. Remove the lid from the specimen cup and place it flat side down. *Do not* touch the inside of the cup or lid.

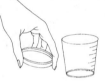

3. Prepare to urinate. (If you're uncircumcised, first pull back your foreskin.) Using a disposable wipe, clean the head of your penis from the urethral opening toward you, as shown. Then discard the used wipe.

4. Urinate a small amount into the toilet. After 1 or 2 seconds, catch about 1 ounce (30 milliliters) of urine in the specimen cup.

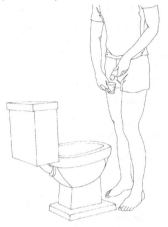

The nurse will tell you how far to fill the cup. As a rule, you'll fill it about one-fourth or more full.

Don't allow the cup to touch your penis at any time. When you're done, place the lid on the cup and return it to the nurse.

Note: Don't drink a lot of water before the test. This could affect the accuracy of test results.

Collecting a urine specimen: For females

Dear Patient:
Your doctor has asked you to provide a urine specimen for testing. The specimen can tell whether you have an infection or whether you have too much or too little of certain substances in your body.

To make sure that the test results are accurate, your urine shouldn't contain "outside germs" from your hands, labia, or urethral opening. *Note:* Don't drink a lot of water before the test. This could affect the accuracy of test results.

Follow the instructions below carefully. Read them through to the end before collecting your specimen.

1. Wash your hands thoroughly. Open the package of disposable wipes that the nurse gave you, and place it on a clean, dry, surface nearby.

2. Remove the lid from the specimen cup and place it flat side down. *Do not* touch the inside of the cup or lid.

3. Sit as far back on the toilet as possible. Spread your labia apart with one hand, keeping the folds separated for the rest of the procedure.

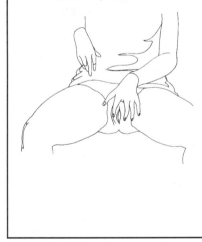

4. Using the disposable wipes, clean the area between the labia and around the urethra thoroughly from front to back. Use a new wipe for each stroke.

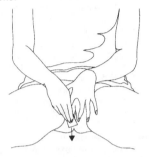

5. Urinate a small amount into the toilet. After 1 or 2 seconds, hold the specimen cup below your urine stream and catch about 1 ounce (30 milliliters) of urine in the cup. Don't allow the cup to touch your skin at any time.

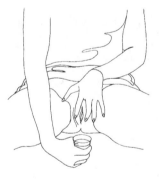

6. Place the lid on the cup and return it to the nurse.

Testing your urine for ketones

Dear Patient:

If your urine contains waste chemicals called ketones, your blood sugar level may be too high.

You should test your urine for ketones when your blood sugar level rises above 240 mg/dl or when you're ill. Even a minor illness can dramatically affect your blood sugar level.

Your doctor will probably recommend testing every 4 hours until your blood sugar level has stabilized or until your illness is over. To test your urine for ketones, follow these steps.

1. First, gather a clean container (a small plastic cup will do), a bottle of reagent strips, and a wristwatch or a clock with a second hand.

2. Collect a urine specimen in the container.

3. Remove one reagent strip from the bottle and replace the cap. Hold the strip so that the test blocks face up, but don't touch the blocks (as shown).

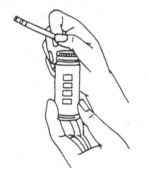

4. Dip the end of the strip with the test blocks into the urine for about 2 seconds. Then remove the strip and shake off excess urine. (Or you can perform the test while you urinate by simply holding the strip under the urine stream for about 2 seconds.)

5. Now hold the reagent strip horizontally and immediately begin timing (as shown), following the manufacturer's directions.

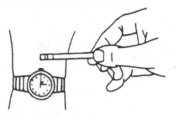

6. After waiting the recommended time, compare the ketone test block with the ketone color chart on the bottle label (as shown).

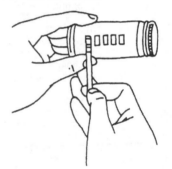

7. Keep a record of your tests, listing the date, the time, the results, and any other pertinent information. Call the doctor if your urine is positive for ketones.

Testing for blood in your stool

Dear Patient:
A home fecal occult blood test is an easy, inexpensive way to detect blood in your stool. For accurate results, follow the directions given by the nurse or doctor, read the instructions included with the test kit, and review these guidelines.

How to get ready
Don't eat red meat or raw fruits and vegetables for 3 days before you take the test and during the test period. Also avoid diet supplements containing iron or vitamin C and painkillers containing aspirin or ibuprofen (such as Advil and Nuprin) for the same time period. All of these substances can affect test results.

Increase your intake of high-fiber foods, such as whole grain breads and cereals. Your doctor may also ask you to eat popcorn or nuts.

How to perform the test
1. Make sure all your supplies are in one place. They may include your test cards (or slides), a chemical developer, a wooden applicator, and a watch with a second hand.
2. Obtain a stool sample from the toilet bowl. Use the applicator to smear a thin film of the sample onto the slot marked "A" on the front of the test card. Smear a thin film of a second sample from *a different area of the same stool* onto the slot marked "B" on the same side of the card.

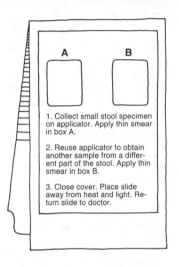

1. Collect small stool specimen on applicator. Apply thin smear in box A.

2. Reuse applicator to obtain another sample from a different part of the stool. Apply thin smear in box B.

3. Close cover. Place slide away from heat and light. Return slide to doctor.

3. *If the doctor or a lab will be analyzing the test samples,* close slots A and B. Put your name and the date on the test kit, and return the card (or slide) to the doctor or lab as soon as possible.

If you're doing the test yourself, turn the card over and open the back window. Apply 2 drops of the chemical developer to the paper covering each sample. Wait 1 minute; then read the results.

If either slot has a bluish tint, the test results are positive for blood in the stool. *If neither slot looks blue,* the test results are normal. Write down the results.

4. Repeat the test on your next two bowel movements. Report the results of all of the tests to the doctor. Even if only one of the six test results is positive, the doctor may recommend other tests.

Discard any unused supplies when you've completed all tests.

Using your Holter monitor

Dear Patient:
Your doctor has ordered a Holter monitor for you to wear for 24 hours. It works like a continuous electrocardiogram (ECG) by recording any irregular heartbeats you may have. The information from this recording will help your doctor determine if these abnormal heartbeats are causing your symptoms, such as chest pain or discomfort, dizziness, or weakness. If you are taking heart medication, the Holter monitor can also help your doctor evaluate how well the medication is working.

The monitor has adhesive patches — called *leads* — that the nurse will attach to your skin. She'll also show you how to wear the monitor on a belt or over your shoulder. If one of the leads becomes loose, secure it with a piece of tape.

While wearing the monitor, you can perform most of your usual activities. You'll even wear it to bed.

Practice these safety measures while you're wearing the Holter monitor.
■ Don't get the monitor wet — don't shower, bathe, or swim with it on.
■ Avoid high-voltage areas, strong magnetic fields, and microwave ovens.

While you're wearing the monitor, you'll write down your activities and feelings. (You can use the diary below as an example.) Your diary will help your doctor establish a connection between your monitor tracing and your activities and feelings. Jot down the time of day when you perform any activity, such as taking medication, eating, drinking, moving your bowels, urinating, engaging in sexual activity, experiencing strong emotions, exercising, and sleeping.

If your monitor has an event button, the nurse will show you how to press it in case you experience anything unusual, such as a sudden, rapid heartbeat.

Day	Time	Activity	Feelings
Tuesday	10:30 am	Rode from hospital in car	Legs tired, some shortness of breath
	11:30 am	Watched TV in living room	Comfortable
	12:15 pm	Ate lunch, took Inderal	Indigestion
	1:30 pm	Walked next door to see neighbor	Shortness of breath
	2:45 pm	Walked home	Very tired, legs hurt
	3:00 - 4:00 pm	Urinated, took nap	Comfortable
	5:30 pm	Ate dinner, slowly	Comfortable
	7:20 pm	Had bowel movement	Shortness of breath
	9:00 pm	Watched TV - drank 1 beer	Heart beating fast for about one minute, no pain
	11:00 pm	Took Inderal, urinated, went to bed	Tired
Wednesday	8:15 am	Awoke, urinated, washed face and arms	Very tired, rapid heartbeat for about 30 seconds
	10:30 am	Returned to hospital	Felt better

Checking your pacemaker by telephone

Dear Patient:
Your doctor wants to check your pacemaker regularly by telephone. Doing this helps him monitor how well the pacemaker is working and the strength of the battery while you stay at home. Here's how to use your pacemaker's transmitter.

Insert the battery
Before using your transmitter for the first time, remove the battery cover and insert the battery supplied by the manufacturer. You'll need to replace the battery every 2 to 3 months.

Set up the transmitter
When you're ready, take the transmitter out of its case. Also remove the electrode cable from the case, and plug the cable into the jack on the transmitter.

Place the electrodes on your fingers or on your wrists. Then turn on the transmitter and listen for the tones indicating that the power is on.

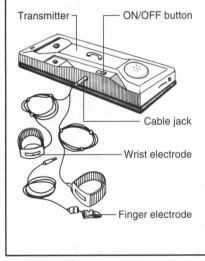

Transmitter — — ON/OFF button

— Cable jack

— Wrist electrode

— Finger electrode

Phone in your electrocardiogram
Dial the telephone number of your doctor's office or the pacemaker clinic, and listen for instructions.

When directed, place the telephone handset in the pacemaker transmitter. Stay still (for up to 60 seconds) to minimize interference with the signals from your heart.

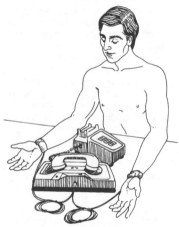

Wait for further instructions. For example, the doctor may ask you to use a special magnet that's in the transmitter's case. To do so, simply hold the magnet over the pacemaker and transmit your electrocardiogram as before.

When you finish transmitting, take off the electrodes and turn off the transmitter. Place the equipment in the storage case until the next time you use it.

Checking your blood cholesterol level

Dear Patient:

Testing your blood cholesterol level can tell you whether you're at risk for heart disease. If you are on a low-cholesterol diet or are taking cholesterol-lowering medication, testing your blood cholesterol level will help you determine whether your cholesterol is under control. If you have any questions about your test results or the risk factors associated with heart disease, *always* consult your doctor.

Follow these steps to learn how to obtain a blood sample and how to perform the test. Remember, because cholesterol levels can change from day to day and can be affected by stress, weight loss, illness, or pregnancy, one cholesterol reading may not be final.

Getting ready

1. Begin by assembling the necessary equipment included in the packet: the test device, the cholesterol test result chart, and a lancet.
2. Read the instructions thoroughly before you stick your finger.

Obtaining blood

1. Wash your hands thoroughly and dry them. Choose a site on the end or side of any fingertip. To enhance blood flow, hold your finger under warm water for a minute or two.
2. Hold your hand below your heart, and milk the blood toward the fingertip you plan to pierce. Squeeze that fingertip with the thumb of the same hand. Place your fingertip (with your thumb still pressed against it) on a firm surface such as a table.
3. Twist off the lancet's protective cap. Then grasp the lancet and

quickly pierce your fingertip just to the side of the finger pad, where you have more blood vessels and fewer nerve endings.
4. Remove your thumb from your fingertip to permit blood flow. Then milk your finger gently until you get a large, hanging drop of blood.
5. Point your finger down directly over the blood well, and place the hanging drop of blood into the blood well, making sure that you fill the black circle completely. Then wait at least 2 but no more than 4 minutes.

Reading the results

When the display windows indicate that the test is complete, read the results. Use the chart included in the packet to identify the exact reading on the test device (as shown). Then compare this reading with the chart to identify your cholesterol level. Remember to inform your doctor about the results.

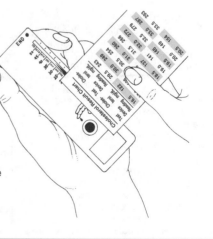

Performing a home ovulation test

Dear Patient:

A home ovulation test helps you determine the best time to try to become pregnant. This test works by monitoring the amount of luteinizing hormone (LH) that's present in your urine.

Normally, during each menstrual cycle, levels of this hormone rise suddenly (LH surge), causing an egg to be released from the ovary 24 to 36 hours later. The release of the egg is known as *ovulation.* Ovulation normally occurs once a month, about 2 weeks before your period, and lasts about 24 hours. This is your most fertile period — the only time each month that you can become pregnant.

Follow these directions to test your urine for the presence of luteinizing hormone and to determine when you are most likely to become pregnant. To know when to begin testing, you'll need to know the length of your menstrual cycle. Count from the beginning of one period to the beginning of the next. (Count the first day of bleeding as day 1). Use the chart below to determine when to begin testing.

Getting ready

1. Read the instructions thoroughly before you perform the test. This test can be performed any time of the day or night but should be performed at the same time each day.

Note: Do not urinate for at least 4 hours before taking this test, and do not drink a lot of liquids for several hours before testing.

2. Remove the test stick from the package and remove the cap.

Performing the test

1. Sit on the toilet. Direct the absorbent tip of the test stick downward and directly into your urine stream for at least 5 seconds or until it is thoroughly wet. *Do not* urinate on the windows. You can also urinate into a clean, dry cup or container and dip the test stick (absorbent tip only) into the urine for at least 5 seconds.

2. Lay the test stick on a clean, dry, flat surface.

Reading the results

1. Wait at least 5 minutes to read the results. When the test is finished, a line will appear in the small window.

2. *If there is no line in the large rectangular window or if the line is lighter than the line in the small rectangular window,* you have not begun your LH surge. You should continue with daily testing.

3. *If you see one line in the large window that is similar to or darker than the line in the small window* (as shown), you have detected an LH surge. This means that you should ovulate within the next 24 to 36 hours.

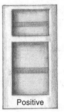

Positive

Once you've determined that you're about to ovulate, you know you're at the start of the most fertile time of your cycle.

Length of cycle	Start test this many days after your last period begins	Length of cycle	Start test this many days after your last period begins
21	5	31	14
22	5	32	15
23	6	33	16
24	7	34	17
25	8	34	18
26	9	36	19
27	10	37	20
28	11	38	21
29	12	39	22
30	13	40	23

Performing a home pregnancy test

Dear Patient:
A home pregnancy test will detect a hormone in your urine that your body produces only if you are pregnant. The test can detect this hormone — human chorionic gonadotropin, or hCG — as early as 1 day after you miss your period. If you have been pregnant or had a miscarriage within the last 8 weeks, or if you are taking a medication that contains hCG or that's used in combination with hCG, the test may produce a false-positive result. In any case, *always* consult your doctor before and after taking this test.

Follow these steps to learn how to perform the test.

Getting ready
1. Read the instructions thoroughly before you perform the test. This test can be performed any time of the day or night — it does not need to be done first thing in the morning.
2. Remove the test stick from the package, and slide the clear splash guard back to expose the absorbent tip.

Performing the test
1. Sit on the toilet and hold the test stick by the thumb grip.
2. Direct the absorbent tip downward and directly into your urine stream for at least 5 seconds or until it is thoroughly wet (as shown above). *Do not* urinate on the windows.
3. You can also urinate into a clean, dry cup or container and dip the test stick (absorbent tip only) into the urine for at least 5 seconds.
4. Lay the test stick on a clean, dry, flat surface.

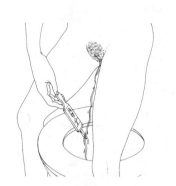

Reading the results
1. Wait at least 3 minutes to read the results. When the test is finished, a line will appear in the small rectangular window.
2. *If you see one line in the round and rectangular windows* (as shown below), the test has indicated that you are pregnant. You should consult your doctor as soon as possible to discuss your pregnancy.

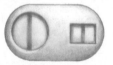

3. *If the only visible line is in the control (rectangular window),* the test has indicated that you are not pregnant. You can perform a repeat test with a new test kit if your period does not start within a week.

Note: If results appear in the round window but not in the rectangular control window, do not read the results because they may be inaccurate. Call the toll-free number located on the test box or package insert.

Performing a home HIV test

Dear Patient:

Human immunodeficiency virus (HIV) is a virus that attacks your immune system and causes acquired immunodeficiency syndrome (AIDS). By testing your blood, you can determine if you've been infected with HIV. Remember that even if you've been exposed to the HIV virus, it may not become evident in your blood for 6 months. If you have any questions about your test results or the risk factors associated with HIV, *always* consult a doctor. Follow these steps to learn how to obtain a blood sample and how to perform the test.

Getting ready

1. Begin by assembling the necessary equipment included in the packet: a lancet, a test card with your personal identification number (to receive the confidential and anonymous test results), and the envelope in which to send the test card to the laboratory.

2. Read the instructions thoroughly before you stick your finger. (They appear in English and Spanish.) Remove the personal identification card from the bottom of the test card and place it in a safe place.

Obtaining blood

1. Wash your hands thoroughly and dry them. Choose a site on the end or side of any fingertip. To enhance blood flow, hold your finger under warm water for a minute or two.

2. Hold your hand below your heart, and milk the blood toward the fingertip you plan to pierce. Squeeze that fingertip with the thumb of the same hand. Place your fingertip (with your thumb still pressed against it) on a firm surface such as a table.

3. Twist off the lancet's protective cap. Then grasp the lancet and quickly pierce your fingertip just to the side of the finger pad, where you have more blood vessels and fewer nerve endings.

4. Remove your thumb from your fin-

gertip to permit blood flow. Then milk your finger gently until you get a large, hanging drop of blood.

5. Point your finger down directly over the three circles on the test card. Completely fill each circle with blood.

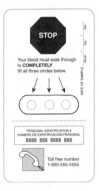

6. Place any used lancets in the containers attached to the mailing card. Slip the test card in the postage-paid mailer, seal the mailer, and send it to the address printed on the front. Save the part of the card that lists the toll-free phone number to call for results.

Obtaining the results

In about 1 week, call the toll-free number on the identification card. Give the person who answers your identification number and wait for the results. *If your test is positive for HIV,* a specially trained counselor will advise you what to do next and will tell you about HIV and AIDS organizations nationwide. *If your test results are negative for HIV,* the trained counselor will advise you how to maintain your negative HIV status.

Remember, a negative test result doesn't necessarily mean you're free from HIV infection. It may simply mean that the antibodies are not yet present in your blood. To be certain, repeat the test in 6 months.

Photo acknowledgments

Collection techniques
p. xxx to xxxiii John Gallagher

Chapter 1: Hematology
pp. 2, 3 Ann Bell, MS, SH(ASCP), CLS, University of Tennessee Center for Health Sciences, Memphis

Chapter 5: Hormones
p. 140 Sterling Publishing Co.

p. 142 Arthur C. Guyton, *Textbook of Medical Physiology,* 8th ed. (Philadelphia: W.B. Saunders Co., 1991).

p. 174 Paul A. Cohen

Chapter 18: Histology
p. 477 © Carroll H. Weiss, RBP, 1981

Chapter 19: Microbes and parasites
p. 505 William G. Leibowitz (formerly Eliot Scientific), New York

p. 515 John Gallagher

Chapter 21: Eye
pp. 563, 575, 576 David Silva, Ophthalmic Photographer, Wills Eye Hospital, Philadelphia

p. 566 Joel I. Hamburger, MD, Northland Radioisotope Lab, Southfield, Mich.

p. 569 © Carroll H. Weiss, RBP, 1981

p. 579 © Joe Savoy, Ophthalmic Photographer, Detroit Institute of Ophthalmology, Grosse Point Park, Mich.

Chapter 22: Ear
pp. 598, 599 John Gallagher

Chapter 23: Respiratory system
pp. 675, 678 Marc S. Lapayowker, MD, Department of Radiology, Abington (Pa.) Memorial Hospital

Chapter 24: Skeletal system
pp. 687, 689 Marc S. Lapayowker, MD, Department of Radiology, Abington (Pa.) Memorial Hospital

p. 696 John J. Joyce, III, MD, University of Pennsylvania, Philadelphia

Chapter 26: Nervous system
p. 764 Marc S. Lapayowker, MD, Department of Radiology, Abington (Pa.) Memorial Hospital

p. 783 (top) Hobson, "Comparison of Pulsed Doppler and Real-time B-mode Echocardiography for Non-invasive Imaging of the Extracranial Carotid Arteries," *Surgery,* Vol. 87, No. 311, March 1980; (bottom left) David S. Sumner, MD; (bottom right) Blackshear, et al., "Detection of Carotid Occlusive Disease by Ultrasonic Imaging and Pulsed Doppler Spectrum Analysis," *Surgery,* Vol. 86, No. 5, November 1979

pp. 781, 782 Donna Blackburn, RN, Northwestern Memorial Hospital, Chicago

p. 788 Marc S. Lapayowker, MD, Department of Radiology, Abington (Pa.) Memorial Hospital

Chapter 27: Gastrointestinal system
pp. 832, 835 (left) Olympus Corporation of America, Medical Instrument Division, New Hyde Park, N.Y.

pp. 835 (right), 855 American Society for Gastrointestinal Endoscopy, Postgraduate Course, May 1976

pp. 850, 853, 871, 880 Marc S. Lapayowker, MD, Department of Radiology, Abington (Pa.) Memorial Hospital

p. 879 Bill Baker

Photo acknowledgments *(continued)*

Chapter 28: Cardiovascular system
pp. 896, 918, 919, 920, 942, 961 Marc S. Lapayowker, MD, Department of Radiology, Abington (Pa.) Memorial Hospital

Chapter 29: Urinary system
pp. 975, 983, 991, 1010 Marc S. Lapayowker, MD, Department of Radiology, Abington (Pa.) Memorial Hospital

Chapter 30: Miscellaneous tests
pp. 1019, 1020 John Gallagher

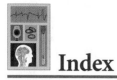

Index

Boldface page numbers indicate major entries; t refers to a table, i to an illustration.

Antioxidants, 249
Antiplatelet antibodies, 46
Anti-Rh₀(D) (Rh-positive) antibody, maternal, 277
Anti-Smith antibodies, test for, 312
Anti-smooth-muscle antibodies, 314t
Anti-smooth-muscle antibody tests, 313, **315**
Antistreptolysin-O, **338-340**
Antithrombin III test, 61
Antithyroglobulin antibodies, 316, 316t
Antithyroid antibody tests, **316-317**
Anuria, 360-361
Aorta, 885
Aortic aneurysm, 676
Aortic arch aneurysm, 677
Aortic disorders, 921, 922
Aortic insufficiency, 917
Aortic pressure, 886
Aortic stenosis
  Doppler ultrasonography for, 923
  ECG for, 918
Aortic valve abnormalities, 917
Aplastic anemia
  bone marrow biopsy for, 494, 497
  fecal urobilinogen test for, 826
  LAP stain in, 35
  platelets in, 46
Aplitest skin test, 1017
  findings in, 1021
  reading, 1021
Apolipoprotein E genotype, 795
Apolipoproteins, 205
Apoproteins, 198
  in blood, 206
Appendicitis
  barium enema for, 844
  WBC count in, 34
Applanation tonometry, 571, 572
Apt test, 734
APTT. *See* Activated partial thromboplastin time.
Aqueous humor, 551
Arachnoiditis, 798, 799
Argentaffin cells, 384
  serotonin secretion by, 406i
Arginine test, **144-145**
Arrhythmia. *See also specific type.*
  calcium serum levels and, 79, 80
  with cardiac catheterization, 943t
  ECG for, 902
  electrophysiology studies for, 891, 947

Arrhythmia *(continued)*
  during exercise ECG, 907
  Holter monitoring for, 912
  intermittent, 888
  potassium serum levels in, 85
ARS A. *See* Arylsulfatase A.
Arterial blood, xv
  collection of, xix-xxv
  puncture sites for, xvi
Arterial blood gas analysis, **74-78**
Arterial blood gases, 70-71
  clinical significance of, 72
  values of, 70
Arterial bypass grafting
  Doppler ultrasonography for monitoring, 923
  locating vein for, 894
Arterial embolization, 858
  with cardiac catheterization, 945t
Arterial encasement, types of, 860i
Arterial ischemia index, 925
Arteries, 885
  occlusion of
    arteriogram of, 942i
    Doppler ultrasonography for, 923, 926, 927
    ocular, 580
  reconstruction of, Doppler monitoring in, 923
  stenosis of, Doppler ultrasonography for, 926, 927
  trauma to, 923
Arteriography, celiac and mesenteric, **857-861**
Arterioles, 885
Arteriosclerosis, 787
Arteriovenous malformation, 786, 787
Arteriovenous occlusion, 790
Arteriovenous shunting, 859
Arthritis
  synovial fluid analysis for, 699
  traumatic, synovial fluid analysis in, 700-701t
  vertebral radiography for, 684, 685
Arthrocentesis, 683, 699
Arthrogram, normal vs. abnormal, 687i
Arthrography, 683, **685-688**
Arthropods, 504
  testing procedures for, 505-506
Arthroscopic surgery, 697
Arthroscopy, **695-697**
  of knee, 696i
Arylsulfatase A, 374, 376
  test for, **376-377**
Ascaris, in stool, 532

Ascaris lumbricoides, in sputum, 535-536
Ascending contrast phlebography. *See* Venography.
Ascites
  CT scan of pancreas for, 871
  D-xylose absorption test for, 1034
  peritoneal fluid analysis for, 818, 819
Ascorbic acid, dietary sources of, 452t
ASO. *See* Antistreptolysin-O.
Asparaginase, 443
Aspartate aminotransferase
  in hepatobiliary disease, 110t
  levels of, 96-97
  after myocardial infarction, 100i
  serum levels of, **104-106**
Aspergillosis, 343-344t
Aspergillus, culture sites for, 507t
Aspermatogenesis, 146
Aspiration biopsy
  bone marrow, 493-496
  liver, 482
  sites of, 494-495i
  target tissue for, 468-469t
Aspirin, 53
AST. *See* Aspartate aminotransferase.
Asthma
  anti-smooth-muscle antibody test for, 315
  arterial blood gas analysis in, 76
  basophils in, 11
  serum antibodies in, 314t
Astigmatism, refractive test for, 565
Astrocytoma, 799
Ataxia-telangiectasia, 354, 355
Atelectasis
  chest X-ray for, 661
  ventilation lung scan for, 675
Atheroma, 861
Atherosclerotic plaque, 861
Athletes, erythropoietin abuse by, 177-178
Atomic absorption spectroscopy, 248
ATP. *See* Adenosine triphosphate.
Atrial kick, 888i
Atrial muscle, 886
Atrial natriuretic factor
  plasma levels of, **178-179**
  role of, 179
Atrial pacing, 948

1098

Blood transfusion *(continued)*
nursing considerations in, 268-269
platelet refractoriness with, 279
preventing hemolytic reactions in, 268-269
tests required for, 266
universal donor and recipient in, 267
urine hemosiderin in, 463
Blood urea nitrogen, **221**
B-lymphocyte assays, **292-294**
B lymphocytes
activation of, 284
in cell-mediated immune response, 285
function of, 11, 283
in immune system, 292-293
origin and role of, 286-287
Body fluids, 74
Bone
biopsy of, **492-493**
densitometry, **690-691**
cancer of, 690
conduction testing, 603
degenerative disorders of, 688
flat, 681
fractured, calcium serum levels in, 80
histology of, 680
hydroxyproline urine test for resorption of, 418, 419
irregular, 681
long, 681
malignancy of, 688
pain in, 683
short, 681
sites of formation of, 690
structure of, 680-681
trauma to, 688
types of, 681, 682i
Bone marrow
aspiration of, **493-497**
hematopoiesis in, 493
normal and abnormal values in, 498-499t
plasma fibrinogen quantitation for lesions of, 63
platelet count in diseases of, 50
red, 493, 681
red blood cell production by, 2-5
WBC differential in depression of, 38t
yellow, 496, 681
Bone marrow biopsy
complications of, 493-494

Bone marrow biopsy *(continued)*
contraindication for, 496
sites of, 494-495i
WBC count in, 34
Bone matrix turnover, 418
Bone mineral density, 690, 691
Bone mineral tracer, 689
Bone pain
bone biopsy for, 492
bone scan for, 688
Bone scan, 683, **688-690**
hot spots in, 689
normal vs. abnormal, 689i
Bone tumor
alkaline phosphatase levels in, 108
bone biopsy for, 492, 493
paranasal sinus X-ray findings in, 667t
skeletal CT scan for, 691, 692
skeletal MRI for, 693, 694
thoracic CT scan for, 676
Bordetella pertussis
nasopharyngeal culture for, 512
throat culture for, 510-511
Borrelia burgdorferi, 246-247
Bowel resection, 83
Bowman's capsule, 358
Bradyarrhythmia, 912
Bradycardia
external fetal monitoring for, 742
internal fetal monitoring for, 746
Bradycardia-tachycardia syndrome, 912
Brain
blood flow in, 757
cells of, 757
CSF analysis for abscess of, 793
tumors of
fasting plasma glucose test in, 234
gamma glutamyl transpeptidase in, 111
postprandial plasma glucose levels in, 237
ventricles of, 757, 758i
Brain death, 770
Brain stem, 757
disorders of, 759
Brain tissue
creatine kinase levels in injury of, 99
hypoglycemia and, 230
Breast
adenocarcinoma of, 471
biopsy of, **469-472,** 747, 749
latest advance in, 470
needle, 470-471
open, 471

Breast *(continued)*
cancer of
mammography for, 747, 748-749
ultrasonography for, 748
cystosarcoma of, 471
cysts of, 749
masses in
biopsy for, **469-472**
histological examination of, 469
tissue analysis of, 469-470
tumors of
biopsy for, 470-472
mammography for, 747, 748-749
ultrasonography of, patient preparation for, 1072
Breast-feeding, 150
Breath hydrogen analysis, 809
Bronchial dilation, 670
Bronchial obstruction, 671
Bronchial tumor, 671
Bronchial wall abnormalities, 656
Bronchiectasis, 670
Bronchiolar obstruction, 668
Bronchioles, 636, 637i
Bronchoalveolar lavage, 655
Bronchogenic carcinoma, 654, 656
bronchoscopy of, 656
gallium scanning for, 1030
mediastinoscopy for, 657
Bronchography, 638t, **670-671**
Bronchopleural fistula, 676
Bronchoscope, 654
features of, 655i
Bronchoscopy, 487, **653-656**
fluoroscopic guidance of, 655
of pulmonary function, 638t
sputum culture for, 515, 516
Bronchus, 636, 637i
chest X-ray of, 665t
structure of, 656
Brucella infections
agglutinins, 341
antigen of, 342
blood culture for, 519
Brucellosis
delayed hypersensitivity skin tests for, 1022, 1025
febrile agglutination test for, 340-342
Brush biopsy, urinary tract, 484
Bruton's agammaglobulinemia, 288

Boldface page numbers indicate major entries; t refers to a table, i to an illustration.

Boldface page numbers indicate major entries; t refers to a table, i to an illustration.

Boldface page numbers indicate major entries; t refers to a table, i to an illustration.

Boldface page numbers indicate major entries; t refers to a table, i to an illustration.

1114

Heart disease *(continued)*
lipoprotein-cholesterol fractionation for, 205
postmenopausal, 200
risk factors for, 205
Heat stability test, 28
Heavy metal poisoning
copper reduction test for, 443
porphyrin urine levels in, 429
Heinz bodies, 28
identifying, 29i
staining for, 124
Heinz body test, **28-30**
for unstable hemoglobins, 27
Helminth infections, 504
stool examination for ova of, 532
testing procedures for, 505-506
Hemagglutination inhibition, 394-396
Hemangioma, 585
Hematest reagent tablet test, 821-822
Hematocrit, **14-16**
normal values of, by age, 15i
of pericardial fluid, 960
Hematologic disorders, 433
Hematology, **1-39**
Hematoma
with cardiac catheterization, 944t
with hematocrit, 15
liver ultrasound for, 876
with red blood cell count, 14
subhepatic and subphrenic, 867
Hematopoiesis, 493
Hematopoietic cells, 496
Hematoxylin stain, 467
Hematuria, 363-365
drugs causing, 366t
free hemoglobin in urine in, 426
hemoglobin in, 425
Heme, 424
fraction breakdown of, 413
metabolic defects in biosynthesis of, 411-413
synthesis of, 428-429
Hemianopia, complete bitemporal, 560i
Hemidiaphragm, 665t
Hemoccult slide test, 822
Hemochromatosis
synovial membrane biopsy for, 500
urine hemosiderin in, 462-463
Hemocytoblasts, 5

Hemodilution, 23
Hemoflagellates, 504
Hemoglobin, 5, 411
abnormal, 6t
hemoglobin electrophoresis in, 23
distinguishing from myoglobin, 215
distribution of, 24t
electrophoresis, **23-25**
fetal, 734
iron in synthesis of, 31
low concentration of, 7
normal values of, by age, 22i
in red blood cells, 2
tests of, **21-33**
total, **21-23**
types of, 5-6, 24t
unstable, **27-28**, 28-29
Heinz body test in, 29
signs and symptoms of, 28
urine levels of, 413
variants of, 6
Hemoglobin C-thalassemia disease, 1032
Hemoglobin electrophoresis
with sickle cell test, 26
for unstable hemoglobins, 27
Hemoglobinopathy
chorionic villi sampling for, 735
sickling phenomenon in, 25
Hemoglobin S-C disease, 3i
Hemoglobin S test. *See* Sickle cell test.
Hemoglobinuria
free hemoglobin in urine in, 426
paroxysmal nocturnal, 35
Hemoglobin urine tests, **424-426**
Hemolysis index, 215, 216
Hemolytic anemia
antibody screening for, 277
autoimmune, 317
cold agglutinins in, 324
direct antiglobulin test for, 276, 277
free hemoglobin in urine in, 424, 425
G6PD in, 123
Heinz body test in, 29
hemoglobin electrophoresis in, 24
PK-deficient, 124, 125
red blood cell survival time in, 1031, 1032
serum bilirubin in, 223, 225
serum ferritin in, 33
serum uric acid in, 223
urine hemosiderin in, 463

Hemolytic disease of newborn, 276, 277
Hemolytic disorders
amniotic fluid analysis for, 732
fecal urobilinogen test for, 435, 825, 826
Hemolytic jaundice, 435
Hemolytic transfusion reactions, 268
direct antiglobulin test for, 276, 277
preventing, 274-275
serum haptoglobin in, 215, 216
Hemophilia, 332
Hemophilia A, 45
Hemophilia B, 45
Hemophilia C, 45
Hemophilic factor A, 44t
Hemorrhage. *See also* Gastrointestinal bleeding.
with bone marrow biopsy, 493-494
with cardiac catheterization, 944t
catecholamine levels in, 176
cortisol levels in, 173
platelet count in, 50
total hemoglobin in, 23
Hemorrhoids, 808
proctosigmoidoscopy for, 833, 835
Hemosiderin, 496
levels of, 497
Hemosiderin urine test, **462-463**
Hemostasis, **41-67**
Henle, loop of, 359i, 360
Heparan sulfate, 441
Heparin
APTT with, 54
lipoproteins and, 208
neutralization assay of, 55
plasma thrombin time with, 61, 62
Hepatic abscess
CT scan for, 868
liver ultrasound for, 874, 875-876
urine amylase test for, 375
Hepatic carcinoma, 430
Hepatic cysts
CT scan for, 868
liver ultrasound for, 874, 875-876
Hepatic disease
alanine aminotransferase levels in, 106
alkaline phosphatase levels in, 108
ammonia levels in, 220

Boldface page numbers indicate major entries; t refers to a table, i to an illustration.

1124

Boldface page numbers indicate major entries; t refers to a table, i to an illustration.

Boldface page numbers indicate major entries; t refers to a table, i to an illustration.

1132

Boldface page numbers indicate major entries; t refers to a table, i to an illustration.

1140

Boldface page numbers indicate major entries; t refers to a table, i to an illustration.

Boldface page numbers indicate major entries; t refers to a table, i to an illustration.

Boldface page numbers indicate major entries; t refers to a table, i to an illustration.

Boldface page numbers indicate major entries; t refers to a table, i to an illustration.

Normal laboratory test values

HEMATOLOGY

Activated partial thromboplastin time
25 to 36 seconds

Bleeding time
Modified template: 2 to 10 minutes
Template: 2 to 8 minutes
Ivy: 1 to 7 minutes
Duke: 1 to 3 minutes

Clot retraction
50%

Erythrocyte sedimentation rate
Males: 0 to 10 mm/hour
Females: 0 to 20 mm/hour

Fibrin split products
Screening assay: <10 µg/ml
Quantitative assay: <3 µg/ml

Fibrinogen, plasma
195 to 365 mg/dl

Hematocrit
Males: 42% to 54%
Females: 38% to 46%
Neonates: 55% to 68%

Hemoglobin, total
Males: 14 to 18 g/dl
Males after middle age: 12.4 to 14.9 g/dl
Females: 12 to 16 g/dl
Females after middle age: 11.7 to 13.8 g/dl

Platelet aggregation
3 to 5 minutes

Platelet count
140,000 to 400,000/µl

Platelet survival
50% tagged platelets disappear within 84 to 116 hours; 100% disappear within 8 to 10 days

Prothrombin consumption time
20 seconds

Prothrombin time
10 to 14 seconds; INR for patients on warfarin therapy, 2.0 to 3.0 (those with prosthetic heart valve, 2.5 to 3.5)

Red blood cell count
Males: 4.5 to 6.2 million/µl venous blood
Females: 4.2 to 5.4 million/µl venous blood

Red cell indices
Mean corpuscular volume: 84 to 99 fl
Mean corpuscular hemoglobin: 26 to 32 fl
Mean corpuscular hemoglobin concentration: 30 to 36 g/dl

Reticulocyte count
0.5% to 2% of total red blood cell count count

Thrombin time, plasma
10 to 15 seconds

BLOOD CHEMISTRY

Acid phosphatase, serum
0.5 to 1.9 U/L

Alanine aminotransferase
Males: 10 to 35 U/L
Females: 9 to 24 U/L

Alkaline phosphatase, serum
Males ≥19 years: 98 to 251 U/L
Females 24 to 65 years: 81 to 282 U/L
Females ≥65 years: 119 to 309 U/L

Amylase, serum
≥18 years: 35 to 115 U/L

Arterial blood gases
pH: 7.35 to 7.45
Pao_2: 75 to 100 mm Hg
$Paco_2$: 35 to 45 mm Hg
O_2Ct: 15% to 23%
Sao_2: 94% to 100%
HCO_3^-: 22 to 26 mEq/L

Aspartate aminotransferase
Males: 8 to 20 U/L
Females: 5 to 40 U/L

Bilirubin, serum
Adults: direct, <0.5 mg/dl; indirect, ≤1.1 mg/dl
Neonates: total, 1 to 12 mg/dl

Blood urea nitrogen
8 to 20 mg/dl

Calcium, serum (atomic absorption)
Males ≥22 years: 8.9 to 10.1 mg/dl
Females ≥19 years: 8.9 to 10.1 mg/dl

Carbon dioxide, total, blood
22 to 34 mEq/L

Cholesterol, total, serum
0 to 240 mg/dl

C-reactive protein, serum
Negative

Creatine, serum
Males: 0.2 to 0.6 mg/dl
Females: 0.6 to 1 mg/dl

Creatine kinase, isoenzymes
CK-BB: none
CK-MB: 0 to 7 U/L
CK-MM: 5 to 70 U/L

Creatine kinase, total
Males ≥18 years: 52 to 336 U/L
Females ≥18 years: 38 to 176 U/L

Creatinine, serum
Males: 0.8 to 1.2 mg/dl
Females: 0.6 to 0.9 mg/dl

Free thyroxine, serum
0.8 to 3.3 ng/dl

Free triiodothyronine
0.2 to 0.6 ng/dl

Gamma-glutamyltransferase
Males: 8 to 37 U/L
Females <age 45: 5 to 27 U/L
Women ≥age 45: 6 to 37 U/L

Glucose, plasma, fasting
70 to 100 mg/dl

Glucose, plasma, oral tolerance
Peak at 160 to 180 mg/dl, 30 to 60 minutes after challenge dose

Glucose, plasma, 2-hour postprandial
<145 mg/dl